Naturopathic I & Integrative Inf

A Colorful Guide toward Health and Vitality and Away from the Boredom, Risks, Costs, and inefficacy of Endless Analgesia and Pharmacoimmunosuppression

A Three-Part Learning System of Text, Slides, and Video

Alex Vasquez D.C. N.D. D.O. F.A.C.N.

- Doctor of Osteopathic Medicine, graduate of University of North Texas Health Science Center, Texas College of Osteopathic Medicine (2010)
- Doctor of Naturopathic Medicine, graduate of Bastyr University (1999)
- Doctor of Chiropractic, graduate of University of Western States (1996)
- Fellow of the American College of Nutrition (2013-present)
- Fellow of the Royal Society of Medicine (2013-present)
- Chief Editor, *International Journal of Human Nutrition and Functional Medicine* IntJHumNutrFunctMed.org
- Private practice of integrative and functional medicine in Seattle, Washington (2000-2001), Houston, Texas (2001-2006), Portland, Oregon (2011-2013), consulting practice (present) based in Barcelona, Spain
- Consultant Researcher and Lecturer (2004-present), Biotics Research Corporation
- Teaching and Academics:
  - Director of Programs, International College/Conference on Human Nutrition and Functional Medicine ICHNFM.org
  - Founder and Former Program Director of the world's first accredited university-affiliated graduate-level program in Functional Medicine
  - Former Adjunct Faculty (2009-2013) of Advanced Laboratory Medicine
  - Former Adjunct Faculty (2004-2005, 2010-2013) and Forum Consultant (2003-2007), The Institute for Functional Medicine
  - Former Adjunct Professor (2011-2013) of Pharmacology, Evidence-Based Nutrition, Immune and Inflammatory Imbalances, Principles of Functional Medicine, Psychology of Wellness
  - Former Adjunct Professor of Orthopedics (2000), Radiographic Interpretation (2000), and Rheumatology (2001), Naturopathic Medicine Program, Bastyr University
- Author of more than 100 articles and letters published in *JAMA—Journal of the American Medical Association*, *BMJ—British Medical Journal*, TheLancet.com, *JAOA—Journal of the American Osteopathic Association*, *Annals of Pharmacotherapy*, *Journal of Clinical Endocrinology and Metabolism*, *Alternative Therapies in Health and Medicine*, *Nutritional Perspectives*, *Journal of Manipulative and Physiological Therapeutics*, *Integrative Medicine*, *Current Allergy and Asthma Reports*, *Nutritional Wellness*, *Evidence-based Complementary and Alternative Medicine*, and *Arthritis & Rheumatism: Official Journal of the American College of Rheumatology*

FunctionalInflammology.com
InflammationMastery.com

Title: Vasquez A. *Naturopathic Rheumatology and Integrative Inflammology, Edition 3.5*. Cundinamarca, Colombia

Copyrights: © 2004-2014 by Alex Vasquez. All rights reserved by the author and enforced to the full extent of legal and financial consequences internationally. No part of this book may be reproduced, stored in a retrieval system, used for the creation of derivative works, or transmitted by any means (electronic, mechanical, photocopying, recording, or otherwise) without written permission from the author.

Trademarks: ® 2013 by Alex Vasquez. The functional immunology/inflammology protocol discussed in this series of videos/notes/books/audios is recalled by the F.I.N.D.S.E.X. acronym trademarked™ in association with Dr Vasquez's books and videos including but not limited to *Functional Immunology and Nutritional Immunomodulation* (2012), *F.I.N.D. S.E.X. The Easily Remembered Acronym for the Functional Inflammology Protocol* (2013), *Integrative Rheumatology and Inflammation Mastery, 3rd Edition* (2014). Portland, Oregon & Austin, Texas; Integrative and Biological Medicine Research and Consulting, LLC. All rights reserved and enforced. For additional information and resources, see InflammationMastery.com and/or FunctionalInflammology.com. Of note, additional trademarks referenced/cited in this work include International College of Human Nutrition and Functional Medicine®, International Conference on Human Nutrition and Functional Medicine®, and *International Journal of Human Nutrition and Functional Medicine*®.

Notices: The intended audiences for this book are health science students and doctorate-level licensed medical clinicians. This book has been written with every intention to make it as accurate as possible, and each section has undergone peer-review by an interdisciplinary group of clinicians. In view of the possibility of human error and as well as ongoing discoveries in the biomedical sciences, neither the author nor any party associated in any way with this text warrants that this text is perfect, accurate, or complete in every way, and all disclaim responsibility for harm or loss associated with the application of the material herein. Information and treatments applicable to a specific *condition* may not be appropriate for or applicable to a specific patient; this is especially true for patients with multiple comorbidities and those taking pharmaceutical medications, which are generally associated with multiple adverse effects and drug/nutrient/herb interactions. Given that this book is available on an open market, lay persons who read this material should discuss the information with a licensed medical provider before implementing any treatments and interventions described herein.

Textbooks in this series	Date & Notes
1. Volume 1: Functional Inflammology: Introduction to Clinical Nutrition, Functional Medicine, and Integrative Pain Management for Disorders of Sustained Inflammation	Started in 2004, updated 2014
2. Volume 2: Disorders of Metabolic Inflammation: Hypertension, Diabetes, Fibromyalgia, Migraine, Alzheimer's disease, Parkinson's disease, etc	Earlier versions: 2009, 2011, 2012
3. Volume 3: Disorders of Allergic Inflammation: General Allergy, Atopic Dermatitis, Asthma, etc	Earlier versions: 2005, 2009
4. Volume 4: Disorders of Autoimmune Inflammation / Integrative Rheumatology: Psoriasis, Rheumatoid Arthritis, SLE, MS, Vasculitis, Dermatomyositis, etc	Earlier versions: 2006, 2007, 2014
5. Volume 5: Clinical Mastery of Common Musculoskeletal Disorders: Integrative Orthopedics	Earlier versions: 2004, 2007, 2012

Chapter and Introduction	Pages
• Preamble	i
1. <u>Patient Assessments, Laboratory Interpretation, Clinical Concepts, Patient Management, Practice Management and Risk Reduction</u>: *This chapter introduces/reviews/updates patient assessments, laboratory interpretation, musculoskeletal emergencies, healthcare paradigms; the common and important conditions hemochromatosis and hypothyroidism are also included in this chapter since these need to be considered on a frequent basis in clinical practice*	1
2. <u>Re-Establishing the Foundation for Health: Lifestyle Medicine and Wellness Promotion</u>: *Reviewed here are diet, lifestyle, psychosocial health, and—given the pervasiveness of persistent organic pollutants and their increasingly recognized clinical importance—an introduction to environmental medicine*	187
3. <u>Basic Concepts and Therapeutics in (Nondrug) Musculoskeletal Care and Integrative Pain Management</u>: *Nonpharmacologic management of musculoskeletal problems is preferred over pharmacologic (e.g., NSAID, Coxib, steroid, opioid) management because of the collateral benefits, safety, and cost-effectiveness associated with manual, dietary, botanical, and nutritional treatments. A brief discussion of the current crisis in musculoskeletal medicine is provided for contextualization and emphasis of the importance of expanding clinicians' knowledge of effective nondrug treatments*	243
4. <u>The Major Modifiable Factors in Sustained Inflammation</u>: *Major components of the "Functional Inflammology Protocol" are reviewed here, from concepts and molecular biology to an emphasis on practical clinical applications*	303
5. <u>Clinical Applications: Rheumatology</u>	543
1) Fibromyalgia — 557	
2) Rheumatoid Arthritis — 596	
3) Psoriasis and Psoriatic Arthritis — 616	
4) Systemic Lupus Erythematosus — 630	
5) Scleroderma & Systemic Sclerosis — 650	
6) Vasculitic Diseases, Giant Cell Arteritis & Polymyalgia Rheumatica, Wegener's Granulomatosis — 672	
7) Spondyloarthropathies: Ankylosing spondylitis, Reactive arthritis, Enteropathic spondyloarthropathy — 686	
8) Sjögren Syndrome/Disease — 697	
9) Raynaud's Syndrome/Phenomenon/Disorder — 703	
Essays and additional information, including the anti-viral protocol — 709	
• Index	741
• <u>Presentation Slides: 1) Introduction to the Functional Inflammology Protocol, 2) Review of Dysbiosis</u>: *More than 270 updated presentation slides containing additional information and citations; readers can view the corresponding online videos*	746 Slides and graphics

Dedications: I dedicate this book to the following people in appreciation for their works, their direct and indirect support of this work, and for their contributions to the advancement of true healthcare.
- **To the students and practitioners of naturopathic/functional medicine**, those who continue to learn so that they can provide the best possible care to their patients
- **To the researchers** whose works are cited in this text
- **To Dr Alan Gaby and Dr Jeffrey Bland,** my most memorable and influential *personal* professors and mentors
  - Of additional note, Dr Bland deserves credit for being the primary developer of the American rendition of "functional medicine", a conceptual framework and clinical model used and discussed in this text. Development and continuous maturation of the functional medicine model has depended upon numerous researchers and clinicians; Dr Jeff Bland was clearly the pioneer for this concept circa 1993 and the nucleus around which many of us have worked (at least initially) in this regard.
- **To Henry Rollins**, in particular for his prose book *One from None*, which completely changed my life in 1991
- **To Dr Friedrich Nietzsche and Dr Noam Chomsky,** my most memorable and influential *virtual* professors and mentors, both of whom exemplify profound scholarship and intellectual independence in favor of developing the highest possible human culture on earth
- **To Dr Bruce Ames**[1] **and Dr Roger J Williams**[2], for proving the importance of biochemical individuality
- **To Dr Chester Wilk**[3,4] **and important others**[5,6,7] for documenting and resisting the organized oppression of natural, non-pharmaceutical, non-surgical healthcare
- **To Jorge Strunz and Ardeshir Farah,** for artistic inspiration over the past 20 years

Acknowledgments for Peer and Editorial Review: Most of the sections that comprise the current work have been previously reviewed/published/presented; peer/editorial reviews are acknowledged below. Acknowledgement here does not imply that the reviewer fully agrees with or endorses the material in this text but rather that they were willing to review specific sections of the book for clinical applicability and clarity and to make suggestions to their own level of satisfaction.
- 2014 Edition of *Naturopathic Rheumatology*: Annette D'Armata ND
- 2012 Edition of *Fibromyalgia in a Nutshell*: Lisa Scholl BA, Annette D'Armata ND
- 2012 Edition of *Migraine Headaches, Hypothyroidism, and Fibromyalgia*: Holly Furlong DC
- 2011 Edition of *Integrative Chiropractic Management of High Blood Pressure and Chronic Hypertension*: Barry Morgan MD, Holly Furlong DC, Kris Young DC, Erika Mennerick DC, and J William Beakey DOM
- 2011 Edition of *Integrative Medicine and Functional Medicine for Chronic Hypertension*: Erika Mennerick DC, JoAnn Fawcett DC, Ileana Bourland MSOM LAc, James Bogash DC, J William Beakey DOM
- 2010 Edition of *Chiropractic Management of Chronic Hypertension*: Joseph Paun MS DC, David Candelario OMS4 (TCOM c/o 2010), James Bogash DC, Bill Beakey DOM, Robert Richard DO
- 2009 Edition of *Chiropractic and Naturopathic Mastery of Common Clinical Disorders*: Heather Kahn MD, Robert Richard DO, James Leiber DO, David Candelario (UNT-HSC TCOM OMS4)
- 2007 Edition of *Integrative Orthopedics*: Barry Morgan MD, Dennis Harris DC, Richard Brown DC (DACBI candidate), Ron Mariotti ND, Patrick Makarewich MBA, Reena Singh (SCNM ND4), Zachary Watkins DC, Charles Novak MS DC, Marnie Loomis ND, James Bogash DC, Sara Croteau DC, Kris Young DC, Joshua Levitt ND, Jack Powell III MD, Chad Kessler MD, Amy Neuzil ND
- 2006 Edition of *Integrative Rheumatology*: Amy Neuzil ND, Cathryn Harbor MD, Julian Vickers DC, Tamara Sachs MD, Bob Sager BSc MD DABFM (Clinical Instructor in the Department of Family Medicine, University of Kansas), Ron Mariotti ND, Titus Chiu (DC4), Zachary Watkins (DC4), Gilbert Manso MD, Bruce Milliman ND, William Groskopp DC, Robert Silverman DC, Matthew Breske (DC4), Dean Neary ND, Thomas Walton DC, Fraser Smith ND, Ladd Carlston DC, David Jones MD, Joshua Levitt ND
- 2004 Edition of *Integrative Orthopedics*: Peter Knight ND, Kent Littleton ND MS, Barry Morgan MD, Ron Hobbs ND, Joshua Levitt ND, John Neustadt (Bastyr ND4), Allison Gandre BS (Bastyr ND4), Peter Kimble ND, Jack Powell III MD, Chad Kessler MD, Mike Gruber MD, Deirdre O'Neill ND, Mary Webb ND, Leslie Charles ND, Amy Neuzil ND

---

[1] Ames BN, et al. High-dose vitamin therapy stimulates variant enzymes with decreased coenzyme binding affinity (increased K(m)). *Am J Clin Nutr*. 2002 Apr;75:616-58
[2] Williams RJ. *Biochemical Individuality: The Basis for the Genetotrophic Concept*. Austin and London: University of Texas Press; 1956
[3] Wilk CA. *Medicine, Monopolies, and Malice: How the Medical Establishment Tried to Destroy Chiropractic*. Garden City Park: Avery, 1996
[4] Getzendanner S. Permanent injunction order against AMA. *JAMA*. 1988 Jan 1;259(1):81-2
[5] Carter JP. *Racketeering in Medicine: The Suppression of Alternatives*. Norfolk: Hampton Roads Pub; 1993
[6] Morley J, Rosner AL, Redwood D. A case study of misrepresentation of the scientific literature: recent reviews of chiropractic. *J Altern Complement Med*. 2001;7:65-78
[7] Terrett AG. Misuse of the literature by medical authors in discussing spinal manipulative therapy injury. *J Manipulative Physiol Ther*. 1995 May;18(4):203-10

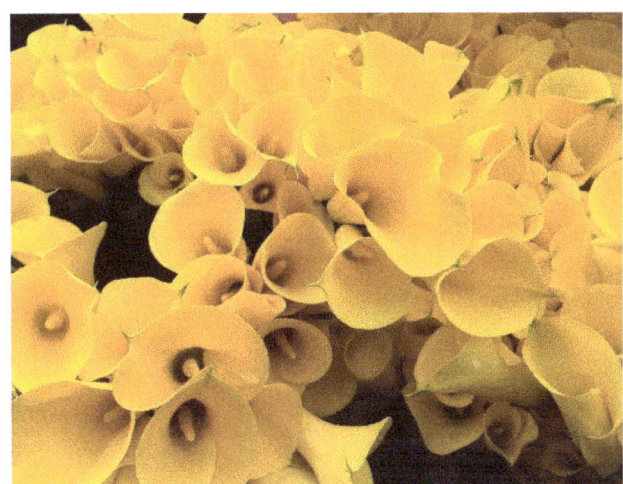

Living color, more vitality: The "colorization" process for the interior of this book began in April 2014 in Bogota (above) and Cartagena Colombia (below).

Format and Layout: The format/layout of this book is designed to efficiently take the reader though the clinically relevant spectrum of considerations for each condition that is detailed. Important topics are given their own section within each chapter, while other less important or less common conditions are only described briefly in terms of the four "clinical essentials" of 1) definition/pathophysiology, 2) clinical presentation, 3) assessment/diagnosis, and 4) treatment/management. Each expanded section which details the more important/common conditions maintains a consistent format, taking the reader through the spectrum of primary clinical considerations: definition/pathophysiology, clinical presentations, differential diagnoses, assessments (physical examination, laboratory, imaging), complications, management, and treatment. As my books have progressed, I am increasingly using an article-by-article review format (especially in the sections on management and treatment) so that readers have more direct access to the information so as to understand and *incorporate* more deeply what the research actually states; the goal and general approach here is to use a *representative sampling* of the research literature.

References and Citations: Citations to articles, abstracts, texts, and personal communications are footnoted throughout the text to provide supporting information and to provide interested readers the resources to find additional information. Many of the cited articles are available on-line for free, and often I have included the website addresses so that readers can easily access the complete article.

Peer-review and Quality Control: Peer-review is essential to help ensure accuracy and clinical applicability of health-related information. Consistent with the importance of these goals, I have employed several "checks and balances" to increase the accuracy and applicability of the information within my textbooks:

- Reliance upon authoritative references: Nearly all important statements are referenced to peer-reviewed biomedical journals or authoritative texts, examples of the latter include *The Merck Manual, Current Medical Diagnosis and Treatment,* and *5-Minute Clinical Consult.* Each citation is provided by a footnote at the bottom of each page so that readers will know quickly and easily exactly where the information was obtained.
- Extensive cross-referencing: Readers will notice the supranormal number of references and citations. Many important statements have several references. Many references (especially textbooks) are referenced several times even on the same page; the purpose of this extensive referencing is three-fold: 1) to guide you the reader to additional information, 2) to help me (as writer) stay organized, and 3) to help you and me (the practicing physicians) employ this information with confidence. In more recent updates/revisions, I have started shortening the number of listed authors by frequent use of *et al* with an interest in keeping each citation to one line of text on the page, likewise reducing mental and eye strain; quite obviously I respect each of the authors—even those whose names are not listed in the citation—and am implementing this solely for the sake of efficient book formatting (aiming for one citation per line) and information density (fewer lines dedicated to citations allows more space for text and images). Given hundreds of pages and thousands of citations, formatting considerations such as these are summatively significant.
- Periodic revision: Any significant errors that are discovered will be posted at InflammationMastery.com/volume1 (…volume2, etc); please check these folders periodically to ensure that you are working with the most accurate information of which I am aware.
- Peer-review: The peer-review process for my books takes several forms. First, colleagues and students are invited to review new and revised sections of the text before publication; every section of the book that you are holding has been independently reviewed by health science students and/or practicing clinicians from various backgrounds: allopathic, chiropractic, osteopathic, naturopathic. Second, you - the reader - are invited to provide feedback about the information in the book, typographical errors, syntax, case reports, new research, etc. If your ideas truly change the nature of the material, I will be glad to acknowledge you in the text (with your permission, of course). If your contribution is hugely significant, such as reviewing three or more chapters or helping in some important way, I will be glad to not only acknowledge you, but to also send you the next edition at a discount or courtesy when your ideas take effect. Third, I keep abreast of new literature by constantly perusing new research and advancements in the health sciences. Having been successful in three separate doctoral programs in the health sciences, I have learned not only to master large amounts of material but to also separate and integrate different viewpoints as appropriate. I also "field test" my protocols with patients in the various clinical arenas in which I work and also with professionals and academicians via presentations and critical dialogue. By implementing these quality control steps, I hope to create a useful text and advance our professions and practices by improving the quality of care that we deliver to our patients.

How to Use This Book Most Effectively: Ideally, these books should be read cover-to-cover within a context of coursework that is supervised by a clinically experienced professor. For post-graduate professionals, they might consider forming a local or virtual "book club" and meeting for weekly or monthly discussions to check their understandings and share their clinical experiences to refine the application of clinical knowledge, perceptions, and skills. Virtual groups and internet forums—such as those hosted by International College of Human Nutrition and Functional Medicine at ICHNFM.ORG—

can provide access to an assembly of international professional peers wherein sharing of clinical questions and experiences are synergistic. This book is not intended to extensively cover all aspects of clinical medicine, such as clinical pharmacology and prescribing (for which I recommend Epocrates.com and its associated app) and medical management (for which I recommend 5-Minute Clinical Consult via book, website, and app).

Video access: Video access is provided via notices and footnotes appropriately placed and indicated throughout the book. Readers actually have to read the book to access the information and gain knowledge.
- Sample: vimeo.com/ichnfm/drv-functional-inflammology-intro2013
- Password: DrVprotocol

Notices: The intention and scope of this text are to provide health science students and doctorate-level clinicians with useful information and a familiarity with available research and resources pertinent to the management of patients in integrative primary care and specialty care settings. Specifically, the information in this book is intended to be used by licensed healthcare professionals who have received hands-on/residential clinical training and supervision at accredited health science colleges. Additionally, information in this book should be used in conjunction with other resources, texts, and in combination with the clinician's best judgment and intention to "*first, do no harm*" and second to provide effective healthcare. Information and treatments applicable to a specific *condition* may not be appropriate for or applicable to a specific *patient* in your office; this is especially true for patients with multiple comorbidities and those taking pharmaceutical medications with multiple adverse effects and drug/nutrient/herb interactions. In my books and articles, I describe treatments—manual, dietary, nutritional, botanical, pharmacologic, and occasionally surgical—and their research support for the clinical condition being discussed; each practitioner must determine appropriateness of these treatments for his/her individual patient and with consideration of the doctor's scope of practice, education, training, skill, and—occasionally—the appropriateness of "off label" use of medications and treatments. This book has been carefully written and checked for accuracy by the author and professional colleagues. However, in view of the possibility of human error and new discoveries in the biomedical sciences, neither the author nor any party associated in any way with this text warrants that this text is perfect, accurate, or complete in every way, and we disclaim responsibility for harm or loss associated with the application of the material herein. With all conditions/treatments described herein, each physician must be sure to consider the balance between what is best for the patient and the physician's own level of ability, expertise, and experience. When in doubt, or if the physician is not a specialist in the treatment of a given severe condition, referral is appropriate. These notes are written with the routine "outpatient" in mind and are not tailored to severely injured patients or "playing field" or "emergency response" situations; consult your First Aid and Emergency Response texts and course materials for appropriate information. These notes represent the author's perspective based on academic education, experience, and post-graduate continuing education and are not inclusive of every fact that a clinician may need to know. This is not an "entry level" book except when used in an academic setting with a knowledgeable professor who can explain the concepts, tests, physical exam procedures, and treatments; this book requires a certain level of knowledge from the reader and familiarity with clinical concepts, laboratory assessments, and physical examination procedures. Suggested doses—if any—are for adults (not infants and children) unless otherwise specified in context; the responsibility for appropriate dosing is of course that of the prescribing clinician in view of the patient's age, weight, overall state, hepatic and renal function, comorbidities, polypharmacy, etc.

Purpose, scope, recommended companion resources

The purpose of this book is not to serve as a stand-alone "recipe book" for the complete management of all reviewed conditions; rather the focus of this book is the delivery of clinically important concepts and facts to enhance the management of various clinical disorders, in particular by documenting and explicating this author's naturopathic, medical, integrative and functional medicine approach. Readers and instructors using this book are encouraged to use whichever additional resources they choose, including but not limited to the supporting videos at Vimeo.com/DrVasquez and Vimeo.com/ICHNFM; in particular, 5-Minute Clinical Consult and Epocrates are excellent and strongly advised companion guides for overall medical diagnosis/management and clinical pharmacology/prescribing, respectively. Clinicians need to have a good understanding of clinical medicine before applying many of the approaches described in this book; cross-referencing and double-checking management strategies and drug doses are essential components of quality care. Both 5-Minute Clinical Consult and Epocrates are available as point-of-care references, and their use is advised.

This work is best used with the relevant videos from DrV available online, some of which are linked and made password-accessible via this book; additional videos by Dr Vasquez are available online (occasionally with accompanying printed presentation slides); please see the following examples and locations:
- vimeo.com/ondemand/ichnfm2013drv and the accompanying 426-page printed book of all slides available createspace.com/4478800,
- vimeo.com/ichnfm
- vimeo.com/drvasquez
- itunes.apple.com/us/artist/dr-alex-vasquez/id475526413
- cdbaby.com/Artist/DrAlexVasquez

Updates, Corrections, and Newsletter: When and if omissions, errata, and the need for important updates become clear, I will post these at the website InflammationMastery.com. A reader might access this page periodically to ensure staying informed of any corrections that might have clinical relevance. This book consists not only of the text in the printed pages you are holding, but also the footnotes and any updates at the website. If any clinically important corrections are made, they will be distributed by newsletter InflammationMastery.com/join_email.html and/or placed in the folder FunctionalInflammology.com/volume1/ (with analogous folders for subsequent volumes, e.g., volume2, etc) for constant availability. Be alerted to new integrative clinical research, updates to this textbook and other news/publications/conferences/videos by registering for the free newsletter at InflammationMastery.com/join_email.html.

Language, Semantics, and Perspective: As a diligent student who previously aspired to be an English professor, I have written this text with great (though inevitably imperfect) attention to detail. Individual words were chosen with care. I confess to knowing, pushing, and creatively breaking several rules of grammar and punctuation. With regard to the he/she and him/her debacle of the English language, I've occasionally mixed singular and plural pronouns for the sake of being efficient and so that the images remain gender-neutral to the extent reasonable. In several previous publications, the subtitle *The art of creating wellness while effectively managing acute and chronic musculoskeletal/health disorders* was chosen to emphasize the intentional creation of wellness rather than a limited focus on disease treatment and symptom suppression; for the 2009 printing of *Chiropractic and Naturopathic Mastery of Common Clinical Disorders*, this subtitle was slightly modified from "creating" to "co-creating" to emphasize the team effort required between physician and patient. *Managing* was chosen to emphasize the importance of treating-monitoring-referring-reassessing, rather than merely *treating*. *Disorders* was chosen to reflect the fact that a distinguishing characteristic of *life* is the ability to regularly create *organized structure* and *higher order* from chaos and *disorder*. For example, plants organize the randomly moving molecules of air and water into the organized structure of biomolecules which eventually take shape as plant structure—fiber, leaves, flowers, petals. Similarly, the human body creates organized structure of increased complexity from consumed plants and other foods; molecules ingested and inhaled from the environment are organized into specific biochemicals and tissue structures with distinct characteristics and definite functions. Injury and disease *result in* or *result from* a lack of order, hence my use of the word "disorders" to characterize human illness and disease. For example, a motor vehicle accident that results in bodily injury, for example, is an example of an external chaotic force, which, when imparted upon human body tissues, results in a disruption (disorder) of the normal structure and organization that previously defined and characterized the now-damaged tissues of the body; likewise, an autoimmune disease process that results in tissue destruction is an *anti-evolutionary* process that takes molecules of higher complexity and reverts them to simpler, fragmented, and non-functional forms. From the perspective of "health" as *organized structure and meaningful function* and "disease" as *the reversion to chaos, destruction of structure, and the loss of function,* the task of healthcare providers is essentially to restore order, and to acutely reduce and proactively prevent/eliminate clinical-biochemical-biomechanical-emotional chaos insofar as it adversely affects the patient's life experience as an individual and our collective experience as an interdependent society. What is required of clinicians then is the ability *first* to create conceptual order from what appears to be chaotic phenomena, and then *second* to materialize—make real and practically applied for patients/people seeking improved health—that conceptual order into our physical world; this is our task, and no small task it is. Also under this heading of Semantics and Language, I will make readers aware of the following additional facts. First, I tend to write very long sentences, both in general and at times when I want to connect two or more complex ideas; rather than be dismayed or discouraged by this occurrence, readers are encouraged to read these longer sentences more than just once and to engage actively, perhaps by asking, "*Why is DrV making an effort to connect these ideas*?" "***What is the conceptual advantage to the binding of these ideas together***?" I am aware of most of the rules of grammar, and I am generally—but not always—compliant. Second, I create new words and phrases as needed; an index of some of these is provided toward the back of the book, whereas some of these new terms are self-explanatory, e.g., *hypoinsulinreception*—underreception or lack of receptor responsiveness to insulin. When possible, I strongly prefer to use single words when discussing concepts, rather than multiple disparate words for singular concepts. I have started to prefer using *italics* rather than "quotation marks" when introducing new terms or when using terms/phrases/words with emphasis; the main purpose of this is to reduce the number of punctuation marks and character spaces, both of which over the course of a multi-volume work of 2,000 pages and hundreds of thousands of words are numerically significant. Last for this section, the *colorization* process that I began in April 2014 for my (larger) books is intended to 1) bring out more detail in my increasingly complex diagrams, 2) bring emphasis and highlighting to areas of particular interest, 3) make the work more visually stimulating/pleasing over the previous black/white/grayscale versions, and—relatedly—4) to keep the work interesting as readers tread through a remarkable amount of complex and detailed information; I realize that some readers may at times find the colorization to be a small distraction, but I think this is better than the alternative of monotony induced by 630 pages of grayscale.

Preface & Introduction

Integrity and Creativity: I have endeavored to accurately represent the facts as they have been presented in texts and research, and to specifically resist any temptation to embellish or misrepresent data as others have done.[8,9] Conversely, I have not endeavored to make this book appeal to the "average" student or reader; my goal is to write and teach to the students at the top of the class, thereby affirming them and pulling the other students forward and upward. While I offer *explanations*, I intentionally resist *simplifications*, except when one simplification might facilitate the comprehension of a more complex phenomenon, or when such a simplification might facilitation the conveyance of information from clinician to patient. I have allowed this text to be unique in format, content, and style, so that the personality of this text can be contrasted with that of the instructor and reader, thus enabling the learner to at least benefit from an intentionally different – and intentionally honest – perspective and approach. Students using this text with the guidance of a qualified professor will benefit from the experience of "two teachers" rather than just one.

Linearity, Nonlinearity, Redundancy, Asynchronicity: Although the overall flow of the text is highly linear and sequential, occasionally I place a conclusion before its introduction for the sake of foreshadowing and therefore for preparing the reader for what is to come. The purpose of this is not simply one of preparation for the sake of allowing the reader to know what is already lying ahead on the path, but more to begin creating new "shelf space" in the reader's intellectual-neuronal "library" so that when the new—particularly if *neoparadigmatic*—information is encountered, a space will already exist for it; it other words: the intent is to make learning easier. Likewise, for the sake of *information retention*— or what is physiologically understood as synaptogenesis—important points are presented more than once, either identically or variantly. Given that *"No one ever reads the same book twice"*[10] (because the "person who starts" the reading of a meaningful book is changed into the "person who finishes" the reading of that book (assuming proper intentionality and application of one's "self"), the person reading these words might consider a second glance after the first. For the sake of efficient use of space I have tried to minimize redundancy; however, in a few locations, redundancy of text and images proved necessary for—for example—viewing the same diagram within two different conversations allows the reader to gain a more profound understanding of the concepts by viewing them from two different conversations/contexts.

Bon Voyage: All artists and scientists—regardless of genre—grapple with the divergent goals of *perfecting* their work and *presenting* their work; the former is impossible in the ultimate sense, while the latter is the only means by which the effort can create the desired effect in the world, whether that is pleasure, progress, or both. At some point, we must all agree

> **Authentic learning is life integration**
> "Ultimately, no one can extract from things—*books included*—more than he already knows. What one has no access to through experience, one has no ear for."
> Nietzsche FW [trans. Hollingdale]. *Ecce Homo*. Penguin; 1979, p70

that it is "good enough" and that it contains the essence of what needs to be communicated. While neither this nor any future edition of this book is likely to be "perfect", I am content with the literature reviewed, presented, and the new conclusions and implications which are described—many for the first time ever—in this text. Firstly in and progressively from my *Integrative Rheumatology* (2006), each chapter achieved/achieves a paradigm shift which distanced/distances us farther from the simplistic pathocentric and pharmacocentric model and toward one which authentically empowers both practitioners and patients. With time, I will make future editions more complete, consistently passionate, and either more or less polemical. I hope you are able to implement these conclusions and research findings *into your own life* and into the *treatment plans for your patients*. Hopefully this work's value and veracity will promote patients' vitality via the vigilant and virtuous clinicians viewing this volume; to the more attentive and thoroughgoing reader, more is revealed (for example, the last sentence is a reference to the descriptive and prophetic movie *V for Vendetta* (2006).

Thank you for engaging with this work, and I wish you and your patients the best of success and health.

Alex Vasquez, D.C., N.D., D.O., F.A.C.N.
September 23, 2014

---

[8] Vasquez A. Zinc treatment for reduction of hyperplasia of prostate. *Townsend Letter for Doctors and Patients* 1996; January: 100
[9] Broad W, Wade N. *Betrayers of the Truth: Fraud and Deceit in the Halls of Science*. New York: Simon and Schuster; 1982
[10] Davies R. *Reading and Writing*. Salt Lake City: University of Utah Press; 1992, page 23

Examples of commonly used abbreviations:

- **25-OH-D** = serum 25-hydroxy-vitamin D(3)
- **ACEi** = angiotensin-2 converting enzyme inhibitor
- **Alpha-blocker** = alpha-adrenergic antagonist
- **ANA** = antinuclear antibodies
- **ARB** = angiotensin-2 receptor blocker/antagonist
- **ARF** = acute renal failure
- **BB** = beta blocker or beta-adrenergic antagonist
- **bHB, BHB** = beta-hydroxy-butyrate
- **BMP** = basic metabolic panel, includes serum Na, K, Cl, CO2, BUN, creatinine, and glucose
- **BP** = blood pressure, relatedly HBP = high blood pressure
- **BUN** = blood urea nitrogen
- **C and S** = culture and sensitivity
- **CAD** = coronary artery disease
- **CBC** = complete blood count
- **CCB** = calcium channel blocker/antagonist
- **CE** = cardiac enzymes, including creatine kinase (CK), creatine kinase myocardial band (CKMB), and troponin-1, with the latter being the most specific serologic marker for acute myocardial injury; for the evaluation of acute MI, these are generally tested 2-3 times at 6-hour intervals with ECG performed at least as often.
- **CHF** = congestive heart failure
- **CHO, carb** = carbohydrate
- **CK** = creatine kinase, historically named creatine phosphokinase (CPK)
- **CKD** = chronic kidney disease, generally stratified into five stages based on GFR of roughly <90, 90-60, 60-30, 30-15, and >15, respectively
- **CMP** = comprehensive metabolic panel, also called a chemistry panel, includes the BMP along with markers of hepatic status albumin, protein, ALT, AST, may also include alkaline phosphatase and rarely GGT; panels vary per laboratory and hospital.
- **CNS** = central nervous system
- **COPD** = chronic obstructive pulmonary disease
- **CRF, CRI** = chronic renal failure/insufficiency
- **CRP** = c-reactive protein, hsCRP = high-sensitivity c-reactive protein

- **CT** = computed tomography
- **CVD** = cardiovascular disease
- **CXR** = chest X-ray
- **DM** = diabetes mellitus
- **DMARD** = disease-modifying antirheumatic drugs
- **ECG** or **EKG** = electrocardiograph
- **Echo** = echocardiography
- **ERS** = endoplasmic reticulum stress
- **GFR** = glomerular filtration rate
- **HDL** = high density lipoprotein cholesterol
- **HTN** = hypertension
- **Ig** = immune globulin = antibodies of the G, A, M, E, or D classes.
- **IHD** = ischemic heart disease
- **I+D** = incision and drainage
- **IM, IV** = intramuscular, intravenous
- **LPS** = bacterial lipopolysaccharide, endotoxin
- **MCV** = mean cell volume
- **MI** = myocardial infarction
- **Mito** = mitochondria(l)
- **MRI** = magnetic resonance imaging, MRI = magnetic resonance angiography
- **mTOR** = mechanistic or mammalian receptor of rapamycin; **TOR** is also reasonable
- **NFkB** = nuclear transcription factor kappa beta
- **PNS** = peripheral nervous system
- **PRN** = from the Latin "pro re nata" meaning "on occasion" or "when necessary"
- **PTH** = parathyroid hormone, iPTH = intact parathyroid hormone
- **PVD** = peripheral vascular disease
- **RA** = rheumatoid arthritis
- **RAD** = reactive airway disease, asthma
- **SIBO** = small intestine bacterial overgrowth
- **SLE** = systemic lupus erythematosus
- **TLR** = Toll-like receptor
- **TRIG(s)** = serum triglycerides
- **UA** = urinalysis
- **UPR** = unfolded protein response
- **US** = ultrasound

Dosing shorthand:

- **bid** = twice daily
- **cc** = with meals
- **hs** = at bedtime
- **ic** = between meals
- **po** = per os = by mouth
- **prn** = as needed

- **q** = each
- **qd** = each day, also /d or /day
- **qid** = four times per day
- **tid** = thrice daily
- **yo** = years old

Begin at the beginning

"He who wishes one day to *fly*, must first learn *standing*
   and *walking*
      and *running*
         and *climbing*
           and *dancing*.
One does not *fly* into *flying*."
 	
Nietzsche FW. *Thus Spoke Zarathustra—A Book for All and None*. 1883-1885

International Journal of Human Nutrition and Functional Medicine ®
- Flexible printing format for authors: free open-access and/or pay-per-access for printed monographs
- Rapid and legitimate peer-review process by international experts
- Authors retain ownership (shared copyrights between author and journal)
- Updates distributed by newsletter via *Int J Hum Nutr Funct Med*. org

Work as love made tangible
"You work that you may keep pace with the earth and the soul of the earth. For to be idle is to become a stranger unto the seasons, and to step out of life's procession. ... Work is love made visible." Kahlil Gibran (1883-1930). *The Prophet*. Publisher Alfred A. Knopf, 1973

Reviews of previous and recent works:

- "I just wanted to tell you how much I appreciate the information I have received from you. I am still digesting most of it. I feel I have learned quite a bit already yet also feel I have barely scratched the surface." *Doctor and Graduate student under Dr Vasquez, 2013*
- "Dr. Vasquez, Thank you for all you do. **Your conference was simply amazing.** No one wanted to leave the room. I met medical professionals and very interesting lay people who were stimulated and invigorated to change their lives and the lives of others. **I am in awe at your intellectual integrity and veracity.** Best of luck to you in all of your future endeavors." *Medical physician and ICHNFM 2013 Conference Attendee*
- "I attended the last ICHNFM conference in Portland (and am still basking in the amazing information received)." *Email from Clinical Oncology Dietitian, in late February 2014*
- "Thanks for a fantastic conference!" *ICHNFM 2013 Conference Attendee*
- "Your discourse today reflected not only your passion and commitment to the wellness of our planet but most importantly the clarity and sincerity of your spirit/ heart/ mind. Always good to be with you and look forward to seeing you soon. Hope we can spend more time then." *Medical physician attendee 2014*
- "I was so refreshed by the 'unfiltered excellence.' What humanness. Breaths of fresh air." *ICHNFM 2013 Attendee*
- "Keep in mind Alex, that humanity is a better place because of you. I know you can't undo it all, but think about how many people would be worse off if it wasn't for your wonderful knowledge being shared with all us docs. Things that I have learned from you have changed peoples' lives for the better." *Naturopathic physician, 2014*
- "Just got back to Guam. Great experience at the International Conference on Human Nutrition and Functional Medicine. Exciting concepts on functional medicine. Thanks Dr. Alex Vasquez and team!" *ICHNFM 2013 Conference Attendee*
- "Already waiting in line to buy next year's ticket! **Dr. Vasquez you crushed it!** The future is looking fun already ☺" *ICHNFM 2013 Conference Attendee*
- "Had an incredible time at the 2013 International Conference on Human Nutrition and Functional Medicine. Got to meet some amazing people and hear from some of the top researchers/health professionals about human nutrition and functional medicine approaches. It was definitely worth every penny and can't wait to go back next year!" *ICHNFM 2013 Conference Attendee*
- "I miss you! Your confidence in a program you believed in. I miss your live classes where we would get off topic on a clinical pearl. I miss your way of teaching in a laid back atmosphere that made me feel comfortable, not intimidated. I just needed to let you know, this program is not the same, I am almost done, otherwise, I would have bailed out! I am grateful for the last 18 months I did have with you at the helm. ... You ignited in me my passion for learning again. You sparked the minds of all of us with your enthusiasm. Don't ever let anyone take that away. It has given birth to your new endeavor, and we will follow where you lead. Enjoy your new surroundings and celebrate your new beginnings. I know I look forward to what is ahead." *Doctor and Graduate student under Dr Vasquez, 2013*
- "Wonderful conference! Thanks so much." *ICHNFM 2013 Conference Attendee*
- "Really wonderful conference! Lots of material ready to implement Monday morning! **Congrats to Alex Vasquez on a herculean job very well done!**" *ICHNFM 2013 Conference Attendee*
- "Thanks for a great conference. I really enjoyed all of the speakers, but your lectures were by far the most useful for implementing ideas into my clinical practice. And the most entertaining." *ICHNFM 2013 Conference Attendee*
- "Thank you for your life-changing work." *Physician, 2011*
- "I want Dr. Vasquez to know that I have just received his book, *Chiropractic and Naturopathic Mastery of Common Clinical Disorders*. **It is a treasure. The best book in my library.** Thank you for the contribution that you are giving to the world of health care." *Clinician, 2010*
- "I appreciate the resources you offer the profession. I use your books and articles regularly." *Doctor, 2011*
- "Dr. Vasquez, I greatly appreciate your efforts. I am a student at ___, 8th trimester, and would like to express my gratitude for your research and works. After coming across your texts in the library, **I quickly found your insight and explanations of the current health care crisis, and in depth coverage and algorithms for inflammatory diseases as a profound inspiration and call to action. I appreciate your attention to detail, and have been taken back several times by the potency and meaning of your sentences. Thank you for your hard work, I will enjoy these books and will surely share with those that have the same drive for true and competent patient care.**" *Health Sciences Student, 2008*
- "I never told you this, but whenever I need to research a particular disease, **besides going on Pubmed and checking some classic Pathophysiology and Clinical Nutrition books, I use your books and I find them extremely well organized, concise, and up-to-date and with the functional/integrative medicine thinking I enjoy and believe it is the future of Health Care.**" *Nutrition Research Consultant and University Faculty in Europe, 2009*

Preface & Introduction

- "Thanks so much. You are a great asset to our profession." *Doctor, 2010*
- "As a 7th trimester student quickly approaching 8th trimester and student clinic, I know I will be utilizing your books often. **Your "Chiropractic and Naturopathic Mastery of Common Clinical Disorders" book is referenced very frequently by many clinicians and faculty members at [our university]. Your work is highly regarded**, and I look forward to clinically utilizing the information I will obtain from your writings." *Health Sciences Student, 2011*
- "I am a chiropractic student at ___ Chiropractic College. I just wanted to drop a quick line thanking you for your thorough and accessible textbook Integrative Orthopedics. We are using it in our Differential Diagnosis class, and **it is the best book I've come across in Chiropractic College bar none. The writing is concise, informative and refreshingly eloquent. The material is super practical. I hope you continue putting out great resources.**" *Health Sciences Student, 2011*
- "I appreciate the resources you offer the profession. **I use your books and articles regularly.**" *Doctor, 2011*
- "**Your Integrated Orthopedics book is magnificent**. I wish all textbooks were structured and as thoughtful as that one." *Health Sciences Student, 2008*
- "By reading the introduction I realize that calling it an orthopedics book; does not do it justice. **It is far more than that. It looks to me that you have created, or are creating, the bible of Integrative Orthopedics and physical medicine**. *Physician, 2007*
- "First of all let me say how honored I am that you have allowed me to review this work. You have done an amazing job! In my opinion **every healthcare provider SHOULD have this on their bookshelf**." *Physician, 2007*
- "Your work on Chapter 12: Hip and Thigh is very good. The chapter is inclusive of the typical pathologies seen in private practice and I particularly liked the separation of juvenile from adult pathologies. Your choice of tests to assess hip and thigh pathology on page 320 is very nice and inclusive. I appreciate your use of algorithms and find them very useful in teaching and in practice. In general, **I thought this chapter represents a quality, state of the art presentation**!" *Clinician and Professor in Clinical Sciences, 2007*
- "I saw your books in a colleague's office and was really impressed. Really appreciate the thoroughness you've put into them." *Doctor, 2010*
- "**It is with great interest and fascination that I have been reading your material both in your two books (Integrative Orthopedics and Integrative Rheumatology) and online. I consider myself very fortunate to have come across your work**, as many of the basic elements of health which you discuss I never learnt or even heard about while in chiropractic college." *Doctor, 2010*
- "I appreciate the resources you offer the profession. I use your books and articles regularly." *Doctor, 2011*
- "**I'm so pleased with your books and was inspired to let you know they have already been incredibly useful! Good index; well organized algorithms. Sometimes I buy educational material and it just sort of sits there... Your books now live on my main desk. Thanks.**" *Physician and Journal Editor, 2009*
- "I just wanted to let you know how much I am enjoying reading **your book Integrative Rheumatology. It is having an extremely positive impact in the way I view health and am having a tough time putting it down. It is very inspirational.** I have long felt that it is very important to set a good example for your patients and now try my best to be one for my future patients. I like how you stress this in your book. In order to be the best example for my patients I am going to need to address some problems with my own health. I look healthy from the outside but I have been suffering from fatigue for about 4 years. It has a very negative impact on my health. People say that doing the same thing and expecting different results is the definition of insanity so I think it is time that I attempt to make some changes. ... **Thanks again for writing such a great book. I feel it is a must have for anyone in a musculoskeletal practice.**" *Health Sciences Student, 2010*
- "My name is [recent graduate], and I've been a fan of your books since I was in chiropractic college at [university] campus. Dr. [Author, Presenter] made your book, Integrative Rheumatology, required reading for his 9th quarter nutrition class. I never looked back, and have since purchased Chiropractic & Naturopathic Mastery of Common Clinical Disorders as well as Chiropractic Management of Chronic Hypertension." *Doctor, 2010*
- "I saw your books in a colleague's office and was really impressed. Really appreciate the thoroughness you've put into them." *Doctor, 2010*
- "Reading the new integrative management of high blood pressure book and I am thoroughly enjoying it; excellent job. **I am feeling so empowered I'm opening another office focusing on 'restoring the foundations of health' for the community** that I open it in. I am looking for a location and networking to find an internist and cardiologist that are forward thinking; I'm very excited!" *Doctor, 2011*
- "Thank you for the presentation at [the university] this past weekend. **My horizons about what can be done to help people were greatly expanded. I am now still studying the notes from the seminar and am looking forward to more study and learning on how to *correctly* manage diabetes and hypertension.**" *Doctor, 2011*

- "Thank you for exposing so many people to the results of our research on the treatment of hypertension. I hope you can pay us a visit during your next trip to our area so we can give you the tour of our new 50+ bed inpatient facility." Dr Alan Goldhamer, Chief of Health Promoting Clinic, 2010
- "**I always enjoy reading your work.** I personally gain a lot of knowledge through being a peer-reviewer for you and am better because of it!" *Doctor, Faculty Member, and Postgraduate Instructor, 2011*
- "**I attended your seminar at [University] in June and have been utilizing your hypertension protocols. In that short time, I have seen some marked progress with various patients.**" *Doctor, 2010*

Chapter 1:
Initial Considerations in Patient Assessment and Management:
An Overview of Key Concepts and Facts in Patient History, Physical Examination, Laboratory Interpretation, Risk Management and Clinical Approach, Common Clinical Considerations

Overview of this chapter

Reviewed herein are the three essential components of patient assessment:
1. History
2. Physical examination
3. Laboratory assessment

Additional concepts and perspectives are provided that will help facilitate risk management and promote and contextualize optimal patient care.

This chapter concludes with two new sections under the title of "Common Clinical Considerations", since these topics—hemochromatosis and hypothyroidism—are both commonly encountered in clinical practice and need to be considered in the routine evaluation of essentially all patients and especially those who present with disorders such as diabetes, depression, fatigue, and musculoskeletal pain. Previously, I had published these as separate chapters in various books, but—again—at this time I think these need to be integrated into basic/daily/routine clinical consideration.

Topics:

- Moving past disease- and drug-centered medicine toward patient-centered health optimization: the goal is *wellness*
- Acute Care and Musculoskeletal Care as Opportunities for Health Optimization
- **Clinical Assessments**
    - History taking & physical examination
    - Orthopedic/musculoskeletal examination: Concepts and goals
    - Neurologic assessment: Review
    - Laboratory assessments: General considerations of commonly used tests
        i. *Routine tests*: Chemistry/metabolic panel, lipid panel, CBC, 25(OH)-vitamin D, ferritin, thyroid stimulating hormone, CRP, ESR
        ii. *Rheumatology/inflammation*: ANA (antinuclear antibodies), ANCA (antineutrophilic cytoplasmic antibodies), RF (rheumatoid factor), CCP (cyclic citrullinated protein antibodies), complement proteins, HLA-B27, additional tests for various immune/inflammatory disorders, tests for chronic infections/dysbiosis
        iii. *Functional assessments*: Lactulose-mannitol assay, comprehensive stool analysis and comprehensive parasitology
- **High-Risk Pain Patients**
- **Clinical Concepts**
    - Not all injury-related problems are injury-related problems
    - Safe patient + safe treatment = safe outcome
    - Four clues to underlying problems
    - Special considerations in the evaluation of children
    - No errors allowed: Differences between primary healthcare and spectator sports
    - "Disease treatment" is different from "patient management"
    - Clinical practice involves much more than "diagnosis and treatment"
    - Clinical Management of Patients with Systemic Inflammatory/Autoimmune Diseases
    - Risk Management, Charting, and Avoiding Medical Errors: Useful Reminders and Acronyms
    - Risk Management: A note especially to students and recent licensees
- **Musculoskeletal Emergencies**
    - Acute compartment syndrome
    - Acute red eye, including acute iritis and scleritis
    - Atlantoaxial subluxation and instability
    - Cauda equina syndrome
    - Giant cell arteritis, temporal arteritis
    - Myelopathy, spinal cord compression
    - Neuropsychiatric lupus
    - Osteomyelitis
    - Septic arthritis, acute nontraumatic monoarthritis
- **Brief Overview of Integrative Healthcare Disciplines**
    - Naturopathic Medicine
    - Functional Medicine
    - Osteopathic Medicine
    - Chiropractic
- **Common Clinical Considerations**
    - Hemochromatosis and Iron Overload
    - Hypothyroidism, particularly Functional/Metabolic/Peripheral Hypothyroidism

> **Moving past diagnosis/disease/drug-centered medicine toward patient-centered health optimization: The goal is *wellness***

Written for students and experienced clinicians, this chapter introduces and reviews many new and common terms, procedures, and concepts relevant to the management of patients with musculoskeletal disorders. Especially for students, the reading of this chapter is essential to understanding the extensive material in this book and will facilitate the clinical assessment and management of patients with various clinical presentations.

Healthcare is currently in a time of significant fluctuation and is ready for changes in the balance of power and the paradigms which direct our therapeutic interventions. For nearly a century, allopathic medicine has hailed itself as "the gold standard", and other professions have either submitted to or been crushed by their ongoing political/scientific manipulations and their continual proclamation of intellectual and therapeutic superiority[1,2,3,4,5,6,7,8,9,10,11,12,13] despite 180,000-220,000 iatrogenic *medically-induced* deaths per year (500-600 iatrogenic deaths per day)[14,15] and consistent documentation that most medical/allopathic physicians are unable to provide accurate musculoskeletal diagnoses due to pervasive inadequacies in medical training.[16,17,18,19] Increasing disenchantment with allopathic *heroic medicine* and its adverse outcomes of inefficacy, exorbitant expenses, and unnecessary death are fostering change, such that allopathic medicine has been dethroned as the leading paradigm among American patients, who spend the majority of their discretionary healthcare dollars on consultations and treatments provided by "alternative" healthcare providers.[20,21] With the ever-increasing utilization of integrative medical services, we must see that our paradigms and interventions keep pace with the evolving research literature and our increasing professional responsibilities so that we can deliver the highest possible quality of care.

> **Medical iatrogenesis kills 493 Americans per day**
>
> "Recent estimates suggest that each year more than 1 million patients are injured while in the hospital and approximately 180,000 die because of these injuries. Furthermore, drug-related morbidity and mortality are common and are estimated to cost more than $136 billion a year."
>
> Holland, Degruy. *Am Fam Physician*. 1997 Nov

While we all readily acknowledge the importance of emergency care for emergency situations, those of us who advocate and practice a more complete approach to healthcare and life readily see the shortcomings of a limited and mechanical approach to healthcare, and we aspire to do more than simply fix problems. The implementation of *multidimensional* (i.e., *comprehensive* and *multifaceted*) treatment plans that address many aspects of pathophysiologic phenomena is a huge step forward in creating improved health and preventing future illness in the patients who seek our professional assistance. However, even complete multidimensional treatment plans still fall short of the goal of creating wellness, if for no other reasons than 1) they are still disease- and problem-

---

[1] Wilk CA. *Medicine, Monopolies, and Malice: How the Medical Establishment Tried to Destroy Chiropractic*. Garden City Park: Avery, 1996
[2] Getzendanner S. Permanent injunction order against AMA. *JAMA*. 1988 Jan 1;259(1):81-2
[3] Carter JP. *Racketeering in Medicine: The Suppression of Alternatives*. Norfolk: Hampton Roads Pub; 1993
[4] Morley J, Rosner AL, Redwood D. A case study of misrepresentation of the scientific literature: recent reviews of chiropractic. *J Altern Complement Med*. 2001 Feb;7:65-78
[5] Terrett AG. Misuse of the literature by medical authors in discussing spinal manipulative therapy injury. *J Manipulative Physiol Ther*. 1995;18(4):203-10
[6] National Alliance of Professional Psychology Providers. AMA Seeks To Control and Restrict Psychologist's Scope of Practice. nappp.org/scope.pdf Accessed Nov 2006
[7] "In an effort to marshal the medical community's resources against the growing threat of expanding scope of practice for allied health professionals, the AMA has formed a national partnership to confront such initiatives nationwide... The committee will use $25,000..." Daly R, American Psychiatric Association. AMA Forms Coalition to Thwart Non-M.D. Practice Expansion. *Psychiatric News* 2006 March; 41: 17 pn.psychiatryonline.org/cgi/content/full/41/5/17-a?eaf Accessed November 25, 2006
[8] Spivak JL. *The Medical Trust Unmasked*. Louis S. Siegfried Publishers; New York: 1961
[9] Trever W. *In the Public Interest*. Los Angeles; Scriptures Unlimited; 1972. This is probably the most authoritative documentation of the illegal actions of the AMA up to 1972; contains numerous photocopies of actual AMA documents and minutes of official meetings with overt intentionality of destroying Americans' healthcare options so that the AMA and related organizations would have a monopoly in national healthcare.
[10] Wenban AB. Inappropriate use of the title 'chiropractor' and term 'chiropractic manipulation' in the peer-reviewed biomedical literature. *Chiropr Osteopat*. 2006;14:16
[11] Orme-Johnson DW, Herron RE. An innovative approach to reducing medical care utilization and expenditures. *Am J Manag Care*. 1997 Jan;3:135-44
[12] van der Steen WJ, Ho VK. Drugs versus diets: disillusions with Dutch health care. *Acta Biotheor*. 2001;49(2):125-40
[13] Texas Medical Association. Physicians Ask Court to Protect Patients From Illegal Chiropractic Activities. texmed.org/Template.aspx?id=5259 Accessed Feb 2007
[14] Starfield B. Is US health really the best in the world? *JAMA*. 2000 Jul 26;284(4):483-5
[15] "Recent estimates suggest that each year more than 1 million patients are injured while in the hospital and approximately 180,000 die because of these injuries. Furthermore, drug-related morbidity and mortality are common and are estimated to cost more than $136 billion a year." Holland EG, Degruy FV. Drug-induced disorders. *Am Fam Physician*. 1997;56(7):1781-8, 1791-2
[16] Freedman KB, Bernstein J. The adequacy of medical school education in musculoskeletal medicine. *J Bone Joint Surg Am*. 1998;80(10):1421-7
[17] Freedman KB, Bernstein J. Educational deficiencies in musculoskeletal medicine. *J Bone Joint Surg Am*. 2002;84-A(4):604-8
[18] Matzkin E, Smith ME, Freccero CD, Richardson AB. Adequacy of education in musculoskeletal medicine. *J Bone Joint Surg Am*. 2005;87-A(2):310-4
[19] Schmale GA. More evidence of educational inadequacies in musculoskeletal medicine. *Clin Orthop Relat Res*. 2005 Aug;(437):251-9
[20] "...Americans made an estimated 425 million visits to providers of unconventional therapy. This number exceeds the number of visits to all U.S. primary care physicians (388 million)." Eisenberg DM, Kessler RC, et al. Unconventional medicine in the United States. Prevalence, costs, and patterns of use. *N Engl J Med*. 1993 Jan 28;328(4):246-52
[21] "Estimated expenditures for alternative medicine professional services increased 45.2% between 1990 and 1997 and were conservatively estimated at $21.2 billion in 1997, with at least $12.2 billion paid out-of-pocket. This exceeds the 1997 out-of-pocket expenditures for all US hospitalizations." Eisenberg DM, Davis RB, Ettner SL, Appel S, Wilkey S, Van Rompay M, Kessler RC. Trends in alternative medicine use in the United States, 1990-1997: results of a follow-up national survey. *JAMA* 1998 Nov 11;280(18):1569-75

oriented, rather than health-oriented, 2) they are prescribed from outside ("The doctor told me to do it.") rather than originating internally and spontaneously by the patient's own direction and affirmation ("I *do* this because I *am* this."), and, finally and most difficult to relay, 3) they are mechanistic rather than organic, they can do no better than the sum of their parts, they flow exclusively from the mind ("do") and not also from the body-soul ("am"). The art of creating wellness takes time to understand, longer to implement clinically, and even longer to apply to one's own life. Wellness is a state of being rather

Ever-increasing popularity of nonallopathic medicine
"...Americans made an estimated 425 million visits to providers of unconventional therapy. This number exceeds the number of visits to all U.S. primary care physicians (388 million)."
Eisenberg DM, et al. Unconventional medicine in the United States. Prevalence, costs, and patterns of use. *N Engl J Med* 1993 Jan

than a checklist of activities in a "preventive health program." The subtle differences that distinguish "wellness" from any "program" or "prescription" are the differences between *leading* versus *following* and *flowing* versus *performing*. Wellness transcends mere health (e.g., vitality and absence of disease) and health (e.g., beyond physical, mental, and psychosocial wellbeing). **True and fully developed authentic wellness is the embodiment of multidimensional health; it is as-complete-as-possible (e.g., asymptotic) self-actualization, full integration of one's life—present, past, and future; it must ultimately be and manifest in physical, mental, emotional, spiritual, sociopolitical, transpersonal and multigenerational dimensions, inclusive of one's shadow[22], work[23], feelings, thoughts, and goals into a cohesive living whole – "a wheel rolling from its own center"[24] and beyond itself, beyond—ultimately—its own place and time.**

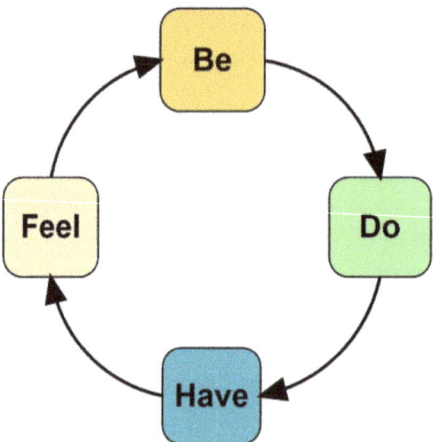

Self-reinforcing cycles of perception, manifestation, action, actualization, and reflection which reinforces (or changes) perception: "Reciprocal causality" is the term popularized by psychologist Nathaniel Branden in his excellent works such as *Psychology of Self-Esteem*. Relatedly, "reciprocal determinism" is the psychosocial theory set forth by psychologist Albert Bandura that a person's behavior both influences and is influenced by personal factors and the social environment.

Authentic Selfhood, Internal Locus of Control, Creativity, Self-Direction

"Innocence is the child, and forgetfulness,
  a new beginning, a game,
    a self-rolling wheel,
      a first movement, a holy *Yea*.
Surely, for the game of creating, there is needed a holy *Yea* unto life."

Nietzsche FW. *Thus Spoke Zarathustra*. Part 1—The Three Metamorphoses.

---

[22] Robert Bly. *The Human Shadow*. Sound Horizons 1991 [audio cassette ISBN: 1879323001] and Bly R. *A Little Book on the Human Shadow*. ISBN: 0062548476
[23] Rick Jarow. *Creating the Work You Love: Courage, Commitment and Career*. Inner Traditions Intl Ltd; 1995. ISBN: 0892815426
[24] Friedrich Wilhelm Nietzsche. Walter Kaufmann (Translator). *Thus Spoke Zarathustra: A Book for None and All*. Penguin USA; 1978, page 27

Acute Care and Musculoskeletal Care: Opportunities for Health Optimization

Clinicians should appreciate that every patient encounter is an opportunity for comprehensive care, disease prevention, and health optimization. This is true whether the presenting complaint is acne, psoriasis, a respiratory infection, or musculoskeletal pain. Given the relatively high frequency of musculoskeletal complaints in clinical practice in general and chiropractic and osteopathic practices in particular, the following section will emphasize the clinical presentation of musculoskeletal complaints as an underappreciated opportunity for wellness care.

Since **approximately 1 of every 7 (14% of total) visits to a primary healthcare provider is for the treatment of musculoskeletal pain or dysfunction**[25], every healthcare provider needs to have 1) knowledge of important concepts related to musculoskeletal medicine, 2) the ability to recognize urgent and emergency conditions, 3) the ability to competently perform orthopedic examination procedures and interpret laboratory assessments, and 4) the knowledge and ability to design and implement effective treatment plans and to coordinate patient management.

In pharmacosurgical allopathic medicine, the goal of musculoskeletal treatment is to address the patient's injury or disorder by alleviating pain with the use of drugs, preventing further injury, and returning the patient to his/her previous status and activities. The most commonly employed interventions are 1) rest and "watchful waiting", 2) non-steroidal anti-inflammatory drugs (NSAIDS) and cyclooxygenase-2-inhibitors (COX-2 inhibitors, or "coxibs"), and 3) surgery. The more action-oriented approaches used by many chiropractic, naturopathic, and osteopathic physicians differs from the allopathic approach because, although avoidance of and "rest" from damaging activities is reasonable and valuable, too much rest without an emphasis on active preventive rehabilitation ❶ encourages patient passivity and ❷ the assumption of the sick role, and it ❸ fails to actively promote tissue healing and ❹ fails to address the underlying proprioceptive deficits that are common in patients with chronic musculoskeletal pain and recurrent injuries.[26,27,28] NSAIDs are considered "first line" therapy for musculoskeletal disorders by allopaths despite the data showing that "There is no evidence that widely used NSAIDs have any long-term benefit on osteoarthritis."[29] What is worse than this lack of efficacy is the evidence showing that NSAIDs *exacerbate* musculoskeletal disease (rather than *cure* it). NSAIDs are known to inhibit cartilage formation and to promote bone necrosis and joint degradation with long-term use[30,31,32,33] and NSAIDs are responsible for more than 16,000 gastrohemorrhagic deaths and 100,000 hospitalizations each year.[34] The "coxibs" were supposed to provide anti-inflammatory benefits with an enhanced safety profile, but the gastrocentric focus of the drug developers failed to appreciate that COX-2 is necessary for the formation of prostacyclin, a prostaglandin created from arachidonic acid via COX-2 that plays an important role in vasodilation and antithrombosis; not surprisingly therefore, use of COX-2-inhibiting drugs has consistently been associated with increased risk for adverse cardiovascular effects including myocardial infarction, unstable angina, cardiac thrombus, resuscitated cardiac arrest, sudden or unexplained death, ischemic stroke, and transient ischemic attacks.[35] Additionally, the use of a COX-2 inhibiting treatment in patients who overconsume arachidonic acid (i.e., most people in America and

> **Allopathic medicine has been described (ie, has described itself) as "scientific" since a time when this was clearly not the case**
>
> "…only about 15% of medical interventions are supported by solid scientific evidence…"
>
> Smith R. Where is the wisdom...? The poverty of medical evidence. *BMJ*. 1991 Oct 5;303:798-9

---

[25] American College of Rheumatology Ad Hoc Committee on Clinical Guidelines. Guidelines for the initial evaluation of the adult patient with acute musculoskeletal symptoms. *Arthritis Rheum*. 1996 Jan; 39(1):1-8 See also: Vasquez A. Musculoskeletal disorders and iron overload disease. *Arthritis Rheum* 1996;39: 1767-8
[26] McPartland JM, Brodeur RR, Hallgren RC. Chronic neck pain, standing balance, and suboccipital muscle atrophy--a pilot study. *J Manipulative Physiol Ther*. 1997;20:24-9
[27] Bullock-Saxton et al. Reflex activation of gluteal muscles in walking. An approach to restoration of muscle function for patients with low-back pain. *Spine* 1993 May;18:704-8
[28] Sinaki M, Brey RH, Hughes CA, Larson DR, Kaufman KR. Significant reduction in risk of falls and back pain in osteoporotic-kyphotic women through a Spinal Proprioceptive Extension Exercise Dynamic (SPEED) program. *Mayo Clin Proc*. 2005 Jul;80(7):849-55
[29] Beers MH, Berkow R (Eds). *The Merck Manual. 17th Edition*. Whitehouse Station; Merck Research Laboratories 1999 page 451
[30] "At…concentrations comparable to those… in the synovial fluid of patients treated with the drug, several NSAIDs suppress proteoglycan synthesis… These NSAID-related effects on chondrocyte metabolism … are much more profound in osteoarthritic cartilage than in normal cartilage, due to enhanced uptake of NSAIDs by the osteoarthritic cartilage." Brandt KD. Effects of nonsteroidal anti-inflammatory drugs on chondrocyte metabolism in vitro and in vivo. *Am J Med*. 1987 Nov 20; 83(5A): 29-34
[31] "The case of a young healthy man, who developed avascular necrosis of head of femur after prolonged administration of indomethacin, is reported here." Prathapkumar KR, Smith I, Attara GA. Indomethacin induced avascular necrosis of head of femur. *Postgrad Med J*. 2000 Sep; 76(899): 574-5
[32] "This highly significant association between NSAID use and acetabular destruction gives cause for concern, not least because of the difficulty in achieving satisfactory hip replacements in patients with severely damaged acetabula."Newman et al. Acetabular bone destruction related to non-steroidal anti-inflammatory drugs. *Lancet* 1985;2:11-4
[33] Vidal y Plana et al. Articular cartilage pharmacology: I. In vitro studies on glucosamine and non steroidal antiinflammatory drugs. *Pharmacol Res Commun*. 1978 Jun;10:557-69
[34] Singh G. Recent considerations in nonsteroidal anti-inflammatory drug gastropathy. *Am J Med*. 1998;105(1B):31S-38S
[35] Mukherjee D, Nissen SE, Topol EJ. Risk of cardiovascular events associated with selective COX-2 inhibitors. *JAMA*. 2001 Aug 22-29;286(8):954-9

other industrialized nations[36]) would be expected to shunt bioavailable arachidonate into the formation of leukotrienes, a group of inflammatory mediators known to promote atherogenesis.[37] Thus, the outcome was entirely predictable: overuse of COX-2 inhibitors should have been expected to create a catastrophe of iatrogenic cardiovascular death, and this is exactly what was allowed to occur—clearly indicating independent but synergistic failures on the part of pharmaceutical companies, the FDA, and the medical profession.[38,39,40,41] According to statements by David J. Graham, MD, MPH, (Associate Director for Science, Office of Drug Safety, FDA) in 2005, an estimated 139,000 Americans who took Vioxx suffered serious complications including stroke or myocardial infarction; between 26,000 and 55,000 Americans died as a result of their doctors' prescribing Vioxx.[42] Additionally, the surgical procedures employed by allopaths for the treatment of musculoskeletal pain do not consistently show evidence of efficacy, safety, or cost-effectiveness. Arthroscopic surgery for osteoarthritis of the knee, for example, costs thousands of dollars to each individual and billions of dollars to the American healthcare system but is no more effective than placebo.[43,44,45] In a review which also noted that only 15% of medical procedures are supported by literature references and that only 1% of such references are deemed scientifically valid, Rosner[46] showed that the risks of serious injury (i.e., cauda equina syndrome or vertebral artery dissection) associated with spinal manipulation are "*400 times lower* than the death rates observed from gastrointestinal bleeding due to the use of nonsteroidal anti-inflammatory drugs and *700 times lower* than the overall mortality rate for spinal surgery."

In integrative/functional medicine, the goal and means of musculoskeletal treatment is to address the patient's injury or disorder by simultaneously alleviating pain with the use of natural, noninvasive, low-cost, and low-risk interventions while improving the patient's overall health, preventing future health problems, and "upgrading" the patient's overall paradigm of health maintenance and disease prevention from one that is passive and reactive to one that is empowered and pro-active. Commonly employed therapeutics include spinal manipulation[47,48,49], exercise[50] and the use of nutritional supplements and botanical medicines[51,52] which have been demonstrated in peer-reviewed clinical trials to be safe and effective for the alleviation of musculoskeletal pain. In order to deliver competent drug-free pain management and to help patients who use nutritional supplements, today's clinicians need to be well-versed in the clinical utilization of such treatments as niacinamide[53], glucosamine and chondroitin sulfates[54], vitamin D[55], vitamin B-12[56], anti-inflammatory diets[57,58], balanced and complete fatty acid therapy[59], proteolytic/pancreatic enzymes[60], and botanical medicines such as *Boswellia*[61], *Harpagophytum*[62], *Uncaria*, and willow bark[63,64]—each of these interventions has been validated in peer-reviewed research for safety and effectiveness.[65] Furthermore, from the perspective of progressive/functional medicine, aiming for such a limited accomplishment as mere "returning the patient to previous status and activities" would be considered substandard, since the patient's overall health was neither addressed nor improved and since returning the patient to his/her previous status and activities would be a direct invitation for the problem to recur indefinitely. Astute physicians

---

[36] Seaman DR. The diet-induced proinflammatory state: a cause of chronic pain and other degenerative diseases? *J Manipulative Physiol Ther*. 2002;25(3):168-79
[37] Dwyer JH, et al. Arachidonate 5-lipoxygenase promoter genotype, dietary arachidonic acid, and atherosclerosis. *N Engl J Med*. 2004 Jan 1;350(1):29-37
[38] Topol EJ. Arthritis medicines and cardiovascular events--"house of coxibs". *JAMA*. 2005 Jan 19;293(3):366-8. Epub 2004 Dec 28
[39] Ray WA, Griffin MR, Stein CM. Cardiovascular toxicity of valdecoxib. *N Engl J Med*. 2004 Dec 23;351(26):2767. Epub 2004 Dec 17
[40] Topol EJ. Failing the public health--rofecoxib, Merck, and the FDA. *N Engl J Med*. 2004 Oct 21;351(17):1707-9
[41] Horton R. Vioxx, the implosion of Merck, and aftershocks at the FDA. *Lancet*. 2004 Dec 4-10;364(9450):1995-6
[42] David J. Graham, MD, MPH, (Associate Director for Science, Office of Drug Safety, USFDA) estimated that 139,000 Americans who took Vioxx suffered serious side effects; he estimated that the drug killed between 26,000 and 55,000 people. commondreams.org/views05/0223-35.htm and fda.gov/cder/drug/infopage/vioxx/vioxxgraham.pdf 2006 Nov
[43] Gina Kolata. A Knee Surgery for Arthritis Is Called Sham. *The New York Times*, July 11, 2002
[44] Moseley JB, et al. A controlled trial of arthroscopic surgery for osteoarthritis of the knee. *N Engl J Med*. 2002;347:81-8
[45] Bernstein J, Quach T. A perspective on the study of Moseley: questioning the value of arthroscopic knee surgery for osteoarthritis. *Cleve Clin J Med* 2003;70:401, 405-6, 408-10
[46] Rosner AL. Evidence-based clinical guidelines for the management of acute low-back pain: response. *J Manipulative Physiol Ther*. 2001;24(3):214-20
[47] Manga P, Angus D, Papadopoulos C, et al. *The Effectiveness and Cost-Effectiveness of Chiropractic Management of Low-Back Pain*. Richmond Hill, Ontario: Kenilworth; 1993
[48] Meade TW, et al. Low-back pain of mechanical origin: randomised comparison of chiropractic and hospital outpatient treatment. *BMJ*. 1990;300(6737):1431-7
[49] Meade TW, et al. Randomised comparison of chiropractic and hospital outpatient management for low-back pain: results from extended follow up. *BMJ*. 1995;311(7001):349-5
[50] Harold Elrick, MD. Exercise is Medicine. *The Physician and Sportsmedicine* - Volume 24 - No. 2 - February 1996
[51] Vasquez A. Revisiting the Five-Part Nutritional Wellness Protocol: The Supplemented Paleo-Mediterranean Diet. *Nutritional Perspectives* 2011 Jan
[52] Vasquez A. Improving overall health while safely and effectively treating musculoskeletal pain. *Nutritional Perspectives* 2005; 28: 34-38, 40-42
[53] Kaufman W. Niacinamide therapy for joint mobility. Therapeutic reversal of a common clinical manifestation of the "normal" aging process. *Conn State Med J* 1953;17:584-591
[54] Reginster JY, et al. Long-term effects of glucosamine sulphate on osteoarthritis progression: a randomised, placebo-controlled clinical trial. *Lancet*. 2001;357(9252):251-6
[55] Vasquez A, Manso G, Cannell J. The clinical importance of vitamin D: a paradigm shift with implications for all healthcare providers. *Altern Ther Health Med* 2004;10:28-36
[56] Mauro GL, et al. Vitamin B12 in low back pain: a randomised, double-blind, placebo-controlled study. *Eur Rev Med Pharmacol Sci*. 2000 May-Jun;4(3):53-8
[57] Seaman DR. The diet-induced proinflammatory state: a cause of chronic pain and other degenerative diseases? *J Manipulative Physiol Ther*. 2002 Mar-Apr;25(3):168-7
[58] Vasquez A. New Insights into Fatty Acid Biochemistry and the Influence of Diet. *Nutritional Perspectives* 2004; October: 5, 7-10, 12, 14
[59] Vasquez A. New Insights into Fatty Acid Supplementation and Its Effect on Eicosanoid Production and Genetic Expression. *Nutritional Perspectives* 2005; January: 5-16
[60] Trickett P. Proteolytic enzymes in treatment of athletic injuries. *Appl Ther*. 1964;30:647-52
[61] Kimmatkar et al. Efficacy and tolerability of Boswellia serrata extract in treatment of osteoarthritis of knee: controlled trial. *Phytomedicine*. 2003 Jan;10(1):3-7
[62] Chrubasik S, et al. Effectiveness of Harpagophytum extract WS 1531 in the treatment of exacerbation of low-back pain. *Eur J Anaesthesiol* 1999 Feb;16(2):118-29
[63] Chrubasik S, et al. Treatment of low-back pain exacerbations with willow bark extract: a randomized double-blind study. *Am J Med*. 2000;109:9-14
[64] Vasquez A, Muanza DN. Comment: Evaluation of Presence of Aspirin-Related Warnings with Willow Bark. *Ann Pharmacotherapy* 2005 Oct;39(10):1763
[65] Vasquez A. Improving overall health while safely and effectively treating musculoskeletal pain. *Nutritional Perspectives* 2005;28:34-42

should appreciate that, especially regarding "chronic" (i.e., sustained) health problems, any treatment plan that allows the patient to resume his/her previous lifestyle is by definition doomed to fail because a return to the patient's previous lifestyle and activities that allowed the onset of the disease/disorder in the first place will most certainly result in the perpetuation and recurrence of the illness or disorder. **Stated more directly: for *healing* to truly be effective, the comprehensive treatment plan must generally result in a permanent and profound change in the patient's lifestyle and emotional climate, which are the primary modifiable determinants of either health or disease.**

Barcelona's tradition of honoring intellectuals—Plaça de George Orwell: George Orwell is best known for his brilliant books *1984* and *Animal Farm* which creatively tell complex tales of herd mentality, politics, and various forms of social control and the manufacture of public consent and conformity. Less well-known is his *Homage to Catalonia*, in which he describes his experience as a volunteer in the Spanish Civil War (during which he was shot in the neck by a sniper) against the fascist regime of Francisco Franco, then supported by Hitler's Nazi Germany and Mussolini's Fascist Italy. His required-reading book *1984* has recently been summarized in a brilliant audio version[66] (and a short free video[67]) to increase its accessibility. In 2014, people protesting government surveillance and unjust imprisonments in Thailand were arrested for reading *1984*.[68]

---

[66] Moustaki N (Author), Podehl N (Narrator). *1984: CliffsNotes*. Audible. cliffsnotes.com/literature/n/1984/book-summary and amazon.com/1984-CliffsNotes/dp/B004S8NFZ2/
[67] Video SparkNotes: Orwell's 1984 Summary. https://youtube.com/watch?v=pTqIVvUPAjw
[68] Associated Press. 23 June, 2014. Protesting Thai reader of Orwell's *1984* dragged off by police in Bangkok. "Police in Thailand yesterday arrested eight people for demonstrating against the nation's increasingly repressive military junta, including a man dragged away by undercover officers for reading a copy of George Orwell's *Nineteen Eighty-Four*. The arrest was the first known case of anyone being detained for reading as a form of protest since the military seized power last month. ... A Thai reporter who witnessed the lone man reading Orwell's classic said he was taken away by half a dozen plainclothes police. The reporter said the man held the book up as officers approached. ... Another of the arrests was of a woman wearing a T-shirt with the words "Respect My Vote" on it." *South China Morning Post* scmp.com/news/asia/article/1538616/protesting-thai-reader-orwells-1984-dragged-police-bangkok. See also Campbell C. A Yellow Shirt Leader Says the Thai Coup Was Planned in 2010. *Time* 2014 Jun 23. time.com/2910484/thai-coup-planned-2010-suthep-thaugsuban/. "My friends told me when they read 1984 for the first time they could never imagine there would be a country like that, but it's happening now in Thailand," says Pimsiri. "People are really watching you, your computers are being monitored... and many people have been detained in undisclosed locations." *Christian Science Monitor* csmonitor.com/World/Asia-Pacific/2014/0530/Orwell-s-1984-suddenly-fashionable-on-Bangkok-streets

Clinical Assessments

The clinical assessments reviewed in the following sections are history-taking, orthopedic/musculoskeletal, and neurologic examinations, and commonly used laboratory tests. **History taking is the art of conducting an *informative* and *collaborative* patient interview.**

The role of the doctor during the interview process is not merely that of a data-collecting machine, spewing out questions and receiving responses. Patient interviews can be a creative, enjoyable, comforting opportunity to build rapport and to establish meaningful connection with another human being. Patients are not simply people with health problems – they are first and foremost our fellow human beings, not so dissimilar from ourselves perhaps, and always full of complexity. Our task is not to fully understand their complexity nor to solve all of their mysteries, but rather to help orchestrate these dynamics into a coordinated if not unified direction that promotes health and healing.

Beyond its diagnostic value, the interview process also provides a key opportunity to gain insight into the patient's psychoepistimology—the patient's operating system for interacting with data and the world and internalizing and metabolizing external inputs in such a way as to merge these with internal experiences (i.e., emotions, feelings, preferences, responses). Epistemology is the branch of philosophy concerned with the nature and scope of knowledge. Per Rand[69], psychoepistimology is a person's "method of awareness"; a person's psychoepistimology creates a "corollary view of existence" and in turn, "A man's method of using his consciousness determines his method of survival." By understanding how the patient views him/herself in the world, understanding his/her goals, and—in essence—what "drives" the patient and what "makes him/her tick", clinicians can shape the nuances of the conversation and the treatment plan to promote the desired cognitive-conceptual-behavioral changes in behavior that are prerequisite for the attainment of optimized health outcomes.

History & Assessment

History of the primary complaint: "D.O.P.P. Q.R.S.T."
- Description/location
- Onset
- Provocation: exacerbates
- Palliation: alleviates
- Quality
- Radiation of pain
- Severity
- Timing

Associated complaints
- Additional manifestations
- Concomitant diseases

Review of systems
- Head-to-toe inventory of health status, associated health problems, and complications

Past health history
- Surgeries
- Hospitalizations
- Traumas
- Vaccinations and medications
- Successful and failed treatments for the current complaint(s)

Family health history
- Genotropic illnesses and predispositions
- Lifestyle patterns
- Emotional expectations

Social history
- Hobbies, work, exposures
- Relationships and emotional experiences
- Interpersonal support
- Malpractice litigation

Health Habits
- Diet: appropriate intake of protein, fruits, vegetables, fats, sugars
- Sleep
- Stress management
- Exercise / Sedentary Lifestyle
- Spirituality / Centeredness
- Caffeine and tobacco
- Ethanol and recreational drugs

Medication and supplements
- Reason, doses, duration, cost
- Side-effects
- Interactions

Responsibility and Compliance
- Ability and willingness to comply with prescribed treatment plan and to incorporate the necessary diet-exercise-relationship-emotional-lifestyle modifications
- *Internal* versus *external* locus of control

---

[69] Rand A. *For the New Intellectual*. New York; Signet:1961, page 16

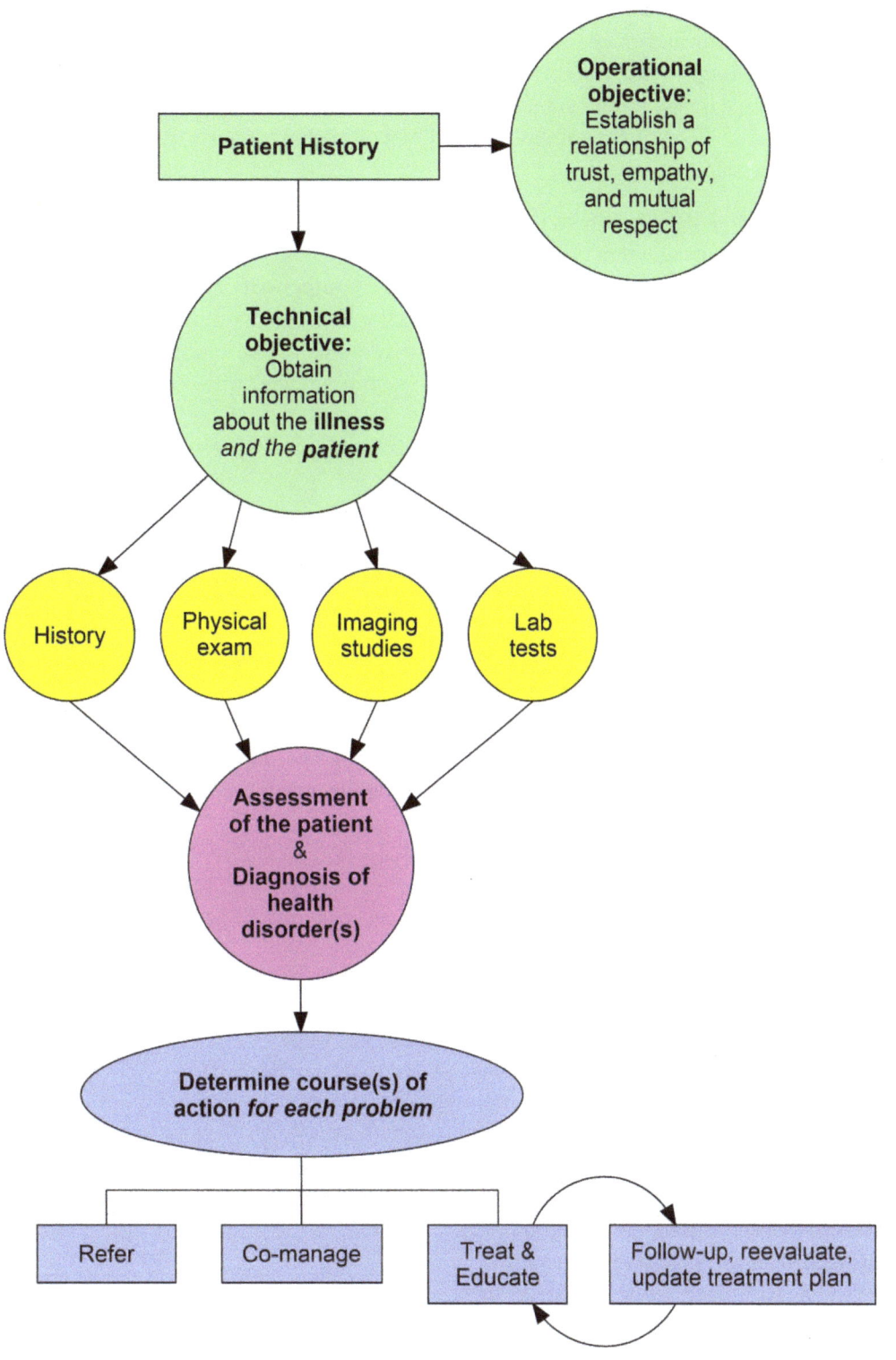

Key components of patient assessment and management: Patient assessment and management is an on-going process that begins with the initial history taken at the first clinical encounter and continues through the physical examination and laboratory assessments and thereafter by monitoring the patient's implementation of and response to the treatment plan. The plan is complete when the desired outcome of health optimization is achieved and sustained.

Clinical acronyms: Outlined here are some of my preferred and—in the case of D.I.R.T. and F.I.N.D.S.E.X.™—unique acronyms which help all of us—students and seasoned clinicians alike—to develop a system of thought which then frees us to apply our higher intellectual functions to the nuances of the clinical case/condition/situation we are considering. Interestingly (and with a bit of Dionysian humor), the sequential use of DIRT, SOAP, and FINDSEX creates an intuitive image to which most adults can relate; from a more Apollonian perspective, we—as mentioned above—can apply this structure of thought to direct our behavior and attain higher levels of clinical care with greater ease and consistency.

Risk management acronym—DIRT: Start with the conscious intention to practice defensively and effectively.
- Defensive mindset: Risk management must be pro-active,
- Duration of treatment: Define and limit the duration of each component of the treatment plan; define the next steps of care (e.g., continued care or laboratory tests) and the date of the return visit,
- Interactions—drugs and diseases: Double-check for interactions of the treatment plan with drugs and the patient's disease(s), especially renal insufficiency. Three commonly encountered clinical examples follow:
  - High-potassium diet ≠ renal insufficiency
  - Vitamin D ≠ hydrochlorothiazide or other hypercalcemic predisposition/state
  - Calcium and magnesium ≠ tetracycline antibiotics
- Referral: Determine the need for additional consultation,
- Return visit: Specify and chart timeframe or date of next visit,
- Treatment plan, charted, dated, signed: Treatment plan must be archived in chart and should be given to patient; the clinician must sign and date the chart note and treatment plan.

Patient management acronym—SOAP: Competent care starts with an open-minded, compassionate, information-seeking excellence-aspiring clinician.
- Subjective: History of presenting complaints; patient's concerns,
- Objective: Physical exam, lab tests: always assess renal function and other basic biochemical parameters; more complex cases require evaluation of more sensitive markers of metabolic and immune imbalance, imaging, biopsy, procedures—as necessary,
- Assessment: Reach an assessment of the entire constellation of patient's situation; diagnosis and appropriate management of each true disease and concern,
- Plan: Informed consent (PARBQ): procedures, alternatives, risks, benefits, questions answered; treatments; follow-up, rescheduling, referral, co-management.

Functional medicine/inflammology treatment acronym—FINDSEX®
- Food: Diet and nutrition: input, metabolism, utilization, unique needs, excretion,
- Infections: Persistent microbial colonization, dysbiosis,
- Nutritional Immunomodulation: Integrative "shaping" of the immune system in favor of Treg at the expense of Th1/2/17. This clinical system has been organized and refined by Dr Vasquez since its first publication in *Functional Immunology and Nutritional Immunomodulation* (2012)
- Dysmetabolism and dysfunctional organelles: Originally in this protocol, dysfunctional mitochondrial was the focus; this has since been expanded to include much broader considerations of dysmetabolism in general and endoplasmic reticulum stress in particular.
- Special considerations, sleep, style of living: This section is intended to cover the basics of sleep, stress management, social considerations, special supplementation, surgery, somatic medicine and spinal manipulation, spirituality, etc.
- Endocrine: Hormonal imbalances must be assessed and corrected/optimized if metabolic and inflammatory balance are to be restored.
- Xenobiotics: Due mostly to the synergistic effects of failure of governmental regulatory agencies combined with careless and reckless corporate production of pollution and toxic chemicals, our world has become highly contaminated with chemicals that alter our hormonal, neurological, reproductive, and immune health. Because this phenomena is subtle, nonacute, and ubiquitous, it is easily overlooked despite its importance.

These considerations will be detailed and developed in the sections that follow.

Components of a Complete Patient History: "D.O.P.P. Q.R.S.T."

Category	Patient history questions and implications
Description, Location: Always start with open-ended questions	• What is it like for you? • What do you experience? • What are you feeling? • Where is the pain/sensation/problem? • Ask about specifics: **Pain, numbness, weakness, tingling**, fatigue, recent or chronic infections, burning, aching, dull, sharp, cramping, stretching, pins and needles, weakness, changes in function (i.e., bowel and bladder continence, sexual function).
Onset	• When did it begin? Have you ever had anything like this before? • Was there a specific event associated with the onset of the problem, such as an injury or an illness, or did the problem start gradually or insidiously? • How has it changed over time? • Prior injuries to site? • Why are you seeking care for this now (rather than last week or last month)? • What has changed? How is the pain/problem developing over time—getting worse or getting better?
Palliation	• How have you tried treating it? Does anything make it go away? • What makes it better? What relieves the pain? • Ask about prior and current treatments, radiographs, medications, supplements (herbs, vitamins, minerals), injections, surgery, massage, manipulation, and counseling. • Knowing response/resistance to previous treatments can provide clinical insight.
Provocation	• Are your symptoms constant, or does the problem come and go? • What makes it worse? What makes the pain worse? • When during the day/week/month/year are your symptoms the worst?
Quality	• Can you describe the pain to me? • What does it feel like? • What do you experience? • Get a clear understanding of the type of sensation(s): stabbing, shooting pain, pins and needles, sharp pain, electric sensation, numbness, burning, aching, throbbing, weakness, tingling, gel phenomenon (stiffness worsened by inactivity), dizziness, confusion, fatigue, shortness of breath.
Radiation	• Does the pain stay localized or does it move to your arm/leg/head/face? • Do you feel pain in other areas of your body?
Severity	• How bad is it? How would you rate it on a scale of one to ten if one were almost no pain and ten was the worst pain you could imagine? Use the validated VAS—visual analog scale—to quantify the level of pain and impairment. • Does this problem prevent you from engaging in your daily activities, such as work, exercise, or hobbies? This is a very important question for determining functional impairment and internal consistency; if the patient is "too injured to work" yet is still able to fully participate in recreational activities that are physically challenging, then malingering is likely.
Timing	• When do you notice this problem? • Is it constant, or does it come and go? Where are you when you notice it the most? • Is it worse in the morning, or worse in the evening? • Does anyone else in your [home/office/worksite] have this same problem? • What times of the day or what days of the week is it the worst?

Components of a Complete Patient History: "D.O.P.P. Q.R.S.T."—*continued*

Category	Patient history questions and implications
Associated manifestations and constitutional symptoms	- *Have you noticed any other problems associated with this problem?* - *Fatigue?* - *Fever?* - *Weight loss? Weight gain?* - *Night sweats?* - *Diarrhea? Constipation?* - *Weakness?* - *Nausea?* - *Bowel or bladder difficulties or changes? Difficulty with sexual function?* These could be related to hormonal imbalances, drug side-effects, relationship problems, nutritional deficiencies, nerve compression, and/or depression. - *Change in sensation near your anus/genitals?* Cauda equina syndrome is an important consideration in patients with low-back pain. - *Loss of appetite?* - *Difficulty sleeping?* - *Skin rash or change in pigmentation?*
ROS: review of systems	- <u>General constitution</u>: fatigue, malaise, fever, chills, weight gain/loss… - *"Now we are going to conduct a head-to-toe inventory just to make sure that we have covered everything."* - <u>Head</u>: headaches, head pain, pressure inside head, difficulty concentrating, difficulty remembering, mental function - <u>Ears:</u> ringing in ears, dizziness, hearing loss, hypersensitivity to noise, ear pain, discharge from ear, pressure in ears - <u>Eyes</u>: eye pain, loss of vision or decreased vision or ability to focus, redness or irritation, seeing flashing lights or spots, double vision - <u>Nose</u>: sinus problems, chronically stuffy nose, difficulty smelling things, nose bleeds, change or decrease in sense of smell or taste - <u>Mouth</u>, teeth, TMJ, pain or sores in mouth, difficulty chewing, sensitive teeth, bleeding gums, pain in jaw joint, change or decrease in sense of taste - <u>Neck</u>: pain at the base of skull, pain in neck, stiffness - <u>Throat:</u> difficulty swallowing, pain in throat, feeling like things get stuck in throat, change in voice, difficulty getting air or food in or out - <u>Chest and breasts</u>: any chest pain, difficult breathing, wheezing, coughing, pain, lumps, or discharge from nipple - <u>Shoulders:</u> pain or aching in your shoulders, restricted motion or stiffness - <u>Arms, elbows, hands:</u> pain or problems with your arms, elbows, hands …in the joints or the muscles…, numbness, tingling, weakness, swelling, changes in fingernails, cold hands? - <u>Stomach, abdomen, pelvis, genitals, urinary tract, rectum, :</u> pain in stomach or abdomen, difficulty with digestion, gas, bloating, regurgitation, ulcer, any problems lower down in your abdomen—near your lower intestines? Pain, lumps, swelling, difficulty passing stool, pain or itching near your anus, genitalia; any genital pain, burning, discharge, redness, irritation, sexual dysfunction or impotence, loss of bowel or bladder control? Diarrhea or constipation? How often do you have a bowel movement? - <u>Hips, legs, knees, ankles, feet:</u> numbness, weakness, pain or tingling in the hips, knees, ankles, or feet; pain in calves with walking, swelling of ankles, cold feet - *Are you aware of anything else that you think I should know in order to help you?*

Components of a Complete Patient History: "D.O.P.P. Q.R.S.T." —*continued*

Category	Patient history questions and implications

Medical history	• *Are you taking any **medications**? What medications have you taken in the past few years?* Finding out that your new patient recently discontinued his 20-year regimen of valproic acid, lithium, and risperidone may significantly change your interpretation of the clinical interview. Likewise, a patient may not be taking immunosuppressive drugs on the day of your first clinical encounter—he or she may have discontinued such drugs against medical advice (AMA) the week prior to consulting with you.
	• *Have you been **treated for any medical conditions** or health problems?*
	• *Have you ever been **hospitalized**?*
	• *Have you ever had **surgery**?*
	• *Have you ever been **diagnosed with any health problems** such as high blood pressure or diabetes?*
	• Investigate for specific problems in the past health history that would be a major oversight to miss:
	   ○ Current or past diseases: cancer, diabetes, psychosis, infections, immune disorders
	   ○ Hypertension or high cholesterol
	   ○ Medications, especially corticosteroids
	   ○ Surgeries, hospitalizations, trauma or previous injuries

Social history	• **Work**—*What do you do for work? Are you exposed to chemicals or fumes at your workplace?* • **Hobbies**—*What do you do for recreation or hobbies? Are you exposed to chemicals or fumes at home or with your hobbies (e.g., painting, gardening)?* • **Eat**—*Tell me about your breakfast, lunch, dinner, snacks… Do you consume foods or drinks that contain aspartame* (linked to increased incidence of brain tumors[70]) *or carrageenan* (possibly linked to increased risk of breast cancer and inflammatory bowel disease[71,72])? • **Exercise**—*What do you do for exercise or physical activity?* • **Drink**—*Do you **drink alcohol**? Coffee/caffeine? Water?* • **Drugs**—*Do you use recreational **drugs**? **Now or in the past?*** • **Smoke**—*Do you **smoke**? Have you ever smoked on a regular basis?* • **Sex**—*Are you **sex**ually active? If so, do you practice safer sex practices? For all women: Is there any chance you could be pregnant right now?* A "yes" reply may contraindicate radiographic assessment and the use of certain nutrients, botanicals, and/or drugs. • **Emotional support, family contact, relationships**: The typical American has no-one in whom to confide and has a social network of two people[73]; in all; Americans are the most medicated/drugged and most socially isolated society that has ever existed.
Family health history	• *Does anyone in your family have any health problems, especially your parents and siblings?* • *Do you have any children? Do they have any health problems?* • *Do any diseases "run in the family" such as cancer, diabetes, arthritis, heart disease?*
Additional questions	• *Do you have any other information for me? Is there anything that I did not ask?* • *What is your opinion as to why you are having this health problem?* • *Are you in litigation for your illness or injuries?*

---

[70] "In the past two decades brain tumor rates have risen in several industrialized countries, including the United States... Compared to other environmental factors putatively linked to brain tumors, the artificial sweetener aspartame is a promising candidate to explain the recent increase in incidence and degree of malignancy of brain tumors." Olney JW, Farber NB, Spitznagel E, Robins LN. Increasing brain tumor rates: is there a link to aspartame? *J Neuropathol Exp Neurol* 1996 Nov;55(11):1115-23
[71] Tobacman JK. Review of harmful gastrointestinal effects of carrageenan in animal experiments. *Environ Health Perspect*. 2001 Oct;109(10):983-94
[72] "However, the gum carrageenan which is comprised of linked, sulfated galactose residues has potent biological activity and undergoes acid hydrolysis to poligeenan, an acknowledged carcinogen." Tobacman JK, Wallace RB, Zimmerman MB. Consumption of carrageenan and other water-soluble polymers used as food additives and incidence of mammary carcinoma. *Med Hypotheses*. 2001 May;56(5):589-98
[73] "Discussion networks are smaller in 2004 than in 1985. The number of people saying there is no one with whom they discuss important matters nearly tripled. The mean network size decreases by about a third (one confidant), from 2.94 in 1985 to 2.08 in 2004. The modal respondent now reports having no confidant; the modal respondent in 1985 had three confidants." McPherson M, Smith-Lovin L, Brashears ME. Social Isolation in America. *American Sociological Review* June 2006 71: 353-375

Patients can be asked to localize and describe their pain/discomfort on drawings such as these. *Examples of descriptions*:

- Numb
- Hypersensitive
- Tingling
- Shooting pain
- Electrical pain
- Stabbing pain
- Burning pain
- Dull ache
- Muscle weakness

FRONT OF BODY

BACK OF BODY

On the lines below, indicate which pain/discomfort you are referring to and then quantify it by placing an "X" on the line.

Location of pain:_____

|—————————————————————————————|
No pain at all   Worst pain imaginable

Location of pain:_____

|—————————————————————————————|
No pain at all   Worst pain imaginable

Review of Systems—checklist: Patients/clients are asked to provide more information by the arrow "→", also at the bottom of each page, and/or whereever more detail is warranted. This form can be completed by the clinician and/or by the client.

GENERAL HEALTH	Very rare-None	Occasional-Mild	Intermittent-Moderate	Frequent-Severe
Fatigue, lack of energy, lack of stamina	☐ 0	☐ 1	☐ 2	☐ 3
Need to decrease or alter activities of daily living due to fatigue, pain, or illness	☐ 0	☐ 1	☐ 2	☐ 3
Insomnia, lack of sleep	☐ 0	☐ 1	☐ 2	☐ 3
Excessive tiredness and increased need for sleep	☐ 0	☐ 1	☐ 2	☐ 3
Tired and/or not hungry after waking	☐ 0	☐ 1	☐ 2	☐ 3
Pain at night, night sweats	☐ 0	☐ 1	☐ 2	☐ 3
Enlarged lymph nodes	☐ 0	☐ 1	☐ 2	☐ 3
Frequent infections	☐ 0	☐ 1	☐ 2	☐ 3
Undesired weight loss	☐ 0	☐ 1	☐ 2	☐ 3
Undesired weight gain, difficulty losing weight	☐ 0	☐ 1	☐ 2	☐ 3
Cold hands or feet	☐ 0	☐ 1	☐ 2	☐ 3
Compulsive/binge eating, increased appetite	☐ 0	☐ 1	☐ 2	☐ 3
Decreased appetite	☐ 0	☐ 1	☐ 2	☐ 3
Hypoglycemia, low blood sugar	☐ 0	☐ 1	☐ 2	☐ 3
Allergies to food or environment	☐ 0	☐ 1	☐ 2	☐ 3
Sensitivity to fumes, chemicals, odors, exhaust	☐ 0	☐ 1	☐ 2	☐ 3
Have you been tested for iron disorders?	☐ NO	☐ YES	☐ ?	
Past diagnosis of serious illness or chronic health condition such a systemic disease, cancer, HIV, mental condition, heart disease, infection, kidney problems, or other condition	☐ NO	☐ YES→		

MUSCLES and JOINTS	Very rare-None	Occasional-Mild	Intermittent-Moderate	Frequent-Severe
Pain, swelling, or limited motion in joint(s)	☐ 0	☐ 1	☐ 2	☐ 3
Pain, swelling, or weakness in muscle(s)	☐ 0	☐ 1	☐ 2	☐ 3
Cramps in muscles, grind teeth at night?	☐ 0	☐ 1	☐ 2	☐ 3
Other problem, concerns, or questions in this area?	☐ NO	☐ YES→		

HEAD and MIND	Very rare-None	Occasional-Mild	Intermittent-Moderate	Frequent-Severe
Headaches	☐ 0	☐ 1	☐ 2	☐ 3
Feeling of pressure inside head	☐ 0	☐ 1	☐ 2	☐ 3
Faintness, loss of consciousness	☐ 0	☐ 1	☐ 2	☐ 3
Dizziness	☐ 0	☐ 1	☐ 2	☐ 3
Seizures, epilepsy	☐ 0	☐ 1	☐ 2	☐ 3
Difficulty thinking or processing information; confusion	☐ 0	☐ 1	☐ 2	☐ 3
Difficulty with concentrating or maintaining attention	☐ 0	☐ 1	☐ 2	☐ 3
Poor memory	☐ 0	☐ 1	☐ 2	☐ 3
Difficulty speaking or talking, slurred speech	☐ 0	☐ 1	☐ 2	☐ 3
Hyperactivity	☐ 0	☐ 1	☐ 2	☐ 3
Learning difficulties, dyslexia	☐ 0	☐ 1	☐ 2	☐ 3
Other problem, concern, or question in this area?	☐ NO	☐ YES→		

Additional notes or comments:

EMOTIONS and SOCIAL HEALTH	Very rare-None	Occasional-Mild	Intermittent-Moderate	Frequent-Severe
Depression, sadness	❏ 0	❏ 1	❏ 2	❏ 3
Anger, irritability, anxiety	❏ 0	❏ 1	❏ 2	❏ 3
Stressful situations	❏ 0	❏ 1	❏ 2	❏ 3
Apathy, lack of interest or concern	❏ 0	❏ 1	❏ 2	❏ 3
Use of alcohol, herbs, drugs, or medications to help manage emotions	❏ 0	❏ 1	❏ 2	❏ 3
Isolation, few friends, distant family	❏ 0	❏ 1	❏ 2	❏ 3
Problems with parents or family	❏ 0	❏ 1	❏ 2	❏ 3
Problems with employer(s) or coworker(s)	❏ 0	❏ 1	❏ 2	❏ 3
Sadness or recurrent problems from childhood or past events	❏ 0	❏ 1	❏ 2	❏ 3
Recent or current thoughts of suicide?	❏ NO	❏ YES→		
Diagnosed mental condition such as bipolar, schizophrenia, or other condition	❏ NO	❏ YES→		
Other problem, concern, or question in this area?	❏ NO	❏ YES→		

EYES	Very rare-None	Occasional-Mild	Intermittent-Moderate	Frequent-Severe
Watery, red, or itchy eyes	❏ 0	❏ 1	❏ 2	❏ 3
Dark circles under eyes	❏ 0	❏ 1	❏ 2	❏ 3
Decrease or loss of vision; cataracts, or glaucoma	❏ 0	❏ 1	❏ 2	❏ 3
Poor night vision, night blindness	❏ 0	❏ 1	❏ 2	❏ 3
Pain in eye(s)	❏ 0	❏ 1	❏ 2	❏ 3
Pain near or behind eye(s)	❏ 0	❏ 1	❏ 2	❏ 3
Other problem, concern, or question in this area?	❏ NO	❏ YES→		

EARS	Very rare-None	Occasional-Mild	Intermittent-Moderate	Frequent-Severe
Earaches, pain in ear(s)	❏ 0	❏ 1	❏ 2	❏ 3
Ringing in ear(s)	❏ 0	❏ 1	❏ 2	❏ 3
Ear infections	❏ 0	❏ 1	❏ 2	❏ 3
Decrease or loss of hearing	❏ 0	❏ 1	❏ 2	❏ 3
Other problem, concern, or question in this area?	❏ NO	❏ YES→		

MOUTH, NOSE, and THROAT	Very rare-None	Occasional-Mild	Intermittent-Moderate	Frequent-Severe
Swollen or tender tongue or gums	❏ 0	❏ 1	❏ 2	❏ 3
Decreased sense of taste or smell	❏ 0	❏ 1	❏ 2	❏ 3
Stuffy nose, nasal congestion	❏ 0	❏ 1	❏ 2	❏ 3
Sinus infections, sinus pain	❏ 0	❏ 1	❏ 2	❏ 3
Nasal polyps	❏ 0	❏ 1	❏ 2	❏ 3
Ulcers or sores in mouth or lips, oral herpes	❏ 0	❏ 1	❏ 2	❏ 3
Allergies/ sneezing/ runny nose	❏ 0	❏ 1	❏ 2	❏ 3
Excessive mucus formation	❏ 0	❏ 1	❏ 2	❏ 3
Drainage to back of throat	❏ 0	❏ 1	❏ 2	❏ 3
Sore throat	❏ 0	❏ 1	❏ 2	❏ 3
Cough or wheeze	❏ 0	❏ 1	❏ 2	❏ 3
Change in voice	❏ 0	❏ 1	❏ 2	❏ 3
Hoarseness, loss of voice	❏ 0	❏ 1	❏ 2	❏ 3
Other problem, concern, or question in this area?	❏ NO	❏ YES→		

LUNGS and HEART	Very rare-None	Occasional-Mild	Intermittent-Moderate	Frequent-Severe
Pain in left arm and/or left side of neck or face	❏ 0	❏ 1	❏ 2	❏ 3
Shortness of breath, difficulty breathing	❏ 0	❏ 1	❏ 2	❏ 3
Irregular heartbeat	❏ 0	❏ 1	❏ 2	❏ 3
Rapid or pounding heartbeat	❏ 0	❏ 1	❏ 2	❏ 3
Chest congestion, bronchitis	❏ 0	❏ 1	❏ 2	❏ 3
Asthma	❏ 0	❏ 1	❏ 2	❏ 3
Medications for lungs or heart	❏ 0	❏ 1	❏ 2	❏ 3
Current or past cigarette smoking or tobacco use	❏ 0	❏ 1	❏ 2	❏ 3
Pain in chest	❏ NO	❏ YES→		
High blood pressure, high cholesterol, or high triglycerides?	❏ NO	❏ YES→		
Other problem, concern, or question in this area?	❏ NO	❏ YES→		
SKIN, HAIR, and NAILS	Very rare-None	Occasional-Mild	Intermittent-Moderate	Frequent-Severe
Acne	❏ 0	❏ 1	❏ 2	❏ 3
Eczema	❏ 0	❏ 1	❏ 2	❏ 3
Psoriasis	❏ 0	❏ 1	❏ 2	❏ 3
Dry skin	❏ 0	❏ 1	❏ 2	❏ 3
Oily skin	❏ 0	❏ 1	❏ 2	❏ 3
Flushing, hot flashes	❏ 0	❏ 1	❏ 2	❏ 3
Itchy skin (with or without redness) or hives	❏ 0	❏ 1	❏ 2	❏ 3
Decrease in body or facial hair	❏ 0	❏ 1	❏ 2	❏ 3
Decrease in head hair (not male pattern baldness)	❏ 0	❏ 1	❏ 2	❏ 3
Increase in body or facial hair	❏ 0	❏ 1	❏ 2	❏ 3
Excessive sweating	❏ 0	❏ 1	❏ 2	❏ 3
Insufficient sweating when hot or active	❏ 0	❏ 1	❏ 2	❏ 3
Area(s) of numbness	❏ 0	❏ 1	❏ 2	❏ 3
Area(s) of tingling	❏ 0	❏ 1	❏ 2	❏ 3
Area(s) of pain	❏ 0	❏ 1	❏ 2	❏ 3
Weak or ridged fingernails	❏ NO	❏ YES		
Change in skin color or pigmentation, vitiligo	❏ NO	❏ YES		
Small rough bumps on back of upper arms	❏ NO	❏ YES		
Other problem, concerns, or questions in this area?	❏ NO	❏ YES→		
STOMACH and DIGESTIVE TRACT	Very rare-None	Occasional-Mild	Intermittent-Moderate	Frequent-Severe
Heartburn	❏ 0	❏ 1	❏ 2	❏ 3
Poor digestion	❏ 0	❏ 1	❏ 2	❏ 3
Nausea	❏ 0	❏ 1	❏ 2	❏ 3
Vomiting	❏ 0	❏ 1	❏ 2	❏ 3
Diarrhea	❏ 0	❏ 1	❏ 2	❏ 3
Constipation	❏ 0	❏ 1	❏ 2	❏ 3
Belching, intestinal bloating, gas or flatulence	❏ 0	❏ 1	❏ 2	❏ 3
Pain in stomach, intestines, colon	❏ 0	❏ 1	❏ 2	❏ 3
Rectal itching, pain, or bleeding	❏ 0	❏ 1	❏ 2	❏ 3
Hemorrhoids	❏ 0	❏ 1	❏ 2	❏ 3
Loss of bowel control, incontinence	❏ 0	❏ 1	❏ 2	❏ 3
Other problem, concern, or question in this area?	❏ NO	❏ YES→		

KIDNEYS and GENITALS	Very rare-None	Occasional-Mild	Intermittent-Moderate	Frequent-Severe
Kidney stones	❏ 0	❏ 1	❏ 2	❏ 3
Other kidney problems	❏ 0	❏ 1	❏ 2	❏ 3
Difficulty controlling urination, incontinence	❏ 0	❏ 1	❏ 2	❏ 3
Bladder problems (other than infections)	❏ 0	❏ 1	❏ 2	❏ 3
Frequent urination	❏ 0	❏ 1	❏ 2	❏ 3
Pain or burning with urination	❏ 0	❏ 1	❏ 2	❏ 3
Discharge or blood in urine	❏ 0	❏ 1	❏ 2	❏ 3
Urinary tract (kidney, bladder, urethra) infection(s)	❏ 0	❏ 1	❏ 2	❏ 3
Sexually transmitted disease(s)	❏ 0	❏ 1	❏ 2	❏ 3
Genital herpes	❏ 0	❏ 1	❏ 2	❏ 3
Low sex drive, low libido	❏ 0	❏ 1	❏ 2	❏ 3
Have you been tested for HIV?	❏ Negative	❏ Positive	❏ Not tested	
Other problem, concern, or question in this area?	❏ NO	❏ YES→		

For **WOMEN** only	Very rare-None	Occasional-Mild	Intermittent-Moderate	Frequent-Severe
Irregular menses	❏ 0	❏ 1	❏ 2	❏ 3
Painful menses	❏ 0	❏ 1	❏ 2	❏ 3
Pain between menses	❏ 0	❏ 1	❏ 2	❏ 3
Painful, swollen, or fibrocystic breasts	❏ 0	❏ 1	❏ 2	❏ 3
Water retention	❏ 0	❏ 1	❏ 2	❏ 3
Premenstrual syndrome	❏ 0	❏ 1	❏ 2	❏ 3
Excessive bleeding	❏ 0	❏ 1	❏ 2	❏ 3
Abnormal uterine bleeding	❏ NO	❏ YES→		
Missed menses	❏ 0	❏ 1	❏ 2	❏ 3
Vaginal dryness, irritation, painful intercourse	❏ 0	❏ 1	❏ 2	❏ 3
Yeast infections	❏ 0	❏ 1	❏ 2	❏ 3
Uterine fibroids	❏ NO	❏ YES		
Menopausal symptoms or concerns	❏ NO	❏ YES→		
Infertility	❏ NO	❏ YES		
Annual Pap smear, breast examination, and health checkup?	❏ NO	❏ YES		
Family history of breast, uterine, or ovarian cancer	❏ NO	❏ YES→		
Other problem, injury, concern in this area?	❏ NO	❏ YES→		

For **MEN** only	Very rare-None	Occasional-Mild	Intermittent-Moderate	Frequent-Severe
Pain or difficulty obtaining or maintaining erection	❏ 0	❏ 1	❏ 2	❏ 3
Pain or difficulty with ejaculation	❏ 0	❏ 1	❏ 2	❏ 3
Pain or mass in testicles	❏ 0	❏ 1	❏ 2	❏ 3
Slow stream of urine or frequent urination	❏ 0	❏ 1	❏ 2	❏ 3
Undescended testis, testis in abdomen or pelvis	❏ NO	❏ YES		
Men over 50: annual PSA test and prostate exam?	❏ NO	❏ YES		
Family history of prostate cancer	❏ NO	❏ YES→		
Other problem, injury, concern in this area?	❏ NO	❏ YES→		

Additional notes or comments:

Physical Examination

Goals and purpose of the orthopedic/musculoskeletal/neurologic examination:
1. To establish an **accurate diagnosis (or diagnoses)**,
2. To assess the patient's **functional status** and current condition,
   a. Range of motion,
   b. Muscle strength,
   c. Ability to perform activities/actions of daily living such as standing, walking, climbing stairs, reaching for overhead objects, etc.
3. To assess, quantify (amount), and qualify (type[s]) of **pain**—if present,
4. To assess for **concomitant and/or underlying and preexisting problems**,
5. To exclude ("rule out") **emergency situations** and occult-yet-impending **disasters**,
6. To **contextualize/integrate** all of the above into a cohesive multidimensional assessment and plan.
- *Example*: If your patient presents with low back and leg pain, and you determine that his fall off a horse resulted in ischial bursitis, have you also excluded a lumbar compression fracture? You can send the patient home with anti-inflammatory treatments and icepacks for the bursitis; but if you missed the spinal fracture, your patient could suffer neurologic injury resultant from your "failure to diagnose." Don't assume that the patient has only one problem until you have proven with your history and examination that other likely problems do not exist.

Functional assessment: When working with patients with acute injuries and systemic diseases, take a wider view of the patient than simply diagnosing the problem.
- Will she be able to return to work?
- Will he be able to drive home safely?
- Will she need help with activities of daily living?
- Is there an occult disease, infection, malignancy, or toxic exposure that is causing these problems?
- Is this an acute presentation of a new problem, or an acute exacerbation of a chronic problem?

Neurologic examination: One of the most important areas to assess when a patient presents with a musculoskeletal complaint is the neurologic system, especially if the complaint is related to a recent traumatic injury. Blood circulation is essential for life; but lack of circulation is only a major consideration in a small number of injuries, and it is usually readily apparent when severe because the problem will become acute quickly. Nerve injuries, however, can be subtle. All patients with spine (neck, thoracic, low back) pain must be questioned thoroughly for evidence of neurologic compromise. Neurologic insults—such as cauda equina syndrome and transverse myelitis—can be painless, can progress rapidly, and can lead to permanent functional disability from muscle weakness or paralysis. Every patient with pain, weakness, or recent trauma must be evaluated for neurologic deficits before the patient is treated and released from care. Neurologic examinations are briefly reviewed in the pages that follow; citations can be used for sources of additional information.

Resources for students on neurologic assessment:
- Goldberg S. *The Four-Minute Neurologic Exam*. Medmaster medmaster.net/
- neuroexam.com/neuroexam/ Information and free videos of a neurologic exam.
- Excellent interactive simulation of assessment of extraocular muscles in a neurologic examination: rad.usuhs.mil/rad/eye_simulator/eyesimulator.html
- Excellent review, noteworthy for its description of a "+5" level of reflex grading denoting sustained clonus: emedicine.medscape.com/article/1147993-overview

Orthopedic Musculoskeletal Examination: Concepts and Goals

Orthopedic tests are detailed or reviewed in each respective chapter of *Integrative Orthopedics*[74] (i.e., shoulder exams are in the chapter on shoulders, knee exams in the chapter on knees). This section reviews the concepts and goals that provide the rationale for performing these tests. Orthopedic tests are designed to place particular types of stress on specific body tissues. Types of stress include tension/distraction, compression/pressure, shear force, vibration, friction, and percussion. Each type of stress is applied to elicit specific information about the exact tissue or structure that is being tested. If you understand the reason for the type of stress that you are applying, and you are aware of the tissue/structure that you are testing, then you will find it much easier to perform the dozens of tests that are required in clinical practice. If you understand the "how" and the "why" then you won't be overwhelmed with named tests that otherwise appear illogical or superfluous.

The tests that are described in *Integrative Orthopedics* meet at least one of the following two criteria: 1) it is a common test that all doctors know and which is needed for the sake of communication and for passing academic and licensing examinations, or 2) it is going to be a useful test in clinical practice.

Always remember that abnormalities found during the physical examination—particularly the neurologic examination—are often indicative of an underlying *nonmusculoskeletal* problem that must be identified or—at the very least—considered and then excluded by additional testing. For example, a patient shoulder pain and neurologic deficits found during the neuromusculoskeletal portion of your examination could have a herniated cervical disc as the underlying cause; but the cause could also be syringomyelia, or an apical lung tumor that is invading local bone and destroying the nerves of the brachial plexus.[75]

Types of stress applied during the physical examination for specific purposes

- **Tension, traction**: To provoke pain from injured/compromised tissues: tendons, muscles, ligaments, and nerves
- **Compression, pressure**: To provoke pain from inflamed tissues; also used to assess for swelling and fluid accumulation in subcutaneous tissue, bursa, and joint spaces such as the knee
- **Shearing force**: To test the integrity of ligaments and intervertebral discs
- **Vibration (using ultrasound or 128 Hz tuning fork)**: To assess vibration sense (neurologic: peripheral nerves and dorsal columns) and screen for broken bones (orthopedic)
- **Friction, grinding**: To elicit pain from injured tissues (cross-fiber friction) and articular surfaces (grinding tests)
- **Percussion, over bone and discs**: To assess for bone fractures, bone infections, and acute disc injuries
- **Percussion, over peripheral nerves**: To assess hypesthesia/tingling suggesting reduced threshold for depolarization secondary to nerve irritation or compression, i.e., Tinel's sign
- **Fulcrum tests**: To assess for bone fractures: commonly the doctor's arm or a firm object is placed centrally under the bone in question and increasingly firm downward stress is applied to both ends of the bone to test for occult fracture
- **Torque, twisting**: To test joint integrity (restriction or laxity) or for occult bone fracture (particularly of the digits)

As a clinician, the successful management and treatment of your patients depends in large part on the following: ❶ knowledge: your ability to conceptualize broadly and to consider many *functional* and *pathologic* causes of your patient's complaints, ❷ tact: the efficiency and accuracy with which you assess, accept, and exclude the various differential diagnoses into your final working diagnosis from which your treatment, management, referral, and co-management decisions are made, ❸ art: your ability to create the changes in your patient's outlook, lifestyle, biochemistry, biomechanics/anatomy, and physiology to effect the desired outcome.

---

[74] Vasquez A. *Integrative Orthopedics*. InflammationMastery.com
[75] "Pancoast tumor has long been implicated as a cause of brachial plexopathy...The possibility of Pancoast lesion should be considered not only in the presence of brachial plexopathy, but also when C8 or T1 radiculopathy is found." Vargo et al. Pancoast tumor presenting as cervical radiculopathy. *Arch Phys Med Rehabil*. 1990 Jul;71(8):606-9

Neurologic Assessment

Clinical neurology is a complex area of study. However, for most doctors, knowledge of clinical neurology hinges on answering three questions:
- Is this patient's presentation normal or abnormal?
- If it is abnormal, does it indicate a specific disease or lesion?
- Does this condition require referral to a specialist or emergency care?

Every clinician needs thorough training in anatomy and clinical neurology to be competent in the management of patients, because even common problems such as "pain" and "fatigue" and "headache" may herald devastating neurologic illness that must be assessed accurately and managed skillfully. While a complete review of clinical neurology is beyond the scope of this text, the following section provides a basic review of the clinical essentials. Clinicians needing a refresher course in clinical neurology are encouraged to read the concise reviews by Goldberg.[76,77]

Reliable indicators of organic (real) neurologic disease:
These cannot be feigned and must be assumed to reveal organic neurologic illness that must be evaluated by a neurologist:
- Significant asymmetry of pupillary light reflex,
- Ocular divergence,
- Papilledema,
- Marked nystagmus,
- Muscle atrophy and fasciculation,
- Muscle weakness with neurologic deficit; upper motor neuron lesions (UMNL) indicate a central nervous system (CNS) lesion and need to be fully evaluated by a specialist; the need for referral is less necessary in cases of peripheral neuropathy of known cause.

Purpose of Neurologic Examination and *Principle of Neurologic Localization*:

The purpose of the neurologic examination is to qualify ("yes" or "no") the presence of a neurologic deficit, and—if present—to localize the lesion so that it can be further assessed with the proper laboratory, imaging, electrodiagnostic, or biopsy techniques. The following 9-point summary of localized lesions does not supplant independent studies of neurology and neuroanatomy but is useful for a quick clinically-relevant review:

1. **Cerebral cortex and internal capsule**: Neurologic deficit depends on location of lesion but is typically a combination of sensory/motor deficit and impaired higher neurologic function such as comprehension (superior temporal gyrus) or socially appropriate behavior (frontal lobe, ventral frontal gyri).
2. **Basal ganglia and striatal system**: Athetosis (lentiform nucleus: putamen and globus pallidus), (hemi)ballism (subthalamic nucleus), chorea (putamen), akinesia, bradykinesia, hypokinesia (lack of nigrostriatal dopamine).
3. **Cerebellum**: Ataxia, awkward clumsy execution of *intentional* motions; may have nystagmus, hypotonia.
4. **Brainstem**: Cranial nerve deficit(s) with contralateral distal sensory and/or UMN motor deficits.
5. **Spinal cord**: Cranial nerves and higher cortical functions are intact; lesion can be a combination of sensory and motor (UMN and LMN) deficits and the pattern distal to lesion may be a complete or incomplete pattern of sensory and motor deficits on one or both sides of body depending on area of spinal cord affected.
6. **Nerve root**: Segmental unilateral motor deficit; dermatomal distribution pain or sensory disturbance.
7. **Peripheral nerve**: Localized combination of sensory and motor deficits; may be bilateral or unilateral.
8. **Neuromuscular junction**: Painless weakness and "fatigable weakness": weakness that *worsens* with repeated testing; typically involves cranial nerves first in myasthenia gravis; also consider Lambert-Eaton Syndrome (LES: autoimmune neuromuscular junction disorder associated with occult malignancy; contrasts with myasthenia gravis in that in LES strength *increases* with repeated testing).
9. **Muscle disease**: Painless weakness, typically involving proximal hip/shoulder muscles first; test for elevated serum aldolase and (phospho)creatine kinase (aka, creatine phosphokinase, CK, CPK).

---

[76] Goldberg S. *Clinical Neuroanatomy Made Ridiculously Simple*. Miami, Medimaster, Inc, 1990. Now in a third edition with interactive CD.
[77] Goldberg S. *The Four-Minute Neurologic Exam*. Miami, Medimaster, Inc, 1992

Clinical assessments of neurologic function and structures

Cortex	Cerebellum
<ul><li>Orientation: Person, place, time, situation</li><li>Mood and cooperation: E.g., calm vs agitated, cooperative vs noncooperative.</li><li>Level of consciousness: Alert, lethargic, stupor, coma (indirect assessment of reticular system in brainstem)</li><li>Memory: Remember objects or numbers; *recent* memory is most commonly affected by brain lesions: *What day of the month is it? How did you get here?*</li><li>Mentation: *Count backward from 100 by 7's.*</li><li>Spelling: *Spell the word "hand" backwards.*</li><li>Stereognosis: Identify by touch a familiar object such as a key or coin.</li><li>Hoffman's reflex: Doctor rapidly extends distal joint of patient's middle finger and watches for patient's hand to perform grasp reflex; this test is performed for motor tract lesions involving the cerebral cortex, cerebellum, and upper motor neurons of the spinal cord.</li><li>Pronator drift: Supinated hands and arms outstretched forward for 30 seconds; doctor taps on palms; falling of hands and arms into pronation suggests UMNL.</li><li>Babinski reflex: Scraping the bottom of the foot results in splaying and flexing of the toes and extension (dorsiflexion) of the big toe; normal in infants.</li></ul>	<ul><li>Gait (lesion: ataxia)</li><li>Heel-to-toe walk</li><li>Tandem gait</li><li>Hand flip, foot tap (lesion: dysdiadochokinesia)</li><li>Finger-to-nose: Patient reaches out to doctor's finger, then patient touches patient nose, then back to new location of doctor's finger.</li><li>Heel-to-shin: Slide heel along shin.</li><li>Walk in circle around chair</li><li>Move eyes in a rapid "figure 8": Technique for provoking latent nystagmus</li><li>Rhomberg's test: Patient stands with feet close together and eyes closed; tests proprioception (peripheral nerves, dorsal columns, spinocerebellar tracts); vision (eyes open tests optic righting reflex) and coordinated motor activity (cerebellum).</li></ul>

Several of the above '"cerebral" deficits may also result from intoxicative, nutritional, or metabolic disorders rather than an organic irreversible physical lesion. Likewise "cerebellar" deficits may also result from lesion of the brainstem tracts/nuclei and cerebellar peduncles, rather than the cerebellum itself.

Brainstem and Cranial Nerves	Spinal Cord, Roots, Nerves

1. Olfactory: **smell**
• Smell: Test with strong and common odors such as coffee; do not use ammonia or other irritants which are perceived via trigeminal nerve (cranial nerve 5)
• This is a worthwhile test in patients with recent head trauma (direct or indirect) such as from motor vehicle accidents (MVA); any violent motion of the head may result in injury to the olfactory fibers passing through the cribiform plate; patients may have associated anosmia or altered sense of flavor; frontal lobe disorders such as altered social behavior may be noted in lesioned patients
2. Ophthalmic: **reading, peripheral vision, fundoscopic**
• Snellen chart for far vision, Rosenbaum card for near vision
• Peripheral vision
• Fundoscopic examination
3. Oculomotor: **move eyes and constrict pupils**
• Eye motion in cardinal fields of gaze
• Pupil contraction to light
• Pupil contraction to accommodation
4. Trochlear: **motor to superior oblique**
• Look "down and in" toward nose
5. Trigeminal: **bite, sensory to face and eyes**
• Bite (motor to muscles of mastication)
• Feel (sensory to face, eyes, and tongue)
6. Abducens: **motor to lateral rectus**
• Looks laterally to the ear
7. Facial: **face muscles and taste to anterior tongue**
• Furrow forehead, close eyes forcefully, smile and frown
• Taste to anterior tongue
8. Vestibulocochlear: **hearing and balance**
• Hearing, Rinne-Weber tests[78]
• Balance: observe gait and Romberg test
9. Glossopharyngeal: **swallowing, and gag reflex**
• Swallow
• Gag reflex (sensory component)
10. Vagus: **motor to palate**
• Say "ahh" to raise uvula
• Gag reflex (motor component)
11. Spinal accessory: **motor to SCM and trapezius**
• Raise your shoulders (against resistance)
• Turn your head (against resistance)
12. Hypoglossal: **motor to tongue**
• Stick out tongue to front
	Motor and reflex
	• Strength: Specific muscles are tested and rated 0-5
	• Plantar (Babinski) reflex: Signifies UMNL
	• Abdominal reflexes: "Present" or "absent" (not rated 0-4); superficial reflexes are lost (rather than hyperactive) with UMNL
	    ○ Upper abdominal: T8-10
	    ○ Lower abdominal: T10-12
	• Anal reflex: Cauda equina and sacral nerve roots
	• Reflexes: Rate 0-4; asymmetric reflexes are more significant than finding absent or hyperactive (+3) reflexes; +4 reflex with sustained clonus is almost always pathologic and requires neurologist referral. Deep tendon reflexes with main spinal root levels are as follows:
	    ○ Biceps: C5
	    ○ Brachioradialis: C6
	    ○ Triceps: C7
	    ○ Patellar: L3-L4
	    ○ Hamstring: L5
	    ○ Achilles: S1
	Sensory
	• Light touch
	• Two-point discrimination
	• Vibration (use 128 Hz tuning fork)
	• Joint position sense and proprioception (eyes closed, locate position of joint)
	• Sharp and dull
	• Hot and cold
	• Sensory loss mapping (if deficits are found)
	• Romberg (peripheral nerves, dorsal columns, vestibular, cerebellar)
	• Nerve root tension tests such as straight leg raising
	• **Subjective pain and discomfort can be indicated on pain diagrams and VAS (visual analog scale) as shown on the following page**

---

[78] "The Rinne and Weber tuning fork tests are the most important tools in distinguishing between conductive and sensorineural hearing loss." Ruckenstein MJ. Hearing loss. A plan for individualized management. *Postgrad Med*. 1995 Oct;98(4):197-200, 203, 206

Deep tendon reflexes are summarized below and on the following page. Hyperreflexia is noted with upper motor neuron lesions (UMNL) in the cortex, subcortical nuclei, brainstem, or corticospinal tracts of the spinal cord, whereas hyporeflexia can result from lesions of lower motor neurons (LMNL) in spinal cord, peripheral nerves, as well as from sensory/afferent defects including diabetic neuropathy, vitamin B-12 deficiency, and Guillain-Barre disorder. Muscle strength should always be "five over five" to be considered normal, whereas in the testing of reflexes, symmetry/asymmetry is generally more important than the grade of response (except with sustained clonus). **Asymmetry of reflex or strength (especially when seen together) is never normal and requires clinical correlation and investigation.** Reflexes and strength are evaluated and graded per details in the following table.

Grading of deep tendon reflexes (DTR) and muscle strength

Deep tendon reflexes	Muscle strength
+5 <u>Hyperreflexia with sustained clonus</u>: Sustained clonus strongly suggests UMNL and requires investigation; most textbooks use a 0-4 scale, yet this 0-5 scale facilitates clear communication of observed lesions.[79]	**5/5 <u>Normal</u>: Full strength: able to withstand gravity and full resistance.**
+4 <u>Marked hyperreflexia</u>: Up to 4 beats of unsustained clonus may be normal[80]; suggests UMNL but may be caused by medications, electrolyte disturbances, etc.	4/5 <u>Partial strength</u>: Able to withstand gravity and partial resistance.
+3 <u>Hyperreflexia</u>: More than normal.	3/5 <u>Partial strength</u>: Only able to resist gravity.
+2 <u>Normal</u>: Neither hyporeflexia nor hyperreflexia.	2/5 <u>Partial strength</u>: Able to contract muscle but unable to resist gravity.
+1 <u>Hyporeflexia</u>: Less than normal	1/5 <u>Slight flicker of muscle contraction</u>: Does not result in joint movement.
0 <u>No reflex</u>: Requires clinical correlation for lesion of sensory receptors, peripheral nerve, spinal cord, anterior horn, or neuromuscular junction; this is a common finding in normal individuals.	0/5 <u>No clinically detectable contraction</u>: Correlate with lesion of peripheral nerve, cord, cerebrum, anterior horn, or neuromuscular junction.

---

[79] Oommen K, edited by Berman SA, et al. Neurological History and Physical Examination. Last Updated: October 4, 2006. *eMedicine* emedicine.com/neuro/topic632.htm
[80] "...three to four beats of clonus can be elicited at the ankles in some normal individuals." Waxman SG. *Clinical Neuroanatomy 25th Edition*. McGraw Hill, 2003, p 325

Laboratory Assessments: General Considerations of Commonly Used Tests

"The laboratory evaluation of patients with rheumatic disease is often informative but rarely definitive."[81]

Laboratory tests are immensely important in evaluating patients with musculoskeletal pain, as these tests allow the clinician to 1) assess for infection (e.g., subacute osteomyelitis), 2) quantify the degree of inflammation (i.e., with CRP or ESR), 3) assess or exclude other disease processes that may be the cause of pain or dysfunction, and 4) assess for concomitant diseases (e.g., septic arthritis complicating rheumatoid arthritis). Additionally, 5) these tests open the door to more complete patient care and holistic management of the whole person because they allow for a more comprehensive and complete understanding of the patient's underlying physiology. **The recommended routine is to use the following panel of tests when assessing patients with musculoskeletal pain: 1) CBC, 2) CRP, 3) chemistry/metabolic panel, and preferably also 4) ferritin, 5) 25(OH)-vitamin D, and 6) thyroid assessment, minimally including TSH** and optimally including free T4, total T3, reverse T3 and anti-thyroid antibodies. The use of a screening evaluation on a routine basis helps identify patients with occult diseases and also allows for more comprehensive management of the patient's overall health. Other tests are indicated in specific situations. *Orthopedics* relies heavily upon physical examination and imaging, whereas *Rheumatology* relies more heavily upon laboratory analysis. In Orthopedics, laboratory tests are used mainly for the purposes of discovering or excluding rheumatic and systemic diseases. In Rheumatology, lab tests are used to specifically identify the type of illness, quantify the severity of the condition, and to assess for concomitant illnesses and complications.

<u>Essential Tests</u>: These tests are <u>required</u> for <u>basic</u> patient assessment

Test	Purpose	Clinical application
CRP (or ESR)	Screening for infection, inflammation, and possibly cancer; if inflammation is present, then these tests allow for a generalized quantification of severity.	Useful in all new patients for helping to differentiate systemic/inflammatory disorders from those which are noninflammatory and mechanical. Also very helpful as a general "barometer" of health since higher values correlate with increased risk for diabetes mellitus and cardiovascular disease; thus this test helps bridge the gap between acute care and wellness promotion.
CBC	Screening for anemia, infection, certain cancers (namely leukemia).	Useful in any patient with nontraumatic musculoskeletal pain or systemic manifestations, especially fever or weight loss; occasionally detects occult B-12 and folate deficiencies.
Chemistry panel	Screening for diabetes, liver disease, kidney failure, bone lesions (alkaline phosphatase), electrolyte disturbances, adrenal insufficiency (hyponatremia with hyperkalemia), hypercalcemia, hyperparathyroidism, et al.	Use this panel in any patient with nontraumatic musculoskeletal pain or systemic manifestations; all patients with hypertension, diabetes, or who use medications that cause hepatotoxicity, nephrotoxicity, etc.
Thyroid assessments	Hypothyroidism is a common problem and is an often overlooked cause of musculoskeletal pain.[82]	This is a reasonable test panel (detailed later) for any patient with fatigue, cold extremities, depression, "arthritis", muscle pain, hypercholesterolemia, or other manifestations of hypothyroidism.
Serum ferritin	Determine iron status	Best test for iron overload and deficiency, both of which are of major importance—detailed in following sections

---

[81] Klippel JH (ed). *Primer on the Rheumatic Diseases. 11th Edition*. Atlanta: Arthritis Foundation. 1997 page 94
[82] "Hypothyroidism is frequently accompanied by musculoskeletal manifestations ranging from myalgias and arthralgias to true myopathy and arthritis." McLean RM, Podell DN. Bone and joint manifestations of hypothyroidism. *Semin Arthritis Rheum*. 1995 Feb;24(4):282-90

Overview of Important Tests: Additional Components of Routine Evaluation

Test	Purpose	Clinical Application
Ferritin—*recommended for all patients given the high prevalence and major significance of both iron overload and iron deficiency*	Important for assessing for iron overload (e.g., hemochromatoic polyarthropathy), and iron deficiency (e.g., low back pain due to colon cancer metastasis). Ferritin values less than 20 in adults (e.g., iron deficiency) or greater than 200 in women and 300 in men (e.g., iron overload) necessitate evaluation and effective treatment.	**Ferritin is the ideal test for both iron overload and iron deficiency.** All patients should be screened for hemochromatosis and other hereditary forms of iron overload regardless of age, gender, or ethnicity.[83] Iron deficiency—particularly in adults—may be the first clue to gastric/colon cancer and generally necessitates referral to gastroenterologist.
Serum 25-hydroxy-vitamin D, 25(OH)D	Vitamin D deficiency is a common cause of musculoskeletal pain and inflammation[84,85], and vitamin D deficiency is a significant risk factor for numerous serious health problems.[86,87,88]	Measurement of serum 25(OH) vitamin D (or empiric treatment with 2,000 – 4,000 IU vitamin D3 per day for adults) is indicated in patients with chronic musculoskeletal pain.[89,90] Optimal vitamin D status correlates with serum 25(OH)D levels of 50 – 100 ng/mL.[91]
Antinuclear antibodies (ANA)	Sensitive (but not specific) for the detection of several autoimmune diseases, especially systemic lupus erythematosus (SLE).	This test is particularly valuable for assessing patients with polyarthropathy, facial rash, and/or fatigue.
Rheumatoid factor (RF)	The primary value of this test is in supporting a diagnosis of rheumatoid arthritis; specificity is low.	RF may be positive in normal health, iron overload, chronic infections, hepatitis, sarcoidosis, and bacterial endocarditis.
Cyclic citrullinated protein (CCP) antibodies	Cyclic citrullinated protein (CCP) antibodies are currently the single best laboratory test for rheumatoid arthritis (RA) and have largely replaced RF.	Citrullinated protein antibodies are rapidly becoming *the test* for diagnosing and confirming RA; used with RF for highly specific "conjugate seropositivity."
Lactulose-mannitol assay	Assesses for malabsorption and excess intestinal permeability—"leaky gut."	Diagnostic test for intestinal damage; excellent nonspecific screening test for pathology or pathophysiology such as celiac and Crohn's disease.
Comprehensive parasitology, stool analysis	Identification and quantification of intestinal yeast, bacteria, and other microbes.	Extremely valuable test when working with patients with chronic fatigue syndromes, fibromyalgia, or autoimmunity.

---

[83] Vasquez A. Musculoskeletal disorders and iron overload disease: comment on the American College of Rheumatology guidelines for the initial evaluation of the adult patient with acute musculoskeletal symptoms. *Arthritis Rheum* 1996;39: 1767-8   InflammationMastery.com/reprints
[84] Masood et al. Persistent limb pain and raised serum alkaline phosphatase earliest markers subclinical hypovitaminosis D Kashmir. *Indian J Physiol Pharmacol* 1989;33:259-61
[85] Al Faraj S, Al Mutairi K. Vitamin D deficiency and chronic low back pain in Saudi Arabia. *Spine*. 2003 Jan 15;28(2):177-9
[86] Grant WB. An estimate of premature cancer mortality in the U.S. due to inadequate doses of solar ultraviolet-B radiation. *Cancer*. 2002;94(6):1867-75
[87] Zittermann A. Vitamin D in preventive medicine: are we ignoring the evidence? *Br J Nutr*. 2003 May;89(5):552-72
[88] Holick MF. Vitamin D: importance in the prevention of cancers, type 1 diabetes, heart disease, and osteoporosis. *Am J Clin Nutr*. 2004;79(3):362-71
[89] Plotnikoff GA, Quigley JM. Prevalence of severe hypovitaminosis D in patients with persistent, nonspecific musculoskeletal pain. *Mayo Clin Proc*. 2003 Dec;78(12):1463-70
[90] Al Faraj S, Al Mutairi K. Vitamin D deficiency and chronic low back pain in Saudi Arabia. *Spine*. 2003 Jan 15;28(2):177-9
[91] Vasquez A, et al. The Clinical Importance of Vitamin D (Cholecalciferol). *Alternative Therapies in Health and Medicine* 2004;10:28-37 and *Integrative Medicine* 2004;3:44-54

Chemistry/metabolic panel	
Overview and interpretation:	▪ Accurate interpretation requires knowledge and pattern-recognition by the doctor to translate numbers into differential diagnoses that are correlated with the clinical presentation, examination, and imaging findings to arrive at probable diagnoses. ▪ Variation exists in the components and ranges offered by different laboratories.
Advantages:	▪ Inexpensive and easy to perform—venipuncture + serum separator tube. ▪ Provides a quick screen for diabetes, hepatitis, renal insufficiency, suggestions of alcohol abuse, hyperparathyroidism, electrolyte imbalances, etc.

Limitation and considerations:	▪ Individual tests and the most common clinical considerations for low and high values are listed in the following section. These values and considerations are provided with the routine adult outpatient in mind and are not inclusive of every possible differential diagnosis and therapeutic consideration. Consult your laboratory texts and reference manuals as needed per patient.
	▪ Abnormal laboratory results are always due to one of four problems:
	  1. Technical error: Error with the laboratory analysis, improper patient identification correlating with the sample, alteration of the sample before delivery to the laboratory (e.g., too much time, too much heat, lysis of cells). Given the importance of laboratory accuracy and the life-and-death decisions that are based upon such reports, this type of error is inexcusable, however, it does occur, occasionally producing results that defy physiologic possibility or which contradict the clinical picture. Repeating the test is appropriate. *Example*: Hypercalcemia (elevated serum calcium) may be reported in error by the laboratory due to problems with the analyzing machinery.
	  2. Drug effect: An otherwise healthy patient may develop a laboratory abnormality due to a drug effect. *Example*: Hypercalcemia can be secondary to the effect of a calcium-sparing diuretic, such as hydrochlorothiazide (HCTZ).
	  3. Pathology: The patient has a diagnosable disease causing the laboratory abnormality. *Example*: Hypercalcemia can be secondary to a parathyroid adenoma which secretes abnormally high amounts of parathyroid hormone; hypercalcemia can also be a presentation of malignancy such as breast cancer or prostate cancer, or from a granulomatous disease such as sarcoidosis.
	  4. Physiologic abnormality: The patient has a physiologic abnormality causing the laboratory abnormality. *Example*: Hypercalcemia can be secondary to excess intake of vitamin D. In practice, hypercalcemia from hypervitaminosis D is very rare because vitamin D has a wide safety margin; but for the sake of this discussion, vitamin D toxicity will be listed as a possible cause of hypercalcemia.

Comments:	▪ All abnormalities require follow-up—repeat test within 2-4 weeks as part of routine follow-up along with additional investigation and clinical re-assessment. Extraordinary abnormalities and those with life-threatening implications should of course be retested immediately; often, the laboratory will hold the blood sample for 7 days and the repeat analysis can be performed on the same blood sample to exclude technical error. ▪ Many ill patients (such as those with chronic fatigue syndrome, fibromyalgia, etc) will have normal results with the metabolic panel and other basic routine laboratory assessments. Therefore, normal results do not ensure that the patient is healthy nor without life-threatening illness. ▪ Generally, laboratory tests are performed in the morning under fasting conditions; such is the standard but is not necessarily required depending on the nature of the test, convenience, and the clinical situation.

Practical overview of common abnormalities on the chemistry/metabolic panel

Low values—considerations	Analyte: range[92]	High values—considerations
Technical error due to faulty processing of sample (i.e., hemolysis); insulinoma, exogenous insulin administration (test serum C-peptide), overdose of anti-hyperglycemic drugs, hypopituitarism and adrenal insufficiency.	**Glucose**: 65-99 mg/dL *Clinical pearl*: Fasting glucose levels can miss mild type-2 diabetes mellitus; a better test for long-term glucose status is hemoglobin A1c.	Postprandial sample, diabetes mellitus type-1 or type-2, Cushing disease or syndrome, acromegaly, pheochromocytoma, glucagonoma, hyperthyroidism. Fasting glucose >126 mg/dL on two or more occasions is consistent with the diagnosis of diabetes mellitus, as is the finding of nonfasting glucose >200 mg/dL on any one occasion. If glucose is >300 mg/dL and patient is unstable (e.g., tachypnic or stuporous), evaluate for diabetic ketoacidosis or hyperosmolar state. Optimal fasting serum glucose is in the range of 70-75 up to 85 mg/dL, since levels >85 mg/dL have been associated with increased mortality.
Hyponatremia[93,94] is potentially fatal and is also a cause of permanent neurologic injury (e.g., pontine myelinolysis). Clinicians should be particularly concerned when the sodium level drops below 125 mmol/L. Symptomatic hyponatremia is worthy of treatment in hospital setting; mild cases due to a recent event such as excess diaphoresis (e.g., prolonged sweating and exercise) or excess fluid intake (e.g., beer potomania [i.e., binge drinking], overhydration with unmineralized water) might be managed with sodium replacement and water restriction. Adrenal insufficiency classically presents with fatigue, hypotension, and hyponatremia with hyperkalemia; ACTH challenge test is the most sensitive and specific laboratory assessment. Older patients, patients with pulmonary disease, and patients taking certain drugs such as serotonin-reuptake inhibitors may develop a chronic and relatively benign mild hyponatremia associated with "reset osmostat syndrome." Sodium levels can be altered downward by conditions that introduce osmotically active substances into the serum, such as immunoglobulins (e.g., multiple myeloma), hyperglycemia, and hypertriglyceridemia; corrective equations are available for such situations.	**Sodium**: 136 to 144 mEq/L (mmol/L)	Hypernatremia in outpatients is rare; assess for drug effect and dehydration with hemoconcentration. Some clinicians will determine the free water deficit, while others will treat with oral or IV hydration with plain water or half-normal saline, respectively. Electrolyte abnormalities—particularly involving sodium—should generally be corrected slowly and with close supervision.

---

[92] The reference range for this table and some provisional information was derived from Medline Plus provided by the U.S. Department of Health and Human Services and National Institutes of Health. nlm.nih.gov/medlineplus/ency/article/003468.htm Accessed June 28, 2011. However, the majority of the information in this table comes from the author's (Dr Vasquez's) clinical training and experience. Editorial and peer reviews were provided by colleagues Barry Morgan MD, William J Beakey DOM, et al.
[93] Goh KP. Management of hyponatremia. *Am Fam Physician*. 2004;69:2387-94 aafp.org/afp/2004/0515/p2387.html Accessed June 2011.
[94] Decaux G, Musch W. Clinical laboratory evaluation of the syndrome of inappropriate secretion of antidiuretic hormone. *Clin J Am Soc Nephrol*. 2008 Jul;3(4):1175-84

Practical overview of common abnormalities on the chemistry/metabolic panel—continued

Low values—considerations	Analyte	High values—considerations
Hypokalemia can cause fatal cardiac arrhythmias and needs to be taken seriously. Replacement is generally via oral administration of potassium-rich foods, juices, or supplements such as potassium citrate (best option) or potassium chloride (KCl, inexpensive and therefore commonly used in medical settings even though KCl is clearly not optimal therapy due to the acidifying effect of the chloride anion). Recalcitrant hypokalemia is often a sign of magnesium depletion.[95] Causes of hypokalemia include diarrhea, vomiting, diuretics, Cushing disease/syndrome, dietary insufficiency, overhydration with mineral-free fluids, hyperaldosteronism and renal artery stenosis. Acute metabolic acidosis should cause relative or absolute elevations in serum K; the finding of normal or low serum K in a patient with acidosis (e.g., diabetic ketoacidosis) indicates (severe) potassium depletion.	**Potassium**: 3.6 to 5.2 mEq/L (mmol/L)	**Hyperkalemia is defined as a potassium level greater than 5.5 mmol/L. Severe hyperkalemia (>7 mmol/L) can be fatal and needs to be taken seriously.** In severe hyperkalemia, treatment and emergency management should be implemented before a complete evaluation and differential diagnosis are performed.[96] ❶ Ensure that blood sample was not hemolyzed. Repeat test if patient is stable and time allows. ❷ If hyperkalemia is severe or patient is symptomatic or has electrocardiographic changes, treat hyperkalemia with intravenous calcium, beta-adrenergic agonists (e.g., albuterol), bicarbonate, insulin and glucose; magnesium sulfate may also help alleviate arrhythmias; oral sodium polystyrene sulfonate (SPS, also known as Kayexalate) is a frequently used potassium-binding agent. ❸ DDX includes adrenal insufficiency, potassium-sparing diuretics, ACE-inhibitors and ARBs, NSAIDs, rhabdomyolysis, renal failure, and massive cell necrosis such as with tumor lysis syndrome.
Evaluate hypocalcemia clinically with Chvostek's sign (~30% sensitive) and Trousseau sign (~90% sensitive) which may also be present in hypomagnesemia; evaluate clinically for arrhythmia, muscle spasm/hypertonicity, and hyperreflexia. Measure serum albumin and perform equation for "corrected calcium" if albumin is low. DDX includes renal failure, hypoparathyroidism, malabsorption, and drug effect (e.g., rarely a loop diuretic such as furosemide). Chronic mild hypocalcemia is treated with oral vitamin D and calcium supplementation; subacute symptomatic hypocalcemia can be treated with intravenous calcium gluconate especially if cardiac arrhythmias are present.	**Calcium**: 8.6 to 10.2 mg/dL	Outpatient hypercalcemia is potentially serious and needs to be evaluated in a stepwise manner: ❶ repeat the test to rule out lab error unless you are confident in the performance of the laboratory and stability of the submitted sample, ❷ review drug list for adverse effect, such as from hydrochlorothiazide (HCTZ) or rarely from excess cholecalciferol intake, ❸ test intact parathyroid hormone (iPTH) to evaluate for hyperparathyroidism, ❹ evaluate for possible granulomatous disease such as sarcoidosis, tuberculosis, Crohn's disease, and possible leukemia or lymphoma, ❺ consider metabolic bone disease such as Paget disease of bone or metastatic bone disease, ❻ evaluate for cancer, ❼ test urine calcium for familial hypocalciuric hypercalcemia, ❽ refer to specialist such as internist or endocrinologist if hypercalcemia persists and answer is not forthcoming.

Corrected calcium (cCa) equations: Used when both serum calcium and albumin are low
American units: cCa (mg/dL) = serum Ca (mg/dL) + 0.8 (4.0 − serum albumin [g/dL])
International units: cCa (mmol/L) = measured total Ca (mmol/L) + 0.02 (40 − serum albumin [g/L])

---

[95] "Herein is reviewed literature suggesting that magnesium deficiency exacerbates potassium wasting by increasing distal potassium secretion." Huang CL, Kuo E. Mechanism of hypokalemia in magnesium deficiency. *J Am Soc Nephrol.* 2007;18:2649-52 jasn.asnjournals.org/content/18/10/2649

[96] "If the hyperkalemia is severe (potassium >7.0 mEq/L) or if the patient is symptomatic, begin treatment before diagnostic investigation of the underlying cause." Garth D. Hyperkalemia in emergency medicine treatment and management. *Medscape Reference* emedicine.medscape.com/article/766479-treatment#a1126 Accessed June 2011

Practical overview of common abnormalities on the chemistry/metabolic panel—*continued*

Low values—considerations	Analyte	High values—considerations
Clinically meaningful hypochloremia is rare among outpatients. Hypochloremic metabolic alkalosis is commonly seen after persistent vomiting. Consider syndrome of inappropriate diuretic hormone (SIADH) secretion, cardiopulmonary disease, and adrenal insufficiency.	**Chloride**: 97 to 111 mmol/L	Hyperchloremia in outpatients is rare; assess for drug effect and dehydration with hemoconcentration; assess for acid-base disturbance, especially acidosis.
Reduced CO2 correlates with hyperventilation; consider acid-base disturbance, salicylate overdose, asthma. Slight decrements in healthy outpatients are probably due to anxious hyperventilation at time of venipuncture.	**CO2 (carbon dioxide)**: 20 - 30 mmol/L	Elevated CO2 can suggest cardiopulmonary compromise and/or acid-base disturbance; assess clinically. Slight elevations in otherwise healthy outpatients are probably due to breath-holding at time of venipuncture.
Reduced total protein with normal albumin suggests hypogammaglobulinemia; evaluate for nephrotic syndrome, liver disease, protein deficiency and malabsorption/enteropathy, immunosuppressive syndromes and consider intravenous gammaglobulin therapy.	**Total protein (albumin + globulins)**: 6.3 - 8.0 g/dL	Elevated total protein with normal albumin suggests hypergammaglobulinemia, such as due to infection or plasma cell dyscrasia (e.g., multiple myeloma and Waldenstrom's disease). Evaluate within the clinical context; order serum protein electrophoresis if cause remains elusive, especially if patient has immune complex disease, neuropathy, or nephropathy.
Assess for liver disease, nephrotic syndrome, protein deficiency, malabsorption (consider celiac disease).	**Albumin**: 3.9 - 5.0 g/dL	Assess for dehydration/hemoconcentration.
Loss of hepatic mass due to cirrhosis, possible pyridoxine deficiency.	**ALT (alanine aminotransferase)**: 10 - 40 IU/L	Hepatocellular liver injury due to chemical toxicity, viral hepatitis, hemochromatosis, metastatic or infectious disease, muscle injury. ALT is preferentially elevated over AST in viral hepatitis.
Loss of hepatic mass due to cirrhosis, possible pyridoxine deficiency.	**AST (aspartate aminotransferase)**: 10 - 40 IU/L	Hepatocellular liver injury due to chemical toxicity, viral hepatitis, hemochromatosis, metastatic or infectious liver disease, myocardial infarct, muscle injury. AST is preferentially elevated over ALT in alcoholic hepatitis and rhabdomyolysis.
Consider zinc deficiency, malnutrition.	**Alkaline phosphatase (abbreviated as ALK PHOS or ALP)**: 44 - 147 IU/L	Metabolic bone disease, metastatic bone disease, vitamin D deficiency, congestive liver disease. Test isoenzymes to differentiate bone versus hepatic origin if cause of elevation remains unclear.

Practical overview of common abnormalities on the chemistry/metabolic panel—*continued*

Low values—considerations	Analyte	High values—considerations
GGT levels are reduced in hypothyroidism, likely as a reflection of total reduction in protein synthesis. Oral contraceptive agents and clofibrate may also reduce levels. **GGT as a possible marker of oxidative stress and xenobiotic exposure** "It is possible that recently reported associations between serum GGT and various health outcomes may be explained by **increases in serum GGT due to the exposure to various environmental pollutants**." Lim et al. *Clin Chem* 2007 Jun	**GGT (Gamma-glutamyl transpeptidase):** 0 to 51 IU/L Discussion of HgbA1c and serum insulin is discussed in the chapters and presentations on diabetes, hypertension, and metabolic syndrome.	Because the GGT enzyme is highly represented in cells of the hepatobiliary tract, it is especially elevated in disorders of this region, especially obstructive jaundice, intrahepatic cholestasis, cholestasis of pregnancy, pancreatitis, liver metastases, alcohol/toxin/drug-induced liver disease, infectious mononucleosis, congestive heart failure, primary biliary cirrhosis, or biliary atresia. Clinicians should search for—when assessing a patient with possible/confirmed hepatobiliary obstruction—a triad of elevated GGT, ALP, and (conjugated) bilirubin. Combined elevations of GGT reflecting hepatic congestion and of MCV suggesting folate-cobalamin deficiency and/or bone marrow toxicity may suggest alcohol abuse. Milder elevations of GGT may be seen with systemic lupus erythematosus (SLE) or hyperthyroidism. GGT is considered the most sensitive laboratory marker for hepatobiliary obstruction; leucine aminopeptidase (LAP) or 5' nucleotidase are additional/confirmatory tests. Unlike ALP which can be elevated in disorders of either liver or bone (thus possibly contributing to a diagnostic dilemma), GGT has no origin in bone. The correlation between elevated GGT and insulin resistance / diabetes mellitus type-2 / metabolic syndrome[97] may be mediated via increased activity of the glutathione and detoxification systems[98] appropriately upregulated in response to the increased body burden of persistent organic pollutants.[99]
Low values are rare but might be noted with severe chronic anemia.	**Total bilirubin:** 0.2 to 1.5 mg/dL **Direct (conjugated) bilirubin:** 0 to 0.3 mg/dL **Indirect (unconjugated) bilirubin:** Determined by subtracting the *direct* from the *total* bilirubin.	Indirect/unconjugated bilirubin is elevated with hemolysis (e.g., hemolytic anemia) and impaired enzymatic conjugation (e.g., Gilbert's syndrome) or both (e.g., neonates). Direct/conjugated bilirubin has been enzymatically conjugated with glucuronic acid but is blocked from hepatobiliary excretion; consider performing liver and gall bladder sonogram (or CT or MRI) to evaluate for causes of biliary obstruction in addition to a careful abdominal exam. In patients with advanced liver disease, perform the Model for End-Stage Liver Disease (MELD) score and/or the MELD-Na score to predict 3-month mortality.[100] Fluoridated water inhibits glucuronidation in some patients with Gilbert's syndrome; biochemical improvement follows avoidance of fluoridated water.[101]

---

[97] Grundy SM. Gamma-glutamyl transferase: another biomarker for metabolic syndrome and cardiovascular risk. *Arterioscler Thromb Vasc Biol*. 2007 Jan;27(1):4-7
[98] McLennan SV et al .Changes in hepatic glutathione metabolism in diabetes. *Diabetes*. 1991 Mar;40(3):344-8
[99] Lim et al. A strong interaction between serum gamma-glutamyltransferase and obesity on the risk of prevalent type 2 diabetes. *Clin Chem* 2007;53:1092-8
[100] MELD calculations are best performed electronically, such as with mayoclinic.org/meld/mayomodel8.html or other medical calculator.
[101] Lee J. Gilbert's disease and fluoride intake. *Fluoride* 1983; 16: 139-45

Practical overview of common abnormalities on the chemistry/metabolic panel—*continued*

Low values—considerations	Analyte	High values—considerations
Liver disease, nephrotic syndrome, protein deficiency and malabsorption.	**BUN (blood urea nitrogen)**: 7 to 20 mg/dL	Consider renal underperfusion (e.g., due to heart failure, GI bleeding, renal artery stenosis, and dehydration), intrinsic renal failure, and post-renal urinary tract obstruction. When renal disease is initially considered, order a urinalysis with microscopic analysis—see following section on urinalysis (UA).
BUN-to-creatinine ratio (normal = ~10) ≥10-20: Renal underperfusion, post-renal obstruction ≤10: Suggests intrinsic renal disease		
Sarcopenia (insufficient muscle mass), protein deficiency and malabsorption.	**Creatinine**: 0.8 to 1.3 mg/dL	Excess dietary protein, creatine supplementation, renal hypoperfusion; the most important consideration is intrinsic renal failure. Creatinine production (from arginine and creatine) is proportional to muscle mass. A rise in creatinine does not become evident until renal function (measured by glomerular filtration rate [GFR]) has fallen by approximately 50%. Creatinine levels indicative of impaired renal function to such an extent that modifications in diet, medications, and co-management become relevant are 1.4 mg/dL in women and 1.5 mg/dL in men. In the evaluation of renal function, the patient's age is a crucial determinant of how the serum creatinine is interpreted for the estimation of renal function (via GFR—see the Cockcroft-Gault equation). Cystatin C is more sensitive than are singular or conjugate interpretations of BUN and creatinine. If drug-induced nephritis is suspected, test urine eosinophils.
Laboratory assessment of renal function, creatinine clearance, glomerular filtration rate (GFR) 1. Routine urinalysis 2. Random urine albumin:creatinine ratio 3. Modification of Diet in Renal Disease (MDRD) equation*, 4. 24-hour urine creatinine measurement, 5. Serum cystatin-C measurement, 6. Cockcroft-Gault equation (below): $$\text{GFR} = \frac{(140 - \text{age years}) \times \text{wt kg} \times (0.85 \text{ if female})}{72 \times \text{serum creatinine in mg/dL}}$$ Clinical pearls for managing the chronic kidney disease (CKD) patient with declining renal function: • <u>When the GFR ≤ 60 (CKD stage 3)</u>: Modify dosages or withdraw certain drugs. Treat the causative problem and/or begin specialist co-management. • <u>When the GFR ≤ 30 (CKD stage 4)</u>: The patient needs to consult a nephrologist. • <u>When the GFR ≤ 15 (CKD stage 5)</u>: The patient needs a transplant or dialysis. *National Institute of Diabetes and Digestive and Kidney Diseases (NIDDK). GFR MDRD Calculator for Adults (Conventional units). Accessed June 2011 nkdep.nih.gov/professionals/gfr_calculators/idms_con.htm		

Cystatin C	

Overview and interpretation:	- Cystatin C is gaining acceptance as studies confirm and define its usefulness, especially as an early, sensitive marker for chronic kidney disease. Concentrations of cystatin C are not affected by gender, age, or race, and cystatin C is not affected by most drugs (prednisone increases; cyclosporine decreases), infections, diet, or inflammation.[102]
	- Produced at a constant rate by all nucleated cells.
	- Freely filtered by the glomerulus.
	- Elevated in: renal disorders.
	   ○ Cystatin C rises more rapidly than creatinine (Cr) in early renal impairment.
	   ○ Good predictor of the severity of ATN (acute tubular necrosis).
	   ○ The cystatin C concentration is an independent risk factor for heart failure, mortality, CVD and non-CVD outcomes in older adults and appears to provide a better measure of risk assessment than the serum Cr concentration.

Advantages:	- More accurate assessment of renal function than creatinine-based assessments. - Can be used to accurately assess renal function when creatinine-based assessments suggest impending renal impairment inconsistent with clinical presentation.
Limitations:	- Cost is approximately US $80. - False "non-renal" elevations may occur with cancer and/or rheumatic disease.

Clinical Case **40yo male presenting for follow-up on abnormal renal function assessment—use of cystatin C to confirm normal kidney function**: This apperantly healthy and athletic 40yo man displays consistently elevated creatinine and an estimated glomerular filtration rate (eGFR) that is close enough at 62 to warrant concern. Clinicians must appreciate that eGFR <60 is consistent with stage 3 chronic kidney disease (CKD) which warrants monitoring and which often necessitates changes in drug dosing (e.g., to avoid metformin-induced lactic acidosis) and diet (e.g., to avoid hyperkalemia).

```
Date and Time Collected   Date Entered    Date and Time Reported   Physician Name        NPI              Physician ID
12/07/11 11:10            12/08/11        12/13/11 04:07ET         VASQUEZ    , A

                                          Tests Ordered
Comp. Metabolic Panel (14); FSH+TestT+LH+DHEA S+Prog+E2...; Chlamydia pneumoniae(IgG/M);
Venipuncture

             TESTS                  RESULT        FLAG        UNITS         REFERENCE INTERVAL     LAB
Comp. Metabolic Panel (14)
Glucose, Serum                        89                      mg/dL              65 - 99            01
BUN                                   18                      mg/dL               6 - 24            01
Creatinine, Serum                   1.41         High         mg/dL            0.76 - 1.27          01
eGFR If NonAfricn Am                  62                      mL/min/1.73            >59
eGFR If Africn Am                     72                      mL/min/1.73            >59
     Note: A persistent eGFR <60 mL/min/1.73 m2 (3 months or more) may
     indicate chronic kidney disease. An eGFR >59 mL/min/1.73 m2 with an
     elevated urine protein also may indicate chronic kidney disease.
     Calculated using CKD-EPI formula.
BUN/Creatinine Ratio                  13                                          9 - 20
```

In this situation, cystatin C was performed and confirmed normal renal function despite persistently elevated creatinine, which is probably attributable to this patient's athleticism and muscle mass.[103]

```
Date and Time Collected   Date Entered    Date and Time Reported   Physician Name        NPI              Physician ID
12/07/11 11:10            12/12/11        12/15/11 07:14ET         VASQUEZ    , A

                                          Tests Ordered
Cystatin C; Written Authorization

             TESTS                  RESULT        FLAG        UNITS         REFERENCE INTERVAL     LAB
Cystatin C                           0.71                     mg/L             0.53 - 0.95          01
```

---

[102] labtestsonline.org/understanding/analytes/cystatin-c/tab/test Accessed April 2012
[103] Thank you, William J Beakey DOM of Professional Co-op Services, Inc. professionalco-op.com for provision of these laboratory services.

Clinical Case 69yo asymptomatic female presenting for routine visit found to have life-threatening hyperkalemia: Review the following labs and outline your treatment plan before reading the discussion below.

PATIENT NAME	PATIENT ID	ROOM NUMBER	AGE	SEX	PHYSICIAN
			69 Y 1941	F	Vasquez

REQUISITION NO	ACCESSION NO	ID.NO.	COLLECTION DATE & TIME	LOG-IN-DATE	REPORT DATE & TIME
			09/22/10 08:00 AM	09/22/10 06:37 PM	09/23/10 03:36AM

NOTES: PT FASTING

TEST	RESULTS OUT OF RANGE	RESULTS WITHIN RANGE	UNITS	EXPECTED RANGE	LAB
BASIC METABOLIC PROFILE					
GLUCOSE		98	MG/DL	65-100	
BUN		19	MG/DL	8-25	
CREATININE		1.2	MG/DL	0.6-1.3	
EGFR AFRICAN AMER.	54		ML/MIN/1.73	>60	
EGFR NON-AFRICAN AMER.	45		ML/MIN/1.73	>60	
SODIUM		136	MEQ/L	133-146	
POTASSIUM	8.5		MEQ/L	3.5-5.3	

RESULTS RECHECKED AND VERIFIED
NOTE: NO VISIBLE HEMOLYSIS OBSERVED.

CHLORIDE		100	MEQ/L	97-110	
CARBON DIOXIDE		27	MEQ/L	18-30	
CALCIUM		10.0	MG/DL	8.5-10.5	
LIPID PANEL					
CHOLESTEROL		193	MG/DL	<200	
TRIGLYCERIDES		129	MG/DL	<150	
HDL CHOLESTEROL		52	MG/DL	>39	
CALCULATED LDL CHOL	115		MG/DL	<100	
RISK RATIO LDL/HDL		2.22	RATIO	<3.22	
HEMOGLOBIN A1C	7.0		%	4.0-5.6	

AMERICAN DIABETES ASSOCIATION GUIDELINES FOR HGB A1C:
GLYCEMIC GOAL IN DIABETES . . . . . . <7.0%
DIAGNOSIS OF DIABETES . . . . >/=6.5%
   CONFIRMED ON REPEAT ANALYSIS OR
   WITH APPROPRIATE SYMPTOMS.
INCREASED RISK FOR DIABETES 5.7-6.4%

| TSH | 10.6 | | UIU/ML | 0.3-5.1 | |

PERFORMING LAB(S) LEGEND:

> Chemistry/metabolic panels should be performed on all new patients prior to treatment and periodically on all established patients to monitor for disease emergence and response to treatment
>
> Treating this diabetic patient with a potassium-rich diet emphasizing low-carbohydrate fruits and vegetables would exacerbate her already life-threatening hyperkalemia. Note also that her hypothyroidism would be expected to contribute to her obesity which is exacerbating her diabetes and that (somewhat theoretically since we don't have her vital signs here) hypothyroid bradycardia could also reduce renal perfusion and contribute to her low GFR and hyperkalemia.

Assessments and plan: ❶ Life-threatening hyperkalemia: The clinician must focus on the emergency issue(s). Many books quote a potassium of 6 mEq/L as a panic value; note that the laboratory already excluded technical error and checked for hemolysis, which are the two most common causes of spurious hyperkalemia. This patient should be called at home and advised to immediately seek transportation by a secondary driver (e.g., taxi, ambulance, friend, neighbor, or relative) to the nearest hospital. If the patient is demented or otherwise incompetent, the clinician should contact the patient's caretaker or call directly for an ambulance. Attention must be given to the reliability of the driver, the urgency of the situation, and the speed by which the driver can get the patient to the hospital; failure by the clinician to ensure proper patient care—which in this case and most situations is best ensured by enrolling the ambulance service—could easily result in medicolegal complications. Hospital treatment for hyperkalemia will include assessment for electrocardiographic changes and treatment of hyperkalemia with intravenous calcium to stabilize cardioelectroconductivity, beta-adrenergic agonists, bicarbonate, diuretics, insulin and glucose; magnesium may also help alleviate arrhythmias; oral sodium polystyrene sulfonate (Kayexalate) is a potassium-binding agent. ❷ Diabetes mellitus: Notice that this patient's fasting glucose level is "normal" and yet the patient is clearly diabetic per the hemoglobin A1c value >6.5%. This patient needs a comprehensive nutritional plan for diabetes management. Promoting dependence on drugs at this early point should be considered inappropriate. ❸ Hypothyroidism: The TSH >10 indicates primary hypothyroidism by any standard; in all probability, unless major contraindications exist (of which very few exist), this patient should be started on a thyroid hormone combination as discussed in the section on thyroid assessment. ❹ Renal insufficiency: This patient has stage-3 chronic kidney disease and should begin a renoprotective and renorestorative program—beyond the basics of hypertension and hyperglycemia control—as discussed in *Chiropractic and Naturopathic Mastery of Common Clinical Disorders*. Use of ACE-inhibitor or ARB is contraindicated due to hyperkalemia. ❺ Dyslipidemia: LDL cholesterol and triglycerides should both be below 100 mg/dL. Diet is key, followed by fatty acid therapy, niacin, and berberine.

Lipid panel:	
Overview and interpretation:	- "High cholesterol" was a buzz phrase many years ago indicating an unfavorable lipid profile causally associated with accelerated atherogenesis and the resultant CVD in its myriad forms. The next step was to identify low-density lipoprotein (LDL) cholesterol as the most obvious kingpin of vascular villains. Advances over the past decade include: 1. Appreciation that other non-lipid molecules such as homocysteine and c-reactive protein (CRP) are important contributors to the atherogenic process, 2. Renewed interest in the beneficial effects of high-density lipoprotein (HDL) cholesterol in mediating vasculoprotection, 3. "Non-standard" CVD risk factors such as very-low-density lipoprotein (VLDL), β-VLDL, intermediate-density lipoprotein (IDL) cholesterol, and lipoprotein-a (Lp-a) are also clinically important. For the sake of this introductory section on the basics of laboratory interpretation, the discussion will be limited to the components of the standard lipid panel; additional tests and details are provided in disease-specific chapters on metabolic/inflammatory disorders.

	Lipids: Goals	**Clinical notes:**
	Total cholesterol: < 200 mg/dL	- Higher cholesterol levels correlate with increased risk for CVD. Except in very rare cases of genotropic disease, the vast majority of humans should be able to achieve a total cholesterol <200 mg/dL via nutritional optimization, exercise, and proper endocrine (especially thyroid) status. The so-called "statin" drugs which block HMG-CoA reductase (3-hydroxy-3-methyl-glutaryl-CoA reductase, the rate-limiting enzyme for the endogenous production of cholesterol) would and should be *orphan drugs*. Reducing serum levels of insulin—the primary inducer of HMG-CoA reductase—is the most rational means by which to reduce total cholesterol levels. Thyroid hormone downregulates HMG-CoA reductase; this explains the well-established association of hypothyroidism with dyslipidemia and hypercholesterolemia.
	LDL: <100 mg/dL	- O'Keefe and Cordain and colleagues[104] have noted that optimal LDL is 50-70 mg/dl and that lower is better and is physiologically normal for humans who eat appropriate diets and who are physically active.
	HDL: >50-60 mg/dL	- Per the American Heart Association[105], "An HDL of 60 mg/dL and above is considered protective against heart disease." Of note, a recent report linked accumulation of persistent organic pollutants (POP) with elevated HDL levels.[106]
	Triglycerides: <100 mg/dL	- Elevated serum triglycerides—except in rare cases of genotropic disease—are indicators of dietary carbohydrate excess and/or alcohol excess and/or insulin resistance. Hypertriglyceridemia is associated with increased CVD risk, higher body mass index (BMI), vitamin D deficiency, and increased risks of breast cancer and prostate cancer. Extreme hypertriglyceridemia (500 mg/dL or more) can cause pancreatitis; administration of omega-3 fatty acids from fish oil is protective.
Advantages		- Allows for the monitoring of established cardiovascular risk factors and a surrogate marker for dietary compliance and lifestyle optimization.
Limitations:		- Other non-lipid risk factors should also be monitored and optimized.
Comments:		- Important panel for overall patient management and disease prevention.

---

[104] O'Keefe JH Jr, Cordain L, et al. Optimal low-density lipoprotein is 50 to 70 mg/dl: lower is better and physiologically normal. *J Am Coll Cardiol*. 2004 Jun 2;43(11):2142-6
[105] American Heart Association. heart.org/HEARTORG/Conditions/What-Your-Cholesterol-Levels-Mean_UCM_305562_Article.jsp Accessed June 2011
[106] "However, unlike the findings with p,p'-DDE, after the initial decrease of HDL-cholesterol from the 1st to 2nd quartile, HDL-cholesterol increased from the 2nd to 4th quartile of these PCBs." Lee DH, Steffes MW, Sjödin A, Jones RS, Needham LL, Jacobs DR Jr. Low dose organochlorine pesticides and polychlorinated biphenyls predict obesity, dyslipidemia, and insulin resistance among people free of diabetes. *PLoS One*. 2011 Jan 26;6(1):e15977

CBC: complete blood count	
Overview and interpretation:	This test measures numbers and indices of white and red blood cells and platelets. A routine "CBC with differential" is affordable, practical, and thus preferred for the vast majority of situations (step 1); the next step when the clinical picture remains unclear is—generally—to order a peripheral blood smear (step 2) before proceeding to a hematologist referral (step 3). Additional tests—more components of step 2—are listed below per topic. If all three blood cell populations are reduced (pancytopenia) consider nutritional anemia, hypersplenism (especially secondary to hepatic cirrhosis), autoimmunity (especially systemic lupus erythematosus), or bone marrow disorder such as myelofibrosis or aplastic anemia.

- WBC (white blood cells): The three most commonly encountered disorders that cause an abnormal WBC count are ❶ bone marrow suppression (causing low WBC count) and conditions associated with elevated WBC count including ❷ leukemia/lymphoma and ❸ response to infection. An elevated WBC count suggests the possibility of infection (especially bacterial infection) or leukemia/lymphoma and therefore requires the clinician's attention. However, relying on the WBC count for the assessment of serious infection is potentially misleading, particularly since, for example, it is elevated in less than 50% of patients with acute and chronic musculoskeletal infections; per Shaw et al[107] "Therefore, it [the WBC count] is helpful when it is high, but potentially misleading when it is normal." Clinicians can gain additional information by assessing percentage and quantitative indices of neutrophils, lymphocytes, and eosinophils, elevations of which may suggest bacterial infections, viral infections, or allergic or parasitic conditions, respectively. Primary care clinicians may also choose to perform lymphocyte immunophenotyping by flow cytometry in patients with unexplained lymphocytosis prior to hematologist consult.
  - Neutropenia: Severe suppression of WBC count resulting in neutropenia can occur in liver disease, viral infections (including but not limited to HIV), autoimmune disorders, bone marrow infiltration/failure, and toxin/alcohol exposure. For severe neutropenia, hospitalization, isolation precautions, prophylactic antibiotics, and marrow-stimulating agents are often indicated. Neutropenia is defined by an absolute neutrophil count (ANC) less than 1500 neutrophilic cells per mm3. Neutropenia is most commonly due to use of anti-cancer cytotoxic agents; other drugs that can cause neutropenia include anticonvulsants (e.g., carbamazepine, valproic acid, diphenylhydantoin), thyroid inhibitors (carbimazole, methimazole, propylthiouracil), antibacterial drugs (penicillins, cephalosporins, sulfonamides, chloramphenicol, vancomycin, trimethoprim-sulfamethoxazole), antipsychotic drugs (clozapine), antiarrhythmics (procainamide), antirheumatic drugs (penicillamine, gold salts, hydroxychloroquine), and NSAIDs.[108] The ANC is calculated with "segs" (segmented neutrophils) and "bands" (band neutrophils) reported on CBC with differential: ANC = Total WBC x (% Segs + % Bands).

> **Absolute neutrophil count (ANC) = Total WBC x (% "Segs" + % "Bands")**
> - Normal value: ≥ 1500 cells/mm3,
> - Mild neutropenia: 1000-1500/mm3,
> - Moderate neutropenia: 500-1000/mm3,
> - Severe neutropenia: ≤ 500/mm3; hospitalization is generally advised

---

[107] Shaw BA, Gerardi JA, Hennrikus WL. How to avoid orthopedic pitfalls in children. *Patient Care* 1999; Feb 28: 95-116
[108] Tefferi A, Hanson CA, Inwards DJ. How to interpret and pursue an abnormal complete blood cell count in adults. *Mayo Clin Proc*. 2005 Jul;80(7):923-36 mayoclinicproceedings.com/content/80/7/923.long This article serves as the main review for this section on CBC interpretation.

CBC: complete blood count—*continued*	

Overview and interpretation —continued:	- RBC (red blood cells and associated indices): Since polycythemia is relatively rare, in most situations the clinician is looking for anemia, most often related to the categories in the subsections that follow this paragraph. The first step is to classify the anemia based on the mean corpuscular volume (MCV) as microcytic (MCV, <80 fL), normocytic (MCV, 80-95 fL), or macrocytic (MCV, >95 fL)—details on following page.
	- Clinical notes on the most common anemias:
	   ○ Nutritional deficiency of B-12 or folate: My approach is to critique the mean corpuscular volume (MCV) and to interpret MCV values greater than 90 with an increased suspicion for folate and/or B-12 deficiency. Clinical experience has shown that MCV values greater than 95 correlate with increased homocysteine levels, and a clinical response (improvement in mood, energy, and a reduction in MCV) is commonly seen following three months of nutritional supplementation. Deficiency of vitamin B-12 can easily be treated with oral administration of 2,000 mcg per day of vitamin B-12.[109] I generally use 5 mg (rarely up to 20 mg) per day of oral folate for the treatment of probable or documented folic acid deficiency; this is safe for most patients, excluding those on antiepileptic drugs.[110] Vitamin B-12 and folic acid *function together* and should be *administered together*. Cyanocobalamin should be avoided due to its cyanide; hydroxocobalamin, methylcobalamin, adenosylcobalamin are better.
	   ○ Iron deficiency (confirmed with assessment of serum ferritin): While inadequate intake, malabsorption, or menstrual bleeding may cause iron deficiency, **adult patients with iron deficiency are at higher probability for gastrointestinal pathology and should therefore be evaluated with endoscopy or other comprehensive assessment** *beyond fecal occult-blood testing* **to rule out gastrointestinal disease.**[111,112] **The standard of care for all healthcare professionals is that adult patients with inexplicable iron deficiency are referred for gastroenteroscopic evaluation to assess for occult gastrointestinal pathology; the major concerns are gastric/colon carcinoma, but malabsorptive conditions and bleeding noncancerous polyps are also worthy of diagnosis.** Iron supplementation should be administered and can reasonably be withheld during acute viral and bacterial infections as it promotes bacterial and viral replication and pathogenicity.
	   ○ The anemia of chronic disease: Generally associated with a corresponding disease history such as long-term RA or renal insufficiency and often associated with increased ESR, CRP, and ferritin. **Do not assume that an anemic patient has iron deficiency until proven with measurement of serum ferritin**. Anemia of chronic kidney disease (CKD) is associated with reduced renal production of erythropoietin, thereby resulting in understimulation of bone marrow.
	   ○ Anemia caused by hemolysis or splenic sequestration: Autoimmune hemolytic anemia most commonly occurs in patients with systemic lupus erythematosus (SLE). Pancytopenia—reduced numbers of RBC, WBC, and platelets—is seen with chronic liver disease that has progressed to cirrhosis and has resulted in hemolysis and splenic sequestration of blood cells; such patients are at risk for esophageal varicies, encephalopathy, and ascites with spontaneous bacterial peritonitis and should be screened and treated appropriately.

---

[109] Kuzminski AM, et al. Effective treatment of cobalamin deficiency with oral cobalamin. *Blood* 1998 Aug 15;92(4):1191-8
[110] "PGA administered in doses up to 1,000 mg orally a day... The folate was well absorbed, as reflected by marked increases in the serum and erythrocyte folate concentrations... There was no evidence of clinical or laboratory toxicity at these high doses of folate." Boss GR, Ragsdale RA, Zettner A, Seegmiller JE. Failure of folic acid (pteroylglutamic acid) to affect hyperuricemia. *J Lab Clin Med* 1980 Nov;96(5):783-9
[111] Rockey DC, Cello JP. Evaluation of the gastrointestinal tract in patients with iron-deficiency anemia. *N Engl J Med*. 1993;329(23):1691-5
[112] "Endoscopy revealed a clinically important lesion in 23 (12%) of 186 patients. ... CONCLUSIONS: Endoscopy yields important findings in premenopausal women with iron deficiency anemia, which should not be attributed solely to menstrual blood loss." Bini EJ, Micale PL, Weinshel EH. Evaluation of the gastrointestinal tract in premenopausal women with iron deficiency anemia. *Am J Med*. 1998 Oct;105(4):281-6

Anemia—the most common considerations in outpatient practice: Always assess patient for tachycardia, hypovolemia, orthostasis, and adequate perfusion; always test serum ferritin during the initial evaluation then perform peripheral blood smear (PBS) if diagnosis remains unclear

- Microcytic anemia:
    - Iron deficiency anemia (IDA): Test serum ferritin. The confirmation of iron deficiency in adults generally requires gastroenterologic consultation to assess for occult gastrointestinal blood loss; this is especially true for all men and post-menopausal women but also applies to premenopausal women.* Testing for celiac disease and hematuria is advised.**
    - Thalassemia: Check for polycythemia, test Hgb electrophoresis; because the diagnosis of the various thalassemias can be complex, consider consulting a hematologist,
    - Anemia of chronic disease (ACD): Assess patient, inflammatory markers, and renal function. The most common causes of ACD are temporal (giant cell) arteritis and polymyalgia rheumatica, rheumatoid arthritis, chronic infection, Hodgkin lymphoma, renal cell carcinoma, myelofibrosis, and Castleman disease (a noncancerous lymphoproliferative disorder).
- Normocytic anemia:
    - Nutritional anemia: Iron deficiency and vitamin B-12 deficiency can both cause normocytic anemia.
    - Bleeding: Assess patient for tachycardia, hypovolemia, and shock; consider transfusion and/or volume repletion as needed. Assess serum ferritin and the reticulocyte count.
    - Chronic renal failure (CRF): Anemia associated with elevated BUN and creatinine.
    - Hypersplenism: Assess for chronic hepatitis and cirrhosis. Cirrhotic patients are at increased risk for gastroesophageal hemorrhage and ascites with spontaneous bacterial peritonitis.
    - Hemolysis: Expect to see elevated reticulocytes (chronic) and lactate dehydrogenase (acute); expect high indirect bilirubin and low serum haptoglobin with intravascular hemolysis; assess for autoimmunity (ANA, direct Coombs test [direct antiglobulin test]), glucose-6-phosphate dehydrogenase (G6PD) deficiency, drug-induced hemolysis, and other causes as case warrants.
    - Bone marrow disorder: Correlate lab findings with patient presentation; consult hematologist if solution is not forthcoming.
- Macrocytosis:
    - Induced by toxins, drugs, alcohol: Assess per patient history and other findings; the most notorious offenders are hydroxyurea, zidovudine, and alcohol.
    - Vitamin B-12 and/or folate deficiency: Consider testing serum methylmalonate and homocysteine followed by empiric supplementation with B-12 at 2,000 or more micrograms per day and folate at 1-5 milligrams per day; determine cause of problem and strongly consider autoimmune gastritis, bacterial overgrowth, and celiac disease. Test serum ferritin because nutritional deficiencies commonly occur together. Administration of vitamin B-12 is advised in all patients suspected of having B-12 deficiency.*** Regarding the clinical presentation of vitamin B-12 deficiency, clinicians should remember the adage that one-third of patients will present with anemia, one-third with peripheral neuropathy, and one-third with central neurologic problems such as depression, psychosis, and/or other disturbances of mood, memory, or personality. Failure to diagnose and treat vitamin B-12 deficiency in a timely manner will result in permanent neurologic damage.
    - Hypothyroidism: Measure TSH and free T4 at a minimum; assess basal body temperature, and speed of Achilles reflex return.

* "A gastrointestinal source of chronic blood loss was identified in a substantial proportion of premenopausal women with iron deficiency anemia." Green BT, Rockey DC. Gastrointestinal endoscopic evaluation of premenopausal women with iron deficiency anemia. *J Clin Gastroenterol*. 2004 Feb;38(2):104-9
** Goddard AF, James MW, McIntyre AS, Scott BB; on behalf of the British Society of Gastroenterology. Guidelines for the management of iron deficiency anaemia. *Gut*. 2011 Jun epocrates.com/dacc/1106/irondefbmj1106.pdf
*** "Thus, therapeutic trials of Cbl are warranted when clinical findings consistent with Cbl deficiency are present..." Solomon LR. Cobalamin-responsive disorders in the ambulatory care setting: unreliability of cobalamin, methylmalonic acid, and homocysteine testing. *Blood* 2005 Feb:978-85 bloodjournal.hematologylibrary.org/content/105/3/978.full.pdf

CBC: complete blood count—continued	
Overview and interpretation—continued:	▪ <u>Platelets</u>: Elevated platelet count (thrombocytosis) can be due to malignant primary thrombocytosis, iron-deficiency anemia, hemolysis, asplenia, and reactive thrombocytosis due to cancer, infection, or chronic inflammation. Low platelet count (thrombocytopenia, fewer than 150,000 platelets per microliter) increases risk for spontaneous bleeding and can—rarely but importantly—be associated with serious and potentially life-threatening disorders such as thrombotic thrombocytopenic purpura/hemolytic uremic syndrome (TTP/HUS) and disseminated intravascular coagulation (DIC). In relatively asymptomatic and nonacute outpatients, the most common causes of thrombocytopenia are hypersplenism due to liver cirrhosis, idiopathic thrombocytopenic purpura (ITP), and drug reaction, most notoriously secondary to trimethoprim-sulfamethoxazole ("Bactrim"), cardiac medications (e.g., quinidine, procainamide, thiazide diuretics), antirheumatic drugs (gold salts [rarely used these days]), and heparin. Heparin-induced thrombocytopenia (HIT, type-2) is potentially fatal and requires immediate cessation of heparin administration. Patients with unexplained persistent thrombocytopenia should be tested for HIV, autoimmunity (ANA), and lymphoproliferative disorders (PBS, immunophenotyping, serum protein electrophoresis, and serum immunofixation). Isolated mild to moderate thrombocytopenia (75,000 – 150,000 platelets per microliter) during pregnancy generally is considered nonpathologic.
Advantages:	▪ The **CBC with differential** is inexpensive and easy to perform and is appropriate for asymptomatic patients. The "CBC with diff" is an appropriate first test for patients who are symptomatic (e.g., fatigue, fever) or have an ongoing history of health problems. In certain healthcare settings where cost containment is a major priority, CBC *without* differential is commonly ordered; however, in outpatient private practice, the additional expenditure of $2 for the CBC *with* differential is the preferred evaluation. It provides a quick screen for anemia, leukemia, infection, and for provisional evidence of B-12/folate and iron deficiencies. The CBC can also identify more complex conditions such as pancytopenia and thereby promote comprehensive patient management; for example, pancytopenia may unmask hepatic cirrhosis which may necessitate use of nadolol for prophylaxis against gastroesophageal variceal hemorrhage as well as use of prophylactic antibiotics against spontaneous bacterial peritonitis. ▪ The **peripheral blood smear (PBS)** is used to further evaluate leukocytosis, anemias, and other abnormalities. In the investigation of persistent leukocytosis, the PBS is of limited value and therefore, while the PBS should certainly be performed, it is generally followed by **immunophenotyping by flow cytometry** if not a direct referral to a hematologist. An excellent review by Tefferi et al[113] concluded, "In general, it is prudent to perform a PBS in most instances of abnormal CBC, along with basic tests that are dictated by the type of CBC abnormalities. The latter may include, for example, serum ferritin in patients with microcytic anemia or lymphocyte immunophenotyping by flow cytometry in patients with lymphocytosis..."
Limitations:	▪ WBC count may be normal even in patients with serious infections. ▪ RBC indices may be normal in people with severe iron deficiency. o **Dr Vasquez's experience**—*Many outpatients with no evidence of anemia on the CBC will be grossly iron deficient with ferritin values less than 6 mcg/L, clearly indicating iron deficiency. Nonanemic iron deficiency contributes to fatigue, depression, RLS, attention deficit.*
Comments:	▪ The **CBC** is a foundational part of the assessment for all new patients. Generally, "CBC *with* differential" should be ordered.

---

[113] Tefferi A, Hanson CA, Inwards DJ. How to interpret and pursue an abnormal complete blood cell count in adults. *Mayo Clin Proc* 2005;80(7):923-3

Clinical Case **Classic iron insufficiency in a healthy 32yo athletic female**: This limited laboratory report is from a 32yo athletic female whose primary complaint is that of "less endurance than expected" given her healthy lifestyle and frequent participation in physical exercise of various types such as running, biking, hiking, and kayaking. Her TSH is on the low end of normal consistent with her taking 17 mcg daily of liothyroinine (T3); note however that the total T3 level remains on the low end of the normal range, suggesting that she may benefit from additional T3 supplementation. The RBC parameters Hgb and Hct are on the low end of the normal range consistent with recent menstruation; the response of the bone marrow to recent blood loss is noted with the RDW being toward the high end of normal, refecting increased marrow production of reticulocytes. Ferritin is suboptimal at 25 ng/mL, given that the optimal range is approximately 40-70 ng/mL. Although various iron supplements are available on the market and high-iron foods such as beef and blackstrap molasis can be used, typical treatment is with iron 18 mg per day often provided as ferrous sulfate 90 mg; note that 5 mg ferrous sulfate = 1 mg elemental iron. Other forms of iron such as ferrous aspartate may be better tolerated. Daily iron supplementation for 2-3 months should elevate the ferritin level and improve the feeling of energy not simply by ❶ improving oxygen delivery to tissues but also by ❷ improving function of the electron transport chain where iron is a required cofactor, ❸ improving the conversion of thyroid hormone (T4) into the active form of T3, and by ❹ improving the production of dopamine and norepinephrine, since iron is a required cofactor for the enzyme tyrosine hydroxylase which converts the amino acid tyrosine into L-DOPA which is converted to dopamine and then partially to norepinephrine. Given that this patient menstruates monthly and has no significant medical history and—specifically—no gastrointestinal complaints; the probability is high that her state of iron insufficiency is due to physiologic blood loss; however, a case could be made for endoscopic evaluation[114], and in the event that the patient suffered from an diagnosed intestinal lesion such as colon cancer, the practitioner who did not refer for gastroenterologic evaluation would be challenged to produce effective medicolegal defense. Guidelines[115] published in 2011 support testing for celiac disease, *H. pylori* infection, and hematuria while reserving endoscopy in premenopausal women to those aged 50 years or older, or with symptoms of gastrointestinal disease, or those with a strong family history of colorectal cancer.

Reported: 07/07/2011 / 06:02 CDT

Test Name	In Range	Out Of Range	Reference Range
TSH, 3RD GENERATION	0.54		mIU/L
	Reference Range		
	> or = 20 Years 0.40-4.50		
	Pregnancy Ranges		
	First trimester 0.20-4.70		
	Second trimester 0.30-4.10		
	Third trimester 0.40-2.70		
T3, TOTAL	97		76-181 ng/dL
CBC (INCLUDES DIFF/PLT)			
WHITE BLOOD CELL COUNT	7.1		3.8-10.8 Thousand/uL
RED BLOOD CELL COUNT	4.28		3.80-5.10 Million/uL
HEMOGLOBIN	12.1		11.7-15.5 g/dL
HEMATOCRIT	36.2		35.0-45.0 %
MCV	84.5		80.0-100.0 fL
MCH	28.4		27.0-33.0 pg
MCHC	33.6		32.0-36.0 g/dL
RDW	14.8		11.0-15.0 %
PLATELET COUNT	248		140-400 Thousand/uL
ABSOLUTE NEUTROPHILS	3586		1500-7800 cells/uL
ABSOLUTE LYMPHOCYTES	2854		850-3900 cells/uL
ABSOLUTE MONOCYTES	525		200-950 cells/uL
ABSOLUTE EOSINOPHILS	107		15-500 cells/uL
ABSOLUTE BASOPHILS	28		0-200 cells/uL
NEUTROPHILS	50.5		%
LYMPHOCYTES	40.2		%
MONOCYTES	7.4		%
EOSINOPHILS	1.5		%
BASOPHILS	0.4		%
FERRITIN	25		10-154 ng/mL

---

[114] "A gastrointestinal source of chronic blood loss was identified in a substantial proportion of premenopausal women with iron deficiency anemia." Green BT, Rockey DC. Gastrointestinal endoscopic evaluation of premenopausal women with iron deficiency anemia. *J Clin Gastroenterol*. 2004 Feb;38(2):104-9
[115] Goddard AF, James MW, McIntyre AS, Scott BB; on behalf of the British Society of Gastroenterology. Guidelines for the management of iron deficiency anaemia. *Gut*. 2011 Jun 6. [Epub ahead of print] epocrates.com/dacc/1106/irondefbmj1106.pdf

Clinical Case **Vitamin B-12 deficiency without hematologic abnormality**—report and discussion: This elderly patient shows no signs of anemia; note also that the MCV is perfectly normal. Given that the psychiatric literature supports a minimal serum vitamin B-12 level of 600 pg/ml, the advocation by medical reference laboratories of a lower "normal" limit of 200 pg/ml is scientifically absurd and ethically indefensible; this is yet another example of the importance of clinicians' knowledge of the literature overriding the laboratory's reference range. The consistent documentation of the rapid reversibility of severe neuropsychiatric illness with vitamin B-12 therapy as the only intervention[116,117] provides additional justification for empiric vitamin B-12 administration in patients with clinical symptoms consistent with vitamin B-12 deficiency regardless of hematologic and serologic findings.[118] Vitamin B-12 deficiency is very serious because it can lead to permanent brain damage, resulting in personality changes, memory impairment, and overt psychotic disorders, including catatonia; mechanisms of neurologic injury may include homocysteine toxicity, autoimmune neuronal demyelinization, and axonal degeneration and nerve-sheath demyelination especially in the median forebrain bundle.[119]

HEMATOLOGY

CBC - WBC STUDIES

Procedure:	WBC 10E3
Reference:	[4.50-11.00]
Units:	/CMM
07DEC06 0926 THU	7.32

CBC - RBC STUDIES

Procedure:	RBC 10E6	HEMOGLOBIN	HEMATOCRIT	MCV	MCH	MCHC	RDW-CV
Reference:	[4.50-5.90]	[13.5-17.5]	[41.0-53.0]	[80.0-94.0]	[27.0-31.0]	[32.0-36.0]	[11.0-16.0]
Units:	/CMM	G/DL	%	FL	PG	%	%
07DEC06 0926 THU	5.16	15.7	46.3	89.7	30.4	33.9	14.1

CBC - PLATELET STUDIES

Procedure:	PLATELET 10E3	MPV
Reference:	[150-500]	[9.0-13.0]
Units:	/CMM	FL
07DEC06 0926 THU	308	11.2

CHEMISTRY PROFILES

ROUTINE CHEMISTRY PROFILES

Procedure:	SODIUM	POTASSIUM	CHLORIDE	CO2	GLUCOSE	BUN	CREATININE	CALCIUM
Reference:	[133-145]	[3.5-5.3]	[100-110]	[22.0-29.0]	[70-110]	[5-25]	[0.5-1.4]	[8.3-10.3]
Units:	MMOL/L	MEQ/L	MMOL/L	MMOL/L	MG/DL	MG/DL	MG/DL	MG/DL
07DEC06 0926 THU	137	4.3	101	27.0	90	16	0.9	9.9

Procedure:	ANION GAP	OSMOLARITY	BUN/CREAT
Reference:	[6-14]	[272-305]	
Units:	MEQ/L	MOSM/K	MG/DL
07DEC06 0926 THU	13	275	17.8

SPECIAL CHEMISTRY

CHEMISTRY SPECIAL/MISCELLANEOUS

Procedure:	FOLATE	VITAMIN B-12
Reference:	[2.0-18.0]	[193-982]
Units:	NG/ML	PG/ML
07DEC06 0926 THU	14.7	182 L

---

[116] Berry N, Sagar R, Tripathi BM. Catatonia and other psychiatric symptoms with vitamin B12 deficiency. *Acta Psychiatr Scand*. 2003 ;108(2):156-9
[117] Newbold HL. Vitamin B-12: placebo or neglected therapeutic tool? *Med Hypotheses*. 1989 Mar;28(3):155-64
[118] Solomon LR. Cobalamin-responsive disorders in the ambulatory care setting. *Blood*. 2005;105:978-85. Very important article supporting empiric vitamin B12 supplementation.
[119] Catalano G, et al. Catatonia. Another neuropsychiatric presentation of vitamin B12 deficiency? *Psychosomatics*. 1998;39:456-60 psy.psychiatryonline.org/cgi/reprint/39/5/456

Nutritional deficiency, diet-responsive disorders, and the allopathic medical paradigm: Review and commentary with emphases on diabetes mellitus and vitamins D and B-12

<u>Consequences of vitamin B-12 deficiency</u>: Initially the manifestations are mild and reversible, but over time they become more severe and strongly refractory to treatment to the point that permanent damage (particularly in the CNS) is anticipated:
- "Bipolar disorder"—Vitamin B12 deficiency can result in a condition indistinguishable from a bipolar disorder,
- Organic brain syndrome, delirium, confusion, poor memory, impaired cognition,
- Dementia and erroneous diagnosis of "Alzheimer's disease",
- Mood disorders, depression, catatonia, paranoia, paranoid psychosis, violent behavior,
- Peripheral neuropathy, "combined degeneration" of anterior and posterior columns of the spinal cord,
- As a result of the above problems, patients who are mismanaged by doctors unknowledgeable about basic nutrition often suffer directly from these effects but also suffer from the medical management from these problems. Mood disorders and psychosis may result from B-12 deficiency, and the medical management of mood disorders and psychosis includes medicalization, electroconvulsive therapy (ECT), and institutionalization.

The medical profession's failure to train its students and doctors in nutrition is widely and consistently documented; given that such a profession-wide policy can do nothing other than result in patient harm and/or drug dependency under the guise of "healthcare", it is—borrowing a phrase from Nietzsche—"the highest of all conceivable corruptions."

- <u>Nutritional deficiencies and the medical paradigm</u> (*J Clin Endocrinol Metab* 2003 Nov): "But public health measures in the first half of the 20th century eradicated the most extreme of the vitamin deficiencies in the industrialized nations, and the physician's actual experience of [obvious] deficiency disease dropped to near zero. Perhaps as a result, the medical profession's approach to nutrition today is still dominated by the external agent paradigm, as witnessed in the national campaigns for cholesterol, saturated fat, and salt. Those who think more seriously in terms of the continuing importance of deficiency per se are often derogated or relegated to the quackery fringe. The result, at the very least, is inattention to the real deficiencies that may masquerade as other disorders, or that may simply be ignored altogether."
- <u>Failure of surgical treatment for low-back pain caused by vitamin D deficiency</u> (*J Am Board Fam Med* 2009 Jan): The author of this case series describes six cases of chronic debilitating back pain—three of which "required surgery"—which were greatly relieved or completely cured by correction of vitamin D deficiency. The author notes, "Chronic low back pain and failed back surgery may improve with repletion of vitamin D from a state of deficiency/insufficiency to sufficiency. Vitamin D insufficiency is common; repletion of vitamin D to normal levels in patients who have chronic low back pain or have had failed back surgery may improve quality of life or, in some cases, result in complete resolution of symptoms."

That nutritional deficiencies can cause mood disorders and mental disease is well-known; in contrast to what patients actually need, the general allopathic approach to these clinical presentations is founded upon the administration of drugs, followed by ECT, institutionalization, and psychosurgery and—lately, instead of scalpel-induced brain damage—radiofrequency heating (thermocapsulotomy) or gamma radiation (radiosurgery, gammacapsulotomy) for the destruction of brain structures, and the surgical implantation of brain electrostimulators. **Meanwhile, thousands of these psychiatrically-labeled patients simply need nutritional supplementation.** Minor exceptions noted, the medical profession as a whole chooses to remain blind to the value of nutrition so that the pharmacosurgical paradigm can remain dominant by continuing to *appear* omnipotent. The dual illusions that are maintained are "Drugs and surgery are the answers to all major health problems" and "If no drug exists for a condition, then it is idiopathic and no curative treatment is available."

Notable/additional publications relevant to this section:
1. Catalano G, Catalano MC, Rosenberg EI, Embi PJ, Embi CS. Catatonia. Another neuropsychiatric presentation of vitamin B12 deficiency? *Psychosomatics*. 1998 Sep-Oct;39(5):456-60
2. Newbold HL. Vitamin B-12: placebo or neglected therapeutic tool? *Med Hypotheses*. 1989 Mar;28(3):155-64
3. Solomon LR. Cobalamin-responsive disorders in the ambulatory care setting: unreliability of cobalamin, methylmalonic acid, and homocysteine testing. *Blood*. 2005 Feb 1;105(3):978-85
4. Christmas D, Eljamel MS, Butler S, et al. Long term outcome of thermal anterior capsulotomy for chronic, treatment refractory depression. *J Neurol Neurosurg Psychiatry*. 2011 Jun;82(6):594-600
5. Malone DA Jr. Use of deep brain stimulation in treatment-resistant depression. *Cleve Clin J Med*. 2010 Jul;77 Suppl 3:S77-80
6. Heaney RP. Vitamin D, nutritional deficiency, and the medical paradigm. *J Clin Endocrinol Metab*. 2003;88:5107-8
7. Schwalfenberg G. Improvement of chronic back pain or failed back surgery with vitamin D repletion: a case series. *J Am Board Fam Med*. 2009 Jan-Feb;22(1):69-74

Nutritional deficiency, diet-responsive disorders, and the allopathic medical paradigm: Review and commentary with emphases on diabetes mellitus and vitamins D and B-12—*continued*

The diabetes deception: Type-2 diabetes mellitus (T2DM) has burgeoned into an epidemic under the dominance of the allopathic disease model, and patients are told that the condition is genetic, progressive and incurable; a review published in the May 2011 issue of *Journal of the American Osteopathic Association* admonished physicians to (mis)educate their patients as follows, with Dr Vasquez's comments in brackets: "Be absolutely clear that T2DM is a lifelong disease [false statement] that will require lifelong treatment [false statement fostering dependency]. Success in controlling the disease and preventing future complications will depend on the patient and physician working together [creation of dependency under the guise of "working together"]. There is often a fatalistic attitude in patients with T2DM [perhaps because they have been lied to and disempowered], so it is important to establish a relationship that on one hand offers hope [creating the illusion of hope while enforcing drug dependency] and on the other does not suggest that the disease will be cured [although the diseases is generally curable with appropriate nutritional intervention]. Be up front with the patient from the first visit and make it clear that T2DM is a chronic illness [enforce drug dependency starting at the first visit]..." This babble was published in a peer-reviewed medical journal despite clear multi-decade evidence showing that T2DM is reversible with nutritional intervention.

T2DM is rapidly reversible with diet (*Diabetologia* 2011 Jun): "Normalization of both beta cell function and hepatic insulin sensitivity in type 2 diabetes was achieved by dietary energy restriction alone. This was associated with decreased pancreatic and liver triacylglycerol stores. **The abnormalities underlying type 2 diabetes are reversible by reducing dietary energy intake.**"

- Diet therapy effective, safe, and is at least as effective as injected insulin for reducing chronic hyperglycemia in T2DM (*Nutr Metab* 2009 May): "The number of patients on sulfonylureas decreased from 7 at baseline to 2 at 6 months. No patient required inpatient care or insulin therapy. In summary, the 30%-carbohydrate diet over 6 months led to a remarkable reduction in HbA1c levels, even among outpatients with severe type 2 diabetes, without any insulin therapy, hospital care or increase in sulfonylureas. **The effectiveness of the [low-carbohydrate] diet may be comparable to that of insulin therapy.**"

Ironically (or not), the first-line drug for T2DM—metformin—causes vitamin B-12 (cobalamin, Cbl) deficiency and exacerbation of the often debilitating peripheral neuropathy of T2DM which is often treated with the drugs gabapentin/Neurontin or pregabalin/Lyrica, which exacerbates obesity and T2DM, thereby promoting a vicious cycle.

- Pregabalin/Lyrica and gabapentin/Neurontin promote fat-weight gain, thereby exacerbating T2DM (*Prescrire Int* 2005 Dec): "Pregabalin, like gabapentin, can lead to weight gain and peripheral edema especially in elderly patients."
- Metformin causes vitamin B-12 deficiency and exacerbates diabetic peripheral neuropathy (*Diabetes Care* 2010 Jan): "Metformin-treated patients had depressed Cbl levels and elevated fasting MMA and Hcy levels. Clinical and electrophysiological measures identified more severe peripheral neuropathy in these patients; the cumulative metformin dose correlated strongly with these clinical and paraclinical group differences. CONCLUSIONS: Metformin exposure may be an iatrogenic cause for exacerbation of peripheral neuropathy in patients with type 2 diabetes."
- Vitamin B-12 deficiency secondary to metformin prescription (*Rev Assoc Med Bras* 2011 Jan): "The present findings suggest a high prevalence of vitamin B12 deficiency in metformin-treated diabetic patients [n=144]. Older patients, patients in long term treatment with metformin and low vitamin B12 intake are probably more prone to this deficiency."
- Metformin-induced vitamin B12 deficiency presenting as a peripheral neuropathy (*South Med J* 2010 Mar): "Chronic metformin use results in vitamin B12 deficiency in 30% of patients. ... **Vitamin B12 deficiency, which may present without anemia and as a peripheral neuropathy, is often misdiagnosed as diabetic neuropathy, although the clinical findings are usually different. Failure to diagnose the cause of the neuropathy will result in progression of central and/or peripheral neuronal damage which can be arrested but not reversed with vitamin B12 replacement.**"
- Low vitamin B-12 status correlates with expedited brain atrophy (*Neurology* 2008 Sep): "The decrease in brain volume was greater among those with lower vitamin B(12) and holoTC levels and higher plasma tHcy and MMA levels at baseline. ... Using the upper (for the vitamins) or lower tertile (for the metabolites) as reference in logistic regression analysis and adjusting for the above covariates, vitamin B(12) in the **bottom tertile (<308 pmol/L)** was associated with increased rate of brain volume loss (odds ratio 6.17)."

Notable/additional publications relevant to this section:
1. Gavin et al. Type 2 diabetes mellitus: practical approaches for primary care physicians. *J Am Osteopath Assoc* 2011;111(5s4):S3-S12
2. Lim EL, et al. Reversal of type 2 diabetes: normalisation of beta cell function. *Diabetologia*. 2011 Jun 9
3. Haimoto et al. Effects of a low-carbohydrate diet on glycemic control in outpatients with severe type 2 diabetes. *Nutr Metab* 2009:6;21
4. Gabapentin/Neurontin causes "Gains of up to 15 kg (33lbs) during 3 months of treatment." pacmedweightloss.com/docs/medications_that_cause_weight_gain.pdf Accessed July 2011.
5. Vogiatzoglou et al. Vitamin B12 status and rate of brain volume loss in community-dwelling elderly. *Neurology*. 2008;71(11):826-32
6. Wile DJ, Toth C. Association of metformin, elevated homocysteine, and methylmalonic acid levels and clinically worsened diabetic peripheral neuropathy. *Diabetes Care*. 2010 Jan;33(1):156-61
7. Nervo M, Lubini A, Raimundo FV, Faulhaber GA, Leite C, Fischer LM, Furlanetto TW. Vitamin B12 in metformin-treated diabetic patients: a cross-sectional study in Brazil. *Rev Assoc Med Bras*. 2011 Jan-Feb;57(1):46-9
8. Bell DS. Metformin-induced vitamin B12 deficiency presenting as a peripheral neuropathy. *South Med J*. 2010 Mar;103(3):265-7
9. [No authors listed] Pregabalin: new drug. Very similar to gabapentin. *Prescrire Int*. 2005 Dec;14(80):203-6

Nutritional deficiency, diet-responsive disorders, and the allopathic medical paradigm: Review and commentary with emphases on diabetes mellitus and vitamins D and B-12—*continued*

Nutritional inertia: consequences for the clinician: Given that the evidence in favor of early and empiric treatment for possible vitamin B-12 deficiency is stronger than evidence in favor of allowing vitamin B-12 deficiency or dependency to persist with potentially catastrophic outcomes, no scientific argument can be made in favor of failing to diagnose and treat vitamin B-12 deficiency/dependency. However, since, in general, the allopathic and osteopathic medical professions have failed to educate their students and doctors about nutrition, these professions have established ignorance as their defense and therefore no standard of care exists for the treatment or failure of treatment of chronic nutritional deficiencies. Ethically, the results are failure to achieve beneficence via failure to diagnose and treat, and the widespread implementation of malfeasance via diagnostic/therapeutic failure complicated by the unnecessary expenses and adverse effects of drugs/surgeries/interventions used in place of nutritional supplementation. ==The enforcement of a standard of care is meaningless when nutritional incompetence is the standard.== Fortunately for patients, the biomedical literature uses increasingly strong language in favor of mandating standards for nutritional evaluation and treatment:

- Nutritional deficiencies and the medical paradigm (*J Clin Endocrinol Metab* 2003 Nov): "J. Cannell (submitted for publication) has written that measures such as this editorial will not change the situation, and that only tort litigation will work. One can only hope that he is wrong. Either way, something needs to change"
- Physicians should routinely use vitamin supplementation as treatment for patients (*JAMA* 2002 Jun): "Physicians should make specific efforts to ensure that patients are taking vitamins they should..."
- Testing and treating for vitamin D deficiency among patients with chronic nonspecific musculoskeletal pain should be the standard of care (*Mayo Clin Proc* 2003 Dec): "Because osteomalacia is a known cause of persistent, nonspecific musculoskeletal pain, screening all outpatients with such pain for hypovitaminosis D should be standard practice in clinical care."
- Testing and treating for vitamin D deficiency among patients with chronic low-back pain should be the standard of care (*Spine* 2003 Jan): "Screening for vitamin D deficiency and treatment with supplements should be mandatory in this setting."

Notable/additional publications relevant to this section:
1. Fletcher RH, Fairfield KM. Vitamins for chronic disease prevention in adults: clinical applications. *JAMA*. 2002;287:3127-9
2. Plotnikoff et al. Prevalence of severe hypovitaminosis D in patients persistent musculoskeletal pain. *Mayo Clin Proc*. 2003;78:1463-70
3. Al Faraj S, Al Mutairi K. Vitamin D deficiency and chronic low back pain in Saudi Arabia. *Spine* 2003 ;28:177-9

UA: Urinalysis	
Overview and interpretation:	- Collection: Unless catheterized, patients are advised to pass approximately one-third of their available urine into the toilet, then pass approximately the middle-third of their urine into the specimen container. Use of an antiseptic to clean the urethral meatus was once advocated to avoid/reduce specimen contamination, but this step is ineffective and therefore unnecessary because contamination rates remain similar at 32% and 29% whether or not, respectively, urethral meatus cleansing is performed.[120]
- Analysis: Analysis should be performed on fresh urine, preferably within 1-2 hours; in outpatient clinical practice this two-hour timeframe is consistently possible only if the clinician performs in-office dipstick analysis (and perhaps microscopic visualization). Samples that cannot be analyzed within 1-2 hours or those which are destined for a reference laboratory should be refrigerated. Dipstick UA can be performed in office and is simple, inexpensive, and—when performed and interpreted with a modicum of competence—sufficiently accurate. Per Klatt[121], "The color change occurring on each segment of the strip is compared to a color chart to obtain results. However, a careless doctor, nurse, or assistant is entirely capable of misreading or misinterpreting the results." Urine samples can be sent to a reference laboratory for more accurate chemical analysis as well as microscopic analysis, culture and sensitivity. Whether infection is clinically suspected or not, clinicians might chose to order "UA with reflex to microscopy and culture" to ensure that urine samples are appropriately processed if the laboratory finds suspicion of UTI upon dipstick analysis.
- Scope of this review: The purpose of this brief review is to concisely refresh clinicians' appreciation of the components of the routine urinalysis, one that is generally performed in-office with a dipstick reagent stick or that is performed by a reference laboratory. This is not an exhaustive review, and microscopic findings have not been detailed here because most clinicians do not perform microscopy in their offices; additional details on UA and microscopic assessment is available in articles such as the excellent review by Simerville, Maxted, and Pahira published in *American Family Physician* 2005 and available on-line at aafp.org/afp/2005/0315/p1153.html as of July 2011.
- Components of routine urinalysis:
o Visual inspection: Urine should be clear with a color ranging from faint yellow (well hydrated, dilute urine) to bright yellow (especially with B-vitamin supplementation). An amber-brown hue might be due to dehydration or a pathologic process resulting in myoglobinuria (i.e., rhabdomyolysis) or the presence of bile pigments (i.e., biliary tract obstruction). A red color to urine suggests hematuria, recent beet consumption, or use of certain drugs or food dyes; the antibiotic rifampin/rifampicin is notorious for adding a red-orange color to the urine (and to a lesser extent to sweat and tears). The urine of patients with porphyria cutanea tarda will be red-brown in natural light and pink-red in fluorescent light.[122] Cloudy urine is due to pyruia (infection), proteinuria, or precipitated phosphate crystals in alkaline urine.
o Strong odor: Odiferous or malodorous urine suggests infection, recent ingestion of foods such as asparagus or nutritional supplements such as lipoic acid, certain medications, concentrated urine due to dehydration or underperfusion of the kidneys.
o Specific gravity: Specific gravity is a measure of solute concentration and thus is proportional to urine osmolality; as such it reflects renal perfusion, hydration, and the ability of the kidneys to perform their critical function of concentrating filtrate. Dilute urine has a specific gravity <1.010 and is seen with adequate/excessive hydration,

---

[120] Simerville JA, Maxted WC, Pahira JJ. Urinalysis: a comprehensive review. *Am Fam Physician*. 2005 Mar 15;71(6):1153-62 aafp.org/afp/2005/0315/p1153.html
[121] Klatt EC. WebPath. Savannah, Georgia, USA. library.med.utah.edu/WebPath/tutorial/urine/urine.html Accessed July 1, 2011
[122] Rich MW. Porphyria cutanea tarda. Don't forget to look at the urine. *Postgrad Med*. 1999 Apr;105(4):208-10, 213-4

UA: Urinalysis

diuretic use, diabetes insipidus, adrenal insufficiency, hyperaldosteronism, and impaired renal function (i.e., failure of the kidneys to concentrate urine). Concentrated urine has a specific gravity >1.020 and correlates with dehydration, renal artery stenosis, hypoperfusion/shock, glucosuria, and syndrome of inappropriate anti-diuretic hormone secretion (SIADH), which is often associated with hyponatremia.

- pH: Urine pH may range from 4.5 (very acidic) to as high as 8.5 (very alkaline). Urine pH correlates with serum pH except in patients with renal tubular acidosis (RTA type-1, a condition associated with chronically alkaline urine). Therefore, urine pH can be used to screen for various conditions of systemic alkalosis and acidosis. The Western diet—also called the standard American diet or S.A.D.—causes mild diet-induced metabolic acidosis[123] which promotes degenerative diseases; in contrast, a diet rich in fruits and vegetables such as the Paleo-Mediterranean diet[124] promotes mild systemic and urinary alkalinization.[125] From a wellness perspective, urine pH should be 7.5 up to 8.0 because urinary alkalinization facilitates xenobiotic excretion[126], promotes urinary retention of minerals such as potassium, magnesium, and calcium, and causes a reduction in serum cortisol.[127] Urine pH—like urine sodium:potassium ratio—can be used as a marker of compliance for intake of fruits, vegetables, and alkalinizing supplements such as potassium citrate. For some patients (mostly female), urine alkalinization may encourage urinary tract infection, especially if gastrointestinal dysbiosis[128] is present; in such situations, the often causative GI dysbiosis should be treated, and consistent or transient urinary acidification can be achieved with oral ascorbic acid. Urea-splitting bacteria can cause the urine to be alkaline, and such bacteria can also promote development of magnesium-ammonium phosphate crystals and so-called staghorn nephrolithiasis. Acidic urine promotes development of uric acid nephrolithiasis; therapeutic urinary alkalinization such as by use of supplemental potassium citrate or an alkalinizing diet is preventive and therapeutic. On this topic, Cicerello et al[129] wrote, "In conclusion urinary alkalization with maintaining continuously high urinary pH values, could be the treatment of choice for stone dissolution and prevention of uric acid stones."
- Bilirubin in urine: If present, bilirubin in urine is of the direct/conjugated fraction (rather than indirect/unconjugated, which is nonhydrosoluble) and indicates the need to evaluate for biliary tract obstruction.
- Urobilinogen: Urobilinogen is (direct) bilirubin that has been conjugated in the liver, passed through the biliary system into the intestine, partially metabolized by bacteria, then reabsorbed via the portal circulation and filtered by the kidney. Elevated urobilinogen is associated with liver disease and hemolytic diseases.
- Glucose: Glucose is found in the urine when the serum glucose exceeds approximately 190 mg/dL and overwhelms the reabsorptive/resorptive capacity of the proximal tubule. Glucose in the urine is presumptive evidence supporting the diagnosis of diabetes mellitus. Rare non-diabetic causes of glucosuria/glycosuria include liver disease, pancreatic disease, and Fanconi's syndrome (characterized by a failure of the proximal renal tubules to reabsorb glucose, amino acids, uric acid, phosphate and bicarbonate).

---

[123] "The modern Western-type diet is deficient in fruits and vegetables and contains excessive animal products, generating the accumulation of non-metabolizable anions and a lifespan state of overlooked metabolic acidosis, whose magnitude increases progressively with aging due to the physiological decline in kidney function." Adeva MM, Souto G. Diet-induced metabolic acidosis. *Clin Nutr*. 2011 Aug;30(4):416-21. Epub 2011 Apr 9.
[124] Vasquez A. Revisiting the Five-Part Nutritional Wellness Protocol: The Supplemented Paleo-Mediterranean Diet. *Nutritional Perspectives* 2011 Jan
[125] Cordain L, Eaton SB, Sebastian A, et al. Origins and evolution of the Western diet: health implications for the 21st century. *Am J Clin Nutr*. 2005 Feb;81(2):341-54
[126] Proudfoot AT, Krenzelok EP, Vale JA. Position Paper on urine alkalinization. *J Toxicol Clin Toxicol*. 2004;42(1):1-26
[127] Maurer et al. Neutralization of Western diet inhibits bone resorption independently of K intake, reduces cortisol secretion in humans. *Am J Physiol Renal Physiol* 2003;:F32-40
[128] Vasquez A. Nutritional and Botanical Treatments Against "Silent Infections" and Gastrointestinal Dysbiosis, Commonly Overlooked Causes of Neuromusculoskeletal Inflammation and Chronic Health Problems. *Nutritional Perspectives* 2006; Jan
[129] Cicerello E, Merlo F, Maccatrozzo L. Urinary alkalization for the treatment of uric acid nephrolithiasis. *Arch Ital Urol Androl*. 2010 Sep;82(3):145-8

UA: Urinalysis

- o Ketones: Most UA dipsticks detect acetic acid; other products of fatty acid metabolism found in urine include acetone and beta-hydroxybutyric acid. Ketonuria indicates either metabolic disturbance such as diabetes mellitus or normal physiology in the fasting or lipolytic state. Many clinicians—particularly medical students and physicians[note 130]—have been taught to view ketonuria as synonymous with ketoacidosis; this is obviously inaccurate since lipolysis and the resulting ketonuria are normal *and quite desirable* physiologic states. Ketonuria can be measured with ketone-specific dipsticks as a marker of weight-loss efficacy and compliance with diet and exercise programs.
- o Protein: Urine should not contain measurable protein on routine urinalysis. Any finding of protein in the urine—even a "trace" amount—requires follow-up; specifically, the test should be repeated within 2-4 weeks and consistently positive results require more detailed testing including serum BUN and creatinine. Urine protein can also be measured in 24-hour urine collections and should not exceed 150 mg/day; greater than this amount is diagnostic of proteinuria, while ≥ 3.5 gm/day is consistent with nephrotic syndrome, mandating a much more comprehensive *and urgent* patient evaluation. Testing for "protein" with a routine urinalysis will not detect all forms of clinically relevant proteinuria; specifically and classically, routine UA is insensitive for the microalbuminuria of diabetes mellitus (detected with the urinary albumin:creatinine ratio) and also the Bence-Jones proteinuria seen with multiple myeloma.

Evaluation of persistent proteinuria
1. Comprehensive evaluation of patient history, physical exam, and overall clinical impression,
2. Measurement of serum BUN, creatinine, albumin, and lipids; consider measuring cystatin c,
3. Microscopic examination of urinary sediment,
4. Assessment for conditions that commonly cause proteinuria, especially hypertension (sphygmomanometry), diabetes (hemoglobin A1c), autoimmune conditions (screen with ANA);
5. Measurement of 24-hour urinary creatinine excretion (or spot urinary albumin-creatinine ratio),
6. Urinary protein electrophoresis,
7. If the above measures are pathoetiologically unfruitful, refer to an internist or nephrologist.

---

[130] One of the arguments most commonly leveled against the ketogenic diet—in particular the Atkins diet—is that the induction of ketosis, as measured by ketonuria, is a potentially problematic state that should be avoided. This is an example of selective medical ignorance since mild ketosis is physiologically normal is clinically advantageous for weight loss and seizure control. In our osteopathic medical school, one lecturer advised our student body of 170 that ketosis was evidence of the "danger from diet therapies." On the contrary, given that most of my medical school professors were obese, they should have more carefully considered the benefits of rational dietary therapy, including low-carbohydrate versions of the Paleo-Mediterranean diet (described in this text) which can produce mild ketosis en route to alleviating diabetes mellitus and hypertension. Examples of selective medical ignorance and bias against low-carbohydrate ketogenic diets abound from allopathic institutions. "One diet that has raised safety concerns among the scientific community is the low-carbohydrate, high-protein diet." Tapper-Gardzina Y, Cotugna N, Vickery CE. Should you recommend a low-carb, high-protein diet? *Nurse Pract.* 2002 Apr;27(4):52-3, 55-6, 58-9. "High Protein / Low Carb (Carbohydrate) Diets. Long term, these fad diets can be harmful. Many of the health claims about these diets are not based on scientific proof. Low carb diets are still just that – a diet. Most people find maintaining a low carb diet difficult if not impossible long term. Even if weight is lost, 90% of fad dieters gain all or most of the weight back in five years." Ohio State University. medicalcenter.osu.edu/PatientEd/Materials/PDFDocs/nut-diet/nut-other/high-pro.pdf 2011 Jul.

UA: Urinalysis—*continued*		
Overview and interpretation:	○	<u>Nitrite</u>: Urinary nit<u>ri</u>te is most often the result of bacterial action on excreted urinary nit<u>ra</u>te; students and clinicians can remember this by recalling that nit<u>ra</u>te is consumed in foods via the <u>a</u>limentary tract, while nit<u>ri</u>te in the urine generally indicates urinary tract <u>i</u>nfection (UTI). A small amount of nitrate is naturally present in some foods, including tap water, beer, some cheese products, cured meats and bacon. Additional environmental sources of nitrate include the nitrates that are intentionally added to foods as preservatives, those which are contaminants from nitrate-containing fertilizers, and those which are present in our polluted environment from pesticides and the manufacture of rubber and latex. Not all bacteria can convert nitrate to nitrite; generally, this reaction indicates the presence of Gram-negative rods such as *Escherichia coli*, the causative agent in the vast majority of UTIs in both men and women. Much less commonly, Gram-positive bacteria may also cause nitrite-positive UTI. A negative urine nitrite does not exclude UTI as it may be due to either a low-nitrate diet, diuretic use, or infection with bacteria that are incapable of reducing nitrate to nitrite. **UTI management** Finding evidence of a UTI requires the clinician to determine the nature of that UTI—urethritis, prostatitis/vaginitis, cystitis, pyelonephritis—and to evaluate the severity of the infection in the context of the patient's age and comorbidities.
	○	<u>Leukocyte esterase</u>: Leukocyte esterase—as its name suggests—is an enzyme produced by white blood cells and is therefore associated with urinary tract infection. Up to five minutes is required for the enzyme to fully react with the dipstick reagent. Obviously, a positive dipstick leukocyte esterase does not itself distinguish between benign infectious cystitis and life-threatening pyelonephritis.
	○	<u>Red blood cells (RBC)</u>: On a dipstick urinalysis (in contrast to a legitimate microscopic exam), "RBC" are reported not because of the presence of cells but because of the peroxidase activity of erythrocytes, which is also noted with myoglobinuria or hemoglobinuria. Thus, a dipstick analysis "positive for RBC" could indicate legitimate hematuria, or the presence of hemoglobin or myoglobin such as from marked intravascular hemolysis or rhabdomyolysis, respectively. Red blood cells in urine are not "normal" per se, but are not necessarily pathologic. Microhematuria can be induced by many benign events, including sexual intercourse, exercise, and sample contamination from menstruation. Conversely, pathologic causes of hematuria include urinary tract infections, glomerulonephritis, IgA nephropathy, and nephrolithiasis; overt hematuria is often the first sign of renal or bladder carcinoma. Thus, when consistently present over 2-3 samples, overt or microscopic hematuria—just like any degree of proteinuria—always requires the clinician's attention. **Overt hematuria and cancer** "Up to 20 percent of patients with gross hematuria have urinary tract malignancy; a full work-up with cystoscopy and upper-tract imaging is indicated in patients with this condition." Simerville JA, Maxted WC, Pahira JJ. Urinalysis: a comprehensive review. *Am Fam Physician*. 2005 Mar;71(6):1153-62
Advantages:	▪	Allows point-of-care testing and thereby facilitates assessment and treatment.
Limitations:	▪	Noted above, e.g., insensitivity to microalbuminuria and mild Bence-Jones proteinuria
Comments:	▪	For additional information, please see any of several excellent clinically-oriented reviews such as Simerville JA, Maxted WC, Pahira JJ. Urinalysis: a comprehensive review. *Am Fam Physician* 2005 Mar aafp.org/afp/2005/0315/p1153.html

Clinical Case Routine lab evaluation in an asymptomatic elderly female—part 1: Whereas a healthy young adult might be treated nonpharmacologically such as with fluid loading and cranberry juice for a routine UTI, clinicians should appreciate several nuances of this case that add to the complexity of appropriate management. This female patient presented for a routine annual examination. Note the patient's date of birth and the date of examination in the lower right-hand corner of the report. Because of the patient's advanced age, additional considerations are warranted. This patient was also noted to be vitamin D deficient and diabetic at the time of the exam—how does this change the overall management? Clinicians must appreciate that elderly patients are less likely to mount a symptomatic and febrile response to advanced urinary tract infections; therefore consideration to the possiblity of pyelonephritis (life-threatening) in contrast to a simple cystitis (benign) must be considered. If the patient has dementia or clinically significant forgetfulness (both of which are easily tested during the office visit), compliance with treatment is much less likely, particularly if the patient does not have access to home nursing and/or does not have a spouse, relative, friend or neighbor who can aid with the supervision of care. Urinary tract infections tend to be more aggressive in elderly patients, especially those who are diabetic, especially those with micronutrient deficiencies.

Questions:
1. What additional assessments are warranted?
2. Would fluid-loading and use of cranberry juice be appropriate treatment for this patient's UTI?
3. What follow-up is recommended?

```
URINALYSIS              01/06/10
                        11:21
U COLOR                 YELLOW
U CLARITY               CLOUDY**
U GLUCOSE               NEGATIVE
U BILE                  NEGATIVE
U KETONES               NEGATIVE
U SPEC GRAVITY          1.012
U BLOOD                 NEGATIVE
U PH                    6.0
                        (NOTE06)
U PROTEIN QUAL          20**
U UROBILINOGEN          0.2
U NITRITE               NEGATIVE
U LEUK ESTERASE         MODERATE**
U WBC                   53*H
U WBCC                  RARE**
U RBC                   5*H
U SQUAM EPITH           13
U HYALINE CAST          2
U MUCOUS                RARE
(NOTE06)
URINE SAMPLES SUBMITTED FOR TESTING MORE THAN 2 HOURS AFTER COLLECTION MAY
YIELD UNRELIABLE RESULTS WHICH INCLUDE INCREASED pH, INCREASED CRYSTAL
FORMATION AND BACTERIAL CONTENT, AND DEGRADATION OF CELLULAR ELEMENTS.
-----------------------------------------------------------------------
                              BDATE: 03/20/1926 SEX: F RACE:
                              13:59 01/29/10
```

Answers:
1. Assessments: Clinical examination must include cardiac auscultatory exam, careful pulmonary auscultation for basilar crackles, distal extremity examination for edema and peripheral vascular disease, assessment for tenderness of the flanks, abdomen, and back. Vital signs are assessed: ❶ temperature, ❷ pulse, ❸ blood pressure, ❹ respiratory rate, and ❺ pain. A chemistry panel, CBC with differential, and CRP or ESR should be performed. The urinalysis is sent for microbial culture and sensitivity. Review patient's current drug regimen. If WBC casts were noted on the microscopic exam, then suspected pyelonephritis would warrant hospitalization.
2. Treatments: Fluid-loading would not be appropriate in an elderly patient who might have cardiopulmonary failure, renal insufficiency, or plasma electrolyte imbalance. Cranberry juice is not universally effective and is generally used for UTIs in younger patients who have evidence of *E coli* infection as evidenced by positive urinary nitrite; because this patient's nitrite is negative, a more likely probability exists that the UTI is due to Gram-positive bacteria and thus cranberry juice is less likely to be effective. A clinician could reasonably label this a complicated UTI due to the patient's advanced age and diabetes; thus, either an extended course of Bactrim DS (po b.i.d. for 7-10 days), or Ciprofloxacin (250-500 mg po b.i.d. for 3 days), or Nitrofurantoin (50-100 mg po q6h x7 days or 100 mg ER po q12h x7 days; give w/ food) would be considered. Drug choice depends on patient's tolerance, recent exposure, renal status, drugs, and results of culture and sensitivity.
3. Follow-up: Review laboratory results as soon as possible; if this visit is occurring at the end of the week, the lab should be alerted to phone the clinician with results over the weekend because concomitant leukocytosis or severe acute phase response (suggesting possible pyelonephritis or urosepsis) would change the management on an urgent basis. Patient should return to the office within 24-48 hours for reassessment and repeat UA. Patient is advised to return to office or go to hospital if symptoms develop— especially fever, chills, dizziness, or persistent nausea.

Clinical Case | **Routine laboratory evaluation in an asymptomatic elderly female—part 2**: Readers should review the lab report in the left side of the page before reading the discussion on the right side of the page. *Write the appropriate interpretation and intervention before looking at the answers in the column on the right.* Normal ranges were not provided with the original report.

```
CBC                     01/06/10
                        11:21
WBC 10E3                7.50
NRBC %                  0.0
NRBC 10E3               0.00
RBC 10E6                4.08*L
HGB                     11.7*L
HCT                     35.1*L
MCV                     86.0
MCH                     28.7
MCHC                    33.3
RDW-CV                  13.7
RDW-SD                  43.1
PLATELET 10E3           175
MPV                     12.3
-----------------------------------
CHEM PANEL              01/06/10
                        11:21
SODIUM                  140
POTASSIUM               4.2
CHLORIDE                102
CO2 VENOUS              27.0
GLUCOSE                 248*H
BUN                     22
SER CREATININE          1.2
CALCIUM                 9.5
GLOBULIN                3.2
TOTAL PROTEIN           7.3
ALBUMIN TOT             4.1
BILI TOTAL              0.5
ALKALINE PHOSPHA        63
SGOT (AST)              15
CHOLESTEROL             186
                        (NOTE01)
TRIGLYCERIDES           122
SGPT (ALT)              11
ANION GAP               11
OSMOLRTY CALC           291
BUN/CREAT               18.3
ALB/GLOB RATIO          1.30
HDL                     31
                        (NOTE02)
LDL CALC                131*H
                        (NOTE03)
(NOTE01)
BORDERLINE HIGH RISK = 200-239
HIGH RISK = 240 AND ABOVE.
(NOTE02)
12-16 HR FASTING:
(NOTE03)
NORMAL = LESS THAN 130 MG/DL
130-159 BORDERLINE/HIGH RISK
>/= 160 HIGH RISK
-----------------------------------
CHEM SPECIAL            01/06/10
                        11:21
HEMOGLOBIN A1C          7.6*H
                        (NOTE04)
25-OHD TOTAL            29
-----------------------------------
BDATE: 03/20/1926 SEX: F
13:59 01/29/10 FROM E585
```

This patient is anemic. The anemia is not of a severity that would be expected to cause cardiopulmonary/perfusion deficits, but the patient should be assessed, particularly if he/she has history of heart failure or lung disease such as emphysema. The MCV is not elevated, nor is it low. This could be due to combined B-12/folate and iron deficiencies; the patient should be tested and treated appropriately. Assuming that the ferritin is low, what is the next mandatory step in the management of this patient? [Answer: Treat the iron deficiency with iron supplementation but be sure to refer the patient for gastrointestinal endoscopy because of the increased probability of intestinal lesion, especially colon cancer.]

This patient is diagnosed with diabetes mellitus because the glucose is above 200. Cardioprotective measures must be implemented, ophthalmologist eye exam initiated, and foot exam performed. An integrative anti-diabetes plan[131] should be implemented.

Clinicians must appreciate the importance of the MDRD equation in this case. The answer is provided below. Perform the Cockcroft-Gault equation on paper (with use of a calculator if necessary), then perform the MDRD equation. Does this change the management of this patient's UTI? Does this change the overall management of this patient? [Answer: This patient has renal insufficiency (GFR 48-55 if African-American and 42-45 if "other race") and therefore some drugs are now contraindicated. Patient is at increased risk of hyperkalemia, especially if taking ACEi or ARB medications. The wise clinician would consider referral to an internist or nephrologist in order to ensure that the patient receives proper monitoring; for example, if the diabetes and renal insufficiency progress, the patient may require dialysis and—possibly—renal transplant, although transplant is unlikely in a patient of this advanced age.][Note 132]

Triglycerides and LDL are higher than optimal. Diet therapy and combination fatty acid supplementation (described later in this text) is indicated. Berberine might be considered as an adjunct.

HgbA1c greater than 6.5% diagnoses diabetes mellitus.

The vitamin D level is low and should be supported with oral administration of 2,000 - 10,000 IU/d and retested at 2-6 months. Serum calcium should be tested after 2-4 weeks of therapy—sooner if the patient is taking a calcium-sparing drug such as hydrochlorothiazide—and again at about 6 and 12 months.

---

[131] Vasquez A. *Chiropractic and Naturopathic Mastery of Common Clinical Disorders, 2009*. See InflammationMastery.com for details and replacements starting in 2014.
[132] Review of this case by Dr Barry Morgan (MD, emergency medicine) is acknowledged and appreciated.

Clinical Case 45yo HLA-B27+ woman with recurrent UTIs and a 7-year history of ankylosing spondylitis treated with anti-TNF drugs: Positive urine culture and positive stool culture demonstrating bacteria (*Escherichia coli* and *Klebsiella pneumoniae*) known to share molecular mimicry and cross-reactivity with HLA-B27: The Gram-negative bacterium *E. coli* produces a protein named "hypothetical protein 168" (Protein Identification Resource [PIR] data bank access code #jp0612) which shares the amino acid sequence "**RRYLE**" with HLA-B27, which contains the sequence "EWL**RRYLE**IGKETLQRVDP."[133] Per the same citation, *Klebsiella pneumoniae*'s protein (PIR s01840) nitrogenase (reductase) molybdenum-iron protein NifN contains the sequence "EWLRR." This amino acid homology confers validation to the phenomenon of molecular mimicry and thus that immune system components such as immunoglobulins and activated T-cells can cross-react between microbial peptides and human tissue antigens.[134] This patient was treated with the combination pharmaceutical antibiotic trimethoprim and sulfamethoxazole commonly referred to as "Bactrim DS" in addition to dietary optimization, hormonal optimization, and nutritional supplementation. Antimicrobial treatment with amoxicillin-clavulanate would have been reasonable, too, except for this patient's prior allergic reaction to the drug.

```
Urine Culture, Routine
  Urine Culture, Routine          Final Report
  Result 1
      Escherichia coli
      50,000-100,000 colony forming units per mL
  Antimicrobial Susceptibility
         ***** S = Susceptible; I = Intermediate; R = Resistant *****
                    P = Positive; N = Negative
         MICS are expressed in micrograms per mL
```

Antibiotic	RSLT#1
Amoxicillin/Clavulanic Acid	S
Ampicillin	S
Cefazolin	S
Cefepime	S
Ceftriaxone	S
Cefuroxime	S
Cephalothin	I
Ciprofloxacin	R
ESBL	N
Ertapenem	S
Gentamicin	S
Imipenem	S
Levofloxacin	R
Nitrofurantoin	S
Piperacillin	S
Tetracycline	S
Tobramycin	S
Trimethoprim/Sulfa	S

Comprehensive Stool Analysis / Parasitology x3

BACTERIOLOGY CULTURE

Expected/Beneficial flora	Commensal (Imbalanced) flora	Dysbiotic flora
4+ Bacteroides fragilis group	3+ Alpha hemolytic strep	3+ Klebsiella pneumoniae ssp pneumoniae
3+ Bifidobacterium spp.		
4+ Escherichia coli		
3+ Lactobacillus spp.		
NG Enterococcus spp.		
2+ Clostridium spp.		
NG = No Growth		

PRESCRIPTIVE AGENTS

	Resistant	Intermediate	Susceptible
Amoxicillin-Clavulanic Acid			S
Ampicillin	R		
Cefazolin			S
Ceftazidime			S
Ciprofloxacin			S
Trimeth-sulfa			S

Susceptible results imply that an infection due to the bacteria may be appropriately treated when the recommended dosage of the tested antimicrobial agent is used.
Intermediate results imply that response rates may be lower than for susceptible bacteria when the tested antimicrobial agent is used.
Resistant results imply that the bacteria will not be inhibited by normal dosage levels of the tested antimicrobial agent.

---

[133] Scofield RH, Warren WL, Koelsch G, Harley JB. A hypothesis for the HLA-B27 immune dysregulation in spondyloarthropathy: contributions from enteric organisms, B27 structure, peptides bound by B27, and convergent evolution. *Proc Natl Acad Sci U S A*. 1993 Oct 15;90(20):9330-4
[134] Rashid T, Ebringer A. Ankylosing spondylitis is linked to Klebsiella—the evidence. *Clin Rheumatol*. 2007 Jun;26(6):858-64

CRP: C-reactive protein	
Overview and interpretation:	- CRP is a protein made by the liver in response to the immunologic activation characteristic of infectious and inflammatory conditions. Generally, any tissue injury or inflammatory process especially that involves the immune system's increased production of IL-6 will result in increased production of CRP.[135] High sensitivity CRP (hsCRP) is preferred over regular CRP due to its greater sensitivity and use in assessing cardiovascular risk. - Elevated values are seen with: 　- <u>Infections</u>: Bacterial, fungal, parasitic, viral diseases; some patients with dysbiosis[136] will have mildly-moderately elevated CRP, 　- <u>Inflammatory bowel disease</u>: Crohn's disease and ulcerative colitis (higher in CD than UC), 　- <u>Autoimmune disease</u>: Rheumatoid arthritis, polymyalgia rheumatica, giant cell arteritis, polyarteritis nodosa, (not always SLE), 　- <u>Acute myocardial infarction or other tissue ischemia</u> 　- <u>Organ transplant rejection</u>: Renal, (not cardiac), 　- <u>Trauma</u>: Burns, surgery, 　- <u>Obesity</u>: Leads to modest elevations in CRP.
Advantages:	- This is an excellent screening test for differentiating "serious problems" (e.g., inflammatory and infectious arthropathy) from "benign problems" such as osteoarthritis. - Since higher values of CRP are a well-recognized risk factor for cardiovascular disease, screening "musculoskeletal patients" with hsCRP provides data for cardiovascular risk assessment and a more comprehensive and holistic treatment approach, thus bridging the gap between acute care and preventive care.
Limitations:	- Elevations in CRP are completely nonspecific, requiring clinical investigation to determine the underlying cause of the immune activation. - CRP may be normal in some patients with severe systemic diseases (such as lupus or cancer), and therefore a normal CRP does not entirely exclude the presence of significant illness.
Comments:	- Writing in *The New England Journal of Medicine*, authors Gabay and Kushner[137] note that measurements of plasma or serum **C-reactive protein can help differentiate inflammatory from non-inflammatory conditions and are useful in managing the patient's disease, since "the concentration often reflects the response to and the need for therapeutic intervention."** Additionally, they note, "Most normal subjects have plasma C-reactive protein concentrations of 2 mg per liter or less, but some have concentrations as high as 10 mg per liter." Deodhar[138] noted that **"Any clinical disease characterized by tissue injury and/or inflammation is accompanied by significant elevation of serum CRP..."** and that **CRP should replace ESR as a method of laboratory evaluation.** Deodhar also noted that **some patients with severe SLE will have normal CRP levels.**

---

[135] Deodhar SD. C-reactive protein: the best laboratory indicator available for monitoring disease activity. *Cleve Clin J Med* 1989 Mar-Apr;56(2):126-30
[136] See Chapter 4 of *Integrative Rheumatology* and Vasquez A. Nutritional and Botanical Treatments Against "Silent Infections" and Gastrointestinal Dysbiosis, Commonly Overlooked Causes of Neuromusculoskeletal Inflammation and Chronic Health Problems. *Nutr Perspect* 2006; Jan InflammationMastery.com/reprints
[137] Gabay C, Kushner I. Acute-phase proteins and other systemic responses to inflammation. *N Engl J Med* 1999 Feb 11;340(6):448-54
[138] Deodhar SD. C-reactive protein: the best laboratory indicator available for monitoring disease activity. *Cleve Clin J Med* 1989 Mar-Apr;56(2):126-30

Clinical Case Elevated hsCRP (high-sensitivity c-reactive protein) in a male patient with metabolic syndrome and rheumatoid arthritis—response to treatment protocol in *Integrative Rheumatology*: This 52-year-old male patient presented with a 4-year history of rheumatoid arthritis which was unresponsive to prednisone and anti-TNF (tumor necrosis factor alpha) drugs, ie, "biologics." As expected, the prednisone exacerbated the patient's insulin resistance and hypertension; the drug failed to produce an anti-inflammatory benefit for this patient. At a cost of several thousand dollars per treatment, the anti-TNF "biologic" drugs failed to provide any benefit. At the intial visit in July 2005, the hsCRP level was 124 mg/L (normal range 0-3 mg/L), as shown in these lab results.

DATE OF SPECIMEN	TIME	DATE RECEIVED	DATE REPORTED	TIME		Houston	TX 77036-0000
7/08/2005	16:19	7/08/2005	7/11/2005	7:38	419	ACCOUNT NUMBER:	42407150

TEST	RESULT	LIMITS	LAB
C-Reactive Protein, Cardiac			
> C-Reactive Protein, Cardiac	124.00H mg/L	0.00 - 3.00	HD
Relative Risk for Future Cardiovascular Event			
Low		<1.00	
Average		1.00 - 3.00	
High		>3.00	

The patient was treated with the protocol outlined in Chapter 4 of *Integrative Rheumatology*.[139] Stool testing showed *Citrobacter freundii* (renamed *Citrobacter rodentium*) which was addressed with botanical medicines; the insufficiency dysbiosis was also corrected per the five-part protocol. Slightly low testosterone and slightly elevated estradiol was optimized with a pharmaceutical aromatase inhibitor (Arimidex) given twice weekly. The five-part nutritional wellness protocol (supplemented Paleo-Mediterranean diet [SPMD]) was implemented.[140]

Comprehensive Parasitology, stool, x2

MICROBIOLOGY

Bacteriology Culture

Beneficial flora		Imbalances		Dysbiotic flora	
Bifidobacter	0+	Gamma strep	1+	Citrobacter freundii	1+
E. coli	2+	Enterobacter sp.	1+		
Lactobacillus	0+				

Mycology (Yeast) Culture

Normal flora	Dysbiotic flora
No yeast isolated	

PARASITOLOGY

	Sample 1		Sample 2
No	Ova or Parasites	No	Ova or Parasites

No anti-inflammatory drugs or botanicals were used. Within five weeks of treatment, the patient's hsCRP dropped from 124 mg/L to 7.58 mg/L—a reduction of approximately 95%—far superior to any previoius response to corticosteroid and biologic drugs. Patient experienced significant alleviation of pain and improved mobility.

8/17/2005	11:06	8/18/2005	8/18/2005	12:32	738	ACCOUNT NUMBER:	42407150

TEST	RESULT	LIMITS	LAB
C-Reactive Protein, Cardiac			
C-Reactive Protein, Cardiac	7.58H mg/L	0.00 - 3.00	HD

---

[139] Vasquez A. *Integrative Rheumatology*. See InflammationMastery.com for newest edition, which in 2014 is *Naturopathic Rheumatology v3.5*.
[140] Vasquez A. Revisiting the Five-Part Nutritional Wellness Protocol. *Nutritional Perspectives* 2011 Jan Reprinted and updated in Chapter 4.

ESR: erythrocyte sedimentation rate	
Overview and interpretation:	<ul><li>Values may be elevated even when no pathology is present because ESR increases with anemia and with age.</li><li>Much more sensitive than WBC count when screening for infection.[141]</li><li>May be normal in about 10% of patients who have pathology such as **giant cell arteritis** and **polymyalgia rheumatica** (conditions where it is generally the only lab abnormality, besides anemia); may also be normal in several other diseases.</li><li>**May be normal in patients with septic arthritis and patients with crystal-induced arthritis: joint aspiration for synovial fluid analysis is indicated if septic arthritis is suspected.**[142]</li><li>Increased with age, anemia, inflammation; higher in women than men. Age-adjusted normal ranges: any value over 25 is considered high in young people, or 40 in elderly women.</li><li>Age-related adjustments for men and women are as follows:<ul><li>Men: age divided by 2</li><li>Women: (age + 10) divided by 2</li></ul></li></ul>
Advantages:	<ul><li>Inexpensive and easy to perform—use the same lavender-topped tube that you use for CBC.</li><li>Provides a quick screen for infection, inflammation, and multiple myeloma—the most common primary bone tumor in adults.</li><li>In patients with elevated levels, ESR can be used to monitor progression of disease and response to treatment.[143] However, a negative/normal test result does not exclude the presence of significant disease; some noteworthy examples include the following: 1) elderly—due to diminished ability to mount an inflammatory response, 2) patients taking anti-inflammatory drugs and immunosuppressants, 3) a significant proportion of patients with lupus will have normal ESR despite aggressive disease, and 4) some cancer patients with clinically significant tumor burden will not show signs of systemic inflammation.</li><li>ESR may be more reliable than CRP for multiple myeloma.[144]</li></ul>
Limitations:	<ul><li>ESR may be normal in a subset of patients with clinically significant infection or inflammation.</li><li>Values are elevated in the elderly and patients with anemia and are thus not necessarily indicative of disease in these populations.</li></ul>
Comments:	<ul><li>This test is generally considered *outdated* and has been replaced in most circumstances by CRP for the evaluation of inflammation and infection.</li><li>The only time I use this test clinically is when I am highly suspicious of inflammation and the CRP is normal. Further, this test may be preferred when assessing for temporal arteritis and for multiple myeloma, two conditions which are classically associated with elevated ESR.</li></ul>

---

[141] Shaw BA, Gerardi JA, Hennrikus WL. How to avoid orthopedic pitfalls in children. *Patient Care* 1999; Feb 28: 95-116
[142] Klippel JH (ed). *Primer on the Rheumatic Diseases. 11th Edition*. Atlanta: Arthritis Foundation. 1997 page 94
[143] Shojania K. Rheumatology: 2. What laboratory tests are needed? *CMAJ*. 2000 Apr 18;162(8):1157-63 cmaj.ca/cgi/content/full/162/8/1157
[144] "ESR, a simple and easily performed marker, was found to be an independent prognostic factor for survival in patients with multiple myeloma." Alexandrakis et al. Clinical and prognostic significance of erythrocyte sedimentation rate (ESR), serum interleukin-6 (IL-6), acute phase protein levels in multiple myeloma. *Clin Lab Haematol*. 2003;25:41-6

Ferritin	
Overview and interpretation:	▪ Ferritin levels are directly proportional to body iron stores, except in patients with inflammation, infection, hepatitis, or cancer. Therefore, measuring ferritin allows assessment for iron deficiency (a cause of fatigue, or early manifestation of GI cancer) and allows for assessment of iron overload (as a cause of joint pain and arthropathy). This test should be performed in all African Americans[145,146], white men over age 30 years[147], diabetics[148], and patients with peripheral arthropathy[149], and exercise-associated joint pain[150,151] The research also justifies testing children[152], women[153], young adults[154] and the general asymptomatic public.[155] ▪ <u>Low ferritin = iron deficiency</u> ▪ <u>High ferritin = iron overload, cancer, inflammation, infection, and/or hepatitis (viral, alcoholic, or toxic)</u>
Advantages:	▪ Reliable screening test for iron overload when used in conjunction with patient assessment and evidence (e.g., normal CRP) of no infection or acute phase response. ▪ This is the blood test of choice for iron deficiency *and* iron overload.
Limitations:	▪ Iron-deficient patients with an acute phase response may have a falsely normal level of ferritin since ferritin is an acute phase reactant and will be elevated *disproportionate to iron status* during inflammation. ▪ Elevations of ferritin (i.e., >200 mcg/L in women and >300 mcg/L in men) need to be retested along with CRP (to rule out false elevation due to excessive inflammation) before making the presumptive diagnosis of iron overload. **In the absence of significant inflammation, ferritin values >200 mcg/L in women and >300 mcg/L in men indicate iron overload and the need for treatment regardless of the absence of symptoms or end-stage complications.**[156]
Comments:	▪ Note that since ferritin is an acute-phase reactant, a high level of serum ferritin by itself does not allow differentiation between iron overload, infection, and the inflammation associated with tissue injury or metastatic disease. Ferritin must be evaluated within the context of the patient's clinical condition and the assessment of at least one other marker for inflammation such as CRP. If the patient is not acutely ill or has not recently suffered tissue injury (e.g., myocardial infarction) and the CRP is normal, then an elevated ferritin value indicates iron overload until proven otherwise with diagnostic phlebotomy, which is safer and less expensive than liver biopsy or MRI. Transferrin saturation can also be measured when the interpretation of ferritin is unclear. By itself, serum iron is unreliable.

---

[145] Barton JC, Edwards CQ, Bertoli LF, Shroyer TW, Hudson SL. Iron overload in African Americans. *Am J Med.* 1995 Dec;99(6):616-23
[146] Wurapa RK, Gordeuk VR, Brittenham GM, et al. Primary iron overload in African Americans. *Am J Med.* 1996;101(1):9-18
[147] Baer DM, Simons JL, et al. Hemochromatosis screening in asymptomatic ambulatory men 30 years of age and older. *Am J Med.* 1995 May;98:464-8
[148] Phelps G, Chapman I, Hall P, Braund W, Mackinnon M. Prevalence of genetic haemochromatosis among diabetic patients. *Lancet* 1989; 2: 233-4
[149] Olynyk J, Hall P, Ahern M, KwiatekR, MackinnonM. Screening for hemochromatosis in a rheumatology clinic. *Aust NZ J Med* 1994; 24: 22-5
[150] McCurdie I, Perry JD. Haemochromatosis and exercise related joint pains. *BMJ.* 1999 Feb 13;318(7181):449-5
[151] "RESULTS: Our findings indicate a high prevalence of HFE gene mutations in this population (49.2%) compared with sedentary controls (33.5%). No association was detected in the athletes between mutations and blood iron markers. CONCLUSIONS: The findings support the need to assess regularly iron stores in elite endurance athletes." Chicharro JL, Hoyos J, Gomez-Gallego F, et al. Mutations in the hereditary haemochromatosis gene HFE in professional endurance athletes. *Br J Sports Med.* 2004 Aug;38(4):418-21. Erratum in: *Br J Sports Med.* 2004 Dec;38(6):793 bjsm.bmjjournals.com/cgi/content/full/38/4/418 Accessed September 12, 2005
[152] Kaikov Y, et al. Primary hemochromatosis in children: report of three newly diagnosed cases and review of the pediatric literature. *Pediatrics* 1992; 90: 37-42
[153] Edwards CQ, Kushner JP. Screening for hemochromatosis. *N Engl J Med* 1993; 328: 1616-20
[154] Gushusrt TP, Triest WE. Diagnosis and management of precirrhotic hemochromatosis. *W Virginia Med J* 1990; 86: 91-5
[155] Balan V, et al. Screening for hemochromatosis: a cost-effectiveness study based on 12, 258 patients. *Gastroenterology* 1994; 107: 453-9
[156] Barton JC, McDonnell SM, Adams PC, Brissot P, Powell LW, Edwards CQ, Cook JD, Kowdley KV. Management of hemochromatosis. Hemochromatosis Management Working Group. *Ann Intern Med.* 1998 Dec 1;129(11):932-9—one of the best papers ever written on this topic.

Ferritin—*Interpretation of serum levels*

Ferritin	Categorization and management
≥ 800 mcg/L	Practically diagnostic of iron overload[157]: Repeat tests; rule out inflammation or occult pathology. Initiate phlebotomy and consider liver biopsy or MRI.
≥ 300 mcg/L	Probable iron overload[158]: Repeat tests; rule out inflammation or occult pathology. In men, initiate phlebotomy and consider liver biopsy or MRI.[159]
≥ 200 mcg/L	*In women*: Suggestive of iron overload[160]: Repeat tests, rule out inflammation or occult pathology. In women, initiate phlebotomy and consider liver biopsy or MRI.[161] *In men*: High-normal *unhealthy* iron status with increased risk of myocardial infarction[162]: Rule out inflammation or occult pathology. No follow-up is mandated, yet blood donation and/or abstention from dietary iron are recommended preventative healthcare measures.
≥ 160 mcg/L	*In women*: Abnormal iron status[163]: Repeat tests, rule out inflammation or occult pathology. Consider phlebotomy and liver biopsy or MRI.
≥80-120 mcg/L	High-normal unhealthy iron status[164,165]: No follow-up is mandated; blood donation and abstention from dietary iron are suggested preventative healthcare measures. A subset of patients with restless leg syndrome (RLS, a condition also causally associated with intestinal bacterial overgrowth dysbiosis) have impaired transport of iron into the brain and therefore require slightly elevated ferritin/iron levels (up to 120) to enhance cerebral iron uptake.
40-70 mcg/L	**Optimal iron status for most people**[166,167]
< 20 mcg/L	Iron deficiency: Search for occult gastrointestinal blood loss with endoscopy or imaging assessments in adults; refer to gastroenterologist.[168,169]

Ferritin is an acute-phase reactant, which means that its production is increased during the acute phase of inflammatory and/or infectious disorders. Therefore the numeric value and hence its clinical meaning can be interpreted only within a context that also includes assessment of the patient's inflammatory status, which is best assessed with either ESR or CRP. If CRP/ESR is high, then the physician might assume that the ferritin value is "falsely elevated"—disproportionately elevated with respect to body iron stores. *Common clinical examples requiring use and skillful interpretation of ferritin*:

- **Elderly or arthritic patient with iron deficiency despite normal serum ferritin**: An elderly patient with normal ferritin and elevated CRP/ESR is probably iron deficient; retesting of ferritin and measurement of transferrin saturation and CBC should be performed promptly. If iron deficiency is confirmed or cannot be excluded, referral for endoscopic examination must be implemented. In a patient with known inflammatory arthropathy, the ferritin may appear normal even though the patient is iron deficient and in need of supplementation and endoscopy.
- **Non-anemic iron deficiency**: A middle-aged patient (commonly a premenopausal woman) presents with fatigue and during the course of evaluation is found to have a normal CBC. Do not let a normal CBC prevent you from assessing ferritin; many nonanemic patients are impressively iron deficient with ferritin values of 2-6 mcg/L and are in need of iron replacement as well as evaluation for conditions including celiac disease, *H. pylori* infection, hematuria, and gastrointestinal bleeding/lesions.

---

[157] Milman N, Albeck MJ. Distinction between homozygous and heterozygous subjects with hemochromatosis using iron status markers and receiver operating characteristic (ROC) analysis. *Eur J Clin Biochem* 1995; 33: 95-8. See also Milman N. Iron status markers in hereditary hemochromatosis. *Eur J Haematol* 1991;47:292-8
[158] Olynyk JK, Bacon BR. Hereditary hemochromatosis: detecting and correcting iron overload. *Postgrad Med* 1994;96: 151-65
[159] "Therapeutic phlebotomy is used to remove excess iron and maintain low normal body iron stores, …initiated in men with serum ferritin levels of 300 microg/L…and in women with serum ferritin levels of 200 microg/L…regardless of the presence or absence of symptoms." Barton et al. Management of hemochromatosis. *Ann Intern Med*. 1998;129:932-9
[160] Barton JC, Edwards CQ, Bertoli LF, Shroyer TW, Hudson SL. Iron overload in African Americans. *Am J Med* 1995; 99: 616-23
[161] Barton JC, McDonnell SM, Adams PC, et al. Management of hemochromatosis. *Ann Intern Med*. 1998 Dec 1;129(11):932-9
[162] Salonen JT, Nyyssonen K, Korpela H,et al. High stored iron levels are associated with excess risk of myocardial infarction in eastern Finnish men. *Circulation* 1992; 86: 803-11
[163] Nicoll D. Therapeutic drug monitoring and laboratory reference ranges. In: Tierney LM, McPhee SJ, Papadakis MA. *Current Medical Diagnosis and Treatment 1996 (35th Edition)*. Stamford: Appleton and Lange, 1996: 1442
[164] Lauffer, RB. *Iron and Your Heart*. New York: St. Martin's Press, 1991: 79-8, 83-88, 162
[165] Sullivan JL. Iron and the sex difference in heart disease risk. *Lancet*. 1981 Jun 13;1(8233):1293-4
[166] Lauffer, RB. *Iron and Your Heart*. New York: St. Martin's Press, 1991: 79-8, 83-88, 162
[167] Vasquez A. High body iron stores: causes, effects, diagnosis, and treatment. *Nutritional Perspectives* 1994; 17: 13, 15-7, 19, 21, 28 and Vasquez A. Men's Health: Iron in men: why men store this nutrient in their bodies and the harm that it does. *MEN Magazine* 1997; Jan:11,21-23 vix.com/menmag/alexiron.htm
[168] Rockey DC, Cello JP. Evaluation of the gastrointestinal tract in patients with iron-deficiency anemia. *N Engl J Med*. 1993;329(23):1691-5
[169] "Endoscopy revealed a clinically important lesion in 23 (12%) of 186 patients. … CONCLUSIONS: Endoscopy yields important findings in premenopausal women with iron deficiency anemia, which should not be attributed solely to menstrual blood loss." Bini EJ, Micale PL, Weinshel EH. Evaluation of the gastrointestinal tract in premenopausal women with iron deficiency anemia. *Am J Med*. 1998 Oct;105(4):281-6

Arthritis & Rheumatism

Official Journal of the American College of Rheumatology

VOLUME 39   OCTOBER 1996   NO. 10

Musculoskeletal disorders and iron overload disease: comment on the American College of Rheumatology guidelines for the initial evaluation of the adult patient with acute musculoskeletal symptoms

To the Editor:

The recent clinical guidelines for the initial evaluation of the adult patient with acute musculoskeletal symptoms, proposed by the American College of Rheumatology (1), provide useful information and a good review for clinicians. However, there is one important omission in these guidelines. Nowhere in the guidelines is hemochromatosis mentioned. Such a prevalent and potentially life-threatening disease certainly deserves to be considered in the evaluation of patients with musculoskeletal disorders.

Hereditary hemochromatosis is now thought to be the most common genetic disorder in the white population (2). Approximately 1 in 250 persons is homozygous for this disorder and will develop the characteristic clinical manifestations such as diabetes, cardiomyopathy, liver disease, endocrine dysfunction, and, most notable for this discussion, arthropathy or other musculoskeletal disorders (2). Although hereditary iron overload disorders have traditionally been thought of as occurring exclusively in whites, recent research by Barton et al (3) indicates that approximately 1 in 67 African-Americans is affected by an etiologically distinct and severe form of iron overload. Hereditary iron overload disorders have been detected in persons of every ethnic background.

Arthropathy affects up to 80% of iron-overloaded patients and is often the only manifestation of this disease (4). Joint pain is a common and early symptom of iron overload, and "bone pain" has also been described as a common initial complaint (5). Clinically and radiographically, hemochromatoic arthropathy can resemble osteoarthritis, calcium pyrophosphate dihydrate deposition disease, pseudogout, rheumatoid arthritis, ankylosing spondylitis, or generalized osteopenia with osteoporotic fractures (4,6,7). Since iron overload can cause such a wide array of musculoskeletal manifestations and because definitive clinical differentiation of iron overload from other arthropathies is very difficult, patients with peripheral arthropathy should be screened for iron overload. Indeed, recent research by Olynyk et al (8) indicates that the prevalence of iron overload is 5 times higher in patients with peripheral arthropathy than in the general population. Therefore, screening of patients with peripheral arthropathy for the possible presence of iron overload is justified.

Thus, since iron overload affects such a large portion of the population and arthropathy is a common manifestation of this disorder, patients with musculoskeletal symptoms should be screened for iron overload (4,8). The current literature suggests that everyone should be screened for iron overload even if there are no symptoms (8–10).

Alex Vasquez, DC
Seattle, WA

1. American College of Rheumatology Ad Hoc Committee on Clinical Guidelines: Guidelines for the initial evaluation of the adult patient with acute musculoskeletal symptoms. Arthritis Rheum 39:1–8, 1996
2. Olynyk JK, Bacon BR: Hereditary hemochromatosis: detecting and correcting iron overload. Postgrad Med 96:151–165, 1994
3. Barton JC, Edwards CQ, Bertoli LF, Shroyer TW, Hudson SL: Iron overload in African Americans. Am J Med 99:616–623, 1995
4. Faraawi R, Harth M, Kertesz A, Bell D: Arthritis in hemochromatosis. J Rheumatol 20:448–452, 1993
5. Adams PC, Kertesz AE, Valberg LS: Clinical presentation of hemochromatosis: a changing scene. Am J Med 90:445–449, 1991
6. Bywaters EGL, Hamilton EBD, Williams R: The spine in idiopathic hemochromatosis. Ann Rheum Dis 30:453–465, 1971
7. Eyres KS, McCloskey EV, Fern ED, Rogers S, Beneton M, Aaron JE, Kanis JA: Osteoporotic fractures: an unusual presentation of hemochromatosis. Bone 13:431–433, 1992
8. Olynyk J, Hall P, Ahern M, Kwiatek R, Mackinnon M: Screening for hemochromatosis in a rheumatology clinic. Aust N Z J Med 24:22–25, 1994
9. Baer DM, Simmons JL, Staples RL, Runmore GJ, Morton CJ: Hemochromatosis screening in asymptomatic ambulatory men 30 years of age and older. Am J Med 98:464–468, 1995
10. Adams PC, Gregor JC, Kertesz AE, Valberg LS: Screening blood donors for hereditary hemochromatosis: decision analysis model based on a 30-year database. Gastroenterology 109:177–188, 1995

Vasquez A. Musculoskeletal disorders and iron overload disease: comment on the American College of Rheumatology guidelines for the initial evaluation of the adult patient with acute musculoskeletal symptoms. *Arthritis Rheum.* 1996 Oct;39(10):1767-8 ncbi.nlm.nih.gov/pubmed/8843875

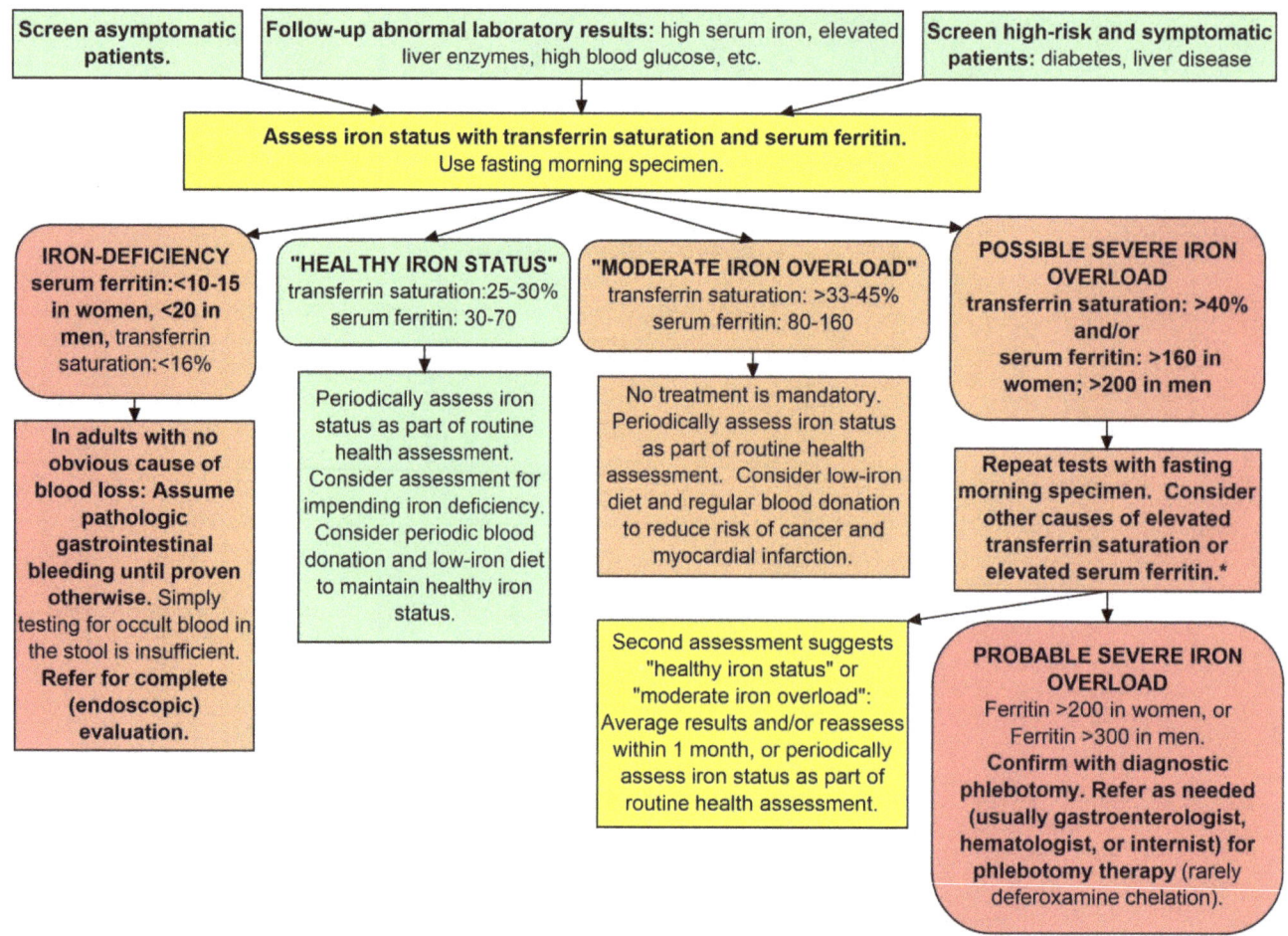

Algorithm for the comprehensive management of iron status: The above flow-chart delineates patient management per iron status.

Basic treatments for severe iron overload:
- **Iron-removal therapy is mandatory**: Phlebotomy therapy is generally performed weekly or twice-weekly; deferoxamine chelation is reserved for patients who do not withstand phlebotomy (due to cardiomyopathy, severe anemia, or hypoproteinemia) or may be used concurrently with phlebotomy in some patients. Periodically assess hematologic and iron indexes. Continue with weekly iron removal therapy until patient reaches mild iron-deficiency anemia, then decrease frequency and continue phlebotomy as needed (e.g., 4 times per year).
- **Laboratory tests and physical examination:** Assess general physical condition and hepatic, cardiac, endocrine, and general health status.
- **Confirm diagnosis:** Liver biopsy ("gold standard") or diagnostic phlebotomy; perhaps MRI.
- **Assess liver status:** Liver biopsy or perhaps MRI. Cirrhosis indicates increased risk of hepatocellular carcinoma and reduced life expectancy. Consider liver ultrasound, serum liver enzyme measurement, and serum alpha-fetoprotein to screen for hepatocellular carcinoma every 6 months. Hepatoma surveillance is mandatory in cirrhotic patients.
- **Implement dietary modifications and nutritional therapies:** Avoid iron supplements, multivitamin supplements with iron, iron-fortified foods, liver, beef, pork, alcohol, and excess vitamin C. Ensure adequate protein intake to replace protein lost during phlebotomy. Diet modifications are not substitutes for iron removal therapy. Consider antioxidant therapy.
- **Screen all blood relatives of patients with primary iron overload**. *Mandatory!*
- **Monitor patient condition, and compliance** with lifelong phlebotomy therapy
- **Assess and address psychoemotional issues/concerns**

25(OH)D: serum 25(OH) vitamin D	
Overview and interpretation:	- **Vitamin D deficiency is a common cause of musculoskeletal pain**[170,171,172], and vitamin D deficiency is a significant risk factor for cancer, autoimmunity, diabetes, mental illness, chronic pain and physical disability.[173,174,175]
- Measurement of serum 25(OH) vitamin D (or empiric treatment with 2,000 – 10,000 IU vitamin D3 per day for adults) is indicated in patients with chronic musculoskeletal pain, particularly low-back pain.[176] Optimal vitamin D status correlates with serum 25(OH)D levels of 50 – 100 ng/mL (125 - 250 nmol/L)—see our review article for more details[177]; levels greater than 100 ng/mL are unnecessary and increase the risk of hypercalcemia.

Excess vitamin D
> 100 ng/mL (250 nmol/L) with hypercalcemia

Optimal range
50 - 100 ng/mL (125 - 250 nmol/L)

Insufficiency range
< 20- 40 ng/mL (50 - 100 nmol/L)

Deficiency
< 20 ng/mL (50 nmol/L)

Interpretation of serum 25(OH) vitamin D levels. Modified from Vasquez et al, *Alternative Therapies in Health and Medicine* 2004 and Vasquez A. *Musculoskeletal Pain: Expanded Clinical Strategies* 2008. |
| Advantages: | - Accurate assessment of vitamin D status. |
| Limitations: | - Patients with certain granulomatous conditions such as sarcoidosis or Crohn's disease and patients taking certain drugs such as thiazide diuretics (hydrochlorothiazide) can develop hypercalcemia due to "vitamin D hypersensitivity" or drug side effects—these patients require frequent monitoring of serum calcium while taking vitamin D supplements. |
| Comments: | - **Routine measurement and/or empiric treatment with vitamin D3 needs to become a routine component of patient care.**[178]
- Periodic assessment of 25(OH)D and serum calcium are required to ensure effectiveness and safety of treatment, respectively.
- I'm increasingly convinced of the merit of measuring 1,25-dihydroxyvitamin D3, at least for the initial assessment of patients with inflammatory/autoimmune conditions. |

---

[170] Masood et al. Persistent limb pain, raised serum alkaline phosphatase earliest markers of subclinical hypovitaminosis D Kashmir. *Indian J Physiol Pharmacol*. 1989;33:259-61
[171] Al Faraj S, Al Mutairi K. Vitamin D deficiency and chronic low back pain in Saudi Arabia. *Spine*. 2003 Jan 15;28(2):177-9
[172] Plotnikoff GA, Quigley JM. Prevalence of severe hypovitaminosis D in patients with persistent, nonspecific musculoskeletal pain. *Mayo Clin Proc*. 2003 Dec;78(12):1463-70
[173] Grant WB. An estimate of premature cancer mortality in the U.S. due to inadequate doses of solar ultraviolet-B radiation. *Cancer* 2002;94(6):1867-75
[174] Zittermannn A. Vitamin D in preventive medicine: are we ignoring the evidence? *Br J Nutr*. 2003 May;89(5):552-72
[175] Holick MF. Vitamin D: importance in the prevention of cancers, type 1 diabetes, heart disease, and osteoporosis. *Am J Clin Nutr*. 2004;79(3):362-71
[176] Al Faraj S, Al Mutairi K. Vitamin D deficiency and chronic low back pain in Saudi Arabia. *Spine*. 2003 Jan 15;28(2):177-9
[177] Vasquez A, et al. Clinical Importance of Vitamin D (Cholecalciferol): A Paradigm Shift with Implications for All Healthcare Providers. *AlternTherap Heal Med* 2004;10:28-37
[178] Heaney RP. Vitamin D, nutritional deficiency, and the medical paradigm. *J Clin Endocrinol Metab*. 2003;88:5107-8 jcem.endojournals.org/cgi/content/full/88/11/5107

THE CLINICAL IMPORTANCE OF VITAMIN D (CHOLECALCIFEROL): A PARADIGM SHIFT WITH IMPLICATIONS FOR ALL HEALTHCARE PROVIDERS

Alex Vasquez, DC, ND, Gilbert Manso, MD, John Cannell, MD

Alex Vasquez, DC, ND is a licensed naturopathic physician in Washington and Oregon, and licensed chiropractic doctor in Texas, where he maintains a private practice and is a member of the Research Team at Biotics Research Corporation. He is a former Adjunct Professor of Orthopedics and Rheumatology for the Naturopathic Medicine Program at Bastyr University. **Gilbert Manso**, MD, is a medical doctor practicing integrative medicine in Houston, Texas. In practice for more than 35 years, he is Board Certified in Family Practice and is Associate Professor of Family Medicine at University of Texas Medical School in Houston. **John Cannell**, MD, is a medical physician practicing in Atascadero, California, and is president of the Vitamin D Council (Cholecalciferol-Council.com), a non-profit, tax-exempt organization working to promote awareness of the manifold adverse effects of vitamin D deficiency.

InnoVision Communications is accredited by the Accreditation Council for Continuing Medical Education to provide continuing medical education for physicians. The learner should study the article and its figures or tables, if any, then complete the self-evaluation at the end of the activity. The activity and self-evaluation are expected to take a maximum of 2 hours.

OBJECTIVES
Upon completion of this article, participants should be able to do the following:

1. Appreciate and identify the manifold clinical presentations and consequences of vitamin D deficiency
2. Identify patient groups that are predisposed to vitamin D hypersensitivity
3. Know how to implement vitamin D supplementation in proper doses and with appropriate laboratory monitoring

Reprint requests: InnoVision Communications, 169 Saxony Rd, Suite 501, Encinitas, CA 92024; phone, (760) 633-3910 or (866) 828-2962; fax, (760) 633-3918; e-mail, alternative.therapies@innerdoorway.com. Or visit our online CME Web site by going to http://www.alternative-therapies.com and selecting the Continuing Education option.

While we are all familiar with the important role of vitamin D in calcium absorption and bone metabolism, many doctors and patients are not aware of the recent research on vitamin D and the widening range of therapeutic applications available for cholecalciferol, which can be classified as both a vitamin and a pro-hormone. Additionally, we also now realize that the Food and Nutrition Board's previously defined Upper Limit (UL) for safe intake at 2,000 IU/day was set far too low and that the physiologic requirement for vitamin D in adults may be as high as 5,000 IU/day, which is less than half of the >10,000 IU that can be produced endogenously with full-body sun exposure.[1,2] With the discovery of vitamin D receptors in tissues other than the gut and bone—especially the brain, breast, prostate, and lymphocytes—and the recent research suggesting that higher vitamin D levels provide protection from diabetes mellitus, osteoporosis, osteoarthritis, hypertension, cardiovascular disease, metabolic syndrome, depression, several autoimmune diseases, and cancers of the breast, prostate, and colon, we can now utilize vitamin D for a wider range of preventive and therapeutic applications to maintain and improve our patients' health.[3] Based on the research reviewed in this article, the current authors believe that assessment of vitamin D status and treatment of vita-

---

Vasquez A et al. The clinical importance of vitamin D (cholecalciferol): a paradigm shift with implications for all healthcare providers. *Altern Ther Health Med* **2004 Sep-Oct**: This article indexed on Medline at ncbi.nlm.nih.gov/pubmed/15478784 and is archived by the author online ICHNFM.ORG/faculty/vasquez/profile.html

Overview of Clinical Approach, Assessments, and Therapeutics

Proof of the cause-and-effect relationship between vitamin D deficiency and chronic musculoskeletal pain comes from clinical trials among deficient patients showing that vitamin D monotherapy alleviates pain. The exemplary study by Al Faraj and Al Mutairi[35] showed that among patients with "idiopathic chronic low back pain," 83% (n = 299) were vitamin D deficient, and supplementation with 5000 to 10 000 IU/d of cholecalciferol for 3 months alleviated or cured the low back pain in more than 95% of patients. The authors concluded that, in the evaluation of chronic musculoskeletal pain among populations with a sufficiently high prevalence of vitamin D deficiency, "Screening for vitamin D deficiency and treatment with supplements should be mandatory in this setting."

Vitamin D has a wide range of safety according to an extensive review of the literature performed by Vieth.[228] Doses of 2000 IU/d of vitamin D3 have been given to children starting at 1 year of age and were not associated with toxicity but led to a reduction in the incidence of type 1 diabetes by 80%, consistent with the vitamin's anti-infective and immunomodulatory roles.[229] A 2004 review[36] on the clinical importance of vitamin D proposed that optimal vitamin D status is defined as 40 ng/mL to 65 ng/mL (100–160 nmol/L) and that "until proven otherwise, the balance of the research indicates that oral supplementation in the range of 1000 IU per day for infants, 2000 IU per day for children and 4000 IU per day for adults is safe and reasonable to meet physiological requirements, to promote optimal health, and to reduce the risk of several serious diseases. Safety and effectiveness of supplementation are assured by periodic monitoring of serum 25(OH)D and serum calcium." Current data and laboratory reference ranges support a higher top limit for serum 25(OH)D of approximately 100 ng/mL (250 nmol/L). Vitamin D hypersensitivity is seen with primary hyperparathyroidism, granulomatous diseases (such as sarcoidosis, Crohn's disease, and tuberculosis), adrenal insufficiency, hyperthyroidism, hypothyroidism, and various forms of cancer, as well as adverse drug effects, particularly with thiazide diuretics. Thiazide diuretics are known to potentiate hypercalcemia.

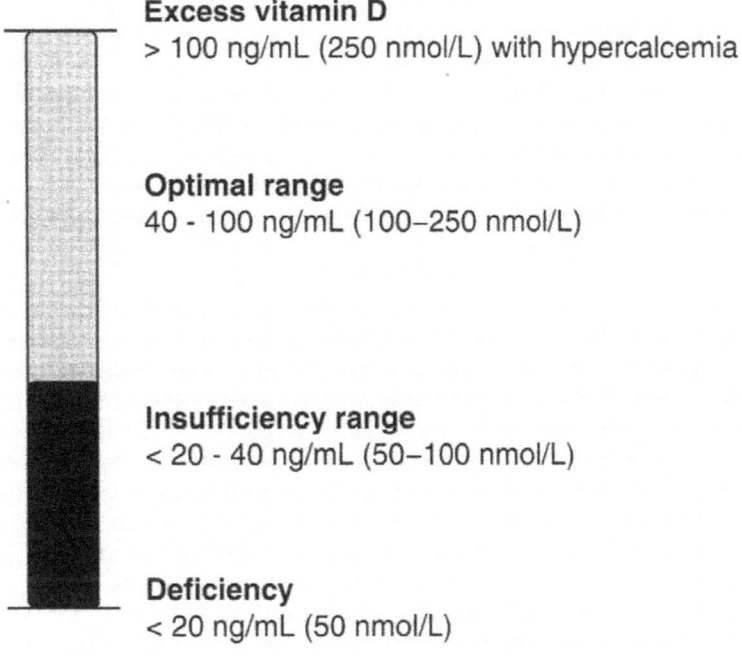

Figure 2.1—Interpretation of Serum 25(OH)D Levels
Adapted from Vasquez A, Manso G, Cannell J. *Altern Ther Health Med.* 2004;10:28-37.36

35

Vasquez A. *Musculoskeletal Pain: Expanded Clinical Strategies*. Institute for Functional Medicine, 2008: This peer-reviewed monograph on common pain syndromes was approved for continuing medical education (CME).

THE LANCET.com

May 6, 2005

Subphysiologic Doses of Vitamin D are Subtherapeutic: Comment on the Study by The Record Trial Group

Dear Editor,

Based on recently published research, it is clear that the study by The Record Trial Group [1] on vitamin D and calcium in the prevention of fractures suffered from at least four important shortcomings which negatively skewed their results.

First, and most important, the dose of vitamin D used in their study (800 IU/d) is subphysiologic and would therefore not be expected to produce a clinically meaningful effect. The physiologic requirement for vitamin D was determined scientifically in a recent study by Heaney and colleagues [2], who showed that healthy men utilize 3,000 to 5,000 IU of cholecalciferol per day, and several recent clinical trials have been published documenting the safety and effectiveness of administering vitamin D in physiologic doses of at least 4,000 IU per day.[3-5] In fact, studies have shown a dose-response relationship with vitamin D supplementation [6], and low doses (e.g., 600 IU) are clearly less effective than higher doses in the physiologic range (e.g., 4,000 IU).[5] It is important to note that the commonly used dose of vitamin D at 800 IU per day was not determined scientifically; rather this amount was determined arbitrarily before sufficient scientific methodology was available.[2,7] Given that the commonly recommended daily intake of vitamin D in the range of 200-800 IU is not sufficient for maintaining adequate serum levels of vitamin D [8], it is therefore incumbent upon modern researchers and clinicians to use doses of vitamin D that are consistent with the physiologic requirement as established in current research.

Second, the authors recognize that patient compliance in their study population was quite poor. This poor compliance obviously contributed to the purported lack of treatment efficacy.

Third, and consistent with recent data published elsewhere [8], virtually all of their patients were still vitamin D deficient at the end of one year of treatment, thereby affirming the inadequacy of the treatment dose. Vitamin D deficiency is common in industrialized nations, particularly those of northern latitudes [9-11], including the UK, where this study was performed. By modern criteria for serum vitamin D levels [12], virtually all of the patients in this study were vitamin D deficient at the beginning of the study, and the insufficient treatment dose of 800 IU/d failed to correct this deficiency even after 1 year of treatment. Given that vitamin D levels must be raised to approximately 40 ng/mL (100 nmol/L) in order to maximally reduce parathyroid hormone levels and bone resorption [13,14], supplementation that does not accomplish the goal of raising serum vitamin D levels into the optimal physiologic range cannot be considered adequate therapy.[12]

Fourth, and finally, there is reason to question the bioavailability of their vitamin D3 supplement, as the authors note that their dose-response was generally lower than that seen in other studies. Bioavailability is a prerequisite for treatment efficacy, and the elderly have higher likeliness of comorbid conditions that impair digestion and absorption of nutrients. Specifically, it is well documented that vitamin D absorption is decreased in elderly patients compared to younger controls [15,16], and this is complicated by an age-related reduction in renal calcitriol production [17,18] and intestinal vitamin D receptors [19], thereby further impairing vitamin D metabolism and calcium absorption. Since emulsification of fat soluble vitamins is required for their absorption [20], and since pre-emulsification of nutrients has been shown to increase absorption and dose-responsiveness of the fat-soluble nutrient coenzyme Q [21, 22], it seems apparent that attention to the form (not merely the dose) of nutrient supplementation is clinically important, particularly when working with elderly patients.

These shortcomings, when combined, could have led to an additive or synergistic reduction in treatment potency that skewed their results toward a conclusion of inefficacy. In order to produce more meaningful results in clinical trials, our group published guidelines [12] recommending that future studies 1) ensure patient compliance, 2) use physiologic doses of vitamin D (e.g., 4,000 IU per day), and 3) ensure that serum levels are raised to a minimum of 40 ng/mL (100 nmol/L), since levels below this threshold are associated with increased parathyroid hormone levels, increased bone resorption, and recalcitrance to bone-building interventions.[23,24]

Alex Vasquez
Biotics Research Corporation
Rosenberg, Texas, USA 77471

Competing Interests: Dr. Vasquez is a researcher at Biotics Research Corporation, an FDA-licensed drug manufacturing facility in the USA.

References:
1. Record Trial Group. Oral vitamin D3 and calcium for secondary prevention of low-trauma fractures in elderly people (Randomised Evaluation of Calcium Or vitamin D, RECORD): a randomised placebo-controlled trial. *Lancet* (Early Online Publication), 28 April 2005
2. Heaney RP, Davies KM, Chen TC, Holick MF, Barger-Lux MJ. Human serum 25-hydroxycholecalciferol response to extended oral dosing with cholecalciferol. *Am J Clin Nutr* 2003;77:204-10
3. Vieth R, Chan PC, MacFarlane GD. Efficacy and safety of vitamin D3 intake exceeding the lowest observed adverse effect level. *Am J Clin Nutr.* 2001;73:288-94
4. Al Faraj S, Al Mutairi K. Vitamin D deficiency and chronic low back pain in Saudi Arabia. *Spine.* 2003;28:177-9
5. Vieth R, Kimball S, Hu A, Walfish PG. Randomized comparison of the effects of the vitamin D3 adequate intake versus 100 mcg (4000 IU) per day on biochemical responses and the wellbeing of patients. *Nutr J.* 2004 Jul 19;3(1):8 nutritionj.com/content/pdf/1475-2891-3-8.pdf
6. Van den Berghe G, Van Roosbroeck D, Vanhove P, Wouters PJ, De Pourcq L, Bouillon R. Bone turnover in prolonged critical illness: effect of vitamin D. *J Clin Endocrinol Metab.* 2003;88:4623-32
7. Vieth R. Vitamin D supplementation, 25-hydroxyvitamin D concentrations, and safety. *Am J Clin Nutr.* 1999;69:842-56 ajcn.org/cgi/reprint/69/5/842.pdf
8. Glerup H, Mikkelsen K, Poulsen L, Hass E, Overbeck S, Thomsen J, Charles P, Eriksen EF. Commonly recommended daily intake of vitamin D is not sufficient if sunlight exposure is limited. *J Intern Med.* 2000;247:260-8
9. Thomas MK, Lloyd-Jones DM, Thadhani RI, Shaw AC, Deraska DJ, Kitch BT, Vamvakas EC, Dick IM, Prince RL, Finkelstein JS. Hypovitaminosis D in medical inpatients. *N Engl J Med* 1998;338:777-83
10. Dubbelman R, Jonxis JH, Muskiet FA, Saleh AE. Age-dependent vitamin D status and vertebral condition of white women living in Curacao (The Netherlands Antilles) as compared with their counterparts in The Netherlands. *Am J Clin Nutr* 1993;58:106-9
11. Kauppinen-Makelin R, Tahtela R, Loyttyniemi E, Karkkainen J, Valimaki MJ. A high prevalence of hypovitaminosis D in Finnish medical in- and outpatients. *J Intern Med.* 2001;249:559-63
12. Vasquez A, Manso G, Cannell J. The clinical importance of vitamin D (cholecalciferol): a paradigm shift with implications for all healthcare providers. *Altern Ther Health Med.* 2004;10:28-36; quiz 37, 94
13. Kinyamu HK, Gallagher JC, Rafferty KA, Balhorn KE. Dietary calcium and vitamin D intake in elderly women: effect on serum parathyroid hormone and vitamin D metabolites. *Am J Clin Nutr* 1998;67:342-8
14. Dawson-Hughes B, Harris SS, Dallal GE. Plasma calcidiol, season, and serum parathyroid hormone concentrations in healthy elderly men and women. *Am J Clin Nutr* 1997;65:67-71
15. Harris SS, Dawson-Hughes B, Perrone GA. Plasma 25-hydroxyvitamin D responses of younger and older men to three weeks of supplementation with 1800 IU/day of vitamin D. *J Am Coll Nutr.* 1999;18:470-4
16. Barragry JM, France MW, Corless D, Gupta SP, Switala S, Boucher BJ, Cohen RD. Intestinal cholecalciferol absorption in the elderly and in younger adults. *Clin Sci Mol Med.* 1978;55:213-20
17. Tsai KS, Heath H 3rd, Kumar R, Riggs BL. Impaired vitamin D metabolism with aging in women. Possible role in pathogenesis of senile osteoporosis. *J Clin Invest.* 1984;73:1668-72
18. Gallagher JC, Riggs BL, Eisman J, Hamstra A, Arnaud SB, DeLuca HF. Intestinal calcium absorption and serum vitamin D metabolites in normal subjects and osteoporotic patients: effect of age and dietary calcium. *J Clin Invest* 1979;64:729-36
19. Ebeling PR, Sandgren ME, DiMagno EP, Lane AW, DeLuca HF, Riggs BL. Evidence of an age-related decrease in intestinal responsiveness to vitamin D: relationship between serum 1,25-dihydroxyvitamin D3 and intestinal vitamin D receptor concentrations in normal women. *J Clin Endocrinol Metab.* 1992;75:176-82
20. Gallo-Torres HE. Obligatory role of bile for the intestinal absorption of vitamin E. *Lipids.* 1970;5:379-84
21. Bucci LR, Pillors M, Medlin R, Henderson R, Stiles JC, Robol HJ, Sparks WS. Enhanced uptake in humans of coenzyme Q10 from an emulsified form. *Third International Congress of Biomedical Gerontology*; Acapulco, Mexico: June 1989
22. Bucci LR, Pillors M, Medlin R, Klenda B, Robol H, Stiles JC, Sparks WS. Enhanced blood levels of coenzyme Q-10 from an emulsified oral form. In Faruqui SR and Ansari MS (editors). *Second Symposium on Nutrition and Chiropractic Proceedings.* April 15-16, 1989 in Davenport, Iowa
23. Stepan JJ, Burckhardt P, Hana V. The effects of three-month intravenous ibandronate on bone mineral density and bone remodeling in Klinefelter's syndrome: the influence of vitamin D deficiency and hormonal status. *Bone* 2003;33:589-596
24. Vasquez A. Health care for our bones: a practical nutritional approach to preventing osteoporosis. [letter] *J Manipulative Physiol Ther.* 2005;28:213

Citation: Vasquez A. Subphysiologic Doses of Vitamin D are Subtherapeutic: Comment on the Study by The Record Trial Group. *Lancet* 2005 published online May 6

Internet: Originally posted at thelancet.com/journals/lancet/article/PIIS0140673605630139/comments

Calcium and vitamin D in preventing fractures

Data are not sufficient to show inefficacy

EDITOR—The study by Porthouse et al had two major design flaws.[1] Firstly, the dose of vitamin D (800 IU per day) is subphysiological and therefore subtherapeutic. Secondly, their use of "self report" as a measure of compliance is unreliable.

The dose of vitamin D at 800 IU daily was not determined scientifically but determined arbitrarily before sufficient scientific methodology was available.[2-4] Heaney et al determined the physiological requirement of vitamin D by showing that healthy men use 4000 IU cholecalciferol daily,[2] an amount that is safely attainable with supplementation[3] and often exceeded with exposure of the total body to equatorial sun.[4]

We provided six guidelines for interventional studies with vitamin D.[5] Dosages of vitamin D must reflect physiological requirements and natural endogenous production and should therefore be in the range of 3000-10 000 IU daily. Vitamin D supplementation must be continued for at least five to nine months. The form of vitamin D should be D_3 rather than D_2. Supplements should be assayed for potency. Effectiveness of supplementation must include measurement of serum 25-hydroxyvitamin D. Serum 25(OH)D concentrations must enter the optimal range, which is 40-65 ng/ml (100-160 nmol/l).

Since the study by Porthouse et al met only the second and third of these six criteria, their data cannot be viewed as reliable for documenting the inefficacy of vitamin D supplementation.

Alex Vasquez, *researcher*

Biotics Research Corporation, 6801 Biotics Research Drive, Rosenberg, TX 77471, USA avasquez@bioticsresearch.com

John Cannell, *president*

Vitamin D Council, 9100 San Gregorio Road, Atascadero, CA 93422, USA

Competing interests: AV is a researcher at Biotics Research Corporation, a drug manufacturing facility in the United States that has approval from the Food and Drug Administration.

References

1. Porthouse J, Cockayne S, King C, Saxon L, Steele E, Aspray T, et al. Randomised controlled trial of calcium and supplementation with cholecalciferol (vitamin D3) for prevention of fractures in primary care. *BMJ* 2005;330: 1003. (30 April.)[Abstract/Free Full Text]
2. Heaney RP, Davies KM, Chen TC, Holick MF, Barger-Lux MJ. Human serum 25-hydroxycholecalciferol response to extended oral dosing with cholecalciferol. *Am J Clin Nutr* 2003;77: 204-10.[Abstract/Free Full Text]
3. Vieth R, Chan PC, MacFarlane GD. Efficacy and safety of vitamin D3 intake exceeding the lowest observed adverse effect level. *Am J Clin Nutr* 2001;73: 288-94.[Abstract/Free Full Text]
4. Vieth R. Vitamin D supplementation, 25-hydroxyvitamin D concentrations, and safety. *Am J Clin Nutr* 1999;69: 842-56.[Abstract/Free Full Text]
5. Vasquez A, Manso G, Cannell J. The clinical importance of vitamin D (cholecalciferol): a paradigm shift with implications for all healthcare providers. *Altern Ther Health Med* 2004;10: 28-36.[ISI][Medline]

Related Article

Randomised controlled trial of calcium and supplementation with cholecalciferol (vitamin D₃) for prevention of fractures in primary care
Jill Porthouse, Sarah Cockayne, Christine King, Lucy Saxon, Elizabeth Steele, Terry Aspray, Mike Baverstock, Yvonne Birks, Jo Dumville, Roger Francis, Cynthia Iglesias, Suezann Puffer, Anne Sutcliffe, Ian Watt, and David J Torgerson
BMJ 2005 330: 1003. [Abstract] [Full Text]

Vasquez A, Cannell J. Calcium and vitamin D in preventing fractures: Data are not sufficient to show inefficacy. *BMJ*. 2005 Jul 9;331:108-9 ncbi.nlm.nih.gov/pubmed/16002891 InflammationMastery/reprints

Thyroid status—laboratory assessments

Overview and interpretation:

- <u>Context</u>: Thyroid disorders are common in clinical practice and thus all clinicians need to have a clear understanding of the clinical presentations and laboratory assessments. Although various aspects of thyroid dysfunction, laboratory tests and clinical presentations will be reviewed here, the primary emphasis will be upon hypothyroidism, which is the most common and *unnecessarily* enigmatic of the thyroid disorders.

- <u>Controversy</u>: In the allopathic medical paradigm, much confusion exists regarding a common but "mysterious" and "enigmatic" condition known as hypothyroidism—low thyroid function. Its converse—**hyper**thyroidism and Graves disease—is well understood, easily diagnosed, and readily treated. Because the medical treatment for **hyper**thyroidism often leaves patients in a **hypo**thyroid state, affected patients thus transition from *clarity* (hyperthyroidism) wherein they feel ill due to the disease process into "*mystery*" (hypothyroidism) wherein they feel ill due to incomplete/inaccurate treatment. The basis for the confusion within the allopathic medical community about hypothyroidism is primarily two-fold: ❶ first, they rely on the wrong test (TSH) as the main basis for laboratory assessment, ❷ second, they use incomplete treatment (T4 without T3) which defies the known physiology of the thyroid gland, which makes at least two hormones rather than one. One might get the impression that perpetual confusion is at times the goal of the medical profession; we certainly see this with the management of hypertension, depression, diabetes mellitus, psoriasis and other inflammatory/autoimmune conditions. For people who seek clarity, it is available.

- <u>Basic physiology</u>: The hypothalamus produces thyrotropin-releasing hormone (TRH) which stimulates the anterior pituitary gland to make thyroid-stimulating hormone (TSH), which stimulates the thyroid gland to produce thyroxine (T4, approximately 85% of thyroid gland hormone production) and triiodothyronine (T3, approximately 15% of thyroid gland hormone production). In the periphery, the prohormone T4 is converted to active T3 by deiodinase enzymes. Stress, glucagon, and environmental toxins (halogenated phenolics, plastic monomers, flame retardants[179]) impair production of T3 and/or increase production of reverse T3, which is either inert or inhibitory to the action of T3. If the thyroid gland begins to fail, then TSH levels increase as the body attempts to stimulate production of thyroid hormones from a failing gland, which typically fails due to autoimmune attack (Hashimoto's thyroiditis); hence the association of elevated blood TSH levels with "primary hypothyroidism." Thyroid hormones have many different functions in the body, and one of the chief effects is contributing to maintenance of the basal metabolic rate, or the speed of reactions within and the temperature of the body. An insufficiency of thyroid hormone adversely effects numerous biochemical reactions and body/organ functions; hence the myriad of clinical presentations reflecting variations in biochemical and physiologic individuality. Conversely yet similarly, excess thyroid hormone (whether endogenously produced or exogenously administered) also affects numerous body systems.

- <u>Clinical presentation of *hyper*thyroidism</u>: The clinical pattern of thyroid excess is more narrowly-focused and thus more predictable and consistent than is the presentation of low thyroid function. The clinical manifestations of hyperthyroidism generally fall into three categories: hyper-adrenergic, hypermetabolic, and ophthalmologic/ocular. ❶ <u>hyper-adrenergic</u>: tachycardia, tremor, diaphoresis, insomnia and a feeling of nervousness and psychomotor agitation due to upregulation of adrenergic tone and generally some degree of relative or absolute hyperthermia; increased dopaminergic and noradrenergic tone in the brain accounts for the neuropsychiatric manifestations, such as mania, psychosis, and

---

[179] "All studied contaminants inhibited DI activity in a dose-response manner… This study suggests that some halogenated phenolics, including current use compounds such as plastic monomers, flame retardants and their metabolites, may disrupt thyroid hormone homeostasis through the inhibition of DI activity in vivo." Butt CM, Wang D, Stapleton HM. Halogenated Phenolic Contaminants Inhibit the In Vitro Activity of the Thyroid Regulating Deiodinases in Human Liver. *Toxicol Sci*. 2011 May 11. [Epub ahead of print]

Thyroid status—laboratory assessments

hypersexuality, ❷ hyper-metabolic: fecal frequency often described as "diarrhea" due to expedited intestinal transit, elevated temperature, and weight loss due to increased overall metabolic rate, ❸ ophthalmologic/ocular: in chronic cases particularly of the autoimmune variety, exophthalmos develops secondary to retro-orbital connective tissue proliferation and autoimmunity directed toward the extraocular muscles; the histologic abnormalities are chiefly characterized by increased accumulation of collagen (behind the eye and within the extraocular muscles, leading to muscle weakness), accumulation of glycosaminoglycans (GAGs), and the attendant edema.

- Clinical presentation of *hypo*thyroidism: In his classic book *Biochemical Individuality*, Williams[180] noted that "a wide variation in thyroid activity exists among 'normal' human beings." Clearly, some patients do not make enough thyroid hormone to function optimally[181]; or, perhaps more precisely, they make enough thyroid hormone (T4) but do not efficiently convert it to the active form (T3) in the periphery. Further complicating the picture is that some patients make appropriate amounts of TSH, T4, and T3 but they make excess of inactive reverse T3 (rT3) which puts them into a physiologic state of hypothyroidism despite adequate glandular function. Patients may have one or more of the following: fatigue, depression, **cold hands and feet** (excluding Raynaud's syndrome, peripheral vascular disease), dry skin, menstrual irregularities, infertility, premenstrual syndrome (PMS), uterine fibroids, excess menstrual bleeding, **low basal body temperature**, weak fingernails, sleep apnea and increased need for sleep (hypersomnia), slow heart rate (relative or absolute **bradycardia**), easy weight gain and difficult weight loss (thus, predisposition to overweight and obesity), hypercholesterolemia, slow healing, decreased memory and concentration, frog-like husky voice, low libido, recurrent infections, hypertension especially diastolic hypertension, poor digestion (due to insufficient gastric production of hydrochloric acid), **delayed Achilles return** (due to delayed muscle relaxation), carotenodermia, vitamin A deficiency, and gastroesophageal acid reflux, constipation, and predisposition to small intestine bacterial overgrowth (SIBO) due to slow intestinal transit. Of these manifestations, cold hands and feet, low basal body temperature, bradycardia, and delayed Achilles return are the most specific; some very competent physicians will—following proper patient evaluation—treat with thyroid hormone based on the clinical presentation of the patient and *with proper consideration of* and *without dependency upon* laboratory findings.
- Overview of thyroid tests:
  - Thyrotropin-releasing hormone (TRH): The hypothalamus releases TRH to stimulate pituitary production of TSH. TRH is not routinely tested in clinical practice, although abnormalities of TRH secretion are noted in patients with mental "depression."
  - Thyroid-stimulating hormone (TSH: 0.4 - 5.0 mIU/L [milli-international units per liter]): TSH is the most commonly performed test for evaluating thyroid status; its frequent (over)use owes more to habit and inexpensiveness than to aspirations for clinical excellence. TSH values greater than 2 mIU/L represent a disturbance of the thyroid-pituitary axis and an increased risk for future thyroid problems[182], and the American Association of Clinical Endocrinologists states, "The target TSH level should be between 0.3 and 3.0 μIU/mL."[183] Clinical rationale is available to support implementation of a therapeutic trial of thyroid hormone treatment in patients who are clinically hypothyroid even if they are biochemically euthyroid (per TSH) provided that treatment is implemented cautiously, in appropriately selected

---

[180] Williams RJ. *Biochemical Individuality: The Basis for the Genetotrophic Concept*. Austin and London: University of Texas Press, 1956 page 82
[181] Broda Barnes MD, Lawrence Galton, *Hypothyroidism: The Unsuspected Illness*. Ty Crowell Co; 1976
[182] Weetman AP. Fortnightly review: Hypothyroidism: screening and subclinical disease. *BMJ: British Medical Journal* 1997;314: 1175
[183] American Association of Clinical Endocrinologists. "The target TSH level should be between 0.3 and 3.0 μIU/mL." AACE Medical Guidelines for Clinical Practice for Evaluation and Treatment of Hyperthyroidism and Hypothyroidism. 2002, 2006 Amended Version. aace.com/sites/default/files/hypo_hyper.pdf Accessed Aug 2011

Thyroid status — laboratory assessments

patients, and patients are appropriately informed.[184,185] If the clinical world were as perfect as it is portrayed in basic physiology textbooks, then a clinician might fancifully rely on TSH to perform the diagnosis *prima facie*, with reduced TSH values correlating with glandular overperformance and negative feedback suppressing TSH secretion, whilst an underperforming gland would require greater stimulation with elevated TSH levels; however, TSH has never been thus vested with infallible reliability, which explains in part why doctors need brains of their own and why better clinicians have developed the capacity for independent thought.

- Free thyroxine (free T4: 4.5 - 11.2 mcg/dL): Unbound T4 is tested to provide evidence of glandular production of thyroid hormone(s). Because T4 is the major thyroid hormone produced by the thyroid gland it serves as an excellent marker for glandular productivity but it reveals nothing about peripheral conversion of T4 to the active thyroid hormone triiodothyronine (T3); in the practice of medicine, conversion of T4 to the active T3 is assumed to reliably occur unabated despite evidence to the contrary, especially among symptomatic patients.

- Triiodothyronine (T3: 100 - 200 ng/dL[186]): In textbook-perfect physiology, T4 is converted by deiodinase enzymes type-1 and type-2 to the active thyroid hormone T3; in reality, this is only part of the story. Because T3 is the active form of the hormone responsible for the physiologic functions of thyroid physiology, a clinician desiring to assess a patient's thyroid status might reasonably ask the proper question by performing the proper test. T3 is tested as "total T3" or "free T3" in large part based on the clinician's preference; the current author prefers total T3 because it can be compared to the total level of reverse T3 (rT3) in a ratio, the optimal range of which is generally considered to be 10-14 as originally presented by McDaniel[187] and reviewed in the following pages. Patients with psychiatric depression have lower levels of T3 than do healthy controls and have been described as having "low T3 syndrome"[188]; very obviously — whether cause or effect — the low T3 levels in these patients would serve to promote and perpetuate their state of mental depression. Although the focus of this review within the subject of laboratory evaluation is not to describe the implementation of thyroid hormone treatment, clinicians should be aware that T3 administration increases hepatic production of sex hormone binding globulin (SHBG) and that therefore T3 administration can reduce cellular bioavailability of protein-bound hormones. Many authoritative and clinically-experienced sources recommend using a time-released (e.g., sustained-release) form of T3 due to its shorter half-life compared with T4. However, obtaining time-released T3 via a compounding pharmacy can be cumbersome and expensive for the patient; clearly some patients respond to once daily dosing of *non*-time-released preparations with good effects and without adverse effects. Some patients can divide the immediate-release dose into two servings per day for enhanced effect and lessened physiologic fluctuations, if necessary. Per Drugs.com[189] in August 2011, "Since liothyronine sodium (T3) is not firmly bound to serum protein, it is readily available to body tissues. The onset of activity of liothyronine sodium is rapid, occurring within a few hours. Maximum pharmacologic response occurs within 2 or 3 days, providing early clinical response. The biological half-life is about 2.5 days." Very

---

[184] Skinner GR, et al. Thyroxine should be tried in clinically hypothyroid but biochemically euthyroid patients. *BMJ: British Medical Journal* 1997 Jun 14; 314(7096): 1764
[185] McLaren EH, Kelly CJ, Pollack MA. Trial of thyroxine treatment for biochemically euthyroid patients has been approved. *BMJ* 1997; 315: 1463
[186] U.S. National Library of Medicine (NLM) and National Institutes of Health (NIH) nlm.nih.gov/medlineplus/ency/article/003687.htm Accessed August 2011
[187] McDaniel AB. Thyroid Assessment: Controversies and Conundrums. Institute for Functional Medicine 14th International Symposium. Tucson, Arizona. May 23-26, 2007
[188] "Out of 250 subjects with major psychiatric depression, 6.4% exhibited low T3 syndrome (mean serum T3 concentration 0.94 nmol/l vs normal mean serum concentration of 1.77 nmol/l)." Premachandra BN, Kabir MA, Williams IK. Low T3 syndrome in psychiatric depression. *J Endocrinol Invest*. 2006 Jun;29(6):568-72
[189] drugs.com/pro/cytomel.html Accessed August 2011.

Thyroid status—laboratory assessments

clearly, a significant portion of hypothyroid patients respond to T3 alone (either time-released, divided-dosing, or once-daily dosing) or a combination of T4 and T3 when other treatments have failed.[190,191]

- Reverse triiodothyronine (rT3: 90 - 320 pg/mL[192]): T4 is converted by deiodinase enzymes type-1 and type-3 to the inactive thyroid hormone rT3; per a standard endocrinology textbook, "Approximately 70–80% of released T4 is converted by deiodinases to the biologically active T3, the remainder to reverse-T3 (rT3) which has no significant biological activity."[193] Clinicians must know that, "The prohormone T4 must be converted to T3 in the body before it can exert biological effects. **During periods of illness or stress, this conversion is often inhibited and can be diverted to the inactive reverse T3 (rT3) moiety.**"[194] Furthermore and very importantly, clinicians should appreciate that rT3 is not simply inactive but that it may actually impair production/utilization of normal T3; "T4-T3 and T4-rT3 conversion are provoked by different enzymes. The **elevation of rT3 might be a cause of the observed decrease in peripheral T3 generation** in old [elderly] subjects, acting via **inhibition of the T4-T3 conversion**."[195] During times of psychologic/physiologic stress and specific types of pharmacologic stress (e.g., propanolol[196] and corticosteroids), T4 metabolism is preferentially shunted away from T3 toward rT3; an anthropocentric explanation holds that by making less of the active T3 and more of the inactive rT3, the body is better able to conserve energy during times of stress by reducing overall metabolic rate, particularly resting energy expenditure and protein utilization. For example, caloric restriction and fasting result in a decrease in resting metabolic rate (RMR), and the reduced RMR persists for months after the fasting has ended and a normal diet is resumed.[197] This author (AV) terms this stress-induced impairment of thyroid hormone conversion "**metabolic hypothyroidism**" or "**functional hypothyroidism**" because the defect is in the metabolism (not the production) of thyroid hormone into its most active form; "**peripheral hypothyroidism**" might also be used to distinguish the fact that the defect is in the peripheral metabolism rather than located more centrally, within the thyroid gland itself. Because psychologic stress and certain pharmacologic exposures—as well as the thyro-metabolic stress of fasting and caloric restriction in which the counterregulatory hormone glucagon appears to trigger enhanced rT3 production—reduce T3 while simultaneously increasing rT3 levels, clinicians can appreciate that calculation of the T3/rT3 ratio will be more significantly altered (and thus a more sensitive indicator of metabolic disruption) than will be the isolated measurements of T3 or rT3 alone. Functional medicine clinicians[198] note the importance of the ratio of total T3 to reverse T3 (tT3:rT3 ratio) and consider the optimal range to be 10-14 with lower ratios indicating impaired formation or T3 and/or excess production of rT3.[199] Contrary to the previous view which held that rT3 was simply inactive, we now appreciate that rT3 actually impairs normal thyroid hormone metabolism thus functioning as an thyrometabolic monkeywrench or "brake" on normal metabolism.

---

[190] Bunevicius R, et al. Effects of thyroxine as compared with thyroxine plus triiodothyronine in patients with hypothyroidism. *N Engl J Med.* 1999 Feb 11;340(6):424-9
[191] Kelly T, Lieberman DZ. The use of triiodothyronine as an augmentation agent in treatment-resistant bipolar II and bipolar disorder NOS. *J Affect Disord.* 2009;116(3):222-6
[192] The reference range provided here for rT3 is a compilation from the laboratory reference ranges from the sample reports on the following pages, each of which is performed by either Quest Diagnostics or LabCorp, the two largest medical laboratories in the United States.
[193] Nussey S, Whitehead S. *Endocrinology: An Integrated Approach*. Oxford: BIOS Scientific Publishers, 2001. See also Box 3.29 Metabolism of thyroid hormones. ncbi.nlm.nih.gov/books/NBK28/box/A270/?report=objectonly Accessed July 2011
[194] *1998 Mosby's GenRX. Sixth Edition*. St. Louis Missouri; Mosby-Year Book, 1998
[195] Szabolcs I, Weber M, Kovács Z, et al. The possible reason for serum 3,3'5'-(reverse) triiodothyronine increase in old people. *Acta Med Acad Sci Hung.* 1982;39(1-2):11-7
[196] "Propranolol administration (40 mg t.i.d. for a week) caused a similar rT3 elevation in old persons (n = 18) as in 12 young ones." Szabolcs I, Weber M, Kovács Z, Irsy G, Góth M, Halász T, Szilágyi G. The possible reason for serum 3,3'5'-(reverse) triiodothyronine increase in old people. *Acta Med Acad Sci Hung.* 1982;39(1-2):11-7
[197] Elliot DL, Goldberg L, Kuehl KS, Bennett WM. Sustained depression of the resting metabolic rate after massive weight loss. *Am J Clin Nutr* 1989 Jan;49(1):93-96
[198] The conclusion of this paragraph is derived from Vasquez A. *Musculoskeletal Pain: Expanded Clinical Strategies*. Institute for Functional Medicine, 2008
[199] McDaniel AB. Thyroid Assessment: Controversies and Conundrums. Institute for Functional Medicine 14th International Symposium. Tucson, Arizona. May 23-26, 2007

Thyroid status—laboratory assessments	
	Elevated rT3 levels predict mortality among critically ill patients.[200] Aberrancies in thyroid hormone levels may reflect organic disease, psychoemotional stress, or nutritional deficiency[201], and therefore such serologic abnormalities warrant consideration of underlying problems and direct treatment when possible. If no underlying cause is apparent, then a trial of thyroid hormone/hormones is reasonable in appropriately selected patients. Beyond stress reduction, allergen/gluten avoidance, and nutritional supplementation with iodine, selenium, and zinc (as indicated per patient), correction of overt, subclinical, and functional hypothyroidism generally centers on the administration of natural or synthetic thyroid hormones in the form of T4 and T3. Correction of functional hypothyroidism (relatively reduced total T3 and increased rT3) is accomplished with either time-released or twice-daily dosing of T3 *without* T4 to suppress endogenous T4 conversion to T3, thereby allowing rT3 levels to fall precipitously. T3 administration allows temporary downregulation of transforming enzymes so that rT3 production is reduced following withdrawal of T3 replacement; thus, short-term and/or periodic T3 administration helps normalize or "reset" peripheral thyroid metabolism so that, following withdrawal of T3 administration, T4 can be converted to T3 without excess production of rT3. The safety and effectiveness of this approach—using T3 administration (often twice daily or in a sustained-release compounded tablet or capsule) to recalibrate peripheral thyroid hormone metabolism—has documented safety and effectiveness.[202] Alleviation of symptoms, restoration of morning body temperature to 98.6° F (oral or axillary) and other clinical objective improvements achieved by the judicious and safe administration of T3 are the criteria of success; physiologic improvement following T3 administration retrospectively confirms the diagnosis. ○ <u>Antithyroid antibodies—antithyroglobulin (anti-TG) and anti-thyroid peroxidase (anti-TPO)</u>: Autoimmune thyroiditis (also called Hashimoto's disease or chronic lymphocytic thyroiditis) or is the most common cause of overt primary hypothyroidism. The diagnosis of autoimmune thyroiditis can be made clinically (i.e., without biopsy) upon detection of elevated blood levels of antibodies against thyroglobulin (anti-thyroglobulin antibodies) and anti-thyroid peroxidase (anti-TPO) antibodies. Autoimmune thyroiditis may present asymptomatically and with normal thyroid hormone levels; classically, patients may have a slightly hyperthyroid presentation as the inflamed gland releases extra thyroid hormone before becoming atrophic and hypofunctional.
Advantages:	▪ Thyroid disorders are quite common in general practice and are often undiagnosed, undertreated, or inappropriately treated. ▪ Consistent with the principle of beneficence, patients and doctors benefit when thyroid disorders are diagnosed and treated appropriately.
Limitations:	▪ A properly interpreted TSH may overlook problems of T4 production or conversion to active T3. Additionally, in some patients, all of these tests are normal but they may have thyroid autoimmunity (i.e., thyroid peroxidase antibodies, anti-TPO) and should receive

---

[200] Peeters RP, Wouters PJ, van Toor H, Kaptein E, Visser TJ, Van den Berghe G. Serum 3,3',5'-triiodothyronine (rT3) and 3,5,3'-triiodothyronine/rT3 are prognostic markers in critically ill patients and are associated with postmortem tissue deiodinase activities. *J Clin Endocrinol Metab.* 2005 Aug;90(8):4559-65
[201] Kelly GS. Peripheral metabolism of thyroid hormones: a review. *Altern Med Rev.* 2000 Aug;5(4):306-33
[202] Friedman M, et al. Supraphysiological cyclic dosing of sustained release T3 in order to reset low basal body temperature. *P R Health Sci J.* 2006 Mar;25(1):23-9

Thyroid status—laboratory assessments	
	treatment with thyroid hormone[203] or some other corrective treatment (e.g., selenium supplementation[204,205] and a gluten-free diet[206]) to normalize thyroid status.
Comments:	- Comprehensive thyroid laboratory testing includes ❶ history, ❷ TSH, ❸ free T4, ❹ total T3, ❺ rT3, ❻ antithyroid antibodies, should be evaluated alongside the ❼ heart rate, ❽ cold extremities and basal body temperature, ❾ Achilles' return speed, and ❿ response to treatment.
- The combination of T3 and T4 (as in the prescription Liotrix/Thyrolar or Armour thyroid) appears to have similar safety to T4 alone (Levothyroxine, Synthroid) and may result in greater improvements in mood and neuropsychological function.[207]
- Glandular thyroid supplements and Armour thyroid generally should *not* be used in patients with thyroid autoimmunity (Hashimoto's thyroiditis) because the bovine/porcine antigens will exacerbate the anti-thyroid immune response as evidenced by increased anti-TPO antibodies.

Optimal thyroid status

<u>Concept by Dr Vasquez</u>: Optimal thyroid status is not defined by basic laboratory testing with TSH and free T4. It is defined *per patient* based on the levels and ratios of all major thyroid-related hormones and antibodies—in association with other hormonal, psychologic, dysbiotic, nutritional and environmental factors— that work best for that particular unique biochemically-individual patient. If a patient may benefit from a therapeutic trial of thyroid hormone (a substance produced naturally within the human body) and if no contraindications such as mania or cardiovascular disease are present, then a therapeutic trial of thyroid hormone is indeed quite likely reasonable and is arguably much more reasonable than the administration of foreign substances that do not correct or support normal physiologic functions.

<u>Laboratory interpretation by Dr McDaniel</u>: "Optimal hormone balance is debatable. My observations: A few "well" people and patients treated successfully with T4 and T3 seem best with:
- TSH around 0.7–0.9µIU/mL
- fT4 around 0.7–0.8ng/dL
- fT3 optimally 3.4–3.8pg/mL
- **Total T3-RT3 ratio 12 +/-2**"

McDaniel AB. Thyroid Assessment: Controversies and Conundrums. Institute for Functional Medicine Fourteenth International Symposium. Tucson, Arizona. May 23-26, 2007

---

[203] Beers MH, Berkow R (eds). *The Merck Manual. 17th Edition*. Whitehouse Station; Merck Research Laboratories 1999 page 96
[204] Duntas LH, Mantzou E, Koutras DA. Effects of a six month treatment with selenomethionine in patients with autoimmune thyroiditis. *Eur J Endocrinol*. 2003 Apr;148(4):389-93 eje-online.org/cgi/reprint/148/4/389
[205] Gartner R, Gasnier BC. Selenium in the treatment of autoimmune thyroiditis. *Biofactors*. 2003;19(3-4):165-70
[206] Sategna-Guidetti C, Volta U, Ciacci C, Usai P, Carlino A, De Franceschi L, Camera A, Pelli A, Brossa C. Prevalence of thyroid disorders in untreated adult celiac disease patients and effect of gluten withdrawal: an Italian multicenter study. *Am J Gastroenterol*. 2001 Mar;96(3):751-7
[207] "CONCLUSIONS: In patients with hypothyroidism, partial substitution of triiodothyronine for thyroxine may improve mood and neuropsychological function; this finding suggests a specific effect of the triiodothyronine normally secreted by the thyroid gland." Bunevicius R, Kazanavicius G, Zalinkevicius R, Prange AJ Jr. Effects of thyroxine as compared with thyroxine plus triiodothyronine in patients with hypothyroidism. *N Engl J Med*. 1999 Feb 11;340(6):424-9

Chapter 1: Clinical Assessments and Concepts

Clinical Case 31yo female with fatigue, a recent history of extreme emotional stress, maternal history of Hashimotos thyroiditis—testing performed in 2010 by Quest Diagnostics: Outline plan before reading discussion.

Test Name	In Range	Out of Range	Reference Range
THYROGLOBULIN ANTIBODIES	<20		<20 IU/mL
THYROID PEROXIDASE ANTIBODIES		38 H	<35 IU/mL
T3, TOTAL	89		76-181 ng/dL
T3 UPTAKE		37 H	22-35 %
T4, FREE	1.6		0.8-1.8 ng/dL
T4 (THYROXINE), TOTAL T4 (THYROXINE), TOTAL	10.9		4.5-12.5 mcg/dL
FREE T4 INDEX (T7)		4.0 H	1.4-3.8
TSH, 3RD GENERATION	0.82		mIU/L

Reference Range

> or = 20 Years   0.40-4.50

Pregnancy Ranges
First trimester   0.20-4.70
Second trimester   0.30-4.10
Third trimester   0.40-2.70

| T3, FREE | 318 | | 230-420 pg/dL |
| **T3, REVERSE** | | 43 H | 11-32 ng/dL |

This test was performed using a kit that has not been approved or cleared by the FDA. The analytical performance characteristics of this test have been determined by Quest Diagnostics Nichols Institute, San Juan Capistrano. This test should not be used for diagnosis without confirmation by other medically established means.

Discussion: Note that the TSH is completely normal and thus would give the impression of normalcy and "health" if the clinician had not ordered the additional tests. Thyroid peroxidase antibodies are minimally elevated; this is consistent with thyroid autoimmunity but titers this low are of limited clinical importance. Note that the rT3 level is abnormally elevated. Note that because the units provided for total T3 (89 ng/dL) and rT3 (43 ng/dL) are identical, no unit conversion is required, thereby making the calculation of the ideal ratio (range: 10-14) very simple. In this patient's case, the ratio comes to 2.06 which is obviously significantly lower than the proposed optimal of 10-14; the patient responded well to liothyronine/Cytomel supplementation with 15 mcg/d. Patients with thyroid autoimmunity often benefit from a gluten-free diet[208] and supplementation with selenium 200 mcg/d.[209] Finally, note that the reference range for total T3 provided by this laboratory is 76-181 ng/dL which contrasts significantly from the range recommended by the US National Institutes of Health (NIH) 100 to 200 ng/dL[210]; using the NIH's reference range, this patient's T3 production is inadequate.

---

[208] "Hypothyroidism, diagnosed in 31 patients (12.9%) and nine controls (4.2%), was subclinical in 29 patients and of nonautoimmune origin in 21. ... In most patients who strictly followed a 1-yr gluten withdrawal (as confirmed by intestinal mucosa recovery), there was a normalization of subclinical hypothyroidism. The greater frequency of thyroid disease among celiac disease patients justifies a thyroid functional assessment. In distinct cases, gluten withdrawal may single-handedly reverse the abnormality." Sategna-Guidetti et al. Prevalence of thyroid disorders in untreated adult celiac disease patients and effect of gluten withdrawal: an Italian multicenter study. *Am J Gastroenterol*. 2001 Mar;96(3):751-7
[209] "Patients with HT assigned to Se supplementation for 3 months demonstrated significantly lower thyroid peroxidase autoantibodies (TPOab) titers (four studies, random effects weighted mean difference: −271.09, 95% confidence interval: −421.98 to −120.19, p< 10⁻⁴) and a significantly higher chance of reporting an improvement in well-being and/or mood (three studies, random effects risk ratio: 2.79, 95% confidence interval: 1.21-6.47, p= 0.016) when compared with controls. ... On the basis of the best available evidence, Se supplementation is associated with a significant decrease in TPOab titers at 3 months and with improvement in mood and/or general well-being."Toulis et al. Selenium supplementation in the treatment of Hashimoto's thyroiditis: a systematic review and a meta-analysis. *Thyroid*. 2010 Oct;20(10):1163-73
[210] U.S. National Library of Medicine and NIH nlm.nih.gov/medlineplus/ency/article/003687.htm Accessed Aug 2011

Toxic metal testing—emphasis on lead and mercury	
Overview and application:	- <u>Introduction</u>: Per the US Department of Labor's Occupational Safety and Health Administration (OSHA)[211], toxic metals, including "heavy metals", are individual metals and metal compounds that negatively affect people's health. While lists of toxic metals can vary per source, OSHA names the following: arsenic, beryllium, cadmium, hexavalent chromium, lead, and mercury; of these, lead and mercury are the most commonly observed problematic toxic metals in outpatient practice. The three most important clinical concepts with regard to testing for "heavy metals" or "toxic metals" are as follows: 1. <u>Heavy metal toxicity/accumulation is not uncommon in clinical practice</u>: Toxic/heavy metal accumulation is clinically important due both to its frequency and its pathophysiologic consequences. An article published in *Journal of the American Medical Association (JAMA)*[212] showed that approximately 8% of [1,709 American] women had [blood mercury] concentrations higher than the US Environmental Protection Agency's recommended reference dose (5.8 µg/L), below which exposures are considered to be without adverse effects; stated more plainly, 8% of American women have (potentially) toxic levels of mercury *even when evaluated by the least sensitive of laboratory methods—blood mercury*, which represents only 5% of total body mercury. Another study, also published in *JAMA*[213], showed a positive relationship between blood lead levels and hypertension, even at blood lead levels considered within the normal range; the authors wrote, "At levels well below the current US occupational exposure limit guidelines (40 µg/dL), blood lead level is positively associated with both systolic and diastolic blood pressure and risks of both systolic and diastolic hypertension among women aged 40 to 59 years." 2. <u>The clinical presentation of heavy metal toxicity/accumulation is generally diverse and nonspecific</u>: Clinical presentations due to or associated with toxic metal accumulation can include dyscognition, fatigue, anemia, chronic pain from myalgia or neuropathy, hypertension, autism, and immune disorders including autoimmunity and allergy. In particular, autism[214,215,216] and hypertension[217,218] are noteworthy for their consistent associations with mercury and with mercury and lead, respectively. 3. <u>Therefore, clinicians should test for and treat toxic metal accumulation</u>: When problems are clinically significant and not extremely unlikely, clinicians have an obligation to test for and treat such problems for the benefit of the patient. Therefore, because toxic metal accumulation is common, clinically significant, and because it is a reversible cause of numerous symptoms, syndromes, and a contributing factor in the development/perpetuation of many other diagnosable conditions commonly labeled as "idiopathic" (e.g., hypertension, immune disorders, mood disorders), clinicians have an obligation to consider and test for toxic metals among their patients. - <u>Additional details—mercury</u>: Mercury is an established neurotoxin, immunotoxin, and nephrotoxin. Because pathophysiologic effects are noted even with very small doses of exposure, one could reasonably argue that no safe amount exists and therefore that any

---

[211] osha.gov/SLTC/metalsheavy/index.html Accessed July 2011.
[212] Schober et al. Blood mercury levels in US children and women of childbearing age, 1999-2000. *JAMA* 2003;289:1667-74 jama.ama-assn.org/content/289/13/1667.long
[213] Nash D, Magder L, Lustberg M, Sherwin RW, Rubin RJ, Kaufmann RB, Silbergeld EK. Blood lead, blood pressure, and hypertension in perimenopausal and postmenopausal women. *JAMA*. 2003 Mar 26;289(12):1523-32. See also Muntner P, He J, Vupputuri S, Coresh J, Batuman V. Blood lead and chronic kidney disease in the general United States population: results from NHANES III. *Kidney Int*. 2003 Mar;63(3):1044-50 nature.com/ki/journal/v63/n3/pdf/4493526a.pdf
[214] Stamova B, Green PG, Tian Y, Hertz-Picciotto I, Pessah IN, Hansen R, Yang X, Teng J, Gregg JP, Ashwood P, Van de Water J, Sharp FR. Correlations between gene expression and mercury levels in blood of boys with and without autism. *Neurotox Res*. 2011;19:31-48. Epub 2009 Nov 24.
[215] "The results of the study indicated that the participants' overall ATEC scores and their scores on each of the ATEC subscales (Speech/Language, Sociability, Sensory/Cognitive Awareness, and Health/Physical/Behavior) were linearly related to urinary porphyrins associated with mercury toxicity. The results show an association between the apparent level of mercury toxicity as measured by recognized urinary porphyrin biomarkers of mercury toxicity and the magnitude of the specific hallmark features of autism as assessed by ATEC." Kern JK, Geier DA, Adams JB, Geier MR. A biomarker of mercury body-burden correlated with diagnostic domain specific clinical symptoms of autism spectrum disorder. *Biometals*. 2010 Dec;23(6):1043-51
[216] Kempuraj D, Asadi S, Zhang B, Manola A, Hogan J, Peterson E, Theoharides TC. Mercury induces inflammatory mediator release from human mast cells. *J Neuroinflammation*. 2010 Mar 11;7:20 jneuroinflammation.com/content/7/1/20
[217] Schober et al. Blood mercury levels in US children and women of childbearing age, 1999-2000. *JAMA* 2003;289:1667-74 jama.ama-assn.org/content/289/13/1667.long
[218] Nash D, et al. Blood lead, blood pressure, and hypertension in perimenopausal and postmenopausal women. *JAMA*. 2003 Mar 26;289(12):1523-32

Toxic metal testing—emphasis on lead and mercury

detected mercury is an indication for therapeutic intervention to remove this toxicant. According to an article by Schober et al[219] published in *JAMA—Journal of the American Medical Association* in 2003, "Approximately 8% of [1,709 American] women had [blood mercury] concentrations higher than the US Environmental Protection Agency's recommended reference dose (5.8 μg/L), below which exposures are considered to be without adverse effects." Sources of exposure include dental amalgams, vaccinations, airborne pollution, deep-water fish such as tuna, some cosmetics[220], and selected herbicides, fungicides, and germicides; recently, high-fructose corn syrup was shown to contain mercury in clinically meaningful amounts.[221] Mercury impairs catecholamine degradation and can thereby cause a clinical syndrome that can include hypertension, tremor, tachycardia, diaphoresis, and neurocognitive changes.[222] Per Shih and Gartner[223], "Mercury combines with the sulfhydryl group of S-adenosylmethionine, which is a cofactor for catecholamine-O-methyltransferase (COMT), and this inhibition of COMT allows accumulation of norepinephrine, epinephrine, and dopamine." The clinical presentation of mercury toxicity can include any of the following: diffuse erythematosus rash, dermatitis (acrodynia), anorexia, malaise, fatigue, muscle pain, proximal and/or distal muscle weakness, tremor, weight loss, insomnia, night sweats, burning peripheral neuropathy (axonal neuropathy), renal insufficiency/failure, inattention, neurocognitive compromise, personality changes, depression, diaphoresis, tachycardia, and hypertension. Mercury poisoning/accumulation can occur in humans as a result of consumption of contaminated foods—especially seafood such as shark, swordfish, king mackerel, tilefish, and albacore ("white") tuna.[224] The immunologic effects of organic and/or inorganic mercury include immunosuppression, immunostimulation, formation of antinucleolar antibodies targeting fibrillarin, and formation and deposition of immune-complexes, resulting in a syndrome called "mercury-induced autoimmunity" which can be induced by exposure of susceptible animals to mercury.[225] Mercury/"silver" amalgam dental fillings rank highly among the most significant source of mercury exposure in humans, and implantation of mercury-silver dental amalgams in susceptible animals causes chronic stimulation of the immune system with induction of systemic autoimmunity.[226] Besides being a neurotoxin with no safe exposure limit[227], mercury is known to modify/antigenize/haptenize endogenous proteins to promote autoimmunity[228], and mercury may also promote autoimmunity by contributing to a pro-inflammatory environment that awakens quiescent autoreactive immunocytes via bystander activation.[229] For example, administration of mercury to "susceptible" mice induces autoimmunity via modification of

---

[219] Schober SE, et al. Blood mercury levels in US children and women of childbearing age, 1999-2000. *JAMA*. 2003 Apr 2;289(13):1667-74
[220] "Most makeup manufacturers have phased out the use of mercury, but it's still added legally to some eye products as a preservative and germ-killer, said John Bailey, chief scientist with the Personal Care Products Council in Washington." Associated Press. Minnesota Bans Adding Mercury To Cosmetics. February 11, 2009. cbsnews.com/stories/2007/12/14/health/main3618048.shtml Accessed August 2011
[221] "Average daily consumption of high fructose corn syrup is about 50 grams per person in the United States. With respect to total mercury exposure, it may be necessary to account for this source of mercury in the diet of children and sensitive populations." Dufault R, LeBlanc B, Schnoll R, Cornett C, Schweitzer L, Wallinga D, Hightower J, Patrick L, Lukiw WJ. Mercury from chlor-alkali plants: measured concentrations in food product sugar. *Environ Health*. 2009 Jan 26;8:2. See also: "High fructose corn syrup has been shown to contain trace amounts of mercury as a result of some manufacturing processes, and its consumption can also lead to zinc loss." Dufault R, et al. Mercury exposure, nutritional deficiencies and metabolic disruptions may affect learning in children. *Behav Brain Funct*. 2009 Oct 27;5:44.
[222] Wössmann W, Kohl M, Grüning G, Bucsky P. Mercury intoxication presenting with hypertension and tachycardia. *Arch Dis Child*. 1999 Jun;80(6):556-7 ncbi.nlm.nih.gov/pmc/articles/PMC1717944/pdf/v080p00556.pdf
[223] Shih H, Gartner JC Jr. Weight loss, hypertension, weakness, and limb pain in an 11-year-old boy. *J Pediatr*. 2001 Apr;138(4):566-9
[224] See fda.gov/Food/FoodSafety/Product-SpecificInformation/Seafood/FoodbornePathogensContaminants/Methylmercury/ucm115662.htm for the white-washed version; see ewg.org/news/bamboozled-fish for a more accurate and complete perspective.
[225] Havarinasab S, Hultman P. Organic mercury compounds and autoimmunity. *Autoimmun Rev*. 2005;4(5):270-5 generationrescue.org/pdf/havarinasab.pdf Dec 2005
[226] "We hypothesize that under appropriate conditions of genetic susceptibility and adequate body burden, heavy metal exposure from dental amalgam may contribute to immunological aberrations, which could lead to overt autoimmunity." Hultman P, Johansson U, Turley SJ, Lindh U, Enestrom S, Pollard KM. Adverse immunological effects and autoimmunity induced by dental amalgam and alloy in mice. *FASEB J*. 1994 Nov;8(14):1183-90
[227] University of Calgary Faculty of Medicine. How Mercury Causes Brain Neuron Degeneration. commons.ucalgary.ca/mercury/ Current Aug 2011
[228] Havarinasab S, Hultman P. Organic mercury compounds and autoimmunity. *Autoimmun Rev*. 2005 Jun;4(5):270-5. generationrescue.org/pdf/havarinasab.pdf Dec 2005
[229] "It is therefore theoretically possible that compounds present in vaccines such as thiomersal or aluminium hydroxyde can trigger autoimmune reactions through bystander effects." Fournie et al. Induction of autoimmunity through bystander effects. Lessons from immunological disorders induced by heavy metals. *J Autoimmun*. 2001 May;16:319-26

Toxic metal testing—emphasis on lead and mercury

the nucleolar protein *fibrillarin*[230]; noteworthy in this regard is the fact that antifibrillarin antibodies are characteristic of the human autoimmune disease scleroderma.[231] The mercury-based preservative thimerosol is a type-IV (delayed hypersensitivity) sensitizing agent[232], and recent research implicates mercury as a contributor to autism[233,234] and eczema.[235] A review and clinical report published by Bains et al[236], stated, "Eczematous eruptions may be produced through topical contact with mercury and by systemic absorption in mercury sensitive individuals. Mercury...may cause hypersensitivity leading to contact dermatitis or Coomb's Type IV hypersensitivity reactions. The typical manifestation is an urticarial or erythematous rash, and pruritus on the face and flexural aspects of limbs, followed by progression to dermatitis." Thus, this survey of the literature supports the notions that mercury toxicity—i.e., a level of mercury in human patients sufficient to cause adverse health effects—is ❶ <u>common</u> (e.g., 8% of American women), ❷ <u>problematic</u> via causation of or contribution to various health problems commonly encountered in clinical practice, ❸ <u>diagnosable</u> via laboratory testing followed by monitoring response to treatment, and ❹ <u>treatable</u>, most notably with DMSA but also to a lesser extent with potassium citrate, selenium, and phytochelatins.

- Additional details—lead: The International Agency for Research on Cancer (IARC, part of the World Health Organization [WHO]) classified lead as a "possible human carcinogen" in 1987. A 2003 review published in *British Medical Bulletin* by Järup[237] noted that lead exposure (which comes equally from air and food, particularly food served via lead-contaminated ceramics) should be avoided as much as possible because physiologic toxicity occurs with low-level exposure; "Blood levels in children should be reduced below the levels so far considered acceptable, recent data indicating that there may be neurotoxic effects of lead at lower levels of exposure than previously anticipated." Occupational exposure to lead occurs in mines, smelting plants, glass-manufacturing facilities, battery plants, and among workers who weld metals already painted with lead-containing paints; air emissions near such facilities and activities may also contaminate nonworkers. Air contamination frequently leads to water contamination, threatening wildlife and humans who are exposed to contaminated water. Children are particularly vulnerable to lead exposure due to very efficient (compared with adults) gastrointestinal absorption and a more permeable ("leaky") blood-brain barrier. Organic lead compounds such as tetramethyl-lead and tetraethyl lead easily penetrate skin and blood-brain barrier of children as well as adults. Classic, large-dose, acute and subacute lead poisoning manifests as anemia, renal tubular damage, and dark blue line of lead sulphide at the gingival margin; clinicians awaiting this classic presentation prior to considering lead toxicity should fortify their knowledge of and reconsider their perspective on this topic. Other symptoms of acute lead poisoning are headache, irritability, abdominal pain and various neurologic-psychiatric symptoms generally referred to as "lead encephalopathy" characterized by sleeplessness, restlessness, confusion/dyscognition, behavioral disturbances, particularly learning and concentration difficulties in children; more extreme manifestations can include acute psychosis and stupor. Per the previously

---

[230] Nielsen JB, Hultman P. Mercury-induced autoimmunity in mice. *Environ Health Perspect*. 2002 Oct;110 Suppl 5:877-81 ehp.niehs.nih.gov/docs/2002/suppl-5/877-881nielsen/abstract.html

[231] "Since anti-fibrillarin antibodies are specific markers of scleroderma, the present animal model may be valuable for studies of the immunological aberrations which are likely to induce this autoimmune response." Hultman P, Enestrom S, Pollard KM, Tan EM. Anti-fibrillarin autoantibodies in mercury-treated mice. *Clin Exp Immunol*. 1989;78(3):470-7

[232] "Thimerosal is an important preservative in vaccines and ophthalmological preparations. The substance is known to be a type IV sensitizing agent. High sensitization rates were observed in contact-allergic patients and in health care workers who had been exposed to thimerosal-preserved vaccines." Westphal et al. Homozygous gene deletions of the glutathione S-transferases M1 and T1 are associated with thimerosal sensitization. *Int Arch Occup Environ Health*. 2000 Aug;73(6):384-8

[233] Vojdani A, Pangborn JB, Vojdani E, Cooper EL. Infections, toxic chemicals and dietary peptides binding to lymphocyte receptors and tissue enzymes are major instigators of autoimmunity in autism. *Int J Immunopathol Pharmacol*. 2003 Sep-Dec;16(3):189-99

[234] Geier DA, Geier MR. A comparative evaluation of the effects of MMR immunization and mercury doses from thimerosal-containing childhood vaccines on the population prevalence of autism. *Med Sci Monit*. 2004 Mar;10(3):PI33-9. medscimonit.com/pub/vol_10/no_3/3986.pdf

[235] Weidinger et al. Body burden of mercury is associated with acute atopic eczema and total IgE in children from southern Germany. *J Allergy Clin Immunol*. 2004;114(2):457-9

[236] Bains VK, Loomba K, Loomba A, Bains R. Mercury sensitisation: review, relevance and a clinical report. *Br Dent J*. 2008 Oct 11;205(7):373-8 intolsante.com/documents/publications/-mercury-sensitisation-review-relevance-and-clinical-report-22.pdf Accessed August 2011

[237] Järup L. Hazards of heavy metal contamination. *Br Med Bull*. 2003;68:167-82

Toxic metal testing—emphasis on lead and mercury	
	cited review by Järup, "Individuals [chronically exposed to lead] with average blood lead levels under 3 μmol/l may show signs of peripheral nerve symptoms with reduced nerve conduction velocity and reduced dermal sensibility."
Overview and application:	- No universally accepted consensus exists for the most accurate testing methodology. However, from the science-based perspectives that toxic metals have been proven to cause harm at levels previously believed to be "acceptable" and that—very importantly—toxic metals are exponentially more toxic when in combination than when present alone, reasonable clinicians can therefore conclude that the best test for clinical use is the one that is most sensitive, along with being reasonably convenient for the patient as well as affordable. For these reasons, the current author and many other clinicians chose DMSA-provoked urine toxic metal testing. Hair and nails can also be tested for chronic exposure, as can blood which is generally only useful for recent and relatively high-level exposure. Our clinical concern in general outpatient practice is not with recent and relatively high-level exposure, and therefore blood is not necessarily optimal. Our clinical concern in general outpatient practice is with chronic low-level exposure which leads to adverse cellular effects despite the failure to "spike" the serum level into the detectable toxic range. Arguments in favor of allowing symptomatic patients to persist untreated in a state of toxic metal accumulation would be difficult to justify scientifically and ethically.
Advantages:	- Toxic metal accumulation is ❶ <u>sufficiently common to warrant testing in selected patients—such testing should be used frequently with a low threshold for implementation</u>, ❷ <u>problematic</u> via causation of or contribution to various health problems commonly encountered in clinical practice, ❸ <u>diagnosable</u> via laboratory testing followed by monitoring response to treatment, and ❹ <u>treatable</u>. Therefore, clinicians should establish pathways for the assessment and treatment of metal toxicity.
Limitations:	- Patients with toxic metal accumulation frequently have accumulation of chemical xenobiotics as well; thus testing for and treating toxicity due to metals only relieves one type of toxicity.
Comments:	- Clinicians should establish pathways for the assessment and treatment of toxic metal accumulation.

Clinical Case **Widespread musculoskeletal pain resembling fibromyalgia secondary to lead and mercury accumulation**: This 54yo athletic female with healthy diet, lifestyle, and supportive relationship presented with chronic diffuse musculoskeletal pain. Health history was sigificant for decades of environmental illness/intolerance (EI) also known as multiple chemical sensitivity (MCS). Family history was positive for maternal temporal (giant cell) arteritis. Physical examination revealed numerous tender points consistent with fibromyalgia; yet the history and stool analysis with comprehensive bacteriology and parasitology were unsupportive of gastrointestinal dysbiosis, particularly of the subtype small intestine bacterial overgrowth, which is causal for fibromyalgia.[238] Laboratory investigations revealed normal results for hsCRP (high-sensitivity c-reactive protein), CK (creatine kinase, a marker of muscle damage and myositis), ANA (anti-nuclear antibodies), vitamin D, calcium, phosphorus, and comprehensive thyroid evaluation. The patient was then (defensively) referred to an osteopathic internist who diagnosed fibromyalgia.

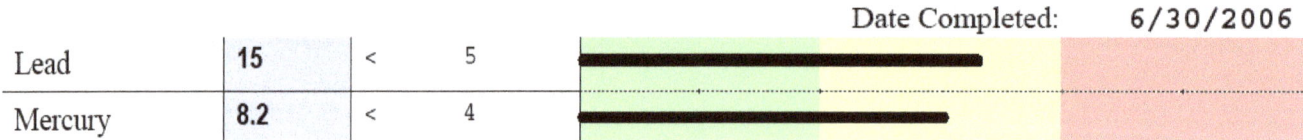

Discussion: The patient, unsatisfied with the diagnosis of fibromyalgia, returned to the current author, who then performed urine heavy metal testing provoked with 10 mg per kilogram of dimercaptosuccinic acid (DMSA). Results revealed the highest levels of lead and mercury encountered in the author's practice at that time. As shown above, lead levels were 6x above the reference range and mercury levels were 7x above the reference range. The patient was commenced on DMSA 10 mg/kg/d on alternating weeks to avoid toxicity in general and bone marrow toxicity (neutropenia) in particular, selenium 800 mcg/d to promote excretion of toxic metals and to support renal and antoxidant protection, vegetable juices to provide potassium and citrate for urinary alkalinization and enhanced excretion of xenobiotics[239], and a proprietary phytochelatin (metal-binding peptides from plants[240]) concetrate to bind toxic metals in the gut and thereby promote their fecal excretion by blocking enterohepatic recycling/recirculation. The use of DMSA for children and adults is supported by peer-reviewed literature.[241,242,243,244,245] DMSA chelation is approved by the US Food and Drug Administration (FDA) for the treatment of marked lead toxicity in children.[246] After approximately 8 months of treatment, the patient was completely free of pain, and the clinical improvement was associated with a reduction in both lead and mercury of approximately 50% as demonstrated by follow-up laboratory testing. Testing was performed by Doctors Data. This case was previously published in peer-reviewed literature for continuing education credits.[247]

---

[238] Vasquez A. *Integrative Orthopedics* and *Integrative Rheumatology* and *Fibromyalgia in a Nutshell* and newer versions in the *Inflammation Mastery* series.
[239] Crinnion WJ. Environmental medicine, part three: long-term effects of chronic low-dose mercury exposure. *Altern Med Rev*. 2000 Jun;5(3):209-23 thorne.com/altmedrev/.fulltext/5/3/209.pdf
[240] Cobbett CS. Phytochelatins and their roles in heavy metal detoxification. *Plant Physiol*. 2000;123:825-32 plantphysiol.org/content/123/3/825
[241] Bradstreet J, Geier DA, Kartzinel JJ, Adams JB, Geier MR. A case-control study of mercury burden in children with autistic spectrum disorders. *Journal of American Physicians and Surgeons* 2003; 8: 76-79 jpands.org/vol8no3/geier.pdf
[242] Crinnion WJ. Environmental medicine, part three: long-term effects of chronic low-dose mercury exposure. *Altern Med Rev*. 2000 Jun;5(3):209-23
[243] Forman J, Moline J, Cernichiari E, Sayegh S, Torres JC, Landrigan MM, Hudson J, Adel HN, Landrigan PJ. A cluster of pediatric metallic mercury exposure cases treated with meso-2,3-dimercaptosuccinic acid (DMSA). *Environ Health Perspect*. 2000 Jun;108(6):575-7 ehp.niehs.nih.gov/docs/2000/108p575-577forman/abstract.html
[244] Miller AL. Dimercaptosuccinic acid (DMSA), a non-toxic, water-soluble treatment for heavy metal toxicity. *Altern Med Rev*. 1998 Jun;3(3):199-207 thorne.com/altmedrev/.fulltext/3/3/199.pdf
[245] DMSA. *Altern Med Rev*. 2000 Jun;5(3):264-7 thorne.com/altmedrev/.fulltext/5/3/264.pdf
[246] "The Food and Drug Administration has recently licensed the drug DMSA (succimer) for reduction of blood lead levels >/= 45 micrograms/dl. This decision was based on the demonstrated ability of DMSA to reduce blood lead levels. An advantage of this drug is that it can be given orally." Goyer RA, Cherian MG, Jones MM, Reigart JR. Role of chelating agents for prevention, intervention, and treatment of exposures to toxic metals. *Environ Health Perspect*. 1995 Nov;103(11):1048-52 ehp.niehs.nih.gov/docs/1995/103-11/meetingreport.html
[247] Vasquez A. *Musculoskeletal Pain: Expanded Clinical Strategies*. Institute for Functional Medicine. 2008

Clinical Case Chronic "idiopathic" hypertension associated with lead and mercury accumulation (per DMSA-provoked urine testing): This 43yo male presents with recalcitrant stage-1 hypertension. His cardiologist prescribed drugs to "treat" (some would say "mask") his elevated blood pressure. Since hypertension always has an underlying cause, the ethical and appropriate course of action is to determine the cause of the problem rather than silencing the alarm that is alerting to an underlying dysfunction. While this case is currently in progress at the time of this writing (the patient's medical records arrived in July 2011), it does offer a model case for clinical decision-making. Clinicians should be aware that, per animal studies, the toxicity of lead and mercury are greatly enhanced when both toxins are present at the same time.

Date Collected: 6/3/2010

Lead	8.5	< 2
Mercury	17	< 3

Mercury and hypertension: Mercury is an established neurotoxin, immunotoxin, and nephrotoxin. Because pathophysiologic effects are noted even with very small doses of exposure, one could reasonably argue that no safe amount exists and therefore that any detected mercury is an indication for therapeutic intervention to remove this toxicant. Sources of exposure include dental amalgams, vaccinations, airborne pollution, and fish; recently, high-fructose corn syrup was shown to contain mercury.[248] Mercury impairs catecholamine degradation and can thereby cause a clinical syndrome that can include hypertension, tremor, tachycardia, diaphoresis, and neurocognitive changes.[249] Per Shih and Gartner[250], "Mercury combines with the sulfhydryl group of S-adenosylmethionine, which is a cofactor for catecholamine-O-methyltransferase (COMT), and this inhibition of COMT allows accumulation of norepinephrine, epinephrine, and dopamine."

Lead and hypertension: In the United States, a consistent correlation has been found between body burden of lead and HTN, even when blood lead levels are well below the current US occupational exposure limit guidelines (40 microg/dl).[251] Harlan et al[252] analyzed data from the second National Health and Nutrition Examination Survey (1976-1980) and thereby found a direct relationship between blood lead levels and systolic and diastolic pressures for men and women and for white and black persons aged 12 to 74 years; they concluded, "Blood lead levels were significantly higher in younger men and women (aged 21 to 55 years) with high blood pressure, but not in older men or women (aged 56 to 74 years)." Schwartz and Stewart[253] found that blood lead was the assessment that most strongly correlated with HTN; they concluded, "Systolic blood pressure was elevated by blood lead levels as low as 5 microg/dl." Thus, clinicians might first measure blood lead levels, which do not measure total body burden but rather the lead that is mobile or *in transit* within the body and which appears to have the best correlation with HTN; the finding of normal blood lead results could then be followed with the more sensitive DMSA-provoked heavy metal testing before concluding that heavy metals are noncontributory to that particular patient's HTN. For heavy metal testing in various clinical scenarios, this author's preference is to use DMSA-provoked measurement of urine toxic metals. After a minimal test dose of DMSA (e.g., in the range of 50-100 mg) to screen for hypersensitivity, patients take oral DMSA 10 mg/kg as a single oral dose in the morning on an empty stomach after emptying the bladder and send a sample from the next urination for laboratory analysis; follow laboratory protocol if different from these instructions. Use of DMSA for lead and mercury chelation/detoxification and for diagnostic purposes is generally safe and effective.[254,255,256]

---

[248] "Average daily consumption of high fructose corn syrup is about 50 grams per person in the United States. With respect to total mercury exposure, it may be necessary to account for this source of mercury in the diet of children and sensitive populations." Dufault R, LeBlanc B, Schnoll R, Cornett C, Schweitzer L, Wallinga D, Hightower J, Patrick L, Lukiw WJ. Mercury from chlor-alkali plants: measured concentrations in food product sugar. *Environ Health*. 2009 Jan 26;8:2. See also: "High fructose corn syrup has been shown to contain trace amounts of mercury as a result of some manufacturing processes, and its consumption can also lead to zinc loss." Dufault R, et al. Mercury exposure, nutritional deficiencies and metabolic disruptions may affect learning in children. *Behav Brain Funct*. 2009 Oct 27;5:44.
[249] Wössmann W, Kohl M, Grüning G, Bucsky P. Mercury intoxication presenting with hypertension and tachycardia. *Arch Dis Child*. 1999 Jun;80(6):556-7 ncbi.nlm.nih.gov/pmc/articles/PMC1717944/pdf/v080p00556.pdf
[250] Shih H, Gartner JC Jr. Weight loss, hypertension, weakness, and limb pain in an 11-year-old boy. *J Pediatr*. 2001 Apr;138(4):566-9
[251] Nash D, Magder L, Lustberg M, Sherwin RW, Rubin RJ, Kaufmann RB, Silbergeld EK. Blood lead, blood pressure, and hypertension in perimenopausal and postmenopausal women. *JAMA*. 2003 Mar 26;289(12):1523-32 jama.ama-assn.org/cgi/content/full/289/12/1523
[252] Harlan WR, et al. Blood lead and blood pressure. Relationship in the adolescent and adult US population. *JAMA*. 1985 Jan 25;253(4):530-4
[253] "Systolic blood pressure was elevated by blood lead levels as low as 5 microg/dl." Schwartz BS, Stewart WF. Different associations of blood lead, meso 2,3-dimercaptosuccinic acid (DMSA)-chelatable lead, and tibial lead levels with blood pressure in 543 former organolead manufacturing workers. *Arch Environ Health*. 2000 Mar-Apr;55(2):85-92
[254] Bradstreet J, Geier DA, Kartzinel JJ, Adams JB, Geier MR. A case-control study of mercury burden in children with autistic spectrum disorders. *Journal of American Physicians and Surgeons* 2003; 8: 76-79 jpands.org/vol8no3/geier.pdf
[255] Miller AL. Dimercaptosuccinic acid (DMSA), a non-toxic, water-soluble treatment for heavy metal toxicity. *Altern Med Rev*. 1998 Jun;3(3):199-207
[256] DMSA. *Altern Med Rev*. 2000 Jun;5(3):264-7 thorne.com/altmedrev/.fulltext/5/3/264.pdf

Antinuclear antibody: ANA	
Overview and interpretation:	- Good screening test for autoimmune conditions: SLE, Sjogren's syndrome, and various other "connective tissue" inflammatory/rheumatic/autoimmune diseases.
- Good and "highly sensitive" for initial assessment of SLE; positive in 95-98% of SLE patients; negative result strongly suggests against diagnosis of SLE.[257] Only 2% of patients with SLE have a negative ANA test—these patients may be identified by testing with anti-RO antibodies and CH50 (complement levels).
- This test measures for the presence of antibodies that react to nucleoproteins. Some labs report titers of 1:20 or 1:40 as "positive"; however, low levels of ANA are common (5-15%) in the general population. Thus, ANA is not specific for any one disease; may be positive in SLE, RA, scleroderma, Sjogren's, also seen with elderly, infected patients, cancer, and with certain medications. Titers less than 1:160 may not indicate the presence of *clinical* autoimmunity[258]; titers >=1:160 usually indicate the presence of active SLE, or other autoimmunity.[259] Titers greater than 1:320 are considered indicative of clinically significant autoimmunity.
- Methodologies (indirect immunofluorescence is most popular), subtypes, and patterns reported for ANA results may be irrelevant or clinically meaningful; the most common descriptors are provided in the table below. Clinicians should order quantitative ANA with reflex to FANA staining patterns

ANA patterns and descriptions[260,261]	*Clinical correlation*
Homogeneous, diffuse nuclear staining	SLE, lupus nephritis, and other autoimmunity
Speckled	SLE, scleroderma, Sjogren's, other autoimmunity
Rim or peripheral staining	Correlates with SLE and lupus nephritis
Anti-centromere: selective staining of the centromeres of nuclei in metaphase	Highly specific for the limited scleroderma subtype associated with **CREST** syndrome
Nucleolar	Correlated with diffuse scleroderma (systemic sclerosis), Sjögren's syndrome, SLE
FANA: fluorescent ANA	The standard ANA test in the US
Anti-Sm: anti-Smith[262]	**Highly specific for SLE**; insensitive: positive in 20-30% of SLE patients
Anti-dsDNA: anti-double stranded DNA	**Highly specific for SLE** and indicative of an increased likelihood of poor prognosis with major organ involvement[263] especially active renal disease
Anti-Ro (anti-SS-A)	Correlates with SLE, Sjögren's syndrome, and neonatal SLE
Anti-La (anti-SS-B)	Sjögren's syndrome or low risk of SLE nephritis
Anti-RNP	SLE and/or mixed connective tissue disease (MCTD)
Anti-Jo-1	Specific but not sensitive for polymyositis/dermatomyositis
Antihistone	SLE and especially drug-induced SLE
Antitopoisomerase (Scl-70)	**Correlates with diffuse scleroderma, especially with interstitial lung disease**

---

[257] Shojania K. Rheumatology: 2. What laboratory tests are needed? *CMAJ*. 2000 Apr 18;162(8):1157-63 cmaj.ca/cgi/content/full/162/8/1157
[258] Hardin JG, Waterman J, Labson LH. Rheumatic disease: Which diagnostic tests are useful? *Patient Care* 1999; March 15: 83-102
[259] Antinuclear Antibodies (ANA), Synonyms: FANA, Test Number: 164947, CPT Code: 86038. https://labcorp.com March 2013
[260] Shojania K. Rheumatology: 2. What laboratory tests are needed? *CMAJ*. 2000 Apr 18;162(8):1157-63 cmaj.ca/cgi/content/full/162/8/1157
[261] Ward MM. Laboratory testing for systemic rheumatic diseases. *Postgrad Med*. 1998 Feb;103(2):93-100.
[262] Lane SK, Gravel JW Jr. Clinical utility of common serum rheumatologic tests. *Am Fam Physician*. 2002;65:1073-80 aafp.org/afp/20020315/1073.html
[263] Shojania K. Rheumatology: 2. What laboratory tests are needed? *CMAJ*. 2000 Apr 18;162(8):1157-63 cmaj.ca/cgi/content/full/162/8/1157

Antinuclear antibody: ANA—continued	
Advantages:	- ANA has 98% sensitivity and 90% specificity for SLE in an unselected population. - The negative predictive value in an unselected population is greater than 99%. ANA is therefore an excellent test for *excluding* the diagnosis of SLE.
Limitations:	- The positive predictive value in an unselected population is about 30%; only 30% of unselected people with a positive result will have SLE—this fact underscores the importance of patient selection and judicious interpretation of this test. - Positive ANA is seen in patients with conditions other than SLE, including rheumatoid arthritis, Sjogren's syndrome, scleroderma, polymyositis, vasculitis, juvenile rheumatoid arthritis (JRA), and infectious diseases.
Comments:	- ANA is most often used to support the diagnosis of SLE in a patient with multisystemic illness and a clinical picture compatible with SLE. Nearly all patients with SLE will have positive ANA. **A positive ANA does not mean that the patient necessarily has SLE; be weary of paraneoplastic syndromes and viral hepatitis as underlying causative processes in patients with an unclear clinical picture.** - I view any "positive ANA" as an indicator of poor health in general and immune dysfunction in particular. The goal, then, is to restore health. I have seen ANA show a trend toward normalization or completely normalize with effective health restoration as detailed in <u>Integrative Rheumatology</u> (Chapter 4). I realize that my experience in this regard contrasts sharply with the allopathic view that serial measurements of ANA are worthless because the result never normalizes once a patient is ANA-positive[264]; I consider this evidence of the effectiveness of my integrative-functional approach and the comparable failure of the allopathic approach.

Antineutrophilic cytoplasmic antibodies: ANCA	
Overview:	- ANCA are autoantibodies to the cytoplasmic constituents of granulocytes and are characteristically found in vasculitic syndromes and also in (Chinese) patients with inflammatory bowel disease[265] and nearly all patients with hepatic amebiasis due to *Entamoeba histolytica*.[266] Two types: - <u>Cytoplasmic ANCA (C-ANCA)</u>: classically seen in Wegener's granulomatosis; also seen in some types of glomerulonephritis and vasculitis; this test is highly sensitive and specific for these conditions. In fact, a positive C-ANCA result can replace biopsy in a patient with a clinical picture of Wegener's granulomatosis.[267] - <u>Perinuclear ANCA (P-ANCA)</u>: considered a nonspecific finding[268] that correlates with SLE, drug induced lupus, and some types of glomerulonephritis and vasculitis. Shojania[269] stated that this test must be confirmed with antimyeloperoxidase antibodies to evaluate for Churg–Strauss syndrome, crescentic glomerulonephritis, and microscopic polyarteritis.
Advantages, limitations, and comments	- Not to be used as a screening test, except in patients with idiopathic vasculitis or glomerulonephritis. - The fact that hepatic amebiasis due to *Entamoeba histolytica* induces production of C-ANCA antibodies in nearly 100% of infected patients may support the hypothesis that autoimmunity can be induced or exacerbated by parasitic infections.

---

[264] Shojania K. Rheumatology: 2. What laboratory tests are needed? *CMAJ*. 2000 Apr 18;162(8):1157-63 cmaj.ca/cgi/content/full/162/8/1157
[265] "Fourteen patients (73.5%) were positive, of which six (31.5%) showed a perinuclear staining pattern and eight (42%) demonstrated a cytoplasmic pattern." Sung JY, Chan KL, Hsu R, Liew CT, Lawton JW. Ulcerative colitis and antineutrophil cytoplasmic antibodies in Hong Kong Chinese. *Am J Gastroenterol*. 1993 Jun;88(6):864-9
[266] "ANCA was detected in 97.4% of amoebic sera; the pattern of staining was cytoplasmic, homogeneous, without central accentuation (C-ANCA)." Pudifin DJ, Duursma J, Gathiram V, Jackson TF. Invasive amoebiasis is associated with the development of anti-neutrophil cytoplasmic antibody. *Clin Exp Immunol*. 1994 Jul;97(1):48-5
[267] Shojania K. Rheumatology: 2. What laboratory tests are needed? *CMAJ*. 2000 Apr 18;162(8):1157-63 cmaj.ca/cgi/content/full/162/8/1157
[268] Shojania K. Rheumatology: 2. What laboratory tests are needed? *CMAJ*. 2000 Apr 18;162(8):1157-63 cmaj.ca/cgi/content/full/162/8/1157
[269] Shojania K. Rheumatology: 2. What laboratory tests are needed? *CMAJ*. 2000 Apr 18;162(8):1157-63 cmaj.ca/cgi/content/full/162/8/1157

	RF: Rheumatoid Factor
Overview and application:	▪ Rheumatoid factor—"anti-IgG antibodies"—are antibodies directed to the Fc portion of the patient's own IgG. Rheumatoid factors are anti-immunoglobulin antibodies, classically anti-IgG IgM. RF are found in low levels in most patients, and despite the "rheumatoid" name, RF is not specific for rheumatoid arthritis.[270] Current tests (latex fixation or nephelometry) detect IgM anti-immunoglobulin antibodies; however IgA-RF appears to have clinical superiority over other forms of RF because it correlates more strongly with clinical status.[271] ▪ This test is most commonly used to support the diagnosis of rheumatoid arthritis in a patient with a compelling clinical picture: peripheral polyarthritis lasting >6 weeks.[272] A negative result with a compelling clinical presentation of RA is termed "seronegative rheumatoid arthritis" by allopathic textbooks whereas a more appropriate term might be oligoarthritis, a condition described as "idiopathic" by allopathic text books despite the clear evidence that the majority of patients have one or more subsets of dysbiosis.[273] ▪ Titers (latex fixation) of 1:160 are considered clinically significant, favoring the diagnosis of RA.[274] However the positive predictive value is low—only 20-34% of people in an unselected population with a positive test result actually have RA.[275,276]
Advantages:	▪ Supports the diagnosis of rheumatoid arthritis: about 60-85% positive/sensitive in patients with rheumatoid arthritis (RA).[277,278] Quantitative titers of RF correlate with prognosis: a very high RF value portends a poor prognosis.
Limitations:	▪ Positive findings are common in the following conditions: rheumatoid arthritis, viral hepatitis, Sjögren's syndrome, endocarditis, scleroderma, mycobacteria diseases, polymyositis and dermatomyositis, syphilis, systemic lupus erythematosus, old age, mixed connective tissue disease, sarcoidosis; positive results may also been noted in: cryoglobulinemia, parasitic infection, interstitial lung disease, asymptomatic relatives of people with autoimmune diseases. ▪ Febrile patients with arthralgia are more likely to have endocarditis than RA.[279] ▪ Patients with iron overload present with a similar clinical picture (i.e., polyarthropathy with systemic complaints) and may have a positive RF. Thus, patients with positive RF and polyarthropathy should be tested for iron overload; use serum ferritin.[280]
Comments:	▪ This test should only be used to confirm the diagnosis of rheumatoid arthritis in patients with a compelling clinical picture of the disease: inflammatory peripheral polyarthropathy with systemic complaints for > 6 weeks. A negative result does not mean that the patient *does not* have rheumatoid arthritis; a positive result does not mean that the patient *does* have rheumatoid arthritis.[281] ▪ CCP (cyclic citrullinated protein) antibodies appear to be more specific and sensitive for RA and is becoming the test of choice for RA as described on the following page.

---

[270] Shojania K. Rheumatology: 2. What laboratory tests are needed? *CMAJ*. 2000 Apr 18;162(8):1157-63 cmaj.ca/cgi/content/full/162/8/1157
[271] Jonsson T, Valdimarsson H. What about IgA rheumatoid factor in rheumatoid arthritis? *Ann Rheum Dis*. 1998 Jan;57(1):63-4
[272] Shojania K. Rheumatology: 2. What laboratory tests are needed? *CMAJ*. 2000 Apr 18;162(8):1157-63 cmaj.ca/cgi/content/full/162/8/1157
[273] See Chapter 4 of *Integrative Rheumatology* and Vasquez A. Reducing Pain and Inflammation Naturally. Part 6: Nutritional and Botanical Treatments Against "Silent Infections" and Gastrointestinal Dysbiosis, Commonly Overlooked Causes of Neuromusculoskeletal Inflammation and Chronic Health Problems. *Nutr Perspect* 2006; Jan
[274] Beers MH, Berkow R (eds). *The Merck Manual. Seventeenth Edition*. Whitehouse Station; Merck Research Laboratories 1999 Page 417
[275] Ward MM. Laboratory testing for systemic rheumatic diseases. *Postgrad Med*. 1998 Feb;103(2):93-100.
[276] Shojania K. Rheumatology: 2. What laboratory tests are needed? *CMAJ*. 2000 Apr 18;162(8):1157-63 cmaj.ca/cgi/content/full/162/8/1157
[277] Tierney ML. McPhee SJ, Papadakis MA (eds). *Current Medical Diagnosis and Treatment 2002, 41st Edition*. New York: Lange Medical, 2002 p854
[278] Shojania K. Rheumatology: 2. What laboratory tests are needed? *CMAJ*. 2000 Apr 18;162(8):1157-63 cmaj.ca/cgi/content/full/162/8/1157
[279] Klippel JH (ed). *Primer on the Rheumatic Diseases. 11th Edition*. Atlanta: Arthritis Foundation. 1997 page 96
[280] Bensen WG, Laskin CA, Little HA, Fam AG. Hemochromatoic arthropathy mimicking rheumatoid arthritis. A case with subcutaneous nodules, tenosynovitis, and bursitis. *Arthritis Rheum* 1978; 21: 844-8
[281] Shojania K. Rheumatology: 2. What laboratory tests are needed? *CMAJ*. 2000 Apr 18;162(8):1157-63 cmaj.ca/cgi/content/full/162/8/1157

CCP: Cyclic citrullinated protein antibody; Citrullinated protein antibodies (CPA); anti-CCP antibodies	
Overview and use:	- CCP—cyclic citrullinated protein antibodies; anticitrullinated protein antibodies: this is a relatively new auto-antibody marker that shows great promise and specificity for the early diagnosis of rheumatoid arthritis (RA). The test often becomes positive/present in asymptomatic patients years before the onset of clinical manifestations of RA.
- As of the first inclusion of this information in my books in December 2006, the information on anti-CCP antibodies is so new that it is not even included in most 2006-edition medical and rheumatology reference textbooks; nonetheless, doctors nationwide are already starting to use this test for the early diagnosis of RA. This may be particularly important because some research has shown that *early* and *aggressive* treatment of RA has an important impact on long-term prognosis[282]; however, the importance of early intervention is debatable.[283]
- Anti-CCP antibodies are directed toward several native proteins (e.g., filaggrin, fibrinogen, and vimentin) that have become posttranslationally modified by an uncharged citrulline in contrast to the normal positively charged arginine. This "citrullination" is catalyzed by a calcium-dependent enzyme, peptidylarginine deiminase (PAD). These changes in protein charge and sequence make the native protein a target of auto-antibody attack by IgG antibodies in RA.[284] However, this does not necessarily imply that citrullination of native proteins is "the cause" of RA because citrullination of native proteins can also occur *de novo* in inflamed joints, which are then further targeted for inflammatory destruction. Until more information is available, we should withhold final judgment as to the ultimate role and origin of anti-CCP antibodies and in the meanwhile view them as a very strong and sensitive association with RA that facilitates the early diagnosis of this disease.
Advantages:	- Anti-CCP antibodies have 98% specificity for RA[285] and is likely to become the future laboratory standard in the diagnosis and prognosis of RA.[286] Anti-CCP antibodies with a positive rheumatoid factor (RF) is termed "composite seropositivity" and appears to be more specific than isolated anti-CCP antibodies or RF.[287]
Limitations:	- The best current data indicates that anti-CCP antibodies are sensitive and specific for RA[288], and clinicians should use this test to diagnose and confirm RA.
Comments:	- Healthy people do not generally have anti-CCP antibodies. Asymptomatic patients with anti-CCP antibodies are at increased risk for clinical RA and are probably *en route* to the manifestation of clinical autoimmunity—RA, Sjogren's disease, or SLE. *Holistically intervene.*
- I hypothesize that PAD may become upregulated in synovial joints exposed to allergens, xenobiotics, bacterial debris/toxins/lipopolysaccharides and that the subsequent citrullination of joint proteins may lead to an autoimmune arthropathy that persists, perhaps despite removal of the inciting immunogen. More obviously (or perhaps more theoretically), given that PAD is calcium-dependent, it may be upregulated secondary to intracellular hypercalcinosis secondary to vitamin D deficiency, magnesium deficiency, or fatty acid imbalance.[289]

---

[282] "CONCLUSION: An initial 6-month cycle of intensive combination treatment that includes high-dose corticosteroids results in sustained suppression of the rate of radiologic progression in patients with early RA, independent of subsequent antirheumatic therapy." Landewe RB, et al. COBRA combination therapy in patients with early rheumatoid arthritis: long-term structural benefits of a brief intervention. *Arthritis Rheum*. 2002 Feb;46:347-56
[283] "By 5 years patients receiving early DMARDs had similar disease activity and comparable health assessment questionnaire scores to patients who received DMARDs later in their disease course." Scott DL. Evidence for early disease-modifying drugs in rheumatoid arthritis. *Arthritis Res Ther*. 2004;6(1):15-18 arthritis-research.com/content/6/1/15
[284] Hill J, Cairns E, Bell DA. The joy of citrulline. *J Rheumatol*. 2004 Aug;31(8):1471-3 jrheum.com/subscribers/04/08/1471.html
[285] Hill J, Cairns E, Bell DA. The joy of citrulline. *J Rheumatol*. 2004 Aug;31(8):1471-3
[286] "We conclude that, at present, the antibody response directed to citrullinated antigens has the most valuable diagnostic and prognostic potential for RA." van Boekel et al. Autoantibody systems in rheumatoid arthritis: specificity, sensitivity and diagnostic value. *Arthritis Res*. 2002;4(2):87-93 arthritis-research.com/content/4/2/87
[287] "…our findings suggest that a positive anti-CCP antibody result does not necessarily exclude SLE in African American patients presenting with inflammatory arthritis. In such patients, the additional assessment of IgA-RF or IgM-RF isotypes may be of added value since composite seropositivity appears to be nearly exclusive to patients with RA." Mikuls et al. Anti-cyclic citrullinated peptide antibody and rheumatoid factor isotypes in African Americans with early rheumatoid arthritis. *Arthritis Rheum*. 2006 Sep;54:3057-9
[288] "Serum antibodies reactive with citrullinated proteins/peptides are a very sensitive and specific marker for rheumatoid arthritis." Migliorini P, Pratesi F, Tommasi C, Anzilotti C. The immune response to citrullinated antigens in autoimmune diseases. *Autoimmun Rev*. 2005 Nov;4(8):561-4
[289] naturopathydigest.com/archives/2006/sep/vasquez.php

Clinical Case **Exemplary case of clinical and laboratory evidence of reversal of "severe, aggressive, drug-resistant" rheumatoid arthritis in a 51yoWF following implementation of the Functional Inflammology Protocol**: This summarizes the 13-month clinical outcome of the first patient treated with the updated functional inflammology protocol after its revision and expansion in March 2012.[290] After being diagnosed accurately by a rheumatologist—for this patient very clearly met diagnostic criteria—this patient presented for care following notably inefficacious treatment with the full medicopharmaceutical antirheumatic protocol comprised of NSAIDs, prednisone (she had only minimal response to prednisone >60mg/d), methotrexate, hydroxychloroquine, and "biologics" including etanercept/Enbrel; she was now being recommended to start newer "experimental" drugs. Following the failure of medical treatment, the patient was treated at the teaching clinic of a naturopathic college where her treatments included a clinician-supervised 26-day water-only fast, which resulted in the loss of 30 pounds (13.6 kilograms) but provided no clinical benefit for the rheumatoid arthritis. [Note: I/Dr Vasquez treat this patient at no charge. Dr William J Beakey of Professional Co-Op Services (Professionalco-op.com) generously donated these laboratory tests for collaborative/research purposes. Biotics Research Corporation (BioticsResearch.com) generously donates nutritional supplements for this patient.]

March 2012—severe symptoms and CCP >250: Patient reports suffering significantly with joint pain and lower extremity edema; foundational nutritional protocol[291] is implemented with antidysbiotic/antimicrobial intervention limited to emulsified oregano oil 600mg/d, mitochondrial support and the nutritional immunomodulation protocol. CCP level at this time is beyond laboratory testing limits, measured simply as "greater than" 250 units.

CCP Antibodies IgG/IgA	>250	High	units	0 – 19
			Negative	<20
			Weak positive	20 – 39
			Moderate positive	40 – 59
			Strong positive	>59

January 2013—mild symptoms and CCP 195: Few modifications are made for the first 9 months and patient feels progressively better, but wants to "move to the next level of improvement" because—despite feeling and functioning significantly better solely with dietary and nutritional interventions—patient still notes exacerbations of pain, particularly following extended manual farm labor. At this time, labs are drawn showing an impressive reduction in CCP levels from "greater than" 250 units to 195 units, correlating with a reduction of at least 22%. At this time, patient was commenced on additional treatments including cabergoline, oral vancomycin, and azithromycin.

CCP Antibodies IgG/IgA	195	High	units	0 – 19
			Negative	<20
			Weak positive	20 – 39
			Moderate positive	40 – 59
			Strong positive	>59

April 2013—virtually normal, CCP 54: Patient continues to improve clinically; her subjective and objective clinical improvements (including additional loss of 30 pounds [13.6 kilograms] and reduction in hand swelling necessitating resizing of wedding ring) correlate nicely with the reduction in CCP levels, which have reduced from >250 units to 54 units, for a reduction of more than 78%. Thus, by objective physical and laboratory criteria, this patient appears to be experiencing authentic reversal—cure—of her disease due to the functional inflammology protocol.

CCP Antibodies IgG/IgA	54	High	units	0 – 19
			Negative	<20
			Weak positive	20 – 39
			Moderate positive	40 – 59
			Strong positive	>59

---

[290] Vasquez A. *Functional Immunology and Nutritional Immunomodulation*. 2012 createspace.com/3899760 and updated as *F.I.N.D. S.E.X® The Easily Remembered Acronym for the Functional Inflammology Protocol*. 2013 createspace.com/4234627
[291] Vasquez A. Revisiting the Five-Part Nutritional Wellness Protocol: Supplemented Paleo-Mediterranean Diet. *Nutr Perspect* 2011 Jan ichnfm.org/faculty/vasquez/profile.html

HLA-B27: Human leukocyte antigen B-27	
Overview and interpretation:	<ul><li>A common (5-10% of general population) genetic marker strongly associated with seronegative* spondyloarthropathy (all of which occur more commonly in men[292]):<ul><li>Ankylosing spondylitis (90-95% of 'whites' and 50% of 'blacks')[293]</li><li>Reactive arthritis [formerly called Reiter's syndrome] (85%)</li><li>Enteropathic spondyloarthropathy</li><li>Psoriatic spondylitis (<60%)</li></ul></li></ul> * Recall that "seronegative" in this context implies that the *rheumatoid factor is negative*, even though *the HLA-B27 may be positive.*
Advantages: Limitations: Comments:	<ul><li>*From a diagnostic perspective*: The clinical application and significance of this test is of limited value. All of the above-listed conditions are better assessed with the combination of clinical assessment and radiographs. In a patient with early and mild disease, this test may add evidence either supporting or refuting the diagnosis; but the test itself is not diagnostic of anything other than a genetic/histologic marker associated with various types of infection-induced arthropathy and autoimmunity (dysbiotic arthropathy[294]).</li><li>*From an integrative/functional medicine perspective*: This test can be of some value if the result is positive and the patient has evidence of a systemic inflammatory/autoimmune disorder since it therefore more strongly suggests that a dysbiotic locus is the cause of disease.[295] A consistent theme in the rheumatology literature is that of "molecular mimicry"—the phenomenon by which structural similarities between human and microbial structures lead to targeting of human tissues by immune responses aimed at microbial antigens. This topic is explored in considerable detail in the section on multifocal dysbiosis in *Integrative Rheumatology*. The important link between microbe-induced autoimmunity and HLA-B27 is that many dysbiotic bacteria produce an HLA-B27-like molecule that appears to trigger an immune response which then erroneously affects human tissues, leading to the clinical picture of autoimmune inflammation. Many of these HLA-B27-producing bacteria colonize the gastrointestinal and genitourinary tracts, promoting musculoskeletal inflammation via molecular mimicry and other mechanisms.[296,297] A strong and growing body of research shows that HLA-B27 is a risk factor for microbe-induced autoimmunity. "Autoimmune" patients positive for HLA-B27 are presumed to have an occult infection—especially gastrointestinal, genitourinary, or sinorespiratory—until proven otherwise.</li><li><u>Keep in mind that HLA-B27 itself is not a "disease"</u> and therefore a "positive" result merely means that the patient has this particular human leukocyte antigen; this test is not and will never be diagnostic of a specific disease—it simply correlates with increased propensity toward dysbiotic arthropathy and suggests the need for dysbiosis testing and the (re)establishment of eubiosis.[298]</li></ul>

---

[292] "The major diseases associated with HLA-B27 (Reiter's disease, ankylosing spondylitis, acute anterior uveitis, and psoriatic arthritis) all occur much more commonly in men." James WH. Sex ratios and hormones in HLA related rheumatic diseases. *Ann Rheum Dis*. 1991 Jun;50(6):401-4

[293] Shojania K. Rheumatology: 2. What laboratory tests are needed? *CMAJ*. 2000 Apr 18;162(8):1157-63 cmaj.ca/cgi/content/full/162/8/1157

[294] See Chapter 4 of *Integrative Rheumatology* and Vasquez A. Nutritional and Botanical Treatments Against "Silent Infections" and Gastrointestinal Dysbiosis, Commonly Overlooked Causes of Neuromusculoskeletal Inflammation and Chronic Health Problems. *Nutr Perspect* 2006; Jan InflammationMastery.com/reprints

[295] "The association between HLA-B27 and reactive arthritis (ReA) has also been well established... In a similar way, microbiological and immunological studies have revealed an association between Klebsiella pneumoniae in AS and Proteus mirabilis in RA." Ebringer et al. HLA molecules, bacteria and autoimmunity. *J Med Microbiol*. 2000 Apr;49:305-11

[296] Inman RD. Antigens, the gastrointestinal tract, and arthritis. *Rheum Dis Clin North Am*. 1991 May;17(2):309-21

[297] Hunter JO. Food allergy--or enterometabolic disorder? *Lancet*. 1991 Aug 24;338(8765):495-6

[298] Dysbiotic arthropathy—joint inflammation and destruction as a result of a neuroimmune inflammatory response to microorganisms. Phrase coined by Alex Vasquez on December 15, 2005. No matching term on Medline or Google search.

Complement levels: CH50, C3, and C4	
Overview and interpretation:	- Complement proteins are consumed in the complement cascades (typically activated by immune complexes) and thus low levels of complement proteins provide indirect evidence of extensive consumption due to immune complex-mediated inflammation. *Low* levels of complement are seen with *increased* disease activity in immune complex disorders (such as SLE, vasculitis, mixed cryoglubulinemia, rheumatoid vasculitis, glomerulonephritis). As expected, low levels of complement are also seen with inherited complement deficiencies; 10%–15% of Caucasian patients with SLE have an inherited complement deficiency.[299] - "CH50" is a screening test for complement levels whereas "C3" and "C4" are more specific for the monitoring of disease activity in autoimmune diseases hallmarked by immune complex deposition, most typically systemic lupus erythematosus (SLE) but also chronic active hepatitis, some chronic infections, poststreptococcal and membranoproliferative glomerulonephritis, and others. Given the wide range of diseases that can cause alterations in complement levels, clinical correlation and differential diagnosis are essential.
Advantages:	- Low complement levels—if not due to genotropic deficiency—provide indirect evidence of immune complex-mediated inflammation. - Elevated levels of complement are seen in conditions of infection or inflammation.
Limitations:	- Some patients have a hereditary absence of complement proteins and thus their levels are always abnormally low; obviously the test cannot be used in these patients for monitoring inflammatory disease.

CIC: Circulating immune complexes	
Overview:	- Antibodies/immunoglobulins are produced in several different "classes": IgG, IgA, IgM, IgE, IgD. IgA antibodies are produced mostly in response to mucosal infections, such as from gastrointestinal dysbiosis or overt infections. When antibodies (in the shape of the letter "Y" with 2 antigen-binding sites on one end and the immuno-reactive site on the other) combine with the target antigen (depicted here in the shape of an oval, such as a bacteria or globular protein), "immune complexes" are formed which are chain-like links of antigens and antibodies. - Although formed in small amounts in healthy persons, in certain disease states, immune complexes may accumulate and initiate complement-dependent injury in various organs and tissues. This activation of complement may begin a series of potentially destructive events in the host, including anaphylatoxin production, cell lysis, leukocyte stimulation, and activation of macrophages and other cells. When immune complexes become fixed to vessel walls, destruction of normal tissue can occur, as in some types of glomerulonephritis and vasculitis. Predisposed to deposition in joints, vessels, and kidneys, immune complexes contribute directly to tissue injury in several autoimmune-inflammatory diseases.[300] **Immune Complexes, (Raji Cell), Quantitative** Reference Range: (Enzyme immunoassay [EIA]; cost $130) - <u>Normal</u>: ≤ 15.0 µg Eq/mL - <u>Equivocal</u>: 15.1-19.9 µg Eq/mL - <u>Positive</u>: ≥20.0 µg Eq/mL
Advantages:	- This test allows for direct quantification of immune-complex production.
Limitations:	- This test has only recently become available to practicing clinicians; however, it is very well supported by many publications in peer-reviewed research.[301]

---

[299] Shojania K. Rheumatology: 2. What laboratory tests are needed? *CMAJ*. 2000 Apr 18;162(8):1157-63 cmaj.ca/cgi/content/full/162/8/1157
[300] Jancar S, Sánchez Crespo M. Immune complex-mediated tissue injury: a multistep paradigm. *Trends Immunol*. 2005 Jan;26(1):48-55
[301] Davies KA, et al. Immune complex processing in patients with systemic lupus erythematosus. *J Clin Invest* 1992;90:2075-83 jci.org/articles/view/116090

Other tests for autoimmunity and immune dysfunction		
Overview and interpretation:	▪ The table below is a quick reference guide to additional clinical disorders and *additional* laboratory tests; diagnostic criteria and lab tests change from time to time. Evaluation should always include history, physical exam, and basic labs such as CBC, UA, and chemistry panel.	
	Disease	**Laboratory (or other) assessment**
	Autoimmune thyroid disease	• Anti(TPO) thyroid peroxidase antibodies: Hashimoto's thyroiditis • Antithyroglobulin antibodies: Hashimoto's thyroiditis • Thyroid stimulating immunoglobulins (TSI, 78%) and thyrotropin receptor antibodies (90%) are noted in Grave's disease
	Latent autoimmune diabetes in adults (LADA), diabetes mellitus type 1.5	• Islet cell antibodies (ICA, also known as antipancreatic islet antibodies) and glutamic acid decarboxylase (GAD) antibodies • LADA/DM1.5 accounts for roughly 10 percent of cases of adult diabetes mellitus; has characteristics of type-1 (autoantibodies) and type-2 (insulin resistance); progresses to insulin-dependence within 6 years of diagnosis; assess beta-cell failure with C-peptide • Consider also tyrosine phosphatase (IA2) antibodies—positive in DM type-1 if this diagnosis is suspected
	Autoimmune hepatitis	• Serum antinuclear antibodies (ANA) • Anti–smooth muscle antibodies (SMA) • Liver-kidney microsomal (type-1 [LKM-1]) antibodies • Anti–liver cytosol-1 (anti-LC1) antibodies • Consider also serum protein electrophoresis (SPEP) and quantitative immunoglobulin analysis; confirm with biopsy
	Primary sclerosing cholangitis (PSC)	• ANA (53%), (p)ANCA (87%), anticardiolipin (66%) and anti-smooth muscle antibodies • Imaging of the bile duct, usually endoscopic retrograde cholangiopancreatography (ERCP)
	Primary biliary cirrhosis (PBC)	• Anti-mitochondrial antibodies (AMA): 93% sensitivity, 98% specificity • ANA: positive in 20-50% of PBC patients • Imaging and biopsy; consider autoimmune cholangitis
	Celiac disease	• IgA Anti-tissue Transglutaminase antibodies (anti-tTG) • IgG and IgA Anti-Gliadin antibodies (AGA) • IgA Deamidated Gliadin Peptide (DGP) antibodies • Quantitative immunoglobulin A (IgA)—performed to exclude selective sIgA deficiency, one of the most common immune deficiency disorders • > 95% of celiac patients have HLA-DQ2 or HLA-DQ8
	Inflammatory bowel disease (IBD)	• IgA and IgG antibodies for *Saccharomyces cerevisiae*—nearly 80% of Crohn's disease patients are positive for either IgA or IgG. "In ulcerative colitis, <15% are positive for IgG, and <2% are positive for IgA. Fewer than 5% of healthy controls are positive for either IgG or IgA antibody, and no healthy controls had antibody for both."[302] • "Atypical ANCA"—positive in a significant percentage of patients with ulcerative colitis, primary sclerosing cholangitis, autoimmune hepatitis • P-ANCA antibodies—"found in 50-70% of ulcerative colitis (UC) patients, but in only 20% of Crohn disease (CD) patients"[303]
	Antiphospholipid/ anticardiolipin/ Hughes syndrome	• IgA, IgG, IgM cardiolipin antibody and IgG, IgM (preferably with IgA) Beta-2 glycoprotein-I antibodies; lupus anticoagulant(s) • Clinical correlation is essential to determine significance
Advantages:	▪ Labs always provide additional data, some of which may be diagnostic.	
Limitations:	▪ Laboratory data must be interpreted within a clinical context in order to properly inform clinical decision-making, diagnostic criteria, and therapeutic intervention.	

---

[302] Inflammatory Bowel Disease (IBD) Profile. https://labcorp.com March 2013
[303] Inflammatory Bowel Disease Differentiation Profile . aruplab.com/guides/ug/tests/0050567.jsp March 2013

Testing for Occult Infections and Dysbiosis—A Practical Introduction and Clinical Approach		
Conceptual overview, advantages and limitations:	<ul><li>With the publication of my *Integrative Rheumatology* textbook in 2006/2007, I was the first to promote the ideas that patients with systemic inflammation in general and autoimmunity in particular <u>*always*</u> have occult "infections" or microbial colonization—dysbiosis—and that this dysbiotic foci is general not singular, nor due to only one offending microbe; rather, inflammatory dysbiosis tends to be multifocal and polymicrobial—what I have termed "multifocal polydysbiosis." In the ensuing years, additional research has consistently proven this model to be correct. I have further defined dysbiosis as "a relationship of non-acute host-microorganism interaction that adversely affects the human host", and I have more recently subdivided the general effects of dysbiosis on the human host as either inflammatory/immunogenic ("inflammatory dysbiosis") or metabolic ("metabolic dysbiosis") although overlap clearly exists.</li><li>Microbial colonization is *necessary but not sufficient* for the existence of the host-microbe relationship that characterizes dysbiosis; the host must be susceptible to the effects of the microbes, and the</li></ul>	**DrV's dysbiosis terminology** <u>Dysbiosis</u>: A relationship of non-acute non-infectious host-microorganism interaction that adversely affects the human host. <u>Dysbiosis subtypes (based on location)</u>: 1. Orodental 2. Sinorespiratory 3. Gastrointestinal 4. Parenchymal, Tissue 5. Genitourinary 6. Cutaneous 7. Environmental 8. Microbial <u>Multifocal dysbiosis</u>: A clinical condition characterized by a patient's having more than one foci/location of dysbiosis; generally the adverse physiologic and clinical consequences are additive and synergistic. <u>Polydysbiosis</u>: Concurrent dysbiosis with several different microbes <u>Main treatment approaches for dysbiosis</u>: ❶ antimicrobial, ❷ immunorestorative, ❸ tolerogenic via nutritional immunomodulation

hosts defense system must be sufficiently impaired to allow the microbial biomass to become qualitatively sufficient (and diverse) to surpass the host's threshold of immunologic and metabolic tolerance. Nevertheless, despite the tripartite requirements for the establishment of dysbiotic inflammation—microbes, immunoincompetence, and intolerance—the fact remains clear that dysbiosis requires microbes. Equally clear is the fact that microbes alone are insufficient for dysbiotic inflammation.

- One of the first questions that arises for clinicians that of choosing methodology for the detection of the offending microbe(s). Briefly, the quest for the identification of the offending microbe(s) is simultaneously wise and sophomoric (soph-, "wise," and moros, "fool"). This approach is wise because the quest for identification and thereafter targeted eradication of the offending microbe is intellectually "clean", clinically efficient, and—most legitimately—allows for precise use of antimicrobial therapy; in reality, this approach is based on numerous erroneous presuppositions including:
    - <u>Presumed physiologic reliability</u>: A common error is that of using antibody assays for the detection of current "infections", especially of the dysbiotic type. Antigen detection is preferable to antibody measurement, given that antibodies may be present even when an infection is presently absent, and that infection/colonization may be present even when antibodies are absent.
    - <u>Presumed equivalence of tests for acute infections and tests for chronic dysbiotic colonizations</u>: Another common error is that of using testing methods developed for the detection of acute infections (e.g., the rapid strep test for acute [extracellular] streptococcal pharyngitis) when seeking to detect dysbiotic infections (e.g., chronic [intracellular] streptococcal pharyngeal colonization of psoriasis).
        - <u>Concept: Microbial phenotype varies per type and chronicity of infection/colonization (*Clinical and Experimental Immunology* 2004 Jan[304]):</u>

---

[304] Gudjonsson JE, Johnston A, Sigmundsdottir H, Valdimarsson H. Immunopathogenic mechanisms in psoriasis. *Clin Exp Immunol*. 2004 Jan;135(1):1-8

"Although streptococci have traditionally been viewed as *extracellular pathogens, they are able to invade several eukaryotic cell types* [i.e., manifest an intracellular phenotype] including squamous epithelium and macrophages, and this has been associated with persistent streptococcal carriage and recurrent infections."

- Presumed performance reliability: Culture-based methodology is notoriously insensitive for anaerobic bacteria, and it is impractical for the detection and identification of complex microbial quorums and biosystems. DNA-based tests exist as numerous methodologies—many of which are patented for research use and are therefore not commercially available; DNA-based testing is impractical for the detection and identification of complex microbial quorums and biosystems with thousands of different microbes.
- Presumed stability of identity of microbes: Microbes have historically been presumed to have stable identities and microbe-disease associations; what we now know is that microbes readily exchange genetic material and that microbial phenotype and metabolic and inflammatory/immunogenic properties can change for example in response to the host's diet or psychoemotional state (the latter described as the study of "microbial endocrinology"[305]).
    - Concept: The emerging irrelevance of microbial identification (*Autoimmune Reviews* 2009 Jul[306]): "These [human-colonizing] bacteria rapidly and frequently share their DNA with their fellow species – even distantly related species – through horizontal gene transfer. ... Some argue that the number of microbes created through genetic recombination is so high that the concept of distinct bacterial species may become obsolete."
- Identification and eradication of a singular offending microbe is noted in the research literature and in clinical practice to occasionally produce brilliant and stunning clinical responses; more commonly—and even more powerfully supported by major trends in the research literature—what we find is a positive clinical response to the combination of ❶ nonspecific antimicrobial therapy (e.g., drugs or botanicals, often and preferably both synthetic and natural agents at the same time), ❷ immunorestorative interventions such as stress reduction and immunonutrition, and ❸ nutritional immunomodulation (detailed in my protocol) to induce immunotolerance. Therefore, the expense and pursuit of identifying the offending microbe(s) is not necessary for a therapeutic response; indeed, the expense and pursuit of identifying the offending microbe(s) may actually deter or delay implementation of effective therapy. However—and finally, the use of testing to determine the presence and persistence of dysbiotic microbial infections/colonizations is occasionally helpful to direct antimicrobial drug therapy especially when more dangerous antimicrobial agents are being employed and/or when previous empiric approaches have not been useful; clinicians can use these and other tests with consideration of the discussion provided above and the more extended discussion in Chapter 4 of *Integrative Rheumatology / Inflammation Mastery*. For the sake of organization, this author's more common test considerations will be listed here by location, with the appreciation that the concept of location is itself somewhat misleading, given that microbes may apparently affect/infect one location (e.g., herpes simplex virus infection of the oral mucosa and associated cranial nerve body) while occultly affecting/infecting a distant location (e.g., the hippocampus).[307]

---

[305] Freestone PP, Sandrini SM, Haigh RD, Lyte M. Microbial endocrinology: how stress influences susceptibility to infection. *Trends Microbiol*. 2008 Feb;16(2):55-64
[306] Proal AD, Albert PJ, Marshall T. Autoimmune disease in the era of the metagenome. *Autoimmun Rev*. 2009 Jul;8(8):677-81
[307] "HSV-1, for example, can infect oral and nasal mucosa and then travels through retrograde axonal transport to the trigeminal ganglion or the olfactory bulb, respectively, where it establishes a latent infection or may rapidly enter the CNS. ... Periodic reactivations from latency are followed by axonal transport of newly produced HSV-1 virions either back to the site of primary infection, where they cause new skin vesicles or mucosal ulcers, or onward to the CNS, where they can cause a productive, but usually mild infection, which may later become latent, as described for rodents. In particular, newly produced virions may target the limbic system, which includes the hippocampus, thalamus and amygdala." De Chiara G, Marcocci ME, Sgarbanti R, et al. Infectious agents and neurodegeneration. *Mol Neurobiol*. 2012 Dec;46(3):614-38

Laboratory tests per location of dysbiotic microbial colonization:	▪ Per the above discussion and context, some of the more common and/or more useful laboratory tests are listed here; these are listed per location for organizational purposes only, with the full appreciation that the location itself is mostly irrelevant, with the possible exception of the gastrointestinal tract which harbors the greatest quantity and diversity of microbes and which harbors these microbes in intimate contact with the bulk of the human immune system—the gut-associated lymphoid tissue (GALT) possesses the largest mass of lymphoid tissue in the human body. In sum, testing for microbes provides either direct and specific evidence of microbes or indirect evidence (both with varying levels of sensitivity), or—at the opposite extreme—empiric evidence (i.e., monitoring response to antimicrobial or immunorestorative interventions) which is completely nonspecific yet much more clinically meaningful. ❶ <u>Direct testing—culture/DNA/antigen</u>: Swab for culture and sensitivity (C-S), DNA-based testing such as polymerase chain reaction (PCR), or antigen detection, ❷ <u>Indirect testing—most commonly antibody assays</u>: Various antibody tests against microbes are available and clinically meaningful, ❸ <u>Empiric testing</u>: Monitoring response to therapeutic-diagnostic intervention with antimicrobial therapy. ▪ Orodental dysbiosis/colonization—introduction to assessment: 　❶ <u>Direct testing—culture/DNA/antigen</u>: Swabs of mucosa, gingiva, teeth, and dentures can be used for culture, DNA, and antigen testing. 　❷ <u>Indirect testing—antibody assays</u>: Antibody titers specific for oral/dental/periodontal microbes correlate with numerous inflammatory disorders, ranging from insulin resistance to rheumatoid arthritis (RA). 　❸ <u>Empiric observation</u>: Oral exam may reveal tooth and gum disease. *Example—rheumatoid arthritis*: "Control of periodontal infection and gingival inflammation by scaling/root planing and plaque control in subjects with periodontal disease may reduce the severity of RA."[308] ▪ Sinorespiratory dysbiosis/colonization—introduction to assessment: 　❶ <u>Direct testing—culture/DNA/antigen</u>: Swabs of nasal and pharyngeal mucosa can be used for culture, DNA, and antigen testing. Sputum can be submitted for culture and direct microscopic analysis. *Example—atopic dermatitis*: In eczema, skin cultures yielded *Staphylococcus aureus* from lesional skin in 87.1% of patients and from the nares in 80.6% of patients. 　❷ <u>Indirect testing—antibody assays</u>: Antibody titers specific for respiratory microbes correlate with numerous inflammatory disorders, ranging from cardiovascular disease to oligoarthritis. 　❸ <u>Empiric observation</u>: *Example—Wegener's granulomatosis/vasculitis*: Treatment with trimethoprim-sulfamethoxazole (co-trimoxazole, a broad-spectrum antibiotic) reduces the incidence of relapses in patients with Wegener's granulomatosis in remission.[309,310] ▪ Gastrointestinal dysbiosis/colonization—introduction to assessment: 　❶ <u>Direct testing—culture/DNA/antigen</u>: Jejunal aspiration is the gold standard for diagnosis of SIBO—small intestinal bacterial overgrowth; similarly, aspiration with or without biopsy followed by direct microscopy or culture is generally the gold standard for the identification of most infections. Stool tests are available using culture, DNA, and antigen-detecting methodology; routine pathogens such as *Salmonella, Shigella, Campylobacter*, and enterohemorrhagic *E coli* (EHEC) can be

---

[308] Al-Katma MK, Bissada NF, Bordeaux JM, et al. Control of periodontal infection reduces the severity of active rheumatoid arthritis. *J Clin Rheumatol*. 2007 Jun;13(3):134-7
[309] Zycinska K, et al. Co-trimoxazole and prevention of relapses of PR3-ANCA positive vasculitis with pulmonary involvement. *Eur J Med Res*. 2009 Dec 7;14 Suppl 4:265-7
[310] Stegeman CA, et al. Trimethoprim-sulfamethoxazole (co-trimoxazole) for the prevention of relapses of Wegener's granulomatosis. *N Engl J Med*. 1996 Jul 4;335(1):16-20

detected by routine (i.e., standard, hospital-based) medical reference laboratories. When testing for dysbiotic-type colonizations, clinicians should utilize a specialty laboratory that presents the results within a context of additional markers for clinical decision-making as discussed in a following section on stool testing.

❷ <u>Indirect testing—antibody assays, lactulose:mannitol assay, inflammatory markers, sIgA, breath hydrogen and methane</u>: Antibody assays specific for gastrointestinal yeast, bacteria, and protozoans are available. In specific situations, very indirect testing such as the lactulose:mannitol assay can be used to determine increased intestinal permeability which can provide indirect evidence of intestinal dysbiosis; likewise, inflammatory markers such as calprotectin, lactoferrin, and lysozyme can also indicate intestinal inflammation which is commonly caused by intestinal microbial overgrowth/colonization. Secretory IgA is also measured in fecal samples and can be interpreted in clinical context; elevated levels suggest immunologic response to intraluminal antigens, the most offensive of which are microbial/dysbiotic. Exhaled hydrogen and methane can be measured following a carbohydrate challenge to assess for nonspecific SIBO. *Example*—fibromyalgia: "3/15 (20%) controls had an abnormal breath test compared with 93/111 (84%) subjects with IBS (p<0.01) and 42/42 (100%) with fibromyalgia (p<0.0001 v controls, p<0.05 v IBS). … The degree of somatic pain in fibromyalgia correlated significantly with the hydrogen level seen on the breath test. An abnormal lactulose breath test is more common in fibromyalgia than IBS. In contrast with IBS, the degree of abnormality on breath test is greater in subjects with fibromyalgia and correlates with somatic pain."[311]

❸ <u>Empiric observation</u>: Response to antimicrobial therapy confirms intestinal microbial overgrowth/dysbiosis/parasitosis; the retrospective diagnosis is made most clearly with observation of a positive clinical response following treatment with orally-administered nonabsorbed antimicrobial agents, such as oregano oil, berberine, nystatin, rifaxamin, and vancomycin. *Example*—empiric diagnosis and treatment of small intestinal bacterial overgrowth: "For cases in which a firm diagnosis cannot be made, but clinical symptoms favor SIBO, empirical antibiotic use may be a more cautious approach to prevent delay of treatment and to prevent increases in symptom severity."[312]

- Genitourinary dysbiosis/colonization—introduction to assessment:
    ❶ <u>Direct testing—culture/DNA/antigen</u>: Reactive/inflammatory arthritis secondary to genitourinary infection is well known, formerly called Reiter's syndrome; a similar association is established in chronic oligoarthritis. *Example*—reactive arthritis: "Urogenital swab cultures showed a microbial infection in 44% of the patients with oligoarthritis (15% *Chlamydia*, 14% *Mycoplasma*, 28% *Ureaplasma*), whereas in the control group only 26% had a positive result (4% *Chlamydia*, 7% *Mycoplasma*, 21% *Ureaplasma*) (P < 0.001). … Urogenital swab culture is the only useful diagnostic method for the detection of the arthritogenic infection in extra-articularly asymptomatic patients with undifferentiated oligoarthritis."[313]
    ❷ <u>Indirect testing—antibody assays</u>: Antibody assays specific for genitourinary microbes are available. *Example*—oligoarthritis: "A Chlamydia IgG-antibody titer >

---

[311] Pimentel M, Wallace D, Hallegua D, Chow E, Kong Y, Park S, Lin HC. A link between irritable bowel syndrome and fibromyalgia may be related to findings on lactulose breath testing. *Ann Rheum Dis*. 2004 Apr;63(4):450-2

[312] Malik BA, Xie YY, Wine E, Huynh HQ. Diagnosis and pharmacological management of small intestinal bacterial overgrowth in children with intestinal failure. *Can J Gastroenterol*. 2011 Jan;25(1):41-5. This is a very excellent article—highly recommended.

[313] Erlacher L, Wintersberger W, Menschik M, et al. Reactive arthritis: urogenital swab culture is the only useful diagnostic method for the detection of the arthritogenic infection in extra-articularly asymptomatic patients with undifferentiated oligoarthritis. *Br J Rheumatol*. 1995 Sep;34(9):838-42

or = 1:256 was found in 22% of the patients in the oligoarthritis group and in 9% of the controls (P < 0.01). However, for only half of *Chlamydia* IgG-positive patients could a *Chlamydia* infection be confirmed by urogenital swab culture."[314]

❸ **Empiric observation:** Response to antimicrobial and immunorestorative interventions. *Example*—rheumatoid arthritis: "We propose that sub-clinical *Proteus* urinary tract infections are the main triggering factors and that the presence of molecular mimicry and cross-reactivity between these bacteria and RA-targeted tissue antigens assists in the perpetuation of the disease process through production of cytopathic auto-antibodies. Patients with RA especially during the early stages of the disease could benefit from *Proteus* anti-bacterial measures involving the use of antibiotics, vegetarian diets and high intake of water and fruit juices such as cranberry juice in addition to the currently employed treatments."[315]

- Cutaneous dysbiosis/colonization—introduction to assessment:
    ❶ **Direct testing—culture/DNA/antigen:** For bacterial infections/colonizations, culture and DNA methods can be used; for fungi, skin scraping followed by KOH wet-mount and microscopic examination is commonly used. *Example*—atopic dermatitis: In eczema, skin cultures yielded *Staphylococcus aureus* from lesional skin in 87.1% of patients and from the nares in 80.6% of patients.[316]
    ❷ **Indirect testing—antibody assays:** Antibodies to dermal microbes can be measured. *Example*—atopic dermatitis: Eczema patients commonly have serum IgE antibodies specific for *Malassezia sympodialis, Candida albicans,* and *Staphylococcus aureus*, and these antibody levels correlate with disease severity.[317]
    ❸ **Empiric observation:** *Example*—atopic dermatitis: "Patients with AD can have sudden exacerbations of AD attributable to overgrowth of *S aureus* that can be independent of true secondary bacterial infection, a notion supported by the clinical response of patients with severe AD to anti-staphylococcal antibiotics [*Dr Vasquez*: and other antimicrobial measures]."

- Environmental dysbiosis/colonization—introduction to assessment:
    ❶ **Direct testing—culture/DNA/antigen:** Home, work, and recreational environments can be surveyed for microbial contamination, particularly mold. Pier-and-beam homes should be inspected for mold and water in the crawlspace; likewise, attics should be inspected for occult leaks and mold. Mold plates, Petri dishes, and filter cartridges can be used to identify airborne microbes. *Fusarium, Trichoderma,* and *Stachybotrys* produce mycotoxins.[318]
    ❷ **Indirect testing—antibody assays:** Tests can be performed for evidence of microbial exposure and immune response (e.g., antibodies specific for microbes); correlative tests can also be performed to assess the clinical and immunological significance of the exposure (e.g., RF, ANA, CCP, and other autoantibodies). *Example*— inflammatory disease associated with working/living in moisture-damaged building: *Chlamydophila pneumoniae* antibodies may be elevated in correlation with clinical symptoms and environmental exposure to microbes.[319] *Example*—

---

[314] Erlacher L, Wintersberger W, Menschik M, et al. Reactive arthritis: urogenital swab culture is the only useful diagnostic method for the detection of the arthritogenic infection in extra-articularly asymptomatic patients with undifferentiated oligoarthritis. *Br J Rheumatol*. 1995 Sep;34(9):838-42

[315] Ebringer A, Rashid T. Rheumatoid arthritis is an autoimmune disease triggered by Proteus urinary tract infection. *Clin Dev Immunol*. 2006 Mar;13(1):41-8

[316] Huang JT, Abrams M, Tlougan B, Rademaker A, Paller AS. Treatment of Staphylococcus aureus colonization in atopic dermatitis decreases disease severity. *Pediatrics*. 2009 May;123(5):e808-14

[317] Sonesson A, Bartosik J, Christiansen J, et al. Sensitization to Skin-associated Microorganisms in Adult Patients with Atopic Dermatitis is of Importance for Disease Severity. *Acta Derm Venereol*. 2012 Oct 16. doi: 10.2340/00015555-1465. medicaljournals.se/acta/content/?doi=10.2340/00015555-1465

[318] Am Acad Pediatrics. Toxic effects of indoor molds. Committee on Environ Health. *Pediatrics* 1998;101(4 Pt1):712-4 aappolicy.aappublications.org/cgi/content/full/pediatrics;101/4/712

[319] Seuri M, Paldanius M, Leinonen M, Roponen M, Hirvonen MR, Saikku P. Chlamydophila pneumoniae antibodies in office workers with and without inflammatory rheumatic diseases in a moisture-damaged building. *Eur J Clin Microbiol Infect Dis*. 2005 Mar;24(3):236-7

biochemical changes noted in persons exposed to microbial contamination: An article co-authored by Vojdani[320] noted, "biochemical abnormal concentrations in creatinine, uric acid, phosphorus, alkaline phosphatase, cholesterol, LDH [*Dr Vasquez*: LDH here is corrected from "HDH" per data in Table 1 of the full-text article], SGOT/AST, segmented neutrophils, lymphocytes, total T3, IgG and IgA immunoglobulins with significant differences between patients and controls."; the authors note an increased prevalence of renal disorders among such patients. *Example*—increased serum autoantibodies in patients exposed to environmental molds: "Abnormally high levels of ANA, ASM, and CNS myelin (immunoglobulins [Ig]G, IgM, IgA) and PNS myelin (IgG, IgM, IgA) were found; odds ratios for each were significant at 95% confidence intervals, showing an increased risk for autoimmunity."[321] *Example*—elevated mold counts, and elevations of non-IgE antibodies in mold-exposed persons: "Detection of high levels (colony-forming units per cubic meter) of molds—which, in this study, strongly suggested that there existed a reservoir of spores in the building at the time of sampling—along with a significant elevation in IgG, IgM, or IgA antibodies against molds and mycotoxins, could be used in future epidemiologic investigations of fungal exposure. In addition to IgE, measurements of IgG, IgM, and IgA antibodies should be considered in mold-exposed individuals."

❸ Empiric observation: Alleviation of clinical symptoms and signs following building evacuation or remediation substantiates the exposure-immunopathology link.

- Parenchymal dysbiosis/colonization—introduction to assessment: Many different "internal" infections/colonizations can contribute to chronic inflammatory disease and—at its most extreme—autoimmunity. Some of these situations are perhaps best described/characterized as true "infections" such as noted with hepatitis C infection contributing to immune-complex-mediated dermatitis and arthritis; infection in this context is noted to have the classic pathologic manifestations of histologic observability and tissue damage (e.g., viral hepatitis and cirrhosis). In other situations, the microbe is neither consistently observable in tissue nor does microbe-induced tissue damage characterize the clinical condition; these situations are perhaps better defined as "parenchymal dysbiosis"—a state of microbe-induced inflammation lacking the classic pathological findings of histologic observability and microbe-induced tissue damage. An example of the latter includes chronic systemic inflammation and—occasionally—inflammatory arthritis (but not septic arthritis) triggered by *Chlamydia/Chlamydophila pneumoniae*. See the following tables for microbe-specific assessments and disease associations.

    ❶ Direct testing—culture/DNA/antigen: *Example*—hepatitis C: Hepatitis C virus RNA detected by quantitative or qualitative PCR.
    ❷ Indirect testing—antibody assays: *Example*—chronic fatigue, chronic oligoarthritis: IgG antibodies specific for *Chlamydia/Chlamydophila pneumonia*.
    ❸ Empiric observation: *Example*—psoriasis: Beneficial response to empiric antimicrobial treatment with penicillin[322] or azithromycin[323] confirms the microbial basis of the disease.

---

[320] Anyanwu E, Campbell AW, Vojdani A, Ehiri JE, Akpan AI. Biochemical changes in the serum of patients with chronic toxigenic mold exposures: a risk factor for multiple renal dysfunctions. *ScientificWorldJournal*. 2003 Nov 3;3:1058-64
[321] Gray MR, Thrasher JD, Crago R, Madison RA, Arnold L, Campbell AW, Vojdani A. Mixed mold mycotoxicosis: immunological changes in humans following exposure in water-damaged buildings. *Arch Environ Health*. 2003 Jul;58(7):410-20
[322] Saxena VN, Dogra J. Long-term use of penicillin for the treatment of chronic plaque psoriasis. *Eur J Dermatol*. 2005 Sep-Oct;15(5):359-62
[323] Saxena VN, Dogra J. Long-term oral azithromycin in chronic plaque psoriasis: a controlled trial. *Eur J Dermatol*. 2010 May-Jun;20(3):329-33

Parenchymal/internal/occult dysbiotic microbes and/or occult infections that can contribute to chronic inflammation, metabolic impairment, or autoimmunity

Viruses	Laboratory assessment	Disease association(s)
Cytomegalovirus (CMV)	IgM antibodies may not peak until 4-7 weeks after onset; IgG antibodies increase by 4x during acute infection; in immunosuppressed patients, PCR and antigen testing is preferred over antibody testing	Fatigue, mononucleosis-like illness, retinopathy in immunosuppressed
Epstein-Barr virus (EBV)	IgG and IgM antibodies to viral antigens are specific and include EBV-early antigen (EA) IgG, EBV-viral capsid antigen (VCA) IgG; EBV-VCA IgM; Epstein-Barr nuclear antigen antibodies (EBNA); IgG titers >1:640 appear to correlate with increased fatigue and clinical response to antiviral treatment in patients with chronic fatigue syndrome[324]	Fatigue, chronic fatigue syndrome, mononucleosis
Hepatitis B virus (HepB, HBV)	HepB surface antigen and DNA are most specific	Liver disease, immune complex (IC)-mediated vasculitis and arthritis
Hepatitis C virus (HepC, HCV)	HCV RNA becomes positive 1-3 weeks postexposure	Liver disease, immune complex (IC)-mediated vasculitis and arthritis
Human herpes virus type-6 (HHV-6)	IgG antibody titers >1:320 correlate with increased fatigue and clinical response to antiviral treatment in patients with chronic fatigue syndrome[325]; IgM and viral DNA levels are elevated in patients with multiple sclerosis[326]	Fatigue, chronic fatigue syndrome, multiple sclerosis
Human immunodeficiency virus (HIV)	Typical protocol is ELISA antibody testing (and/or Western blot) followed by PCR for viral load; for acute infection (prior to [antibody] seroconversion) and severe immunosuppression, DNA-based testing is preferred	Fatigue, peripheral neuropathy, opportunistic infections, severe acute psoriasis
Herpes simplex virus types 1 and 2 (HSV1, HSV2)	Measured by chemiluminescence (CI) or enzyme immunoassay (EIA), IgG antibody titers correlate with exposure/infection and level of viral replication (i.e., higher titers indicate higher viral replication); Western blot methodology is considered the epidemiologic gold standard[327] but IgG measurements by CI/EIA are clinically very reliable and are more widely available.	Fatigue, acute encephalitis, Alzheimer's disease, multiple sclerosis

---

[324] "Nine out of 12 (75%) patients experienced near resolution of their symptoms, allowing them all to return to the workforce or full time activities. In the nine patients with a symptomatic response to treatment, EBV VCA IgG titers dropped from 1:2560 to 1:640 (p = 0.008) and HHV-6 IgG titers dropped from a median value of 1:1280 to 1:320 (p = 0.271)." Kogelnik AM, Loomis K, Hoegh-Petersen M, et al. Use of valganciclovir in patients with elevated antibody titers against Human Herpesvirus-6 (HHV-6) and Epstein-Barr Virus (EBV) who were experiencing central nervous system dysfunction including long-standing fatigue. *J Clin Virol*. 2006 Dec;37 Suppl 1:S33-8

[325] "Nine out of 12 (75%) patients experienced near resolution of their symptoms, allowing them all to return to the workforce or full time activites. In the nine patients with a symptomatic response to treatment, EBV VCA IgG titers dropped from 1:2560 to 1:640 (p = 0.008) and HHV-6 IgG titers dropped from a median value of 1:1280 to 1:320 (p = 0.271)." Kogelnik AM, Loomis K, Hoegh-Petersen M, et al. Use of valganciclovir in patients with elevated antibody titers against Human Herpesvirus-6 (HHV-6) and Epstein-Barr Virus (EBV) who were experiencing central nervous system dysfunction including long-standing fatigue. *J Clin Virol*. 2006 Dec;37 Suppl 1:S33-8

[326] "Results demonstrate increased levels of anti-HHV6-IgG (78.2% versus 76.4% in controls; P = NS), and IgM (34.6% versus 6.5% in controls; P < 0.05) in MS patients. ... Moreover, load of cell-free viral DNA was higher in RRMS and SPMS patients and detected in 60.2% (47/78) of MS patients, compared with 14.6% (18/123) of healthy controls (P < 0.001)." Ramroodi N, Sanadgol N, Ganjali Z, Niazi AA, Sarabandi V, Moghtaderi A. Monitoring of active human herpes virus 6 infection in Iranian patients with different subtypes of multiple sclerosis. *J Pathog*. 2013;2013:194932

[327] Accessed in March 2013. "The Western Blot, the most accurate of these blood tests, is done at the University of Washington." depts.washington.edu/herpes/faq.php#faqCat-3. "The Western blot assay is the most validated method for identifying type-specific antibodies and is considered the gold standard. ... The Western blot assay is conducted exclusively at the University of Washington where clinical specimens can be sent and processed. Two type-specific glycoprotein G serological tests are commercially available in the United States. Sensitivity and specificity of these tests are comparable to the Western blot assay. These tests cost $10 to $40 (U.S. dollars)." uspreventiveservicestaskforce.org/uspstf05/herpes/herpesup.htm

Parenchymal/internal/occult dysbiotic microbes and/or occult infections that can contribute to chronic inflammation, metabolic impairment, or autoimmunity—*continued*

Viruses—continued	Laboratory assessment	Disease association(s)
Parvovirus B19	IgG and IgM antibodies are commonly used; however, "high-level viremia in acutely infected persons may cause virus-antibody complexes, which will result in a false-negative IgM test result. In this setting, polymerase chain reaction (PCR) may be a better diagnostic modality."[328]	Arthritis/arthralgia, which can mimic rheumatoid arthritis[329]
Bacteria, protozoa, etc.	**Assessment**	**Disease association(s)**
Infectious agents well-known to cause reactive/inflammatory arthritis: *Chlamydia trachomatis* and various species in the genera *Salmonella, Shigella, Campylobacter,* and *Yersinia*	Direct microscopy, culture, DNA-based testing; antibody testing is less commonly used for these acute and subacute infections; empiric antimicrobial treatment without laboratory testing is reasonable with a compelling clinical picture of infection and associated inflammopathy/arthropathy	Reactive arthritis, chronic arthritis, autoimmune thyroiditis (especially *Yersinia*, in which case anti-*Yersinia* antibodies are strongly correlated with thyroid disease[330])
Borrelia burgdorferi, Babesia species including *microti, divergens,* MO1, *duncani* (WA-1)	IgG and IgM antibodies, Western blot, PCR; many experienced clinicians prefer IGeneX testing; much controversy exists about the "best" testing method(s)	Fatigue, Lyme disease (erythema chronicum migrans, myocarditis, arthritis, meningitis, neuropathies)
Chlamydia/Chlamydophila pneumoniae	IgG titers > 1:64 correlate with chronic/persistent infection/colonization[331]; likewise, IgA titers > 1:20 correlate with chronic/persistent infection/colonization; IgA positivity and/or PCR positivity correlate with myocardial infarction[332]; as expected PCR is considered best evidence of current active infection, since antibody levels do not always correlate with active infection whereas nuclear material is rapidly degraded by human restriction endonucleases and therefore when present provides clear proof of current infection/colonization	Chronic fatigue, chronic inflammatory arthritis (responds to prolonged combination therapy with azithromycin and rifampin[333]), multiple sclerosis[334], myocardial infarction

---

[328] Cennimo DJ, Steele RW. Parvovirus B19 Infection Workup. emedicine.medscape.com/article/961063-workup Accessed March 2013
[329] Sabella C, Goldfarb J. Parvovirus B19 infections. *Am Fam Physician*. 1999 Oct 1;60(5):1455-60
[330] "In contrast to the low prevalence of antibodies in controls (less than 8%), 48 of 67 patients (75%) with a variety of thyroid disorders had titers greater than 1:8. Antibodies were found in 24 of 36 patients with Graves' disease, five of six with autonomous adenoma, seven of seven with Hashimoto's thyroiditis, three of five with idiopathic primary hypothyroidism, four of 11 with nontoxic nodular goiter, and one of two with thyroid carcinoma." Shenkman L, Bottone EJ. Antibodies to Yersinia enterocolitica in thyroid disease. *Ann Intern Med*. 1976 Dec;85(6):735-9
[331] "Because there is as yet no standardisation of serological criteria for persistent infection, we considered antibody titres of > 1/20 in the IgA fraction, together with IgG titres of 1/64 to 1/256, to be indicative of persistent infection." Ben-Yaakov M, Eshel G, Zaksonski L, Lazarovich Z, Boldur I. Prevalence of antibodies to Chlamydia pneumoniae in an Israeli population without clinical evidence of respiratory infection. *J Clin Pathol*. 2002 May;55(5):355-8
[332] Haider M, et al. Acute and chronic Chlamydia pneumoniae infection and inflammatory markers in coronary artery disease patients. *J Infect Dev Ctries*. 2011 Aug;5:580-6
[333] Carter JD, Espinoza LR, Inman RD, Sneed KB, Ricca LR, Vasey FB, Valeriano J, Stanich JA, Oszust C, Gerard HC, Hudson AP. Combination antibiotics as a treatment for chronic Chlamydia-induced reactive arthritis: a double-blind, placebo-controlled, prospective trial. *Arthritis Rheum*. 2010 May;62(5):1298-307
[334] "In clinically definite MS patients, the VUMC and USF detection rates were 72 and 61%, respectively, and in patients with monosymptomatic MS, the VUMC and USF detection rates were 41 and 54%, respectively. The PCR signal was positive for 7% of the OND controls at VUMC and for 16% at USF. These studies confirm our previous reports concerning the high prevalence of C. pneumoniae in the CSF of MS patients." Sriram S, Yao SY, Stratton C, et al. Comparative study of the presence of Chlamydia pneumoniae in cerebrospinal fluid of Patients with clinically definite and monosymptomatic multiple sclerosis. *Clin Diagn Lab Immunol*. 2002 Nov;9(6):1332-7.

Parenchymal/internal/occult dysbiotic microbes and/or occult infections that can contribute to chronic inflammation, metabolic impairment, or autoimmunity—*continued*

Bacteria, protozoa, etc.	Assessment	Disease association(s)
Helicobacter pylori	Serum IgA, IgM, IgG antibodies—IgG antibodies are the most useful *serologic* test (>90% sensitive and specific) for monitoring response to eradication therapy despite the fact that antibody titer may remain elevated for a long time after *H pylori* eradication; urea breath test (gives false-negative results with coccoid forms of *H pylori* that do not produce urease, use of antibiotics, bismuth, histamine-2 blockers, or proton pump inhibitors), stool antigen shows excellent specificity (98%) and sensitivity (94%) and is highly responsive to the presence or absence of the infection[335]	Chronic gastritis and gastroduodenal ulceration, hypochlorhydria and subsequent maldigestion and small intestine bacterial overgrowth (SIBO), Sjogren syndrome, GI lymphoma, migraine, reactive/chronic arthritis, Raynaud's phenomenon
Mycoplasma species including *pneumoniae*, *fermentans*, *hominis*, *penetrans*, *genitalium*	IgG and IgM antibodies to various subspecies; PCR showed positivity in patients with fatigue/fibromyalgia: *M. pneumoniae* (54/91), *M. fermentans* (44/91), *M. hominis* (28/91) and *M. penetrans* (18/91)[336]	Chronic fatigue syndrome and fibromyalgia, Gulf War Illness[337], autoimmunity
Pseudomonas aeruginosa, *Acinetobacter* spp	Culture of site (urine, stool, sputum, wounds, cerebrospinal fluid) as indicated, otherwise, use stool culture and urine culture if investigating neuronal autoimmunity; serum IgA and IgG antibodies against *Pseudomonas aeruginosa* and *Acinetobacter* spp antigens are elevated in patients with multiple sclerosis[338,339], however such testing is not widely commercially available for routine clinical use; the current author has found stool testing and culture for *Pseudomonas aeruginosa* to be valuable in the treatment of neuronal autoimmunity	Neuronal autoimmunity including peripheral neuropathy and multiple sclerosis
Streptococcal infections: *Streptococcus pyogenes*, streptococci hemolytic groups A, B, D, and G	Acute pharyngeal infections are generally diagnosed clinically, with or without the use of "rapid Strep tests" or throat culture and treated with short-term penicillin-based antibiotic. However, with chronic infections/colonizations, the microbiologic phenotype of the bacteria changes from the extracellular form prototypical of acute infections to that of an intracellular form; as a general guideline, acute/extracelluar infections respond more rapidly to treatment than do chronic/intracellular infections. Standard laboratory testing includes culture, and serum measurements of antistreptolysin-O (ASO), antihyaluronidase, anti-DNase-B, and Streptozyme; diagnosis can also be supported by response to treatment.	Psoriasis, rheumatoid arthritis, polymyositis, dermatomyositis, rheumatic fever, and many other chronic inflammatory disorders

---

[335] Santacroce L, Katz J. Helicobacter Pylori Infection Workup. emedicine.medscape.com/article/176938-workup#a0719 Updated: Feb 15, 2013
[336] Nasralla M, Haier J, Nicolson GL. Multiple mycoplasmal infections detected in blood of patients with chronic fatigue syndrome and/or fibromyalgia syndrome. *Eur J Clin Microbiol Infect Dis*. 1999 Dec;18(12):859-65
[337] "In studies on hundreds of U.S. and British veterans with Gulf War Illness, approximately 40-50% of Gulf War Illness patients show evidence of mycoplasmal infections compared to 6-9% in non- deployed, healthy subjects." Nicolson GL, Nasralla MY, Nicolson NL, Haier J. High Prevalence of Mycoplasmal Infections in Symptomatic (Chronic Fatigue Syndrome) Family Members of Mycoplasma-Positive Gulf War Illness Patients. *J Chronic Fatigue Syndrome* 2003; 11(2): 21-36
[338] Hughes LE, Smith PA, Bonell S, et al. Cross-reactivity between related sequences found in Acinetobacter sp., Pseudomonas aeruginosa, myelin basic protein and myelin oligodendrocyte glycoprotein in multiple sclerosis. *J Neuroimmunol*. 2003 Nov;144(1-2):105-15
[339] Hughes LE, Bonell S, Natt RS, et al. Antibody responses to Acinetobacter spp. and Pseudomonas aeruginosa in multiple sclerosis: prospects for diagnosis using the myelin-acinetobacter-neurofilament antibody index. *Clin Diagn Lab Immunol*. 2001 Nov;8(6):1181-8

Clinical Case Polymicrobial positivity in a patient diagnosed with systemic lupus erythematosus (SLE), mixed connective tissue disease (MCTD), Raynaud's syndrome, and secondary amyloidosis (inaccurately diagnosed as bilateral carpal tunnel syndrome and peripheral edema)—positivity toward *Mycoplasma*, *Chlamydia/Chlamydophila*, and parvovirus: Of these three results, the positivity against *Chlamydia/Chlamydophila pneumoniae* is the most actionable per published research; antibody titers against *Mycoplasma* and parvovirus are may indicate past "extinguished" or current "smouldering" infection/colonization—only a clinical trial with antibacterial and antiviral interventions (respectively) followed by monitoring 1) clinical response to treatment, 2) reduction in other markers of autoimmune disease activity, such as Sjogren's antibodies and anti-double-stranded DNA antibodies in this case, and 3) reduction in microbe-specific antibody titers would be able to prove or refute the microbe-autoimmunity links in this particular case. Negative results for anti-dsANA and CCP not shown.

DATE OF COLLECTION	TIME	DATE RECEIVED	DATE REPORTED	TIME
11/02/2012	13:15	11/03/2012	11/05/2012	14:11

TEST	RESULT	LIMITS
Antiextractable Nuclear Ag		
> RNP Antibodies	5.6H AI	0.0 - 0.9
> Smith Antibodies	1.8H AI	0.0 - 0.9

Test	Result	Units	Flag	Reference Range
Sjorgren's Ant-SS-A	2.0	AI	H	0.0-0.9
Sjorgren's Ant-SS-B	<0.2			-

Account Number	Patient ID	Control Number	Date and Time Collected	Date Reported	Sex	Age(Y/M/D)	Date of Birth
		0	04/26/13 09:46	04/30/13	F	69	

TESTS	RESULT	FLAG	UNITS	REFERENCE INTERVAL	LAB

Mycoplasma pneu. IgG/IgM Abs
  M pneumoniae IgG Abs   203   High   U/mL   0 - 99
                                                Negative: <100
                                                Indeterminate: 100 - 320
                                                Positive: >320

The reference interval established is intended as a baseline only. Values >100 may indicate a recent infection with Mycoplasma pneumoniae and need to be confirmed either by a positive IgM result and/or an additional specimen drawn 2-4 weeks later showing a significant increase in antibody levels.

  M pneumoniae IgM Abs   <770   U/mL   0 - 769
                                                Negative   <770

Clinically significant amount of M. pneumoniae antibody not detected.

Chl. pneumoniae (IgG/IgM/IgA)
  Chlamydia pneumoniae IgG   >1:256   High   Neg:<1:16
  Chlamydia pneumoniae IgM   <1:10   Neg:<1:10
  Chlamydia pneumoniae IgA   >1:256   High   Neg:<1:16

Parvovirus, Antibody   Stage: Final   Resulted: 11/2/2012

Test	Result	Units	Flag	Reference Range
Parvo IgG 163303	5.7	index	H	0.0-0.8
Negative <0.9				
Equivocal 0.9 - 1.1				
Positive >1.1				
Parvo IgM 163303	0.1	index		0.0-0.8
Negative <0.9				
Equivocal 0.9 - 1.1				
Positive >1.1				

Clinical Case Multiple laboratory abnormalities and polydysbiosis in a patient diagnosed with RA, psoriasis, and Hashimoto's thyroiditis—positivity toward *Proteus* (most likely urogenital), inflammatory gastrointestinal dysbiosis (markedly elevated lysozyme and lactoferrin with no obviously dysbiotic microbes detected), and high-"normal" titers against ASO (most likely pharyngeal): Patient has three different autoimmune diseases, HTN, and severe obesity.

Date and Time Collected	Date Entered	Date and Time Reported	Physician Name	NPI	Physician ID
05/24/12 14:42	05/24/12	05/30/12 15:39ET	VASQUEZ, A		

Tests Ordered
Testosterone, F Eqlib+T LC/MS; Thyroid Antibodies; Hemoglobin A1c; Thyroxine (T4) Free, Direct, S; DHEA-Sulfate; TSH; Prolactin; Estradiol; Reverse T3, Serum; Vitamin D, 25-Hydroxy; t-Transglutaminase (tTG) IgA; Triiodothyronine (T3); Ferritin, Serum; Venipuncture

TESTS	RESULT	FLAG	UNITS	REFERENCE INTERVAL	LAB
Testosterone, F Eqlib+T LC/MS					
Testosterone, Total, LC/MS	334.1	Low	ng/dL	348.0 - 1197.0	
Testosterone, Free	7.85		ng/dL	5.00 - 21.00	
% Free Testosterone	2.35		%	1.50 - 4.20	
Thyroid Antibodies					
Thyroid Peroxidase (TPO) Ab	235	High	IU/mL	0 - 34	
	Please note reference interval change				
Antithyroglobulin Ab	<20		IU/mL	0 - 40	
Siemens (DPC) ICMA Methodology					
Hemoglobin A1c	5.4		%	4.8 - 5.6	

Increased risk for diabetes: 5.7 - 6.4
Diabetes: >6.4
Glycemic control for adults with diabetes: <7.0

Thyroxine (T4) Free, Direct, S					
T4, Free (Direct)	1.12		ng/dL	0.82 - 1.77	
DHEA-Sulfate	267.7		ug/dL	160.0 - 449.0	
TSH	3.510		uIU/mL	0.450 - 4.500	
Prolactin	5.6		ng/mL	4.0 - 15.2	
Estradiol	28.4		pg/mL	7.6 - 42.6	
Roche ECLIA methodology					
Reverse T3, Serum	25.5		ng/dL	13.5 - 34.2	
Vitamin D, 25-Hydroxy	19.4	Low	ng/mL	30.0 - 100.0	

Date and Time Collected	Date Entered	Date and Time Reported	Physician Name	NPI	Physician ID
08/27/12 14:06	08/27/12	08/29/12 15:09ET	VASQUEZ, A		679

Tests Ordered
Anticardiolipin Ab, IgG/M, Qn; Immunoglobulin A, Qn, Serum; Antistreptolysin O Ab; Venipuncture

TESTS	RESULT	FLAG	UNITS	REFERENCE INTERVAL	LAB
Antistreptolysin O Ab	199.5		IU/mL	0.0 - 200.0	

PROTEUS OX - 19	POSITIVO 1:80	(This appears to be an antibody titer.)	
ESTUDIO	**RESULTADO**	**UNIDAD**	**REFERENCIA**
Acs. ANTI PEPTIDO CICLICO CITRULINADO (Ac. CCP) IgG	✱200.0	U/mL	0.00-5.00
Ac. ANTI-NUCLEARES	NEGATIVOS		NEGATIVOS

RHEUMATOID FACTOR	183 (H)	0 - 14 IU/mL
SED RATE WESTERGREN	28 (H)	0 - 15
C-REACTIVE PROTEIN	1.3 (H)	0 - 0.8 mg/dL
ANA TITER	1:80 (Abnl)	Negative
ANA PATTERN	Homogeneous (Abnl)	Negative
Result Narrative		
ANA TITER 2	1:160 (Abnl)	Negative
ANA PATTERN 2	Speckled (Abnl)	Negative

Clinical Case—continued Multiple laboratory abnormalities and multifocal polydysbiosis in a patient diagnosed with RA, psoriasis, and Hashimoto's thyroiditis (continued): Inflammatory gastrointestinal dysbiosis, presumably due to low-level *Klebsiella* and nonculturable yeast

Comprehensive Stool Analysis / Parasitology x3

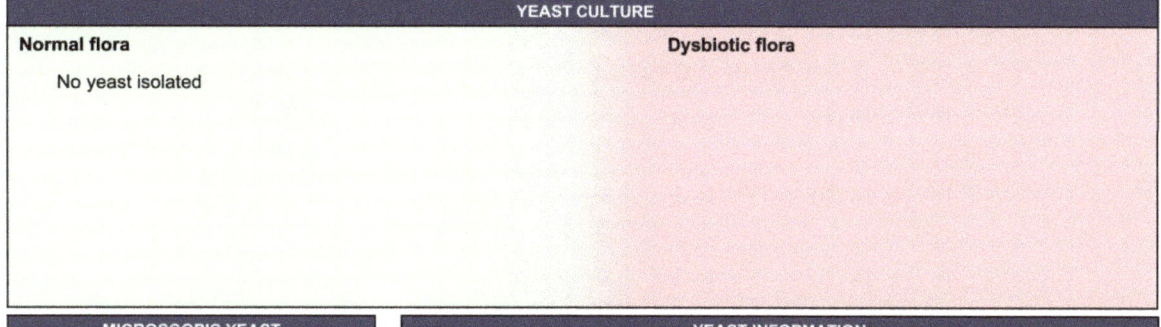

BACTERIOLOGY CULTURE		
Expected/Beneficial flora	**Commensal (Imbalanced) flora**	**Dysbiotic flora**
2+ Bacteroides fragilis group	1+ Klebsiella pneumoniae ssp pneumoniae	
3+ Bifidobacterium spp.		
4+ Escherichia coli		
3+ Lactobacillus spp.		
4+ Enterococcus spp.		
NG Clostridium spp.		
NG = No Growth		

BACTERIA INFORMATION

Expected /Beneficial bacteria make up a significant portion of the total microflora in a healthy & balanced GI tract. These beneficial bacteria have many health-protecting effects in the GI tract including manufacturing vitamins, fermenting fibers, digesting proteins and carbohydrates, and propagating anti-tumor and anti-inflammatory factors.

Clostridia are prevalent flora in a healthy intestine. Clostridium spp. should be considered in the context of balance with other expected/beneficial flora. Absence of clostridia or over abundance relative to other expected/beneficial flora indicates bacterial imbalance. If *C. difficile* associated disease is suspected, a Comprehensive Clostridium culture or toxigenic *C. difficile* DNA test is recommended.

Commensal (Imbalanced) bacteria are usually neither pathogenic nor beneficial to the host GI tract. Imbalances can occur when there are insufficient levels of beneficial bacteria and increased levels of commensal bacteria. Certain commensal bacteria are reported as dysbiotic at higher levels.

Dysbiotic bacteria consist of known pathogenic bacteria and those that have the potential to cause disease in the GI tract. They can be present due to a number of factors including: consumption of contaminated water or food, exposure to chemicals that are toxic to beneficial bacteria; the use of antibiotics, oral contraceptives or other medications; poor fiber intake and high stress levels.

YEAST CULTURE	
Normal flora	**Dysbiotic flora**
No yeast isolated	

MICROSCOPIC YEAST		YEAST INFORMATION
Result: **Expected:**		Yeast normally can be found in small quantities in the skin, mouth, intestine and mucocutaneous junctions. Overgrowth of yeast can infect virtually every organ system, leading to an extensive array of clinical manifestations. Fungal diarrhea is associated with broad-spectrum antibiotics or alterations of the patient's immune status. Symptoms may include abdominal pain, cramping and irritation. When investigating the presence of yeast, disparity may exist between culturing and microscopic examination. Yeast are not uniformly dispersed throughout the stool, this may lead to undetectable or low levels of yeast identified by microscopy, despite a cultured amount of yeast. Conversely, microscopic examination may reveal a significant amount of yeast present, but no yeast cultured. Yeast does not always survive transit through the intestines rendering it unvialble.
Many None - Rare		
The microscopic finding of yeast in the stool is helpful in identifying whether there is proliferation of yeast. Rare yeast may be normal; however, yeast observed in higher amounts (few, moderate, or many) is abnormal.		

Despite lackluster results in the microbiologic section of this comprehensive stool/microbiology text, results show markedly elevated lysozyme and lactoferrin, most likely attributable to exaggerated "dysbiotic" immune response against *Klebsiella pneumoniae* and nonculturable yeast. This case exemplifies the importance of interpreting microbiologic tests in patient-specific context.

INFLAMMATION			
	Within	Outside	Reference Range
→ Lysozyme*		1280	<= 600 ng/mL
→ Lactoferrin		29.2	< 7.3 µg/mL
White Blood Cells	None		None - Rare
Mucus	Neg		Neg

Lysozyme* is an enzyme secreted at the site of inflammation in the GI tract and elevated levels have been identified in IBD patients. **Lactoferrin** is a quantitative GI specific marker of inflammation used to diagnose and differentiate IBD from IBS and to monitor patient inflammation levels during active and remission phases of IBD. **White Blood Cells** (WBC): in the stool are an indication of an inflammatory process resulting in the infiltration of leukocytes within the intestinal lumen. WBCs are often accompanied by mucus and blood in the stool. **Mucus** in the stool may result from prolonged mucosal irritation or in a response to parasympathetic excitability such as spastic constipation or mucous colitis.

Clinical Case—continued Multiple laboratory abnormalities and multifocal polydysbiosis in a patient diagnosed with RA, psoriasis, and Hashimoto's thyroiditis: Urinalysis showing mild metabolic acidosis along with asymptomatic bacteruria/bacteriuria; urinary leukocytes (not normal) is noted.

FECHA 20/08/2011   # 200037

EXAMEN GENERAL DE ORINA

EDAD 33 AÑOS   **Sexo** M

PRUEBA	RESULTADO		REFERENCIA	
Densidad	+1.030		1.01 - 1.03	
pH	5.5		5.00 8.00	
Proteinas	0	mg/dl	0	mg/dl
Glucosa	0	mg/dl	0	mg/dl
Cetonas	0	mg/dl	0	mg/dl
Bilirrubinas	0		0	
Urobilinogeno	NORMAL		0.2	E.U./dl.
Hemoglobina	0		0	
Nitritos	NEGATIVO		Negativo	

Examen Microscopico 40x

Leucocitos:	0 A 1 POR 3 CAMPOS		Piocitos:	0
Eritrocitos:	0		Cilindros:	0
Cristales:	0		Bacterias:	MODERADAS
Filamento Moco:	MODERADO		Levaduras:	0

Clinical Case Multiple laboratory abnormalities in a patient diagnosed with multiple sclerosis: Elevated IgE corresponding with food allergies and immune dysfunction/activation; oxidative stress clearly indicated by low levels of glutathione.

Test Name	In Range	Out Of Range	Reference Range
HOMOCYSTEINE, CARDIOVASCULAR	5.2		<10.4 umol/L
IMMUNOGLOBULIN E		862 H	<OR=114 kU/L
GLUTATHIONE		526 L	544-1228 umol

Immune reactiviy suggesting chronic *Chlamydia/Chlamydophila pneumoniae* colonization; the particular relevance of this finding in this case is the correlation between *Chlamydia/Chlamydophila pneumoniae* infection and multiple sclerosis.[340]

```
CHLAMYDIA/CHLAMYDOPHILA
  ANTIBODY PANEL 1 (IGG)
  C. TRACHOMATIS IGG            <1:64
  C. PNEUMONIAE IGG                          1:256 H
  C. PSITTACI IGG               <1:64
     REFERENCE RANGE:   <1:64
```

Elevated IL-6 at 5.85 pg/ml (range 0.31-5.0) indicating immune activation; one might question the value of this test (ordered by another physician) except possibly for use in monitoring responsiveness to treatment.

```
INTERLEUKIN 6, HIGHLY
   SENSITIVE, ELISA                  5.85 H        0.31-5.00 pg/mL
```

Low intracellular red blood cell magnesium at 3.9 mg/dl (range 4.0-6.4) correlates with 1) insufficient magnesium intake, 2) increased renal loss and metabolic acidosis, and 3) oxidative stress in general and gluathone depletion in particular.

```
MAGNESIUM, RBC                         3.9 L        4.0-6.4 mg/dL
```

Clinical Case Normalization of antibody titers against *Streptococcus* following antibiotic-immunorestorative treatment in a patient with difficult-to-treat rheumatoid arthritis: Elevated anti-Streptococcal antibodies showing reduction/normalization following nutritional supplementation with immunorestorative vitamins, minerals and fatty acids and administration of azithromycin, emulsified oregano oil, and oral vancomycin. Patient also positive for *Chlamydia/Chlamydophila pneumoniae* at a titer of 1:256 (data not shown). Streptococcal bacteria can be involved in acute and chronic infections; typically the acute infection phenotype is extracellular while the chronic "dysbiotic" phenotype can be either/both extracellular and intracellular. Streptococcal bacteria are associated with numerous inflammatory and autoimmune diseases, particularly psoriasis, rheumatoid arthritis, and dermatomyositis. In brilliant research publshed by Svartz[341] rheumatoid arthritis was induced in animals by innoculating them with group B streptococci isolated from the nasopharynx of RA patients. Note also in the example below that in the intial testing, only 1 of the 3 tests was positive.

Account Number	Patient ID	Control Number	Date and Time Collected	Date Reported	Sex	Age(Y/M/D)	Date of Birth
			12/22/12 09:22	12/26/12	F		

TESTS	RESULT	FLAG	UNITS	REFERENCE INTERVAL	LAB
Anti-DNase B Strep Antibodies	134	High	U/mL	0 - 120	
Streptozyme	Negative			Neg:<1:100	
Antistreptolysin O Ab	63.3		IU/mL	0.0 - 200.0	

Date and Time Collected	Date Entered	Date and Time Reported	Physician Name	NPI	Physician ID
07/13/13 00:00	07/17/13	07/22/13 04:05ET			

Tests Ordered
Anti-DNase B Strep Antibodies; Written Authorization

TESTS	RESULT	FLAG	UNITS	REFERENCE INTERVAL	LAB
Anti-DNase B Strep Antibodies	99		U/mL	0 - 120	

Results verified by repeat testing

---

[340] Sriram S, et al. Comparative study of the presence of Chlamydia pneumoniae in cerebrospinal fluid of Patients with clinically definite and monosymptomatic multiple sclerosis. *Clin Diagn Lab Immunol*. 2002 Nov;9(6):1332-7 cvi.asm.org/content/9/6/1332.long

[341] "In experimental arthritis, produced by streptococci group B (Svartz), there appears in rats the same type of joint disease as in human RA and, besides, a rheumatoid factor (RF)-like macroglobulin, which cannot be distinguished by available methods from human RF macroglobulin. ...The streptococci B used in our investigations were mostly isolated from the nasopharynx of RA patients. Svartz N. The origin of rheumatoid arthritis. *Rheumatology*. 1975;6:322-8

DrV's perspective on the relativity of microbial activity—herpes simplex virus (HSV) as an example: Too often, doctors and clinicians seem to misunderstand the complexity and relativity of human microbial colonization, which—in this conversation—very clearly includes occult viral activity, even and specifically that which is not clinically manifest, that which is nonacute, and/or which is commonplace. Distinctions will be presented in the following table with clinical examples of HSV infection to follow.

Common (mis)perceptions	More accurate perceptions
• Patients either have infections that are clinically apperant or they are unaffected by microbes.	• In the human metaorganism/superorganism, microbial cells outnumber human cells by a ratio of 10 to 1, meaning that for each human cell, the body harbors ~10 microbes, allowing the statement that "humans" are really 90% microbes/bacteria.[342] • "Each person is host to some 100 trillion microbes, predominantly bacteria."[343] Thus, the total microbial load (TML) and total antigenic immunostimulatory load (TAIL) is quite considerable, whether or not a patient has an obvious "infection".
• If a patient has had a common infection such as HSV-1 or *Chlamydophila/Chlamydia pneumoniae*, then — when the infection is not appearant even though it might be persistent— it is considered to be irrelevant.	• Just because an infection is common does not mean that it is benign; HSV-1 is an example of a common infection (seen in approximately 50% of people worldwide) which has been correlated with several chronic health problems ranging from multiple sclerosis to Alzheimer's disease. • Just because the infection is not clinically *appearant* does not mean that the infection is "cleared" or clinically *irrelevant*; many chronic and persistent infections/colonizations remain subclinically active despite — or perhaps because of— the absense of an obvious vigorous immunological response.
• Chronic infections are seen quantitatively (ie, "you either had/have it or you don't").	• Chronic infections are both quantitative (ie, present or absent) and qualitative with respect to the impact that they have on metabolic processes and immunological/inflammatory reponses. Thus, the degree of the microbal load and microbial activity/replication is important, not simply the presence or absense of the microbe(s).
• Chronic inflammatory disorders are idiopathic; they result from "a combination of genetic predisposition with unidentified environmental triggers."	• Total microbial load (TML) and total antigenic immunostimulatory load (TAIL) contribute to activation of the innate immune response and the subsequent development of inflammatory diseases, the pattern of which will depend on other pro- and anti-inflammatory and immuno-regulatory and –dysregulatory balances.
• Microbial colonizations—like nutritional defiencies—are primarily singular.	• Microbial colonizations—like nutritional defiencies—are nearly always multiple—not singular. • The patterns of inflammatory responses are primarily secondary to the TML and TAIL of the patient's genetic, nutritional, microbial, immunological, mitochondrial, psychosocial, hormonal and xenobiotic statuses.

Clinical Cases—HSV1 positivity with varying antibody levels correlating with clinical outbreaks Lower antibody titers correlate with less viral activity: Here we see evidence of HSV seropositivity with a relatively low titer in a patient who has never experienced a clinical herpetic outbreak.

```
HSV I/II, IgG/Rfx Type II IgG
   HSV I/II IgG                        21.6    High      index       0.0 - 0.8
```

Higher antibody titers correlate with more viral activity: Here we see evidence of HSV seropositivity with a relatively high titer in a patient who experiences frequent clinical (oral) herpetic outbreaks.

```
HSV I/II, IgG/Rfx Type II IgG
   HSV I/II IgG                        36.5    High      index       0.0 - 0.8
                                                         Negative      <0.9
                                                         Equivocal  0.9 - 1.0
                                                         Positive      >1.0
```

---

[342] Dizikes C. 'We are 90% bacteria,' says researcher for Hospital Microbiome Project. *Chicago Tribune* 2013, Jan 02 articles.chicagotribune.com/2013-01-02/news/ct-met-microbiome-20130102_1_human-microbiome-bacteria-human-life
[343] Betts KS. A study in balance: how microbiomes are changing the shape of environmental health. *Environ Health Perspect*. 2011 Aug;119(8):A340-6

Lactulose-mannitol assay: assessment for intestinal hyperpermeability and malabsorption	
Overview and interpretation:	- The lactulose-mannitol assay is a highly validated assessment for the accurate determination of small intestine permeability. This test is used to diagnose "leaky gut", which is a common problem and contributor to systemic inflammation in patients with inflammation and immune dysfunction—see Chapter 4 of *Integrative Rheumatology*. Intestinal hyperpermeability reflects inflammation of and damage to the small intestine mucosa and is seen in patients with parasite infections, food allergies, celiac disease, malnutrition, bacterial infections, systemic ischemia or inflammation, ankylosing spondylitis, Crohn's disease, eczema, psoriasis, and those who consume enterotoxins such as NSAIDs and excess ethanol.[344]
- Elevations of **lactulose** indicate increased **paracellular** permeability caused by intestinal damage and are diagnostic of "leaky gut." *Clinical pearl*: remember that the "L" in *lactulose* rhymes with *leaky*. Decrements in **mannitol** suggest impaired **transcellular** absorption and suggest malabsorption in general and villous atrophy in particular. *Clinical pearl*: remember that the "M" in *mannitol* rhymes with *malabsorption*. Classically, in patients with damaged intestinal mucosa, we see a combined *increase* in *paracellular* permeability (measured with lactulose) and a *reduction* in *transcellular* transport (measured with mannitol); these divergent effects result in an increased lactulose-to-mannitol ratio.
Advantages:	- This test is safe and affordable for the assessment of small intestine mucosal integrity. Abnormal results—"leaky gut" and/or malabsorption—generally indicate one or more of following, which can be recalled by the acronym M.E.D. F.I.T.[345]
  1. <u>Malnutrition</u>: Such as due to poor intake, catabolism, or malabsorption; we might also consider in particular: zinc, glutamine, and vitamin D3.
  2. <u>Enterotoxins</u>: Such as NSAIDs or ethanol.
  3. **<u>Dysbiosis</u>: including yeast, bacteria, protozoa, amebas, worms, etc.****
  4. **<u>Food allergies</u>: Including celiac disease, but also with milder food allergies.****
  5. <u>Inflammatory bowel disease</u>: Crohn's disease, ulcerative colitis, or family history of IBD.
  6. <u>Trauma or major injury/inflammation (sufficient to induce a catabolic response)</u>: Tissue hypoxia, trauma, recent surgery, etc.

  **Note that of these six items, all but two can be excluded by history and patient assessment; therefore, a clinician could very reasonably perform specialized stool testing to assess for dysbiosis since negative results in a patient with increased intestinal permeability would then point toward food allergy. |
| *Limitations:* | - Abnormalities and the identification of "leaky gut" are nonspecific and do not point to a specific or single diagnosis or treatment. |
| *Comments:* | - The value of this test is two-fold: 1) as a screening test for the above-mentioned disorders, and 2) as a method for determining the efficacy of treatment once the cause of the problem has been putatively identified and treated.
- This test can be used to promote compliance and to encourage the use of additional testing in patients who are otherwise prone to noncompliance or who resist other tests, such as stool testing. In other words, the clinician can gain an advantage by showing the patient an objective abnormality which then validates the need for treatment and additional testing.
- I only use this test on rare occasions because I more commonly either assume that a patient has leaky gut if he/she has one of the aforementioned conditions or we move directly to stool testing and comprehensive parasitology—clearly one of the most valuable tests in the management and treatment of systemic inflammation and immune dysfunction—otherwise known as "autoimmunity" and "allergy." |

---

[344] Miller AL. The Pathogenesis, Clinical Implications, and Treatment of Intestinal Hyperpermeability. *Alt Med Rev* 1997:2(5):330-345
[345] Credit to Angelique Marquez for the MEDFIT acronym and proving that great teachers inspire genious in their students ☺

Clinical Case **Highly abnormal lactulose-mannitol ratio in a patient with idiopathic peripheral neuropathy prior to comprehensive stool analysis and parasitology showing intestinal dysbiosis**: This 40-yo man presented with a multiyear history of periodic febrile exacerbations of peripheral neuropathy that would cause severe paresthesias and motor deficits. Patient had been evaluated by several board-certified medical neurologists to no avail. Laboratory, imaging, electrodiagnostic studies, and cerebrospinal fluid (CSF) analysis revealed nonspecific abnormalities that did not lead to an established diagnosis. From an integrative naturopathic and functional medicine perspective, food allergy and intestinal dysbiosis are the most obvious probable etiologies; these clinical suspicions were confirmed with laboratory testing showing increased intestinal permeability and gastrointestinal dysbiosis.

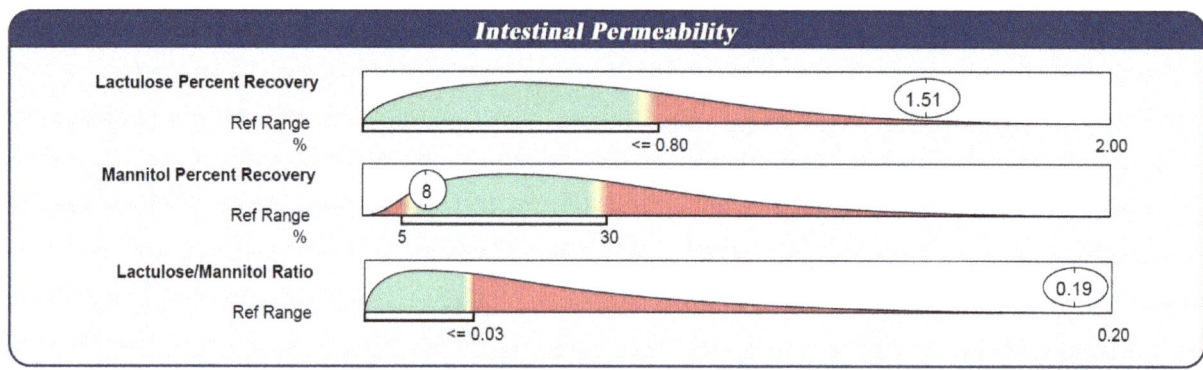

As expected, comprehensive parasitology showed intestinal dysbiosis, including insufficiency of *Lactobacillus* and presence of *Psuedomonas* and abnormal yeast species. Of particular note, *Psuedomonas aeruginosa* shows cross-reactivity with human neuronal tissues.[346,347] Eradication of the dysbiotic condition with a combination of dietary improvement, nutritional supplementation, hormonal optimization, and antimicrobial drugs and herbs lead to rapid and sustained remission of this "idiopathic peripheral neuropathy" which had defied standard medical diagnosis and treatment for many years.

Comprehensive Stool Analysis / Parasitology x3

MICROBIOLOGY

Bacteriology Culture

Beneficial flora		Imbalances		Dysbiotic flora	
Bifidobacter	4+	Haemolytic E. coli	4+	Pseudomonas sp.	4+
E. coli	4+	Gamma strep	2+		
Lactobacillus	2+				

Mycology (Yeast) Culture

Normal flora		Dysbiotic flora
Candida glabrata	1+	
Rhodotorula sp.	1+	

---

[346] Hughes LE, Bonell S, Natt RS, et al. Antibody responses to Acinetobacter spp. and Pseudomonas aeruginosa in multiple sclerosis: prospects for diagnosis using the myelin-acinetobacter-neurofilament antibody index. *Clin Diagn Lab Immunol.* 2001 Nov;8(6):1181-8 cvi.asm.org/content/8/6/1181.full.pdf
[347] Hughes LE, Smith PA, Bonell S, Natt RS, Wilson C, Rashid T, Amor S, Thompson EJ, Croker J, Ebringer A. Cross-reactivity between related sequences found in Acinetobacter sp., Pseudomonas aeruginosa, myelin basic protein and myelin oligodendrocyte glycoprotein in multiple sclerosis. *J Neuroimmunol.* 2003 Nov;144(1-2):105-15

Comprehensive stool analysis and comprehensive parasitology	
Overview and interpretation:	- **This is clearly one of the most valuable tests in clinical practice when working with patients with chronic fatigue, systemic inflammation, and autoimmunity. Second only to routine laboratory assessments such as CBC, chemistry panel, and CRP, the importance of stool testing and comprehensive parasitology assessments must be appreciated by progressive clinicians of all disciplines.**
- Stool testing must be performed by a specialty laboratory because the quality of testing provided by most standard "medical labs" and hospitals is completely inadequate. Initial samples should be collected on three separate occasions by the patient and each sample should be analyzed separately by the laboratory.
- Important qualitative and quantitative markers include the following:
- **Beneficial bacteria ("probiotics")**: Microbiological testing should quantify and identify various beneficial bacteria, which should be present at "+4" levels on a 0-4 scale.
- **Harmful and potentially harmful bacteria, protozoans, amebas, etc.**: Questionable or harmful microbes should be eradicated even if they are not identified as true pathogens in the Paleo-classic Pasteurian/Kochian sense.[348]
- **Yeast and mycology**: At least two tests must be performed for a complete assessment: 1) yeast culture, and 2) microscopic examination for yeast elements. Both tests are necessary because some patients—perhaps those with the most severe symptomatology and the most favorable response to anti-yeast treatment—will have a negative yeast culture and positive findings on the microscopic examination. In other words, these patients have intestinal yeast that contributes to their disease/symptomatology but which does not grow on culture despite being clearly visible with microscopy; a similar pattern (using a swab of the rectal mucosa rather than microscopy) is referred to as "negative culture with positive smear."[349]
- **Microbial sensitivity testing**: An important component to parasitology testing is the determination of which anti-microbial agents (natural and synthetic) the microbe is sensitive to. This helps to guide and enhance the effectiveness of anti-microbial therapy.
- **Secretory IgA**: SIgA levels are elevated in patients who are having an immune response to either food or microbial antigens.[350] Thus, in a patient with minimal dysbiosis, say for example with *Candida albicans*, an elevated sIgA can indicate that the patient is having a hypersensitivity reaction to an otherwise benign microbe—in this case, eradication of the microbe is warranted and may result in a positive clinical response. Low sIgA suggests either primary or secondary immune defect such as selective sIgA deficiency[351] or malnutrition, stress, prednisone/corticosteroids, or possibly mycotoxicosis (immunosuppression due to fungal immunotoxins). In addition to addressing any systemic causative factors, a low sIgA may be addressed with the administration of bovine colostrum, glutamine, vitamin A, and *Saccharomyces boulardii*; the following doses may be considered for use in adults with proportionately smaller doses for children:
- Bovine colostrum: 2.4 – 3.6 grams per day in divided doses for adults. No drug interactions are known. Side effects may include increased energy, insomnia, and stimulation. One study in particular used very large doses of 10 grams per

---

[348] Vasquez A. Reducing Pain and Inflammation Naturally. Part 6: Nutritional and Botanical Treatments Against "Silent Infections" and Gastrointestinal Dysbiosis, Commonly Overlooked Causes of Neuromusculoskeletal Inflammation and Chronic Health Problems. *Nutr Perspect* 2006; Jan

[349] "According to Galland, the best predictor of who will respond to anticandida medication is a negative stool culture combined with a positive smear of the rectal mucosa (for the identification of intracellular hyphal forms of the organism); however, even that test is not 100% reliable." Gaby AR. Before you order that lab test: part 2. *Townsend Letter for Doctors and Patients*. 2004; January findarticles.com/p/articles/mi_m0ISW/is_246/ai_112728028

[350] Quig DW, Higley M. Noninvasive assessment of intestinal inflammation: inflammatory bowel disease vs. irritable bowel syndrome. *Townsend Letter for Doctors and Patients* 2006;Jan:74-5

[351] "Selective IgA deficiency is the most common form of immunodeficiency. Certain select populations, including allergic individuals, patients with autoimmune and gastrointestinal tract disease and patients with recurrent upper respiratory tract illnesses, have an increased incidence of this disorder." Burks AW Jr, Steele RW. Selective IgA deficiency. *Ann Allergy*. 1986;57:3-13

> **Comprehensive stool analysis and comprehensive parasitology**
>
> day for four days in children and found no adverse effects[352]; another case report of a child involved the use of 50 grams per day for at least two weeks and showed no adverse effects.[353]
> - **Glutamine**: 6 grams 3 times per day (18 grams per day) is a common dosage with significant literature support.
> - **Vitamin A**: Correction of subclinical vitamin A deficiency improves mucosal integrity and increases sIgA production in humans.[354] Common doses used by integrative clinicians are in the range of 200,000 IU to 300,000 for a limited amount of time, generally 1-4 weeks; thereafter the dose is tapered. Patients are educated as to manifestations of toxicity (see the chapter on *Therapeutics* toward the end of this book) and the importance of limited duration of treatment.
> - *Saccharomyces boulardii*: Common dose for adults is 250 mg thrice daily; ability of this treatment to increase sIgA levels and its anti-infective efficacy have been documented in human and animal studies.
>
> - **Short-chain fatty acids**: These are produced by intestinal bacteria. Quantitative excess indicates bacterial overgrowth of the intestines, while insufficiency indicates a lack of probiotics or an insufficiency of dietary substrate, i.e., soluble fiber. Abnormal patterns of individual short-chain fatty acids indicate qualitative/quantitative abnormalities in gastrointestinal microflora, particularly anaerobic bacteria that cannot be identified with routine bacterial cultures.
> - **Beta-glucuronidase**: This is an enzyme produced by several different intestinal bacteria. High levels of beta-glucuronidase in the intestinal lumen serve to nullify the benefits of detoxification (specifically glucuronidation) by cleaving the toxicant from its glucuronide conjugate. This can result in re-absorption of the toxicant through the intestinal mucosa which then re-exposes the patient to the toxin that was previously detoxified ("enterohepatic recirculation" or "enterohepatic recycling"[355]). This is an exemplary aspect of "auto-intoxication" that results in chronic fatigue and upregulation of Phase 1 detoxification systems (Chapter 4 of *Integrative Rheumatology*).
> - **Lactoferrin**: The iron-binding glycoprotein lactoferrin is an inflammatory marker that helps distinguish functional disorders (i.e., IBS) from more serious diseases (i.e., IBD). Approximate values are as follows:
>   - Healthy and IBS: 2 mcg/ml
>   - Severe dysbiosis: up to 120 mcg/ml
>   - Inactive IBD: 60-250 mcg/ml
>   - Active IBD: > 400 mcg/ml.
> - **Lysozyme**: Elevated in proportion to intestinal inflammation in dysbiosis and IBD.
> - **Other markers**: Other markers of digestion, inflammation, and absorption are reported with the more comprehensive panels performed on stool samples. These tests are not always necessary, but such additional information is always helpful when working with complex patients. These markers are relatively self-explanatory and/or are described on the results of the test by the laboratory.

---

[352] "In this double blind placebo-controlled trial, 80 children with rotavirus diarrhea were randomly assigned to receive orally either 10 g of IIBC (containing 3.6 g of antirotavirus antibodies) daily for 4 days or the same amount of a placebo preparation." Sarker SA, Casswall TH, Mahalanabis D, Alam NH, Albert MJ, Brussow H, Fuchs GJ, Hammerstrom L. Successful treatment of rotavirus diarrhea in children with immunoglobulin from immunized bovine colostrum. *Pediatr Infect Dis J*. 1998 Dec;17(12):1149-54

[353] Lactobin-R is a commercial hyperimmune bovine colostrum with some specificity for cryptosporidiosis; administration to a 4 year old child with AIDS and severe diarrhea resulted in significant clinical improvement in the diarrhea and "permanent elimination of the parasite from the gut as assessed through serial jejunal biopsy and stool specimens." Shield et al. Bovine colostrum immunoglobulin concentrate for cryptosporidiosis in AIDS. *Arch Dis Child*. 1993 Oct;69(4):451-3

[354] "It can increase resistance to infection by increasing mucosal integrity, increasing surface immunoglobulin A (sIgA) and enhancing adequate neutrophil function. If infection occurs, vitamin A can act as an immune enhancer, increasing the adequacy of natural killer (NK) cells and increasing antibody production." Faisel H, Pittrof R. Vitamin A and causes of maternal mortality: association and biological plausibility. *Public Health Nutr*. 2000 Sep;3(3):321-7

[355] Parker RJ, Hirom PC, Millburn P. Enterohepatic recycling of phenolphthalein, morphine, lysergic acid diethylamide (LSD) and diphenylacetic acid in the rat. Hydrolysis of glucuronic acid conjugates in the gut lumen. *Xenobiotica*. 1980 Sep;10(9):689-70

Comprehensive stool analysis and comprehensive parasitology	
Advantages:	- **Stool analysis in general and parasitology assessments in particular provide supremely valuable information in the comprehensive assessment and treatment of patients with complex illnesses such as chronic fatigue, irritable bowel syndrome, fibromyalgia, and all of the autoimmune/rheumatic diseases.**
Limitations:	- Tests vary in price from $250-$400. - Anaerobic bacteria are difficult to culture. - Specialty examinations, such as for *Helicobacter pylori* antigen and enterohemorrhagic *E. coli* cytotoxin, must be requested specifically at additional cost.
Comments:	- I have found stool testing to be the single most powerful diagnostic tool for helping chronically ill patients to attain improved health. Insights from stool/parasitology testing can be used to implement powerfully effective treatments. The value of this test in the treatment of patients with rheumatic disease must be appreciated.

Concepts, facts, and tools to promote safe clinical practice

Concept: Not all "Injury-related Problems" are "Injury-related Problems"

In the case of most acute injuries, the underlying problem is often the injury itself. However, the physician must conduct a thorough history and examination to assess for possible underling pathologies that cause or contribute to the problem that "appears" to be injury-related. Congenital anomalies, underlying pathology, previous injury, occult infections, and psychoemotional disorders may have been present *before* the "injury."

> "Pediatric infections and neoplasms are notorious for masquerading as sport injuries."
>
> "...Take the relevant history directly from the patient, and keep tumors and infections high on your list of differential diagnoses... For example, about 15% of children with leukemia present with musculoskeletal complaints..."
>
> Shaw BA, Gerardi JA, Hennrikus WL. How to avoid orthopedic pitfalls in children. *Patient Care* 1999 Feb

Just because the patient reports a problem such as pain following an injury does not mean that the injury is the *sole* cause of the pain. *Do not let a biased history lead you down the wrong path*. **In children and young adults, 5% of "sports-related" injuries are associated with preexisting infection, anomalies, or other conditions.** In adult women, "…between 9% and 20% of women with breast cancer attribute their symptoms to previous trauma to the breast. In these cases, the association of the breast mass with a traumatic event resulted in a delay in diagnosis ranging from four months to one year."[356]

A group of German physicians describe a man who presented with a soft-tissue pain following a soccer game; he was later diagnosed with a malignant tumor—synovial sarcoma.[357] Similarly, Wakeshima and Ellen[358] describe a young athletic woman who presented with chronic hip pain. The woman's history was significant for ulcerative colitis, but otherwise her radiographs were normal and her history and examination lead to a diagnosis of trochanteric bursitis. However, the patient's condition did not respond to routine treatment, and additional investigation over several months lead to a diagnosis of giant cell carcinoma. The authors concluded, "This case shows **the importance of repeat radiographic studies in patients whose joint pain does not respond or responds slowly to conservative therapy, despite initial normal findings.**"

What you expect to find and hear when taking a trauma-related history is that **1) a healthy patient** with no previous health concerns was **2) exposed to a traumatic event**, the history and consequences of which perfectly coincide with the injury you are assessing in your office, and that **3) your physical examination findings are all consistent** and lead to a specific diagnosis, which then **4) responds to your treatment**. If you find discrepancies between the history of the injury and your physical examination findings (e.g., fever after a "sports-related" injury), if the patient appears unhealthy in disproportion to the presenting complaint, or if the patient does not respond to your treatment, then you must consider the possibility of preexisting or concomitant disease.

When treating children, be very careful to get an accurate history—this is difficult since your two sources of information are not very reliable: parents often think that they already have the problem figured out, and so their history will be biased toward convincing you of what they think is the problem and solution; children are often not good historians and can form illogical relationships between events that can be misleading.

Astute doctors search for and rule-out/exclude preexisting and underlying pathology before ascribing the problem to the "obvious cause." Always assess for consistency between the history, examination findings, and response to treatment—inconsistencies suggest the need for additional investigation.

---

[356] Seifert S. Medical Illness Simulating Trauma (MIST) syndrome: case reports and discussion of syndrome. *Fam Med* 1993 Apr;25(4):273-6
[357] Engel C, Kelm J, Olinger A. Blunt trauma in soccer. The initial manifestation of synovial sarcoma. [Article in German] *Zentralbl Chir* 2001 Jan;126(1):68-71
[358] Wakeshima Y, Ellen MI. Atypical hip pain origin in a young athletic woman: a case report of giant cell carcinoma. *Arch Phys Med Rehabil* 2001 Oct;82(10):1472-5

Chapter 1: Clinical Assessments and Concepts

> **Previous health history**
> **+**
> **History of the present complaint**
> **+**
> **Clinical observations and physical examination findings**
> **+**
> **Response to treatment**
>
> *If all 4 parts of the story do not add up perfectly, then you need to consider alternate diagnoses and take appropriate steps to ensure patient care.*

- **Abuse:** child abuse, adult abuse, elder abuse → Assess and report to authorities as indicated
- **Systemic illness:** cancer, infection, rheumatic
- **Preexisting condition:** metabolic disorder or congenital anomaly
- **Inadequate compliance with treatment** → Discover and address cause of non-compliance

If you have a specific condition in mind, then test specifically for it. If you suspect preexisting/concomitant illness but are unsure of exact nature of the condition, gather additional information by:

1) **Taking a more detailed history,**
2) **Ordering lab tests:** CBC, chemistry panel, ferritin, hsCRP, UA
3) **Obtaining diagnostic imaging:** radiographs, bone scan, MRI, CT, US
4) **Reassessing patient** within two weeks for progression of disease or crossing diagnostic threshold.
5) **Referral or co-management:** if the patient does not respond to your treatment and/or you suspect an underlying serious pathology, refer the patient to another physician at least for co-management. Put your referral in writing and chart appropriately. "When in doubt, refer it out."

Clinical management: Inconsistencies between the history, exams, and response to treatment indicate the need for additional investigation and additional diagnostic considerations.

Clinical management: Inconsistencies between the history, exams, and response to treatment indicate the need for additional investigation and additional diagnostic considerations.

High-Risk Pain Patients

When a patient has musculoskeletal pain and any of the following characteristics, radiographs should be considered as an appropriate component of comprehensive evaluation. These considerations are particularly—though not exclusively—relevant for spine and low-back pain.[359]

1. More than 50 years of age
2. Physical trauma (accident, fall, etc.)
3. Pain at night
4. Back pain not relieved by lying supine
5. Neurologic deficits (motor or sensory)
6. Unexplained weight loss
7. Documentation or suspicion of inflammatory arthropathy[360]
    - Ankylosing spondylitis
    - Lupus
    - Rheumatoid arthritis
    - Juvenile rheumatoid arthritis
    - Psoriatic arthritis
8. Drug or alcohol abuse (increased risk of infection, nutritional deficiencies, anesthesia)
9. History of cancer
10. Intravenous drug use
11. Immunosuppression, due to illness (e.g., HIV) or medications (e.g., steroids or cyclosporine)
12. History of corticosteroid use (causes osteoporosis and increased risk for infection)
13. Fever above 100° F or suspicion of septic arthritis or osteomyelitis
14. Diabetes (increased risk of infection, nutritional deficiencies, anesthesia)
15. Hypertension (abdominal aneurysm: low back pain, nausea, pulsatile abdominal mass)
16. Recent visit for same problem and not improved
17. Patient seeking compensation for pain/ injury (increased need for documentation)
18. Skin lesion (psoriasis, melanoma, dermatomyositis, the butterfly rash of lupus, scars from previous surgery, accident, etc....)
19. Deformity or immobility
20. Lymphadenopathy (suggests cancer or infection)
21. Elevated ESR/CRP (cancer, infection, inflammatory disorder)
22. Elevated WBC count
23. Elevated alkaline phosphatase (bone lesions, metabolic bone disease, hepatopathy, vitamin D deficiency)
24. Elevated acid phosphatase (occasionally used to monitor prostate cancer)
25. Positive rheumatoid factor and/or CCP—cyclic citrullinated protein antibodies
26. Positive HLA-B27 (propensity for inflammatory arthropathies)
27. Serum gammopathy (multiple myeloma is the most common primary bone tumor)
28. "High-risk for disease" *examples*:
    - Long-term heavy smoking of cigarettes
    - Long-term exposure to radiation
    - Obesity
29. Strong family history of inflammatory, musculoskeletal, or malignant disease
30. Others:_____
_____
_____
_____

---

[359] Remember that metastasis often travel first from the primary site to bone, therefore bone pain may be an early manifestation of occult cancer. Most of the above are from "Table 1: The high-risk patient: clinical indications for radiography in low back pain patients." J Taylor, DC, DACBR, D Resnick, MD. Imaging decisions in the management of low back pain. *Advances in Chiropractic*. Mosby Year Book. 1994; 1-28

[360] Radiographs are often essential for diagnosis or to rule out complications of the disease. For example, in patients with inflammatory arthropathies such as these, spontaneous rupture of the transverse ligament (at the odontoid process) has been reported; although rare, this complication could be life-threatening if mismanaged or undiagnosed.

Concept: Safe Patient + Safe Treatment = Safe Outcome

The purpose of performing the history and physical examination on a new *or established* patient is to determine their current health status—including their mental and emotional health and their physical health, particularly as this relates to important and life-threatening possibilities such as cancer, infections, fractures, systemic diseases, and neurologic compromise. The questions that lead this investigation are: "**What is this patient's current status?**" "**Does this patient have a serious disease, neurologic injury, or are they at high risk for developing a serious complication in the near future that can be prevented with appropriate care *now*?**"

Is your patient safe?

- The question to ask yourself is, "Is this patient's health problem or current complaint/exacerbation a manifestation of an underlying condition that could result in a negative outcome?
- If a patient comes to you with a headache, and you neglect to find that their blood pressure is 230/130, then you missed the opportunity to help them avoid the stroke that they could have after leaving your office.
- If a patient comes to you with a complaint of low back pain, and you neglect to perform a neurologic examination to find that *the patient already has a neurologic deficit even before you treated them*, then you have lost the opportunity to defend yourself in court when the patient later claims that *your* treatment and *your* management of their case is the reason that they now have a permanent neurologic deficit.

Is your treatment safe?: Have you been perfectly clear with the patient about the risks and benefits of your treatment plan? **Have you obtained informed consent**? Have you charted **"PAR-B"** to indicate that you have discussed the **P**rocedures, **A**lternatives, **R**isks, and **B**enefits of your treatment plan? Have you been clear about the duration of treatment and the need for appropriate follow-up? If you are prescribing nutrition or botanical medicines, have you informed the patient about the duration of treatment? **Have you looked for contraindications to your otherwise brilliant treatment plan**? What about the fact that this patient was on corticosteroids for the past 15 years and only discontinued prednisone 2 months before arriving at your office? *The patient may have steroid-induced osteoporosis even though he/she is no longer on prednisone.* When you recommend that your patient take 100,000 IU of vitamin A to treat her throat infection, what happens when she presents to your office 8 months later with signs of vitamin A toxicity because she continued her treatment plan indefinitely rather than using it only for 7 days as you had intended?

> **Check your work**
> Double-check to ensure that your patient is safe (no forthcoming complications or predictable emergencies) and that your treatment is safe (appropriate, effective, clearly communicated, and time-limited with instructions to return for office visit).

==Be sure to put a time limit on your treatment plans.== Every treatment plan should be 1) given to the patient in legible print and clear statements, 2) be copied for the chart, 3) include "what to do if things get worse" in the event of adverse treatment effect or exacerbation of problem, and 4) include patient's responsibility for returning to office/clinic for follow-up and reassessment.

Informed consent: From a legal standpoint, doctors can only treat a patient after the patient has given *consent to treatment*. Patients can only authoritatively consent to treatment after they have been educated about the treatment—thereafter, they can provide *informed consent*. Educating the patient requires discussion (and documentation) of each of the following:

- Procedures—what may take place, what is required; duration, costs, follow-up,
- Alternatives—what options are available,
- Risks—what risks are involved,
- Benefits—what benefits can be reasonably expected,
- Questions—allow for the patient to ask questions and receive answers.

This is commonly charted as "**PARB—no questions**" or "**PARB—questions answered**" once the patient gives consent to treatment; alternatively and more humorously, this may be charted as "**PAR-B-Q**".

Concept: Four Clues to Discovering Underlying Problems

When I taught Orthopedics at Bastyr University I encouraged students to search for specific **sets of clues** when evaluating patients. These clues—often insignificant in isolation but meaningful in combination—were often the "red flags" that could help make the difference between an accurate diagnosis and a missed diagnosis. These four categories can be recalled with the mnemonic "*S.C.I.N.*" or "*S.C.I.M.*" These four areas of assessment/safety emphasis differ from the "vindicates" mnemonic which is used for differential diagnosis.

Vindicates: a popular mnemonic acronym for differential diagnosis	
V	Vascular / Visceral referral
I	Infectious / Inflammatory / Immunologic
N	Neurologic / Nutritional / New growth: neoplasia or pregnancy
D	Deficiency / Degenerative
I	Iatrogenic (drug related) / Intoxication / Idiosyncratic
C	Congenital / Cardiac or circulatory
A	Allergy / Autoimmune / Abuse: drugs, alcohol, physical
T	Trauma / Toxicity
E	Endocrine / Exposure
S	Subluxation / Somatic dysfunction / Structural / Stress / Secondary gain

- **Systemic symptoms and signs**: Ask about systemic signs and symptoms such as fever, weight loss, lymphadenopathy, or skin rash in patients who present with pain because these "whole body" manifestations might indicate an underlying or concomitant disease that deserves attention, either independently from the musculoskeletal pain, or as a cause of the musculoskeletal pain. For example, "headache" may appear benign, whereas "headache with fever and skin rash" suggests meningitis—a medical emergency. "Low-back pain" is a common occurrence; yet "low-back pain with weight loss and fever" might suggest occult malignancy, osteomyelitis, or other systemic disease.

- **Complications:** We *ask about* and *look for* already existing complications, such as "numbness, weakness, tingling in the arms or hands, legs or feet" to rapidly screen for neurologic deficits and we follow this up with screening assessments such as "squat and rise", toe walk, heel walk, and reflexes for spinal cord and lower extremity neuromuscular integrity. Additionally, when dealing with patients with spine-related complaints or injuries, we also ask about changes or loss of function in bowel and bladder control and numbness near the anus or genitals, which may be the *only* clinical clues to cauda equina syndrome—a medical emergency. Ask about effects of the condition on ADL (activities of daily living) to attain a more comprehensive view of the condition and to ensure that the patient's story is consistent.

- **Indicators from the history**: We look for specific "red flags" and "yellow flags" such as trauma, risk factors (such as smoking, prednisone, alcohol), or a positive history of chronic infections or cancer. Nonmechanical musculoskeletal pain in a patient with a history of or high risk for cancer is highly suspicious and mandates thorough investigation.

- **Non-Mechanical pain**: Non-mechanical pain suggests a pathologic etiology rather than simple joint dysfunction. Pain at night, pain that occurs without an inciting injury, pain that is not strongly affected by motion and is not powerfully provoked by your physical examination assessments suggests the possibility of underlying disorder such as cancer, neuropathy, or infection. However, the ability to elicit an exacerbation of pain with "mechanical" maneuvers does not indicate that the pain is "mechanical" and therefore "non-pathologic." Mechanical pain can still be pathologic pain, such as the exquisite pain felt by patients with spinal fractures—they may be neurologically intact, they do have pain worse with motion, but they are not safe to manipulate, and they require appropriate treatment and referral on an urgent basis.

Check your work
Keeping these four assessment categories in mind can serve as a useful "checkpoint" to ensure that your patient is safe, and that your treatment is appropriate and therefore safe, too.

Concept: Special Considerations in the Evaluation of Children

> "Pediatric infections and neoplasms are notorious for masquerading as sport injuries. … There is only one way to avoid this trap: Take the relevant history directly from the patient, and keep tumors and infections high on your list of differential diagnoses."[361]

- **Consider the possibility of child abuse when a child presents with an injury:** As a non-naïve physician, you always have to consider the possibility of child abuse when a child presents with an injury. Be detailed in your history taking, and be sure to search for discrepancies between 1) the child's version of the incident, 2) the adult's version of the incident, and 3) what is realistic (based on your practical life experience and clinical training). As a primary care physician, you are obligated to report your *suspicion* of child abuse to law enforcement agencies and/or child protective services.
- **Children heal quickly:** This rapid healing is good as long as tissues are approximated. But if a fractured bone is displaced and not correctly replaced, then problematic malunion deformities may result *within **days***.
- **Children are more susceptible to rapidly progressing infections than are adults:** Soft tissue, joint, and bone infections need to be diagnosed expeditiously and treated aggressively.
- **Children are radiographically different from adults:** Make sure that your radiographs are interpreted by a competent radiologist with experience in the interpretation of *pediatric radiographs*. Radiographic considerations specific to children include:
    - **Epiphyseal growth plates**
    - **Secondary ossification centers**
    - **Variants in trabecular patterns and bone densities**
    - **Specific conditions that happen only in children, such as slipped capital femoral epiphysis**
    - **Congenital anomalies**
    - **Difficulty following directions with positioning** (applies to some adults, too!)
    - **Bone scans can be difficult to interpret in children:** Bone scans derive their value from the demonstration of a focal increase in uptake of radioactive isotopes, which demonstrates and localizes an area of increased metabolic activity. In adults, this increased and localized activity generally indicates pathology, especially malignant disease in bone (primary or metastatic) and recent fracture. In children, however, since their bones are already highly metabolically active due to the normal growth process, bone scans are difficult to interpret and are not highly reliable for the demonstration of focal lesions.

Playground injury or child abuse? Infection or cancer? Undiagnosed developmental disorder, congenital anomaly, or metabolic illness?
Always consider the possibility of abuse, cancer, infection, or congenital anomaly as a cause of musculoskeletal pain in children, even if the injury appears to be related to injury or trauma. Strongly consider lab tests, as well as radiographs (interpreted by a pediatric radiologist). When in doubt, refer for second opinion. If you suspect abuse, you have a legal and ethical obligation to report your <u>suspicion</u>.

---

[361] Shaw BA, Gerardi JA, Hennrikus WL. How to avoid orthopedic pitfalls in children. *Patient Care* 1999; Feb 28: 95-116

Concept: Differences between Primary Healthcare and Spectator Sports

In baseball, "errors" have been defined as "a defensive mistake that allows a batter to stay at the plate or reach first base, or that advances a base runner."[362] In baseball, a few errors can make the difference between winning and losing a particular game or season. However, a few errors in a game are to be expected, and ultimately the team can start over at the next game or season and try to do better.

Healthcare, however, is not a game, and even relatively minor errors such as the doctor's forgetting to ask a particular question or perform a specific test can result in a patient's catastrophic injury or death. In healthcare, when we are dealing with serious injuries and illnesses, even a single "error" is not allowed. "Failure to diagnose" is one of the biggest reasons for malpractice claims against doctors; such judgments often result in loss of licensure and awards of hundreds of thousands of dollars. "Failure to treat" results

> **Don't be naïve**
> While your compassion for human suffering and your love of nutrition and exercise may have directed you into healthcare, your professional success and survival will depend in large part on your ability to manage the technical and defensive aspects of clinical practice.
>
> Neuromusculoskeletal disorders and autoimmune diseases are "big league" clinical problems, and they need to be taken seriously.

when the patient is injured because the doctor failed to effectively treat the patient or when the doctor failed to provide the appropriate referral to a specialist in a timely manner. Such failures are not only capable of destroying a physician's career and forcing the liquidation of his/her possessions, but such cases can also greatly damage the integrity of whole professions, especially the naturopathic and chiropractic professions which are generally *guilty until proven innocent* due to the double standards imposed by those adherent to the "always right" dogma of the medical paradigm.[363] Stated differently, **if the doctor does not ask the right questions and perform the right tests, then the doctor may miss an emergency diagnosis. Missing an emergency diagnosis can result in patient death. Patient death may result in litigation, loss of license for the doctor, and irreparable harm to the profession.** The upcoming section on **Musculoskeletal Emergencies** represents *core competencies* that every clinician must keep present in his/her mind during each interaction with a patient with musculoskeletal complaints, especially patients who are elderly, on medications such as prednisone, and those with known autoimmune or immunosuppressive disorders.

Concept: "Disease Treatment" is Different from "Patient Management"

> "The key to successful intervention for orthopedic problems in a primary care practice is to know what conditions to refer and when and to whom to refer the refractory patient."[364]

Treating a problem is one thing, managing a patient is something different. "Problems" such as "low back pain" are abstract concepts, and we automatically form mental lists of treatments for problems that are irrespective of the patient who has the condition. However this list may be of only very limited applicability to the individual patient with whom you are working. Management of patients includes ❶ assessing and reassessing the differential diagnoses, ❷ monitoring compliance with treatments, including the treatments of other healthcare providers, ❸ co-treating with other healthcare providers, ❹ assessing for contraindications, ❺ monitoring patient status and effectiveness of treatments, and also ❻ the office-related tasks of charting, documentation, billing, and correspondence. The management of emergency conditions often involves transport to the nearest hospital. In some situations, the patient will be able to drive himself/herself without difficulty. In other situations, the patient should be driven by friend, family, or taxi. In the most extreme, the patient should be transported by ambulance. When in doubt about the mode of transport, do not hesitate to call 911 for an ambulance. If the taxi driver gets lost on the way to the hospital, or your patient goes into shock while being driven by a friend, the liability will come back to haunt the ***doctor***, not the *friend* or the *taxi driver*.

---

[362] nocryinginbaseball.com/glossary/glossary.html Accessed November 11, 2006
[363] Micozzi MS. Double standards and double jeopardy for CAM research. *J Altern Complement Med.* 2001 Feb;7(1):13-4
[364] Brier S. *Primary Care Orthopedics*. St. Louis: Mosby, 1999 page ix

Concept: Clinical Practice Involves Much More than "Diagnosis and Treatment"

Emergency room and hospital-based physicians are appropriately able to focus solely on diagnosis and treatment as their primary spheres of activity and interaction with patients. However, those of us in private practice learn that *healthcare* involves much more than simply being a "good doctor." From an integrative perspective we have to go beyond diagnosis and treatment *for each health disorder* with each patient. Beyond *diagnosis* and *treatment* are *understanding* and *integration*. Orchestrating all of this into a treatment plan that the patient can actually implement requires creativity, resourcefulness, and the ability to enroll patients in the process of *redesigning*—often *rebuilding*—their lives.

Components of Patient Care and Practice Management: Recall that **28% of malpractice claims involve mistakes made by medical office staff**; this includes unreturned phone calls which can culminate in malpractice by way of "patient abandonment." Similarly, inability to get a timely consultation may result in sufficient "sense of harm" that a patient may decide to sue; this is a factor in 10% of malpractice cases.[365]

---

[365] James R. Hall, Ph.D., L.Psych., FABMP, FGICPP. Departments of Internal Medicine and Psychology, UNT Health Science Center at Fort Worth. "Communication and Medico-Legal Issues." October 19, 2006

Clinical Management of Patients with Systemic Inflammatory/Autoimmune Diseases

In *Integrative Rheumatology* (2006, 2007, 2014), other peer-reviewed publications[366,367,368], and later the *Inflammation Mastery* multivolume series starting in 2014, I provide—what is to the best of my knowledge—an original conceptualization of rheumatic diseases:

1) Autoimmunity is a manifestation of immune dysfunction.
2) "Different" autoimmune diseases have much in common despite the different labels applied and manifestations observed. The commonalities in their etiologies and pathogenesis provides the rationale for the similarities in their treatments and a focus on identifying and ameliorating the underlying causes of autoimmunity as detailed: 1) food allergies/incompatibilities, 2) multifocal dysbiosis, 3) hormonal imbalances, 4) xenobiotic immunotoxicity, and 5) a pro-inflammatory diet and lifestyle. The new additions to this list starting in 2012[369] and 2013[370] are 6) mitochondrial dysfunction—in 2014 endoplasmic reticulum stress was added, and 7) nutritional immunomodulation.
3) Autoimmunity can be *ameliorated* (not always eliminated) in the majority of patients with combined and coordinated effort on the part of the physician and the patient to address the most common cause**s** of immune dysfunction, which rarely operate in isolation and are generally found in synergistic combination.
4) Since the etiopathogenesis is generally complex and multifaceted, treatment must be assertive and likewise multifaceted. Only rarely will a simple "silver bullet" cure be effective and sustainable.

Of the four major healthcare paradigms in Western medicine—i.e., osteopathic, chiropractic, naturopathic, and allopathic—the naturopathic paradigm is uniquely—and perhaps *solitarily*—well-suited for the successful assessment of and intervention for most autoimmune diseases. For it is only in naturopathic medicine that we find the specific admonishment to *Treat the Cause*, and this is a critical differentiation from the allopathic model which codifies and compels the use of symptom-suppressing and immune-suppressing medications. The original chiropractic model acknowledges the multifaceted nature of health and disease but is too vague in this context to direct assessment and treatment. The original osteopathic model did not include an appreciation of biochemical/nutritional considerations and environmental contributions which are essential for the treatment of autoimmunity. Obvious to any student of rheumatology is that the allopathic paradigm turns to symptom-suppressing drugs as "first line treatment" for rheumatic disease; this is—in the long-term—an abysmal failure except for suppression of acute inflammation and that it reduces symptomatology. Drug-only management of autoimmunity protracts the disease while imposing an impressive array of medication side-effects and nearly unbearable financial burdens. The failure of the modern allopathic medical paradigm is evidenced in the increased utilization of high-dose chemotherapy and stem-cell transplantation for the treatment of autoimmune diseases[371], an action which seems to confess, "Since we were unsuccessful with our first use of a hammer, instead of trying a different approach, we will just use a bigger hammer." The data is quite clear that even with "optimal drug therapy" and subspecialist management, the majority of patients with rheumatoid arthritis are "poorly controlled" with regard to disease activity—in other and more direct terms: medical management fails.[372]

> **Failure of long-term drug management of rheumatic disease**
> - < 50% of subjects remained in remission 1 year later.
> - Other studies have described sustained remission in daily practice as uncommon, being reached by only 17% to 36% of RA patients for up to 6 months. These studies did not evaluate time in remission beyond 6 months. A recent study…also concluded that long-term remission is rare, considering that the probability of a remission lasting 2 years was 6% to 14%.
> - Conclusions: This study shows that in clinical practice, a minority of RA patients are in sustained remission.
>
> Prince et al. Sustained rheumatoid arthritis remission is uncommon in clinical practice. *Arthritis Res Ther* 2012 Mar arthritis-research.com/content/14/2/R68

---

[366] Vasquez A. "Inflammation and Autoimmunity: A Functional Medicine Approach." David S. Jones, MD (Editor-in-Chief). *Textbook of Functional Medicine*. Gig Harbor, WA; Institute for Functional Medicine: 2006, pages 409-417
[367] Vasquez A. Web-like Interconnections of Physiological Factors. *Integrative Medicine: A Clinician's Journal* 2006, April/May, 32-37
[368] Vasquez A. Reducing Pain and Inflammation Naturally. Part 6: Nutritional and Botanical Treatments Against "Silent Infections" and Gastrointestinal Dysbiosis, Commonly Overlooked Causes of Neuromusculoskeletal Inflammation and Chronic Health Problems. *Nutritional Perspectives* 2006; January
[369] Vasquez A. *Functional Immunology and Nutritional Immunomodulation*. 2012
[370] Vasquez A. *Integrative Rheumatology, Nutritional Immunomodulation, and Functional Inflammology*. 2013
[371] "Hematopoietic stem cell transplantation is an increasingly used therapy for treatment of autoimmune diseases and severe immune-mediated disorders." Burt RK, Verda L, Statkute L, Quigley K, Yaung K, Brush M, Oyama Y. Stem cell transplantation for autoimmune diseases. *Clin Adv Hematol Oncol*. 2004 May;2(5):313-9
[372] Prince et al. Sustained rheumatoid arthritis remission is uncommon in clinical practice. *Arthritis Res Ther* 2012 Mar arthritis-research.com/content/14/2/R68

Parc de la Ciutadella, Venus, and Quadriga de l'Aurora: Grandeur of this scale reflects and reinforces true culture—a society's aspiration toward higher ideals, and a progressively better life. Societal aspirations are virtually nonexistent in modern times, wherein indifference, inertia, and ignorance are more apparent than are concern, progress, and knowledge. *What would be the characteristics of a modern aspirational culture?* An aspirational human culture seeks to develop the positive potentialities of life in general and human life in particular. As such, it provides for the maximal development of human intellectual, creative, and social potential, thus allowing people to achieve the maximal development of those qualities that are generally considered to be "most truly human." Consistent with these goals, systems of education, work, production, transportation are orchestrated to maximize learning, participation, efficient implementation, and sustainability (etc). Democratic and meritocratic ideas and ideals pervade educational, occupational, and political systems. From an early age, students are taught intellectual skills, history, health/physicality, practical life skills, at least two languages, and effective communication and conflict resolution skills. How is that for a start?[373]

> **Culture: humanity with a goal**
> "There is lacking the one goal. As yet humanity has not a goal. But pray tell me, my brethren, if the goal of humanity be still lacking, is there not also still lacking *humanity itself?*"
>
> Nietzsche FW. *Thus Spoke Zarathustra, The Thousand and One Goals*

---

[373] This is not an exhaustive treatise on the possible positive future of humanity; I wrote it on my phone to assuage boredom while waiting on air cargo to be released in Spain. Have you ever waited on a government process in Spain that requires more than 1 person and more than one piece of paper? It's like standing still in slow motion, like sleeping in frozen oatmeal, like moving at glacial speed. Actually, with the government-facilitated melting of the ice caps, glacial speed these days is becoming a metaphor for speed. ... For a more developed discussion of this topic, see Largent C, Breton D. *The Paradigm Conspiracy: Why Our Social Systems Violate Human Potential—And How We Can Change Them Paperback*. Hazelden Publishing: 1998

Risk Management, Charting, and Avoiding Medical Errors: Useful Reminders & Acronyms

This page conveniently summarizes the most important acronyms for risk management, documentation, treatment, and patient education.

Acronym	Components	Exegesis
D.I.R.T.	Defensive mindset	Start with the conscious intention to practice defensively and effectively
	Duration of treatment	Define and limit the duration of each component of the treatment plan; define the next steps of care (e.g., continued care or laboratory tests) and the date of the return visit
	Interactions with disease and drugs	Double-check for interactions of the treatment plan with drugs and the patient's disease(s), especially renal insufficiency
	Referral	Determine the need for additional consultation
	Treatment plan, charted, dated, signed	Treatment plan must be archived in chart and should be given to patient; the clinician must sign and date the chart note and treatment plan
S.O.A.P.	Subjective	Patient's concerns, goals, changes in status
	Objective	Clinician's findings, including physical examination, reports from laboratory, imaging, biopsy, and consultations
	Assessments	Global assessments, firm diagnoses
	Plan	Treatments—definitions, durations for each concern, goal, assessment, diagnosis
F.I.N.D. S.E.X.®[374]	Food and nutrition	5-part nutritional wellness protocol—supplemented Paleo-Mediterranean diet: low-carbohydrate Paleo diet, multivitamin/mineral, physiologic doses of cholecalciferol, combination fatty acid therapy (CFAT), probiotics, allergy elimination-challenge, avoid genetically modified pseudofoods
	Infections and dysbiosis	Assess or treat empirically; components of treatment include antimicrobial, immunomodulation, immunorestoration
	Nutritional immunomodulation	See *Integrative Rheumatology, Inflammation Mastery* (2014 and beyond) for the latest update to the protocol—component #10 added in 2014 Jan.
	Dysfunctional mitochondria	Optimize mitochondrial function via mitophagy, resuscitation, and interventional disinhibition
	Stress, sleep, spinal health, sociology, sweat/exercise	Stress management and lifestyle/psychosocial optimization, sleep, spinal manipulation as indicated, sweat via daily exercise
	Endocrine/hormonal optimization	Especially assess and correct thyroid, prolactin, estradiol, insulin, DHEA, testosterone, and cortisol
	Xenobiotics and toxins	Toxicity is pandemic, therefore daily detoxification is mandatory and should target metals and organic/carbon-based toxins
P.A.R.B.Q.	Procedures	Explain the components of the treatment plan
	Alternatives	Explain what options and modifications exist
	Risks	Explain the risks of treatment, consider the aforementioned components of drug-interactions, disease-interactions, referral, and duration of treatment
	Benefits	Explain the anticipated benefits in realistic terms; never guarantee efficacy since "Each patient is different and each patient's response to treatment is unique."
	Questions answered	Document that questions—if any—were answered

---

[374] The FINDSEX acronym is a registered trademark by Dr Vasquez associated with *Functional Immunology and Nutritional Immunomodulation* (2012), "*F.I.N.D. S.E.X®" The Easily Remembered Acronym for the Functional Inflammology Protocol* (2013), and updated books in the Inflammation Mastery series from InflammationMastery.com

Risk Management: A Note Especially to Students and Recent Licensees

Even if you are a board-certified rheumatologist and an assertive and astute clinician with years of experience, the consideration of these guidelines may help protect **you** from malpractice liability and **your patient** from harm. Practicing "good medicine" is inherently defensive and in the best interests of the patient and the doctor.

1. **Document the specifics of your treatment plan and the rationale behind it**.
2. **Do not tell your patient to discontinue their anti-rheumatic drugs unless these drugs are in your scope of practice *and* discontinuing such drugs is therapeutically appropriate.**
3. **Give your patient written instructions, and specifically delineate time parameters for the next visit to monitor for therapeutic effectiveness, adverse effects, and disease progression/regression.**
4. **Always have an internist or rheumatologist (or appropriate specialist) on-board as part of the clinical team** in case the patient experiences an exacerbation and needs to be hospitalized or acutely immunosuppressed.
5. **When working with patients that have potentially serious diseases such as most of the autoimmune diseases, you should have a back-up plan integrated into your treatment plan from day one.** You might consider having patients sign a consent form that includes language consistent with the following:
   - *"Due to the uniqueness of each disease and each individual, including his or her willingness and ability to implement the treatment plan, no guarantees of successful treatment can be offered."*

   "Dr.___ is not available on a 24-hour basis at all times. If you have a serious health problem that requires immediate attention, you should call your other doctors(s), call 911, or have someone take you to the nearest hospital emergency room. If you notice an adverse effect from one of the components of your health plan, you should discontinue it then call Dr.__ and inform him/her of what occurred."
   - *"Treatments with other physicians or healthcare providers are not necessarily to be discontinued. Please let Dr.__ know if you are being treated by other healthcare providers (physicians, counselors, therapists, etc.). Consult your prescribing doctor before discontinuing medications."*
6. **Test responsibly.**
7. **Treat responsibly.**
8. **Re-test to document effectiveness of your intervention.**
9. **When in doubt, refer the patient for co-management.** If you are working with a serious life-threatening disease, and *your plan* or *the patient's implementation of it* is unable to produce ***documentable results***, then you should refer the patient for allopathic/osteopathic/specialist co-management for the sake of protecting the patient from harm and for protecting yourself from undue liability.
10. **Practice defensively.** You will thereby safeguard your patient and your livelihood.

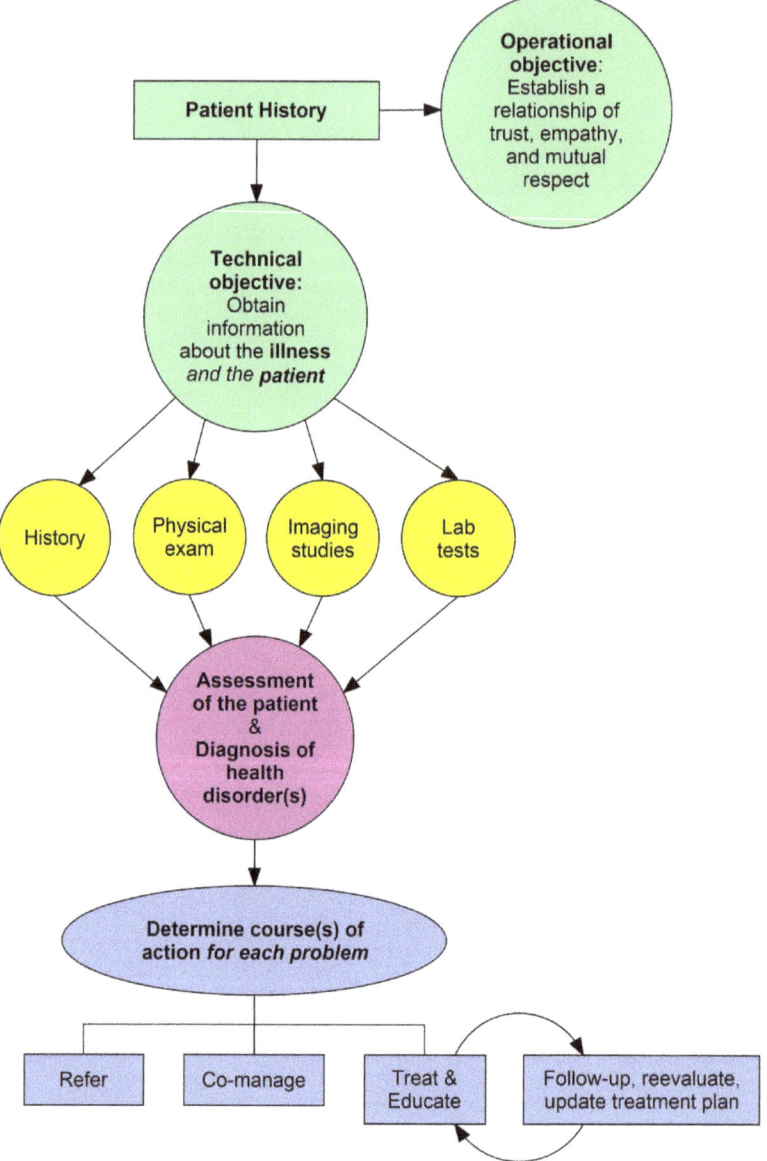

Musculoskeletal Emergencies

These are some of the "core competencies" that clinicians can never afford to miss, and these are pertinent to patients with musculoskeletal disorders, whether structural/orthopedic or metabolic/rheumatic. With these conditions, clinicians are wise to err on the side of caution— *"When in doubt, refer out"*—and implement the appropriate referral on an expedient basis. These are organized in a clinical/logical manner rather than listed alphabetically.

Neurovascular Disorders

Problem	Presentation	Assessment	Management
Neuropsychiatric lupus	<ul><li>Psychosis</li><li>Seizures</li><li>Transient ischemic attacks</li><li>Severe depression</li><li>Delirium, confusion</li></ul>	<ul><li>Neuropsychiatric manifestations with history of lupus</li></ul>	<ul><li>Emergency or prompt referral as indicated</li></ul>
Giant cell arteritis, Temporal arteritis: Considered a medical emergency since it may rapidly progress to blindness due to associated involvement of the ophthalmic artery: *"Loss of vision is the most feared manifestation and occurs quite commonly."*[375]	Presentation typically includes the following:<ul><li>Headache, scalp tenderness</li><li>Jaw claudication</li><li>Changes in vision</li><li>Systemic manifestations of rheumatic disease: fever, weight loss, muscle aches</li></ul>	<ul><li>Palpation of the temporal artery may reveal a "cord-like" artery</li><li>Elevated ESR</li><li>CBC may show anemia</li><li>Temporal artery biopsy is diagnostic</li></ul>	<ul><li>Standard medical treatment is with immediate prednisone</li><li>Implement treatment that is immediately effective or refer patient for medical treatment</li></ul>
Acute red eye: General term including acute iritis and scleritis; despite the name of this condition, redness may actually be rather minimal, and it is typically accompanied by cloudy changes in region of the iris and lens	<ul><li>Eye pain and redness</li><li>May have facial pain</li><li>May be the presenting manifestation of rheumatic disease</li></ul>	<ul><li>Red eye</li><li>Photophobia</li><li>Reduced vision</li><li>May have fixed pupil</li><li>Differential diagnosis includes acute glaucoma, bacterial/amebic/viral conjunctivitis or keratitis, allergy, and irritation due to contact lens</li></ul>	<ul><li>"The **acute** onset of a **painful, red** eye, even in the absence of visual upset, should be regarded primarily as an ophthalmological emergency."[376]</li><li>**Granulomatous uveitis** occurs in 15% of patients with sarcoidosis and can result in bilateral blindness—this must be managed as a medically urgent condition</li></ul>

---

[375] Tierney ML. McPhee SJ, Papadakis MA (eds). *Current Medical Diagnosis and Treatment, 41st Edition*. New York: Lange Medical; 2002. P999-1005
[376] McInnes I, Sturrock R. Rheumatological emergencies. *Practitioner*. 1994 Mar;238(1536):220-4

Neural canal compression

Problem	Presentation	Assessment	Management
Atlantoaxial instability: Excess mobility between the atlas and axis (commonly due to lesion of the dens or transverse ligament) makes the spinal cord vulnerable to compressive injury when the atlas translates anteriorly on the axis especially during cervical flexion; may progress to neurologic compromise including respiratory and somatic paralysis	• Post-traumatic neck injury • Down's syndrome • May present spontaneously (without trauma) in patients with inflammatory rheumatic disease, especially rheumatoid arthritis and ankylosing spondylitis • May have gradual or sudden onset of myelopathy: upper motor neuron lesion (UMNL) signs (e.g., spastic weakness), changes in bowel-bladder function, numbness	• Clinical suspicion is followed by lateral cervical and APOM (anteroposterior open mouth) radiographs to assess ADI (atlantodental interval) and dens • MRI should be performed in patients with suspected myelopathy • Neurologic examination of the upper and lower extremities • Do not force neck flexion; do not perform the Soto Hall test	• **Urgent neurosurgical consultation is recommended; stabilizing surgery is the best option for the prevention of neurologic catastrophes**[377] • Onset of myelopathy mandates referral to ER and/or neurosurgeon; immobilize with spine board or hard cervical collar and transport appropriately • Asymptomatic and mild increases in ADI (< 5mm) might be managed conservatively with activity restriction, exercises, and bracing/collars) • PAR discussion and referral for surgical consultation is necessary for informed consent and safe management
Myelopathy, spinal cord compression or lesion: May occur due to infection, edema, tumor, spinal fracture, stenosis, or inflammatory disease	• **Spastic weakness** • Bowel-bladder dysfunction • Numbness • Problems are distal to cord lesion	• Hyperreflexia • Rigidity • Muscle weakness • MRI (with and without contrast) should be performed in patients with suspected myelopathy; CT may also be indicated	• Obtain MRI to confirm diagnosis • Immobilize spine and transport if necessary • Acute myelopathy is a medical emergency that can result in rapid-onset paralysis
Cauda equina syndrome: Compression of the sacral nerve roots due to lumbar disc herniation **Cauda equina syndrome is a surgical emergency.**	• History of sciatic low back pain • Urinary retention, perineal numbness, and fecal incontinence are common • May have lower extremity weakness	• Assess for bladder distention • Assess anal sphincter strength with rectal exam • Lower extremity neurologic examination	• Urgent referral for CT/MRI to confirm diagnosis • If diagnosis is confirmed or strongly suspected clinically, urgent referral for surgical decompression is mandatory

---

[377] "When atlantoaxial stability is lost...it is thought that surgical stabilisation of the atlantoaxial joint is more reasonable and beneficial than conservative management. Minimal trauma of an unstable atlantoaxial joint can lead to serious neurological injury." Moon MS, Choi WT, Moon YW, Moon JL, Kim SS. Brooks' posterior stabilization surgery for atlantoaxial instability: review of 54 cases. *J Orthop Surg* (Hong Kong). 2002 Dec;10(2):160-4. josonline.org/PDF/v10i2p160.pdf

Acute peripheral nerve compression

Problem	Presentation	Assessment	Management
Acute compartment syndrome: acute onset of *potentially irreversible* muscle and/or nerve compression injury due to inflammation, swelling, or bleeding within a fascial compartment **Acute compartment syndrome is a surgical emergency.**	▪ Most commonly occurs in the anterior leg; may also occur in the posterior leg as well as forearm—these are the areas most notable anatomically for the investment of muscle in tight and resilient fascial sheaths ▪ Onset generally follows strenuous exercise that leads to reactive hyperemia and secondary edema ▪ May occur following trauma or fracture	Assess for: ▪ Pulselessness ▪ Palor ▪ Painful passive stretch ▪ Weakness ▪ **Numbness** ▪ Assessment and treatment should be performed on an emergency basis since irreversible nerve damage begins within 6 hours of intracompartmental hypertension	▪ Decompressive fasciotomy is the standard treatment for acute compartment syndrome that could result in permanent muscle necrosis and/or permanent nerve death ▪ Acute compartment syndrome can be fatal if rhabdomyolysis precipitates renal failure[378]

Musculoskeletal infections

Problem	Presentation	Assessment	Management
Septic arthritis: intraarticular bacterial infection; complications of septic arthritis are 1) articular destruction and 2) **death in 5-10% of patients**[379] **Septic arthritis is a medical emergency**	▪ **Febrile** patient has **acute/subacute mono/oligo-arthritis** ▪ Some patients may not have fever ▪ Other possible findings: Immuno-suppression due to medications, concomitant disease (RA, DM), elderly ▪ In some patients with concomitant disease or medications, the clinical picture can be blurred.	▪ **Warm, swollen, tender joint** ▪ Clinical assessment with **immediate referral for joint aspiration**, which reveals manifestations of infection such as WBC's and bacteria ▪ Differential diagnosis includes trauma, gout, CPPD, hemochromatosis	▪ **Immediate referral for joint aspiration** ▪ **An aggressive and prolonged course of IV and oral antimicrobials** ▪ "Immune support" such as vitamin A and glutamine and general measures to improve health and prevent recurrence
Osteomyelitis, infectious discitis: considered a medical emergency[380] **Osteomyelitis—especially vertebral osteomyelitis—is a medical emergency**	▪ Febrile patient with bone pain ▪ Assess for constitutional manifestations such as weight loss, night sweats, and malaise	▪ Exacerbation of bone pain when stress/percussion is applied to the bone ▪ Lab: CRP & WBC may be elevated ▪ MRI is more sensitive than CT, bone scan, or radiography[381]	▪ Emergency referral for vertebral osteomyelitis, since **up to 15% of patients will develop nerve lesions or cord compression**[382] ▪ Urgent referral for other types of osteomyelitis

---

[378] Paula R. Compartment Syndrome, Extremity. *eMedicine* June 22, 2006 emedicine.com/emerg/topic739.htm Accessed November 26, 2006
[379] Tierney ML. McPhee SJ, Papadakis MA. *Current Medical Diagnosis and Treatment. 35th edition*. Stamford: Appleton & Lange, 1996 page 759
[380] American College of Rheumatology Ad Hoc Committee on Clinical Guidelines. Guidelines for the initial evaluation of the adult patient with acute musculoskeletal symptoms. *Arthritis Rheum*. 1996;39(1):1-8. Also note my accompanying reply in *Arthritis Rheum*. 1996 Oct;39(10):1767-8
[381] Tierney ML. McPhee SJ, Papadakis MA (eds). *Current Medical Diagnosis and Treatment 2002, 41st Edition*. New York: Lange Medical; 2002. p 883
[382] King RW, Johnson D. Osteomyelitis. Updated July 13, 2006. *eMedicine* emedicine.com/emerg/topic349.htm Accessed Dec 24, 2006

Acute Nontraumatic Monoarthritis and Septic Arthritis

- "Acute monoarthritis is a potential medical emergency that must be investigated and treated promptly."[383]
- "Monoarthropathies should initially be investigated to exclude sepsis. ... Diagnostic joint aspiration ... should be carried out immediately."[384]
- "In acute monoarthritis, it is essential that infection of a joint be diagnosed or excluded, and this can only be done by joint aspiration and synovial fluid culture."[385]
- "Acute monoarthritis should be considered infectious until proven otherwise."[386]

Clinical presentations:
- Patient presents with acute joint pain in one joint (occasionally more than one joint may be involved).
- May or may not have fever and other systemic manifestations of infection.

> **Clinical Pearl**
>
> The primary goal of this section is to solidify your awareness of septic arthritis, its differential diagnoses, and the method and importance of assertive diagnosis and management.
>
> Septic arthritis is a medical emergency, and some authoritative textbooks report a mortality rate of 5-10%.
>
> Septic arthritis must be diagnosed urgently with joint aspiration, and it must be treated with antibiotics in order to preserve the joint and prevent spread of the infection.

Major Differential Diagnoses for Nontraumatic Monoarthritis

Problem	Presentation	Assessment & Management
Septic arthritis: intraarticular bacterial infection; complications of septic arthritis are 1) articular destruction and 2) **death in 5-10% of patients**[387]	▪ **Febrile** patient has **acute/subacute mono/oligo-arthritis** ▪ **Onset over hours or days** Other possible findings: ▪ Immuno-suppression due to medications, concomitant disease (RA, DM), elderly ▪ Some patients may not have fever ▪ In some patients with a previous or concomitant disease process, the clinical picture can be blurred	▪ **Warm, swollen, red, painful joint** ▪ Clinical assessment with **immediate referral for joint aspiration**, which reveals characteristic manifestations of infection such as WBCs and bacteria ▪ **Immediate joint aspiration** ▪ An aggressive and prolonged course of IV and oral antimicrobials ▪ "Immune support" and general measures to improve health and prevent recurrence

> **Septic arthritis is life-threatening**
>
> "Septic arthritis is still a life-threatening disease with a mortality of 2–5% and high morbidity."
>
> Zacher J, Gursche A. Regional musculoskeletal conditions: 'hip' pain. *Best Practice & Research Clinical Rheumatology*. 2003 Feb;17:71-85

---

[383] Cibere J. Rheumatology: 4. Acute monoarthritis. *CMAJ (Canadian Medical Association Journal)*. 2000;162(11):1577-83 cmaj.ca/cgi/content/full/162/11/1577 Jan 2004
[384] McInnes I, Sturrock R. Rheumatological emergencies. Practitioner. 1994 Mar;238(1536):220-4
[385] American College of Rheumatology Ad Hoc Committee on Clinical Guidelines. Guidelines for the initial evaluation of the adult patient with acute musculoskeletal symptoms. *Arthritis Rheum*. 1996 Jan;39(1):1-8
[386] Cibere J. Rheumatology: 4. Acute monoarthritis. CMAJ (*Canadian Medical Association Journal*). 2000;162(11):1577-83 cmaj.ca/cgi/content/full/162/11/1577 Jan 2004
[387] Tierney ML. McPhee SJ, Papadakis MA. *Current Medical Diagnosis and Treatment, 35th edition*. Stamford: Appleton and Lange, 1996 page 759

Major differential diagnoses for non-traumatic monoarthritis—*continued*

Problem	Presentation	Assessment & Management
Osteochondritis dissecans: A disorder of unclear etiology (trauma and/or avascular necrosis) which results in the death and subsequent fragmentation of subchondral bone[388]	- Primarily affects ages 10-30 years - **Most common in the knees and elbows** - Locking and crepitus due to intraarticular loose bodies ("joint mice") - Some patients are almost asymptomatic, while others have acute pain - Swelling of the affected joint	- Radiographs—consider to assess both knees as the condition is bilateral in 30% - MRI is used to assess severity and need for surgical intervention - Stable and nondisplaced lesions may be managed nonsurgically; larger and displaced fragments require surgical repair to reduce long-term complications[389]
Transient synovitis, irritable hip: Non-specific short-term inflammation and effusion of the hip joint	- Acute onset of painful hip and limp - Decreased pain with hip in flexion and abduction - Considered the most common cause of hip pain in children[390] - More common in boys, age 3-6 years and generally younger than 10 years - May have recent history of viral infection, and some children (1.5-10%) eventually manifest RA or AVN[391]	- May have slight elevation of ESR - Normal WBC - No fever; the child appears healthy - "…radiography is indicated to exclude osseous pathological conditions…"[392] - **Joint aspiration is indicated if septic arthritis is suspected**[393] - Conservative treatment, restricted exertion and weight-bearing for several weeks
Legg-Calve-Perthe's disease: Idiopathic ischemic necrosis of the femoral head occurring in children **Avascular necrosis (AVN) of the femoral head, osteonecrosis**: Ischemic necrosis of the femoral head	Perthe's disease: - 80% occur in children generally between ages of 4-9 years; more common in boys; may present with hip pain or knee pain AVN: - Ages 20-40 years - Unilateral hip pain - May have knee pain - History of trauma is common AVN associations: - Steroid use, prednisone - Hyperlipidemia - Alcoholism - Pancreatitis - Hemoglobinopathies - Smoking - Fatty liver disease: "fat globules from the liver"[394]	- Limited ROM - **Radiographs**; if normal and clinical suspicion is high order MRI or bone scan - **Crutches** - **Orthopedic referral is recommended** although not all patients will require surgery and some may be managed conservatively[395]

---

[388] Tatum R. Osteochondritis dissecans of the knee: a radiology case report. *J Manipulative Physiol Ther* 2000 Jun;23(5):347-51
[389] Browne RF, Murphy SM, Torreggiani WC, Munk PL, Marchinkow LO. Radiology for the surgeon: musculoskeletal case 30. Osteochondritis dissecans of the medial femoral condyle. *Can J Surg*. 2003;46(5):361-3 cma.ca/multimedia/staticContent/HTML/N0/l2/cjs/vol-46/issue-5/pdf/pg361.pdf
[390] Maroo S. Diagnosis of hip pain in children. *Hosp Med* 1999 Nov;60(11):788-93
[391] Souza TA. *Differential Diagnosis for the Chiropractor: Protocols and Algorithms*. Gaithersberg, Maryland: Aspen Publications. 1997 page 265
[392] Maroo S. Diagnosis of hip pain in children. *Hosp Med* 1999 Nov;60(11):788-93
[393] Maroo S. Diagnosis of hip pain in children. *Hosp Med* 1999 Nov;60(11):788-93
[394] Skinner HB, Scherger JE. Identifying structural hip and knee problems. *Postgrad Med* 1999;106(7):51-2, 55-6, 61-4
[395] Souza TA. *Differential Diagnosis for the Chiropractor: Protocols and Algorithms*. Gaithersberg, Maryland: Aspen Publications. 1997 page 263

Major differential diagnoses for non-traumatic monoarthritis—*continued*

Problem	Presentation	Assessment & Management
Gout	• **Febrile** patient has **acute/subacute mono/oligo-arthritis** • **Onset over hours or days** • "A history of discreet attacks, usually affecting one joint, that precede the onset of fixed symmetric arthritis is the major clue."[396] • May have fever, chills, tachycardia, leukocytosis—just like septic arthritis	• Clinical presentation may be sufficient for DX; however septic arthritis should be excluded • Serum uric acid is generally meaningless for the diagnosis of gout since many gout patients will have normal serum uric acid • Medical treatment is rest, NSAID's, and allopurinol • Fluid loading: >3 liters per day; monitor for electrolyte imbalances and hyponatremia as needed • Integrative assessment and treatment for insulin resistance, hormonal imbalances, and nutritional deficiencies
CPPD: Calcium pyrophosphate dihydrate deposition disease	• Idiopathic • May be caused by iron overload in some patients • Presentation may be acute or subacute	• Medical diagnosis is by synovial biopsy • Radiographs reveal chondrocalcinosis • Allopathic treatment is NSAIDs; phytonutritional anti-inflammatory treatments may also be used (see Chapter 3 of *Integrative Orthopedics/Rheumatology*) • Oral colchicine 0.5 to 1.5 mg per day prevents attacks[397]
Hemarthrosis: Generally associated with trauma, anticoagulation (i.e., coumadin), leukemia, hemophilia	• Monoarthralgia with limited motion • May follow direct trauma • Nontraumatic hemarthrosis may be due to anticoagulation, leukemia, hemophilia	• Synovial fluid analysis reveals blood • Treatment of underlying disorder; refer as indicated
Slipped capital femoral epiphysis (SCFE): The most common cause of hip pain in adolescents[398]	• Seen in adolescents generally 8-17 years of age • Classic presentation is a tall overweight boy with **hip pain**, knee pain, and/or a painful limp: "*Slipped femoral capital epiphysis is a developmental injury that must be considered in any adolescent who presents with hip pain.*"[399]	• **Radiographs** of both hips (bilateral SCFE in 40%): "**AP and frog lateral views are recommended in all children over age of 9 years with hip pain**."[400] • Orthopedic referral—"*…the patient should be referred immediately to an orthopedist for surgical stabilization.*"[401]

---

[396] Hardin JG, Waterman J, Labson LH. Rheumatic disease: Which diagnostic tests are useful? *Patient Care* 1999; March 15: 83-102
[397] Beers MH, Berkow R (eds). *The Merck Manual. Seventeenth Edition*. Whitehouse Station; Merck Research Laboratories 1999 Page
[398] Maroo S. Diagnosis of hip pain in children. *Hosp Med* 1999 Nov;60(11):788-93
[399] O'Kane JW. Anterior hip pain. *Am Fam Physician* 1999 Oct 15;60(6):1687-96
[400] Maroo S. Diagnosis of hip pain in children. *Hosp Med* 1999 Nov;60(11):788-93
[401] O'Kane JW. Anterior hip pain. *Am Fam Physician* 1999 Oct 15;60(6):1687-96

Clinical assessment of non-traumatic monoarthritis:
- History and orthopedic assessment of the joint
- Laboratory tests must be performed if you have a suspicion of infection

History/subjective:
- Acute or subacute joint pain with or without systemic manifestations and fever.
- History or may not be significant; other than the obvious risk factor of immunosuppression, septic arthritis can occur with impressive spontaneity and randomness

Differential physical examination and objective findings:
- **Septic arthritis**: pain and limitation of motion, swelling, redness; patient may have systemic symptoms of fever and malaise
- **Gout**: pain and limitation of motion, swelling, redness; patient may have systemic symptoms of fever and malaise
- **Pseudogout and calcium pyrophosphate dihydrate deposition disease (CPDD/CPPD)**: pain and limitation of motion, swelling, redness; patient may have systemic symptoms of fever and malaise
- **Ischemic necrosis**: pain and limitation of motion; swelling, redness and systemic symptoms are less likely.
- **Hemarthrosis**: pain and limitation of motion; often associated with trauma, use of anticoagulant medications[402], or hemophilia and other hematologic abnormalities[403]
- **Tumor**: assess with history, imaging, and biopsy if possible
- **Injury**: Meniscal injury, fracture, ligament injury; physical examination procedures are described in the chapters that follow

Imaging and laboratory assessments:
- **Septic arthritis**: joint aspiration; STAT CBC (for WBC count) and CRP
- **Gout**: joint aspiration; CBC (for WBC count) and CRP
- **Pseudogout and PPDD**: rule out septic arthritis with joint aspiration, CBC, and CRP; radiographs often show chondrocalcinosis
- **Ischemic necrosis**: radiographs are diagnostic
- **Hemarthrosis**: joint aspiration and assessment for underlying disease or medication, especially if the condition was not trauma-induced
- **Tumor**: assess with radiographs
- **Injury**: rule out infection; consider imaging with radiography or MRI.

Establishing the diagnosis:
- The aforementioned examinations and lab assessments should establish the exact diagnosis. **The priorities are 1) first exclude life-threatening illness (i.e., septic arthritis), then 2) to exclude serious injury or illness,** and finally 3) to help manage the exact problem.

Complications:
- **Septic arthritis can result in death in 5-10% of patients. "Five to 10 percent of patients with an infected joint die, chiefly from respiratory complications of sepsis. The mortality rate is 30% for patients with polyarticular sepsis. Bony ankylosis and articular destruction commonly also occur if the treatment is delayed or inadequate."**[404] Complications vary per location, infecting organism, severity, and patient.

---

[402] Riley SA, Spencer GE. Destructive monarticular arthritis secondary to anticoagulant therapy. *Clin Orthop*. 1987 Oct;(223):247-51
[403] Jean-Baptiste G, De Ceulaer K. Osteoarticular disorders of haematological origin. *Baillieres Best Pract Res Clin Rheumatol*. 2000 Jun;14(2):307-23
[404] Tierney ML. McPhee SJ, Papadakis MA. *Current Medical Diagnosis and Treatment. 35th edition*. Stamford: Appleton & Lange, 1996 page 759

Clinical management of non-traumatic monoarthritis:
- **Suspected septic arthritis requires referral for joint aspiration and antimicrobial drugs.**
- Referral if clinical outcome is unsatisfactory or if serious complications are evident.
- Treatment of other conditions that cause acute monoarthritis (such as gout and calcium pyrophosphate dihydrate deposition disease) is based on the problem and individual patient.

Treatments:
- **Septic arthritis requires IV/oral antimicrobial drugs:** Intravenous antibiotics are generally started before culture results are available. After results and culture from synovial fluid analysis have been considered, the dose, combination, and administration of antibiotics can be fine-tuned. Frequently, antibiotics are administered intravenously for at least 3-4 weeks. Surgical/endoscopic drainage/debridement and immobilization during the acute phase may also be implemented.[405]
- **Immunonutrition considerations:** Immunonutritional considerations are listed below; doses listed are for adults. Although studies have not been performed specifically in patients with bone/joint infections, general benefits derived from the use of immunonutrition are reductions in severity/frequency/duration of major infections, abbreviated hospitalization (i.e., early discharge due to expedited healing and recovery), reductions in the need for medications, significant improvements in survival, and hospital savings.[406,407,408,409,410,411,412]
    - Paleo-Mediterranean diet: as detailed later in this text and elsewhere[413,414]
    - Vitamin and mineral supplementation: anti-infective benefits shown in elderly diabetics[415]
    - High-dose vitamin A: Vitamin A shows potent immunosupportive benefits, and vitamin A stores are depleted by the stress of infection and injury. Consider 200,000-300,000 IU per day of retinol palmitate for 1-4 weeks, then taper; reduce dose or discontinue with onset of toxicity symptoms such as skin problems (dry skin, flaking skin, chapped or split lips, red skin rash, hair loss), joint pain, bone pain, headaches, anorexia (loss of appetite), edema (water retention, weight gain, swollen ankles, difficulty breathing), fatigue, and/or liver damage.
    - Arginine: Dose for adults is in the range of 5-10 grams daily
    - Fatty acid supplementation: In contrast to the higher doses used to provide an anti-inflammatory effect in patients with autoimmune/inflammatory disorders, doses used for immunosupportive treatments should be kept rather modest to avoid the *relative* immunosuppression that has been controversially

---

[405] Brusch JL. Septic Arthritis (Last Updated: October 18, 2005). *eMedicine*. emedicine.com/med/topic3394.htm Accessed Nov 25, 2006

[406] "To evaluate the metabolic and immune effects of dietary arginine, glutamine and omega-3 fatty acids (fish oil) supplementation, we performed a prospective study... CONCLUSIONS: The feeding of Neomune in critically injured patients was well tolerated as Traumacal and significant improvement was observed in serum protein. Shorten ICU stay and wean-off respirator day may benefit from using the immunonutrient formula." Chuntrasakul C, Siltham S, Sarasombath S, Sittapairochana C, Leowattana W, Chockvivatanavanit S, Bunnak A. Comparison of a immunonutrition formula enriched arginine, glutamine and omega-3 fatty acid, with a currently high-enriched enteral nutrition for trauma patients. *J Med Assoc Thai*. 2003 Jun;86(6):552-6

[407] "CONCLUSIONS: In conclusion, arginine-enhanced formula improves fistula rates in postoperative head and neck cancer patients and decreases length of stay." de Luis DA, Izaola O, Cuellar L, Terroba MC, Aller R. Randomized clinical trial with an enteral arginine-enhanced formula in early postsurgical head and neck cancer patients. *Eur J Clin Nutr*. 2004;58(11):1505-8

[408] "In this prospective, randomised, double-blind, placebo-controlled study, we randomly assigned 50 patients who were scheduled to undergo coronary artery bypass to receive either an oral immune-enhancing nutritional supplement containing L-arginine, omega3 polyunsaturated fatty acids, and yeast RNA (n=25), or a control (n=25) for a minimum of 5 days... Intake of an oral immune-enhancing nutritional supplement for a minimum of 5 days before surgery can improve outlook in high-risk patients who are undergoing elective cardiac surgery." Tepaske R, et al. Effect of preoperative oral immune-enhancing nutritional supplement on patients at high risk of infection after cardiac surgery: a randomised placebo-controlled trial. *Lancet*. 2001 Sep 1;358(9283):696-701

[409] "The feeding of IMMUNE FORMULA was well tolerated and significant improvement was observed in nutritional and immunologic parameters as in other immunoenhancing diets. Further clinical trials of prospective double-blind randomized design are necessary to address the so that the necessity of using immunonutrition in critically ill patients will be clarified." Chuntrasakul C, et al. Metabolic and immune effects of dietary arginine, glutamine and omega-3 fatty acids supplementation in immunocompromised patients. *J Med Assoc Thai*. 1998 May;81(5):334-43

[410] "enteral diet supplemented with arginine, dietary nucleotides, and omega-3 fatty acids (IMPACT, Sandoz Nutrition, Bern, Switzerland) " Senkal M, et al. Early postoperative enteral immunonutrition: clinical outcome and cost-comparison analysis in surgical patients. *Crit Care Med* 1997;25(9):1489-96

[411] "supplemented diet with glutamine, arginine and omega-3-fatty acids... It was clearly established in this trial that early postoperative enteral feeding is safe in patients who have undergone major operations for gastrointestinal cancer. Supplementation of enteral nutrition with glutamine, arginine, and omega-3-fatty acids positively modulated postsurgical immunosuppressive and inflammatory responses." Wu GH, Zhang YW, Wu ZH. Modulation of postoperative immune and inflammatory response by immune-enhancing enteral diet in gastrointestinal cancer patients. *World J Gastroenterol*. 2001 Jun;7(3):357-62 wjgnet.com/1007-9327/7/357.pdf

[412] "using a formula supplemented with arginine, mRNA, and omega-3 fatty acids from fish oil (Impact)... CONCLUSIONS: Immune-enhancing enteral nutrition resulted in a significant reduction in the mortality rate and infection rate in septic patients admitted to the ICU. These reductions were greater for patients with less severe illness." Galban C, Montejo JC, Mesejo A, Marco P, Celaya S, Sanchez-Segura JM, Farre M, Bryg DJ. An immune-enhancing enteral diet reduces mortality rate and episodes of bacteremia in septic intensive care unit patients. *Crit Care Med*. 2000 Mar;28(3):643-8

[413] Vasquez A. A Five-Part Nutritional Protocol that Produces Consistently Positive Results. *Nutritional Wellness* 2005 Sep. Reprinted and updated in Chapter 4.

[414] Vasquez A. Implementing the Five-Part Nutritional Wellness Protocol for the Treatment of Various Health Problems. *Nutritional Wellness* 2005 November. Reprinted and updated in Chapter 4.

[415] "CONCLUSIONS: A multivitamin and mineral supplement reduced the incidence of participant-reported infection and related absenteeism in a sample of participants with type 2 diabetes mellitus and a high prevalence of subclinical micronutrient deficiency." Barringer TA, Kirk JK, Santaniello AC, Foley KL, Michielutte R. Effect of a multivitamin and mineral supplement on infection and quality of life. A randomized, double-blind, placebo-controlled trial. *Ann Intern Med*. 2003 Mar;138:365-71 annals.org/cgi/reprint/138/5/365

reported in patients treated with EPA and DHA. Reasonable doses are in the following ranges for adults: EPA+DHA: 500-1,500, and GLA: 300-500 mg.

- Glutamine: Glutamine enhances bacterial killing by neutrophils[416], and administration of 18 grams per day in divided doses to patients in intensive care units was shown to improve survival, expedite hospital discharge, and reduce total healthcare costs.[417] Another study using glutamine 12-18 grams per day showed no benefit in overall mortality but significant benefits in terms of reduced healthcare costs (-30%) and significantly reduced need for medical interventions.[418] After administering glutamine 26 grams/d to severely burned patients, Garrel et al[419] concluded that glutamine reduced the risk of infection by 3-fold and that oral glutamine "may be a life-saving intervention" in patients with severe burns. A dose of 30 grams/d was used in a recent clinical trial showing hemodynamic benefit in patients with sickle cell anemia.[420] The highest glutamine dose that the current author is aware of is the study by Scheltinga et al[421] who used 0.57 gm/kg/day in cancer patients following chemotherapy administration; for a 220-lb-pt, this would be approximately 57 grams of glutamine per day.

- Melatonin: 20-40 mg hs (*hora somni*—Latin: sleep time). Immunostimulatory anti-infective action of melatonin was demonstrated in a small clinical trial wherein septic newborns administered 20 mg melatonin showed significantly increased survival over nontreated controls.[422]

---

[416] Furukawa et al. Glutamine-enhanced bacterial killing by neutrophils from postoperative patients. *Nutrition* 1997;13(10):863-9. *In vitro* study.

[417] Griffiths RD, Jones C, Palmer TE. Six-month outcome of critically ill patients given glutamine-supplemented parenteral nutrition. *Nutrition* 1997;13(4):295-302

[418] "There was no mortality difference between those patients receiving glutamine-containing enteral feed and the controls. However, there was a significant reduction in the median postintervention ICU and hospital patient costs in the glutamine recipients $23 000 versus $30 900 in the control patients." Jones C, Palmer TE, Griffiths RD. Randomized clinical outcome study of critically ill patients given glutamine-supplemented enteral nutrition. *Nutrition*. 1999 Feb;15(2):108-15

[419] The glutamine dose in this study was "a total of 26 g/day" administered in four divided doses. CONCLUSION: "The results of this prospective randomized clinical trial show that enteral G reduces blood culture positivity, particularly with P. aeruginosa, in adults with severe burns and may be a life-saving intervention." Garrel D, Patenaude J, Nedelec B, et al. Decreased mortality and infectious morbidity in adult burn patients given enteral glutamine supplements. *Crit Care Med*. 2003 Oct;31(10):2444-9

[420] Niihara Y, Matsui NM, Shen YM, et al. L-glutamine therapy reduces endothelial adhesion of sickle red blood cells to human umbilical vein endothelial cells. *BMC Blood Disord*. 2005 Jul 25;5:4 biomedcentral.com/1471-2326/5/4

[421] "Subjects with hematologic malignancies in remission underwent a standard treatment of high-dose chemotherapy and total body irradiation before bone marrow transplantation. After completion of this regimen, they were randomized to receive either standard parenteral nutrition (STD, n = 10) or an isocaloric, isonitrogenous nutrient solution enriched with crystalline L-glutamine (0.57 g/kg/day, GLN, n = 10)." Scheltinga MR, Young LS, Benfell K, Bye RL, Ziegler TR, Santos AA, Antin JH, Schloerb PR, Wilmore DW. Glutamine-enriched intravenous feedings attenuate extracellular fluid expansion after a standard stress. *Ann Surg*. 1991 Oct;214(4):385-93; discussion 393-5 pubmedcentral.nih.gov/articlerender.fcgi?tool=pubmed&pubmedid=1953094 For additional review, see Ziegler TR. Glutamine supplementation in cancer patients receiving bone marrow transplantation and high dose chemotherapy. J Nutr. 2001 Sep;131(9 Suppl):2578S-84S jn.nutrition.org/cgi/content/full/131/9/2578S

[422] Gitto E, et al. Effects of melatonin treatment in septic newborns. *Pediatr Res*. 2001;50:756-60 pedresearch.org/cgi/content/full/50/6/756

Brief Overview of Integrative Healthcare Disciplines

Naturopathic Medicine, Functional Medicine, Osteopathic Medicine, Chiropractic

Introduction

In these following sections, I provide some review and insights about each of the main integrative healthcare disciplines; these are distinguished by their relatively greater eclecticism contrasted to the narrow range of allopathic medicine, which relies almost exclusively on drugs and surgery and—again in contrast—requires greater passivity on the part of the clinician and the patient.

All institutions and professions have their shadow—that part that is disowned, denied, repressed; to appreciate the whole and maintain honesty and integrity, the totality should be appreciated, lest our apprehension and vision become and remain selective. This closing paragraph for each section will be further developed over the next few years. I might hope that readers were first familiarized with the concept of shadow during previous courses in Psychology, since the concept is well popularized after having originated from the work of the famous psychologist Carl Jung PhD who founded analytical psychology and introduced concepts such as *synchronicity*, *individuation*, *extraversion/extroversion*, *introversion*, *archetypes*, *collective unconscious*, and *shadow* into the psychological and social sciences and eventually common conversation. "In Jungian psychology, the shadow or "shadow aspect" may refer to 1) an unconscious aspect of the personality which the conscious ego does not identify in itself. Because one tends to reject or remain ignorant of the least desirable aspects of one's personality, the shadow is largely negative, or 2) the entirety of the unconscious, i.e., everything of which a person is not fully conscious. ... "Everyone carries a shadow," Jung wrote, "and the less it is embodied in the individual's conscious life, the blacker and denser it is."[423]

---

[423] wikipedia.org/wiki/Shadow_(psychology) 2014

Naturopathic Medicine

> "The work of the naturopathic physician is to elicit healing by helping patients to create or recreate conditions for health to exist within them. Health will occur where the conditions for health exist. Disease is the product of conditions which allow for it." *Jared Zeff, ND*[424]

The diagram on this page is derived from the review by Zeff published in 1997 in *Journal of Naturopathic Medicine* entitled "The process of healing: a unifying theory of naturopathic medicine." By my interpretation, the diagram is important for at least three reasons.

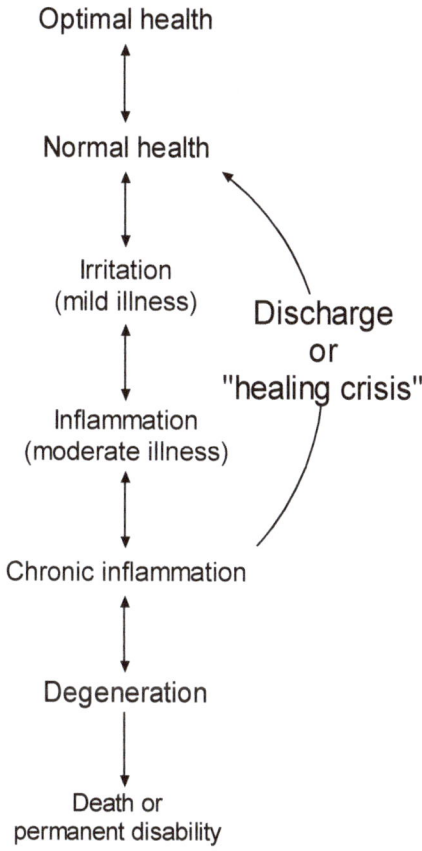

First, whereas the allopathic profession describes the genesis of most diseases as *idiopathic* and therefore [somehow] exclusively serviceable by drugs and surgery, the naturopathic profession describes disease processes as *multifactorial* and *logical* and therefore treatable by the skilled discovery and treatment of the underlying causes. Such underlying causes, which nearly always occur as a plurality, may vary mildly or significantly even within a group of patients with the same diagnosis.

Second, the diagram shows that the development of disease and the restoration of health are both *processes*. The restoration and retention of health requires *intentionality* and *tenacity* in lieu of the simplistic *miracle medicines* and *passive treatments* proffered by the pharmaceutical industry. Generally, disease does not arrive from outside; it is the result of one or more internal imbalances. Chronic illness is generally the result of manifold internal imbalances that culminate in numerous physiologic insults which compromise essential functions to the point that one or more organ systems begin to fail; we as patients and doctors generally label this as some specific "disease" or other, and the general—often erroneous—assumption has been that each *specific disease* (i.e., label, …abstraction, …conceptual entity) requires a *specific treatment* rather than a generalized health-restorative approach. Health is restored through a progressive and stepwise program that addresses as many facets of the illness as possible while vigorously supporting optimal physiologic function.

Third, the fact that Zeff considered the discharge or "healing crisis" so important that it merited inclusion in this diagram shows, indirectly, the naturopathic emphasis on detoxification and the eradication of dysbiosis. Both in the treatment of toxic metal/chemical exposure and in the treatment of chronic infections, patients often go through an acute or subacute phase of feeling ill before experiencing a dramatic alleviation of symptoms; the fact that symptoms may temporarily "get worse before getting better" has been referred to as the "healing crisis." This can occur for at least three reasons. First, in the elimination of chemicals and metals from the body, they must first be released from the tissues; the transition from tissues to blood is similar to a subacute re-exposure which triggers symptoms of toxicity until the toxin is excreted via sweat, urine, bile, or breath. Similarly, improvement in nutritional status—a cornerstone of all naturopathic interventions—expedites/facilitates/restores physiologic processes that have been relatively dormant due to lack of enzymatic cofactors such as vitamins and minerals[425]; optimization of nutritional status provides an opportunity for these pathways (such as detoxification of stored xenobiotics) to function again at which time they must "catch up" on work that has not been performed during the time of nutritional deficiency. The activation of these pathways is an essential step toward health restoration but results in an initial upregulation of hepatic phase-1/oxidative biotransformation which often results in the formation of reactive intermediates that temporarily impair physiologic processes and cause an initial exacerbation of symptoms. Third, whether through immunorestoration or the use of botanical/pharmacologic antimicrobial

---

[424] Zeff JL. The process of healing: a unifying theory of naturopathic medicine. *Journal of Naturopathic Medicine* 1997; 7: 122-5
[425] Ames BN. The metabolic tune-up: metabolic harmony and disease prevention. *J Nutr*. 2003 May;133(5 Suppl 1):1544S-8S

agents, the symptom-exacerbating "die off" reaction—classically called the Jarisch-Herxheimer reaction in the context of treating syphilis—is a result of increased (endo)toxin production/release by bacteria/microbes in response effective antimicrobial processes, whether physiologic or pharmacologic.

Modern naturopathic medicine has grown from deeply rooted European healing traditions reaching back several centuries. Naturopathic physicians have unwaveringly demonstrated respect, love, and appreciation for the healing powers of nature and the process of life itself.[426] Following their coursework in the basic biomedical sciences, naturopathic physicians are trained in urology, oncology, neurology, pediatrics, obstetrics and gynecology, urology, manual physical manipulation (including spinal manipulation), minor surgery, medical procedures, professional ethics, therapeutic diets, clinical and interventional nutrition, botanical medicines, psychological counseling, environmental medicine, and other modalities. Licensed naturopathic physicians commonly practice as generalists and family doctors.[427,428,429,430]

Naturopathic Principles, Concepts, & the *Vis Medicatrix Naturae*

1. **First, Do No Harm** *(Primum Non Nocere)*: Naturopathic physicians use good judgment and compassion to ensure that the treatment does not cause harm to the patient. This contrasts with the effects of allopathic treatment, which collectively kill more than 180,000-220,000 patients per year, at least 493 American patients per day.[432]

2. **Identify and Treat the Causes** *(Tolle Causam)*: "*Illness does not occur without cause.*" Naturopathic physicians focus on identifying and addressing the underlying deficiency, toxicity, impairment, or imbalance that is the cause of the health problem or disease.

> **Vis Medicatrix Naturae: the healing power of nature**
>
> "The healing power of nature is the inherent self-organizing and healing process of living systems... It is the naturopathic physician's role to support, facilitate and augment this process by identifying and removing obstacles to health and recovery, and by supporting the creation of a healthy internal and external environment."[431]

3. **Treat the Whole Person**: "*The multifactorial nature of health and disease requires a personalized and comprehensive approach to diagnosis and treatment.*" On some occasions the illness does take precedence over the person who has it—such in emergency situations like septic arthritis, acute ischemia, and pulmonary edema. In these cases, the situation must be managed appropriately, and these situations are not immediately amenable to long-term lifestyle changes—they require immediate treatment. However, the vast majority of cases in routine outpatient clinical practice will require detailed and bipartite attention to the facets of both **the disease process** and **the person who has the illness**. Our focus as naturopathic physicians on the individual patient is what sets our healing profession apart from others that focus exclusively on the disease and do not consider the manifold intricacies of the individual patient.

4. **The Healing Power of Nature: *Vis Medicatrix Naturae***: Naturopathic medicine recognizes an inherent self-healing process in the person that is ordered and intelligent. The body has many highly efficient mechanisms for sustaining and regaining health. These mechanisms have their specific and necessary components (e.g., nutrients) and means by which they can be impaired (e.g., xenobiotic immunosuppression). Poor health and disease can result from impairment of these self-healing processes and biologic mechanisms, and thus the body's inherent, natural, self-healing mechanisms—the "healing power of nature"—can be diminished to the state of ineffectiveness or harm (e.g., autoimmunity). Recognizing that the body has this inherent goal of and movement toward self-healing, naturopathic physicians start by identifying and removing "obstacles to cure" rather than ignoring these factors and masking the manifestations of dysfunction with symptom-suppressing drugs.

---

[426] Kirchfeld F, Boyle W. *Nature Doctors: Pioneers in Naturopathic Medicine*. Portland, Oregon; Medicina Biologica (Buckeye Naturopathic Press, East Palestine, Ohio), 1994
[427] Boon HS, et al. Practice patterns of naturopathic physicians: results from a random survey of licensed practitioners in two US States. *BMC Complement Altern Med*. 2004;4:14
[428] Smith MJ, Logan AC. Naturopathy. *Med Clin North Am*. 2002 Jan;86(1):173-84
[429] Cherkin DC, et al. Characteristics of visits to licensed acupuncturists, chiropractors, massage therapists, and naturopathic physicians. *J Am Board Fam Pract*. 2002;15:463-72
[430] Cherkin DC, et al. Characteristics of licensed acupuncturists, chiropractors, massage therapists, and naturopathic physicians. *J Am Board Fam Pract*. 2002 Sep-Oct;15:378-90
[431] Quoted from the American Association of Naturopathic Physicians website aanp.net/Basics/h.naturo.philo.html on February 4, 2001. Other italicized quotes in this section are from the same source. This website has since been replaced by naturopathic.org/
[432] "Recent estimates suggest that each year more than 1 million patients are injured while in the hospital and approximately 180,000 die because of these injuries. Furthermore, drug-related morbidity and mortality are common and are estimated to cost more than $136 billion a year." Holland EG, Degruy FV. Drug-induced disorders. *Am Fam Physician*. 1997;56(7):1781-8, 1791-2

5. **Prevention**: Healthy lifestyle, proper nutrition, and emotional hygiene go a long way toward preventing (and treating) most conditions. Specific conditions have specific risk factors and causes that have to be considered per patient and condition.
6. **Doctor as Teacher (*Docere*)**: Naturopathic physicians explain the situation and the proposed solution to the patient so that the patient is empowered with understanding and with the comfort of knowing what has happened, what is happening, and the proposed course of upcoming events. Naturopathic physicians strive to let their own lives serve as a models for our patients. This does not mean that naturopathic doctors have to feign perfection; the task is to live the best and most conscious life that we can, to be present with our emotions, qualities, and faults and to treat ourselves with respect and acceptance. We can exemplify health (rather than perfection) to our patients by being who we authentically are and by so doing we can facilitate their own acceptance of their current health situation, which is a prerequisite to self-initiated change.

> **Physician, heal thyself.**
> "Physician, heal thyself; thus you help your patient, too.
> Let this be his best medicine
> that he beholds with his eyes:
> the doctor who heals himself."
>
> Nietzsche FW. *Thus Spoke Zarathustra* (1892). [Kaufmann W, translator]. Viking Penguin: 1954, page 77

7. **Re-Establish the Foundation for Health**: An overview of this important naturopathic concept is provided throughout this chapter.
8. **Removing "obstacles to cure"**: *examples*

Obstacle to the optimization of health	Example of possible intervention
o Toxic exposures, medication side-effects	▪ Reduce drug use and dependency
o Toxic relationships, emotional obstacles, past events, unfulfilling occupation,	▪ Improve self-esteem, develop conflict resolution skills, determine life goals and values and a plan for their pursuit
o Social isolation: the typical American has only two friends no-one in whom to confide[433]	▪ Encourage social interaction
o Diet with excess fat, arachidonate, sugar, additives, colorants, and insufficiency of protein, fiber, phytonutrients, and health-promoting fatty acids: ALA, GLA, EPA, DHA, and oleic acid	▪ Diet improvement and nutritional supplementation
o Sedentary lifestyle, lack of exercise	▪ Encourage exercise
o Weight gain/loss as necessary for weight optimization	▪ Encourage self-valuing
o Epidemic exposure to mercury, lead, and xenobiotics	▪ Support detoxification process as a lifestyle

Hierarchy of Therapeutics: This naturopathic concept articulates the importance of addressing *the underlying cause* rather than simply focusing on *the presenting problem*, which is the *symptom of the cause*. Further, interventions are **prioritized**, *for example*:
- Patient-implemented *before* doctor-implemented.
- Removal of harming agent *before* addition of a therapeutic agent: e.g., stop smoking *before* investing in respiratory therapy; implement healthy diet and exercise before higher-risk and higher-cost drugs for hypertension and hypercholesterolemia.
- Low-force interventions *before* high-force interventions.
- Generally: Diet *before* nutritional supplements; nutrients *before* botanicals; botanicals *before* drugs; modulatory drugs *before* suppressive/inhibitory drugs; integrative care *before* surgery.
- See examples below.

---

[433] McPherson M, Smith-Lovin L, Brashears ME. Social Isolation in America: Changes in Core Discussion Networks over Two Decades. *American Sociological Review* 2006; 71: 353-75 asanet.org/galleries/default-file/June06ASRFeature.pdf

Hierarchy of Therapeutics (specifically sequential)	Example of possible intervention
1. <u>Reestablishing the foundation for health</u>	<ul><li>Mental/emotional/spiritual health</li><li>Meditation, freeze-frame, "time out", relaxation</li><li>Positive visualization, positive expectation, affirmation</li><li>Counseling, social contact, group work</li><li>Family contact and resolution</li><li>Dietary intake and nutritional health which addresses the patient's biochemical individuality[434] and correction of deficiencies or excesses</li><li>Identification and elimination of food allergies/sensitivities</li><li>Reduce toxin exposure, promote detoxification</li><li>Identification and elimination of exposure to xenobiotics</li><li>Remove or reduce specific "obstacles to cure"</li></ul>
2. <u>Stimulation of the "healing power of nature" and the "vital force"</u>	<ul><li>Constitutional hydrotherapy</li><li>Homeopathy, Botanical adaptogens</li><li>Tai Chi, Qigong: "energy-cultivation"</li><li>Acupuncture, Spinal manipulation</li><li>Meditation, rest</li></ul>
3. <u>Tonification of weakened systems</u>	<ul><li>Botanical medicines and nutritional supplementation to help restore normal cellular/tissue function</li><li>Spinal manipulation to address the primary somatovisceral dysfunction and/or secondary musculoskeletal disorders</li><li>Hormonal supplementation, exercise, hydrotherapy</li></ul>
4. <u>Correction of structural integrity</u>	<ul><li>Spinal manipulation, deep tissue massage, visceral manipulation, lymphatic pump to promote immune surveillance[435], stretching, balancing, muscle strengthening, and proprioceptive retraining</li><li>Surgery, as a last resort</li></ul>

<u>The shadow of the naturopathic profession</u>: I would say that the weakness of the naturopathic profession is simply that—its lack of power *internally* to translate to power *externally*. Naturopathic physicians are few in number, and their incomes do not rival those of allopathic/osteopathic physicians (and thus cannot collectively afford powerful state organizations and paid lobbyists as can allopathic-pharmaceutical groups); they do not have the cultural authority of allopathic physicians, and they do not have the *carte blanche* backing of the pharmaceutical industry, whose financial power and thus political influence are both massive in the United States.[436] Naturopathic physicians have faced in the past and continue to face in recent/current times opposition/oppression by groups such as the AMA whose deep pockets and political contacts are used for legal/legislative initiatives such as marshalling "the medical community's resources against the growing threat of expanding scope of practice for allied health professionals."[437] The

> **Physician-philosophers of the future**
>
> "*Where must we reach with our hopes?* We have no option: we must reach for new philosophers, for those spirits strong and original enough to provide the stimuli for an opposing way of estimating current values [seeing things anew] and to initiate a revaluation and [if necessary] reversal of 'eternal values'."
>
> Nietzsche FW. <u>Beyond Good and Evil: Prelude to a Philosophy of the Future</u> (1886). Essay #203. Cambridge Texts in the History of Philosophy, page 91

---

[434] Williams RJ. <u>Biochemical Individuality: The Basis for the Genetotrophic Concept</u>. Austin and London: University of Texas Press, 1956
[435] "Lymph flow in the thoracic duct increased from 1.57±0.20 mL·min-1 to a peak TDF of 4.80±1.73 mL·min-1 during abdominal pump, and from 1.20±0.41 mL·min-1 to 3.45±1.61 mL·min-1 during thoracic pump." Knott EM, Tune JD, Stoll ST, Downey HF. Increased lymphatic flow in the thoracic duct during manipulative intervention. *J Am Osteopath Assoc*. 2005 Oct;105(10):447-56 jaoa.org/cgi/content/full/105/10/447
[436] This is only one of many documented examples. "The legislation was the cornerstone of Republican's domestic agenda and would extend limited prescription drugs coverage under Medicare to 41 million Americans, including 13 million who had never been covered before. At an estimated cost of just under $400 billion over 10 years, it was the largest entitlement program in more than 40 years, and the debate broke down along party lines." Under the Influence: Steve Kroft Reports On Drug Lobbyists' Role in Passing Bill That Keeps Drug Prices High cbsnews.com/news/under-the-influence/ Originally broadcast on April 1, 2007, updated on July 23, 2007. 2014 Jun
[437] "In an effort to marshal the medical community's resources against the growing threat of expanding scope of practice for allied health professionals, the AMA has formed a national partnership to confront such initiatives nationwide… The committee will use $25,000…" Daly R, American Psychiatric Association. AMA Forms Coalition to Thwart Non-M.D. Practice Expansion. Psychiatric News 2006 March; 41: 17 pn.psychiatryonline.org/cgi/content/full/41/5/17-a?eaf Accessed November 25, 2006

nutritional supplement and whole foods industries have failed to provide adequate support for the naturopathic profession in proportion to the increase in nutrition supplement sales and the public's increasing appreciation for *and purchase of* whole and organic foods, both of which have been supported by the naturopathic profession. Naturopathic schools are not without some occasional administrative incompetence and political pettiness; notable events during 2013 within two schools caused the unnecessary loss of intellectual power and internationally-respected irreplaceable academic/clinical/intellectual leadership from the profession in ways that clearly violate the profession's social, humanitarian, and intellectual values, despite administrative declarations to the opposite. Overall, the naturopathic profession continues to make positive albeit slow progress. Because the naturopathic profession's philosophy of healthcare stems from and extends back to life itself, naturopathic medicine is, at present and without any legitimate question, the only philosophy and model of primary healthcare (contrasted to allopathic and osteopathic) capable of salvaging, reforming, and optimizing healthcare outcomes in particular and human life in general.

Barefoot physician (Wahkeena Falls, Oregon): "Let us spend one day as deliberately as Nature, and not be thrown off the track by every nutshell and mosquito's wing that falls on the rails [train tracks]. Let us rise early and fast, or let us break the fast gently and without perturbation; let company come and let company go, let the bells ring and the children cry—determined to make a day of it. Why should we knock under and go with the stream? ... Let us settle ourselves, and work and wedge our feet downward through the mud and slush of opinion, and prejudice, and tradition, and delusion, and appearance, that alluvion which covers the globe, through Paris and London, through New York and Boston and Concord, through Church and State, through poetry and philosophy and religion, until we come to a hard bottom and rocks in place, which we can call *reality*." Thoreau HD. *Walden*. 1854

Functional Medicine

Introduction and personal experiences/perspectives: "Functional Medicine" as most of us know and appreciate it was developed from initial concepts that spawned from the genius of Dr Jeffrey Bland, a PhD biochemist drawn into the world of nutrition by a project of one of his graduate students, and who later made many paradigm-shifting contributions to the fields of clinical biochemistry and clinical practice of physicians world-wide. I (DrV) consider myself to have been a student and apprentice of Dr Bland starting in 1994, when I started attending his *Nutritional Biochemistry* presentations (vicariously, via audio cassettes) and every post-graduate conference and symposium I could attend, which was a considerable number (more than 300 hours of post-graduate training by the time I was 25yo), since I had by then relocated to the Pacific Northwest region of the United States, a few hours from where Dr Bland had HealthComm, the Functional Medicine Research Center, and later the Institute for Functional Medicine. Dr Bland's work quite obviously influenced me greatly, along with the work of Jonathan Wright MD (also in the Pacific Northwest), Leo Galland MD, and especially Alan Gaby MD; under their "nutritional influences", I basically "grew up" in an intellectual house of clinical nutrition and functional medicine. I would basically listen to audios of their lectures constantly, until the tapes wore out. Dr Bland's presentation *Advancement in Clinical Nutrition* in 1994 (cherished audio cassette pictured below)

Dr Vasquez was selected by the Institute for Functional Medicine to write its peer-reviewed CME monograph on disorders of pain and inflammation: *Musculoskeletal Pain: Expanded Clinical Strategies*, published by the Institute for Functional Medicine in 2008. Parts of this section were originally derived from the pre-edited draft of the introduction to that book, and any variations are used here with permission. Modifications were made to this section during revisions in 2011 and again in 2014. *Musculoskeletal Pain* contained an introduction to functional medicine and a review of assessments and therapeutics, followed by the clinical topics: migraine headaches, fibromyalgia, back pain, and rheumatoid arthritis. As would be expected, all of these topics have been discussed to a higher level of detail in more recent editions of *Integrative Orthopedics* (3rd Edition and later), *Integrative Rheumatology* (3rd Edition and later), *Fibromyalgia in a Nutshell* (2012), and the *Inflammation Mastery* series starting in 2014.

struck me with particular profundity; I listened to it so often that I had parts of it memorized because of the combination of verbal eloquence for which Dr Bland is famous and for the intellectual independence and lucidity with which Dr Bland articulated a new vision for medicine: that of moving beyond the *static* pathology-based models of disease toward appreciating illnesses as disorders of impaired *function*. Most people familiar with my work know that nutritional biochemistry and functional medicine are best described as my second interests following psychology and philosophy; indeed, I spent most of any "free time" during my 20s while completing two consecutive doctorates engaged with athletics, philosophy/psychology, and functional nutrition/medicine. The combination(s) of studying Gaby, Wright, Bland, Galland simultaneously with Rollins, Nietzsche, Bradshaw, Bly, Hillman, Lee, Meade, Kipnis, Moore, Miller, Deida, Branden, professionals and various personal groups gave me a unique view of health(care) and human potential; what appeared clear and obvious from these eclectic viewpoints was unknown or unspeakable among the majority of professors and students in the classes and clinics where I studied and learned.

Dr Bland's declaration that health and disease are *dynamic states of function* and *not static states of determinism* is powerful because Dr Bland uniquely had the ability to communicate his model with articulate clarity and the scientific knowledge to support every component. His model of *health as a dynamic entity* clearly opposed the static Pathology-based view of disease upon which allopathic medicine is founded: generally that disease states are constant and require life-long drug treatment (or surgery). The idea that clinicians should focus on improving *dynamic* function (mostly via nutrition and lifestyle) rather than treating *static* disease (always with drugs and surgery) was about as radical in Western medicine as analogous scientific landmarks such as the earth is round (Aristotle, et al), that the sun is the center of our planetary system (Aristarchus, Copernicus, Galileo), the evolution and interconnection of species (Darwin), and the denial of metaphysics and affirmation of earthly life (Nietzsche).

Evolution of medicine, from metaphysical determinism to dynamic molecular biology: Historically, prevailing views of disorders of pain and inflammation were conceptually similar to those of most other diseases and premodern accounts of life in general. Our clinical predecessors did the best they could to understand, describe, and treat the health problems with which their patients presented, and the paradigms from which these clinical entities were viewed and addressed were shaped by the social, religious, and scientific views and limitations of their time. Lacking a molecular and physiologic understanding of disease origination, and restrained by metaphysical and simplistic models of "cause and effect", premodern clinicians devised models for the understanding and treatment of disease that generally appear unsatisfactory today in light of the advances in our understanding in disparate yet interrelated fields such as psychoneuroimmunology, molecular biology, nutrigenomics, environmental medicine and toxicology. Despite these advances, we as a human society and as healthcare providers still carry many of these previous conceptualizations and misconceptualizations with us as we move forward toward a future wherein our views and interventions will be much more precise and "objective" in contrast to the generalized and phenomenalistic approaches that typified premodern medicine and which still permeate certain aspects of clinical care today. For example, we still use the term "stroke" to describe acute cerebrovascular insufficiency, although the term originated from the view that affected patients had been "struck" by the gods or fates perhaps as a form of punishment for some ethical or religious transgression. Even today, patients and clinicians commonly interpret disease as some form of punishment or as an extension of spiritual or intrapersonal shortcoming. Advancing science allows us to disassemble complex events that were previously experienced as *phenomena*, that is, as undecipherable and enigmatic events that overwhelmed comprehension. Dr Bland's functional medicine concept and the clinical tools that were developed from it began the process of helping clinicians grasp a science-based and systems-based multidimensional and decipherable view of diseases and corresponding treatments; as such, it has facilitated the achievement of higher clinical efficacy, improved patient outcomes, and more favorable safety and cost-effectiveness profiles.

Whereas the advancement of our scientific knowledge often leads us to discard previous models and interventions, occasionally modern science helps us to understand and revisit previous interventions that may have been prematurely or unduly discarded. For example, Hippocrates' admonition to "Let thy food be thy medicine, and thy medicine be thy food" experienced decades of devaluation when dietary, nutritional, and other natural interventions were misbranded as "quackery." On the contrary to these premature and unsubstantiated condemnations, simple natural interventions such as therapeutic fasting and augmentation of vitamin D3 status (via nutritional supplementation or exposure to ultraviolet-B radiation) have shown remarkable safety and efficacy in the mitigation of chronic hypertension, musculoskeletal pain, and autoimmunity.[438,439,440,441,442,443,444,445,446] Relatedly, newer research has also shown that the appropriate use of vitamin supplementation helps prevent

---

[438] Goldhamer A, et al. Medically supervised water-only fasting in the treatment of hypertension. *J Manipulative Physiol Ther* 2001 Jun;24(5):335-9
[439] Goldhamer AC, et al. Medically supervised water-only fasting in the treatment of borderline hypertension. *J Altern Complement Med*. 2002 Oct;8(5):643-50
[440] Goldhamer AC. Initial cost of care results in medically supervised water-only fasting for treating high blood pressure and diabetes. *J Altern Complement Med* 2002 Dec;8:696-7
[441] Krause R, Bühring M, Hopfenmüller W, Holick MF, Sharma AM. Ultraviolet B and blood pressure. *Lancet*. 1998 Aug 29;352(9129):709-10
[442] Pfeifer et al. Effects of a short-term vitamin D(3) and calcium supplementation on blood pressure and parathyroid hormone. *J Clin Endocrinol Metab*. 2001 Apr;86(4):1633-7
[443] McCarty MF. Preliminary fast may potentiate response to a subsequent low-salt, low-fat vegan diet in management of hypertension. *Med Hypotheses*. 2003 May;60(5):624-33
[444] Hyppönen E, Läärä E, Reunanen A, Järvelin MR, Virtanen SM. Intake of vitamin D and risk of type 1 diabetes: a birth-cohort study. *Lancet*. 2001 Nov 3;358(9292):1500-3
[445] Fuhrman J, et al. Brief case reports of medically supervised, water-only fasting associated with remission of autoimmune disease. *Altern Ther Health Med*. 2002;8:112,110-1
[446] Holick MF. Vitamin D deficiency: what a pain it is. *Mayo Clin Proc*. 2003 Dec;78(12):1457-9

chronic disease by numerous mechanisms including modulation of gene transcription, enhancement of DNA repair and stability, and enhancement of metabolic efficiency.[447,448,449]

While all clinicians can appreciate the importance of protocols and clinical practice guidelines, we must also perpetually ratify the preeminence of patient individuality and therefore the importance of tailoring treatment to the patient's unique combination of biochemical individuality, comorbid conditions, drug use, personal goals, and willingness to participate in a health-promoting lifestyle. Standardized protocols and practice guidelines are founded on the fallacy of disease homogeneity and the irrelevance of physiologic, psychosocial, and biochemical individuality.

A clinician who is unaware of the political forces that shape healthcare policy and research is analogous to a captain of an oceangoing ship not knowing how to use a compass, sextant, or coastline map. Medical science and healthcare policy are influenced by a myriad of powerful private interests which are motivated by their own goals, at times different from the stated goals of medicine, which purports to hold paramount the patient's welfare. Scientific objectivity and the guiding ethical principles of informed consent, beneficence, autonomy, and non-malfeasance are subject to different interpretations depending upon the lens through which a dilemma is viewed. When this "dilemma" is the whole of healthcare, what first appears as order and structure now appears as the disarrayed tug-of-war between factions and private interests, with paradigmatic victory often being awarded to those with the best marketing campaigns and political influence with less importance given to safety, efficacy, and the economic burden to consumers.[Compilation footnote 450] To be ignorant of such considerations is to be blind to the nature of research, policy, and our own biased inclinations for and against particular paradigms, assessments, and interventions. Research articles and sources of authority must be approached with an artist's delicacy, and with a

---

[447] Fletcher RH, Fairfield KM. Vitamins for chronic disease prevention in adults: clinical applications. *JAMA*. 2002 Jun 19;287(23):3127-9
[448] Heaney RP. Long-latency deficiency disease: insights from calcium and vitamin D. *Am J Clin Nutr*. 2003 Nov;78(5):912-9
[449] Ames BN. The metabolic tune-up: metabolic harmony and disease prevention. *J Nutr*. 2003 May;133(5 Suppl 1):1544S-8S
[450] Editorial. Drug-company influence on medical education in USA. *Lancet*. 2000 Sep 2;356(9232):781

1. Horton R. Lotronex and the FDA: a fatal erosion of integrity. *Lancet*. 2001 May 19;357(9268):1544-5
2. Editorial. Politics trumps science at the FDA. *Lancet*. 2005 Nov 26;366(9500):1827
3. Topol EJ. Failing the public health--rofecoxib, Merck, and the FDA. *N Engl J Med*. 2004 Oct 21;351(17):1707-9
4. Wolinsky H, Brune T. *The Serpent on the Staff: The Unhealthy Politics of the American Medical Association*. GP Putnam and Sons, New York, 1994
5. Wilk CA. *Medicine, Monopolies, and Malice: How the Medical Establishment Tried to Destroy Chiropractic*. Garden City Park: Avery, 1996
6. Carter JP. *Racketeering in Medicine: The Suppression of Alternatives*. Norfolk: Hampton Roads Pub; 1993
7. National Alliance of Professional Psychology Providers. AMA Seeks To Control and Restrict Psychologist's Scope of Practice. nappp.org/scope.pdf 2006 Nov
8. Daly R, American Psychiatric Association. AMA Forms Coalition to Thwart Non-M.D. Practice Expansion. *Psychiatric News* 2006 March; 41: 17
9. Angell M. *The Truth About the Drug Companies: How They Deceive Us and What to Do About it*. Random House; August 2004
10. Terrett AG. Misuse of the literature by medical authors in discussing spinal manipulative therapy injury. *J Manipulative Physiol Ther*. 1995 May;18(4):203-10
11. Morley et al. A case study of misrepresentation of the scientific literature: recent reviews of chiropractic. *J Altern Complement Med*. 2001 Feb;7(1):65-78
12. Wenban AB. Inappropriate use of title 'chiropractor' and term 'chiropractic manipulation' in peer-reviewed biomedical literature. *Chiropr Osteopat*. 2006 Aug;14:16
13. Spivak JL. *The Medical Trust Unmasked*. Louis S. Siegfried Publishers; New York: 1961
14. Trever W. *In the Public Interest*. Los Angeles; Scriptures Unlimited; 1972. This is probably the most authoritative documentation of the illegal actions of the AMA up to 1972; contains numerous photocopies of actual AMA documents and minutes of official meetings with overt intentionality of destroying Americans' healthcare options so that the AMA and related organizations would have a monopoly in healthcare.
15. Getzendanner S. Permanent injunction order against AMA. *JAMA*. 1988 Jan 1;259(1):81-2
16. "A national study released today reports 20 million American families — or one in seven families — faced hardships paying medical bills last year, which forced many to choose between getting medical attention or paying rent or buying food…" Freeman, Liz. 'Working poor' struggle to afford health care. *Naples Daily News*. naplesnews.com/npdn/news/article/0,2071,NPDN_14940_3000546,00.html
17. "The USA's 5.8 million small companies… Health care costs are rising about 15% this year for those with fewer than 200 workers vs. 13.5% for those with 500 or more… But many small employers cite increases of 20% or more. That's made insurance the No. 1 small business problem…" Jim Hopkins. Health care tops taxes as small business cost drain. *USA TODAY*. usatoday.com/news/health/2003-04-20-small-business-costs_x.htm.
18. "Though the U.S. has slightly fewer doctors per capita than the typical developed nation, we have almost twice as many MRI machines and perform vastly more angioplasties. …at least 31 percent of all the incremental income we'll earn between 1999 and 2010 will go to health care." Regnier P. Healthcare myth: We spend too much. *Money Magazine* October 13, 2003: 11:29 AM EDT money.cnn.com/2003/10/08/pf/health_myths_1/
19. "Although they spend more on health care than patients in any other industrialized nation, Americans receive the right treatment less than 60 percent of the time, resulting in unnecessary pain, expense and even death…" Ceci Connolly. U.S. Patients Spend More but Don't Get More, Study Finds: Even in Advantaged Areas, Americans Often Receive Inadequate Health Care. *Washington Post*, May 5, 2004; Page A15washingtonpost.com/ac2/wp-dyn/A1875-2004May4
20. McGlynn et al. The quality of health care delivered to adults in the United States. *N Engl J Med*. 2003 Jun 26;348(26):2635-45
21. Brennan et al. Incidence of adverse events and negligence in hospitalized patients. *Qual Saf Health Care*. 2004 Apr;13(2):145-51
22. "Basically, you die earlier and spend more time disabled if you're an American rather than a member of most other advanced countries." Christopher Murray MD PhD, Director of World Health Organization's Global Program on Evidence for Health Policy who.int/inf-pr-2000/en/pr2000-life.html Accessed July 12, 2004
23. Shi L. Health care spending, delivery, and outcome in developed countries: a cross-national comparison. *Am J Med Qual* 1997;12(2):83-93
24. Holland EG, Degruy FV. Drug-induced disorders. *Am Fam Physician*. 1997 Nov 1;56(7):1781-8, 1791-2
25. Brennan et al. Incidence of adverse events and negligence in hospitalized patients. *Qual Saf Health Care*. 2004 Apr;13(2):145-51
26. Whitaker R. The case against antipsychotic drugs: a 50-year record of doing more harm than good. *Med Hypotheses*. 2004;62(1):5-13
27. Use of horse estrogens in humans as "hormone replacement therapy" exemplified the application of a strong carcinogen to millions of unsuspecting women: Zhang et al. Major metabolite of equilin, 4-hydroxyequilin, autoxidizes to an o-quinone which isomerizes to potent cytotoxin 4-hydroxyequilenin-o-quinone. *Chem Res Toxicol*. 1999 Feb;12(2):204-13; Pisha et al. Evidence that a metabolite of equine estrogens, 4-hydroxyequilenin, induces cellular transformation in vitro. *Chem Res Toxicol*. 2001;14:82-90; Zhang et al. Equine estrogen metabolite 4-hydroxyequilenin induces DNA damage in rat mammary tissues. *Chem Res Toxicol*. 2001 Dec;14:1654-9
28. Newman NM, Ling RS. Acetabular bone destruction related to non-steroidal anti-inflammatory drugs. *Lancet*. 1985 Jul 6; 2(8445): 11-4
29. "In 1983, 2876 people died from medication errors. ... By 1993, this number had risen to 7,391 - a 2.57-fold increase." Phillips DP, Christenfeld N, Glynn LM. Increase in US medication-error deaths between 1983 and 1993. *Lancet*. 1998 Feb 28;351(9103):643-4
30. Smith R. Medical journals are an extension of the marketing arm of pharmaceutical companies. *PLoS Med*. 2005 May;2(5):e138
31. van der Steen WJ, Ho VK. Drugs versus diets: disillusions with Dutch health care. *Acta Biotheor*. 2001;49(2):125-40

willingness to receive new information as worthy of preeminence over deeply rooted and well ensconced institutionalized fallacies.

Understanding How Interconnected Systems Participate in Health and Disease: When viewed as a diagram, the web of major influences reveals the interconnected nature of causes, effects, and body systems and how imbalance or disruption in one area can lead to problems in another. Once homeostatic reserves and compensatory mechanisms are depleted, the patient experiences progressively worsening health (which may be asymptomatic) and the eventual manifestation of clinical disease.

Although newer versions of this diagram have been developed over the past few years, replacing the previous version provided below, the original diagram—interconnected by Vasquez in 2003—is the most efficient and practical for demonstrating the body systems and external inputs most important to the maintenance of health and genesis of disease. These systems and inputs described in following pages with particular consideration given to pain and inflammation, both of which are leading causes of disability and illness among patients seen in general practice and specialty and subspecialty care on a daily basis.

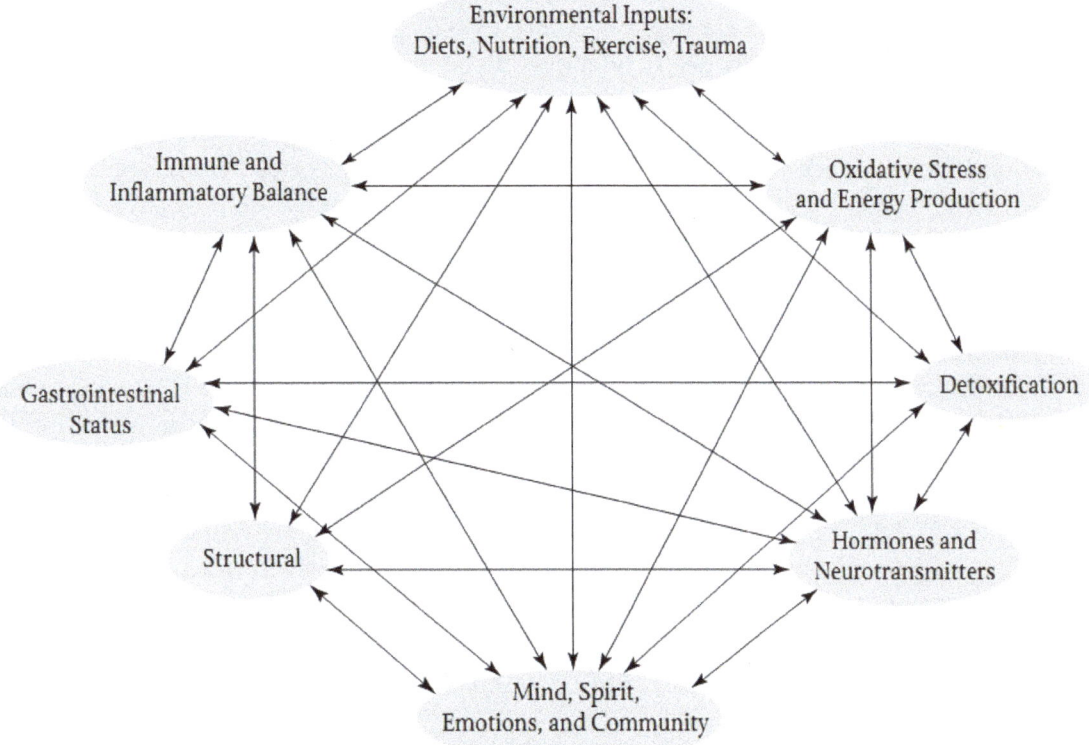

Interconnected Physiologic Web illustrated by Alex Vasquez (circa 2003): This version of "the Functional Medicine Matrix" interconnected by Alex Vasquez provides an illustration of the interdependency of physiologic factors and organ systems; this version was published in Vasquez A. Web-like Interconnections of Physiological Factors. *Integrative Medicine* 2006 Apr/May. The Matrix is owned and has since been completely changed by the Institute for Functional Medicine.

Exploring the Different Aspects of the Interconnected Physiologic Web
1. Hormonal and neurotransmitter imbalances: While most clinicians are aware that neurotransmitters can either transmit pain signals or dampen their reception, many clinicians are not aware that neurotransmitter status is somewhat malleable and can be modulated with nutritional supplementation and botanical medicines. The examples that will be considered here are the tryptophan-serotonin-melatonin and the phenylalanine-tyrosine-dopamine-norepinephrine-epinephrine and enkephalin pathways.

- Tryptophan and 5-hydroxytryptophan (5HTP) are prescription and nonprescription nutritional supplements that are the amino acid precursors for the formation of the neurotransmitter serotonin and the pineal hormone melatonin. Biochemically, these conversions are linear as follows: tryptophan → 5HTP → serotonin → melatonin. Tryptophan depletion and low levels of serotonin are consistently associated with depression, anxiety, exacerbation of eating disorders, and increased sensitivity to acute and chronic pain. Serotonergic pathways are impaired by chronic stress due to increased utilization of serotonin (e.g., serotonin-dependent cortisol release) and increased hepatic degradation of tryptophan by cortisol-stimulated tryptophan pyrrolase.[451] Therapeutically, supplementation with 5HTP augments serotonin and melatonin synthesis and has specific applicability in the alleviation of depression and pain syndromes such as fibromyalgia and headache, including migraine, tension headaches, and juvenile headaches.[452,453] Certainly part of the benefit from 5HTP supplementation is derived from the increased formation of melatonin, as the biological effects of melatonin extend beyond its sleep-promoting role to include powerful antioxidation, anti-infective immunostimulation[454], and preservation of mitochondrial function, a benefit which is of particular relevance to the treatment of fibromyalgia.[455]

- The conditionally essential fatty acids found in fish oil modulate serotonergic and adrenergic activity in the human brain[456], and given the role of serotonin and norepinephrine in the central processing of pain perception[457], a reasonable hypothesis holds that the pain-relieving activity of fish oil supplementation[458] is partly due to central modulation of pain perception and is not wholly due to modulation of eicosanoid production and inflammatory mediator transcription as previously believed.

- Vitamin D3 supplementation may also augment serotonergic activity[459], and this mechanism may partly explain the mood-enhancing and pain-relieving benefits of vitamin D3 supplementation. Attentive readers will note that this brief discussion has already begun to bridge the gaps between nutritional status, neurotransmitter synthesis, pain sensitivity, immune function, and mitochondrial bioenergetics.

- Supplementation with DL-phenylalanine (DLPA; racemic mixture of D- and L-forms of the amino acid phenylalanine derived from synthetic production) has long been used in the treatment of pain and depression.[460] The nutritional L-isomer is converted from phenylalanine → tyrosine → L-dopa → dopamine → norepinephrine → epinephrine. Augmentation of this pathway promotes resistance to fatigue, depression, and pain. The synthetic D-isomer augments pain-relieving enkephalin function by inhibiting enkephalin degradation by the enzyme carboxypeptidase A (enkephalinase); the resultant augmentation of enkephalin levels is generally believed to underlie the analgesic and mood-enhancing benefits of DLPA supplementation.

- Therapeutic massage is yet another means to modulate neurotransmitter synthesis for the alleviation of pain. In a study of patients with chronic back pain, massage increased serotonin and dopamine levels (measured in urine).[461]

Hormonal imbalances are particularly relevant to the discussion of chronic pain caused by inflammation characteristic of autoimmune diseases such as rheumatoid arthritis (RA). Often clinically subtle but nonetheless of extreme importance, these hormonal influences on painful inflammation are worthy of their own detailed discussion and thus will be reviewed later in this textbook. Generally speaking and with a few noted exceptions, the research literature points to a specific pattern of hormonal imbalances among patients with autoimmunity, and this pattern is consistent with the pro-inflammatory and immunodysregulatory effects of estrogens and prolactin and the anti-inflammatory and

---

[451] Sandyk R. Tryptophan availability and the susceptibility to stress in multiple sclerosis: a hypothesis. *Int J Neurosci*. 1996 Jul;86(1-2):47-53
[452] Turner EH, Loftis JM, Blackwell AD. Serotonin a la carte: supplementation with the serotonin precursor 5-hydroxytryptophan. *Pharmacol Ther*. 2006 Mar;109(3):325-38
[453] Birdsall TC. 5-Hydroxytryptophan: a clinically-effective serotonin precursor. *Altern Med Rev*. 1998 Aug;3(4):271-80
[454] Gitto E, et al. Effects of melatonin treatment in septic newborns. *Pediatr Res*. 2001 Dec;50(6):756-60
[455] Acuna-Castroviejo D, Escames G, Reiter RJ. Melatonin therapy in fibromyalgia. *J Pineal Res*. 2006 Jan;40(1):98-9
[456] Hibbeln et al. Omega-3 fatty acid deficiencies in neurodevelopment, aggression and autonomic dysregulation: opportunities for intervention. *Int Rev Psychiatry* 2006;18:107-18
[457] Wise TN, Fishbain DA, Holder-Perkins V. Painful physical symptoms in depression: a clinical challenge. *Pain Med*. 2007 Sep;8 Suppl 2:S75-82
[458] Goldberg RJ, Katz J. A meta-analysis of the analgesic effects of omega-3 polyunsaturated fatty acid supplementation for inflammatory joint pain. *Pain*. 2007;129(1-2):210-23
[459] Lansdowne AT, Provost SC. Vitamin D3 enhances mood in healthy subjects during winter. *Psychopharmacology* (Berl). 1998 Feb;135(4):319-23
[460] Russell AL, McCarty MF. DL-phenylalanine markedly potentiates opiate analgesia. *Med Hypotheses*. 2000 Oct;55(4):283-8
[461] Hernandez-Reif M, Field T, Krasnegor J, Theakston H. Lower back pain is reduced and range of motion increased after massage therapy. *Int J Neurosci* 2001;106(3-4):131-45

immunomodulatory effects of cortisol, dehydroepiandrosterone (DHEA), and testosterone. Patients with autoimmune neuromusculoskeletal inflammation generally display a complete or partial pattern of hormonal disturbances typified by elevated estrogen and prolactin and lowered testosterone, DHEA, and cortisol; appropriate therapeutic correction of these imbalances can safely result in disease amelioration. Rectification of endocrinologic imbalances ("orthoendocrinology") is detailed later in this book.

2. Oxidation-reduction imbalances and mitochondriopathy: Oxidative stress results from the chronic systemic inflammation seen in painful inflammatory disorders such as RA, and oxidative stress contributes to the perpetuation and exacerbation of inflammatory diseases via expedited tissue destruction and alterations in gene transcription and resultant enhancement of inflammatory mediator production.[462] Immune activation increases production of reactive oxygen species (ROS; "free radicals"), and oxidant stress increases activation of pro-inflammatory transcription factors (such as nuclear factor KappaB, NFkB) and also increases spontaneous oxidative modification of endogenous proteins such as cartilage matrix which then undergoes expedited degradation or immunologic attack; thus a vicious cycle of oxidation and inflammation exacerbates and perpetuates various inflammation-associated diseases, resulting in therapeutic recalcitrance and autonomous disease progression.[463,464] A rational clinical approach to breaking this vicious pathogenic cycle can include simultaneous antioxidation and immunomodulation, the former with diet optimization and nutritional supplementation and the latter with allergen avoidance, hormonal correction, xenobiotic detoxification, and specific phytonutritional modulation of pro-inflammatory pathways. Severe and acute inflammation can and often should be suppressed pharmacologically, but sole reliance on pharmacologic immunosuppression leaves the patient vulnerable to iatrogenic immunosuppression and the well-known increased risk for cardiovascular disease, osteoporosis, infection, and clinical malignancy while failing to address the underlying biochemical and immunologic imbalances which generate and maintain all chronic inflammatory and autoimmune diseases. The contribution of mitochondrial dysfunction to chronic recurrent or persistent pain is most plainly demonstrated in migraine and fibromyalgia. An important characteristic of migraine is mitochondrial dysfunction, the severity of which correlates positively with the severity of the headache syndrome.[465] In fibromyalgia, numerous abnormalities in cellular bioenergetics are noted, which correlate clinically with the lowered lactate threshold, persistent muscle pain, reduced functional capacity, and the subjective fatigue that characterize the disorder.[466] Nutritional preservation and enhancement of mitochondrial function was termed "mitochondrial resuscitation" by Jeffrey Bland PhD in the 1990s, and clinical implementation of such an approach generally includes, in addition to diet and lifestyle modification, supplementation with coenzyme Q-10, niacin, riboflavin, thiamin, lipoic acid, magnesium, and other nutrients and botanical medicines which enhance production of adenosine triphosphate (ATP).[467]

3. Detoxification and biotransformational imbalances: As our environment becomes increasingly polluted and as researchers and clinicians expand their appreciation and knowledge of the adverse effects of xenobiotics (toxic metals and chemicals), healthcare providers will need to attend to their patients' detoxification capacity and xenobiotic load as a component of the prevention and treatment of disease. By now, senior students and practicing clinicians should be aware of the association of xenobiotics in prototypic diseases such as Parkinson's disease[468,469], adult-onset diabetes mellitus[470,471,472,473], and attention-

---

[462] Hitchon CA, El-Gabalawy HS. Oxidation in rheumatoid arthritis. *Arthritis Res Ther*. 2004;6(6):265-78
[463] Tak PP, et al. Rheumatoid arthritis and p53: how oxidative stress might alter the course of inflammatory diseases. *Immunol Today*. 2000 Feb;21(2):78-82
[464] Kurien BT, Hensley K, Bachmann M, Scofield RH. Oxidatively modified autoantigens in autoimmune diseases. *Free Radic Biol Med*. 2006 Aug 15;41(4):549-56
[465] Lodi R, et al. Quantitative analysis of skeletal muscle bioenergetics and proton efflux in migraine and cluster headache. *J Neurol Sci*. 1997 Feb 27;146(1):73-80
[466] Park et al. Use of P-31 magnetic resonance spectroscopy to detect metabolic abnormalities in muscles of patients with fibromyalgia. *Arthritis Rheum*. 1998 Mar;41(3):406-13
[467] Pieczenik SR, Neustadt J. Mitochondrial dysfunction and molecular pathways of disease. *Exp Mol Pathol*. 2007 Aug;83(1):84-92
[468] Corrigan FM, et al. Organochlorine insecticides in substantia nigra in Parkinson's disease. *J Toxicol Environ Health A*. 2000 Feb 25;59(4):229-34
[469] Fleming L, Mann JB, Bean J, Briggle T, Sanchez-Ramos JR. Parkinson's disease and brain levels of organochlorine pesticides. *Ann Neurol*. 1994 Jul;36(1):100-3
[470] Fujiyoshi et al. Molecular epidemiologic evidence for diabetogenic effects of dioxin exposure in U.S. Air force veterans of the Vietnam War. *Environ Health Perspect*, 2006 Nov;114(11):1677-83
[471] Lee DH, Lee IK, Song K, Steffes M, Toscano W, Baker BA, Jacobs DR Jr. A strong dose-response relation between serum concentrations of persistent organic pollutants and diabetes: results from the National Health and Examination Survey 1999-2002. *Diabetes Care* 2006 Jul;29(7):1638-44
[472] Lee DH, Lee IK, Jin SH, Steffes M, Jacobs DR Jr. Association between serum concentrations of persistent organic pollutants and insulin resistance among nondiabetic adults: results from the National Health and Nutrition Examination Survey 1999-2002. *Diabetes Care*, 2007 Mar;30(3):622-8
[473] Remillard RB, Bunce NJ. Linking dioxins to diabetes: epidemiology and biologic plausibility. *Environ Health Perspect*, 2002 Sep;110(9):853-8

deficit hyperactivity disorder.[474,475,476] The role of xenobiotic exposure and impaired detoxification in neuromusculoskeletal pain and inflammatory disorders is more subtle and is generally mediated through the resultant immunotoxicity that manifests as autoimmunity. Occasionally, clinicians will encounter patients with musculoskeletal symptomatology that defies standard diagnosis and treatment but which responds remarkably and permanently to empiric clinical detoxification treatment. The numerous roles of xenobiotic exposure in the genesis and perpetuation of chronic health problems and the role of clinical detoxification in the treatment of such problems has been detailed elsewhere by Crinnion[477,478,479,480,481], Rea[482], Bland[483,484], Vasquez[485,486], and others.[487,488]

4. **Immune imbalances**: Immune imbalances have an obvious role in musculoskeletal inflammation when discussed in the context of autoimmune diseases such as rheumatoid arthritis, ankylosing spondylitis, and systemic lupus erythematosus. While the standard medical approach to this pathophysiology has focused almost exclusively on the pharmacologic suppression of resultant inflammation and tissue destruction, other disciplines such as naturopathic medicine and functional medicine have emphasized the importance of determining and addressing the underlying causes of such immune imbalance. While clinicians of all disciplines must appreciate the important role of pharmacologic immunosuppression in the treatment of inflammatory exacerbations as seen with giant cell arteritis or neuropsychiatric lupus, they should also appreciate that sole reliance on immunosuppression for long-term management of inflammatory disorders is destined to therapeutic failure insofar as it does not correct the underlying cause of the disease and creates dependency upon perpetual immunosuppression with its attendant costs (not uncommonly in the range of $20,000 - 50,000 per year) and adverse effects including infection and increased risk for cancer. Rather than presuming that immune dysfunction and the resultant inflammation and autoimmunity are results of spontaneous generation, astute clinicians seek to identify and correct the causes of these immune imbalances. By identifying and correcting the underlying causes of immune imbalance (when possible), clinicians can lessen or obviate the need for chronic polypharmaceutical treatment with anti-inflammatory and immunosuppressive agents. Vasquez[489] proposed that secondary immune imbalances (distinguished from primary congenital disorders) generally arise from one or more of five main problems: ❶ habitual consumption of a pro-inflammatory diet, ❷ food allergies and intolerances, ❸ microbial dysbiosis, including multifocal polydysbiosis, ❹ hormonal imbalances, and ❺ xenobiotic exposure and accumulation resulting in immunotoxicity via bystander activation and enhanced processing of autoantigens as well as haptenization and neoantigen formation. These influences may act singularly or when combined may be additive and synergistic.

5. **Inflammatory imbalances**: Inflammatory imbalances may be distinguished from immune imbalances insofar as inflammatory imbalances connote disorders of inflammatory mediator production in the absence of the immunodysfunction that typifies allergy, autoimmunity, or immunosuppression. Here again, long-term consumption of a pro-inflammatory diet[490] is a primary consideration because such a diet typically oversupplies inflammatory precursors such as arachidonate and undersupplies anti-inflammatory phytonutrients such as vitamin D, zinc, selenium, and the numerous phytochemicals that reduce activation

---

[474] Rauh VA, et al. Impact of prenatal chlorpyrifos exposure on neurodevelopment in the first 3 years of life among inner-city children. *Pediatrics*. 2006 Dec;118(6):e1845-59
[475] Cheuk DK, Wong V. Attention-deficit hyperactivity disorder and blood mercury level: a case-control study in Chinese children. *Neuropediatrics*. 2006 Aug;37(4):234-40
[476] Nigg et al. Low blood lead levels with clinically diagnosed attention-deficit/hyperactivity disorder and mediated by weak cognitive control. *Biol Psychiatry*. 2008;63:325-31
[477] Crinnion W. Results of a Decade of Naturopathic Treatment for Environmental Illnesses: A Review of Clinical Records. *J Naturopathic Medicine* vol. 7; 2, 21-27
[478] Crinnion WJ. Environmental medicine, part 1: the human burden of environmental toxins and their common health effects. *Altern Med Rev*. 2000 Feb;5(1):52-63
[479] Crinnion WJ. Environmental medicine, part 2: health effects of and protection from ubiquitous airborne solvent exposure. *Altern Med Rev*. 2000 Apr;5(2):133-43
[480] Crinnion WJ. Environmental medicine, part 3: long-term effects of chronic low-dose mercury exposure. *Altern Med Rev*. 2000 Jun;5(3):209-23
[481] Crinnion WJ. Environmental medicine, part 4: pesticides - biologically persistent and ubiquitous toxins. *Altern Med Rev*. 2000 Oct;5(5):432-47
[482] Rea WJ, Pan Y, Johnson AR. Clearing of toxic volatile hydrocarbons from humans. *Bol Asoc Med P R*. 1991 Jul;83(7):321-4
[483] Bland JS, et al. A Medical Food-Supplemented Detoxification Program in the Management of Chronic Health Problems. *Altern Ther Health Med*. 1995 Nov 1;1(5):62-71
[484] Minich DM, Bland JS. Acid-alkaline balance: role in chronic disease and detoxification. *Altern Ther Health Med*. 2007 Jul-Aug;13(4):62-5
[485] Vasquez A. *Integrative Rheumatology: Second Edition*. Fort Worth, Texas; Integrative and Biological Medicine Research and Consulting, 2007
[486] Vasquez A. Diabetes: Are Toxins to Blame? *Naturopathy Digest* 2007; April
[487] Kilburn et al. Neurobehavioral dysfunction in firemen exposed to polychlorinated biphenyls (PCBs): improvement after detoxification. *Arch Environ Health* 1989;44:345-50
[488] Cecchini M, LoPresti V. Drug residues store in the body following cessation of use: impacts on neuroendocrine balance and behavior--use of the Hubbard sauna regimen to remove toxins and restore health. *Med Hypotheses*. 2007;68(4):868-79
[489] Vasquez A. *Integrative Rheumatology: Second Edition*. Fort Worth, Texas; Integrative and Biological Medicine Research and Consulting, 2007
[490] Seaman DR. The diet-induced proinflammatory state: a cause of chronic pain and other degenerative diseases? *J Manipulative Physiol Ther*. 2002 Mar-Apr;25(3):168-79

of inflammatory pathways.[491,492,493,494] Three of the best examples of correctable inflammatory imbalances are those due to vitamin D deficiency, fatty acid imbalances, and overconsumption of simple sugars and saturated fats. Vitamin D deficiency is a widespread and serious health problem that spans nearly all geographic regions and socioeconomic strata with several important adverse effects. Vitamin D deficiency results in systemic inflammation[495] and chronic musculoskeletal pain[496] which both resolve quickly upon correction of the nutritional deficiency. Similarly and consistent with the Western/American pattern of dietary intake, overconsumption of alpha-linoleic acid and arachidonate along with underconsumption of alpha-linolenic acid (ALA), gamma-linolenic acid (GLA), eicosapentaenoic acid (EPA), docosahexaenoic acid (DHA), and oleic acid subtly yet powerfully shift nutrigenomic tendency and precursor availability in favor of enhanced systemic inflammation. Correction of this imbalance such as with reduced consumption of arachidonate and increased consumption of EPA and DHA has consistently proven to be of significant clinical value in the management of chronic inflammatory disorders.[497,498] Measurable increases in systemic inflammation and oxidative stress follow glucose challenge[499], consumption of saturated fatty acids as found in cream[500], and consumption of a "fast food" breakfast, which triggers the prototypic inflammatory activator NF-kappaB for enhanced production of inflammatory mediators.[501] This triad (vitamin D deficiency, fatty acid imbalance, and overconsumption of sugars and saturated fats) is typical of the Western/American pattern of dietary intake, and the molecular means and clinical consequences of such dietary choices is quite clear, evidenced by burgeoning epidemics of metabolic and inflammatory diseases.

6. <u>Digestive, absorptive, and microbiological imbalances</u>: The grouping of digestive and absorptive considerations suggests that the alimentary tract and its accessory organs of the liver, gall bladder and pancreas will be the focus of these core clinical imbalances, and the addition of microbiological imbalances should remind current clinicians that gastrointestinal dysbiosis is an important and frequent clinical consideration. Impaired digestion begins neither in the stomach nor in the mouth, but it stems rather from any socioeconomic milieu which deprives people of the means to prepare wholesome health-promoting meals and the time to consume those meals in a relaxed parasympathetic-dominant mode, preferably among good company, stimulating conversation, and appropriate ambiance. Poor dentition, xerostomia, hypochlorhydria, cholestasis or cholecystectomy, pancreatic insufficiency, mucosal atrophy, altered gut motility, and bacterial overgrowth of the small bowel are important and common contributors to impaired digestion and absorption; clinicians should consider these frequently and implement treatment with a low threshold for intervention. The relevance of these problems to pain and the musculoskeletal system is generally that of malnutrition and its macro- and micronutrient consequences. Sunlight-deprived individuals must rely on dietary sources of vitamin D, which are hardly adequate for the prevention of overt deficiency; any impairment in digestion, emulsification, or absorption of this fat-soluble vitamin can readily lead to hypovitaminosis D and its resultant musculoskeletal consequences of osteomalacia and unremitting pain.[502] Consumption of foods to which the individual is sensitized ("food allergies") can trigger migraine and other chronic headaches[503,504] as well as generalized musculoskeletal pain and arthritis.[505,506,507] Avoidance of the offending foods often results in amelioration or complete remission of the painful syndrome at low cost and high efficacy without reliance on expensive or potentially harmful or addictive pain-relieving drugs. Occasionally, gluten enteropathy (celiac disease) presents with arthritic pain

---

[491] Vasquez A. New Insights into Fatty Acid Biochemistry and the Influence of Diet. *Nutr Perspectives* 2004; Oct: 5,7-10,12,14
[492] Vasquez A. New Insights into Fatty Acid Supplementation and Its Effect on Eicosanoid Production and Genetic Expression. *Nutritional Perspectives* 2005; January: 5-16
[493] Vasquez A. Improving overall health while safely and effectively treating musculoskeletal pain. *Nutritional Perspectives* 2005; 28: 34-38, 40-42
[494] Vasquez A. Nutritional and Botanical Inhibition of NF-kappaB, the Major Intracellular Amplifier of the Inflammatory Cascade. *Nutritional Perspectives* 2005;July: 5-12
[495] Timms PM, et al. Circulating MMP9, vitamin D and variation in the TIMP-1 response with VDR genotype. *QJM*. 2002 Dec;95(12):787-96
[496] Al Faraj S, Al Mutairi K. Vitamin D deficiency and chronic low back pain in Saudi Arabia. *Spine*. 2003 Jan 15;28(2):177-9
[497] James MJ, Gibson RA, Cleland LG. Dietary polyunsaturated fatty acids and inflammatory mediator production. *Am J Clin Nutr*. 2000 Jan;71(1 Suppl):343S-8S
[498] James et al. Dietary n-3 fats as adjunctive therapy in a prototypic inflammatory disease. Prostaglandins *Leukot Essent Fatty Acids*. 2003 Jun;68(6):399-405
[499] Mohanty P, et al. Glucose challenge stimulates reactive oxygen species (ROS) generation by leucocytes. *J Clin Endocrinol Metab*. 2000 Aug;85(8):2970-3
[500] Mohanty et al. Both lipid and protein intakes stimulate increased generation of reactive oxygen species. *Am J Clin Nutr*. 2002 Apr;75(4):767-72
[501] Aljada A. Increase in intranuclear nuclear factor kappaB and decrease in inhibitor kappaB in mononuclear cells after a mixed meal. *Am J Clin Nutr*. 2004 Apr;79(4):682-90
[502] Basha B, Rao DS, Han ZH, Parfitt AM. Osteomalacia due to vitamin D depletion: a neglected consequence of intestinal malabsorption. *Am J Med*. 2000 Mar;108(4):296-300
[503] Grant EC. Food allergies and migraine. *Lancet*. 1979 May 5;1(8123):966-9
[504] Millichap JG, Yee MM. The diet factor in pediatric and adolescent migraine. *Pediatr Neurol*. 2003 Jan;28(1):9-15
[505] van de Laar MA, Aalbers M, Bruins FG, et al. Food intolerance in rheumatoid arthritis. II. Clinical and histological aspects. *Ann Rheum Dis*. 1992 ;51(3):303-6
[506] Golding DN. Is there an allergic synovitis? *J R Soc Med*. 1990 May;83(5):312-4
[507] Hvatum M, Kanerud L, Hällgren R, Brandtzaeg P. The gut-joint axis: cross reactive food antibodies in rheumatoid arthritis. *Gut*. 2006 Sep;55:1240-7

and chronic synovitis; the pain and inflammation remit on a gluten-free diet.[508] Alterations in intestinal microbial balance or an individual's unique response to endogenous bacteria (i.e., dysbiosis) can lead to systemic inflammation, arthritis, vasculitis, and musculoskeletal pain; clinical nuances and molecular mechanisms of gastrointestinal dysbiosis will be surveyed later in this monograph based on a previous review by Vasquez.[509] Clinicians should appreciate that dysbiosis can occur at sites other than the gastrointestinal tract, most importantly the nasopharynx and genitourinary tracts. Eradication of the occult infection or mucosal colonization often results in marked reductions in systemic inflammation and its clinical complications. Interested readers are directed to the excellent review by Noah[510] on the relevance of dysbiosis and its treatment relative to psoriasis; additional citations and clinical applications will be discussed later in this book.

7. <u>Structural imbalances from cellular membrane function to the musculoskeletal system</u>: Molecular structural imbalances lie at the heart of the concept of "biochemical individuality" originated by Roger J. Williams[511] in 1956, and this concept was soon thereafter expanded into the theory and practice of "orthomolecular medicine" pioneered by Linus Pauling and colleagues.[512,513] Pauling is considered by many authorities to be the original source of the concept of molecular medicine because he coined the phrase "molecular disease" after his team's discovery in 1949 that sickle cell anemia resulted from a single amino acid substitution that caused physical deformation of the hemoglobin molecule in hypoxic conditions.[514] One of Pauling's students, Jeffery Bland,

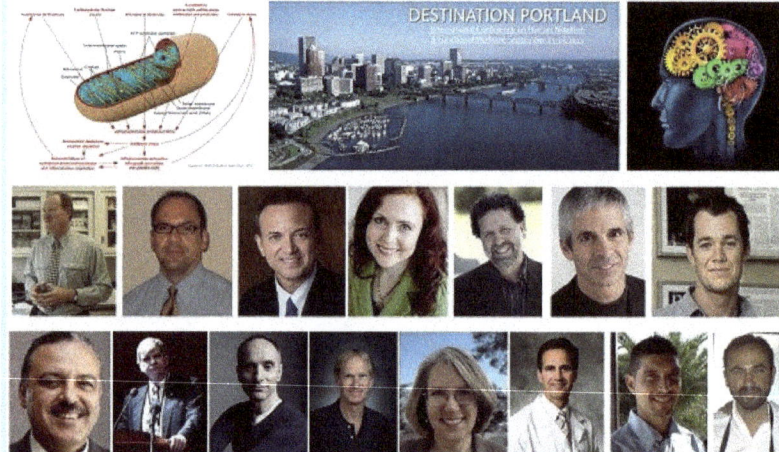

continued this legacy with the organization of "functional medicine.[515] Single nucleotide polymorphisms (SNP; pronounced "snip") are DNA sequence variations that can result in amino acid substitutions that render the final protein (e.g., structural protein or enzyme) abnormal in structure and therefore function. This aberrancy may or may not cause clinical disease (depending on the severity and importance of the variation), and consequences of the dysfunction may be occult, subtle, or obvious. One of the most powerful and effective means for treating diseases resultant from SNPs that result in enzyme defects is the use of high-dose vitamin supplementation, and this forms the scientific basis for "mega-vitamin therapy" as elegantly and authoritatively reviewed by Bruce Ames, et al.[516] SNP-induced alterations in enzyme structure reduce affinity for vitamin-derived coenzyme binding; this reduced affinity can be "overpowered" by administration of high doses of the required vitamin cofactor to increase tissue

---

[508] Bourne JT, Kumar P, Huskisson EC, Mageed R, Unsworth DJ, Wojtulewski JA. Arthritis and coeliac disease. *Ann Rheum Dis*. 1985 Sep;44(9):592-8
[509] Vasquez A. Nutritional and Botanical Treatments against "Silent Infections" and Gastrointestinal Dysbiosis. *Nutr Perspect* 2006; Jan: 5-21
[510] Noah PW. The role of microorganisms in psoriasis. *Semin Dermatol*. 1990 Dec;9(4):269-76
[511] Williams RJ. <u>Biochemical Individuality: The Basis for the Genetotrophic Concept</u>. Austin and London: University of Texas Press, 1956. Page x
[512] Pauling L. On the Orthomolecular Environment of the Mind. In: Williams RJ, Kalita DK. <u>Physician's Handbook on Orthomolecular Medicine</u>. Keats Publishing: 1977. p 76
[513] Pauling L, Robinson AB, Teranishi R, Cary P. Quantitative analysis of urine vapor and breath by gas-liquid partition chromatography. *Proc Natl Acad Sci* 1971 Oct;68:2374-6
[514] Pauling L, Itano HA, Singer SJ, Wells IC. Sickle cell anemia, a molecular disease. *Science*. 1949 Nov 25;110(2865):543-8
[515] Bland JS. Jeffrey S. Bland, PhD, FACN, CNS: functional medicine pioneer. *Altern Ther Health Med*. 2004 Sep-Oct;10(5):74-81
[516] Ames BN, et al. High-dose vitamin therapy stimulates variant enzymes with decreased coenzyme binding affinity (increased K(m)). *Am J Clin Nutr*. 2002 Apr;75(4):616-58

concentrations of the nutrient to promote binding of the enzyme with its ligand for the performance of enzymatic function. Thus, the scientific rationale for nutritional therapy is derived in part from the recognition that altered enzymatic function due to altered enzyme structure can often be corrected by administration of supradietary doses of nutrients. Relatedly, the structure and function of cell membranes is determined by their composition, which is influenced by dietary intake of fatty acids, and which influences production prostaglandins and leukotrienes. This is an important aspect of the scientific rationale for the use of specific fatty acid supplements in the prevention and treatment of painful inflammatory musculoskeletal disease. Cell membrane structure and function can also be altered by systemic oxidative stress; the concomitant alterations in intracellular ions (e.g., calcium) and receptor function along with activation of transcription factors such as NF-kappaB contribute to widespread physiologic impairment which creates a vicious cycle of inflammation, metabolic disturbance, and additional free radical generation.[517,518] Somatic dysfunction, musculoskeletal disorders, and inefficient biomechanics contribute to pain, increased production of inflammatory mediators, and the expedited degeneration of tissues such as collagen and cartilage matrix. Physicians trained in clinical biomechanics and physical medicine appreciate the subtle nuances of musculoskeletal structure-function relationships and address these problems directly with physical and manual means rather than ignoring the physical problem and only treating its biochemical sequelae. While biomechanics, palpatory diagnosis, and manual therapeutics takes years of diligent study for the achievement of proficiency, some of these concepts will be reviewed later in this book, particularly in the section on integrative pain management.

8. Psychological and Spiritual Equilibrium: The connections between physical pain and psychoemotional status and events is worthy of thorough discussion and not merely for the sake of improving upon outdated clinical practices which have typically marginalized these ethereal considerations or considered them only long enough to substantiate psychopharmaceutical intervention. A survey of the literature makes clear the interconnected nature of pain, inflammation, psychoemotional stress, depression, social isolation, and nutritional status; due to space and time limitations, a brief overview must necessarily suffice for the exemplification of representative concepts. Stressful and depressive life events promote the development, persistence, and exacerbation of disorders of pain and inflammation through nutritional, hormonal, immunologic, oxidative, and microbiologic mechanisms. Stated most simply, the perception of stressful events and the resultant neurohormonal cascade results in expedited metabolic utilization and increased urinary excretion of nutrients (e.g., tryptophan , and zinc, magnesium, retinol, respectively) which sum to effect nutritional imbalances and depletion, particularly when the stress response is severe and prolonged.[519,520,521] Specific to the consideration of pain, the depletion of tryptophan (and thus serotonin and melatonin) leaves the patient vulnerable to increased pain from lack of antinociceptive serotonin and to increased inflammation due to impaired endogenous production of anti-inflammatory cortisol, the adrenal release of which requires serotonin-dependent stimulation.[522] Severe stress, inflammation, and drugs used to suppress immune-mediated tissue damage (e.g., cyclosporine) increase urinary excretion of magnesium[523], and the eventual magnesium depletion renders the patient more vulnerable to hyperalgesia, depression, and other central nervous system and psychiatric disorders.[524,525] Furthermore, experimental and clinical data have shown that magnesium deficiency leads to a systemic pro-inflammatory state associated with oxidative stress and increased levels of the nociceptive and proinflammatory neurotransmitter substance P.[526] Stress increases secretion of prolactin, a hormone which plays an important pathogenic role in chronic inflammation and autoimmunity.[527,528] An abundance of experimental

---

[517] Evans JL, Maddux BA, Goldfine ID. The molecular basis for oxidative stress-induced insulin resistance. *Antioxid Redox Signal*. 2005 Jul-Aug;7(7-8):1040-52
[518] Joseph et al. Membrane and receptor modifications of oxidative stress vulnerability in aging. Nutritional considerations. *Ann N Y Acad Sci*. 1998 Nov 20;854:268-76
[519] Stephensen CB, Alvarez JO, et al. Vitamin A is excreted in the urine during acute infection. *Am J Clin Nutr*. 1994 Sep;60(3):388-92
[520] Ingenbleek Y, Bernstein L. The stressful condition as a nutritionally dependent adaptive dichotomy. *Nutrition*. 1999 Apr;15(4):305-20
[521] Henrotte et al. Blood and urinary magnesium, zinc, calcium, free fatty acids, and catecholamines in type A and type B subjects. *J Am Coll Nutr*. 1985;4(2):165-72
[522] Sandyk R. Tryptophan availability and the susceptibility to stress in multiple sclerosis: a hypothesis. *Int J Neurosci*. 1996 Jul;86(1-2):47-53
[523] DiPalma JR. Magnesium replacement therapy. *Am Fam Physician*. 1990 Jul;42(1):173-6
[524] Murck H. Magnesium and affective disorders. *Nutr Neurosci*. 2002 Dec;5(6):375-89
[525] Hashizume N, Mori M. An analysis of hypermagnesemia and hypomagnesemia. *Jpn J Med*. 1990 Jul-Aug;29(4):368-72
[526] Weglicki W, et al. Potassium, magnesium, and electrolyte imbalance and complications in disease management. *Clin Exp Hypertens*. 2005 Jan;27(1):95-112
[527] Imrich R. The role of neuroendocrine system in the pathogenesis of rheumatic diseases (minireview). *Endocr Regul*. 2002 Jun;36(2):95-106
[528] Orbach H, Shoenfeld Y. Hyperprolactinemia and autoimmune diseases. Autoimmun Rev. 2007 Sep;6(8):537-42

and clinical research supports the model that chronic psychoemotional stress reduces mucosal immunity, increases intestinal permeability, and allows for increased intestinal colonization by microbes that then stimulate immune responses that cross-react with musculoskeletal tissues and result in the clinical manifestation of autoimmunity and painful rheumatic syndromes which appear clinically as variants of acute and chronic reactive arthritis[529,530,531,532,533,534,535,536], formerly Reiter' syndrome.[537] Very interestingly, certain intestinal bacteria can sense when their human host is stressed, and they take advantage of the situation by becoming more virulent whereas previously these same bacteria may have been incapable of causing disease.[538,539] Psychoemotional stress also reduces mucosal immunity and increases colonization in locations other than the gastrointestinal tract. Microbial colonization of the genitourinary tract ("genitourinary dysbiosis") appears highly relevant in the genesis and perpetuation of rheumatoid arthritis.[540,541,542,543] Stressful life events also lower testosterone in men and the resultant lack of hormonal immunomodulation can increase the frequency and severity of exacerbations of rheumatoid arthritis[544]; resultant inflammation further suppresses testosterone production and bioavailability[545] leading to a self-perpetuating cycle of hypogonadism and inflammation. Thus, by numerous routes and mechanisms, psychoemotional stress increases the prevalence, persistence, and severity of musculoskeletal inflammation and pain.

Psychiatric codiagnoses are common among patients with painful neuromusculoskeletal disorders, and when the prevailing medical logic cannot solve the musculoskeletal riddle, the disorder is often ascribed to its accompanying mental disorder. The "appropriate" treatment from this perspective is the prescription of psychoactive drugs, generally of the "antidepressant" class. Science-based explanations are needed to expand clinicians' consideration of new possibilities which may someday prevail over commonplace suppositions that leave both clinician and patient trapped within a paradigm of futilely cyclical reasoning and its resultant simplistic symptom-targeting interventions. The following subsections provide alternatives to the "idiopathic pain is caused by its associated depression and both should be treated with antidepressant drugs" hypothesis.

    a. Pain, inflammation, and mental depression are final common pathways for nutritional deficiencies and imbalances: As a scientific community we now know that the epidemic problem of vitamin D deficiency leads to both musculoskeletal pain[546] as well as depression[547], and that supplementation with physiologic doses of vitamin D results in an enhanced sense of well-being[548] and high-efficacy alleviation of musculoskeletal pain and depression while providing other major collateral benefits.[549] Since the existence of vitamin D deficiency is more probable than that of antidepressant deficiency, the appropriate intervention for the former is more scientific and rational than that of the latter. Relatedly, research in various fields has shown that Western/American lifestyle and diet patterns diverge radically from human physiologic expectations and human nutritional

---

[529] Tlaskalová-Hogenová et al. Commensal bacteria (normal microflora), mucosal immunity and chronic inflammatory and autoimmune diseases. *Immunol Lett*. 2004 May 15;93(2-3):97-108
[530] Collins SM. Stress and the Gastrointestinal Tract IV. Modulation of intestinal inflammation by stress. *Am J Physiol Gastrointest Liver Physiol*. 2001 Mar;280(3):G315-8
[531] Hart A, Kamm MA. Review article: mechanisms of initiation and perpetuation of gut inflammation by stress. *Aliment Pharmacol Ther*. 2002 Dec;16(12):2017-28
[532] Farhadi A, Fields JZ, Keshavarzian A. Mucosal mast cells are pivotal elements in inflammatory bowel disease that connect the dots: stress, intestinal hyperpermeability and inflammation. *World J Gastroenterol*. 2007 Jun 14;13(22):3027-30
[533] Yang PC, et al. Chronic psychological stress in rats induces intestinal sensitization to luminal antigens. *Am J Pathol*. 2006 Jan;168(1):104-14
[534] Rashid T, Ebringer A. Ankylosing spondylitis is linked to Klebsiella--the evidence. *Clin Rheumatol*. 2007 Jun;26(6):858-64
[535] Vasquez A. *Integrative Rheumatology*. Fort Worth, Texas; Integrative and Biological Medicine Research and Consulting, 2007 InflammationMastery.com
[536] Samarkos M, Vaiopoulos G. The role of infections in the pathogenesis of autoimmune diseases. *Curr Drug Targets Inflamm Allergy*. 2005 Feb;4(1):99-103
[537] Panush RS, Wallace DJ, Dorff RE, Engleman EP. Retraction of the suggestion to use the term "Reiter's syndrome" sixty-five years later: the legacy of Reiter, a war criminal, should not be eponymic honor but rather condemnation. *Arthritis Rheum*. 2007 Feb;56(2):693-4
[538] Alverdy J, Holbrook C, Rocha F, Seiden L, Wu RL, Musch M, Chang E, Ohman D, Suh S. Gut-derived sepsis occurs when the right pathogen with the right virulence genes meets the right host: evidence for in vivo virulence expression in Pseudomonas aeruginosa. *Ann Surg*. 2000 Oct;232(4):480-9
[539] Wu L, Holbrook C, Zaborina O, Ploplys E, Rocha F, Pelham D, Chang E, Musch M, Alverdy J. Pseudomonas aeruginosa expresses a lethal virulence determinant, the PA-I lectin/adhesin, in the intestinal tract of a stressed host: the role of epithelia cell contact and molecules of the Quorum Sensing Signaling System. *Ann Surg*. 2003;238(5):754-64
[540] Ebringer A, Rashid T. Rheumatoid arthritis is an autoimmune disease triggered by Proteus urinary tract infection. *Clin Dev Immunol*. 2006 Mar;13(1):41-8
[541] Erlacher L, Wintersberger W, Menschik M, et al. Reactive arthritis: urogenital swab culture is the only useful diagnostic method for the detection of the arthritogenic infection in extra-articularly asymptomatic patients with undifferentiated oligoarthritis. *Br J Rheumatol*. 1995 Sep;34(9):838-42
[542] Rashid T, Ebringer A. Rheumatoid arthritis is linked to Proteus--the evidence. *Clin Rheumatol*. 2007 Jul;26(7):1036-43
[543] Ebringer A, Rashid T, Wilson C. Rheumatoid arthritis: proposal for the use of anti-microbial therapy in early cases. *Scand J Rheumatol*. 2003;32:2-11
[544] James WH. Further evidence that low androgen values are a cause of rheumatoid arthritis: the response to seriously stressful life events. *Ann Rheum Dis* 1997;56:566
[545] Karagiannis A, Harsoulis F. Gonadal dysfunction in systemic diseases. *Eur J Endocrinol*. 2005 Apr;152(4):501-13
[546] Plotnikoff GA, Quigley JM. Prevalence of severe hypovitaminosis D in patients with persistent, nonspecific musculoskeletal pain. *Mayo Clin Proc*. 2003 Dec;78(12):1463-70
[547] Wilkins et al. Vitamin D deficiency is associated with low mood and worse cognitive performance in older adults. *Am J Geriatr Psychiatry*. 2006 Dec;14(12):1032-40
[548] Vieth R, Kimball S, Hu A, Walfish PG. Randomized comparison of the effects of the vitamin D3 adequate intake versus 100 mcg (4000 IU) per day on biochemical responses and the wellbeing of patients. *Nutr J*. 2004 Jul 19;3:8
[549] Vasquez et al. The clinical importance of vitamin D (cholecalciferol): a paradigm shift with implications for all healthcare providers. *Altern Ther Health Med*. 2004;10:28-36

requirements.[550] With regard to fatty acid intake and the resultant effects on inflammation and neurotransmission, modernized diets are a "set-up" for musculoskeletal pain and mental depression, which frequently occur concomitantly and which are both alleviated by corrective fatty acid intervention such as fish oil supplementation as a source of EPA and DHA.[551,552] Correction of fatty acid imbalance is therefore more rational in the comanagement of pain and depression than is sole reliance on antidepressant and anti-inflammatory drugs; the latter have their place in treatment but neither addresses the primary cause of the problem and both drug classes have important adverse effects and significant costs in contrast to the safety, affordability, and collateral benefits derived from fatty acid supplementation. Also relevant to this discussion of chronic pain triggered and perpetuated by nutritional imbalances are the pro-inflammatory nature of the Western/American diet[553] and the pain-sensitizing effects of epidemic magnesium deficiency.[554] Therefore, correction of nutritional deficiencies and optimization of nutritional status should generally logically supersede the prescription of drugs in patients with concomitant depression and pain.

b. <u>Pain, inflammation, and depression are final common pathways of physical inactivity</u>: Exercising muscle elaborates cytokines ("myokines") with anti-inflammatory activity; a sedentary lifestyle fails to stimulate this endogenous anti-inflammation and is therefore relatively pro-inflammatory.[555] Further, exercise has antidepressant benefits mediated by positive influences on neurotransmission, growth factor elaboration, endocrinologic function, self-image, skill-building, and social contact.[556] Patients with musculoskeletal pain should be encouraged to exercise to the extent possible given the individual's capacity and type of injury and/or degree of disability. Thus, a prescription for exercise might supersede the prescription of drugs in patients with concomitant depression and pain. Exercise prescriptions must consider frequency, duration, intensity, variety, safety, enjoyment, accountability and objective measures of compliance and progress, as well as appropriate combinations of components which emphasize aerobic fitness, strengthening, flexibility, muscle balancing, coordination, skill-building and functional/practical applications.

c. <u>Pain and depression are final common pathways of inflammation</u>: Several pro-inflammatory cytokines are psychoactive and cause depression, social withdrawal, impaired cognition, and sickness behavior.[557] As an alternative to the use of antidepressant drugs, correction of the underlying inflammatory disorder by natural, pharmacologic, or integrative means may subsequently promote restoration of normal affect and cognitive function.

d. <u>Pain, inflammation, and mental depression are final common pathways for hormonal deficiencies and imbalances</u>: Deficiencies of thyroid hormones, testosterone, cortisol, and DHEA, and/or insufficiency or excess of estrogen can cause depression and impaired neuroemotional status. Hormonal aberrations are common in patients with chronic musculoskeletal pain, particularly of the inflammatory and autoimmune types. Clinical trials have shown that administration of thyroid hormones, testosterone, DHEA, cortisol and suppression prolactin can each provide anti-inflammatory, analgesic, and antidepressant benefits among appropriately selected patients. Thus, identification and correction of hormonal imbalances might supersede the prescription of antidepressant drugs in patients with concomitant depression, inflammation, and pain.

Our cultural and scientific advancements in the knowledge of how the brain and mind function have been paradoxically paralleled by social trends showing increasing depression and social isolation; the typical American has only two friends and no one in whom to confide.[558] In the United States, violent injuries are epidemic, and the level of firearm morbidity and mortality in the US is far higher than anywhere else in the

---

[550] O'Keefe JH Jr, Cordain L. Cardiovascular disease resulting from a diet and lifestyle at odds with our Paleolithic genome. *Mayo Clin Proc*. 2004 Jan;79(1):101-8
[551] Kiecolt-Glaser JK, et al. Depressive symptoms, omega-6:omega-3 fatty acids, and inflammation in older adults. *Psychosom Med*. 2007 Apr;69(3):217-24
[552] Simopoulos AP. Omega-3 fatty acids in inflammation and autoimmune diseases. *J Am Coll Nutr*. 2002 Dec;21(6):495-505
[553] Aljada et al. Increase in intranuclear nuclear factor kappaB and decrease in inhibitor kappaB in mononuclear cells after a mixed meal. *Am J Clin Nutr*. 2004 Apr;79(4):682-90
[554] Park JH, Niermann KJ, Olsen N. Evidence for metabolic abnormalities in the muscles of patients with fibromyalgia. *Curr Rheumatol Rep*. 2000 Apr;2(2):131-40
[555] Petersen AM, Pedersen BK. The anti-inflammatory effect of exercise. *J Appl Physiol*. 2005 Apr;98(4):1154-62
[556] Cotman CW, Berchtold NC, Christie LA. Exercise builds brain health: key roles of growth factor cascades and inflammation. *Trends Neurosci*. 2007 Sep;30(9):464-72
[557] Wilson CJ, Finch CE, Cohen HJ. Cytokines and cognition--the case for a head-to-toe inflammatory paradigm. *J Am Geriatr Soc*. 2002 Dec;50(12):2041-56
[558] McPherson M, Smith-Lovin L, Brashears ME. Social Isolation in America: Changes in Core Discussion Networks over Two Decades. *Am Sociological Rev* 2006; 71: 353-75

industrialized world.[559] This does to some extent beg the question of the value of "scientific knowledge" of the brain and mind within a social structure that is increasingly violent and fragmented. Further, the mental depression resultant from pandemic social isolation would be better served by physicians' admonition for increased social contact than by the continued overuse of drugs which inhibit neurotransmitter reuptake.

Conclusion: The clinical employment of the functional medicine approach to chronic disease management and health promotion rests upon a foundation of competent patient management and then extends to consider the well-documented contributions of the causative *internal and external imbalances* that have allowed the genesis and perpetuation of the problem(s) under consideration. The attainment of wellness, the success of preventive medicine, and the optimization of socioemotional health cannot be attained by pharmacological suppression of the manifestations of dysfunction that result from nutritional and neuroendocrine imbalances, xenobiotic accumulation, sedentary lifestyles, social isolation, and mucosal microbial colonization. Rather, these problems are addressed directly, and these and other causative considerations must remain foremost in the mind of the physician committed to the successful, ethical, and cost-effective long-term prevention and management of chronic health disturbances, particularly those characterized by inflammation and pain.

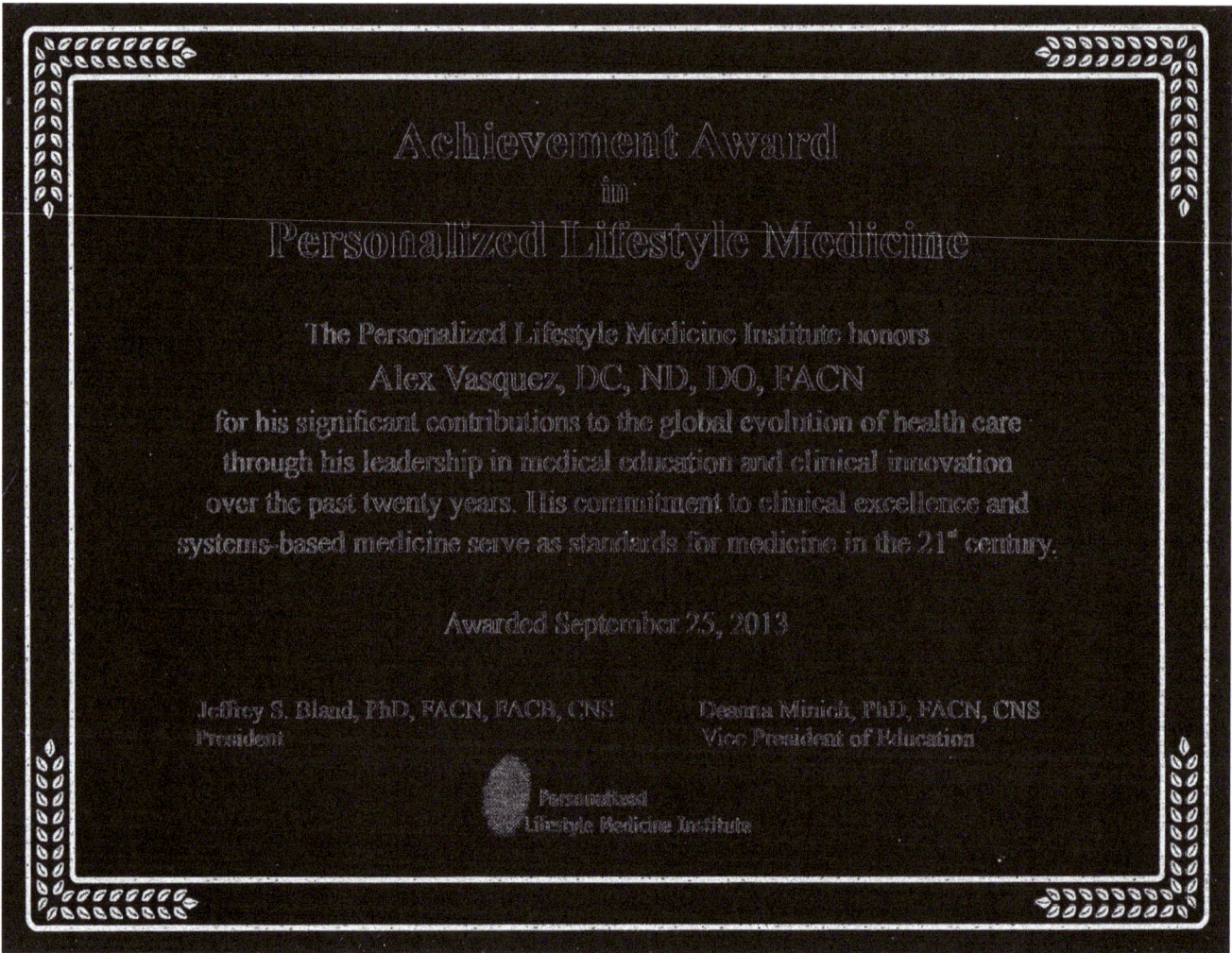

Achievement award: Sincere appreciation was shared at our 2013 International Conference on Human Nutrition and Functional Medicine, wherein Dr Vasquez and Dr Bland received awards for their contributions to the fields of nutrition and functional medicine. vimeo.com/ichnfm/2013keynote or vimeo.com/100562693 **Password:** Keynote

---

[559] Preventing firearm violence: a public health imperative. American College of Physicians. *Ann Intern Med.* 1995 Feb 15;122(4):311-3

The shadow(s) of functional medicine: The single biggest shadow of functional medicine is pretty obvious to those of us who have been involved with what has now been described/degraded by some as a "movement" as if it were a social fad or cult rather than the culmination of biomedicine's potential: it is the *gross profiteering* off of the intellectual foundation provided by Dr Jeffrey Bland and of functional medicine's image as *a more sophisticated alternative to alternative medicine*. Some "authorities" within functional medicine overcharge their clinical patients, and some prominent organizations within functional medicine beg for donations (including occasional crying on stage) under the pretense of working as a "nonprofit organization" while the internal mechanics of the organization overpay a select few administrators and undermine speaking careers and profitability of teaching faculty.

Examples of dysfunction in functional medicine:
- Overpaying a select few: Using nonprofit status to grossly overpay part-time employees, e.g., more than $164,000 in a single year for part-time work or less.[560] Among the consequences of this are the demoralization of expert teaching faculty who are underpaid for their talent and hard work. The other obvious issue is that of integrity, or—more accurately—lack thereof. Personally, I think using "nonprofit status" to pay luxurious salaries to people who work (far) less than part-time is disingenuous and misleading; probably, donors would be less enthusiastic about their donations if they knew the "nonprofit" money was being used to overpay a small group of employees. Other *constantly elevating* salaries of $140,000 and $144,000 are far out of range for their corresponding US national average pay of $54,000-64,000 with a top 10% of $110,000.[561] From experience, I've learned to be wary when I see accountants of organizations being overpaid. At one particular so-called "non-profit" physician-education institution, we note that the accountant's salary exceeds the annual salary of many doctorate-level clinicians and certainly exceeds the salary of most college, university, and medical school professors (including full professors with hard-earned tenure); this is even more noteworthy during a time of major economic recession which particularly impacts the cash-only practices of many functional medicine clinicians.
- Forcing members/attendees to pay *more* to receive *less*: Diluting educational quality for the intentional purpose of enlarging the quantity so that members/attendees will have to pay for additional courses to receive what would have otherwise been more/better information for less cost. Entrapping people in a "certification" process of diluted material makes them pay *more* while the organization works *less*.
- Exploitation of experts: Exploiting expert's knowledge by video-recording their presentations and then selling those presentations to third parties without informing or paying the expert, thus forcing the experts to essentially *compete with themselves* as lecturers. For me as a lecturer, I find it wholly unacceptable that an organization would pay me once for a presentation, and then record and sell my presentation to other audiences without compensating me; in this instance, the organization would be profiting far more from my own work—simply for pushing the "record" button—than would I after decades and long hours of work.
- Laboratory profiteering: A "functional medicine laboratory" used worthless laboratory methods[562] to profiteer millions of dollars from functional medicine clinicians and patients. Likely, the doctors and customers deserve a refund or compensation for this falsity, which likely lead to instances of misdiagnosis, delayed diagnosis, and erroneous treatment. Given the high cost of laboratory assessments in functional medicine—wherein a single panel of tests can cost $500-700 easily—the use of bogus laboratory methods cost patients and any unwitting insurance companies (tens of) millions of dollars in aggregate. This is very hypocritical to occur within the functional medicine community—wherein many of us professors and presenters are on a first name basis together—given that functional medicine was supposedly based on integrity and a commitment to improve healthcare costs and outcomes.

---

[560] guidestar.org/ "Trusted nonprofit information. Search GuideStar for the most complete, up-to-date nonprofit data available." 2013 Jun and rechecked in 2014 Jul
[561] "According to the BLS, the median annual salary for an accountant was $63,550 in 2012, or $30.55 per hour. The best-paid 10 percent earned roughly $111,510," money.usnews.com/careers/best-jobs/accountant/salary
[562] Gingras BA, Duncan SB, Scheuller NJ, Schreckenberber PC. Assessment of diagnostic accuracy of recently introduced DNA stool screening test. *International Journal of Human Nutrition and Functional Medicine* 2014: 2(1);1 intjhumnutrfunctmed.org/publications/

- Standing on the shoulders of giants does not make one a giant: Self-evident but frequently forgotten, this "esteem via association" has caused some people—indeed entire organizations—to consider themselves genius simply because they have worked with a genius. The fallacy is pretty clear from outside the organizational bubble.
- Misguided truths: Misusing the name(s) of intellectual giants such as Jeffrey Bland and Linus Pauling and allowing low performers to undermine standards of excellence; bestowing grand namesake awards to people based on financial return and petty friendships rather scientific contribution or intellectual development or modeling of a life worthy of general aspiration.
- Verbal abuse and internet bullying: I observed an email discussion (2014 Jul) among many prominent "functional medicine experts" wherein one participant assumed the right to character assassinate another person merely for asking questions that were beyond the "bully's" intellectual ability to process and respond. This became a classic demonstration of the well-known Karpman drama triangle, wherein the bully/aggressor was clearly the offender—including using profanity and the insinuation of physical threat—yet he claimed to be the rescuer/defender of some of the more feeble participants and—as is classic and common—the victim. That such a conversation would occur among the highest members of the functional medicine community is an embarrassment to the very idea of functional medicine and how it should manifest in the real world.
- Arrogance, elitism, and profiteering—recent clinical experience: A patient of mine was charged $15,000 by a *prominent functional medicine clinician* for an initial evaluation of a previous diagnosis of rheumatoid arthritis; most of this profiteering was secured via overcharging for laboratory tests, the vast majority of which were unnecessary, as they simply lead to the assessment of inflammation (which we already knew) and need for nutritional supplementation (which we already knew). **Originally, functional medicine was based in part on the idea that we could help patients become healthier in a less costly and more efficient manner by treating the causes of their problems**; in this clinician's case, he chose to exploit the patient's illness, desire for healing, and the fame of functional medicine by cashing-in on her desperation—$15,000 for a one-time consultation and lab tests is pure exploitation, made even worse by the clinician's inefficacy.
- Unfair and unreasonable contracts for faculty: Contract clauses that force employees to resign their intelligence and self-respect by agreeing that the organization has no accountability whatsoever, even if it violates the self-same contract. "Faculty agrees to indemnify, defend, and hold harmless from any and all actions, causes of action, claims, demands, costs, liabilities, expenses, and damages (including attorney's fees) arising out of or in connection with any breach of this Agreement."
- "We care (but we really don't)": Having a touchy-feely appearance and then refusing to accept feedback from paid members and faulty, alienating membership and faculty.
- Firing faculty members who have worked hard for the organization for more than 10 years and not even having the courage to let them know they have been replaced, e.g., faculty members who find out on Facebook that they are no longer employed.
- Telling people how lucky they are to be in attendance: Modeling arrogance while talking humility, e.g., traditions of self-congratulatory behavior: telling audience members how lucky they are to be in attendance, after these same audience members have paid thousands of dollars to travel, attend, lodge, and take time away from clinical practice and family in order to attend educational events. In one example, a lecturer gave 15 self-congratulatory comments in the first 17 minutes of her presentation.
- Submit to my entitlement: In accord with the gross differential between image and reality, I know one notable presenter within the functional medicine movement who lectures on the importance of *the healing/therapeutic power of relationships* and then demanded (from me) free admission to my presentations and teaching materials because he said I had an obligation to "honor" our "relationship"; I'll tell anyone in the world from the highest podium I can find and the biggest PowerPoint screen we can hire that any relationship that includes **haughty demands for submission** and **arrogant assumptions of entitlement** is *not* a healing relationship and *not* one that should be modeled by someone well-positioned in the leadership of a major functional medicine institution.

Osteopathic Medicine

Osteopathy was founded by Andrew Taylor Still, a medical doctor who sought to reform what was then called the "Heroic" paradigm of medicine, which embraced bloodletting and the administration of leeches, purgatives, emetics, and poisons such as mercury as means for "rebalancing" what were perceived to be internal causes of disease, namely the "four humours" of the body which were thought to be blood, phlegm, black bile, and yellow bile. In part because of his training within and identification with the medical profession, Still sought to *reform* rather than *directly oppose* the "mainstream medicine" of his day; in contrast, chiropractic's founder Daniel David Palmer was more strongly opposed to the horrific medicine of his time and thus was more *revolutionary* than *evolutionary* in his approach to forging a new paradigm of health and healthcare. Still's willingness to align with the medical profession and the increasingly powerful and influential pharmaceutical industry unquestionably helped his fledgling profession survive the extinction that otherwise would have been swift at the hands of allopathic groups such as the American Medical Association (AMA), which labeled osteopathic physicians as "cultists" and systematically restricted inclusion of the osteopathic profession into mainstream healthcare by proclamation in 1953 that "…all voluntary associations with osteopaths are unethical." When osteopathic resistance mounted, the AMA and its co-conspirators, who were later found guilty of violating the nation's antitrust laws by illegally suppressing competition and attempting to build a medical monopoly[563], acquiesced and accepted osteopaths into its ranks—a strategy which the medical profession believed would eventually destroy the osteopathic profession by forcing it to resign its ideals and identity. In his review of osteopathic history, Gevitz[564] writes, "…the M.D.'s gradually came to believe that the only way to destroy osteopathy was through the absorption of D.O.'s, much as the homeopaths and eclectics [naturopaths] had been swallowed up early in the century." Even recently, the AMA has listed osteopathic medicine under "alternative medicine"[565] although several osteopathic medical colleges have consistently provided training that is superior to most "conventional" allopathic medical schools.[566] Today, osteopathic physicians practice in most ways similarly to allopaths—i.e., with unlimited scope of practice in all 50 states, full access to the use of drugs and surgery, and with a very pharmacosurgical paradigm of disease and healthcare. Osteopathic medicine is one of the fastest growing healthcare professions in America.

Osteopathic Manipulative Medicine:

Osteopathic manipulative medicine (OMM) is similar to and yet distinct from chiropractic manipulation; the naturopathic profession—true to its eclectic roots—incorporates techniques from all professions. In contrast to chiropractic, OMM terminology and therapeutics focus much more on soft tissues, and the osteopathic lesion—"somatic dysfunction"—is clearly originated from soft tissues in contrast to the chiropractic lesion—the "vertebral subluxation"—which obviously originates from spinal articulations. Whereas the chiropractic intent of correcting or "adjusting" the "subluxation" was historically to improve function of the nervous system, the osteopathic lesion is addressed to more fully improve not only function of the nervous system but also of the vascular, lymphatic, and myofascial systems, too.[567] With regard to the latter, the osteopathic profession has always emphasized the importance of fascia in the genesis of "somatic dysfunction." Indeed, fascia appears to play an important and dynamic (not passive) role in neuromusculoskeletal health, particularly as it is a major contributor to proprioception and may also have a more direct effect through the recently described ability of fascia to actively contract in a smooth-muscle-like manner.[568]

From this author's perspective, two of the most widely used osteopathic texts—*Osteopathic Principles in Practice* (1994) by Kuchera and Kuchera[569], and *Outline of Osteopathic Manipulative Procedures* (2006) by Kimberly[570]—both leave very much to be desired with respect to their clarity, terminology, clinical applicability, and referencing

---

[563] Getzendanner S. Permanent injunction order against AMA. *JAMA*. 1988 Jan 1;259(1):81-2
[564] Gevitz N. *The D.O.'s: Osteopathic Medicine in America*. Johns Hopkins University Press; 1991; pages 100-103
[565] American Medical Association. Report 12 of the Council on Scientific Affairs (A-97) Full Text ama-assn.org/ama/pub/category/13638.html November 23, 2006
[566] Special report. America's best medical schools. Schools of Medicine. The top schools: primary care. *US News World Rep*. 2004 Apr 12;136(12):74
[567] Williams N. Managing back pain in general practice--is osteopathy the new paradigm? *Br J Gen Pract*. 1997 Oct;47(423):653-5
[568] "…the existence of an active fascial contractility could have interesting implications for the understanding of musculoskeletal pathologies with an increased or decreased myofascial tonus. It may also offer new insights and a deeper understanding of treatments directed at fascia, such as manual myofascial release therapies or acupuncture." Schleip et al. Active fascial contractility: Fascia may be able to contract in a smooth muscle-like manner and thereby influence musculoskeletal dynamics. *Med Hypotheses*. 2005;65:273-7
[569] Kuchera WA, Kuchera ML. *Osteopathic Principles in Practice, revised second edition*. Kirksville, MO, KCOM Press; 1994
[570] Kimberly PE. *Outline of Osteopathic Manipulative Procedures.The Kimberly Manual 2006*. Kirksville College Osteopathic Medicine. Walsworth Publish. Co., Marceline, Mo

to the scientific literature. *Manipulation of the Spine, Thorax and Pelvis: An Osteopathic Perspective* (2006) by Gibbons and Tehan[571] is much more accessible and clinically applicable; however the text focuses exclusively on high-velocity low-amplitude (HVLA) techniques and therefore does not provide sufficient background and training for students in the very techniques that distinguish osteopathic from chiropractic techniques, namely heightened attention to the myofascial dysfunction that (appropriately) underlies the osteopathic lesion.

Ironically, the very growth and "allopathicization" of the profession that has threatened the profession's adherence to its holistic tenets has caused a reflexive re-affirmation of these tenets, and the profession has responded with a well-funded and intentional directive to scientifically investigate the mechanisms and efficacy of osteopathic manipulative medicine.[572,573] Recent findings include improved function and reduced pain in patients treated with a comprehensive manipulative technique for the shoulder[574], as well as the significant efficacy of ankle manipulation for patients with recent ankle injuries.[575]

Further, OMM treatment of patients medicated for depression was found to triple the effectiveness of drug monotherapy.[576] Other studies have shown benefit of OMM in the treatment of geriatric pneumonia[577], pediatric asthma[578], pediatric dysfunctional voiding[579], carpal tunnel syndrome[580], low-back pain[581], and recovery from cardiac bypass surgery.[582] Replication and validation of these studies—many of which are small or of nonrigorous design (e.g., open clinical trials with no control group)—is important to further define and establish the value of osteopathic manipulation in clinical care.

> **Osteopathic Interventions need to be Consistent with Osteopathic Philosophy**
>
> "In contrast to the description of the osteopathic medical profession by the American Osteopathic Association, namely, "doctors of osteopathic medicine, or D.O.s, apply the philosophy of treating the whole person to the prevention, diagnosis and treatment of illness, disease and injury," [the authors of the article in question] essentially reviewed only pharmacologic treatment. ...It is hoped that future reviews in this journal can include a more balanced survey of the literature, inclusive of non-pharmacologic and "holistic" interventions that are consistent with osteopathic philosophy."
>
> Vasquez A. Interventions need to be Consistent with Osteopathic Philosophy. [Letter] *JAOA: Journal of the American Osteopathic Association* 2006 Sep
> jaoa.org/cgi/content/full/106/9/528

<u>The shadow of osteopathic medicine</u>: Most insiders will agree that—with all due respect for the tremendous progress made by the osteopathic profession, having gone from *medical oppression* to *medical acceptance* to now *medical parity* and some would argue *medical superiority* due to the equivalent *quality* of education and (with the discipline of osteopathic manipulative medicine) greater *quantity* of medical education compared with allopaths—the challenge for the profession now is that of identity, or—more accurately—integrity. Can and will the osteopathic profession maintain and champion its holistic perspective on health and all that such a perspective entails, or will it continue to genuflect to the pathocentric and pharmacodependent model of allopathic medicine? These are obviously important questions with implications for the educational process, clinical practice, and professional differentiation and post-graduate education. In our osteopathic college at University of North Texas Health Science

---

[571] Gibbons P, Tehan P. *Manipulation of the Spine, Thorax and Pelvis: An Osteopathic Perspective*. Churchill Livingstone; 2006. Isbn: 044310039X
[572] Wisnioski SW 3rd. "Circle Turns Round" to "Allopathic Osteopathy." *J Am Osteopath Assoc* 2006; 106: 423-4 jaoa.org/cgi/content/full/106/7/423
[573] Teitelbaum HS, et al. Osteopathic medical education: renaissance or rhetoric? *J Am Osteopath Assoc*. 2003 Oct;103(10):489-90 jaoa.org/cgi/reprint/103/10/489
[574] Knebl JA, Shores JH, Gamber RG, Gray WT, Herron KM. Improving functional ability in the elderly via the Spencer technique, an osteopathic manipulative treatment: a randomized, controlled trial. *J Am Osteopath Assoc*. 2002 Jul;102(7):387-96 jaoa.org/cgi/reprint/102/7/387
[575] This study shows the rapid onset and benefit of manipulative medicine for the treatment of acute ankle sprains: Eisenhart AW, Gaeta TJ, Yens DP. Osteopathic manipulative treatment in the emergency department for patients with acute ankle injuries. *J Am Osteopath Assoc*. 2003 Sep;103(9):417-21 jaoa.org/cgi/reprint/103/9/417
[576] This study impressively showed that musculoskeletal manipulation improved treatment effectiveness for depression from 33% to 100%. "After 8 weeks, 100% of the OMT treatment group and 33% of the control group tested normal by psychometric evaluation. ... The findings of this pilot study indicate that OMT may be a useful adjunctive treatment for alleviating depression in women." Plotkin et al. Adjunctive osteopathic manipulative treatment in women with depression. *J Am Osteopath Assoc*. 2001 Sep;101(9):517-23
[577] This study showed improved clinical outcomes and reduced antibiotic use in elderly patients with pneumonia when treated with manipulative medicine: "The treatment group had a significantly shorter duration of intravenous antibiotic treatment and a shorter hospital stay." Noll DR, Shores JH, Gamber RG, Herron KM, Swift J Jr. Benefits of osteopathic manipulative treatment for hospitalized elderly patients with pneumonia. *J Am Osteopath Assoc*. 2000 Dec;100(12):776-82 jaoa.org/cgi/reprint/100/12/776
[578] Osteopathic manipulation improved pulmonary function in pediatric patients with asthma: "With a confidence level of 95%, results for the OMT group showed a statistically significant improvement of 7 L per minute to 9 L per minute for peak expiratory flow rates. These results suggest that OMT has a therapeutic effect among this patient population." Guiney PA, Chou R, Vianna A, Lovenheim J. Effects of osteopathic manipulative treatment on pediatric patients with asthma: a randomized controlled trial. *J Am Osteopath Assoc*. 2005 Jan;105(1):7-12 jaoa.org/cgi/content/full/105/1/7
[579] Nemett et al. Randomized controlled trial of effectiveness of osteopathy-based manual physical therapy treating pediatric dysfunctional voiding. *J Pediatr Urol* 2008 Apr:100-6
[580] Sucher BM, Hinrichs RN, Welcher RL, Quiroz LD, St Laurent BF, Morrison BJ. Manipulative treatment of carpal tunnel syndrome: biomechanical and osteopathic intervention to increase the length of the transverse carpal ligament: part 2. Effect of sex differences and manipulative "priming". *J Am Osteopath Assoc*. 2005 Mar;105(3):135-43. Erratum in: *J Am Osteopath Assoc*. 2005 May;105(5):238 jaoa.org/cgi/content/full/105/3/135
[581] "CONCLUSION: OMT significantly reduces low back pain. The level of pain reduction is greater than expected from placebo effects alone and persists for at least three months." Licciardone JC, Brimhall AK, King LN. Osteopathic manipulative treatment for low back pain: a systematic review and meta-analysis of randomized controlled trials. *BMC Musculoskelet Disord*. 2005 Aug 4;6:43 biomedcentral.com/1471-2474/6/43
[582] This study showed benefit from osteopathic manipulation administered immediately after coronary artery bypass graft surgery: "The observed changes in cardiac function and perfusion indicated that OMT had a beneficial effect on the recovery of patients after CABG surgery. The authors conclude that OMT has immediate, beneficial hemodynamic effects after CABG surgery when administered while the patient is sedated and pharmacologically paralyzed." O-Yurvati et al. Hemodynamic effects of osteopathic manipulative treatment immediately after coronary artery bypass graft surgery. *J Am Osteopath Assoc*. 2005 Oct;105(10):475-81 jaoa.org/cgi/content/full/105/10/475

Center Texas College of Osteopathic Medicine, we obviously proved ourselves to be a top medical school in Primary Care Medicine (*U.S. News & World Report*, 2002 through present), Top 15 Specialty Ranking in Rural Medicine, Geriatrics (2013), Top 20 Specialty Ranking in Family Medicine (2013), and our students in particular attained top performance on US Medical Licensing Examination (USMLE) and Comprehensive Osteopathic Medical Licensing Examination (COMLEX) wherein I personally scored in the top 1% and 5% nationally for each of the medical licensing exams I took; but at times we seemed to have nearly paid for our education with our souls: I have never worked so hard in my life as I did in osteopathic medical school, and while I wished some less brutal methods might have been used, I am authentically grateful for the transformative experience. However, when I look at the profession as a reader of the *Journal of American Osteopathic Association* (JAOA), I often get the impression I am looking at a profession that has sold itself for too low a price to the pharmaceutical paradigm; reading the *JAOA* often leaves me with the impression that I just read some very noncomplex articles, many of which seem/are directly authored promotional material from the pharmaceutical industry. I continue to hope that "future reviews in this journal [and perspectives from the profession it represents] can include a more balanced survey of the literature, inclusive of non-pharmacologic and "holistic" interventions that are consistent with osteopathic philosophy."[583]

Political graffiti in Merida Spain 2013 January: Translates from Spanish to English as "Drugs, wars, and junk [garbage] food are killing us." One might wonder if "drogas/drugs" is meant to imply recreational drugs or prescriptions drugs, the latter of which—in the form of "adverse drug effects" and other iatrogenesis—kill 3,500 patients per week in the United States alone; per the excellent clinical review published in *American Family Physician* (1997 Nov): "Recent estimates suggest that each year more than 1 million patients are injured while in the hospital and approximately 180,000 die because of these injuries. Furthermore, drug-related morbidity and mortality are common and are estimated to cost more than $136 billion a year."

---

[583] Vasquez A. Interventions need to be Consistent with Osteopathic Philosophy. [Letter] *JAOA: Journal of the American Osteopathic Association* 2006 Sep. jaoa.org/cgi/content/full/106/9/528

Chiropractic

"The human body represents the actions of three laws—spiritual, mechanical, and chemical—united as one triune. As long as there is perfect union of these three, there is health." Daniel David Palmer—the founder of chiropractic

The basic philosophical model which is taught in many chiropractic colleges is to envision health, disease, and patient care from a conceptual model named the "triad of health" which gives its attention to the three fundamental foundations for well-being: namely, the physical/structural, mental/emotional, and biochemical/nutritional aspects of health. Revolutionary at the time of its inception in the early 1900's, this model now forms the foundation for the increasingly dominant and very popular paradigm of "holistic medicine." It remains a powerful contrast and an attractive alternative to the reductionistic allopathic approach, which generally approaches the human body as if it were simply a conglomerate of independent organ systems that have little or no functional relationship to each other.[584]

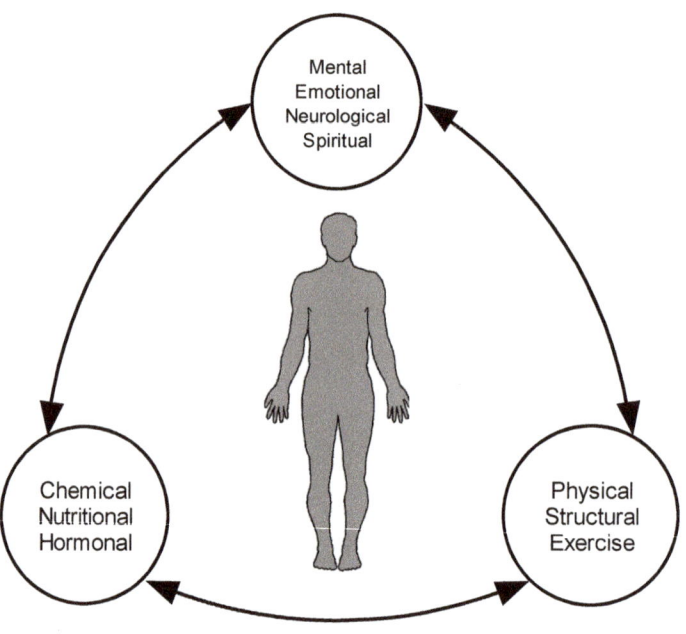

The chiropractic "triad of health"

Using the state of the sciences before the year 1910, chiropractic was founded with a profound appreciation of the integrated nature of health, and the therapeutic focus was on spinal manipulation. In describing the chiropractic model of health, DD Palmer[585] wrote, "The human body represents the actions of three laws—spiritual, mechanical, and chemical—united as one triune. As long as there is perfect union of these three, there is health." While the therapeutic focus of the profession has been spinal manipulation, from its inception the chiropractic profession has emphasized a holistic, integrative model of therapeutic intervention, health, and disease, and chiropractic was the first healthcare profession in America to specifically claim that the optimization of health requires attention to spiritual-emotional-psychological, mechanical-physical-structural, and biochemical-nutritional-hormonal-chemical considerations.

From its inception, chiropractic has been a philosophy of healing that considered the entire health of the patient by addressing the interconnected aspects of our chemical-spiritual-physical being. Later, intraprofessional factions polarized between holistic and vitalistic paradigms; the latter has been presumed to be the philosophy of the entire profession by organizations such as the American Medical Association[586] that have sought to contain and eliminate chiropractic and other forms of natural healthcare[587] by falsifying research[588,589], intentionally misleading the public and manipulating politicians[590,591,592], arriving at illogical conclusions which support the medical paradigm and refute the value of manual therapies[593], and exploiting weaknesses within the profession for its own

---

[584] Beckman JF, Fernandez CE, Coulter ID. A systems model of health care: a proposal. *J Manipulative Physiol Ther*. 1996 Mar-Apr; 19(3): 208-15
[585] Palmer DD. *The Science, Art, and Phiosophy, of Chiropractic*. Portland, OR; Portland Printing House Company, 1910: 107
[586] American Medical Association. Report 12 of the Council on Scientific Affairs (A-97) Full Text. ama-assn.org/ama/pub/category/13638.html Accessed Sep 10, 2005
[587] Getzendanner S. Permanent injunction order against AMA. *JAMA*. 1988 Jan 1;259(1):81-2
[588] Terrett AG. Misuse of the literature by medical authors in discussing spinal manipulative therapy injury. *J Manipulative Physiol Ther*. 1995 May;18(4):203-10
[589] Morley J, Rosner AL, Redwood D. A case study of misrepresentation of the scientific literature: recent reviews of chiropractic. *J Altern Complement Med*. 2001 Feb;7(1):65-78
[590] Spivak JL. *The Medical Trust Unmasked*. Louis S. Siegfried Publishers; New York: 1961
[591] Trever W. *In the Public Interest*. Los Angeles; Scriptures Unlimited; 1972. This is probably the most authoritative documentation of the illegal actions of the AMA up to 1972; contains numerous photocopies of actual AMA documents and minutes of official meetings with overt intentionality of destroying Americans' healthcare options so that the AMA and related organizations would have a monopoly in healthcare.
[592] Wolinsky H, Brune T. *The Serpent on the Staff: The Unhealthy Politics of the American Medical Association*. GP Putnam and Sons, New York, 1994
[593] Mein EA, et al. Manual medicine diversity: research pitfalls and the emerging medical paradigm. *J Am Osteopath Assoc*. 2001 Aug;101(8):441-4

financial profitability and political advantage.[594] Intentional misrepresentation and defamation of chiropractic continues to occur to recent times, as documented by the 2006 review by Wenban.[595]

In accord with the comprehensive chiropractic training in musculoskeletal management, numerous sources of evidence demonstrate that chiropractic management of the most common spinal pain syndromes is safer and less expensive than allopathic medical treatment, particularly for the treatment of low-back pain. In their extensive review of the literature, Manga et al[596] published in 1993 that chiropractic management of low-back pain is superior to allopathic medical management in terms of greater safety, greater effectiveness, and reduced cost; they concluded, "There is an overwhelming body of evidence indicating that chiropractic management of low-back pain is more cost-effective than medical management" and "There would be highly significant cost savings if more management of LBP [low-back pain] was transferred from medical physicians to chiropractors." In a randomized trial involving 741 patients, Meade et al[597] showed, "Chiropractic treatment was more effective than hospital outpatient management, mainly for patients with chronic or severe back pain… The benefit of chiropractic treatment became more evident throughout the follow up period. Secondary outcome measures also showed that chiropractic was more beneficial." A 3-year follow-up study by these same authors[598] in 1995 showed, "At three years the results confirm the findings of an earlier report that when chiropractic or hospital therapists treat patients with low-back pain as they would in day to day practice, those treated by chiropractic derive more benefit and long term satisfaction than those treated by hospitals." In 2004 Legorreta et al[599] reported that the availability of chiropractic care was associated with significant cost savings among 700,000 patients with chiropractic coverage compared to 1 million patients whose insurance coverage was limited to allopathic medical treatments; whether the cost savings associated with chiropractic availability are due to 1) improved overall health and reduced need for pharmacosurgical intervention, 2) greater safety and lower cost of chiropractic treatment versus pharmacosurgical treatment, and/or 3) self-selection by wellness-oriented, perhaps healthier, and higher-income patients, remains to be determined. A literature review by Dabbs and Lauretti[600] showed that spinal manipulation is safer than the use of NSAIDs in the treatment of neck pain; of note beyond NSAIDs is the finding that Coxibs have injured and killed tens of thousands of patients.[601] Contrasting the rates of manipulation-associated cerebrovascular accidents to the dangers of medical and surgical treatments for spinal disorders, Rosner[602] noted, "These rates are 400 times lower than the death rates observed from gastrointestinal bleeding due to the use of nonsteroidal anti-inflammatory drugs and 700 times lower than the overall mortality rate for spinal surgery." Similarly, in his review of the literature comparing the safety of chiropractic manipulation in patients with low-back pain associated with lumbar disc herniation, Oliphant[603] showed that, "The apparent safety of spinal manipulation, especially when compared with other [medically] accepted treatments for [lumbar disk herniation], should stimulate its use in the conservative treatment plan of [lumbar disk herniation]."

Osteopathic medicine, discussed in a following section, shares a few features in common with chiropractic. Osteopathic medicine and chiropractic are American-born healthcare professions and paradigms that started at nearly the same time in history and from many of the same foundational principles. Both professions were started in the late 1800's and early 1900's and were founded upon the philosophical premise that the body functioned as a whole and that therefore healthcare and therapeutic interventions needed to be comprehensive in scope and multifaceted in their application. Further, both professions emphasized the importance of structural integrity as a foundational component of health and thus embraced manual manipulative therapy and spinal manipulation. From their common origins, subtle differences and chance historic events shaped and further separated these professions from each other.

---

[594] Wilk CA. *Medicine, Monopolies, and Malice: How the Medical Establishment Tried to Destroy Chiropractic*. Garden City Park: Avery, 1996
[595] Wenban AB. Inappropriate use of the title 'chiropractor' and term 'chiropractic manipulation' in the peer-reviewed biomedical literature. *Chiropr Osteopat*. 2006;14:16
[596] Manga P, et al. *The Effectiveness and Cost-Effectiveness of Chiropractic Management of Low-Back Pain*. Richmond Hill, Ontario: Kenilworth Publishing; 1993
[597] Meade TW, et al. Low-back pain of mechanical origin: randomised comparison of chiropractic and hospital outpatient treatment. *BMJ*. 1990;300(6737):1431-7
[598] Meade TW, et al. Randomised comparison of chiropractic and hospital outpatient management for low-back pain: results from extended follow up. *BMJ*. 1995;311(7001):349-5
[599] Legorreta et al. Comparative analysis of individuals with and without chiropractic coverage: patient characteristics, utilization, and costs. *Arch Intern Med*. 2004;164:1985-92
[600] Dabbs V, Lauretti WJ. A risk assessment of cervical manipulation vs. NSAIDs for the treatment of neck pain. *J Manipulative Physiol Ther*. 1995;18:530-6
[601] Topol EJ. Failing the public health--rofecoxib, Merck, and the FDA. *N Engl J Med*. 2004 Oct 21;351(17):1707-9
[602] Rosner AL. Evidence-based clinical guidelines for the management of acute low-back pain: response to the guidelines prepared for the Australian Medical Health and Research Council. *J Manipulative Physiol Ther*. 2001;24(3):214-20
[603] Oliphant D. Safety of spinal manipulation in the treatment of lumbar disk herniations: a systematic review and risk assessment. *J Manipulative Physiol Ther*. 2004;27:197-210

The shadow(s) of the chiropractic profession: Coming face-to-face with the shadow(s) of the chiropractic profession has easily been one of the biggest disappointments in my life. Like many young athletic students who are attracted to the profession, I fell in love with the profession's *image* and its *potential*—before I knew about the *realities* within the schools and the larger profession. That I have/had been a major cheerleader for the chiropractic profession—advocating for the profession's scope expansion, for high professional standards, and for greater integrative chiropractic care—is well documented in my many publications for the chiropractic profession starting in 1994[604], including my being the first (to my knowledge) chiropractic doctor published in the American College of Rheumatology's journal *Arthritis & Rheumatism*[605], my writing of the profession's first clinical textbook on the management of hypertension and differential diagnosis of high blood pressure[606], and my numerous other *pro-chiropractic* books, articles, and editorials.[607] However, after working

---

The price of our commitment to truth

"We have had to pay dearly for every atom of truth. We have had to pay for it with almost everything that our hearts, our love, our trust cling to. This requires greatness of soul. The service of truth is the hardest service."

Nietzsche FW. *Cambridge University Texts in the History of Philosophy*; 2005, p. 49

Truth can—and often does—hurt

"Your pain is the breaking of the shell that encloses your understanding. It is the bitter potion by which the physician within you heals your sick self; so therefore, trust the physician and drink his remedy in silence and tranquility."

Kahlil Gibran. *The Prophet*; 1923

---

[604] Vasquez A. High body iron stores: causes, effects, diagnosis, and treatment. *Nutritional Perspectives* 1994
[605] Vasquez A. Musculoskeletal disorders and iron overload disease. [Letter] *Arthritis & Rheumatism* 1996; 39:1767-8
[606] Vasquez A. *Chiropractic Management of Chronic Hypertension 2010, Integrative Chiropractic Management of High Blood Pressure: Updated & Expanded 2nd Edition* 2011
[607] A sample listing of additional pro-chiropractic, chiropractic-specific, and chiropractic-friendly books, articles, and editorials by Dr Vasquez:
1. Vasquez A. *Integrative Orthopedics*: 2004, 2007, 2012
2. Vasquez A. *Integrative Rheumatology*: 2006, 2007, 2014
3. Vasquez A. *Musculoskeletal Pain: Expanded Clinical Strategies*: Printed monograph approved for ACCME PRA-1 Continuing Medical Education. 2008 May
4. Vasquez A. *Chiropractic and Naturopathic Mastery of Common Clinial Disorders*: 2009
5. Vasquez A. *Selected Topics in NeuroMusculoskeletal Medicine*: 2013
6. Vasquez A. Chiropractors Managing Chronic Hypertension An Idea Who's Time Has Arrived. *Dynamic Chiropractic* 2010 Jun
7. Vasquez A. Affirmation and Rebirth of the Chiropractic Profession, Part 1. Setting New Standards in Office-Based Musculoskeletal Care and Health Promotion. *Dynamic Chiropractic* 2007 Apr
8. Vasquez A. Affirmation and Rebirth of the Chiropractic Profession, Part 2. *Dynamic Chiropractic* 2007 Apr
9. Vasquez A. Chiropractic Musculoskeletal Competence: Is Being "Best" Good Enough? *Dynamic Chiropractic* 2007 Mar
10. Vasquez A. Implementing the Five-Part Nutritional Wellness Protocol for the Treatment of Various Health Problems. *Nutritional Wellness*—a chiropractic nutrition magazine 2005 Nov
11. Vasquez A. The Importance of Integrative Chiropractic Health Care in Treating Musculoskeletal Pain and Reducing the Nationwide Burden of Medical Expenses and Iatrogenic Injury and Death: A Concise Review of Current Research and Implications for Clinical Practice and Healthcare Policy. *The Original Internist*—a chiropractic magazine/journal 2005; 12(4): 159-182
12. Vasquez A. Revisiting the Five-Part Nutritional Wellness Protocol: The Supplemented Paleo-Mediterranean Diet. *Nutritional Perspectives*—published by the American Chiropractic Association's Council on Nutrition 2011 January
13. Vasquez A. Five-Part Nutritional Wellness Protocol That Produces Consistently Positive Results. *Nutritional Wellness*—chiropractic nutrition magazine 2005 Sep
14. Vasquez A. The Science of Chiropractic and Spinal Manipulation, Part 2 mercola.com/2005/mar/12/chiropractic_spine.htm 2005, March 12
15. Vasquez A. The Science of Chiropractic and Spinal Manipulation, Part 1 mercola.com/2005/mar/9/chiropractic_spine.htm 2005, March 9
16. Vasquez A. Vitamin D Supplementation in the Treatment of Musculoskeletal Pain. *The Original Internist*—a chiropractic magazine/journal 2004; 11: 7-9
17. Vasquez A, John Cannell, MD. Better Bones and Beyond: Vitamin D Plays Role in Inflammatory and Metabolic Disease. *Holistic Primary Care* 2004; (Fall) 5: 3,6,7
18. Vasquez A. Integrative Orthopedics and Vitamin D: Testing, Administration, and New Relevance in the Treatment of Musculoskeletal Pain. *Townsend Letter for Doctors and Patients* 2004; October, 75-77
19. John Cannell, MD and Vasquez A. Measuring Your Vitamin D Levels: Your Most Important Blood Test? mercola.com/2004/jul/3/vitamin_d_levels.htm 2004, July 3
20. Vasquez A. Interventions Need to Be Consistent with Osteopathic Philosophy. *JAOA: Journal of the American Osteopathic Association* 2006 Sep
21. Vasquez A. Web-like Interconnections of Physiological Factors. *Integrative Medicine: A Clinician's Journal* 2006 Apr/May
22. Vasquez A. Reducing pain and inflammation naturally - Part 6: Nutritional and Botanical Treatments against "Silent Infections" and Gastrointestinal Dysbiosis, Commonly Overlooked Causes of Neuromusculoskeletal Inflammation and Chronic Health Problems. *Nutritional Perspectives*—by ACA Council on Nutr 2006 Jan
23. Vasquez A. "Chapter 10: Organ System Function and Underlying Mechanisms: The Interconnected Web." In Jones DS (Editor-in-Chief). *Textbook of Functional Medicine*. Institute for Functional Medicine. 2005
24. Vasquez A. "Chapter 25: Structural Imbalances." In Jones DS (Editor-in-Chief). *Textbook of Functional Medicine*. Institute for Functional Medicine. 2005
25. Vasquez A. "Chapter 27: Inflammation and Autoimmunity: A Functional Medicine Approach." In Jones DS (Editor-in-Chief). *Textbook of Functional Medicine*. Institute for Functional Medicine. 2005
26. Vasquez A, Murray MT. Chapter 188 "Inflammatory Bowel Diseases: Ulcerative Colitis and Crohn's Disease" in Pizzorno JE, Murray MT (Eds). *Textbook of Natural Medicine: Third Edition*. Churchill Livingstone. 2005 Nov
27. Vasquez A. Reducing pain and inflammation naturally - Part 5: Improving neuromusculoskeletal health by optimizing immune function and reducing allergic reactions: a review of 16 treatments and a 3-step clinical approach. *Nutritional Perspectives*—published by the ACA's Council on Nutrition 2005 Oct
28. Vasquez A, Muanza DN. Comment: evaluation of presence of aspirin-related warnings with willow bark.[letter] *Annals of Pharmacotherapy* 2005 Oct
29. Vasquez A, Cannell J. Calcium and vitamin D in preventing fractures: data are not sufficient to show inefficacy.[letter] *BMJ: British Medical Journal* 2005 May
30. Vasquez A. Reducing pain and inflammation naturally - Part 4: Nutritional and Botanical Inhibition of NFkappaB, the Major Intracellular Amplifier of the Inflammatory Cascade. A Practical Clinical Strategy Exemplifying Anti-Inflammatory Nutrigenomics. *Nutritional Perspectives*—published by the American Chiropractic Association's Council on Nutrition 2005 July
31. Vasquez A. Subphysiologic Doses of Vitamin D are Subtherapeutic: Comment on the Study by The Record Trial Group. *TheLancet.com* 2005 May online
32. Vasquez A. Reducing pain and inflammation naturally - Part 3: Improving overall health while safely and effectively treating musculoskeletal pain. *Nutritional Perspectives*—published by the American Chiropractic Association's Council on Nutrition 2005; 28: 34-38, 40-42
33. Vasquez A. Healthcare for our bones: Practical nutritional approach to preventing osteoporosis. [Letter]. *J.Manipulative and Physiological Therapeutics* 2005;28:213
34. Vasquez A. Reducing Pain and Inflammation Naturally. Part 2: New Insights into Fatty Acid Supplementation and Its Effect on Eicosanoid Production and Genetic Expression. *Nutritional Perspectives*—published by the American Chiropractic Association's Council on Nutrition 2005; January: 5-16
35. Muanza DN, Vasquez A, et al. Isoflavones and Postmenopausal Women. [Letter] *JAMA: Journal of the American Medical Association* 2004; 292: 2337
36. Vasquez A. Reducing Pain and Inflammation Naturally. Part 1: New Insights into Fatty Acid Biochemistry and the Influence of Diet. *Nutritional Perspectives*—published by the American Chiropractic Association's Council on Nutrition 2004 Oct
37. Vasquez A, Gilbert Manso, M.D., John Cannell, M.D. The Clinical Importance of Vitamin D (Cholecalciferol). *Alternative Therapies in Health and Medicine* 2004
38. Vasquez A. A brief review of two potential adverse effects of zinc supplementation. *Nutritional Perspectives*—published by the ACA's Council on Nutrition 1995

within the profession in the post-graduate arena and — very especially— within several chiropractic colleges, I learned more than a few distasteful lessons by direct observation and experience; being the diligent researcher that I am, I've ensured that all of these experiences have been corroborated by other staff and professionals within the school(s) and/or documented with archived emails, internal documents, and meeting transcripts.

The degree of administrative incompetence that I have witnessed within chiropractic academics, and which I have seen other professors abused by, and which has been independently documented in *The Chronicle of Higher Education*[608,609,610] is simply stunning and bewildering; **for those who love academics and education and who hold / have held a high vision for the chiropractic profession, these experiences are particularly painful.** My observations, experiences, and those of others include but are not limited to the following: petty politics carried to the extreme, and repeated and sequential *constructive dismissals* (illegal); lowering of academic standards to lessen the burden on administrators and to increase enrollment; familial and nonfamilial nepotism (e.g., hiring and overpaying unqualified family members and "friends"); misleading the Board of Directors/Trustees by misrepresenting facts about critical institutional issues such as finances, and usurping money from one program to compensate for another program's failings so that the Board would not know the truth; using school money to pay-off fired administrators with *nondisclosure agreements* so that administrative corruption/incompetence remains hidden, and using school attorneys and thus school money to threaten professors who disagree with administrative recklessness; implementing sweeping changes within the faculty, staff, and Board of Directors/Trustees (i.e., administrative *scorched earth policy*) in such a way that institutional accountability becomes a practical impossibility because the "people who know" are excised from the campus and are replaced by newbies just trying to learn the ropes and keep their jobs; allowing email and phone privacy to be breached (e.g., eavesdropping, selective deletion of sensitive emails); lying to students and other faculty about the inappropriate political genesis of administrative changes; intentionally false advertising to attract students; blocking professor's school email during final exam week thus prohibiting communication with students and support staff and then accusing professor of "failing to honor contract obligations and teaching duties"; accepting huge sums of money from corporate interests and misdirecting the educational course –e.g., allowing the insertion of corporate-produced "educational material" into the official doctorate-level clinical curriculum and allowing corporate-friendly "administrators" to replace established expert teachers and clinicians; maintaining appearances (such as with glossy catalogs and visitor gifts) rather than supporting quality education and faculty needs (e.g., radiology departments without basic modern radiology equipment); failing to support basic science and clinical faculty[611]; falsifying meeting minutes and/or the data presented within those meetings; lying to students about

---

Pitfalls and misadventures in chiropractic academics

All-to-common themes in chiropractic academics:
- Administrative mistreatment of teaching faculty
- Gross overpayment of upper administrators: drains monies from academics, demoralizes teaching faculty
- Exclusion of teaching faculty from Board meetings, so that a very "selective truth" can be presented
- Selection of admin-friendly Board members who overlook and remain voluntarily blind to school problems and administrative misbehavior
- Inappropriate firing and constructive dismissal of qualified and performing middle admin and professors for political purposes

Chronicle of Higher Education 2012 Apr15
chronicle.com/article/Chiropractic-Colleges-Ruling/131539/

Some of the biggest problems and challenges for the chiropractic profession—e.g., quality of education, issues of professionalism and ethics, retention of quality faculty and clinicians, maintaining and educating for the desired scope of practice—stem from chiropractic colleges and "university" administrators themselves

"But concerns about management are central to the issues surrounding chiropractic colleges, and overcoming them may be key to the institutions' efforts to build their reputations in mainstream higher education, draw more students, and ultimately, survive."

Fuller A. Chiropractic Colleges Seek Legitimacy Amid Financial Woes. *Chronicle of Higher Education* 2012

The opportunity to make things better is in the hands of chiropractic clinicians, students, teachers, and alumni

Chiropractic clinicians, students, teachers, and alumni have the option to run and hide from these problems, or to acknowledge them and then use the information to demand accountability and authentic professionalism from upper administrators and the weak Boards that have allowed chaos to reign.

---

[608] Fuller A. Chiropractic Colleges Seek Legitimacy Amid Financial Woes. *Chronicle of Higher Education*. 2012 Apr 15.
[609] Stripling J. Presidential Couple at Chiropractic College Draws Fire Over Wife's Role. *Chronicle of Higher Education*. 2012 Apr15.
[610] Stripling J. Dogged by Nepotism Charges, Chiropractic College Reveals Earnings of Chief's Family. *Chronicle of Higher Education*. 2012 Oct 17
[611] Comic video with a lot of painful accuracy about chiropractic academics: "So you're thinking of going to chiropractic college? youtube.com/watch?v=TqpAvaSUnkY

the safety/application of carcinogenic chemicals to the school's landscape; exorbitant and extended presidential vacations abroad during times of institutional initiatives and crises; bypassing criteria for advancement for a select few administrators and thereby undermining the legitimacy of academic titles and effort by honest faculty; ultimately but not exclusively, these result in the repulsion of quality students and faculty from the chiropractic profession, diminution of educational quality, impairment of clinical performance, and retardation of the profession *from within* from delivering the highest quality of care and achieving greater professional success for its members. Any true proponent of the chiropractic profession will acknowledge that these problems need to be addressed *at their sources within chiropractic academics* if the profession is to move forward toward greater authenticity, cultural authority, and professional success; the shame of chiropractic's self-sabotage—and how this blocks the profession *from within* from moving forward—is well reflected in the African proverb, "If there is no enemy within, the enemy outside can do us no harm." Chiropractic clinicians, students, teachers, and alumni have the option to run and hide from these problems, or to acknowledge them and then use the information to demand accountability and authentic professionalism from upper administrators. Smaller minds will get angry at the revelation and realization of inconvenient truths, but the only way to help the situation get better is to address these problems in chiropractic schools—not continue to deny and cover them. These problems are not isolated in one particular chiropractic school or another but are disappointingly common and chronic across several chiropractic schools; greater oversight by regional accreditors is also needed since unfortunately the administrators are often not accountable and the Boards of these schools impose no accountability either, via ignorance, neglect, or the common combination of the two: intentional ignorance. The problem is compounded exponentially when school administrators have positions within the offices of the regional accreditors; this gross conflict of interest creates a situation where *the fox is guarding the henhouse*, and "accountability" is just a joke at the expense of students, professors, and the public who deserve it.

A common experience in chiropractic academics: micromanagement for short-term gain at the expense of the future of the profession and quality of education
"The administration does not care about quality control: they consistently undermine the efforts of the basic science professors and clinical faculty. It is dangerous and irresponsible on the part of the administration of the schools. You will find that the administrations of chiropractic colleges are hell-bent on destroying their own profession in exchange for short-term monetary gains."   To be sure, this is a social rather than scientifically-referenced quote, but it is largely consistent with what I and many other students and faculty in chiropractic colleges have experienced. youtube.com/watch?v=TqpAvaSUnkY

Examples of these problems have been documented in articles published in *The Chronicle of Higher Education* and while this documentation is important, that two of the articles cited refer to a single chiropractic college thereby might contribute to a false impression that similar events are not occurring in other colleges, which is *very* clearly not the situation. Other noteworthy problems are the profession's persistent lack of use of laboratory testing[612] and additional evidence proving that the profession *as a whole* is not engaged in primary care[613], the overuse of radiography[614], and the error in logic that suppression of the profession by medical groups indicates parity with those medical groups. Despite all of this, chiropractic-specific musculoskeletal manipulation—"the adjustment"—remains an impressively potent therapeutic tool: alleviating pain and musculoskeletal dysfunction for many and delivering the occasional "chiropractic miracle" for few. Similarly, some chiropractors with additional post-graduate training and certification deliver clinically brilliant and highly competent primary and specialist care.

Wilk vs American Medical Association: The successful antitrust case against medical monopolization
The following 2 pages provide the transcript of the 1987 judgment that was intended to end AMA's attempt to eliminate chiropractic.

---

[612] National Board of Chiropractic Examiners. *Practice Analysis of Chiropractic 2010*. Chapter 9. "Draw blood, collect urine and/or perform other laboratory tests in your office = 0.3/range 0-5 = Virtually Never." "Order blood, urine, or other laboratory tests from an outside facility = 0.8 = Yearly." "Perform a focused cardiopulmonary examination = 0.9 = Yearly" "Review laboratory studies and interpret the results = 1.6 = Monthly." nbce.org/wp-content/uploads/analysis_chapter_09.pdf

[613] National Board of Chiropractic Examiners. *Practice Analysis of Chiropractic 2010*. Chapter 8, Patient Conditions. nbce.org/wp-content/uploads/analysis_chapter_08.pdf

[614] Some sample citations are provided at ncahf.org/pp/chirop.html#hazardous; note "In addition, across all five vignettes, 25% of chiropractors would take, or order, a full spine plain x-ray. ... There is no evidence that full spine x-rays are warranted in these vignettes and this finding is troubling considering the radiation dose that the patient would receive." Walker et al. Management of people with acute low-back pain. *Chiropr Man Therap*. 2011 Dec 15;19(1):29 While the overuse of radiography within the chiropractic profession has abated in recent years, no reasonable person within the profession will deny that the profession as a whole has overused radiography to assess *functional* rather than *pathologic* problems of the spine and that most of these same functional problems could have been diagnosed *without radiography* and treated successfully *without radiography*. As a gross example, virtually our entire freshman class in chiropractic school received full-spine radiographs and a full set of regional radiographs during our introduction to clinical services in the first year of chiropractic college; generally this means that hundreds and thousands of chiropractic students have been exposed unnecessarily to a significant amount of ionizing radiation, pseudo-justified by minimal or facticious criteria and for the need to give graduating students the radiography credits needed per school accreditation.

Special Communication

IN THE UNITED STATES DISTRICT COURT
FOR THE NORTHERN DISTRICT OF ILLINOIS
EASTERN DIVISION

CHESTER A. WILK, et al.,)
                        Plaintiffs,)
               v.) No. 76 C 3777
AMERICAN MEDICAL ASSOCIATION,)
et al.,)
                       Defendants.)

PERMANENT INJUNCTION ORDER AGAINST AMA

Susan Getzendanner, District Judge

The court conducted a lengthy trial of this case in May and June of 1987 and on August 27, 1987, issued a 101 page opinion finding that the American Medical Association ("AMA") and its members participated in a conspiracy against chiropractors in violation of the nation's antitrust laws. Thereafter an opinion dated September 25, 1987 was substituted for the August 27, 1987 opinion. The question now before the court is the form of injunctive relief that the court will order.

See also p 83.

As part of the injunctive relief to be ordered by the court against the AMA, the AMA shall be required to send a copy of this Permanent Injunction Order to each of its current members. The members of the AMA are bound by the terms of the Permanent Injunction Order if they act in concert with the AMA to violate the terms of the order. Accordingly, it is important that the AMA members understand the order and the reasons why the order has been entered.

The AMA's Boycott and Conspiracy

In the early 1960s, the AMA decided to contain and eliminate chiropractic as a profession. In 1963 the AMA's Committee on Quackery was formed. The committee worked aggressively—both overtly and covertly—to eliminate chiropractic. One of the principal means used by the AMA to achieve its goal was to make it unethical for medical physicians to professionally associate with chiropractors. Under Principle 3 of the AMA's Principles of Medical Ethics, it was unethical for a physician to associate with an "unscientific practitioner," and in 1966 the AMA's House of Delegates passed a resolution calling chiropractic an unscientific cult. To complete the circle, in 1967 the AMA's Judicial Council issued an opinion under Principle 3 holding that it was unethical for a physician to associate professionally with chiropractors.

The AMA's purpose was to prevent medical physicians from referring patients to chiropractors and accepting referrals of patients from chiropractors, to prevent chiropractors from obtaining access to hospital diagnostic services and membership on hospital medical staffs, to prevent medical physicians from teaching at chiropractic colleges or engaging in any joint research, and to prevent any cooperation between the two groups in the delivery of health care services.

Published by order of Susan Getzendanner, US District Judge, Sept 25, 1987.

The AMA believed that the boycott worked—that chiropractic would have achieved greater gains in the absence of the boycott. Since no medical physician would want to be considered unethical by his peers, the success of the boycott is not surprising. However, chiropractic achieved licensing in all 50 states during the existence of the Committee on Quackery.

The Committee on Quackery was disbanded in 1975 and some of the committee's activities became publicly known. Several lawsuits were filed by or on behalf of chiropractors and this case was filed in 1976.

Change in AMA's Position on Chiropractic

In 1977, the AMA began to change its position on chiropractic. The AMA's Judicial Council adopted new opinions under which medical physicians could refer patients to chiropractors, but there was still the proviso that the medical physician should be confident that the services to be provided on referral would be performed in accordance with accepted scientific standards. In 1979, the AMA's House of Delegates adopted Report UU which said that not everything that a chiropractor may do is without therapeutic value, but it stopped short of saying that such things were based on scientific standards. It was not until 1980 that the AMA revised its Principles of Medical Ethics to eliminate Principle 3. Until Principle 3 was formally eliminated, there was considerable ambiguity about the AMA's position. The ethics code adopted in 1980 provided that a medical physician "shall be free to choose whom to serve, with whom to associate, and the environment in which to provide medical services."

The AMA settled three chiropractic lawsuits by stipulating and agreeing that under the current opinions of the Judicial Council a physician may, without fear of discipline or sanction by the AMA, refer a patient to a duly licensed chiropractor when he believes that referral may benefit the patient. The AMA confirmed that a physician may also choose to accept or to decline patients sent to him by a duly licensed chiropractor. Finally, the AMA confirmed that a physician may teach at a chiropractic college or seminar. These settlements were entered into in 1978, 1980, and 1986.

The AMA's present position on chiropractic, as stated to the court, is that it is ethical for a medical physician to professionally associate with chiropractors provided the physician believes that such association is in the best interests of his patient. This position has not previously been communicated by the AMA to its members.

Antitrust Laws

Under the Sherman Act, every combination or conspiracy in restraint of trade is illegal. The court has held that the conduct of the AMA and its members constituted a conspiracy in restraint of trade based on the following facts: the purpose of the boycott was to eliminate chiropractic; chiropractors are in competition with some medical physicians; the boycott had substantial anti-competitive effects; there were no pro-competitive effects of the boycott; and the plaintiffs were injured as a result of the conduct. These facts add up to a violation of the Sherman Act.

In this case, however, the court allowed the defendants the opportunity to establish a "patient care defense" which has the following elements:

(1) that they genuinely entertained a concern for what they perceive as scientific method in the care of each person with whom they have entered into a doctor-patient relationship; (2) that this concern is objectively reasonable; (3) that this concern has been the dominant motivating factor in defendants' promulgation of Principle 3 and in the

conduct intended to implement it; and (4) that this concern for scientific method in patient care could not have been adequately satisfied in a manner less restrictive of competition.

The court concluded that the AMA had a genuine concern for scientific methods in patient care, and that this concern was the dominant factor in motivating the AMA's conduct. However, the AMA failed to establish that throughout the entire period of the boycott, from 1966 to 1980, this concern was objectively reasonable. The court reached that conclusion on the basis of extensive testimony from both witnesses for the plaintiffs and the AMA that some forms of chiropractic treatment are effective and the fact that the AMA recognized that chiropractic began to change in the early 1970s. Since the boycott was not formally over until Principle 3 was eliminated in 1980, the court found that the AMA was unable to establish that during the entire period of the conspiracy its position was objectively reasonable. Finally, the court ruled that the AMA's concern for scientific method in patient care could have been adequately satisfied in a manner less restrictive of competition and that a nationwide conspiracy to eliminate a licensed profession was not justified by the concern for scientific method. On the basis of these findings, the court concluded that the AMA had failed to establish the patient care defense.

None of the court's findings constituted a judicial endorsement of chiropractic. All of the parties to the case, including the plaintiffs and the AMA, agreed that chiropractic treatment of diseases such as diabetes, high blood pressure, cancer, heart disease and infectious disease is not proper, and that the historic theory of chiropractic, that there is a single cause and cure of disease is wrong. There was disagreement between the parties as to whether chiropractors should engage in diagnosis. There was evidence that the chiropractic theory of subluxations was unscientific, and evidence that some chiropractors engaged in unscientific practices. The court did not reach the question of whether chiropractic theory was in fact scientific. However, the evidence in the case was that some forms of chiropractic manipulation of the spine and joints was therapeutic. AMA witnesses, including the present Chairman of the Board of Trustees of the AMA, testified that some forms of treatment by chiropractors, including manipulation, can be therapeutic in the treatment of conditions such as back pain syndrome.

Need for Injunctive Relief

Although the conspiracy ended in 1980, there are lingering effects of the illegal boycott and conspiracy which require an injunction. Some medical physicians' individual decisions on whether or not to professionally associate with chiropractors are still affected by the boycott. The injury to chiropractors' reputations which resulted from the boycott has not been repaired. Chiropractors suffer current economic injury as a result of the boycott. The AMA has never affirmatively acknowledged that there are and should be no collective impediments to professional association and cooperation between chiropractors and medical physicians, except as provided by law. Instead, the AMA has consistently argued that its conduct has not violated the antitrust laws.

Most importantly, the court believes that it is important that the AMA members be made aware of the present AMA position that it is ethical for a medical physician to professionally associate with a chiropractor if the physician believes it is in the best interests of his patient, so that the lingering effects of the illegal group boycott against chiropractors finally can be dissipated.

Under the law, every medical physician, institution, and hospital has the right to make an individual decision as to whether or not that physician, institution, or hospital shall associate professionally with chiropractors. Individual choice by a medical physician voluntarily to associate professionally with chiropractors should be governed only by restrictions under state law, if any, and by the individual medical physician's personal judgment as to what is in the best interest of a patient or patients. Professional association includes referrals, consultations, group practice in partnerships, Health Maintenance Organizations, Preferred Provider Organizations, and other alternative health care delivery systems; the provision of treatment privileges and diagnostic services (including radiological and other laboratory facilities) in or through hospital facilities; association and cooperation in educational programs for students in chiropractic colleges; and cooperation in research, health care seminars, and continuing education programs.

An injunction is necessary to assure that the AMA does not interfere with the right of a physician, hospital, or other institution to make an individual decision on the question of professional association.

Form of Injunction

1. The AMA, its officers, agents and employees, and all persons who act in active concert with any of them and who receive actual notice of this order are hereby permanently enjoined from restricting, regulating or impeding, or aiding and abetting others from restricting, regulating or impeding, the freedom of any AMA member or any institution or hospital to make an individual decision as to whether or not that AMA member, institution, or hospital shall professionally associate with chiropractors, chiropractic students, or chiropractic institutions.

2. This Permanent Injunction does not and shall not be construed to restrict or otherwise interfere with the AMA's right to take positions on any issue, including chiropractic, and to express or publicize those positions, either alone or in conjunction with others. Nor does this Permanent Injunction restrict or otherwise interfere with the AMA's right to petition or testify before any public body on any legislative or regulatory measure or to join or cooperate with any other entity in so petitioning or testifying. The AMA's membership in a recognized accrediting association or society shall not constitute a violation of this Permanent Injunction.

3. The AMA is directed to send a copy of this order to each AMA member and employee, first class mail, postage prepaid, within thirty days of the entry of this order. In the alternative, the AMA shall provide the Clerk of the Court with mailing labels so that the court may send this order to AMA members and employees.

4. The AMA shall cause the publication of this order in JAMA and the indexing of the order under "Chiropractic" so that persons desiring to find the order in the future will be able to do so.

5. The AMA shall prepare a statement of the AMA's present position on chiropractic for inclusion in the current reports and opinions of the Judicial Council with an appropriate heading that refers to professional association between medical physicians and chiropractors, and indexed in the same manner that other reports and opinions are indexed. The court imposes no restrictions on the AMA's statement but only requires that it be consistent with the AMA's statements of its present position to the court.

6. The AMA shall file a report with the court evidencing compliance with this order on or before January 10, 1988.

It is so ordered.

Susan Getzendanner
United States District Judge

Common Clinical Considerations: Hemochromatosis and Hypothyroidism

Iron Overload and Genetic Hemochromatosis:
Identification and Management

Introduction to Iron Overload

In its "classic" form, homozygous genetic hemochromatosis is noted in about 1 per 200-250 Caucasian persons, with a similar incidence among Hispanics. The incidence among persons of African descent is notably higher, reported as high as 1 per 80 among hospitalized African Americans. The heterozygous form of iron overload which is phenotypically milder occurs in as many as 1 per 7 (14% of total) persons; any disorder that is common in the general population will be even more common in a clinical population of symptomatic care-seeking patients, especially those with musculoskeletal disorders and complaints.[615]

Testing serum ferritin on a routine basis in clinical practice allows for the detection of iron deficiency (very common, even among non-anemic patients) and iron overload (quite common, especially among patients with joint pain, diabetes, heart failure, and liver disease as well as many other clinical manifestations—most common of which is asymptomaticity.

Hypothyroidism:
Clinical, Functional, and Practical Considerations

Introduction:

Due mostly to the allopathic medical profession's limited view of hypothyroidism, the condition has remained enigmatic, and both doctors and patients have been rendered ineffective in their ability to understand and treat this common clinical condition. In the following few pages, the illusion of complexity and incomprehensibility will be deflated. This chapter details the most important considerations in the assessment and treatment of various types of low thyroid function. As with the other chapters of the book, information will be presented in an outlined format.

---

[615] Vasquez A. Musculoskeletal disorders and iron overload disease: comment on the American College of Rheumatology guidelines for the initial evaluation of the adult patient with acute musculoskeletal symptoms. *Arthritis & Rheumatism*: Official Journal of the American College of Rheumatology 1996; 39:1767-8

Iron Overload
Primary/Genetic Hemochromatosis
Secondary Hemochromatosis

<u>Description/pathophysiology</u>:
- **Hereditary iron overload disorders are now recognized as being among the most common genetic diseases in the human population.**[616,617,618,619,620,621,622]
- Iron overload is a phenotypic state to which a patient arrives by either genetic or environmental/iatrogenic routes. The severity of iron overload can range from moderate to severe.
- Excess iron catalyzes oxidative stress which damages body tissues and structures in which the iron is stored. In patients with genetic hemochromatosis, two problems exist simultaneously: 1) a disproportionately large amount of iron is absorbed from the gastrointestinal tract (i.e., these patients' iron absorption is "too efficient"), and 2) iron is preferentially deposited in parenchymal tissues such as the heart, liver, pancreas, pituitary gland, and joints rather than being stored safely within the reticuloendothelial system. The deposition of excess iron in parenchymal tissues promotes destruction of these organs/tissues via oxidative mechanisms and subsequent tissue necrosis and fibrosis, leading to the protean manifestations of the disease dependent upon which organs are most affected in the individual patient: heart failure, hepatic fibrosis, hypoinsulinemic diabetes, hypopituarism, and hemochromatoic arthropathy.
- Iron overload can be defined as a state of "iron toxicity" similar to mercury toxicity or poisoning with any other heavy metal or toxin, except that the mechanism is more related to the *quantity* of the iron rather than the unique characteristics or *quality* of iron itself. In other words, whereas the toxicity of mercury can be seen even when only small amounts of the metal are present, the toxicity of iron is directly related to the amount of the excess iron, rather than the inherent toxicity of the iron itself.

> **Iron overload disorders are common in all ethnic/racial populations**
>
> Genetic hemochromatosis is considered one of the most common hereditary disorders in the Caucasian population with a homozygote frequency of 1 per 200-250 (approx 0.5%) and a heterozygote frequency of about 1 in 7 (approx 14%); the condition is at least as common in other ethnic groups except that this predisposition toward iron overload is more common in Africans (as high as 1 in 20) and African-Americans (as high as about 1 in 80 in some series among hospitalized patients). Of course, the expected frequency would be even higher among symptomatic patients than among the general population. **Thus, for a clinician in full-time practice, the only reason for not appreciating this condition among one's patient population several times per year is because one is simply not sufficiently looking and testing for this condition.**

Rationale for screening all patients
1. Hereditary iron-accumulation disorders occur in a large percentage of the population.
2. Persons with the disease usually have no symptoms.
3. Clinical manifestations are often indicative of irreversible organ damage or organ failure.
4. Iron overload can cause death if not treated early.
5. Early treatment ensures normal life expectancy.
6. **Therefore, early detection (before the onset of symptoms and organ damage) requires screening asymptomatic patients.**

<u>Test of choice</u>: **Serum ferritin**, shows the best correlation with body iron stores and thus prognosis and need for treatment.

---

[616] Olynyk JK, Bacon BR. Hereditary hemochromatosis: detecting and correcting iron overload. *Postgrad Med* 1994; 96: 151-65
[617] Phatak PD, Cappuccio JD. Management of hereditary hemochromatosis. *Blood Rev* 1994; 8: 193-8
[618] Rouault TA. Hereditary hemochromatosis. *JAMA* 1993; 269: 3152-4
[619] Crosby WH. Hemochromatosis: current concepts and management. Hosp Pract 1987; 22:173-92
[620] Bloom PD, Gordeuk VR, MacPhail AP. HLA-linked hemochromatosis and other forms of iron overload. *Dermatol Clin* 1995; 13: 57-63
[621] Barton JC, Bertoli LF. Hemochromatosis: the genetic disorder of the twenty-first century. *Nat Med* 1996; 2: 394-5
[622] Lauffer, RB. <u>Iron and Your Heart</u>. New York: St. Martin's Press, 1991

Clinical presentations:
- **Many patients are asymptomatic.**
- **Most patients eventually present with a problem that is attributed to another disorder**:
  - Diabetes: Patients may present with diabetes, which is erroneously attributed to metabolic syndrome or type-2 diabetes.[623]
  - Musculoskeletal pain: Patients may present with joint pain that is erroneously attributed to osteoarthritis[624], rheumatoid arthritis[625], or some other musculoskeletal syndrome.[626]
  - Cardiomyopathy: Patients may present with heart failure that is written off as "idiopathic cardiomyopathy."[627]
  - Liver disease: Hemochromatosis liver disease resembles and exacerbates viral hepatitis, alcoholic hepatitis, and porphyria.
- Fatigue, lethargy, weakness
- Chronic abdominal pain
- Liver damage: Hepatomegaly, elevated serum levels of liver enzymes and alkaline phosphatase, fibrosis and cirrhosis, hepatocellular carcinoma, or other findings such as hematemesis and melena, ascites, hyperbilirubenemia and jaundice, hypoalbuminemia, hepatic encephalopathy, clotting dysfunction, anemia, liver abscess, increased incidence of esophageal carcinoma.
- Abnormal glucose metabolism or diabetes mellitus: Elevated glucose levels. Usually asymptomatic, yet can cause weight loss, polyuria, polyphagia, polydypsia.
- Musculoskeletal disorders: Arthritis and arthralgia, generalized osteoporosis, bone pain, myalgia. Especially arthropathy of the hands and wrists, hips, and knees.
- Cardiac dysfunction: Cardiomyopathy, arrhythmia, fibrillation, congestive heart failure; shortness of breath or dyspnea on exertion, fatigue.
- Cutaneous manifestations: Slate-gray or ashen coloration, increased pigmentation ('tan') of the skin, atrophy of the skin, ichthyosis, koilonychia, loss of body hair, increased incidence of malignant melanoma.
- Endocrine disorders: Hypogonadotrophic hypogonadism, (autoimmune) hypothyroidism, hyperthyroidism; manifest as decreased libido, impotence, testicular atrophy, or sterility in males, amenorrhea or difficulty conceiving in females, loss of body hair.
- Susceptibility to increased frequency and severity of infections: Especially infections due to *Yersinia enterocolitica*, *Vibrio vulnificus*, HIV, and *Mycobacterium tuberculosis*.
- Neurologic symptoms: Blurred vision, sensorineural hearing loss, hyperactivity, dementia, attention deficit disorder, ataxia, lightheadedness, dizziness, anxiety, depression, tinnitus, confusion, lethargy, memory loss, disorientation, headaches and migraine headaches, personality changes, hallucinations, paranoia, chronic treatment-resistant psychiatric illness such as schizophrenia, compulsive disorders, bipolar affective disorder.

Conditions causally associated with iron overload

Primary/genetic disorders
1. Homozygous genetic hemochromatosis
2. Heterozygous genetic hemochromatosis
3. African iron overload
4. African-American hemochromatosis (African-American iron overload)
5. Non-HLA-linked hemochromatosis
6. Juvenile hemochromatosis
7. Neonatal hemochromatosis

Secondary and metabolic disorders
8. Dietary excess of iron
9. Parenteral administration of iron in the form of iron injections and blood transfusions
10. Porphyria cutanea tarda
11. Portacaval shunt
12. Hepatic cirrhosis, portal hypertension, and splenomegaly
13. AIDS
14. Sudden infant death syndrome
15. Alcoholism
16. Metabolic syndrome

Inherited red blood cell abnormalities ("iron-loading anemias", hemoglobinopathies)
17. Alpha-thalassemia
18. Beta-thalassemia
19. Thalassemia intermedia
20. Sideroblastic anemia
21. Aplastic anemia
22. Anemia associated with pyruvate kinase deficiency
23. AC hemoglobinopathy
24. AS hemoglobinopathy
25. X-linked hypochromic anemia
26. Pyridoxine-responsive anemia
27. Atransferrinemia

---

[623] "Most of the patients (95%) had one or more of the following conditions; obesity, hyperlipidaemia, abnormal glucose metabolism, or hypertension. INTERPRETATION: We have found a new non-HLA-linked iron-overload syndrome which suggests a link between iron excess and metabolic disorders." Moirand R, Mortaji AM, Loreal O, Paillard F, Brissot P, Deugnier Y. A new syndrome of liver iron overload with normal transferrin saturation. *Lancet*. 1997 Jan 11;349(9045):95-7
[624] Axford JS, Bomford A, Revell P, et al. Hip arthropathy in genetic hemochromatosis: radiographic and histologic features. *Arthritis Rheum* 1991; 34: 357-61
[625] Bensen et al. Hemochromatoic arthropathy mimicking rheumatoid arthritis. A case with subcutaneous nodules, tenosynovitis, and bursitis. *Arthritis Rheum* 1978; 21: 844-8
[626] Olynyk J, Hall P, et al. Screening for genetic hemochromatosis in a rheumatology clinic. *Australian and New Zealand Journal of Medicine* 1994; 24: 22-25
[627] [No authors listed] Case records of the Massachusetts General Hospital. Weekly clinicopathological exercises. Case 31-1994. A 25-year-old man with the recent onset of diabetes mellitus and congestive heart failure. *N Engl J Med*. 1994 Aug 18;331(7):460-6

- 'Alcoholism': Alcoholism can cause elevated liver enzymes and liver damage, and many iron overload patients are erroneously diagnosed as alcoholics despite their abstinence from alcohol when the clinician fails to consider iron overload as the cause for the hepatopathy.
- Any race, nationality, or ethnic background: Hereditary iron overload conditions have been identified in people of all ethnic backgrounds and nationalities. Secondary iron overload conditions can occur irrespective of genetic predisposition.
- Either gender: Iron overload conditions occur in both men and women
- A family history of, or suggestive of, a hereditary iron overload condition: Family history of iron overload, hereditary anemia or iron-loading anemia, cardiac disorders or "heart disease", arthritis, diabetes, neurologic disorders, liver disease, impotence, amenorrhea, sterility.

Musculoskeletal manifestations of iron overload
Clinical findings may include:
▪ Joint pain
▪ Bone pain
▪ Joint swelling
▪ Loss of motion
▪ Bursitis
▪ Tendonitis
▪ Tenosynovitis
▪ Subcutaneous nodules
Sites of involvement
▪ **Metacarpophalangeal joints**
▪ **Wrist**
▪ **Hip**
▪ **Knee**
▪ Shoulder
▪ Ankle
▪ Metatarsophalangeal joints
▪ Elbow
▪ Spine
▪ Symphysis pubis
▪ Achilles tendon
▪ Plantar fascia
Radiographic findings
▪ **Joint space narrowing**
▪ **Sclerosis**
▪ Cysts
▪ Pseudocysts
▪ Osteophytes
▪ **Hook-like osteophytes at the metacarpal heads (high specificity)**
▪ Flattened or "squared-off" metacarpal heads
▪ Generalized osteopenia
▪ Generalized osteoporosis
▪ Chondrocalcinosis
▪ Subchondral cysts
▪ Carpal erosions
▪ Calcific tendonitis

Differential diagnoses:
- Diabetes mellitus: Remember that the classic presentation of hemochromatosis is "bronze diabetes with cirrhosis." **All patients with diabetes should be tested for iron overload.**[628,629]
- Cardiomyopathy:
- Hepatopathy: **Iron overload is one of the most important rule-outs in patients with liver disease.**[630] Liver biopsy is often indicated to assess condition and disease co-existence.
- Musculoskeletal disorders: **Patients with polyarthropathy should be tested for iron overload.**[631]
    - Degenerative arthritis or osteoarthritis
    - Pseudogout, calcium pyrophosphate dihydrate deposition disease
    - Rheumatoid arthritis[632]
    - Ankylosing spondylitis: The resemblance here is only superficial, related primarily to calcification of the intervertebral discs and ligaments.[633]
- Hyperthyroidism and hypothyroidism[634,635]
- Hypogonadotrophic hypogonadism: Erectile dysfunction in men, subfertility in women[636]
- Porphyria cutanea tarda: "Virtually all patients have increased iron stores; serum iron, iron saturation, and ferritin values."[637] **All patients with porphyria cutanea tarda must be tested for iron overload.**

Clinical assessment:
- **History/subjective:**
    - The manifestations of the condition are so protean that history is generally non-sensitive and non-specific for the disorder. Rarely, a patient will mention that a relative was diagnosed with iron overload or that a relative had an unusual heart or liver disease, and this clue may lead to a diagnosis of iron overload in unsuspecting family members.

---

[628] Czink E, Tamas G. Screening for idiopathic hemochromatosis among diabetic patients. *Diabetes Care* 1991; 14: 929-30
[629] Phelps G, Chapman I, Hall P, Braund W, Mackinnon M. Prevalence of genetic haemochromatosis among diabetic patients. *Lancet* 1989; 2: 233-4
[630] Herrera JL. Abnormal liver enzyme levels: clinical evaluation in asymptomatic patients. *Postgrad Med* 1993; 93: 119-32
[631] M'Seffar AM, Fornasier VL, Fox IH. Arthropathy as the major clinical indicator of occult iron storage disease. *JAMA* 1977; 238: 1825-8
[632] Bensen WG, Laskin CA, Little HA, Fam AG. Hemochromatoic arthropathy mimicking rheumatoid arthritis. *Arthritis Rheum* 1978; 21: 844-8
[633] Bywaters EGL, Hamilton EBD, Williams R. The spine in idiopathic hemochromatosis. *Ann Rheum Dis* 1971; 30: 453-65
[634] Edwards CQ, Kelly TM, Ellwein G, Kushner JP. Thyroid disease in hemochromatosis. Increased incidence in homozygous men. *Arch Intern Med* 1983 Oct;143(10):1890-3
[635] Phillips G Jr, Becker B, Keller VA, Hartman J 4th. Hypothyroidism in adults with sickle cell anemia. *Am J Med* 1992 May;92(5):567-70
[636] Tweed MJ, Roland JM. Haemochromatosis as an endocrine cause of subfertility. *BMJ*. 1998 Mar 21;316(7135):915-6 bmj.bmjjournals.com/cgi/content/full/316/7135/915
[637] "Virtually all patients have increased iron stores; serum iron, iron saturation, and ferritin values." Rich MW. Porphyria cutanea tarda. *Postgrad Med*. 1999;105: 208-10, 213-4

- **Physical examination/objective**:
  o The classic presentation of the fully developed disease is "bronze diabetes with arthritis and cirrhosis."
  o Physical examination should be specific for the patient's complaint(s) of arthritis, cardiomyopathy, diabetes, etc.
- **Imaging & laboratory assessments**:
  o **Routine screening with serum ferritin for iron overload among all patients should be the standard of care in clinical practice**.
    ▪ "In view of the high prevalence of hereditary hemochromatosis, its dire consequences when untreated, and its treatability, screening for the disorder should be performed routinely."[638]
    ▪ "Screening for hemochromatosis is both feasible and cost-effective, and we recommend its use in patients seeking medical care."[639]
    ▪ "The high gene frequency in the general population warrants routine screening tests in asymptomatic healthy young adults."[640]
    ▪ "Primary iron overload occurs in African Americans… Clinicians should look for this condition."[641]
  o Imaging: The radiographic findings are nearly identical to those of osteoarthritis, except more joints are typically involved and that the distribution is typically symmetric (both due to the systemic/metabolic nature of the disease). Hook-like osteophytes at the metacarpal heads—with the "hooks" pointing proximally (rather than distally, as in rheumatoid arthritis) may be the only finding that could be called pathognomonic. Flattened or "squared-off" metacarpal heads are also seen. See previous table labeled *"Musculoskeletal manifestations of iron overload"* for more details.
  o Laboratory evaluation: Serum ferritin is the test of choice when looking for primary iron overload, secondary iron overload, and/or iron deficiency and should be a component of each new patient's evaluation, just as are CBC and the chemistry/metabolic panel. Transferrin saturation is a common test used for the detection of genetic hemochromatosis in research studies because it measures both iron levels but also disordered iron handling; this is why this test is best used in research screening of large populations. For clinicians, serum ferritin is very obviously the superior lab test for iron overload and deficiency.
    ▪ <u>Transferrin saturation</u>: Good test for detecting genetic hemochromatosis before iron overload has occurred; values greater than 40% should be repeated *in conjunction with a measurement of serum ferritin*. Guidelines for screening for genetic hemochromatosis advocate the transferrin saturation test because it is a more sensitive assessment (compared to serum ferritin) for the hemochromatosis genotype which manifests phenotypically not simply as increased iron absorption and accumulation but also as an abnormality in iron handling which preferentially alters the transferrin saturation value, which is the ratio of serum iron to serum transferrin; the former rises due to increased iron absorption while the latter declines due to impaired hepatic synthetic function secondary to the preferential intraparenchymal deposition of iron in genetic hemochromatosis. Thus, genetic hemochromatosis is not simply a disorder characterized by increased iron absorption; it is also a disorder of iron handling/metabolism wherein iron is stored intracellularly in tissue parenchyma rather than (as in non-GH persons) in the reticuloendothelial system.
    ▪ <u>Ferritin</u>: **Routine use of serum ferritin is the most reasonable and cost-effective means for diagnosing this condition in symptomatic and asymptomatic patients**. Elevations of ferritin (i.e., >200 mcg/L in women and >300 mcg/L in men) need to be retested along with CRP (to rule out false elevation due to excessive inflammation) before making the presumptive diagnosis of iron overload. **In the absence of significant inflammation, ferritin values >200 mcg/L in women and >300 mcg/L in men indicate iron**

---

[638] Fairbanks VF. Laboratory testing for iron status. *Hosp Pract* (Off Ed) 1991 Suppl 3:17-24
[639] Balan V, Baldus W, Fairbanks V, et al. Screening for hemochromatosis: a cost-effectiveness study based on 12, 258 patients. *Gastroenterology* 1994; 107: 453-9
[640] Gushusrt TP, Triest WE. Diagnosis and management of precirrhotic hemochromatosis. *W Virginia Med J* 1990; 86: 91-5
[641] Wurapa RK, Gordeuk VR, Brittenham GM, Khiyami A, Schechter GP, Edwards CQ. Primary iron overload in African Americans. *Am J Med*. 1996 Jul;101(1):9-18

overload and the need for treatment/phlebotomy regardless of the absence of symptoms or end-stage complications.[642] Another benefit to the use of serum ferritin is the frequent detection of iron deficiency

Interpretation of iron status based on serum ferritin (in descending order)

Ferritin	Categorization and management
≥ 800 mcg/L	Practically diagnostic of severe iron overload[643]: Repeat tests; rule out inflammation or occult pathology. Initiate phlebotomy and consider liver biopsy or MRI.
≥ 300 mcg/L	Probable iron overload; clear predisposition to iron accumulation[644]: Repeat tests; rule out inflammation or occult pathology. In men, initiate phlebotomy and consider liver biopsy or MRI.[645]
≥ 200 mcg/L	*In women*: Probable iron overload; clear predisposition to iron accumulation[646]: Repeat tests, rule out inflammation or occult pathology. In women, initiate phlebotomy and consider liver biopsy or MRI.[647] *In men*: High-normal *unhealthy* iron status with increased risk of myocardial infarction[648]: Rule out inflammation or occult pathology. No follow-up is mandated, yet blood donation and/or abstention from dietary iron are recommended preventative healthcare measures.
≥ 160 mcg/L	*In women*: Abnormal iron status[649]: Repeat tests, rule out inflammation or occult pathology. Consider phlebotomy and liver biopsy or MRI.
≥80-120 mcg/L	High-normal unhealthy iron status[650,651]: No follow-up is mandated; blood donation and abstention from dietary iron are suggested preventative healthcare measures. A subset of patients with restless leg syndrome (RLS, a condition also causally associated with intestinal bacterial overgrowth dysbiosis) have impaired transport of iron into the brain and therefore require slightly elevated ferritin/iron levels (up to 120) to enhance cerebral iron uptake.
40-70 mcg/L	**Optimal iron status for most people**[652,653]
< 20 mcg/L	Iron deficiency: Search for occult gastrointestinal blood loss with endoscopy or imaging assessments in adults; refer to gastroenterologist.[654,655]

---

[642] Barton JC, McDonnell SM, Adams PC, Brissot P, Powell LW, Edwards CQ, Cook JD, Kowdley KV. Management of hemochromatosis. Hemochromatosis Management Working Group. *Ann Intern Med.* 1998 Dec 1;129(11):932-9
[643] Milman N, Albeck MJ. Distinction between homozygous and heterozygous subjects with hemochromatosis using iron status markers and receiver operating characteristic (ROC) analysis. *Eur J Clin Biochem* 1995; 33: 95-8. See also Milman N. Iron status markers in hereditary hemochromatosis: distinction between individuals being homozygous and heterozygous for the hemochromatosis allele. *Eur J Haematol* 1991;47:292-8
[644] Olynyk JK, Bacon BR. Hereditary hemochromatosis: detecting and correcting iron overload. *Postgrad Med* 1994;96: 151-65
[645] "Therapeutic phlebotomy is used to remove excess iron and maintain low normal body iron stores, ... initiated in men with serum ferritin levels of 300 microg/L or more and in women with serum ferritin levels of 200 microg/L or more, regardless of the presence or absence of symptoms." Barton JC, McDonnell SM, Adams PC, Brissot P, Powell LW, Edwards CQ, Cook JD, Kowdley KV. Management of hemochromatosis. Hemochromatosis Management Working Group. *Ann Intern Med.* 1998 Dec 1;129(11):932-9.
[646] Barton JC, Edwards CQ, Bertoli LF, Shroyer TW, Hudson SL. Iron overload in African Americans. *Am J Med* 1995; 99: 616-23
[647] Barton JC, McDonnell SM, Adams PC, et al. Management of hemochromatosis. *Ann Intern Med.* 1998 Dec 1;129(11):932-9
[648] Salonen JT, Nyyssonen K, Korpela H,et al. High stored iron levels are associated with excess risk of myocardial infarction in eastern Finnish men. *Circulation* 1992; 86: 803-11
[649] Nicoll D. Therapeutic drug monitoring and laboratory reference ranges. In: Tierney LM, et al. *Current Medical Diagnosis and Treatment.* Appleton and Lange, 1996: 1442
[650] Lauffer, RB. *Iron and Your Heart*. New York: St. Martin's Press, 1991: 79-8, 83-88, 162
[651] Sullivan JL. Iron and the sex difference in heart disease risk. *Lancet.* 1981 Jun 13;1(8233):1293-4
[652] Lauffer, RB. *Iron and Your Heart*. New York: St. Martin's Press, 1991: 79-8, 83-88, 162
[653] Vasquez A. High body iron stores: causes, effects, diagnosis, and treatment. *Nutritional Perspectives* 1994; 17: 13, 15-7, 19, 21, 28 and Vasquez A. Men's Health: Iron in men: why men store this nutrient in their bodies and the harm that it does. *MEN Magazine* 1997; Jan:11,21-23 vix.com/menmag/alexiron.htm
[654] Rockey DC, Cello JP. Evaluation of the gastrointestinal tract in patients with iron-deficiency anemia. *N Engl J Med.* 1993;329(23):1691-5
[655] "Endoscopy revealed a clinically important lesion in 23 (12%) of 186 patients. ... CONCLUSIONS: Endoscopy yields important findings in premenopausal women with iron deficiency anemia, which should not be attributed solely to menstrual blood loss." Bini EJ, Micale PL, Weinshel EH. Evaluation of the gastrointestinal tract in premenopausal women with iron deficiency anemia. *Am J Med.* 1998 Oct;105(4):281-6

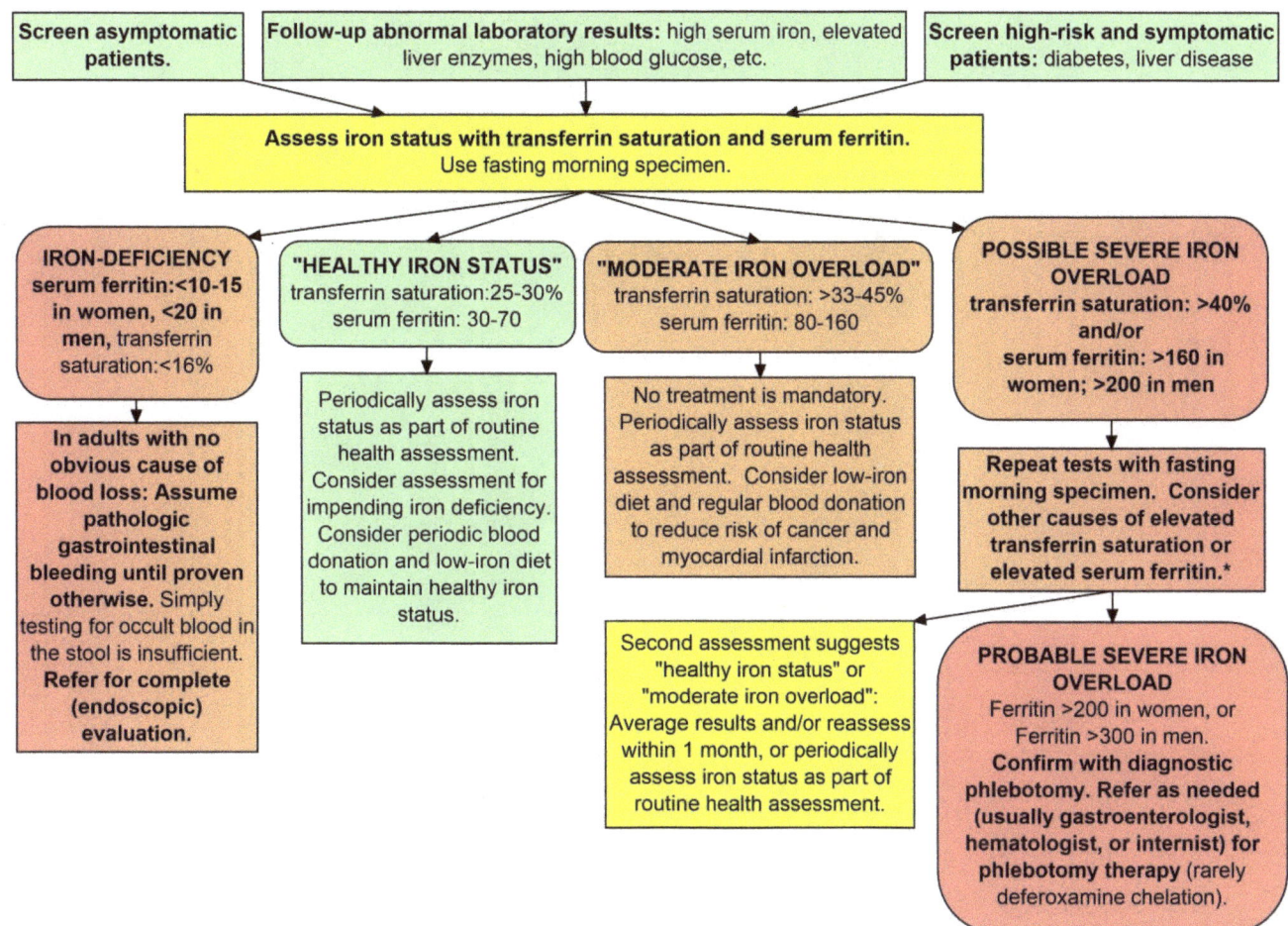

Guide to Patient Management Based on Iron Status:
- Deficiency: Adult patients with iron deficiency must generally be presumed to have occult gastrointestinal blood loss and should therefore be referred for gastrointestinal endoscopy; this is consistent with the standard of care in medicine.
- Optimal: Ferritin levels between 40-70 mcg/L are generally optimal for most men and women; up to 120 mcg/L is reasonable for subsets of patients with restless leg syndrome, perhaps also those with recalcitrant depression and/or Parkinsonian features to allow sufficient iron entry into the brain for maximal dopamine production.
- Excess: Levels greater than 200 mcg/L in a woman or 300 mcg/L in a man are suggestive of iron overload and/or tendency toward accumulation and are physiologically unnecessary and medically unjustifiable, particularly as increased iron stores correlate with increased cancer mortality, increased cardiovascular mortality, and increased all-cause mortality.
- Overload: Diagnosis and treatment for iron overload can occur simultaneously with diagnostic/therapeutic phlebotomy. Genetic testing and liver biopsy are generally inefficient expenditures of financial and medial resources; genetic testing is largely irrelevant in the presence of the hemochromatosis phenotype (i.e., otherwise inexplicable iron accumulation) while liver biopsy exposes the patient to unnecessary treatment delays, risk, and expenses. Identification of idiopathic or genotropic iron overload requires testing of genetic relatives.

Musculoskeletal findings in genetic hemochromatosis: The only specific finding is the retrograde hook-like osteophytes at the metacarpal heads; other findings of intervertebral disc calcification, osteophytosis of the humeral head, and meniscal chondrocalcinosis are nonspecific and therefore easily nondiagnosed or misdiagnosed. Images here are respectfully used with kind permissions of Dr Manfred Harth and *Journal of Rheumatology* (hands and knee) and Dr JD Macfarlane and *Journal of Bone and Joint Surgery* (spine and shoulder) per personal correspondence, written permission, and provision of radiographs.

- **CRP**: Should be relatively normal as iron overload is not inflammatory, per se. If the ferritin is elevated and the CRP is markedly elevated, then inflammatory and hepatic diseases must be considered, namely advanced cancer, viral hepatitis or other hepatopathy, and alcoholic liver disease. If the ferritin is elevated and the CRP is normal, then the most likely diagnosis is iron overload, which should be confirmed either with liver biopsy or diagnostic/therapeutic phlebotomy.
- **CBC**: may show anemia, but the findings here are nonspecific
- **Chemistry panel**: may show evidence of diabetes and hepatopathy
- **Thyroid assessment**: may show hyperthyroidism or hypothyroidism, both of which are more common in patients with iron overload.
- **Bone marrow biopsy**: unnecessary and archaic in this setting, now that serum ferritin is widely available.
- **Liver biopsy**: traditionally considered the "gold standard" for diagnosing iron overload but is now clearly unnecessary for the diagnosis, which can be established by monitoring the response to therapeutic phlebotomy, which is the treatment of choice.[656] **Life-saving diagnostic and therapeutic phlebotomy should never be denied or delayed for lack of liver biopsy in patients with laboratory indicators of iron overload**.[657]
- **Genetic testing, such as for the HFE mutation**: This is a waste of time and money in most clinical situations; these tests should be reserved for research purposes and for evaluation of affected relatives—especially children—of index cases. The only value these tests may have in clinical practice is that of supporting a diagnosis in a patient with elevated serum ferritin who refuses biopsy, liver MRI, or phlebotomy; however, a negative result is meaningless if the ferritin is high and the clinical picture is compatible with iron overload. If the diagnosis is established, genetic relatives must be tested.

Establishing the diagnosis: Any *one* of the following three is sufficient:
- Diagnostic liver biopsy shows heavy iron deposits.
- Characteristic laboratory findings (ferritin >200 in women or >300 in men) *and* the ability to resist intractable anemia with serial/weekly phlebotomies.
- Characteristic MRI of liver *and* the ability to tolerate serial/weekly phlebotomies.

> **Initiation of therapeutic phlebotomy is based on serum ferritin and does not require liver biopsy**
>
> "Therapeutic phlebotomy is used to remove excess iron and maintain low normal body iron stores, and it should be initiated in men with serum ferritin levels of 300 microg/L or more and in women with serum ferritin levels of 200 microg/L or more, regardless of the presence or absence of symptoms."
>
> Barton JC, McDonnell SM, Adams PC, Brissot P, Powell LW, Edwards CQ, Cook JD, Kowdley KV. Management of hemochromatosis. Hemochromatosis Management Working Group. *Ann Intern Med*. 1998 Dec

Complications:
- Patients diagnosed *and effectively treated* before the onset of signs and symptoms have normal life expectancy.
- The most common causes of premature mortality in undiagnosed and untreated patients are related to heart failure, liver failure, infections and/or complications of diabetes.

Clinical management:
- Treatment for severe iron overload is iron-removal therapy. Since blood is high in iron, the removal of blood—therapeutic phlebotomy—is the treatment of choice. Deferoxamine chelation can be administered to patients who refuse or cannot withstand phlebotomy (i.e., patients with cardiomyopathy, severe anemia, hypoproteinemia) but is much less effective, much more expensive, and with side effects such as neurotoxicity. Adjunctive nutritional and lifestyle modifications are no substitute for iron-removal therapy, and weekly phlebotomy is the treatment of choice.
- When a hereditary iron overload disorder is diagnosed, all (first-degree) blood relatives must be screened for iron overload.

---

[656] "Therapeutic phlebotomy is used to remove excess iron and maintain low normal body iron stores, and it should be initiated in men with serum ferritin levels of 300 microg/L or more and in women with serum ferritin levels of 200 microg/L or more, regardless of the presence or absence of symptoms." Barton JC, McDonnell SM, Adams PC, Brissot P, Powell LW, Edwards CQ, Cook JD, Kowdley KV. Management of hemochromatosis. Hemochromatosis Management Working Group. *Ann Intern Med*. 1998 Dec 1;129:932-9
[657] Sullivan JL, as quoted in Crawford R, ed. "The debate." In: *Ironic Blood: information on iron overload*. West Palm Beach: Iron Overload Diseases Association. 1996; 16 (2)

Treatments:
- Medical standard: Iron-removal is accomplished by weekly phlebotomy of 1-2 units (250-500 mL of blood, each of which removes 250 mg of iron), and deferoxamine chelation is used in patients who cannot tolerate phlebotomy. Complications of the disease, such as arthritis, heart failure, hypogonadism, and diabetes are treated appropriately. Cirrhotic patients must be monitored for hepatoma with twice-yearly liver ultrasound and measurement of serum alpha-fetoprotein. Always, when a hereditary iron overload disorder is diagnosed, all (first-degree) blood relatives must be screened for iron overload.
- Diet modifications: These are no substitute for iron-removal therapy with phlebotomy and are weak in their effectiveness by comparison.
  - Decrease consumption of foods and nutritional supplements which are significant sources of iron: Iron supplements, iron-fortified foods and supplements, liver, beef, pork, lamb.
  - Increase consumption of foods that will decrease intestinal absorption of iron from ingested food: tannins in tea, phytates (in whole-grain products, bran, legumes, nuts, and seeds), soy protein, egg, calcium supplements.
  - Ensure adequate protein intake to replace protein lost during phlebotomy.
  - Decrease consumption of excess ascorbic acid (vitamin C); high-dose vitamin C supplementation is clearly contraindicated.[658]
  - Alcohol consumption should be avoided because ethanol exacerbates liver damage and increases iron absorption from the gut.
- Silymarin: Milk thistle has proved benefit in an animal model of iron overload[659] and is probably suitable for use in patients with iron overload, particularly given its ability to reverse cirrhosis.[660] More recently, silybin has been shown to chelate iron in the gastrointestinal tract and reduce its absorption; the more important finding here is that silybin is safe for patients with hemochromatosis.
  - Iron-chelating potential of silybin in patients with hereditary hemochromatosis (*Eur J Clin Nutr* 2010 Oct[661]): "Milk thistle contains silybin, which is a potential iron chelator. … In this crossover study, on three separate occasions, 10 patients who were homozygous for the C282Y mutation in the HFE gene (and fully treated) consumed a vegetarian meal containing 13.9 mg iron with: 200 ml water; 200 ml water and 140 mg silybin (Legalon Forte); or 200 ml tea. Blood was drawn once before, then 0.5, 1, 2, 3 and 4 h after the meal. Consumption of silybin with a meal resulted in a reduction in the postprandial increase in serum iron (AUC±s.e.) compared with water (silybin 1726.6±346.8 versus water 2988.8±167; P<0.05) and tea (silybin 1726.6±346.8 versus tea 2099.3±223.3; P<0.05). In conclusion, silybin has the potential to reduce iron absorption, and this deserves further investigation, as silybin could be an adjunct in the treatment of hemochromatosis."
- Antioxidant supplementation (excluding high-dose ascorbate): Oxidative stress is increased and antioxidant reserves are decreased in patients with iron overload.
- Coenzyme Q10: CoQ-10 probably has a role in the treatment of hemochromatoic cardiomyopathy given its safety and efficacy in other cardiomyopathies.[662,663,664,665,666,667,668,669]

Musculoskeletal disorders and iron overload disease—reminder to review the previous article on page 57
"Approximately one and a 250 persons is homozygous for this disorder and will develop the characteristic clinical manifestations such as diabetes, cardiomyopathy, liver disease, endocrine dysfunction, and, most notable for this discussion, arthropathy or other musculoskeletal disorders. … The current literature suggests that everyone should be screened for iron overload, regardless of the presence or absence of symptoms."
Vasquez A. *Arthritis Rheum.* 1996 Oct

---

[658] Mclarlan et al. Congestive cardiomyopathy and hemochromatosis: rapid progression possibly accelerated by excessive ingestion of ascorbic acid. *Aust NZ J Med* 1982;12:187-8
[659] "CONCLUSIONS: Oral administration of silybin protects against iron-induced hepatic toxicity in vivo. This effect seems to be caused by the prominent antioxidant activity of this compound." Pietrangelo A, et al. Antioxidant activity of silybin in vivo during long-term iron overload in rats. *Gastroenterology*. 1995 Dec;109(6):1941-9
[660] Salmi et al. Effect of silymarin and chemical, functional, and morphological alterations of the liver. A double-blind controlled study. *Scand J Gastroenterol* 1982;17:517-21
[661] Hutchinson et al. The iron-chelating potential of silybin in patients with hereditary haemochromatosis. *Eur J Clin Nutr*. 2010 Oct;64(10):1239-41
[662] Greenberg S, Frishman WH. Co-enzyme Q-10: a new drug for cardiovascular disease. *J Clin Pharmacol* 1990; 30: 596-608
[663] Langsjoen PH, Langsjoen PH, Folkers K. Long-term efficacy and safety of coenzyme Q-10 therapy for idiopathic dilated cardiomyopathy. *Am J Cardiol* 1990; 65: 521-3
[664] Manzoli U, Rossi E, Littarru GP, et al. Coenzyme Q-10 in dilated cardiomyopathy. *Int J Tiss Reac* 1990; 12: 173-8
[665] Langsjoen et al. Pronounced increase of survival of patients with cardiomyopathy when treated with coenzyme Q-10 and conventional therapy. *Int J Tiss Reac* 1990;12:163-8
[666] Folkers K. Heart failure is a dominant deficiency of coenzyme Q-10 and challenges for future clinical research on CoQ-10. *Clin Investig* 1993; 71: s51-s54
[667] Folkers K, et al. Therapy with coenzyme Q-10 of patients in heart failure who are eligible or ineligible for a transplant. *Biochem Biophys Res Commun* 1992;182:247-53
[668] Mortensen SA, et al. Coenzyme Q-10: clinical benefits with biochemical correlates suggesting a scientific breakthrough.... *Int J Tiss Reac* 1990;12:155-62
[669] Langsjoen PH, Langsjoen PH, Folkers K. A six-year clinical study of therapy of cardiomyopathy with coenzyme Q-10. *Int J Tiss Reac* 1990; 12: 169-71

Hypothyroidism:
Clinical, Functional, and Practical Considerations

Description/pathophysiology:
- **Anatomy and normal physiology of thyroid hormone production and function**: The base of the brain contains a region called the hypothalamus, which coordinates many body functions and secretes thyrotropin releasing hormone (TRH) which stimulates the nearby pituitary gland to produce thyroid stimulating hormone (TSH). The TSH produced from the pituitary gland on the underside of the brain provides the stimulating signal to the thyroid gland, located at the front of the neck, for it to produce its hormones. The main hormones secreted by the thyroid gland are thyroxine (also called "T4" because it is the thyroid hormone made from the amino acid tyrosine [T] that has four [4] molecules of iodine) and triiodothyronine, also called "T3" because it has three molecules of iodine. Most of the hormone produced by the thyroid gland is in the form of T4, which is much less biologically active than T3. T4 is converted into T3 in the liver and in the peripheral tissues of the body, with the notable exception of the brain. Although the thyroid gland's production of T3 is quantitatively less than that of T4, because T3 is the active form of the hormone, the direct production of T3 from the thyroid gland itself is important for peripheral tissues such as the brain which are unable to sufficiently convert T4 into T3.

Illustration of thyroid hormone production, stimulation, and peripheral metabolism: Although most doctors have been taught to focus only on thyroid production, updated clinicians realize the importance of considering thyroid production in conjunction with peripheral thyroid metabolism and the differential conversion from the inactive T4 to the reciprocally produced active T3 and reverse T3, the latter of which is either biologically inert or—more likely—counteractive to normal T3 utilization. Conversion of T4 to active T3 is achieved by type-1 and type-2 deiodinase (5' [five prime] iodinase) while conversion of T4 to reverse T3 is achieved by types-2 deiodinase (5-iodinase).[670] Impaired glandular production of thyroid hormones is appropriately termed central or glandular hypothyroidism, while impaired peripheral conversion or utilization of thyroid hormone is appropriately termed metabolic or peripheral or functional hypothyroidism.

---

[670] Kansagra et al. The Challenges and Complexities of Thyroid Hormone Replacement. *Lab Med.* 2010;41(6):229-348 medscape.com/viewarticle/722086_8

- **Hormones and feedback mechanisms**: When thyroid hormone production is insufficient, receptors in the hypothalamus and pituitary sense the hormone deficiency and respond by increasing the production of TSH to stimulate hormone production from the thyroid gland; when thyroid hormone production increases, feedback to the hypothalamus and pituitary reduces TSH production to lower thyroid hormone production. In these ways, as with many other body systems and physiological processes, the body is able to maintain a steady state of thyroid hormone production; most people have heard of this phenomenon of self-regulation referred to as *homeostasis*, even though a more accurate term is *homeodynamics*, because it is an active (not static) process in constant fluctuation and regulation. If a patient is given too much thyroid hormone by prescription, then the TSH level will be reduced; if a patient has hypothyroidism and is undertreated with an insufficient amount of thyroid hormone, then the TSH will remain elevated. Lab tests and optimal hormone levels will be discussed later in this chapter.
- **Problems that may arise in thyroid hormone production and metabolism**: In this section, details will be provided about common problems that can arise in thyroid hormone production and metabolism:
  - Problems of the hypothalamus: Damage to the hypothalamus from an injury such as head trauma, cancer, or infection can result in an inability to produce TRH; these problems are very rare. Doctors do not generally test for TRH production; however, some abnormalities in TRH production have been noted in patients with chronic depression. "Hypothalamic hypothyroidism" is hypothyroidism resulting from a problem in the hypothalamus; this is also called *tertiary hypothyroidism*, because it is two "steps" away from the primary location of thyroid hormone production—the thyroid gland itself.
  - Problems of the pituitary gland: Rarely, the pituitary gland might overproduce TSH and function autonomously from TRH stimulation; this will result in excess thyroid hormone production. More commonly but still rare, damage to the pituitary gland—for example if a nearby tumor compresses the gland, or if the gland is damaged by a disease like iron overload (e.g., hemochromatosis) or by a stroke (e.g., Sheenan's syndrome)—can cause a reduction in TSH production. Problems localized to the pituitary gland resulting in either excess or deficient production of TSH are very rare and are not responsible for the majority of thyroid disorders. Hypothyroidism caused by problems in the pituitary gland is called *secondary hypothyroidism* because it is *secondary* to (i.e., caused by) problems *outside* of the thyroid gland.
  - Problems of the thyroid gland: Several problems can affect the thyroid gland and its ability to produce the proper amount of thyroid hormone. Some of the more relevant disorders are discussed in the following subsections:
    - Graves' disease—autoimmune ***hyper*thyroidism**: Graves' disease is a fairly common autoimmune disease wherein the body's immune system creates antibodies to the TSH receptor. These antibodies stimulate the TSH receptor just as would the normal TSH hormone, and thus the result is an increased production of thyroid hormones from the gland, causing excess thyroid gland function and the clinical manifestations of hyperthyroidism. Common manifestations of the disease are weight loss, excess body heat, diarrhea due to more rapid gastrointestinal transit, and tremor (shakiness) and tachycardia (fast heart rate) due to increased stimulation of the sympathetic nervous system. Another common trademark manifestation of Graves' disease is exophthalmos—"bulging of the eyes"—because excess fibrous tissue is deposited behind the eyes and because the muscles surrounding the outside of the eyes are weakened by immune (antibody) damage. Graves' disease is most commonly treated with drugs that block the metabolism of thyroid hormones, or with other drugs such as radioactive iodine which cause destruction of the thyroid gland, resulting in hypothyroidism which is then treated with prescription thyroid hormone. Graves' disease can be considered a form of *primary* hyperthyroidism because it is hyperthyroidism resulting from abnormal function of the gland *itself*, even though the cause of the problem is the antibodies that are interacting with the gland receptors. With Graves' disease or any other cause of primary hyperthyroidism, lab tests will show that TSH is low and T4 is high. Occasionally noted clinically is a mixed hyper-/hypo- picture, Graves' with Hashimoto's.
      - Nonpharmacologic treatment options for Graves's disease: The best nonpharmacologic treatment for hyperthyroidism is the amino acid L-carnitine 1-4 grams/d orally; carnitine blocks entry of thyroid hormone into the nucleus of the cell, thereby blocking most of the effects of excess thyroid

hormone.[671] Very interestingly, when researchers or we as clinicians use carnitine in patients with normal thyroid status, we do not see adverse effects consistent with "carnitine-induced hypothyroidism", which is to say that carnitine appears to block *excess* thyroid hormone reception but appears to not have a blocking effect on *normal* thyroid function/reception. Since Graves' disease is an autoimmune disorder, attention should be given to normalizing immune function (nutritional immunomodulation) and removing triggers of autoimmunity such as allergenic/immunogenic foods, dysbiotic microbial infections, and xenobiotics—all of these are discussed in Chapter 4 of this book. Finally, patients with the iron-accumulating disease hemochromatosis have an increased risk for developing Graves disease; thus, patients with Graves disease—especially males—should be tested and treated for iron overload, specifically using the blood test serum ferritin, as detailed in Chapter 1.

- <u>Viral infection, acute viral thyroiditis</u>: The thyroid gland can be infected by a viral infection, perhaps as a consequence of an upper respiratory infection; this is called "viral thyroiditis." (Keep in mind that the suffix "-itis" simply means inflammation, so "thyroiditis" just means inflammation of the thyroid gland, whether from infection, trauma [rare], or autoimmune disease [most common].) Classically, the patient has had a recent viral infection—such as a common cold—and the thyroid gland, located at the anterior lower neck just barely above the rib cage, is tender and slightly swollen. In these situations, infection of the gland causes release of thyroid hormone from the gland, temporarily resulting in hyperthyroidism. If the gland is damaged by the infection, then the period of transient *hyper*thyroidism may be followed by *hypo*thyroidism due to failure of the gland to produce sufficient thyroid hormone. This resulting hypothyroidism may be mild or severe, temporary or permanent.

- <u>Hashimoto's disease, autoimmune thyroiditis, autoimmune *hypo*thyroidism</u>: The most common cause of *primary hypothyroidism*—hypothyroidism resulting from failure of the thyroid gland—is autoimmune destruction of the thyroid gland, also called Hashimoto's thyroiditis in recognition of the Japanese medical scientist Hashimoto Hakaru who first described the condition in 1912. The condition is also called lymphocytic thyroiditis because biopsy of the thyroid gland will show infiltration of immune cells called lymphocytes, which cause damage to the glandular tissue. In this condition, the body's own immune system—specifically the T-cells and the antibodies/immunoglobulins made by the B-cells or plasma cells—causes injury to and eventual destruction of the thyroid gland. Autoimmune destruction of the thyroid gland can occur as a solitary phenomenon, or it may occur as part of another autoimmune disorder, such as rheumatoid arthritis (RA), systemic lupus erythematosus (SLE, lupus), or Sjögren's syndrome. If the thyroid gland itself is failing to produce sufficient amounts of thyroid hormone, then feedback mechanisms will cause TSH to increase; thus, what most doctors look for when screening for hypothyroidism is simply an elevated TSH. For many doctors, if they fail to find an elevated TSH, then they will exclude

> **If autoimmune hypothyroidism is the problem, then what is the cause of the problem?**
>
> Given that an autoimmune disease process (involving auto-antibodies and auto-reactive T-cells) can lead to inflammatory destruction of the thyroid gland, a reasonable question becomes "What triggers the immune system to attack the thyroid gland?" The top six answers to this question are:
> ❶ Exposure to the dietary protein gluten, found in grains such as wheat, rye, barley,
> ❷ Nutritional deficiency of selenium, and possibly vitamins D and A,
> ❸ Localized viral infection, noted to result commonly in self-limited thyroid disease,
> ❹ Infection with specific bacteria—such as *Yersinia enterocolitica*—anywhere in the body but especially the gastrointestinal tract,
> ❺ Xenobiotic exposure,
> ❻ Iron overload—patients and especially men with hemochromatosis have a higher risk of developing autoimmune thyroid disease especially Graves disease.
> A genetic predisposition atop any of these other six triggers will increase the probability of developing autoimmune thyroiditis but is by itself insufficient.

---

[671] "In conclusion, L-carnitine is effective in both reversing and preventing symptoms of hyperthyroidism and has a beneficial effect on bone mineralization. Because hyperthyroidism depletes the body deposits of carnitine and since carnitine has no toxicity, teratogenicity, contraindications and interactions with drugs, carnitine can be of clinical use." Benvenga et al. Usefulness of L-carnitine, a naturally occurring peripheral antagonist of thyroid hormone action, in iatrogenic hyperthyroidism: a randomized, double-blind, placebo-controlled clinical trial. *J Clin Endocrinol Metab*. 2001 Aug;86(8):3579-94. "Taken together, all these experiments indicate that L-carnitine decreases the access of thyroid hormone to thyroid hormone receptors by decreasing the amount of hormone having access to cell nuclei, and not by inhibiting thyroid hormone interaction with the nuclear receptors." Benvenga et al. Effects of carnitine on thyroid hormone action. *Ann N Y Acad Sci* 2004 Nov;1033:158-67

hypothyroidism as a diagnosis and will not treat the patient with thyroid hormone even if the patient is *clinically hypothyroid*, that is, showing all the clinical manifestations expected with hypothyroidism. Blood levels of T4 may be normal due to compensatory stimulation by extra TSH; T4 levels might also be reduced. Most often, laboratory tests will also reveal elevated levels of antibodies which specifically target components of the thyroid gland. The two most common antibodies seen in Hashimoto/autoimmune thyroiditis are directed toward thyroglobulin, which is a protein found in the thyroid gland, and against the enzyme peroxidase; these are called anti-thyroglobulin antibodies and anti-thyroid peroxidase (anti-TPO) antibodies, respectively.

- Problems of peripheral metabolism: As reviewed above in the section on normal thyroid metabolism, the thyroid gland's production of thyroid hormone—mostly T4—is followed by conversion of T4 into the active form of thyroid hormone, which is T3. During times of stress, the body's ability to produce and utilize T3 is impaired because the enzymes that catalyze this conversion change in a way that produces a different hormone called "reverse T3" (rT3), which is certainly less active than normal T3 and which appears to actually block the function of the normal T3 that is produced. In these situations, TSH and T4 levels are generally normal, and since most doctors do not test the levels of T3 and rT3, the problem is almost never discovered. Reliable test for T3 and rT3 have been available for many years; the reason that most doctors do not use these tests is that they were not taught to do so in medical school and because most textbooks have not yet incorporated this relatively new information. A well-known paradox is that medical education and clinical training are very slow to change certain ideas despite the clarity of science (such as the importance of optimal nutrition—see extensive reviews in Chapters 2,3,4), and yet are very fast to accept unscientific changes that support drug over-prescribing and nutritional ignorance, such the widespread overuse of unproven drugs (such as rofecoxib/Vioxx, which was a new anti-inflammatory drug that was not very effective for pain but which caused tens of thousands of deaths before its withdrawal[672]) and the American Medical Association's discouragement of GMO labeling—keeping the public ignorant about the food they eat—despite clear scientific evidence of adverse effects.[673]

- **Definitions and descriptions of hypothyroidism**: The American Thyroid Association has described hypothyroidism as follows in a 2003 publication—ATA Hypothyroidism Booklet[674]—available on their website in December 2011: "Hypothyroidism is an underactive thyroid gland ("hypo-"means *under* or below *normal*). Hypothyroidism means that the thyroid gland cannot make enough thyroid hormone to keep the body running normally. People are hypothyroid if they have too little thyroid hormone in their blood." Patients and clinicians should appreciate that while this definition is accurate, it is incomplete because hypothyroidism involves more than the state of insufficient hormone production from the gland; in some situations we see that patients make sufficient thyroid hormone from their thyroid gland, but that the peripheral metabolism of their thyroid hormone is impaired, thereby creating the paradox of hypothyroid manifestations despite normalcy of commonly performed lab tests. Hypothyroidism should therefore be at least partially defined as a clinical syndrome of health problems which are fully or partly reversible with proper replacement of thyroid hormones.

- **A new practical definition of hypothyroidism**: Rather than defining hypothyroidism by "hormone levels in the blood", a wiser and more accurate definition of hypothyroidism holds that the condition should be defined as "an adverse physiological state caused by insufficient function of thyroid hormone at the *cellular* (not *serum*) level, resulting in clinical manifestations consistent with hypothyroidism and which respond wholly or partly to appropriately dosed and formulated thyroid replacement therapy, notably with T4 and T3 in combination, or T3 alone, but generally not T4—the inactive hormone—alone." This definition of hypothyroidism is based on physiology, i.e., the fact that the purpose of thyroid hormone is to effect action and changes at the cellular level to support optimal health and vitality; defining the presence or absence of hypothyroidism on the clinician's

---

[672] Topol EJ. Failing the public health--rofecoxib, Merck, and the FDA. *N Engl J Med.* 2004 Oct 21;351(17):1707-9 nejm.org/doi/pdf/10.1056/NEJMp048286
[673] "…there is no scientific justification for special labeling of bioengineered foods, as a class, and that voluntary labeling is without value unless it is accompanied by focused consumer education." Nestle M. The AMA's Strange Position on GM Foods. *THE ATLANTIC* 2012 Jun theatlantic.com/health/archive/2012/06/the-amas-strange-position-on-gm-foods-test-but-dont-label/258968/ Finamore et al. Intestinal and peripheral immune response to MON810 maize ingestion in weaning and old mice. *J Agric Food Chem.* 2008 Dec 10;56(23):11533-9 pubs.acs.org/doi/abs/10.1021/jf802059w Krüger et al. Detection of Glyphosate Residues in Animals and Humans. *Environmental & Analytical Toxicology* 2014 Jan;4;2 omicsonline.org/open-access/detection-of-glyphosate-residues-in-animals-and-humans-2161-0525.1000210.pdf Gammon C. Weed-whacking herbicide proves deadly to human cells. *Scientific American* 2009 Jun scientificamerican.com/article/weed-whacking-herbicide-p/
[674] American Thyroid Association. ATA Hypothyroidism Booklet. 2003 Available at thyroid.org/patients/brochures/Hypothyroidism%20_web_booklet.pdf on December 2011. "This booklet was prepared by the American Thyroid Association (ATA), a professional society of physicians and researchers specializing in the thyroid gland. Founded in 1923, the ATA fosters excellence and innovation in patient care, research, education, and public advocacy. The recommendations given here are those of the ATA."

measurement of TSH is myopic and doctorcentric/anthropocentric, if not misanthropic. The purpose of the thyroid gland is to make sufficient thyroid hormone to effect normal healthy physiology; the purpose of the thyroid gland is not to produce a level of thyroid hormone that fits within a laboratory reference range defined by a small group of laboratories, researchers, and clinicians based on small numbers of patients, many of whom were likely not optimally healthy. Therefore, any accurate definition of hypothyroidism must be based on physiology rather than on blood tests; again, the purpose of the hormonal system is to create certain physiologic effects consistent with health and vitality, not to produce an amount of hormone considered "normal."

- **One way to explain this to patients**: The way that I have often explained this to patients—verbally or as below from my written patient education materials—is so say something to the effect that, "Thyroid hormones have many different functions in the body, and their chief effect is contributing to the control of the basal metabolic rate, or the *speed of biochemical reactions and physiologic processes* and the *temperature of the body*. For reasons that are not entirely clear, some people do not make enough thyroid hormone to function optimally.[675] Other people make enough to be considered "normal" but they do not feel well, and they often feel better when taking additional thyroid hormone as prescribed by their doctor.[676,677] Indeed, a famous physiology researcher at the University of Texas at Austin—Dr. Roger J Williams—noted in his classic book *Biochemical Individuality*, "a wide variation in thyroid activity exists among 'normal' human beings."[678]

Clinical presentations:
- **Prevalence**: Hypothyroidism is common, affecting about 10% of the population. It is more commonly diagnosed in women than in men; this may be because autoimmune disorders (such as autoimmune thyroiditis) are generally more common in women—some of these reasons (and solutions) are discussed in Chapter 4.
    - Fatigue: Fatigue and "not enough energy" are among the most common complaints of patients with hypothyroidism. Fatigue and low energy are nonspecific subjective complaints that correlate with innumerable health conditions, including depression, existential crisis, anemia, hypothyroidism, infection, cancer, autoimmune diseases, cardiopulmonary disease, nutritional deficiency, and many others.
    - Depression, lack of energy, lack of appetitive drives: Depression is common among patients with hypothyroidism. The most direct explanations for this are ❶ reduced function of the adrenergic nervous system, specifically the reception of neurotransmitters norepinephrine and dopamine, which support energy/attention/vigilance and drive/direction/pleasure, respectively, ❷ reduced metabolic function overall due to lower body temperature (most enzymes function most efficiently within a narrow range of temperatures), ❸ nutritional deficiencies due to reduced stomach acid production (noted in patients with hypothyroidism) and/or bacterial overgrowth of the small bowel (SIBO) secondary to slow intestinal transit, which is well noted in patients with hypothyroidism. Additionally, patients with hypothyroidism often have weight gain, difficult weight loss, reduced appetite and sex drive, various health problems such as hypertension and headaches, and also the experience of being underdiagnosed/undertreated and feeling misunderstood by their doctors and perhaps by friends, family, and intimate/romantic partners as well; these can all contribute to the psychological and social aspects of depression and feelings of sadness, despair, and isolation. Notice from above the combination of reduced food appetite/intake with weight gain and difficult weight loss; this paradox has very few explanations and is therefore a clue in the patient's history suggesting hypothyroidism. Many patients diagnosed with "depression" actually have "depression secondary to hypothyroidism"; rather than being treated with potentially dangerous so-called "anti-depressant drugs" these patients would be better treated for improved mood and enhanced overall health by receiving treatment to optimize thyroid function, namely thyroid hormone.
    - Low body temperature, cold hands and feet: Because T3 increases energy expenditure and therefore increases body heat, patients with an insufficiency of thyroid hormone commonly notice feeling cold and also not tolerating cold weather—a phenomenon referred to as cold intolerance. This can be assessed simply by touching the skin and hands of a person with hypothyroidism; often the initial handshake at the

---

[675] Broda Barnes MD, Lawrence Galton, *Hypothyroidism: The Unsuspected Illness*. Ty Crowell Co; 1976
[676] Skinner GR, et al. Thyroxine should be tried in clinically hypothyroid but biochemically euthyroid patients. *BMJ: British Medical Journal* 1997 Jun 14; 314(7096): 1764
[677] McLaren EH, Kelly CJ, Pollack MA. Trial of thyroxine treatment for biochemically euthyroid patients has been approved. *BMJ* 1997; 315: 1463
[678] Williams RJ. *Biochemical Individuality: The Basis for the Genetotrophic Concept*. Austin and London: University of Texas Press, 1956 page 82

start of the patient's office visit is the first clue to hypothyroidism. Many of these patients have low oral temperatures that never reach the normal temperature of 98.6° Fahrenheit (F) or 37° Celsius (C); often they report that the only time their oral temperature reaches the normal temperature is when they have a "fever" due to an infection. Very few conditions cause low body temperature; therefore, the finding of a consistently low body temperature is a clinical finding that is objective and significant and which warrants evaluation. Low body temperature is most consistent with hypothyroidism; to a lesser extent it is consistent with high estrogen levels, low testosterone levels and—in women and on a menstrual/periodic basis—low progesterone levels. Poor peripheral circulation to the extremities can also produce the feeling of localized coldness; the main conditions to consider in this regard are peripheral arterial disease (PAD, generally seen in elderly patients with other manifestations of cardiovascular disease) and Raynaud's phenomenon (periodic vasoconstriction secondary to vasomotor instability, commonly noted with other autoimmune diseases such as scleroderma and lupus and/or bacterial infections such as with the common bacteria *Helicobacter pylori*, detailed in Chapters 4 (and 5 of DrV's *Naturopathic Rheumatology*).

- Dry skin: Dry skin is commonly noted in patients with hypothyroidism. This may be due to a combination of impaired nutrient absorption and also impaired function of the oil-producing glands of the skin.
- Constipation, poor digestion, acid reflux: Because hypothyroidism leads to a generalized slowing of the body's functions, it commonly leads to slower intestinal transit, which manifests as constipation. Impaired gastrointestinal motility can also promote acid reflux. Approximately 30% of patients with Hashimoto's/autoimmune thyroiditis also make antibodies to the acid-producing cells in the stomach (parietal cells), and this can eventually lead to damage to the stomach lining and reduced stomach acid production, thereby impairing protein digestion. The lack of stomach acid and/or the slowing of intestinal transit promotes excessive growth of bacteria in the intestines because they are not being killed by stomach acid and/or "moved along" by normal peristaltic motions; this small intestinal bacterial overgrowth (SIBO) can lead to other problems such as fatigue, fibromyalgia, chemical sensitivity, and inflammatory arthritis.
- Menstrual irregularities, premenstrual syndrome (PMS), uterine fibroids, excess menstrual bleeding, polycystic ovarian syndrome (PCOS): Women with hypothyroidism commonly have one or more menstrual or reproductive disorders[679]; these are generally reversible or at least partially treatable with normalization of thyroid hormone status and optimization of other health factors. Women with polycystic ovary syndrome have higher-than-normal rates of goiter and autoimmune hypothyroid disease.[680]
- Infertility and the feeling and experience of not having enough sex hormones: Proper thyroid status is needed for the complexities of gonadal function and reproductive success. Men and women with hypothyroidism may have problems with regard to sexual function, desire, and reproduction; infertility and subfertility are common among this patient population. Thyroid hormone is directly necessary for sex hormone production and for the successful maintenance of pregnancy. Primary hypothyroidism associated with elevated TSH levels commonly leads to elevated levels of a pituitary hormone called prolactin, which causes infertility either by direct mechanisms or by secondary mechanisms, such as increasing the liver's production of a protein called sex-hormone-binding globulin (SHBG) which binds to sex hormones (estrogen and testosterone) so tightly that they are unavailable to cells to complete

> **Hypothyroidism is a cause of sexual dysfunction and reproductive disorders in men and women**
>
> "Via its interaction in several pathways, normal thyroid function is important to maintain normal reproduction. ... Male reproduction is adversely affected by both thyrotoxicosis [hyperthyroidism] and hypothyroidism. Erectile abnormalities have been reported. ... In females, thyrotoxicosis and hypothyroidism can cause menstrual disturbances. Thyrotoxicosis is associated mainly with hypomenorrhea and polymenorrhea, whereas hypothyroidism is associated mainly with oligomenorrhea [reduced frequency of menstruation]. Thyroid dysfunction has also been linked to reduced fertility. ... Autoimmune thyroid disease is present in 5-20% of unselected pregnant women. ... Overt hypothyroidism has been associated with increased rates of spontaneous abortion, premature delivery and/or low birth weight, fetal distress in labor, and perhaps gestation-induced hypertension and placental abruption."
>
> Krassas et al. Thyroid function and human reproductive health. *Endocr Rev*. 2010 Oct

---

[679] Weeks AD. Menorrhagia and hypothyroidism. Evidence supports association between hypothyroidism and menorrhagia. *BMJ*. 2000 Mar 4;320(7235):649
[680] "In this case-control study, anti-thyroid antibodies and goiter prevalence were significantly higher in PCOS patients. These data suggest that thyroid exam and evaluation of thyroid function and autoimmunity should be considered in such patients." Kachuei M, Jafari F, Kachuei A, Keshteli AH. Prevalence of autoimmune thyroiditis in patients with polycystic ovary syndrome. *Arch Gynecol Obstet*. 2012 Mar;285(3):853-6

their functions, such as supporting sex drive, sexual function, and reproductive capability.[681] As a cause of low libido, hypothyroidism impairs neurotransmitters such as norepinephrine and dopamine which promote sex drive in men and women. Hypothyroidism also impairs internal production of testosterone, which is a necessary hormone for sex drive and sexual performance.

- Weak fingernails, hair loss: The weak fingernails seen in hypothyroidism are almost certainly due to impaired protein digestion and amino acid and mineral absorption, as well as metabolic impairment of the cells in the nail matrix which produces the toenails and fingernails. Via similar mechanisms, hypothyroidism also causes loss of head hair, which is particularly notable in women. The finding of weak fingernails is a relatively specific finding for a limited number of considerations; generally these are protein deficiency (due to insufficient intake, impaired digestion or absorption, or increased metabolic consumption or increased renal excretion), deficiency of minerals such as zinc, and hypothyroidism. Severe cases of skin diseases such as psoriasis can also affect the nails, but generally these conditions are evident upon observation of the patient; the clinical findings are also different from those seen in hypothyroidism (i.e., flaking of the nails in hypothyroidism versus pitting of the nails with psoriasis).

- Increased need for sleep: An increased need for sleep—termed either hypersomnia or hypersomnolence—is sometimes noted among hypothyroid patients, who might have the experience of needing extra sleep (e.g., > 9 hours per night) and yet not feeling refreshed after a good night's sleep. Other causes of increased need for and/or reduced quality of sleep are heart failure and sleep apnea; these can generally be distinguished from hypothyroidism based on history, physical exam, laboratory tests, and—more accurately but not generally needed—special tests such as echocardiography and sleep tests (polysomnography).

- Overweight, gain weight easily, difficulty losing weight: Thyroid hormone is an important factor energy utilization and thus caloric expenditure and therefore calorie intake-expenditure balance. Any low thyroid condition will promote weight gain and reduced weight loss because the overall metabolic rate is lowered in states of low thyroid status. The caveat to this situation is that patients with hypothyroidism often have reduced appetite, and therefore food intake may be reduced and thereby mask reduced caloric expenditure because body weight may not change much. When present, the paradox of "weight gain despite reduced food intake" strongly suggests hypothyroidism.

- High cholesterol, dyslipidemia, cardiovascular risk: Patients with hypothyroidism commonly have elevated blood cholesterol levels (as well as triglycerides and lipoprotein-a levels), and ridiculously and unfortunately, many patients who need thyroid treatment are forced to take cholesterol-lowering "statin" drugs instead of receiving the proper treatment for hypothyroidism, which is generally thyroid hormone. We now know that the cause of the elevation of cholesterol is not due to an effect on the cholesterol producing enzyme HMG-CoA reductase, but rather the elevated cholesterol levels noted in hypothyroidism are due to reduced uptake/reception and subsequent breakdown/catabolism of LDL cholesterol in the liver, while elevated triglyceride levels are due to reduced activity of the enzyme lipoprotein lipase.[682] Hypothyroidism is also well-known to cause (reversible) hyperhomocysteinaemia. Many patients noted to have high cholesterol levels are prescribed a lifetime of cholesterol-lowering drugs; this is unfortunate because what these patients often need is thyroid hormone.

- Slow heart rate, heart abnormalities (asymmetric septal hypertrophy, similar to and often confused with idiopathic hypertrophic subaortic stenosis): The average adult heart rate of the "textbook-normal" adult is approximately 72 beats per minute (b/m); abnormally slow heart rate (bradycardia) is defined as less than 60 b/m and excessively fast heart rate is greater than 100 b/m. In certain situations, a fast or slow heart rate might be normal for the situation at hand; for example, well-trained athletes may have a "normal" heart rate in the 50s, and an individual who is anxious, severely anemic, sick with an infection, or over-caffeinated might have an elevated heart rate that does not indicate a serious/real disease. If I see a patient with a heart rate <65 b/m and the patient is not athletic and does not have a heart condition or is not taking

---

[681] Hardy KJ, Seckl JR. Endocrine assessment of impotence—pitfalls of measuring serum testosterone without sex-hormone-binding globulin. *Postgrad Med J* 1994 Nov;70:836-7
[682] "Decreased activity of LDL-receptors' resulting in decreased receptor-mediated catabolism of LDL and IDL is the main cause of the hypercholesterolemia observed in hypothyroidism." Liberopoulos EN, Elisaf MS. Dyslipidemia in patients with thyroid disorders. *Hormones* (Athens). 2002 Oct-Dec;1(4):218-23

a medication that slows the heart rate, then I become suspicious of hypothyroidism and will look for other historical, physical, or laboratory evidence of hypothyroidism. Hypothyroidism can also cause a rare heart disorder called asymmetric septal hypertrophy (ASH), which is very similar to and often confused with idiopathic hypertrophic subaortic stenosis (IHSS); treatment with thyroid hormone generally cures this heart problem.[683]

- High blood pressure, diastolic hypertension: Hypothyroidism is a well-known cause of high blood pressure, specifically a type of high blood pressure called diastolic hypertension; treatment with thyroid hormone generally cures this problem.
- Slow healing: Reduced overall metabolic rate and impaired protein digestion and utilization—both of which are noted in patients with hypothyroidism—leads to impaired healing of wounds and injuries.
- Decreased memory and concentration: Reduced overall metabolic rate and impaired protein digestion and utilization—both of which are noted in patients with hypothyroidism—leads to impaired memory and cognition. Protein is the source of amino acids, which are used by the body to make neurotransmitters such as serotonin, dopamine, and norepinephrine. Low thyroid state also impairs the function of the nervous system, specifically the adrenergic aspect of the nervous system which uses dopamine and norepinephrine to promote attention, mood, and pleasure.
- Muscle weakness: In more severe cases, hypothyroidism can cause a muscle disease (hypothyroid myopathy); this can lead to muscle weakness.
- Sleep apnea: Hypothyroidism contributes to sleep apnea (impaired breathing during sleep).
- Frog-like husky voice: Changes in voice is commonly noted among patients with reduced thyroid function.
- Recurrent infections: Hypothyroidism impairs immune function, resulting in more severe and more frequent infections.
- Many other manifestations: Because thyroid hormone is necessary for every body system, its lack or insufficiency thereby also affects all body systems. Thus, *many* adverse health effects and symptoms may result from an insufficiency of thyroid hormone.

Major differential diagnoses for hypothyroidism:

- Because hypothyroidism can result in so many different health problems and subjective symptoms, the list of diagnostic considerations that share similarities with hypothyroidism is virtually endless. Each of the symptoms above has its own list of possible different diagnostic considerations. However, despite the confusion and similarity shared with other diseases, careful study of hypothyroidism from my experience with patients and with the fruits of reflection have revealed a pattern of symptoms in hypothyroidism that is indeed unique:
   - ❶ The symptom cluster of "fatigue, depression, cold hands and feet, dry skin, constipation..."
   - ❷ Weight gain despite reduced appetite and reduced food intake
   - ❸ Persistently low body temperature—described in adjacent text box
   - ❹ Slow or relatively slow heart rate—what I call "relative bradycardia"
   - ❺ Delayed Achilles reflex return (discussed below).

> **How to measure first-morning axillary temperature**
> 1. Shake down mercury thermometer before going to bed; leave thermometer near bedside (but obviously not in the bed where it could be warmed or broken),
> 2. Immediately upon wakening, before any other activity, place thermometer deep in axilla (armpit) and measure temperature for 7-10 minutes,
> 3. Normal is 97.8-98.2°F; less than this temperature warrants consideration of hypothyroidism.

Clinical assessment:

- **History/subjective**: Historical findings and clinical presentations are listed above. The symptom cluster of "fatigue, depression, cold hands and feet, dry skin, constipation" is classic and may be present in whole (rare) or in part (common).
- **Physical examination/objective**: The most relevant clinical findings are discussed here:
   - Low body temperature: Very few conditions result in persistently low body temperature; clearly the most common and important of these conditions is hypothyroidism. Patients who are persistently uncomfortable

---

[683] "In 10 patients who returned to euthyroid state with L-thyroxine therapy, these abnormalities resolved. We conclude that long-standing hypothyroidism leads to a reversible cardiomyopathy, manifested by asymmetric septal hypertrophy with or without other echocardiographic features of a hypertrophic obstructive cardiomyopathy." Santos et al. Echocardiographic characterization of the reversible cardiomyopathy of hypothyroidism. *Am J Med.* 1980 May;68(5):675-82

with cold hands and feet and persistent cold intolerance are worthy of assessment and treatment. Objectively, the physician will note that upon the welcoming handshake, the patient's hands feel cold; this assessment will be invalidated if the patient recently washed hands in hot or cold water, is wearing gloves, or if the physician also has hypothyroidism and is therefore equally cold. A persistently low first-morning *oral* temperature below 98.6° F warrants consideration for hypothyroidism. A persistently low first-morning *axillary* (underarm) temperature below 97.8-98.2° F warrants consideration of hypothyroidism.

- o Delayed Achillies reflex return: The deep tendon reflexes assessed by doctors during most clinical encounters contain two components: the contraction phase and the relaxation phase. Most of the time, we as doctors are primarily concerned with the contraction phase, which tells us about the integrity of the neuromuscular system. However, when we are looking for hypothyroidism, we are more concerned with the relaxation phase of the reflex; patients with hypothyroidism have reduced speed of muscular relaxation, and therefore the relaxation phase of the reflex cycle is prolonged. This finding is highly specific for hypothyroidism; some earlier medical diagnosis textbooks stated that a delayed Achilles reflex return "indicates" hypothyroidism, which is to say it is practically a diagnostic finding.
- o Slow heart rate—bradycardia: A heart rate less than 65 b/m suggests the possibility of hypothyroidism unless the patient is a well-conditioned athlete, has heart conduction problems, or is taking a medication such as a beta-blocking drug which will slow the rate of heart contractions.

- **Imaging & laboratory assessments**:
  - o Imaging: Imaging is not routinely relevant in the assessment and monitoring of hypothyroidism. Ultrasound scans and radionucleotide scans can be used to assess for more serious thyroid diseases, such as thyroid cancer.
  - o Laboratory evaluation: Laboratory evaluation of the patient with clinical manifestations of low thyroid function should be tertiary in importance to 1) the physician's assessment, judgment, and experience and 2) the patient's need for effective treatment for his/her complaints. As is stated with regard to the treatment of hypertension: *the physician's judgment remains paramount*.
    - Thyrotropin-releasing hormone—TRH: TRH is not routinely tested in clinical practice, although abnormalities of TRH secretion are noted in patients with mental "depression."
    - Thyroid-stimulating hormone—TSH (reference range 0.4 - 5.0 mIU/L [milli-international units per liter]): TSH is the most commonly performed test for evaluating thyroid status; its frequent (over)use owes more to habit and inexpensiveness than to aspirations for clinical excellence. TSH values greater than 2 mIU/L represent a disturbance of the thyroid-pituitary axis and an increased risk for future thyroid problems[684], and the American Association of Clinical Endocrinologists stated initially in 2006 (and again in 2011), "The target TSH level should be between 0.3 and 3.0 μIU/mL."[685] Clinical rationale is available to support implementation of a therapeutic trial of thyroid hormone treatment in patients who are *clinically hypothyroid* even if they are *biochemically euthyroid* (per TSH) provided that treatment is implemented cautiously, in appropriately selected patients, and patients are appropriately informed.[686,687] If the clinical world were as perfect as it is portrayed in basic physiology textbooks, then a clinician might fancifully rely on TSH to perform the diagnosis *prima facie*, with reduced TSH values correlating with

> **Optimal thyroid status**
>
> Concept by Dr Vasquez: Optimal thyroid status is not defined by basic laboratory testing with TSH and free T4. It is defined *per patient* based on the levels and ratios of all major thyroid-related hormones and antibodies—in association with other hormonal, psychologic, dysbiotic, nutritional and environmental factors—that work best for that *biochemically unique* patient.
>
> Laboratory interpretation by Dr McDaniel: "Optimal hormone balance is debatable. My observations: A few "well" people and patients treated successfully with T4 and T3 seem best with:
> - TSH around 0.7–0.9 μIU/mL
> - fT4 around 0.7–0.8 ng/dL
> - fT3 optimally 3.4–3.8 pg/mL
> - Total T3-RT3 ratio 12 +/-2"
>
> McDaniel AB. Thyroid Assessment: Controversies and Conundrums. Institute for Functional Medicine Fourteenth International Symposium. Tucson, Arizona. May 23-26, 2007

---

[684] Weetman AP. Fortnightly review: Hypothyroidism: screening and subclinical disease. *BMJ: British Medical Journal* 1997;314: 1175
[685] American Association of Clinical Endocrinologists. "The target TSH level should be between 0.3 and 3.0 μIU/mL." AACE Medical Guidelines for Clinical Practice for Evaluation and Treatment of Hyperthyroidism and Hypothyroidism. 2002, 2006 Amended Version. https://aace.com/sites/default/files/hypo_hyper.pdf Accessed Aug 2011
[686] Skinner GR, et al. Thyroxine should be tried in clinically hypothyroid but biochemically euthyroid patients. *BMJ: British Medical Journal* 1997 Jun 14; 314(7096): 1764
[687] McLaren EH, Kelly CJ, Pollack MA. Trial of thyroxine treatment for biochemically euthyroid patients has been approved. *BMJ* 1997; 315: 1463

glandular overperformance and negative feedback suppressing TSH secretion, whilst an underperforming gland would require greater stimulation with elevated TSH levels; however, TSH has never been thus vested with infallible reliability, which explains in part why doctors need brains of their own and why better clinicians have developed the capacity for independent thought.

- **Free thyroxine—free T4** (reference range 4.5 - 11.2 mcg/dL): Unbound T4 is tested to provide evidence of glandular production of thyroid hormone(s). Because T4 is the major thyroid hormone produced by the thyroid gland, it serves as an excellent marker for glandular productivity but it reveals nothing about peripheral conversion of T4 to the active thyroid hormone triiodothyronine (T3); in the practice of medicine, conversion of T4 to the active T3 is assumed to reliably occur unabated despite evidence to the contrary, especially among symptomatic and ill patients, the exact patients to whom we are providing care.

- **Triiodothyronine—free T3 or total T3, the active form of thyroid hormone** (reference range: 100 - 200 ng/dL[688]): Yes, contrary to what I was taught in medical school, I actually perform and advocate testing for the active form of the thyroid hormone when assessing patients for low thyroid function; some (non)experts/thinkers might consider this heretical or a waste of money, but I consider it to be a manifestation of common sense in the interest of providing efficient and cost-effective care. In textbook-perfect physiology, T4 is converted by the selenium-dependent deiodinase enzymes to the active thyroid hormone T3; in reality, this is only part of the story. Because T3 is the active form of the hormone responsible for the physiologic functions of thyroid physiology, a clinician desiring to assess a patient's thyroid status might reasonably ask the proper question by performing the proper test. T3 is tested as "total T3" or "free T3" in large part based on the clinician's preference; the current author prefers total T3 because it can be compared to the total level of reverse T3 (rT3) in a ratio, the optimal range of which is generally considered to be 10-14 as originally presented by McDaniel[689] and reviewed in the following pages. Patients with psychiatric depression have lower levels of T3 than do healthy controls and have been described as having "low T3 syndrome"[690]; very obviously, the low T3 levels in these patients would serve to promote and perpetuate their state of mental depression. Clinicians should be aware that T3, like estrogens, increases hepatic production of sex hormone binding globulin (SHBG) and that therefore T3 (and estrogen) administration can reduce cellular bioavailability of protein-bound hormones such as testosterone. Many authoritative and clinically-experienced sources recommend using a time-released (e.g., sustained-release) form of T3 due to its shorter half-life compared with T4. However, obtaining time-released T3 via a compounding pharmacy can be cumbersome and expensive for the patient; clearly many patients respond to once daily dosing of *non-time-released T3 preparations—Cytomel or its generic equivalent—with good effects and without adverse effects*. Some patients can divide the immediate-release dose into two servings per day for enhanced effect and lessened physiologic fluctuations, if necessary. Per Drugs.com[691] in August 2011, "Since liothyronine sodium (T3) is not firmly bound to serum protein, it is readily available to body tissues. The onset of activity of liothyronine sodium is rapid, occurring within a few hours. Maximum pharmacologic response occurs within 2 or 3 days, providing early clinical response. The biological half-life is about 2.5 days." Very clearly, a significant portion of hypothyroid patients respond to T3 alone (either time-released, divided-dosing, or once-daily dosing) or a combination of T4 and T3 when other treatments have failed.[692,693]

- **Reverse triiodothyronine—rT3** (reference range: 90 - 320 pg/mL[694]): In addition to its conversion into the active T3 hormone, T4 can also be converted by deiodinase enzymes into the inactive thyroid hormone rT3; per a standard endocrinology textbook, "Approximately 70–80% of released T4 is converted by deiodinases to the biologically active T3, the remainder to reverse-T3 (rT3) which has no

---

[688] U.S. National Library of Medicine (NLM) and National Institutes of Health (NIH) nlm.nih.gov/medlineplus/ency/article/003687.htm Accessed August 2011
[689] McDaniel AB. Thyroid Assessment: Controversies and Conundrums. Institute for Functional Medicine Fourteenth International Symposium. Tucson, Az. May 23-26, 2007
[690] "Out of 250 subjects with major psychiatric depression, 6.4% exhibited low T3 syndrome (mean serum T3 concentration 0.94 nmol/l vs normal mean serum concentration of 1.77 nmol/l)." Premachandra BN, Kabir MA, Williams IK. Low T3 syndrome in psychiatric depression. *J Endocrinol Invest*. 2006 Jun;29(6):568-72
[691] drugs.com/pro/cytomel.html August 2011.
[692] Bunevicius R, et al. Effects of thyroxine as compared with thyroxine plus triiodothyronine in patients with hypothyroidism. *N Engl J Med*. 1999 Feb 11;340(6):424-9
[693] Kelly T, Lieberman DZ. The use of triiodothyronine as an augmentation agent in treatment-resistant bipolar II and bipolar disorder NOS. *J Affect Disord*. 2009;116(3):222-6
[694] The reference range provided here for rT3 is a compilation from the laboratory reference ranges from the sample reports on the following pages, each of which is performed by either Quest Diagnostics or LabCorp, the two largest medical laboratories in the United States.

significant biological activity."[695] Clinicians must know that, "The prohormone T4 must be converted to T3 in the body before it can exert biological effects. **During periods of illness or stress, this conversion is often inhibited and can be diverted to the inactive reverse T3 (rT3) moiety.**"[696] Furthermore and very importantly, clinicians should appreciate that rT3 is not simply inactive but that it may actually impair production/utilization of normal T3; "T4-T3 and T4-rT3 conversion are provoked by different enzymes. The elevation of rT3 might be a cause of the observed decrease in peripheral T3 generation in old [elderly] subjects, acting by an inhibition of the T4-T3 conversion."[697] During times of psychologic/physiologic stress and specific types of pharmacologic stress (e.g., propanolol[698] and corticosteroids), T4 metabolism is preferentially shunted away from T3 toward rT3; an anthropocentric explanation holds that by making less of the active T3 and more of the inactive rT3, the body is better able to conserve energy during times of stress by reducing overall metabolic rate, particularly resting energy expenditure and protein utilization. For example, caloric restriction and fasting result in a decrease in resting metabolic rate (RMR), and the reduced RMR persists for months after the fasting has ended and a normal diet is resumed.[699] This author (AV) terms this stress-induced impairment of thyroid hormone conversion "**metabolic hypothyroidism**" or "**functional hypothyroidism**" because the defect is in the metabolism (not the production) of thyroid hormone into its most active form; "**peripheral hypothyroidism**" might also be used to distinguish the fact that the defect is in the peripheral metabolism rather than located more centrally, within the thyroid gland itself. Because psychologic stress and certain pharmacologic exposures—as well as the thyro-metabolic stress of fasting and caloric restriction in which the counterregulatory hormone glucagon appears to trigger enhanced rT3 production—*reduce* active T3 while simultaneously *increasing* rT3 levels, clinicians can appreciate that calculation of the T3/rT3 ratio will be more significantly altered (and thus a more sensitive indicator of metabolic disruption) than will be the isolated measurements of T3 or rT3 alone. Functional medicine clinicians[700] note the importance of the ratio of total T3 to reverse T3 (tT3:rT3 ratio) and consider the optimal range to be 10-14 with lower ratios indicating impaired formation or T3 and/or excess production of rT3.[701] Contrary to the previous view which held that rT3 was simply inactive, we now appreciate that rT3 actually impairs normal thyroid hormone metabolism thus functioning as an thyrometabolic monkeywrench or "brake" on normal metabolism. Even if rT3 were only *inactive* and not *counteractive*, measuring its levels and the T3:rT3 ratio would still be appropriate. Elevated rT3 levels predict mortality among critically ill patients.[702] Aberrancies in thyroid hormone levels may reflect organic disease, psychoemotional stress, or nutritional deficiency[703], and therefore such serologic abnormalities warrant consideration of underlying problems and direct treatment when possible. If no underlying cause is apparent, then a trial of thyroid hormone/hormones is reasonable in appropriately selected patients. Beyond stress reduction, allergen/gluten avoidance, and nutritional supplementation with iodine, selenium, and zinc (as indicated per patient), correction of overt, subclinical, and functional hypothyroidism generally centers on the administration of natural or synthetic thyroid hormones in the form of T4 and T3. Correction of functional hypothyroidism (relatively reduced total T3 and increased rT3) is accomplished with either time-released or twice-daily dosing of T3 *without* T4 to suppress endogenous T4 conversion to T3, thereby allowing rT3 levels to fall precipitously. T3 administration allows temporary downregulation of transforming enzymes so that rT3 production is reduced following withdrawal of T3 replacement; thus, short-term and/or periodic T3 administration helps normalize or "reset" peripheral thyroid metabolism so that, following

---

[695] Nussey S, Whitehead S. *Endocrinology: An Integrated Approach*. Oxford: BIOS Scientific Publishers; 2001. See also Box 3.29 Metabolism of thyroid hormones. ncbi.nlm.nih.gov/books/NBK28/box/A270/?report=objectonly Accessed July 2011
[696] *1998 Mosby's GenRX. Sixth Edition*. St. Louis Missouri; Mosby-Year Book, Inc., 1998
[697] Szabolcs I, et al. The possible reason for serum 3,3'5'-(reverse) triiodothyronine increase in old people. *Acta Med Acad Sci Hung*. 1982;39(1-2):11-7
[698] "Propranolol administration (40 mg t.i.d. for a week) caused a similar rT3 elevation in old persons (n = 18) as in 12 young ones." Szabolcs I, et al. The possible reason for serum 3,3'5'-(reverse) triiodothyronine increase in old people. *Acta Med Acad Sci Hung*. 1982;39(1-2):11-7
[699] Elliot DL, et al. Sustained depression of the resting metabolic rate after massive weight loss. *Am J Clin Nutr* 1989 Jan;49(1):93-96
[700] The conclusion of this paragraph is derived from Vasquez A. *Musculoskeletal Pain: Expanded Clinical Strategies*. Published 2008 by The Institute for Functional Medicine.
[701] McDaniel AB. Thyroid Assessment: Controversies and Conundrums. Institute for Functional Medicine Fourteenth International Symposium. Tucson, Az. May 23-26, 2007
[702] Peeters RP, et al. Serum 3,3',5'-triiodothyronine (rT3) and 3,5,3'-triiodothyronine/rT3 are prognostic markers in critically ill patients and are associated with postmortem tissue deiodinase activities. *J Clin Endocrinol Metab*. 2005 Aug;90(8):4559-65
[703] Kelly GS. Peripheral metabolism of thyroid hormones: a review. *Altern Med Rev*. 2000 Aug;5(4):306-33

withdrawal of T3 administration, T4 can be converted to T3 without excess production of rT3. The safety and effectiveness of this approach—using T3 administration (often twice daily or in a sustained-release compounded tablet or capsule) to recalibrate peripheral thyroid hormone metabolism—has documented safety and effectiveness.[704] Alleviation of symptoms, restoration of morning body temperature to 98.6° F (oral or axillary) and other clinical objective improvements achieved by the judicious and safe administration of T3 are the criteria of success; physiologic improvement following T3 administration retrospectively confirms the diagnosis of either hypothyroidism generally or functional hypothyroidism in particular.

- Antithyroid antibodies—antithyroglobulin (anti-TG) and anti-thyroid peroxidase (anti-TPO): Autoimmune thyroiditis (also called Hashimoto's disease or chronic lymphocytic thyroiditis) or is the most common cause of overt primary hypothyroidism. The diagnosis of autoimmune thyroiditis can be made clinically (i.e., without biopsy) upon detection of elevated blood levels of antibodies against thyroglobulin (anti-thyroglobulin antibodies) and anti-thyroid peroxidase (anti-TPO) antibodies. Autoimmune thyroiditis may present asymptomatically and with normal thyroid hormone levels; classically, patients may have a slightly hyperthyroid presentation as the inflamed gland releases extra thyroid hormone before becoming atrophic and hypofunctional.

Establishing the diagnosis:
- Hypothyroidism: The diagnosis of hypothyroidism is supported by the constellation of ❶ the patient's history and subjective complaints, ❷ physical examination findings, ❸ laboratory findings, and ❹ response to a clinical trial of thyroid hormone, preferably T3 alone or the combination of T4 and T3 which are consistent with the physiologic production of thyroid hormones from the thyroid gland. Treatment with T4 alone cannot be considered optimal therapy, if for no other reason than *the supremely important reason* that the brain cannot adequately convert T4 to T3; given the importance of the brain for our subjective feelings and perceptions as well as objective homeodynamic regulation, common sense argues against giving the hypothyroid brain a hormone that it cannot use.
- Autoimmune thyroiditis: The diagnosis of Hashimoto's/autoimmune thyroiditis is strongly suggested by the finding of elevated antibody levels against thyroglobulin and/or TPO.

DrV's perspective on the complexity and frequent lack of success in treating autoimmune hypothyroidism
The treatment of hypothyroidism has been a clinical conundrum for doctors for many years; it is the topic of many journal articles, debate and confusion, and well-ensconced views and opinions. Here, I will deconstruct the conundrum: • Errors in testing and treating: From my perspective, the obvious reason for this confusion is that doctors—as medical students and as post-graduate readers of textbooks and journal articles that have inaccurate information—are trying to do the right thing (help patients) with the wrong information about testing (i.e., that TSH is the best [and almost exclusive] test for evaluating thyroid function) and treating (that the inactive T4 hormone should be used). Both of these promulgations are absurdly wrong. The reason that this topic is so confusing and contentious is that doctors have been misled to use the wrong test (TSH only) and the wrong treatment (T4 only); this explains why hypothyroid patients rarely receive any helpful treatment and are even more rarely treated to fully satisfactory result. • Failure to consider, appreciate, and test for the important peripheral metabolism of thyroid hormones: Most doctors do not test for T3 levels; this erudite and unintellectual considering that if they are considering "hypothyroidism" as a diagnosis they should use testing that includes assessment of the active hormone in question. Fewer clinicians test for reverse T3, and fewer still appreciate the importance—conceptual more than mathematical—of the reciprocal T3:rT3 ratio. Given that T3 is the active hormone, doctors should test for and treat with T3—alone or in combination with T4—when working with hypothyroid patients. In my experience, proof that rT3 is *antagonistic* and not merely *inactive* is shown by the tolerance "high rT3 patients" have to treatment with high doses of T3 which should otherwise be and later are excessive, but which are tolerated during initial treatment when rT3 levels are still elevated. • Not knowing how to treat autoimmunity, naively believing that giving thyroid hormone will be sufficient to resolve the immune imbalance that is manifesting as thyroid autoimmunity: If patients have thyroid autoimmunity as the cause of their hypothyroidism, simply giving thyroid hormone appears to me to be a rather ridiculous idea because it leaves the primary disease—the autoimmunity—untreated and therefore persistent. Many integrative doctors have used nonspecific health-improvement measures such as dietary improvement, general nutritional supplementation, and avoidance of common dietary allergens/immunogens to provide better care and alleviate immune dysfunction, but these general measures pale in comparison to what can be achieved with the more contemporary and comprehensive applications of functional inflammology and nutritional immunomodulation (Chapter 4). Thus, the autoimmunity needs to be treated directly, independently from and yet in conjunction with the hypothyroidism.

---

[704] Friedman M, et al. Supraphysiological cyclic dosing of sustained release T3 in order to reset low basal body temperature. *P R Health Sci J.* 2006 Mar;25(1):23-9

Complications:
- Complications of hypothyroidism: The complications of hypothyroidism are mainly continuations of the health problems previously mentioned in the sections on clinical presentations and clinical assessments. The most common and "important" problems from a clinical/medical perspective are depression, cardiovascular/hypertensive/hypercholesterolemic/hyperhomocysteinemic risks, reproductive/sexual problems, and increased susceptibility to infection. From a more personal perspective for the patients with *undiagnosed*, *untreated* or *insufficiently treated* hypothyroidism, the impaired quality of life, the chronic tiredness and fatigue, the lack of mental clarity and chronic low-grade depression, plus the feeling that "something is wrong with me" and the lack of understanding from doctors, friends, family, and intimate partners can be very distressing.

Clinical management:
- Implementation of effective treatment: Patients with laboratory evidence of hypothyroidism and/or a compelling clinical picture of hypothyroid deserve treatment with thyroid hormone—T3 alone, or T3 and T4 in combination—if no important conditions contraindicate its use. Conditions such as mania, seizure disorder, cardiac arrhythmia, coronary artery disease, and adrenal insufficiency are the main—but not absolute—contraindications.
- Consideration of other immune disorders: Patients with autoimmune thyroiditis have higher-than-normal rates of celiac disease (gluten intolerance) and other autoimmune disorders; these should be assessed and treated per the applied functional inflammology protocol with disease-specific considerations.[705]
- Periodic monitoring: Patients should be monitored for safety with clinical assessment and laboratory tests at the initiation of treatment and at approximately 3-6 months after the initiation of treatment and then yearly thereafter.

Treatments:
- **Overall considerations**: Treatment of low thyroid function generally centers on the administration of thyroid hormone(s), although some patients are able to restore normal thyroid function with specific dietary modification (e.g., avoidance of allergens and gluten-containing grains) and nutritional supplementation (e.g., selenium). A few people are able to take thyroid hormone treatment for a few months or years, and then discontinue the medication and yet maintain normal function; these are likely cases of transient thyroiditis and/or peripheral/functional hypothyroidism that either self-resolved or resolved with supportive thyroid treatment. Many people take the hormones for life. As implied previously, my position on this is that hypothyroidism and autoimmunity are separate issues and each needs to be addressed directly and effectively for optimal outcome.
- **Thyroid hormone replacement—physiologically appropriate—with T4 and T3**: Patients with insufficient function of thyroid hormone generally need *more* thyroid hormone to overcome their *hypo*thyroidism expeditiously, which is generally delivered in the form of biologically identical synthetic thyroid hormones, T4 and/or T3. Unfortunately, most (allopathic) doctors have been trained to use T4 without T3; this is nonphysiologic and therefore neither intellectually nor scientifically nor physiologically valid. When patients are hypothyroid, they generally need T4 and T3 together because the thyroid gland makes both of these hormones, and they are both required for optimal and normal thyroid status. Studies that have used T4 alone without T3 may have found "lack of effectiveness" not because the patients did not stand to benefit from thyroid hormone(s) but because the patients were given *inactive* T4 when they needed *active* T3, or a combination of T4 with T3. The three most common types of thyroid hormone replacement are described as follows.

  > **Patients often feel better with combination T4 and T3 rather than T4 alone**
  >
  > "Twelve patients preferred combination treatment, 6 patients preferred the add-on combination treatment, 2 patients preferred standard treatment, and 6 patients had no preference."
  >
  > Escobar-Morreale HF, et al. Thyroid hormone replacement therapy in primary hypothyroidism. *Ann Intern Med*. 2005 Mar

  o Synthetic T4: L-thyroxine, Levothyroxine: L-thyroxine is synthetic T4; it is chemically the same as the hormone produced in the body. Because it is synthetic and not derived from animal tissue, it does not

---

[705] See various and upcoming books on rheumatology, most recent of which in 2014 is Vasquez A. *Naturopathic Rheumatology and Integrative Inflammology—v3.5*. ISBN-13: 978-0990620426. An update to this work is anticipated in 2015/2016 and will be noted at the website InflammationMastery.com

contain antigens that can provoke an immune response. Levothyroxine/T4 must be converted in the body to liothyronine/T3 in order to be active; therefore, T4 administration is more safe and "stable" than is the administration of T3 but it is also generally less effective, especially for neuropsychiatric symptoms of depression, anhedonia, and fatigue. The standard allopathic medical approach is to use T4 *without* T3[706,707] and the presumed—not examined—"logic" of using an inactive hormone when these patients need and benefit from the active form continues to elude ascriptions of logic.

> **Combination T4 and T3 (not T4 alone) provides a mood-elevating antidepressant effect**
>
> "Fourteen of 17 patients showed improvement. ... **This case series shows that T3 may be successfully employed as a long term treatment augmentation of major depression if over time dosage levels are increased beyond the traditional 50 mcg.**"
>
> Kelly TF, Lieberman DZ. Long term augmentation with T3 in refractory major depression. *J Affect Disord*. 2009 May

- Available dose forms (amount per tablet): 25, 50, 75, 88, 100, 112, 125, 137, 150, 175, 200, 300 mcg.
- Conversion equivalents of various forms of thyroid hormone: levothyroxine 100 mcg = liothyronine 25 mcg = Liotrix 1 grain = thyroid (porcine) 1 grain.
- Dose for adults: 50-200 to a max of 300 mcg PO (by mouth) qd (daily) with a starting dose of 12.5-50 mcg PO qd; doses are smaller for children. Levothyroxine appears to be slightly more effective if taken at night rather than in the morning.[708]
- Info: Give on empty stomach between meals; specifically avoid soy products within 2 hours of thyroid hormone administration because constituents of soy bind thyroid hormone in the gastrointestinal tract.
- Contraindications and cautions: Allergy to the preparation, recent heart attack, adrenal insufficiency; caution with cardiovascular disease, cardiac arrhythmia, diabetes mellitus, and elderly patients.
- Drug/botanical/nutrient interactions: L-carnitine 1-4 grams/d can clearly block the hyperthyroid state via blocking thyroid hormone entry into the nucleus[709]; this treatment is effective for Graves disease, iatrogenic hyperthyroidism (thyroid hormone overdose), and thyroid storm. The botanical medicine lemon balm (*Melissa officinalis*) is claimed to block TSH binding to the thyroid gland receptor, but scientific data—let alone a quality clinical trial in humans—is lacking to support this contention.
- Adverse effects—generally not noted with proper dosing: Unmasking of cardiac arrhythmias, angina if cardiovascular disease and arterial stenosis is present. Excessive dosing or overdose can cause palpitations, tachycardia, nervousness, tremor, weight loss (long-term), diaphoresis/sweating, diarrhea/loose stools, abdominal cramps, anxiety.
- Safety/Monitoring: *Pregnancy*: A, *Lactation*: Safe
- Half-life: 6-7 days

o Synthetic T3—Liothyronine, Cytomel: T3 is the active form of thyroid hormone and it is therefore rapidly utilized and thus has a shorter half-life than does T4. T3 is the preferred form of thyroid hormone administration for the treatment of the previously described peripheral/metabolic hypothyroidism, treatment of which must be accomplished via suppressing endogenous T4 production to reduce the amount of rT3 being produced by stress-induced physiologic/enzymatic adaptations.[710]

- Available dose forms (amount per tablet): 5, 25, 50 mcg
- Conversion equivalents of various forms of thyroid hormone: levothyroxine 100 mcg = liothyronine 25 mcg = Liotrix 1 grain = thyroid (porcine) 1 grain.
- Dose for adults: 25-75 mcg PO qd; for severe hypothyroidism start with a low dose of 5-10 mcg PO qd.
- Info: Give on empty stomach between meals; specifically avoid soy products within 2 hours of thyroid hormone administration because constituents of soy bind thyroid hormone in the gastrointestinal tract.

---

[706] Escobar-Morreale HF, et al. Treatment of hypothyroidism with combinations of levothyroxine plus liothyronine. *J Clin Endocrinol Metab*. 2005 Aug;90(8):4946-54
[707] Joffe RT, et al. Treatment of clinical hypothyroidism with thyroxine and triiodothyronine: a literature review and metaanalysis. *Psychosomatics*. 2007 Sep-Oct;48(5):379-84
[708] "Levothyroxine taken at bedtime significantly improved thyroid hormone levels. Quality-of-life variables and plasma lipid levels showed no significant changes with bedtime vs morning intake. Clinicians should consider prescribing levothyroxine intake at bedtime." Bolk N, Visser TJ, Nijman J, Jongste IJ, Tijssen JG, Berghout A. Effects of evening vs morning levothyroxine intake: a randomized double-blind crossover trial. *Arch Intern Med*. 2010 Dec 13;170(22):1996-2003
[709] "In conclusion, L-carnitine is effective in both reversing and preventing symptoms of hyperthyroidism and has a beneficial effect on bone mineralization. Because hyperthyroidism depletes the body deposits of carnitine and since carnitine has no toxicity, teratogenicity, contraindications and interactions with drugs, carnitine can be of clinical use." Benvenga et al. Usefulness of L-carnitine, a naturally occurring peripheral antagonist of thyroid hormone action, in iatrogenic hyperthyroidism: a randomized, double-blind, placebo-controlled clinical trial. *J Clin Endocrinol Metab*. 2001 Aug;86(8):3579-94. "Taken together, all these experiments indicate that L-carnitine decreases the access of thyroid hormone to thyroid hormone receptors by decreasing the amount of hormone having access to cell nuclei, and not by inhibiting thyroid hormone interaction with the nuclear receptors." Benvenga et al. Effects of carnitine on thyroid hormone action. *Ann N Y Acad Sci* 2004 Nov;1033:158-67
[710] Friedman M, et al. Suprahysiological cyclic dosing of sustained release T3 in order to reset low basal body temperature. *P R Health Sci J*. 2006 Mar;25(1):23-9

- **Contraindications and cautions**: Allergy to the preparation, recent heart attack, adrenal insufficiency; caution with cardiovascular disease, cardiac arrhythmia, diabetes mellitus, and elderly patients.
- **Adverse effects—generally not noted with proper dosing**: Unmasking of cardiac arrhythmias, angina if cardiovascular disease and arterial stenosis is present. Excessive dosing or overdose can cause palpitations, tachycardia, nervousness, tremor, weight loss, diaphoresis/sweating, diarrhea, abdominal cramps, anxiety.

> **Contraindications to T3, liothyronine**
> Absolute contraindications:
> - Anaphylaxis or severe hypersensitivity,
> - Acute (current) myocardial infarction,
> - Hyperthyroidism,
> - Untreated adrenal insufficiency.
>
> Relative contraindications and cautions:
> - CAD, angina pectoris, or cardiac arrhythmia,
> - Elderly patients, severe hypothyroidism—start with low dose and titrate as tolerated.

- **Safety/Monitoring**: *Pregnancy*: A, *Lactation*: Safe
- **Half-life**: 1 day; I think this is perfect, since if the dose is not correct—let's say for example, that the dose is too high initially—the patient can skip the dose on the following day and then resume with a lower dose on the following day.
- **Noteworthy proof of safety and remarkable efficacy of T3— triiodothyronine as an augmentation agent in treatment-resistant bipolar II and bipolar disorder NOS** (*J Affect Disord* 2009 Aug[711]): "The charts of 125 patients with bipolar II disorder and 34 patients with bipolar disorder NOS were reviewed. Patients had been unsuccessfully treated with an average of 14 other medications before starting T3. At an average dose of 90.4 mcg (range 13 mcg-188 mcg) the medication was well tolerated. None of the patients experienced a switch into hypomania, and only 16 discontinued due to side effects. Improvement was experienced by 84%, and 33% experienced full remission. … Augmentation with supraphysiologic doses of T3 should be considered in cases of treatment resistant bipolar depression."

o **Synthetic T4 with synthetic T3—Liotrix, Thyrolar**: This is a convenient yet more expensive way to obtain synthetic T4 along with synthetic T3 in an attempt to most closely mimic normal thyroid hormone production. It is dosed orally between meals in strengths of "1", "2", and "3". This product can be very difficult to obtain. Some but not all studies show clinical improvement in patients who use combination T4 and T3 rather than T4 alone.

o **Animal-derived glandular products with either T4 and T3, or T3 alone**: Glandular products derived from the thyroid glands of cows and pigs contain T4 and T3; these preparations of desiccated/dried thyroid gland are available by prescription such as Armour Thyroid generic desiccated thyroid. T3 derived from desiccated thyroid is also available without prescription. Patients who show greater benefit with these products than they did with synthetic T4 alone are probably responding to the T3, but the possibility exists that other nutritive factors or hormones in the whole gland are providing benefit. My preference is to avoid the use of glandular products in patients with thyroid autoimmunity due to the possible/documented exacerbation of the (auto)immune response, which can be monitored by measurement of blood levels of anti-TPO and anti-thyroglobulin antibodies. Furthermore, in these modern times, in America wherein most of the corn and soy fed to cows and pigs is genetically manipulated and overtreated with herbicides like glyphosate, my educated opinion is that the food supply in general and commercially/corporate-raised non-organic animal products are contaminated with GMO toxins (see Chapter 4), some of which are mitochondrial toxins and others of which have been shown to promote pro-inflammatory immune responses in animal experiments. Likewise, I advocate that all patients with inflammatory/autoimmune conditions consume an organic diet, as discussed in Chapter 4.

- **Nonpharmacologic and nonhormonal treatments, including nutritional and botanical supplementation**:
  o **Zinc—15-50 mg per day**: Zinc is necessary for the proper metabolism of thyroid hormones. Many patients—especially the elderly—are deficient in zinc. Zinc supplementation is quite safe and the pill(s) should be taken with food in order to avoid stomach upset. Long-term high-dose zinc supplementation can cause deficiency of copper. I always recommend use of a high-potency multivitamin-multimineral supplement

---

[711] Kelly et al. The use of triiodothyronine as an augmentation agent in treatment-resistant bipolar II and bipolar disorder NOS. *J Affect Disord.* 2009 Aug;116(3):222-6

to patients as part of the foundational treatment plan—see my review[712] which is also reprinted and updated/amended in Chapter 4.

- Selenium—200-800 mcg per day: Selenium, zinc, and iron are all necessary for the biochemical pathways necessary for the peripheral metabolism of thyroid hormones, specifically the conversion of T4 to T3; deficiency of these nutrients can induce a "metabolic hypothyroidism" or "nutritional hypothyroidism" due to impairment of thyroid hormone metabolism and utilization. Further, zinc and selenium support antioxidant defenses; whereas iron is an antioxidant a low doses and a potent pro-oxidant in when present in higher amounts. Several studies have shown that nutritional supplementation with selenium 200 micrograms (mcg) per day for adults lowers the levels of anti-thyroid antibodies within three months and to an even greater extent by the end of nine months[713]; although this simple treatment is not always effective, it is clearly benign, and higher doses of selenium 400-800 mcg/d—especially in combination with the other components of the nutritional immunomodulation protocol detailed in Chapter 4—would very clearly be expected to produce better results.

- Iron—only for patients with iron deficiency documented by the lab test serum ferritin: Iron is necessary for the proper metabolism of thyroid hormones. Iron status is assessed with a lab test called serum ferritin, and the optimal range is 40-70 ng/mL for most people; for patients with restless leg syndrome their ferritin can be up to 100 ng/mL to overcome defects in blood-brain transport. Iron deficiency in adults can be a sign of gastrointestinal blood loss such as from a stomach ulcer or colon cancer and must therefore always be evaluated appropriately.

- Food allergen avoidance, especially gluten: Among food "allergy" disorders (discussed in Chapter 4) associated with thyroid autoimmunity, allergy to the protein gluten found in grains such as wheat, rye, and barley is clearly preeminent. A specific "gluten related disorder"—celiac disease—is associated with autoimmunity in general and thyroid autoimmunity in particular. Approximately 15% of patients with celiac disease have thyroid autoimmunity (i.e., Hashimoto's thyroiditis), and this is reversible in a large percentage of patients following the adoption of a gluten-free diet; however, this simple treatment is not always effective. Furthermore, food allergic reactions in general and celiac disease in particular can cause damage to the absorptive gastrointestinal mucosa, and the resulting malabsorption can reduce uptake of thyroid hormone administration; treatment options include allergen avoidance such as a gluten-free diet (GFD) or—less optimally—use of higher doses of thyroid hormone to overcome the malabsorption.[714]

    - Positive study—Prevalence of thyroid disorders in untreated adult celiac disease patients and effect of gluten withdrawal (*Am J Gastroenterol* 2001 Mar[715]): "241 consecutive untreated patients and 212 controls were enrolled. ... In most patients who strictly followed a 1-yr gluten withdrawal (as confirmed by intestinal mucosa recovery), there was a normalization of subclinical hypothyroidism. ... The greater frequency of thyroid disease among celiac disease patients justifies a thyroid functional assessment. In distinct cases, gluten withdrawal may single-handedly reverse the abnormality."

    - Negative study—Gluten-free diet and autoimmune thyroiditis in patients with celiac disease (*Scand J Gastroenterol.* 2012 Jan[716]): "During the follow-up, the thyroid volume decreased significantly in the patients with celiac disease compared with the controls, indicating the progression of thyroid gland atrophy despite the gluten-free diet. CONCLUSIONS: Celiac patients had an increased risk of thyroid autoimmune disorders. A gluten-free diet seemed not to prevent the progression of autoimmune process during a follow-up of 1 year."

---

[712] Vasquez A. Five-Part Nutritional Wellness Protocol: The Supplemented Paleo-Mediterranean Diet. *Nutritional Perspectives* 2011 Jan InflammationMastery.com/reprints
[713] "We prospectively studied 80 women with HT, median age 37 (range 24-52) years, for 1 year. All patients received 200 microg Se in the form of l-selenomethionine orally for 6 months. ... An overall reduction of 21% (p < 0.0001) compared with the basal values was noted in Group A. ... Our study showed that in HT patients 6 months of Se treatment caused a significant decrease in serum anti-TPO levels, which was more profound in the second trimester. The extension of Se supplementation for 6 more months resulted in an additional 8% decrease, while the cessation caused a 4.8% increase, in the anti-TPO concentrations." Mazokopakis et al. Effects of 12 months treatment with L-selenomethionine on serum anti-TPO Levels in Patients with Hashimoto's thyroiditis. *Thyroid.* 2007 Jul;17(7):609-12 "L-selenomethionine substitution suppresses serum concentrations of TPOAb in patients with AIT, but suppression requires doses higher than 100 microg/day which is sufficient to maximize glutathione peroxidase activities. The suppression rate decreases with time." Turker et al. Selenium treatment in autoimmune thyroiditis: 9-month follow-up with variable doses. *J Endocrinol.* 2006 Jul;190(1):151-6 "We demonstrate that Se administration in our AIT patient's cohort does not induce significant immunological changes, either in terms of cytokine production patterns of peripheral T lymphocytes or of TPOAb levels. Our data suggest that AIT patients with moderate disease activity (in terms of TPOAb and cytokine production patterns) may not (equally) benefit as patients with high disease activity." Karanikas et al. No immunological benefit of selenium in consecutive patients with autoimmune thyroiditis. *Thyroid.* 2008 Jan;18(1):7-12
[714] "Atypical CD increases need for T4. The effect was reversed by GFD or by increasing T4 dose. Malabsorption of T4 may provide opportunity to detect CD that was overlooked until the patients were put under T4 therapy." Virili et al. Atypical celiac disease as cause of increased need for thyroxine. *J Clin Endocrinol Metab.* 2012 Mar;97:E419-22
[715] Sategna-Guidetti et al. Prevalence of thyroid disorders in untreated adult celiac disease patients and effect of gluten withdrawal. *Am J Gastroenterol.* 2001 Mar;96(3):751-7
[716] Metso et al. Gluten-free diet and autoimmune thyroiditis in patients with celiac disease. A prospective controlled study. *Scand J Gastroenterol.* 2012 Jan;47(1):43-8

- o *Coleus forskolii*: *Coleus forskolii* is a useful botanical medicine that is often stated to enhance thyroid function; but the research supporting this effect is weak at best. One recent study showed that the extract forskolin promoted weight loss and muscle gain in overweight and obese men, but these benefits were not attributed to improved thyroid function.
- o 7-keto-DHEA, also called 7-oxo-DHEA: 7-keto-DHEA is a metabolite of the hormone DHEA (dehydroepiandrosterone) which is a weak androgen (i.e. similar to but less potent than testosterone); 7-keto-DHEA metabolite does not have hormonal effects per se. One small study showed that administration of 7-keto-DHEA resulted in an increase in T3 levels.
- o Detoxification and avoidance of chemicals/xenobiotics: Xenobiotic exposure is ubiquitous due to chemical contamination of our food, air, water and surroundings, and thyroid autoimmunity and impaired thyroid function occur early following chemical exposure and bioaccumulation.[717] The common-sense solutions are 1) avoidance of exposure to the extent possible—this obviously includes mandating tighter government-corporate regulations on pollution production, and 2) promotion of optimal detoxification. Detoxification is introduced in Chapter 1 and given more detail in Chapter 4 and the accompanying video presentations.
- **Specific treatment for the autoimmunity—implementation of the functional immunology protocol, especially the nutritional immunomodulation component**: As stated above, my position is that the greatest success is achieved in the treatment of autoimmune hypothyroid thyroiditis by treating the hypothyroidism separately from the autoimmunity. My opinion is that treatment of hypothyroidism has been unnecessarily obfuscated when in reality the treatment options are few, the worst option (generally, although it might be useful for some patients)—T4—is overused, and the best options—T3 alone or combinations of T3 and T4—have been underused. Furthermore, most doctors have not until recently had an effective and comprehensive plan for reversing autoimmunity; I have provided such a plan in my Functional Inflammology Protocol (Chapter 4) and with clinical applications for specific autoimmune disorders in my updated *Rheumatology* textbooks.

Clinical Case 38yo male under extreme psychological stress with constantly cold extremities—testing performed by LabCorp (2010): Clinicians should appreciate the stunning suppression of T3 combined with the marked elevation of rT3; note that the T4 level is normal and that if this had been the only test performed then the patient's underlying and obvious functional/metabolic/peripheral hypothyroidism would have been missed.

TESTS	RESULT	FLAG	UNITS	REFERENCE INTERV
Triiodothyronine (T3)				
Triiodothyronine (T3)	57	Low	ng/dL	71-180
Reverse T3				
Reverse T3	312		pg/mL	90-350
Triiodothyronine, Free, Serum				
Triiodothyronine, Free, Serum	2.5		pg/mL	2.0-4.4

Step-by-step conversion from ng/dL to pg/mL—end result is multiply by 10 (i.e., 10x)

Original units	Convert ng to pg[718]	Convert dL to mL	Simplify the fraction
1 ng / 1 dL	1,000 pg / 1 dL	1,000 pg / 100 mL	10 pg / 1 ml
57 ng / 1 dL	57,000 pg / 1 dL	57,000 pg / 100 mL	570 pg / 1 mL

Discussion: In this case, because the T3 level is low, *prima facie* justification for administration of T3 is provided, assuming that the clinical picture is compatible and that no contraindications to treatment are present. To calculate the total T3/rT3 ratio, equilibrate the units (multiply total T3 in ng/dL x 10 to convert to pg/mL; 1 pg = 0.001 ng [1 ng = 1,000 pg]; 1 dl = 100 ml). The total T3/rT3 ratio should be >10-14 (per McDaniel, op cit), but in this patient's case 570/312 = 1.8. Remember, more T3 than rT3 is better; hence, the higher ratio is better. On-line calculators for this conversion have been developed and surely more will be available in the future. This athletic and otherwise healthy

---

[717] Schmidt MA, Bland JS. Thyroid gland as sentinel: interface between internal and external environment. *Altern Ther Health Med.* 1997 Jan;3(1):78-81 "However, there is now reasonably firm evidence that PCBs have thyroid-disrupting effects, and there is emerging evidence that also phthalates, bisphenol A, brominated flame retardants and perfluorinated chemicals may have thyroid disrupting properties." Boas et al. Thyroid effects of endocrine disrupting chemicals. *Mol Cell Endocrinol.* 2012 May 22;355(2):240-8 "Thyroid autoimmune disease, a multifactorial organ-specific autoimmune disorder, is marking a constant increase worldwide. It is thought to be caused by multiple environmental factors triggering autoimmune response in genetically susceptible individuals, though the exact mechanisms linking environmental factors to thyroid autoimmunity are not as yet well understood. Nevertheless, there is increasing evidence that mainly nutritive factors and environmental pollution by metals and chemicals (e.g. organochlorines, pesticides) are the main factors in the present-day spread of this disease." Duntas LH. Environmental factors and thyroid autoimmunity. *Ann Endocrinol* (Paris). 2011 Apr;72(2):108-13 Zoeller TR. Environmental chemicals targeting thyroid. Hormones (Athens). 2010 Jan-Mar;9(1):28-40

[718] Double-checked with unitconversion.org/weight/nanograms-to-picograms-conversion.html July 2011

220-lb (100 kg) patient responded very well to T3 (liothyronine/Cytomel) with a starting dose of 150 mcg which was eventually tapered to 25 mcg and then to 12.5 mcg; in this patient's case, the initial high dose of T3 was well-tolerated because of the initially low level of T3, the elevated rT3 which appears to block T3 function, and the patient's overall excellent cardiovascular fitness. A reasonable dosage range for liothyronine/Cytomel supplementation is 12.5-50 mcg for most patients tapered to the constellation of patient tolerance, patient preference, heart rate, basal body temperature optimization to 98.6° F, suppression of TSH and T4, resolution of symptoms and objective markers, and clinician's impression and experience.

Clinical Case A **42yo male with fatigue**—testing performed by Quest Diagnostics (2010): Review the labs and outline your treatment plan before reading the discussion below. Note that the "optimal ratio" provided by the laboratory in this example was performed using free T3 rather than total T3 and without converting to equal units; regardless of the mathematics, clinicians should think conceptually and physiologically since doing so makes appropriate treatment very obvious and intuitive.

```
FREE T3/REVERSE T3 RATIO
    FREE T3/REVERSE T3 RATIO                    0.93 L          1.05-1.91**
    FREE T3                              325                    230-420 pg/dL
    REVERSE T3                                   350 H          100-340*** pg/mL
        **Ratio= Free T3 in pg/dL : reverse T3 in pg/mL. Ratio for reference
        range is calculated by dividing the lower and upper end of free T3
        with the mean of reverse T3 (220 pg/mL).

        ***Observed reference range is reported for reverse T3 per client
        request.
```

Step-by-step conversion from pg/dL to pg/mL—end result is divide by 100 (i.e., 0.01x): Provided for the sake of completeness even though the conversion is not necessary per the laboratory interpretation provided above.

Original units	Convert dL to mL	Simplify the fraction
1 pg / 1 dL	1 pg/ 100 mL	0.01 pg/ 1 mL
325 pg/ 1 dL	325 pg / 100 mL	3.25 pg / 1 mL

Discussion: Note that if the T3 had been tested without rT3 the results would have been reported as "normal" and that a "depressed" patient so assessed would have likely been given an "antidepressant" medication and a diagnosis of depression rather than the proper treatment with T3 and a diagnosis of functional hypothyroidism. Luckily for this patient, his clinician tested rT3 and upon finding it impressively elevated treated with patient with T3 to suppress rT3 production by temporarily suppressing T4 production. The ratio calculation is provided and interpreted by the laboratory; notice that the "ideal ratio" for **total** T3/rT3 (>10) differs from that of **free** T3/rT3 (>1.05) *and that per the ratio provided by the labotatory does not equilibriate the measurement units*. This method is acceptable but is not the preferred method for determining functional thyroid status. The preferred method is the one presented by McDaniel (op cit) who advocated using total T3 (not free T3) in comparison with rT3 interpreted by an optimal ratio of 10-14.

Plaza Mayor (Main Square) of Villa de Leyva, Colombia: Several formatting changes and updates to *Rheumatology* v3.5 were made in Villa de Leyva in 2014 Sep. Panoramic photo above by DrV.

Chapter 2:
Wellness Promotion
&
(Re)Establishing the Foundation for Health

> **Introduction to Lifestyle Optimization, Wellness Promotion, and Disease Prevention**
>
> This section details the lifestyle modifications that support a wellness-promoting whole-health program.
>
> Among the four major primary healthcare professions in the United States and most other countries—chiropractic, osteopathy, naturopathy, and allopathy—the naturopathic profession stands preeminent in its emphasis upon wellness promotion and lifestyle optimization. This chapter reviews wellness promotion from the current author's perspective and experience—both personal and professional—which is consistent with but not officially representative of the naturopathic profession's concepts "re-establish the foundation of health" and "hierarchy of therapeutics."
>
> This chapter originated many years ago as a handout for patients wherein it explained and described basic concepts that are foundational to health restoration, preservation, and optimization. Over the years that this handout has evolved into a chapter for my books, it has become more detailed and more relevant for clinicians treating patients. In essence, this chapter is a blueprint for the construction of a healthy lifestyle. While it may not cover every consideration, it covers the basics in sufficient detail so as to allow patients to change tracks from the downward descent of the disease-promoting lifestyle to the upward ascent of the health-promoting lifestyle.
>
> Replacing the passive and disempowering drug-surgery paradigm with an active and empowering integrative/functional model of healthcare is one goal of this section.
>
> This section can be thought of as a collection of essays. The review and consideration of a wide range of topics—which might otherwise appear random and nontopical to a reader accustomed to a more limited scope of discussion—is necessary due to the multifaceted nature of human experience and the widely ranging influences on health and disease outcomes.

<u>Topics</u>:
- **Re-establishing the Foundation for Health**
  - **Healthcare, Health, and Wellness**
  - **Daily living**
    - Lifestyle habits
    - Motivation: background and clinical applications
    - Exceptional living: the key to exceptional results
    - Recognize and affirm individual uniqueness
    - Individuation & conscious living: alternatives to common paradigms
    - Quality and quantity of sleep: concepts and clinical applications
    - Exercise, obesity, BMI, and proinflammatory activity of adipose tissue
  - **Diet is a powerful tool for the prevention and treatment of disease**
    - Make "whole foods" the foundation of the diet
    - Increase consumption of fruits and vegetables
    - Phytochemicals: food-derived anti-inflammatory nutrients
    - Eat the right amount of protein
    - Reducing consumption of sugars: exceptions for supercompensation
    - Avoiding artificial sweeteners, colors, and other additives, reducing caffeine
    - To the extent possible, eat "organic" foods
    - Recognize the importance of avoiding food allergens
    - Supplement your healthy diet with vitamins, minerals, and fatty acids
    - General guidelines for the safe use of nutritional supplements
  - **Advanced concepts in nutrition**
    - "Biochemical Individuality" and "Orthomolecular Medicine"
    - Nutrigenomics: Nutritional genomics
    - Putting it all together: *the supplemented Paleo-Mediterranean diet*
  - **Emotional, mental, and social health**
    - Stress management and authentic living
    - Stress always has a biochemical/physiologic component
    - The body functions as a whole
    - Healing past experiences
    - Autonomization, intradependence, emotional literacy, corrective experience
  - **Environmental health**
    - Environmental exposures and the importance of detoxification
    - Avoid unnecessary chemical medications and medical procedures
    - Intestinal health, bowel function, and introduction to dysbiosis
- **Natural holistic healthcare contrasted to standard medical treatment**
- **Opposite influences of health promotion vs. disease promotion**

Introduction to Wellness Promotion: Re-Establishing the Foundation for Health

> *"The work of the naturopathic physician is to elicit healing by helping patients to create or recreate conditions for health to exist within them.*
> **Health will occur where the conditions for health exist.**
> **Disease is the product of conditions which allow for it."** *Jared Zeff, N.D.*[1]

One of the most important concepts within the philosophy and practice of naturopathic medicine is that of "re-establishing the foundation for health." This means that instead of first looking to a specific treatment or "magic bullet" to solve a health problem, we first look at the environment in which the problem arose to determine if the patient's environment has initiated or perpetuated the problem. The term *environment* as used here means much more than the patient's immediate surroundings at home and work; it includes all modifiable factors that may have an effect on the patient's health, such as lifestyle, diet, exercise, supplementation, chronic and situational stress, medications with positive and negative effects, exposure to toxicants and microbes, nutritionally-modifiable genetic factors[2], emotions, feelings, and unconscious assumptions[3], and many other considerations. Although the genes that we and our patients have inherited cannot be changed, we can very often modulate the expression of those genes (e.g., via nutrigenomics, described later) by modifying the biochemical, microbial, toxicologic, and neurohormonal milieu that bathes our cells and thus our genes; this concept was expressed in a statement by the US Centers for Disease Control and Prevention in its "Gene-Environment Interaction Fact Sheet" available on-line.[4]

"Optimal health" does not and never will come in a pill or tonic—the human body and the interactions that we each have between our genes, outlooks, environments, and lifestyles are far too complex to ever be addressed wholly and completely by a simplistic paradigm or single treatment. Even a superficial observation of the complexity of human physiology and the complexity of our environments (including noise, toxins such as benzene and mercury, chemicals such as formaldehyde from building materials, work stress and multitasking, ionizing and electromagnetic radiation exposure, microwaves, etc) shows that **our modern lifestyles subject the human body to many more "stressors" than ever before in the history of human existence.** Each of these stressors depletes our psychic and physiologic reserves, such that daily replenishment and protection are necessary.

> **Environment—lifestyle, diet, stresses, microbes, toxins—influences genetic expression and the manifestation of health or disease**
>
> "Virtually all human diseases result from the interaction of genetic susceptibility factors and modifiable environmental factors, broadly defined to include infectious, chemical, physical, nutritional, and behavioral factors. ...
>
> "Even so-called single-gene disorders actually develop from the interaction of both genetic and environmental factors. ...
>
> "We do not inherit a disease state per se. Instead, we inherit a set of a susceptibility factors to certain effects of environmental factors and therefore inherit a higher risk for certain diseases."
>
> Gene-Environment Interaction Fact Sheet by the Centers for Disease Control and Prevention, August 2000

Research in nutrition and physiology is revealing the mechanisms by which "simple" lifestyle practices and dietary interventions exert their powerful benefits. For example, whole foods such as fruits and vegetables contain over 8,000 phytochemicals with different physiologic effects[5], and simple practices such as meditation and massage can significantly alter hormone and neurotransmitter levels.[6,7] On the surface, a simple practice such as consumption of fruits and vegetables and a multivitamin/multimineral supplement may seem to be a way to provide merely "good nutrition"; however the clinical effects can include antidepressant[8] and anti-inflammatory

---

[1] Zeff JL. The process of healing: a unifying theory of naturopathic medicine. *Journal of Naturopathic Medicine* 1997; 7: 122-5
[2] Kaput J, Rodriguez LR. Nutritional genomics: the next frontier in the postgenomic era. *Physiol Genomics* 16:166–177 physiolgenomics.physiology.org/cgi/content/full/16/2/166
[3] Miller A. *The truth will set you free: overcoming emotional blindness and finding your true adult self.* New York: Basic Books; 2001
[4] Gene-Environment Interaction Fact Sheet by the US CDC, 2000 ashg.org/pdf/CDC%20Gene-Environment%20Interaction%20Fact%20Sheet.pdf Reviewed 2014 Jun
[5] "We propose that the additive and synergistic effects of phytochemicals in fruit and vegetables are responsible for their potent antioxidant and anticancer activities, and that the benefit of a diet rich in fruit and vegetables is attributed to the complex mixture of phytochemicals present in whole foods." Liu RH. Health benefits of fruit and vegetables are from additive and synergistic combinations of phytochemicals. *Am J Clin Nutr*. 2003 Sep;78(3 Suppl):517S-520S
[6] "The significant decrease of the catecholamine metabolite VMA (vanillic-mandelic acid) in meditators, that is associated with a reciprocal increase of 5-HIAA supports as a feedback necessity the "rest and fulfillment response" versus "fight and flight"." Bujatti M, Riederer P. Serotonin, noradrenaline, dopamine metabolites in transcendental meditation-technique. *J Neural Transm*. 1976;39(3):257-67
[7] "By the end of the study, the massage therapy group, as compared to the relaxation group, reported experiencing less pain, depression, anxiety and improved sleep. They also showed improved trunk and pain flexion performance, and their serotonin and dopamine levels were higher." Hernandez-Reif et al. Lower back pain is reduced and range of motion increased after massage therapy. *Int J Neurosci* 2001;106(3-4):131-45
[8] Benton D, Haller J, Fordy J. Vitamin supplementation for 1 year improves mood. *Neuropsychobiology*. 1995;32(2):98-105

benefits[9] by enhancing the efficiency of biochemical reactions[10] and by reducing excess activity of NF-kappaB[11], respectively. The power of interventional nutrition utilizing high-doses and/or synergistic formulations of nutraceuticals and phytonutraceuticals becomes much more clinically apparent when patients first (re)establish a healthy foundation of diet and lifestyle practices upon which these treatments can be added; **I estimate that the effectiveness of treatments for complex illness such as inflammatory diseases and cancer is *at least* doubled when patients implement these lifestyle changes in addition to specific treatments rather than relying on specific treatments alone without a healthy supportive lifestyle.** In other words, "*foundation for health* + specific treatments" is much more effective than "***un****healthy lifestyle* + specific treatments." This explains, in part, the discrepancy between the relatively lackluster response seen in *single-intervention* clinical trials* compared to the better results that we attain clinically when using a holistic approach characterized by *multicomponent* treatment plans. The biochemical and "scientific" reasons for this positive/negative synergism will become more clear during the course of this chapter and textbook.

    Single-intervention clinical trials (i.e., clinical trials that utilize only one treatment) are the "gold standard" in allopathic drug-based research because in that setting the goal is to quantify and qualify the nature of positive and negative responses to a single intervention, generally a drug. However, this approach loses much of its luster and relevance in clinical settings where neither patients nor their environments and treatment plans can be standardized due to the unique constitution, lifestyle, history, and other nuances of each patient. Single intervention clinical trials have a place in the researching of all treatments, including natural interventions. However, clinicians—especially recent graduates—must pry themselves away from this research tool when it comes to treating individual patients in clinical practice, where **single interventions are the antithesis of holistic treatment**.

Daily Living: Life occurs on a moment-to-moment and daily basis. Choices that we make in relationships, occupations, exercise, and diet have profound and powerful influence over the course of our lives—particularly our health and happiness. Despite the previous and current obfuscation of health information by allopathic groups[12,13,14,15,16] and the pharmaceutical industry[17,18], enough valid information and common sense is available to doctors and the public such that **ignorance is no longer a viable excuse for deferring responsibility for lifestyle-induced disease and misery**.[19] Eating too much sugar and fat while not eating enough fruits and vegetables is making a choice to have an increased probability of developing diabetes, cancer, heart disease, arthritis, and obesity. Exercising regularly, eating a healthy diet, and supplementing the diet with high-quality nutrients and botanicals is making the choice to greatly reduce one's risk of health problems[20,21] and to nurture one's life and one's body so that one can make the most of one's life experience and enjoy life, hobbies, life purpose(s), travel, creativity, community involvement, and time with friends and family.

    When we were children, we looked to other people to provide for us and to "take care of us." **As adults, we have to assume responsibility for the course of our own lives, to make decisions based on long-term considerations rather than instant gratification and selective ignorance.** Of course, this does not mean that we have to abandon enjoyment; but it does mean that we can make decisions based on priorities, and if health is a priority then we should take steps to attain and maintain it. For people who have chosen to make their health a priority, sugar- and fat-laden food begins to lose its appeal, and exploring new health-building experiences such as

---

[9] Church TS, Earnest CP, Wood KA, Kampert JB. Reduction of C-reactive protein levels through use of a multivitamin. *Am J Med*. 2003;115(9):702-7
[10] Ames BN, Elson-Schwab I, Silver EA. High-dose vitamin therapy stimulates variant enzymes with decreased coenzyme binding affinity (increased K(m)): relevance to genetic disease and polymorphisms. *Am J Clin Nutr*. 2002 Apr;75(4):616-58 ajcn.org/cgi/content/full/75/4/616
[11] Vasquez A. Reducing pain and inflammation naturally - part 4: nutritional and botanical inhibition of NF-kappaB, the major intracellular amplifier of the inflammatory cascade. A practical clinical strategy exemplifying anti-inflammatory nutrigenomics. *Nutritional Perspectives*, July 2005:5-12
[12] Wolinsky H, Brune T. *The Serpent on the Staff: The Unhealthy Politics of the American Medical Association*. GP Putnam and Sons, New York, 1994
[13] Wilk CA. *Medicine, Monopolies, and Malice: How the Medical Establishment Tried to Destroy Chiropractic*. Garden City Park: Avery, 1996
[14] Carter JP. *Racketeering in Medicine: The Suppression of Alternatives*. Norfolk: Hampton Roads Pub; 1993
[15] National Alliance of Professional Psychology Providers. AMA Seeks To Control and Restrict Psychologist's Scope of Practice. nappp.org/scope.pdf 2006 Nov
[16] "In an effort to marshal the medical community's resources against the growing threat of expanding scope of practice for allied health professionals, the AMA has formed a national partnership to confront such initiatives nationwide... The committee will use $25,000..." Daly R, American Psychiatric Association. AMA Forms Coalition to Thwart Non-M.D. Practice Expansion. *Psychiatric News* 2006 March; 41: 17 pn.psychiatryonline.org/cgi/content/full/41/5/17-a?eaf Accessed November 25, 2006
[17] Angell M. *The Truth About the Drug Companies: How They Deceive Us and What to Do About It*. Random House; August 2004
[18] "It begins on the first day of medical school... It starts slowly and insidiously, like an addiction, and can end up influencing the very nature of medical decision-making and practice... Attempts to influence the judgment of doctors by commercial interests serving the medical industrial complex are nothing if not thorough." Editorial. Drug-company influence on medical education in USA. *Lancet*. 2000 Sep 2;356(9232):781
[19] "Error is not blindness, error is cowardice. Every acquisition, every step forward in knowledge is the result of courage, of severity towards oneself, of cleanliness with respect to oneself." Nietzsche FW. *Ecce Homo: How One Becomes What One Is*. [Translator: Hollingdale RJ] Penguin Books:1979,34
[20] Orme-Johnson DW, Herron RE. An innovative approach to reducing medical care utilization and expenditures. *Am J Manag Care*. 1997;3(1):135-44
[21] Vasquez A. Five-Part Nutritional Protocol that Produces Consistently Positive Results. *Nutr Wellness* 2005Sep

healthy cooking, outdoor activities, and community involvement can become an empowering lifestyle that can be transformed into an art—one that is particularly amenable to building relationships and connections with other people. **The improved sense of well-being and improved physical and intellectual performance obtained from consumption of a health-promoting Paleo-Mediterranean diet (described later) supersedes any short-term gratification from the disease-promoting diet commonly referred to as the Standard American Diet (SAD).** When people want to be healthy,

> **Health living: lifestyle as living art**
> "What one should learn from artists: How can we make things beautiful, attractive, and desirable for us when they are not?—and I rather think that in themselves they never are! ... This we should learn from artists, while being wiser than they are in other matters. For with them this subtle power usually comes to an end where art ends and life begins; but we want to be the poets of our lives—first of all in the smallest, most everyday matters."
>
> Nietzsche FW. *Joyful Knowledge*, 1882. Essay #299

exercising and spending enjoyable time outdoors becomes more fun than the inactivity and passivity of watching television. When we consider that the average American watches at least 3-4 hours of television per day then we should not be surprised that, with physical inactivity as such a major component of the day, Americans show progressively higher rates of obesity, cancer, heart disease, and diabetes. Such an inactive lifestyle also affects our children: on average, each American child watches more than 23 hours of television per week[22]—a national habit that unquestionably contributes to the high levels of obesity and (social) illiteracy demonstrated by America's youth. Adults who watch average amounts of television are exposed to—some might say "…indoctrinated by…") more than 30 hours of drug advertisements per year—far exceeding their exposure to other, potentially more authentic, health-promoting health information.[23] Not only does television siphon time and energy that could be used more productively, more socially, or more enjoyably, but at a cost of $50-100 per month ($600 to $1,200 per year) **cable television subtracts from the available resources (i.e., time, money, and attention) that could be directed toward health-promoting choices.** Cable television—because of its financial cost and time commitment—is only one of many examples of how everyday lifestyle choices can have an impact on long-term health/disease outcomes. **Clinicians should encourage patients to become mindful of their choices and the impact these choices have on long-term health and vitality.**

<u>Lifestyle habits</u>: Without the conscious decision that **health is a priority** and the realization that **optimal health has to be earned rather than taken for granted**, patients and doctors alike can fall into the belief that healthcare and health maintenance are *burdens* and *inconveniences* rather than opportunities for fulfillment and self-care. Taking an **empowered** and **pro-active** role in one's healthcare may include a coordinated program of diet changes (i.e., eating certain foods, avoiding other foods, modulating total intake), regular exercise, nutritional supplementation, stress reduction, and relationship improvement. Unhealthy habits such as eating junk foods, using tobacco, and watching too much television rob people of the time, energy, motivation, and financial resources that could otherwise be used to improve health and prevent unnecessary illness. As described later in this chapter, the choices that are made on a daily basis from this point forward are the most powerful predictors of future health and are generally more powerful than past habits or genetic inheritance. We can all greatly increase our probability of enjoying a future of high-energy health rather than painful illness by consistently choosing health-promoting options instead of foods, behaviors, and emotional states that promote illness.

---

[22] "American children view over 23 hours of television per week. * Teenagers view an average of 21 to 22 hours of television per week. * By the time today's children reach age 70, they will have spent 7 to 10 years of their lives watching television." American Academy of Pediatrics aapca1.org/aapca1/tv.html accessed September 30, 2003

[23] "...many ads may be targeted specifically at women and older viewers. Our findings suggest that Americans who watch average amounts of television may be exposed to more than 30 hours of direct-to-consumer drug advertisements each year, far surpassing their exposure to other forms of health communication." Brownfield et al. Direct-to-consumer drug advertisements on network television: an exploration of quantity, frequency, and placement. *J Health Commun*. 2004 Nov-Dec;9(6):491-7

One hour of time per day and/or about $2 - $8 per day:

Active self-care lifestyle	*Distraction & inactive lifestyle*
1. Meditation 2. Yoga, stretching 3. Walking, jogging, biking, no-cost calisthenics 4. Martial arts, Tai Chi 5. Hot bath 6. Cooking new healthy meals 7. Herbal teas (especially green tea) provide anti-inflammatory, anticancer, and antioxidant benefits 8. Basic nutritional supplementation (less than $2 per day): 1) High-potency multivitamin and multimineral supplement, 2) Complete balanced, fatty acid supplementation, 3) 2,000 – 4,000 IU vitamin D per day for adults, 4) probiotics and/or symbiotic. **Benefits** 1. Increased flexibility and joint mobility 2. Reduction in blood pressure 3. Reduced risk of cancer 4. Increased strength 5. Improved cognitive function 6. New and enjoyable meals 7. Relaxation 8. New life skills 9. Improved heart health 10. The opportunity to develop social skills and more friends and a better social support network 11. Reduced risk for Alzheimer's and Parkinson's diseases **Cost:** At $2 per day for meditation, stretching, calisthenics, (etc.) and basic supplementation, the total comes to $730 per year.	1. Cable television 2. 1 pack of cigarettes per day 3. Designer coffee such as Grande Café Latte **Results** 1. Cable television: Cost $2 - $4 per day = average $1,095 per year) 2. 1 pack of cigarettes per day ($3 per day = $1,095 per year) 3. Grande Café Latte ($4 per day = average $1,460 per year) **Cost:** For cable television, cafe coffee, and cigarettes, the total comes to approximately $3,600 per year.

Motivation: We all have a combination of reasons, feelings, inclinations, and unconscious influences that support and perpetuate our health behaviors.[24,25,26] Getting in touch with those motivations can help us to better understand the healthy/functional (health-promoting) and unhealthy/dysfunctional (illness-promoting) aspects of our psyches. Uncovering and "upgrading" these motivations can help us and our patients to develop more authentic lives and improved health. Self-defeating behaviors, such as 1) a willingness to remain ignorant of factors which influence health, 2) a willingness to frequently consume disease-promoting processed convenience foods, and 3) submission to confinement within the boundaries of one's insurance coverage (which often confines one to drugs and surgery as the only treatment options), reflect—*at best*—the willingness to settle for mediocrity and—*at worst*—an unconscious movement in the direction of illness and early death—masochism and suicide by lifestyle. Conversely, an unencumbered drive toward health will create the greatest opportunity for wellness. Since **actions originate from beliefs and goals**, we can surmise much about undisclosed beliefs and goals in others and ourselves simply by observing outward behavior. Effectively changing actions (such as diet and lifestyle choices) therefore must include not only behavior modification but also careful examination and reconsideration of largely unconscious goals and beliefs that motivate and underlie those behaviors. **When a fully empowered motivation toward health is matched with accurate informational insight, we have the *potential* for health-promoting change—*potential* which only becomes *manifest* after the habitual application of appropriate *action*.** Patients and doctors alike can benefit from considering the factors that incline them *toward* or *away* from behaviors that promote health or disease.

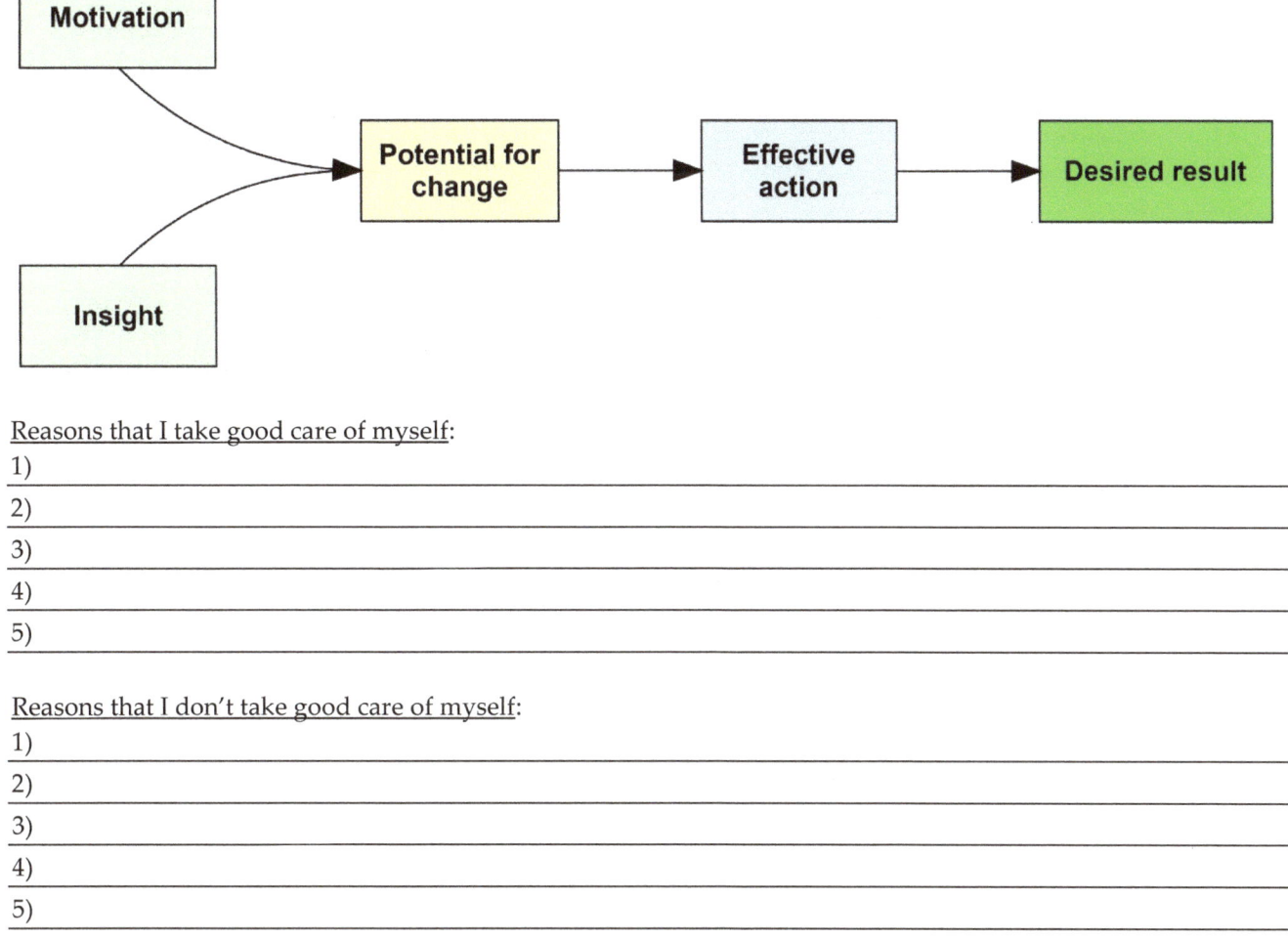

Reasons that I take good care of myself:
1) _____
2) _____
3) _____
4) _____
5) _____

Reasons that I don't take good care of myself:
1) _____
2) _____
3) _____
4) _____
5) _____

---

[24] Bradshaw J. *Healing the Shame that Binds You* [Audio Cassette (April 1990) Health Communications Audio; ISBN: 1558740430]
[25] Miller A. *The Drama of the Gifted Child: The Search for the True Self*. Basic Books: 1981. The book is brilliant, brave, and classic; the audiocassette version is also wonderful.
[26] Prochaska, JO, Norcross, JC, and DiClemente, CC (1994). *Changing for Good*. NY, William Morrow and Company; 1994

Motivation: moving from theory to practice: Many recently-graduated doctors start with the erroneous assumption that all patients actually want to become healthier, and furthermore, that all that the doctor has to do is "enlighten" them to the error of their ways and the patient will be dutifully compliant unto the attainment of his or her health-related goals. In reality, many people are surprisingly indifferent about their health. Many people do not care if they are 30 lbs overweight or have hypertension or will die early as a result of their lifestyle; they often have to be encouraged to begin to *consider* making positive changes.

> **Action determines outcome**
> "Knowing is not enough; we must apply. Willing is not enough; we must do."
> Johann Wolfgang von Goethe, German writer, scientist (1749-1832)

Dr. James Prochaska[27] has elucidated the different stages of patient preparedness, and we note that each of these five levels of thought and action produces specific results and requires different types of support from the doctor. I have summarized and modified Dr. Prochaska's lecture in the following table; for additional discussion and details, see his book *Changing for Good*.[28]

Level of preparedness and readiness for change

Stage: representative statement	Doctor's interventions and social support
1. **Pre-contemplation**: "I am not seriously thinking about making a change to be healthier."	- Outreach - Retainment
2. **Contemplation**: "I am thinking about making a change, but I am not ready for action."	- Resolve resistance - Emphasize benefits - Address ambivalence
3. **Preparation**: "I am getting ready to make a change, but I am not taking effective action yet."	- Ensure adequate preparation - Prevent relapse following initial action
4. **Action**: "I am beginning to make changes to become healthier."	- Support (group support is best) - Encouragement - Reward system
5. **Maintenance**: "I take action every day and on a consistent basis to reach my goals."	- Continued provision for continuation of health changes: facilities, supplements, social support, affirmation

Recognizing the different levels of patient preparedness and addressing individual patients with a customized approach not only for their *disease* but also for their *level of preparedness* for action can help doctors deliver more effective healthcare. Also, patients may have different levels of preparedness for different aspects of their treatment plans. He/she may be ready for *action* with regard to exercise, in *preparation* for dietary change, but in *precontemplation* for the use of supplements and botanicals.

> **Unencumbered commitment to health**
> "It was during the years of my lowest vitality that I ceased to be a pessimist. The instinct of **self-restoration** forbade me a philosophy of poverty and discouragement. This in fact is how that long period of sickness appears go me now. I soon discovered life anew, including myself. **I turned my will to health**, to life, into a philosophy….into the will to power."
> Nietzsche FW. *Ecce Homo: How One Becomes What One Is*, 1888. See also the BBC documentary on Nietzsche in the 3-part series *Human, All Too Human* (1999, free online).

---

[27] Prochaska JO. *Changing for good: motivating diabetic patients*. The Coming Storm: Reversing the Rising Pandemic of Diabetes and Metabolic Syndrome. The Eleventh International Symposium on Functional Medicine. May 13-15, 2004 in Vancouver, British Columbia, Canada. Pages 173-180. Institute for Functional Medicine
[28] Prochaska, JO, Norcross, JC, and DiClemente, CC (1994). *Changing for Good*. NY, William Morrow and Company; 1994

The secret to being exceptionally healthy: *One has to live in an exceptional (unique, personalized) way*. We cannot expect to achieve the goal of being vibrantly healthy or exceptionally happy if we live in the same way as everyone else, particularly when our fellow citizens are likely to be overweight, depressed, socially isolated[29], requiring multiple pharmaceutical medications[30], and experiencing a state of progressively declining health.[31] *Healthy lifestyle* not only includes the basics of adequate sleep, healthy whole-foods diet, supportive relationships, and regular exercise, but it also includes preventive medicine and pro-active healthcare. Despite the fact that we in the United States (US) spend more on medical treatments than does any other country in the world, Americans have the worst health outcomes of all the major industrialized countries.[32,33,34] This is largely because *American medicine* is centered on a *disease-oriented model of medicine* which means that instead of having a healthcare system and social structure that proactively promotes health and prevents disease before it happens, our systems are *reactive*—treating disease *after* it occurs rather than emphasizing the prevention of disease *before* it occurs. The dominant allopathic model in the US is also reductionistic: focusing on the small problem (micromanagement) rather than the big picture (macromanagement).

Clearly, the most effective method for avoiding expensive and potentially dangerous medical procedures and drug treatments is for us as a nation and as individuals to shift our thinking from a *disease treatment* model of healthcare to a more logical program of aggressive *disease prevention* and *wellness promotion* via the use of safe natural treatments rather than heroic interventions.[35,36] Of course, this means that our concept and view of health and healthcare will have to change. As noted by Shi[37], "Redesigning the system of health care delivery in the United States may be the only viable option to improve the quality of health care." In the meantime, while we work for change on a national level, we are wise to change our personal habits and healthcare choices in favor of natural and preventive healthcare.

Americans have poor health outcomes compared to citizens of other industrialized nations
"Basically, you die earlier and spend more time disabled if you're an American rather than a member of most other advanced countries." Christopher Murray MD PhD, Director of World Health Organization's Global Program on Evidence for Health Policy. Jun 4, 2000 who.int/inf-pr-2000/en/pr2000-life.html

Approximately 493 Americans are killed daily by hospital injuries and drug-prescribing errors
"Recent estimates suggest that each year more than 1 million patients are injured while in the hospital and approximately 180,000 die because of these injuries. Furthermore, drug-related morbidity and mortality are common and are estimated to cost more than $136 billion a year." Holland EG, Degruy FV. Drug-induced disorders. *Am Fam Physician*. 1997

Medical drug (in)efficacy
"The vast majority of drugs —more than 90 percent— only work in 30 or 50 percent of the people." Allen Roses, M.D., worldwide vice-president of genetics at GlaxoSmithKline. Published Dec 8, 2003 ttp://commondreams.org/headlines03/1208-02.htm

Healthy lifestyle and *biochemical individuality* credo: Recognize and affirm that you are a unique individual with unique needs: For each of us, our "personality" extends far beyond and far deeper than our sense of humor and our choice of clothing; we are very unique on a physiologic and biochemical level as well. So-called *normal* and *apparently healthy* individuals vary greatly in their biochemical efficiency and nutritional needs. This is the concept of "biochemical individuality" which was first detailed in 1956 by the renowned scientist Roger J Williams from the University of Texas. In his historic work *Biochemical Individuality: The Basis for the Genetotrophic Concept*, Dr.

---

[29] McPherson M, et al. Social Isolation in America: Changes in Core Discussion Networks over Two Decades. *American Sociological Review* 2006; 71: 353-75
[30] "According to the latest available data, total health care costs reached $1.3 trillion in 2000. This represents a per capita health care expenditure of $4,637. The total prescription drug expenditure in 2000 was $121.8 billion, or approximately $430 per person." Presentation to the U.S. Senate Commerce Committee April 23, 2002 "Drug Pricing & Consumer Costs" Kathleen D. Jaeger, R.Ph., J.D. commerce.senate.gov/hearings/042302jaegar.pdf
[31] Zack MM, Moriarty DG, Stroup DF, Ford ES, Mokdad AH. Worsening trends in adult health-related quality of life and self-rated health-United States, 1993-2001. *Public Health Rep*. 2004 Sep-Oct;119(5):493-505 pubmedcentral.nih.gov/articlerender.fcgi?tool=pubmed&pubmedid=15313113
[32] "[America] also has the fewest hospital days per capita, the highest hospital expenditures per day, and substantially higher physician incomes than the other OECD countries. On the available outcome measures, the United States is generally in the bottom half, and its relative ranking has been declining since 1960." Anderson GF, Poullier JP. Health spending, access, and outcomes: trends in industrialized countries. *Health Aff* (Millwood) 1999 May-Jun;18(3):178-92 content.healthaffairs.org/cgi/reprint/18/3/178.pdf
[33] "However, on outcomes indicators such as life expectancy and infant mortality, the United States is frequently in the bottom quartile among the twenty-nine industrialized countries, and its relative ranking has been declining since 1960." Anderson GF. In search of value: an international comparison of cost, access, and outcomes. *Health Aff* 1997 Nov-Dec;16(6):163-71
[34] "Basically, you die earlier and spend more time disabled if you're an American rather than a member of most other advanced countries," says Christopher Murray, MD, PhD, Director of WHO's Global Program on Evidence for Health Policy. who.int/inf-pr-2000/en/pr2000-life.html
[35] "Systematic access to managed chiropractic care not only may prove to be clinically beneficial but also may reduce overall health care costs." Legorreta A, et al N. Comparative Analysis of Individuals With and Without Chiropractic Coverage. *Archives of Internal Medicine* 2004; 164: 1985-1992
[36] Orme-Johnson DW, Herron RE. An innovative approach to reducing medical care utilization and expenditures. *Am J Manag Care*. 1997;3(1):135-44
[37] Shi L. Health care spending, delivery, and outcome in developed countries: a cross-national comparison. *Am J Med Qual* 1997;12(2):83-93

Williams[38] reviews research that conclusively proves that among *apparently healthy* individuals, we can objectively determine great differences in physiology, organ efficiency, enzyme function, and nutritional needs. For example, variables that promote health include increased enzyme efficiency and efficient digestion and assimilation of nutrients, while internal factors that reduce health can include inadequate digestion, inefficient absorption, increased excretion of nutrients, impaired detoxification, poor enzyme function and "partial genetic blocks"—a term now understood to imply single nucleotide polymorphisms[39] and related enzyme defects, which result in **supradietary requirements for specific vitamins and minerals** for the prevention of disease and maintenance of health.[40] What this means for us as doctors and for our patients in practical terms is that in order for us to become as healthy as possible, we will almost certainly have to give attention to each person's unique biochemical abilities/disabilities in order to maximize the function of the various body systems, enzymes, and to optimize genetic expression.[41] This means that what works for one's neighbor, spouse, or best friend in terms of exercise, diet and nutrition may not work for one's unique physiology. We must all muster the courage to affirm that, in order to attain the goal of stable or progressively better health, we will each have to learn about how our unique bodies work—what conditions of health must be created. We will have to learn to make changes in lifestyle and daily routine which reflect and honor our bodies' ways of working. This may mean modifying work, sleep, and exercise schedules, avoiding some foods and eating others, and customizing nutrient intake to meet the body's needs as they are *in the present*—the health program that appears to have worked last year may not be appropriate at the present time. The process of learning how a person's body works requires time, patience, and the process of trial and error—from patient and doctor—but achieving the goal of improved health and increased energy are well worth the effort.

Individuation and the practice of conscious living: Our visions of reality are influenced by religious institutions, large corporations, advertising networks[42], corporate-owned mass media[43], and what Professors Stevens and Glatstein called "the medical-industrial complex."[44] Some of the paradigms that are advocated are both *unhistorical* (having no historical precedent) and *antihistorical* (contrary to the available historical precedent, which includes sustainability). Some of these companies and organizations offer us a view of reality and vision of our individual potentials that is fashioned in such a way as to promote the financial and political interests of the company or organization. Conversely, the actualization of our true physical, emotional, intellectual, and spiritual potentials may require that we separate from or at least attain a conscious appreciation of the (pseudo)reality that we have been advised to follow.[45,46] Critiques of and reasonable alternatives to our current paradigms of school[47], work[48,49], and money[50] have been discussed elsewhere and are worthy of consideration. Becoming mindful of the paradigms and assumptions under which we live is the first step in true individuation, characterized by choosing (*creating* the best option: freedom) rather than deciding (*selecting* one of the offered options: the illusion of freedom). Various conscious thoughts and unconscious assumptions create our "working reality" which represents the way that we see things and the paradigm by which we *act in* and *interact with* the larger world. These layers come from our own families, schools,

> **The importance of living consciously**
> "Consciousness is our basic tool for successful adaptation to reality. The more conscious we are in any situation, the more possibilities we tend to perceive, the more options we have, the more powerful we are — perhaps even the longer we will live.
> Living consciously means **seeking to be aware of everything** that bears on our actions, purposes, values, and goals — and **behaving in accordance** with that which we see and know."
>
> Branden N. *The Art of Living Consciously*.

---

[38] Williams RJ. *Biochemical Individuality: The Basis for the Genetotrophic Concept*. Austin and London: University of Texas Press, 1956
[39] Ames BN. Cancer prevention and diet: help from single nucleotide polymorphisms. *Proc Natl Acad Sci U S A*. 1999 Oct 26;96(22):12216-8
[40] Ames BN, Elson-Schwab I, Silver EA. High-dose vitamin therapy stimulates variant enzymes with decreased coenzyme binding affinity (increased K(m)): relevance to genetic disease and polymorphisms. *Am J Clin Nutr*. 2002 Apr;75(4):616-58 ajcn.org/cgi/content/full/75/4/616
[41] "The combination of biochemical individuality and known functional utilities of allelic variants should converge to create a situation in which nutritional optima can be specified as part of comprehensive lifestyle prescriptions tailored to the needs of each person." Eckhardt RB. Genetic research and nutritional individuality. *J Nutr* 2001;131(2):336S-9S
[42] "Patients' requests for medicines are a powerful driver of prescribing decisions. In most cases physicians prescribed requested medicines but were often ambivalent about the choice of treatment. If physicians prescribe requested drugs despite personal reservations, sales may increase but appropriateness of prescribing may suffer." Mintzes et al. Influence of direct to consumer pharmaceutical advertising and patients' requests on prescribing decisions: two site cross sectional survey. *BMJ*. 2002 Feb 2; 324(7332): 278-9
[43] *Manufacturing Consent: Noam Chomsky and the Media*. Movie directed by Achbar M and Wintonick P. 1992. See also zeitgeistmovie.com/
[44] Stevens CW, Glatstein E. Beware the Medical-Industrial Complex. *Oncologist* 1996;1(4):IV-V theoncologist.alphamedpress.org/cgi/reprint/1/4/190-iv.pdf
[45] Breton D, Largent C. *The Paradigm Conspiracy*. Center City; Hazelden: 1996
[46] Pearce JC. *Exploring the Crack in the Cosmic Egg: Split Minds and Meta-Realities*. New York: Washington Square Press; 1974
[47] Gatto JT. *Dumbing us down: the hidden curriculum of compulsory education*. Gabriola Island, Canada; New Society Publishers: 2005
[48] "No one should ever work. In order to stop suffering, we have to stop working. That doesn't mean we have to stop doing things. It does mean creating a new way of life based on play…" Black B. *The abolition of work and other essays*. Port Townsend: Loompanics Unlimited; 1985, pages 17-33
[49] Jarow R. *Creating the Work You Love: Courage, Commitment and Career*; Inner Traditions Intl Ltd; 1995 [ISBN: 0892815426]
[50] Dominguez JR. *Transforming Your Relationship with Money*. Sounds True; Book and Cassette edition: 2001 Audio tape.

teachers, churches, companies, friends, parents, and ourselves—our previous interpretations and misinterpretations of ourselves and events; in sum, our responses to outer events combined with our internal experiences meld into our perception of ourselves (known as "the genesis of personal identity") and how we as individuals relate to our inner ourselves and [our perception of] the outer world. Becoming conscious of these realities and illusions allows us the opportunity to discard those views that are inaccurate, dysfunctional, and harmful and to accept a truer reality based on what we experience, feel, and know to be real—in the present, as adults. Once we are freed from *unreality*, we can live true to ourselves in a way that is authentically responsible to our own needs *and* the needs of our communities so that we can simultaneously sustain our obligations to society[51,52] while being free to be unique individuals.[53,54]

Examples of commonly accepted paradigms and their reasonable alternatives

Commonly accepted paradigms ↳ Implication and effect	Alternate paradigm ↳ Implication and effect
It is OK to be irresponsible in daily choices and then blame health problems on bad luck, bad genes, or both. ↳ Many people fail to take responsibility for their lives and thereby become victims of circumstances—negative circumstances that they themselves helped to create.	**Lifestyle, especially diet and nutrition, is the most powerful influence on health outcomes. Therefore, an educated patient is empowered to direct his/her health destiny.** ↳ Optimal health *per individual* is attained when people take responsibility for their lives, seek health information, and then incorporate this information into their daily routine in the form of healthy living: health-promoting lifestyle, eating, exercise, supplementation, relationships, and occupational and social activities, including socio-political involvement to protect the environment and resist the privatization of life and the spoliation of the environment in which we live and upon which our lives and health depend.[55,56]
In general, chemical medications are the answer to nearly all health problems. ↳ The belief in medications as the primary treatment of disease creates a patient population that is apathetic, disempowered, and dependent upon the medical-pharmaceutical industry, which grows richer and more powerful despite so-called 'earnest' attempts at cost containment.[57]	**Many acute and chronic problems can be more effectively managed in terms of prevention, safety, efficacy, and cost-effectiveness when phytonutritional interventions are either used as primary therapy or, when necessary, used in conjunction with medications.** ↳ A reduction in disease prevalence via health-promoting diet and lifestyle along with integrative treatments offers the best opportunity for benefit to patients, doctors, and third-party payers.[58]

---

[51] Bly R. *The Sibling Society*. Vintage Books USA; Reprint edition (June 1, 1997) ISBN: 0679781285 (Abridged audio edition (May 1, 1996)
[52] Bly R. *Where have all the parents gone? A talk on the Sibling Society*. New York: Sound Horizons, 1996 Highly recommended.
[53] Bradshaw J. *Healing the Shame that Binds You* [Audio Cassette (April 1990) Health Communications Audio; ISBN: 1558740430]
[54] Miller A. *The truth will set you free: overcoming emotional blindness and finding your true adult self*. New York: Basic Books; 2001
[55] "Your lack of interest in the past, your lack of involvement, your unwillingness to develop coherent strategies, your unwillingness to challenge authority - these have created a vacuum in decision-making, that has been filled by professional groups with close relationships with the chemical industries..." Samuel Epstein MD, 1993. Professor of Occupational and Environmental Medicine at the School of Public Health, University of Illinois Medical Center Chicago. converge.org.nz/pirm/pestican.htm
[56] Kristin S. Schafer, Margaret Reeves, Skip Spitzer, Susan E. Kegley. Chemical Trespass: Pesticides in Our Bodies and Corporate Accountability. Pesticide Action Network North America. May 2004 Available at panna.org/campaigns/docsTrespass/chemicalTrespass2004.dv.html on August 1, 2004
[57] "In this paper I offer four hypotheses to help explain why use of pharmaceuticals has continued to grow even as managed care and other cost containment efforts have flourished." Berndt ER. The U.S. pharmaceutical industry: why major growth in times of cost containment? *Health Aff* (Millwood). 2001 Mar-Apr;20(2):100-14
[58] "Hospital admission rates in the control group were 11.4 times higher than those in the MVAH group for cardiovascular disease, 3.3 times higher for cancer, and 6.7 times higher for mental health and substance abuse. ...MVAH patients older than age 45...had 88% fewer total patients days compared with control patients." Orme-Johnson DW, Herron RE. An innovative approach to reducing medical care utilization and expenditures. *Am J Manag Care*. 1997 Jan;3(1):135-44

Examples of commonly accepted paradigms and their reasonable alternatives — *continued*

Commonly accepted paradigms ↳ Implication and effect	Alternate paradigm ↳ Implication and effect
Work ethic: a belief that "hard work" has moral value and makes a person "better." ↳ Belief in the principle of "work ethic" encourages people to mindlessly engage in work for the sake of engaging in work without considering the implications of their actions or other alternatives that might produce a more beneficial outcome.[59]	Work is the means rather than an end unto itself (except when the "work" is enjoyable, in which case it is no longer "work"). ↳ Occupations and professions can be designed for the enhancement of life (health, pleasure, relationships, the environment, care of the poor) rather than as an end to themselves at the expense of the individual, society, and the environment.
Adults should give 10.5-12 hours per day 5 days per week to work. ↳ In most corporate environments, employee's work at least 8.5 hours per day, with 1 additional hour spent in commuting[60] and another hour spent in preparation, transportation, and maintenance of work-related clothing, preparing work-related meals, maintaining the auto that is used for work-related tasks. With 10.5 hours given directly to work, 0.5-1 additional hours are needed for recuperation from work-related stress ("daily decompression"); thus the average amount of time given to work-related activities is much larger than commonly believed.[61] Because of the time and energies devoted to "work" the vast majority of people feel that they do not have sufficient time for themselves, their families and friends, their creativity, learning about the world, political involvement, and other more important aspects of life. "Not enough time" is the most common reason given by patients for not exercising.	A paradigm of a 4-day workweek is just as valid and perhaps more valid than one that advocates a 5-day workweek. A paradigm of a 6-hour workday is at least as valid as one of an 8-10 hour workday. ↳ Many people in our culture are chronically overworked, undernourished, tired and suffer from an insufficiency of time to simply be in community, to rest, to be creative. Living with such limitations and pressures should be expected to produce a population that is reactively hedonistic, impulsive, and prone to addiction. Behaviors that are addictive (e.g., drugs, alcohol) and destructive (e.g., over-eating, alcohol, sugar, fat) are simply frustrated and maladaptive coping strategies to combat the stress caused by a damaging, unnatural paradigm from which most people cannot escape.[62] Redesigning our societal structures and expectations in ways that conform to our natural humanity and biologic, nutritional, and emotional needs is more rational than forcing *en masse* all of humanity to contort and conform to an artificial posture and cadence of performance, productivity, "professionalism", and other unnatural expectations. Less time dedicated to work and all that it entails leaves more time for 1) healthy cooking, 2) relaxed, conscious, and enjoyable eating, 3) exercise, 4) creativity and hobbies, 5) keeping informed of and involved with political change, and 6) participation in social relationships.[63] ↳ Readers of my books know that I advocated the 4-day workweek since the publication of my *Integrative Orthopedics* in 2004 and *Integrative Rheumatology* in 2006; finally, in 2014 this idea has made headlines: "One of Britain's leading doctors has called for the country to switch to a four-day week to help combat high levels of work-related stress, let people spend more time with their families or exercising, and reduce unemployment. Bringing the standard working week down from five to four days would also help address medical conditions, such as high blood pressure and the mental ill-health associated with overwork or lack of work, Prof John Ashton said."[64]

---

[59] "Conventional wisdom is the habitual, the unexamined life, absorbed into the culture and the fashion of the time, lost in the mad rush of accumulation, lulled to sleep by the easy lies of political hacks and newspaper scribblers, or by priests who wouldn't know a god if they met one." Nisker W. *Crazy Wisdom*. Berkeley; Ten Speed Press: 1990, p 7
[60] Sep 8, 2003: Average daily one-way commute to work in the United States takes just over 26 minutes, according to the Bureau of Transportation Statistics' Omnibus Household Survey. Omnibus Household Survey Shows Americans' Average Commuting Time is Over 26 Minutes. bts.gov/press_releases/2003/bts020_03/html/bts020_03.html
[61] Dominguez JR. *Transforming Your Relationship with Money*. Sounds True; Book and Cassette edition: 2001
[62] Breton D, Largent C. *The Paradigm Conspiracy: Why Our Social Systems Violate Human Potential-And How We Can Change Them*. Hazelden: 1998
[63] "Take back your time" is a major U.S./Canadian initiative to challenge the epidemic of overwork, over-scheduling and time famine that now threatens our health, our families and relationships, our communities and our environment. simpleliving.net/timeday/ on August 3, 2004
[64] Campbell D. UK needs four-day week to combat stress, says top doctor. *The Guardian* 2014 theguardian.com/society/2014/jul/01/uk-four-day-week-combat-stress-top-doctor

Quality and quantity of sleep: A sleep duration of less than 8 hours of deep solid sleep each night is physiologically insufficient for most of people; many people feel best with 9 hours of sleep, yet some people appear to function well on about 6 hours of sleep per night. Not only is it important to get a sufficient *quantity* of sleep, but we need to ensure that the *quality* of the sleep receives appropriate attention, as well. Sleep should be mostly continuous, not "broken" or interrupted. Some experts believe that people should be able to recall their dreams at night, as this may be a sign of proper neurotransmitter status, especially with regard to serotonin, which is affected by pyridoxine[65] as well as other factors. Going to bed at a regular hour (not later than 10 or 11 at night) helps to synchronize the daily schedule with the body's inherent hormonal rhythms and "physiological clock" which expects one to be in deep sleep by midnight and to be waking at approximately 8 o'clock in the morning. Recent research has shown that **sleep deprivation causes a systemic inflammatory response manifested objectively by increases in high-sensitivity C-reactive protein (hsCRP)**.[66] Correspondingly, sleep apnea, a condition associated with repetitive sleep disturbances, is also associated with an elevation of CRP[67], and effective treatment of sleep apnea results in a normalization of CRP levels.[68] We could therefore conclude that **sleep deprivation creates a proinflammatory condition**. Furthermore, **sleep deprivation has been proven to impair intellectual functioning, emotional state, and immune function**, with abnormalities in immune status already evident the morning after sleep deprivation.[69] Wakefulness and exposure to light at night result in a suppression of melatonin production and may therefore contribute to cancer development since melatonin has anticancer actions that would be abrogated by its reduced endogenous production.[70,71] Limited evidence also suggests that melatonin production is altered in patients with the inflammatory conditions eczema[72] and psoriasis[73] and that this sleep-related hormone has anti-inflammatory/anti-autoimmune benefits that may be relevant for the suppression of diseases such as multiple sclerosis[74] and sarcoidosis.[75]

> **The Importance of Sleep**
> Regulation of sleep-wake cycles and the regular satisfaction of sleep needs are important for preservation of immune function, intellectual performance, emotional stability, and the internal regulation of the body's inflammatory tendency.

- Sleep disturbance, immune dysregulation, and disturbed inflammatory regulation (*Am J Geriatr Psychiatry.* 2012 Sep[76]): "Poor sleep diminishes mental and physical health. ... Participants categorized as poor sleepers on the basis of Pittsburgh Sleep Quality Index scores had significantly larger IL-6 responses to the cognitive stressors than good sleepers. The association between poor sleep and heightened IL-6 response to acute stress was not explained by other psychosocial factors previously linked to immune dysregulation, including depressive symptoms, perceived stress, and loneliness. CONCLUSIONS: Findings add to the growing evidence for poor sleep as an independent risk factor for poor mental and physical health. Older adults may be particularly vulnerable to effects of sleep disturbance due to significant age-related changes in both sleep and inflammatory regulation."

---

[65] "...a significant difference in dream-salience scores (this is a composite score containing measures on vividness, bizarreness, emotionality, and color) between the 250-mg condition and placebo over the first three days of each treatment... An hypothesis is presented involving the role of B-6 in the conversion of tryptophan to serotonin." Ebben M, Lequerica A, Spielman A. Effects of pyridoxine on dreaming: a preliminary study. *Percept Mot Skills* 2002 Feb;94(1):135-40
[66] "CONCLUSIONS: Both acute total and short-term partial sleep deprivation resulted in elevated high-sensitivity CRP concentrations... We propose that sleep loss may be one of the ways that inflammatory processes are activated and contribute to the association of sleep complaints, short sleep duration, and cardiovascular morbidity observed in epidemiologic surveys." Meier-Ewert et al. Effect of sleep loss on C-reactive protein, an inflammatory marker of cardiovascular risk. *J Am Coll Cardiol.* 2004 Feb 18;43:678-83
[67] "OSA is associated with elevated levels of CRP, a marker of inflammation and of cardiovascular risk. The severity of OSA is proportional to the CRP level." Shamsuzzaman et al. Elevated C-reactive protein in patients with obstructive sleep apnea. *Circulation.* 2002 May 28;105(21):2462-4
[68] "CONCLUSIONS: Levels of CRP and IL-6 and spontaneous production of IL-6 by monocytes are elevated in patients with OSAS but are decreased by nCPAP." Yokoe T, Minoguchi K, Matsuo H, Oda N, Minoguchi H, Yoshino G, Hirano T, Adachi M. Elevated levels of C-reactive protein and interleukin-6 in patients with obstructive sleep apnea syndrome are decreased by nasal continuous positive airway pressure. *Circulation.* 2003 Mar 4;107(8):1129-34 circ.ahajournals.org/cgi/reprint/107/8/1129.pdf
[69] "Taken together, SD induced a deterioration of both mood and ability to work, which was most prominent in the evening after SD, while the maximal alterations of the host defence system could be found twelve hours earlier, i.e., already in the morning following SD." Heiser P, et al. Alterations of host defense system after sleep deprivation are followed by impaired mood and psychosocial functioning. *World J Biol Psychiatry* 2001 Apr;2(2):89-94
[70] "Observational studies support an association between night work and cancer risk. We hypothesise that the potential primary culprit for this observed association is the lack of melatonin, a cancer-protective agent whose production is severely diminished in people exposed to light at night." Schernhammer ES, Schulmeister K. Melatonin and cancer risk: does light at night compromise physiologic cancer protection by lowering serum melatonin levels? *Br J Cancer.* 2004 Mar 8;90(5):941-3
[71] "This is the first biological evidence for a potential link between constant light exposure and increased human breast oncogenesis involving MLT suppression and stimulation of tumor LA metabolism." Blask DE, Dauchy RT, Sauer LA, Krause JA, Brainard GC. Growth and fatty acid metabolism of human breast cancer (MCF-7) xenografts in nude rats: impact of constant light-induced nocturnal melatonin suppression. *Breast Cancer Res Treat.* 2003 Jun;79(3):313-20
[72] "In 6 patients exhibiting low serum levels of melatonin, the circadian melatonin rhythm was found to be abolished. In 8 patients a diminished nocturnal melatonin increase was observed compared with the controls (n = 40)." Schwarz W, et al. Alterations of melatonin secretion in atopic eczema. *Acta Derm Venereol.* 1988;68(3):224-9
[73] "Our results show that psoriatic patients had lost the nocturnal peak and usual circadian rhythm of melatonin secretion." Mozzanica N, Tadini G, Radaelli A, et al. Plasma melatonin levels in psoriasis. *Acta Derm Venereol.* 1988;68(4):312-6
[74] "This hypothesis is supported by the observation that administration of melatonin (3 mg, orally) at 2:00 p.m., when the patient experienced severe blurring of vision, resulted within 15 minutes in a dramatic improvement in visual acuity and in normalization of the visual evoked potential latency after stimulation of the left eye." Sandyk R. Diurnal variations in vision and relations to circadian melatonin secretion in multiple sclerosis. *Int J Neurosci.* 1995 Nov;83(1-2):1-6
[75] Cagnoni ML, Lombardi A, Cerinic MC, Dedola GL, Pignone A. Melatonin for treatment of chronic refractory sarcoidosis. *Lancet.* 1995;346:1229-30
[76] Heffner et al. Sleep disturbance and older adults' inflammatory responses to acute stress. *Am J Geriatr Psychiatry.* 2012 Sep;20(9):744-52

Helping patients improve quality and quantity of sleep
- Schedule sufficient time for sleep; generally this is 9 hours to allow time for "winding down" and "daily decompression" so that a full 8 hours of sleep can ensue.
- Reduce intake of stimulants such as caffeine, tobacco, and aspartame. Some patients will need to reduce intake only in the evening, while others will need to reduce intake even in the morning in order to have improved quality and quantity of sleep later at night.
- Exercise early in the day (morning or early afternoon) to promote restful sleep at night.[77]
- Avoid aggressive or arousing physical activity in the evening to avoid increases in norepinephrine, epinephrine, and cortisol, which can discourage sleep.
- Dim lights at night to promote melatonin production. Beginning one to two hours before bedtime, turn off bright lights and use only dim lighting. Bright lights reduce melatonin secretion and stimulate neocortical activity and thereby inhibit sleep.
- Have an evening ritual/pattern that helps the psyche recognize that the time for sleep has arrived. Such practices can include relaxing warm tea, meditation, prayer, and daily reflection.
- For patients with a pattern of falling asleep and then waking approximately 4-6 hours later with feelings of hunger or anxiety (nocturnal hypoglycemia), they should eat a small meal or snack of complex carbohydrates, protein, and fat before going to bed. For example, the combination of nuts (or nut butter) with whole fruit such as apples provides protein, fat, and complex carbohydrate with a low glycemic index to provide sustenance throughout the night. Protein powders and other sources of "predigested" amino acids should generally be avoided late at night because an excess consumption of high protein foods can reduce tryptophan entry into the brain and thus reduce serotonin and melatonin synthesis. Most amino acid-derived neurotransmitters such as dopamine, glutamate, and norepinephrine are excitatory/stimulatory in nature.
- Vitamin and mineral supplementation is commonly beneficial, particularly with thiamine[78], methylcobalamin (weak evidence[79]), and magnesium (particularly sleep disturbance associated with restless leg syndrome[80]). Vitamins should be taken earlier in the day (with breakfast and lunch; not before bed); however calcium and magnesium can be taken before bed.
- Earplugs, window covers, and a quiet, snore-free environment are generally conducive to better sleep.
- For patients with difficulty falling asleep, consider 5-hydroxytryptophan consumed with simple carbohydrate (50-200 mg for adults, up to 2 mg/kg[81] for children), melatonin (0.5-10 mg), valerian-hops tea or capsules[82] 60-90 minutes before bedtime.

---

[77] "This is the first report to demonstrate that low intensity activity in an elderly population can increase deep sleep and improve memory functioning." Naylor E, et al. Daily social and physical activity increases slow-wave sleep and daytime neuropsychological performance in the elderly. *Sleep.* 2000 Feb 1;23(1):87-95

[78] Wilkinson TJ, Hanger HC, Elmslie J, George PM, Sainsbury R. The response to treatment of subclinical thiamine deficiency in the elderly. *Am J Clin Nutr.* 1997;66(4):925-8

[79] "However, because the percentage of improvement was low and significant improvement was inconsistent, Met-12 might be considered to have a low therapeutic potency and possible use as a booster for other treatment methods of the disorders." Takahashi K, et al. Double-blind test on the efficacy of methylcobalamin on sleep-wake rhythm disorders. *Psychiatry Clin Neurosci.* 1999 Apr;53(2):211-3

[80] "Our study indicates that magnesium treatment may be a useful alternative therapy in patients with mild or moderate RLS-or PLMS-related insomnia." Hornyak M, Voderholzer U, et al. Magnesium therapy for periodic leg movements-related insomnia and restless legs syndrome: an open pilot study. *Sleep.* 1998 Aug 1;21(5):501-5

[81] Bruni O, Ferri R, Miano S, Verrillo E. 1-5-Hydroxytryptophan treatment of sleep terrors in children. *Eur J Pediatr.* 2004 May 14

[82] "Sleep improvements with a valerian-hops combination are associated with improved quality of life. Both treatments appear safe and did not produce rebound insomnia upon discontinuation during this study. Overall, these findings indicate that a valerian-hops combination and diphenhydramine might be useful adjuncts in the treatment of mild insomnia." Morin et al. Valerian-hops combination and diphenhydramine for treating insomnia: a randomized placebo-controlled clinical trial. *Sleep.* 2005 Nov 1;28:1465-71

Exercise: Human existence has changed radically over the past few millennia, centuries, and decades, and one of the most profound changes has been in our relationship to physical activity. Paleologists and historical scientists agree that physical activity among humans is at its all-time historical low, and that levels of exertion that we now call "vigorous and frequent exercise" would have been *completely normal* in the daily lives of our ancestors, who engaged in at least four times more physical activity than their modern-day progeny.[83] At one time—a time in which vigorous physical activity was a normal part of daily life—probably no word existed for what modern people describe and often resist as "exercise."

Our current mode of compulsory primary and secondary education prioritizes "being still" over physical exertion/expression for the vast majority of students' time. Thus having been separated from their inherent tendency to be physically active and emotionally expressive, many children grow into adults who have to be *retaught to inhabit their bodies* and to engage in physical activity on a daily basis. Basic science has proven that this is true: when animals are restrained, they show less activity when freed and no longer tied down. Conversely, when animals are rigorously exercised, they show higher levels of *spontaneous physical activity* when left to their own discretion. A probable sociological parallel is at work in human cultures where, under the guise of *office work* (sitting still), driving in cars (sitting still), and *spectator entertainment* (sitting still), people are corralled into lifestyles of physical inactivity in a wide range of apparently divergent activities. Watching television, driving a car, seeing a movie, doing computer/desk work at the office, attending a sports event or educational lecture, seeing the opera—all of these are simply different forms of ***sitting***, of physical inactivity. Changing our social structure in a way that prioritizes *life* over *work*, such as moving toward a 4-day work week and/or a 6-hour work day, would allow people more time to live their lives, to pursue healthy diets and relationships, to be creative, and to engage in more physical activity; thus, "escape entertainment" such as fiction books and movies and processed "fast foods"—the latter of which are inherently unhealthy[84]—would become less necessary and less attractive.

Daily exercise is health-promoting and restorative

"The health rewards of exercise extend far beyond its benefits for specific diseases."
1. Exercise reduces blood clotting,
2. ...lowers blood pressure,
3. ...lowers cholesterol,
4. ...improves glucose tolerance and insulin sensitivity,
5. ...enhances self-image, elevates mood,
6. ...reduces stress,
7. ...creates a feeling of well-being,
8. ...reinforces other positive life-style changes,
9. ...stimulates creative thinking,
10. ...increases muscle mass,
11. ...increases basal metabolic rate,
12. ...promotes improved sleep,
13. ...stimulates healthy intestinal function,
14. ...promotes weight loss, and
15. ...enhances appearance.

"Furthermore, **the ability of exercise to restore function to organs, muscles, joints, and bones is not shared by drugs or surgery**."

Harold Elrick, MD. Exercise is medicine. *Physician and Sportsmedicine*. 1996 February: 24; 2

Daily exercise is the body's physiological expectation

"Although modern technology has made physical exertion optional, it is still important to exercise as though our survival depended on it, and in a different way it still does.

We are genetically adapted to live an extremely physically active lifestyle."

O'Keefe JH Jr, Cordain L. Cardiovascular disease resulting from a diet and lifestyle at odds with our Paleolithic genome. *Mayo Clin Proc*. 2004 Jan

---

[83] Eaton SB, Cordain L, Eaton SB. An evolutionary foundation for health promotion. *World Rev Nutr Diet* 2001; 90:5-12
[84] For an additional social-experimental perspective see movie directed by Morgan Spurlock. *Super Size Me*. supersizeme.com released in 2004

Exploring the spectrum of physical activity from inactivity to athleticism

Inactivity	Minimally active	Active	Healthy	Athletic
• Bed-ridden • Chair-ridden • Minimal activity, such as walking to car or bathroom or to buy groceries • Activity in this category is equivalent to or barely above that which is necessary to sustain life	• Periodic performance of more activity than the minimal needed to sustain life, such as walking around the block after dinner, or taking a brief stroll at a park or at the beach	• Regular performance of low/moderate levels of activity at work or leisure, at least 30-60 minutes of physical activity per day	• 60-120 minutes of vigorous activity such as running, swimming, cycling, or other physical training 4-7 days per week	• More than 2 hours devoted to conditioning, strengthening, and skill-building 4-7 days per week

At least 30-45 minutes of exercise four days per week is the *absolute minimum*. Ideally, patients who have been sedentary and are over age 45 years would have a pre-exercise physical exam that might also include electrocardiography before embarking on a program of vigorous exercise. Patients who have been sedentary for many years can start slowly with their new exercise program, gradually increasing the duration and intensity. With the simple addition of regular exercise to their routine, patients will have significantly reduced risk for problems such as depression, chronic pain, cancer, coronary artery disease, stroke, hypertension, diabetes, arthritis, osteoporosis, dyslipidemia, obesity, chronic obstructive pulmonary disease, constipation, and other problems.[85] Furthermore, successful prevention and treatment of health problems with exercise and lifestyle modifications reduces dependency on pharmaceutical drugs, thereby further saving lives. O'Keefe and Cordain[86] report that **during the hunter-gatherer period, humans averaged 5-10 miles of daily running and walking. Additionally, other physical activities such as heavy lifting, digging, and climbing would have been considered "normal" aspects of daily life rather than "exercise"—an achievement for which modern/industrialized people seek recognition.** Thus, when sedentary patients achieve the first-step goal of walking around the block after dinner, we can commend them for making a significant stride forward in ultimately attaining better health, but we cannot stop there nor delude them into believing that this is adequate.

> **Industrialized Westernized societies' disregard/disdain for connection with the body**
>
> "That I deemed it an imposition to have to make use of my perfectly adequate coordination, or resented—from unexamined principle—**the use of time to fill a need**, was an **arbitrary assignment of values** that [this other culture] did not share."
>
> Liedloff J. *The Continuum Concept*, 1977, page 15

- Physical activity can prevent physical and cognitive decline in postmenopausal women (*Maturitas* 2014 Jun[87]): Results of this systematic review of the literature showed that all previous studies found that physical activity was associated with lower rates of cognitive and physical decline and a significant reduction in all-cause mortality; exercise interventions (or lifestyle activities) that improved cardiorespiratory exercise capacity showed the most positive impact on physical health. The authors encouraged the embedding of physical activity programs into public health initiatives, developing home-based exercise programs that require few resources, and creating interventions that can incorporate physical activity within a healthy lifestyle. The review also suggests that clinicians should consider prescribing exercise that it is of a high enough intensity to obtain the positive sustained effects of exercise.

> **The philosophy of physicality**
>
> "There is more wisdom in your body than in your deepest philosophy."
>
> Nietzsche FW, *Thus Spoke Zarathustra*

---

[85] Harold Elrick, MD. Exercise is Medicine. *The Physician and Sportsmedicine* 1996 Feb
[86] O'Keefe JH Jr, Cordain L. Cardiovascular disease resulting from a diet and lifestyle at odds with our Paleolithic genome. *Mayo Clin Proc*. 2004 Jan;79(1):101-8
[87] Anderson et al. Can physical activity prevent physical and cognitive decline in postmenopausal women? A systematic review. *Maturitas*. 2014 Jun. pii: S0378-5122(14)00206-0

Common physical activities: a buffet of options from which to choose
☑ **"Boot camp"-style aerobics classes**: excellent variety and fast-pace maintains oxygen debt for the entire session (generally 60 minutes) even among reasonably well trained "healthy" people
☑ **Aerobic machines such as elliptical runners and stair-climbing machines**: easy on joints; accessible during inclement weather; easy to integrate with weight-lifting which is commonly available at the same facility
☑ **Baseball**: requires some skill in throwing and batting, but otherwise this is a very inactive sport
☑ **Football**: much of the game is spent in inactivity; most of the fitness comes from preparation for the game, not the game itself; high impact activity wherein injuries are expected
☑ **Hiking**: virtually free of expense; allows for conversation, exploration, and time in nature; mountains required
☑ **Indoor aerobics**: excellent for cardiovascular fitness and weight loss, requires and thus promotes coordination and timing
☑ **Indoor cycling**: excellent for cardiovascular fitness and weight loss, easy on the joints; accessible during inclement weather
☑ **Jogging and running**: easy, accessible, virtually free; allows for conversation and exploration; increases endorphin production and promotes a sense of well-being; detoxification via sweating
☑ **Kayaking and canoeing**: excellent combination of relaxation and exertion; develops upper body strength and balance
☑ **Martial arts**: requires more balance, coordination, timing, strategy, endurance; injuries are to be expected, as is enhanced sense of security and confidence
☑ **Outdoor cycling (mountain and trail)**: same as above; requires more balance and coordination
☑ **Outdoor cycling (road)**: same as above with added bonus of being outdoors; promotes independence from automobiles and petroleum products – thereby reducing pollution and sustaining the environment
☑ **Rock-climbing (indoor and outdoor)**: requires upper body and grip strength; promotes agility, resourcefulness, courage, and trust; good for building stronger relationships assuming that your partner does not drop the rope or get distracted; carries some inherent risk
☑ **Skiing, snowboarding, cross-country skiing**: Require balance and coordination, costly equipment, and appropriate season and climate; risk of traumatic injury due to speed in skiing and snowboarding. Cross-country skiing is generally safe from trauma and provides excellent cardiovascular exertion, in addition to exposure to nature
☑ **Soccer**: excellent for lower-body conditioning, teamwork, and coordination, the rapid stops and turns can be hard on joints
☑ **Surfing**: paddling requires upper body endurance and strength; some leg strength is required but is not strongly developed during the riding portion of surfing, which is mostly technique and "style"; excellent proprioceptive training
☑ **Swimming**: requires access to a pool or suitable body of water; excellent for promoting fitness in a way that is generally easy on joints and muscles and is without impact; requires and thus promotes coordination and timing
☑ **Tennis and racket sports**: requires more balance, coordination, timing, strategy, endurance; the rapid stops, starts, and turns can be hard on joints; upper body exertion is asymmetric and can promote muscle imbalance
☑ **Volleyball**: good team activity; not highly exertional in terms of either aerobic fitness nor strength acquisition
☑ **Walking**: easy, accessible, virtually free; allows for conversation and exploration; allows for time outdoors
☑ **Weight lifting, bodybuilding, and powerlifting**: excellent for increasing lean body mass – one of the primary determinants of basal metabolic rate; promotes bone strengthening
☑ **Yoga, Calisthenics**: inexpensive, can be done alone or in groups; does not require much/any equipment, therefore costs are low and access is near universal

Obesity: Obesity is a major risk factor for cardiovascular disease, cancer, diabetes mellitus, depression, joint degeneration and pain. Obese people also commonly report difficulties with performing daily activities, and they also report higher rates of depression and social isolation than do people of normal weight. "Body Mass Index" is a clinically valuable measure of height-weight proportionality and therefore adiposity, since an excess of height-proportionate weight is more commonly due to excess adipose than to excess muscle. To calculate BMI simply chart height and weight in the table below. Numbers greater than 25 correlate with being "overweight" while numbers greater than 30 meet the criteria for "obesity." BMI determinations may not be reflective of disease risk for people who are pregnant, highly muscular, or for young children or the frail elderly. BMI is interpreted as follows:

- Severely underweight: < 16.5
- Underweight: 16.5 - 18.4
- **Normal: 18.5 - 24.9**
- Overweight: 25 - 29.9
- Obese Class 1: 30 - 34.9
- Obese Class 2 (severe obesity): 35 - 39.9
- Obese Class 3 (morbid obesity): 40 - 47.9
- Obese Class 4 (supermorbid obesity): ≥ 48

Weight in kilograms (*derived from pounds and inches from original table below; BMI is approximate)

Height: (cm*)	45	50	55	59	63	68	73	77	82	86	90	95	100	104	109	114
152	20	21	23	25	27	29	31	33	35	37	39	41	43	45	47	49
155	19	21	23	25	26	28	30	32	34	36	38	40	42	43	45	47
157	18	20	22	24	26	27	29	31	33	35	37	38	40	42	44	46
160	18	19	21	23	25	27	28	30	32	34	35	37	39	41	43	44
162	17	19	21	22	24	26	27	29	31	33	34	36	38	39	41	43
165	17	18	20	22	23	25	27	28	30	32	33	35	37	38	40	42
167	16	18	19	21	23	24	26	27	29	31	32	34	36	37	39	40
170	16	17	19	20	22	23	25	27	28	30	31	33	34	36	38	39
173	15	17	18	20	21	23	24	26	27	29	30	32	33	35	36	38
175	15	16	18	19	21	22	24	25	27	28	30	31	32	34	35	37
177	14	16	17	19	20	22	23	24	26	27	29	30	32	33	34	36
180	14	15	17	18	20	21	22	24	25	26	27	28	30	32	33	35
182	14	15	16	18	19	20	22	23	24	26	27	28	30	31	33	34
185	13	15	16	17	18	20	21	22	24	25	26	28	29	30	32	33
188	13	14	15	17	18	19	21	22	23	24	26	27	28	30	31	32
190	12	14	15	16	17	19	20	21	22	24	25	26	27	29	30	31
193	12	13	15	16	17	18	19	21	22	23	24	26	27	28	29	30

Weight in pounds

Height: (Ft'inch")	100	110	120	130	140	150	160	170	180	190	200	210	220	230	240	250
5'0"	20	21	23	25	27	29	31	33	35	37	39	41	43	45	47	49
5'1"	19	21	23	25	26	28	30	32	34	36	38	40	42	43	45	47
5'2"	18	20	22	24	26	27	29	31	33	35	37	38	40	42	44	46
5'3"	18	19	21	23	25	27	28	30	32	34	35	37	39	41	43	44
5'4"	17	19	21	22	24	26	27	29	31	33	34	36	38	39	41	43
5'5"	17	18	20	22	23	25	27	28	30	32	33	35	37	38	40	42
5'6"	16	18	19	21	23	24	26	27	29	31	32	34	36	37	39	40
5'7"	16	17	19	20	22	23	25	27	28	30	31	33	34	36	38	39
5'8"	15	17	18	20	21	23	24	26	27	29	30	32	33	35	36	38
5'9"	15	16	18	19	21	22	24	25	27	28	30	31	32	34	35	37
5'10"	14	16	17	19	20	22	23	24	26	27	29	30	32	33	34	36
5'11"	14	15	17	18	20	21	22	24	25	26	27	28	30	32	33	35
6'0"	14	15	16	18	19	20	22	23	24	26	27	28	30	31	33	34
6'1"	13	15	16	17	18	20	21	22	24	25	26	28	29	30	32	33
6'2"	13	14	15	17	18	19	21	22	23	24	26	27	28	30	31	32
6'3"	12	14	15	16	17	19	20	21	22	24	25	26	27	29	30	31
6'4"	12	13	15	16	17	18	19	21	22	23	24	26	27	28	29	30

Adipose tissue is biologically active, promoting systemic inflammation and "estrogen dominance", thereby promoting the development of inflammatory and malignant diseases such as psoriasis and cancers of the breast, prostate, and colon. The previous view that fat (adipose) tissue was merely serving as an inert and inactive depot for lipid/energy storage is now replaced with the view that adipose tissue is biologically-active, influencing overall health via complex mechanisms that are biochemical-inflammatory-endocrinologic and not merely mechanical (i.e., excess weight, excess mass).[88] **Excess fat tissue—especially visceral/abdominal adipose—creates a systemic proinflammatory state** evidenced most readily by the elevations in hsCRP commonly seen in patients with obesity and the metabolic syndrome.[89] Adipokines are cytokines secreted by adipose tissue and include tumor necrosis factor-alpha, interleukin-6, and leptin—a cytokine derived from fat cells that promotes inflammation and immune activation; levels are higher in obese patients and decrease after weight loss. Obese patients also appear to have "leptin resistance" with regard to the suppression of appetite by leptin. **Adipose creates excess estrogens;** concomitant hyperglycemia increases androgen production[90], and these androgens are subsequently converted to estrogens by aromatase in the adipose tissue. For example, the adrenal gland makes androstenedione, which can be converted by aromatase in adipose tissue into estrone.[91] These proinflammatory and hormonal perturbations manifest clinically as an increased risk for breast, prostate, endometrial, colon and gallbladder cancers, insulin resistance and cardiovascular disease. The combination of inflammation, reduced testosterone, and elevated estrogen is also predisposes toward the development of autoimmune/inflammatory diseases.

Overview of the proinflammatory and endocrinologic activity of adipose tissue: Adipose promotes systemic inflammation via adipokines and expedites the production of estrogens at the expense of androgens via aromatase.

---

[88] "The fat cell is a true endocrine cell that secretes a variety of factors, including metabolites such as lactate, fatty acids, prostaglandin derivatives and a variety of peptides, including cytokines (leptin, tumor necrosis factor, interleukin-1 and -6, adiponectin), angiotensinogen, complement D (adipsin), plasminogen activator inhibitor-1 and undoubtedly many others." Bray GA. The underlying basis for obesity: relationship to cancer. *J Nutr*. 2002 Nov;132(11 Suppl):3451S-3455S

[89] "Our results indicate a strong relationship between adipocytokines and inflammatory markers, and suggest that cytokines secreted by adipose tissue could play a role in increased inflammatory proteins secretion by the liver." Maachi M, et al. Systemic low-grade inflammation is related to both circulating and adipose tissue TNFalpha, leptin and IL-6 levels in obese women. *Int J Obes Relat Metab Disord*. 2004;28:993-7

[90] Christensen et al. Elevated levels of sex hormones and sex hormone binding globulin in male patients with insulin dependent diabetes mellitus. *Dan Med Bull*. 1997;44:547-50

[91] "Conversion of androstenedione secreted by adrenal gland into estrone by aromatase in adipose tissue stroma provides an important source of estrogen for the postmenopausal woman. This estrogen may play an important role in development of endometrial and breast cancer." Bray GA. Underlying basis for obesity. *J Nutr* 2002;3451S-3455S

The Daily Diet—Powerful Intervention for the Prevention and Treatment of Disease: "Whole foods" should form the foundation and majority of the diet. As doctors and patients, we should emphasize whole fruits, vegetables, nuts, seeds, berries, and lean sources of protein. "Whole foods" are foods that are found in nature, and they should be eaten as closely as possible to their natural state—preferably *unprocessed* and *raw*. Creating a diet based on whole, natural foods by emphasizing the consumption of fruits, vegetables, and lean meats and excluding high-fat factory meats, high-sugar foods like white potatoes, and milled grains like wheat and corn is essential for our efforts of promoting health by matching the human *diet* with the human *genome*.[92] Our genetic make-up was co-created over a period of more than 2.6 million years by interaction with the environment as it exists in its natural state. This environment mandated daily physical activity and a diet that was exclusively composed of 1) fresh fruits, 2) fresh vegetables (mostly uncooked), 3) raw nuts, seeds, berries, roots, and 4) generous portions of lean game meat that was rich in omega-3 fatty acids from free-living animals who were lean because they also ran, fasted, and dealt with limited food supplies. Humans have deviated from this original diet for the sake of ease, conformity, and short-term satisfaction at the expense of health and longevity. Peoples who consume traditional, natural diets have dramatically lower incidences *major* health problems such as cancer, cardiovascular disease, diabetes, obesity and also suffer much less from *milder* problems such as acne, psoriasis, dental cavities, oral malocclusion, and chronic sinus congestion. Societies that are free of these disorders become overwhelmed with them *within only one or two generations* as soon as they adopt the American/Western style of eating. These facts were conclusively documented by Weston Price in his famous 1945 masterpiece *Nutrition and Physical Degeneration*[93] and have been reiterated recently in an excellent review by O'Keefe and Cordain in *Mayo Clinic Proceedings*.[94]

The Supplemented Paleo-Mediterranean Diet

My conclusion after reading several hundred articles on epidemiology, nutritional biochemistry, and dietary intervention studies is that the Paleo-Mediterranean diet—particularly its pesco-vegetarian version—is the single most healthy dietary regimen for the broadest range of patients and for the prevention of the widest range of diseases including cancer, hypertension, diabetes, dermatitis, depression, obesity, arthritis and all inflammatory and autoimmune diseases. By definition, this is a diet that helps patients increase their intake of fruits and vegetables (fiber, antioxidants, phytonutrients), increases their intake of fish (for the anti-inflammatory omega-3 fats EPA and DHA) while reducing intake of the pro-cancer and pro-inflammatory omega-6 fats linoleic acid and arachidonic acid), and it is naturally low in sugars and cholesterol (for alleviating hyperglycemia and dyslipidemia). This dietary pattern helps patients avoid grains, particularly wheat (a common allergen), and it reduces the intake of the high-fermentation carbohydrates in breads, pasta, pastries, potatoes, and sucrose which promote overgrowth of bacteria and yeast in the intestines. Supplementing this pesco-vegetarian diet with vitamins, minerals, fatty acids such as fish oil and GLA (from borage oil), and protein from soy and whey makes this diet effective for both the treatment and prevention of many conditions; I have called this "the Supplemented Paleo-Mediterranean Diet."

1. Vasquez A. A Five-Part Nutritional Protocol that Produces Consistently Positive Results. *Nutritional Wellness* 2005 Sep
2. Vasquez A. Implementing the Five-Part Nutritional Wellness Protocol for the Treatment of Various Health Problems. *Nutritional Wellness* 2005 Nov
3. Vasquez A. Revisiting the Five-Part Nutritional Wellness Protocol: The Supplemented Paleo-Mediterranean Diet. *Nutritional Perspectives* 2011 Jan

---

Consuming the right amount of protein: Dietary protein is eaten to provide the body with amino acids, which are the fundamental components that the body uses to create new tissues (such as skin, mucosal surfaces, hair, and nails), heal wounds (e.g., formation of collagen), fight off infections (e.g., formation of immunoglobulin proteins, antibodies), and to create specific hormones (such as insulin and thyroid hormones) and neurotransmitters, such as dopamine, serotonin, norepinephrine, and gamma-aminobutyric acid (GABA). Amino acid profiles in meats, eggs, and milk/dairy/whey is similar to that of the human body and such dietary sources have been described as containing relatively more "complete protein" than most plant-based protein sources. For plant-based diets without concomitant use of animal proteins to provide sufficient quantity and quality of protein, foods must be combined with respect to one another's amino acid profiles; beyond learned attention to *quality*, additional attention is needed to ensure sufficient *quantitative* intake, especially for vegetarian athletes, particularly those engaged in resistance training.

For most people (without kidney or liver problems) the goal for daily protein intake should be 0.50-0.75 grams of protein per pound of lean body weight, depending on activity level and other health needs (see table). Sufficient dietary protein is essential for patients with musculoskeletal injuries because tissue healing relies on the

---

[92] O'Keefe JH Jr, Cordain L. Cardiovascular disease resulting from a diet and lifestyle at odds with our Paleolithic genome. *Mayo Clin Proc*. 2004 Jan;79(1):101-8
[93] Price WA. *Nutrition and Physical Degeneration*. Santa Monica; Price-Pottinger Nutrition Foundation: 1945
[94] O'Keefe JH Jr, Cordain L. Cardiovascular disease resulting from a diet and lifestyle at odds with our Paleolithic genome. *Mayo Clin Proc*. 2004 Jan;79(1):101-8

constant availability of amino acids and micronutrients[95], which should be supplied by a healthy, balanced, whole-foods diet that may be supplemented with specific vitamins, minerals, and phytonutrients. Low-protein diets suppress immune function, reduce muscle mass, and impair healing[96,97] whereas intakes of higher amounts of protein safely facilitate healing and the maintenance of muscle mass. Increased protein intake does not adversely affect bone health as long as dietary calcium intake is adequate.[98] According to the 1998 review by Lemon[99], "Those involved in strength training might need to consume as much as …1.7 g protein x kg(-1) x day(-1)…while those undergoing endurance training might need about 1.2 to 1.6 g x kg(-1) x day(-1)… **…there is no evidence that protein intakes in the range suggested will have adverse effects in healthy individuals.**"

Recommended Grams of Protein per Patient Profile and Body Weight Per Day		
Patient Profile	*Per* **pound** of weight[100]	*Per* **kilogram** of weight
Infants and children ages 1-6 years[101]	0.45-0.68	0.99-1.4
RDA for sedentary adult and children ages 6-18 years[102]	0.4	0.88
Adult recreational exerciser—average for adults	**0.5-0.75**	**1.1-1.65**
Adult competitive athlete	0.6-0.9	1.32-1.98
Adult building muscle mass	0.7-0.9	1.54-1.98
Dieting athlete	0.7-1.0	1.54-2.2
Growing teenage athlete	0.9-1.0	1.98-2.2
Pregnant women need additional protein	Add 15-30 grams/d[103]	Same

For patients who are completely sedentary, multiply body weight in pounds by 0.4 and this will give the number of grams of protein that should be eaten each day.[104] For patients who are very active (frequent weight lifting, or competitive athlete), multiply body weight in pounds by 0.7-0.9 and this will give the number of grams of protein that should be eaten each day.

Again, compared with sedentary people, *sick people, injured people,* and *athletes* need more protein to maintain weight, fight infections, repair injuries, and build and maintain muscle. Not only can insufficient protein intake cause muscle weakness and loss of weight, but recent articles have also suggested that low-protein diets can cause suppression of the immune system[105] and impairment of healing after injury or surgery.[106]

For example, in most instances and according to the data presented in and reviewed for this section, a person weighing 120 pounds should aim for at least 60 grams of protein per day, or 90 grams of protein per day if he/she is more physically active, ill, or injured. A can of tuna has 30 grams of protein; one egg has 6 grams of protein. If she is going to eat eggs as a source of protein for a meal, she might have to eat as many as five eggs to reach a target of 30 grams of protein per meal. When eating meat, visualize the amount of meat in a can of tuna to estimate the amount of protein being eaten—for example, if the portion of meat at a given meal is about the size of a half can of tuna, then we can estimate that the serving contains 15-20 grams of high-quality protein. By knowing the "target intake" for the day, and by estimating the amount of protein eaten with each meal, patients will be able to modify their protein intake to ensure that they reach their protein intake goal.

Protein supplements—most common of which are based on concentrates of or isolated components of egg, soy, or cow's milk— can be used *in conjunction with a healthy diet*. Patients using a protein supplement should eat a healthy diet and then add protein supplements between regular meals. If they substitute a protein supplement for

---

[95] "Supplementation with protein and vitamins, specifically arginine and vitamins A, B, and C, provides optimum nutrient support of the healing wound." Meyer NA, Muller MJ, Herndon DN. Nutrient support of the healing wound. *New Horiz* 1994 May;2(2):202-14
[96] Castaneda et al. Elderly women accommodate to a low-protein diet with losses of body cell mass, muscle function, and immune response. *Am J Clin Nutr* 1995 Jul;62(1):30-9
[97] [No author listed]. Vegetarians and healing. *JAMA* 1995; 273: 910
[98] Heaney RP. Excess dietary protein may not adversely affect bone. *J Nutr* 1998 Jun;128(6):1054-7
[99] Lemon PW. Effects of exercise on dietary protein requirements. *Int J Sport Nutr* 1998 Dec;8(4):426-47
[100] Slightly modified from Nancy Clark, MS, RD. Protein Power. *The Physician and Sportsmedicine* 1996, volume 24, number 4
[101] 1.5-1 g/kg/d (0.68-0.45 grams per pound of body weight. Younger people need proportionately more protein.) Brown ML (ed). *Present Knowledge in Nutrition. Sixth Edition*. Washington DC: International Life Sciences Institute Nutrition Foundation; 1990 page 68
[102] 0.83 g.kg-1.d-1 (equivalent to 0.37 grams per pound of body weight) Pellet PL. Protein requirements in humans. *Am J Clin Nutr* 1990 May;51:723-37
[103] Weinsier RL, Morgan SL (eds). *Fundamentals of Clinical Nutrition*. St. Louis: Mosby, 1993 page 50
[104] Pellet PL. Protein requirements in humans. *Am J Clin Nutr* 1990 May;51(5):723-37
[105] Castaneda et al. Elderly women accommodate to a low-protein diet with losses of body cell mass, muscle function, and immune response. *Am J Clin Nutr* 1995 Jul;62:30-9
[106] Vegetarians and healing. *Journal of the American Medical Association* 1995; 273: 910

a regular meal, then they may not actually increase protein intake. Whole *real* foods should form the foundation for the diet—patients should not rely too heavily on *protein supplements* when patients can get better results *and improved overall health* with *whole foods*. Whey, casein, and lactalbumin are proteins from milk and dairy products, and may therefore be allergenic in people allergic to cow's milk; however, I (DrV) generally enjoy and endorse the use of whey protein isolate given its high-quality protein, convenience, low cost, antioxidant benefits via glutathione precursors, satiating effect via tryptophan provision, gut-healing effects and immune-supporting and anti-dysbiotic immunoglobulins. Soy protein is safe and a source of high-quality protein for adults[107], and research shows that consumption of soy protein can help reduce the risk of cancer and heart disease[108]; however, I do not recommend the use of large quantities of supplemental soy protein for pregnant women, or for children due to the potential for disrupting endocrine function. Patients may have to experiment with different products until they find one that is suitable in regard to taste, texture, digestibility, hypoallergenicity, nutritional effects, ease of preparation, and affordability.

> **Proteins, fruits, vegetables—not grains**
>
> "Historical and archaeological evidence shows hunter-gatherers generally to be lean, fit, and largely free from signs and symptoms of chronic diseases. When hunter-gatherer societies transitioned to an agricultural grain-based diet, their general health deteriorated. ... When former hunter-gatherers adopt Western lifestyles, obesity, type-2 diabetes, atherosclerosis, and other diseases of civilization become commonplace."
>
> O'Keefe JH Jr, Cordain L. Cardiovascular disease resulting from a diet and lifestyle at odds with our Paleolithic genome. *Mayo Clin Proc.* 2004;79:101-8

Recall again that the goal is *improved health*, not simply *adequate protein intake*. If we focus solely on "grams of protein" then we might overlook adverse effects that are associated with certain protein sources. Cow's milk is a high quality protein, but it is commonly allergenic and can exacerbate joint pain in sensitive individuals.[109] Beef, liver, pork and other land animal meats are excellent sources of protein, but they are also generally rich sources of arachidonic acid[110] (if not grass-fed) and iron[111], both of which have been shown to exacerbate joint pain and inflammation. Fish is an excellent source of protein, but fish are often poisoned with mercury and other toxicants, which can be ingested by humans to produce negative health effects.[112,113]

Most patients (and doctors) need to increase consumption of fruits and vegetables: Encourage consumption of collard greens, broccoli, kale, spinach, chard, lettuce, onions, red peppers, green beans, carrots, apples, oranges, nuts, blueberries and other fruits and vegetables. Patients can find or make a good low-carbohydrate dressing (such as lemon-garlic tahini[114]) to make these vegetables taste great. Fresh fruits and vegetables are best; but frozen fruits and vegetables are acceptable. Patients can buy a package of (organic) frozen vegetables; then when they are ready for a healthy-and-fast meal, simply thaw the vegetables or warm/steam them on the stovetop. In just a few minutes and with only minimal effort, by regularly eating vegetables, they will have significantly reduced their risk for heart disease, diabetes, cancer, hemorrhoids, constipation, and many other chronic health problems. Using frozen vegetables and eating vegetables only twice per day is not *optimal*—it is *minimal*. For many patients, consuming two servings of vegetables per day is a major lifestyle change. Ultimately, the goal is for fresh fruits and vegetables to form a major portion of the diet, to be the main course rather than simply a side dish. A diet based on fruits and vegetables is a powerful nutritional strategy for reducing the risk for cancer, heart disease, and autoimmune and inflammatory disorders.[115]

Phytochemicals—important antioxidant and anti-inflammatory nutrients from fruits, vegetables, nuts, seeds, berries, and many herbs and spices: While we have all commonly thought of the benefits of fruits and vegetables as being derived from the vitamins, minerals, and fiber, we are learning from new research that many if not most

---

[107] "These results indicate that for healthy adults, the isolated soy protein is of high nutritional quality, comparable to that of animal protein sources, and that the methionine content is not limiting for adult protein maintenance." Young et al. Evaluation of the protein quality of an isolated soy protein in young men: relative nitrogen requirements and effect of methionine supplementation. *Am J Clin Nutr.* 1984 Jan;39(1):16-24
[108] Lissin LW, Cooke JP. Phytoestrogens and cardiovascular health. *J Am Coll Cardiol.* 2000 May;35(6):1403-10
[109] Golding DN. Is there an allergic synovitis? *J R Soc Med* 1990 May;83(5):312-4
[110] Adam O, et al. Anti-inflammatory effects of a low arachidonic acid diet and fish oil in patients with rheumatoid arthritis. *Rheumatol Int* 2003 Jan;23(1):27-36
[111] Dabbagh AJ, Trenam CW, Morris CJ, Blake DR. Iron in joint inflammation. *Ann Rheum Dis* 1993; 52:67-73
[112] "These fish often harbor high levels of methylmercury, a potent human neurotoxin." Evans EC. The FDA recommendations on fish intake during pregnancy. *J Obstet Gynecol Neonatal Nurs* 2002 Nov-Dec;31(6):715-20
[113] "Geometric mean mercury levels were almost 4-fold higher among women who ate 3 or more servings of fish in the past 30 days compared with women who ate no fish in that period.." Schober SE, et al. Blood mercury levels in US children and women of childbearing age, 1999-2000. *JAMA* 2003 Apr 2;289(13):1667-74
[114] Mollie Katzen. *The New Moosewood Cookbook*, Ten Speed Press; page 103
[115] "...one of the most consistent research findings is that those who consume higher amounts of fruits and vegetables have lower rates of heart disease and stroke as well as cancer..." Seaman DR. The diet-induced proinflammatory state: a cause of chronic pain and other degenerative diseases? *J Manipulative Physiol Ther.* 2002;25(3):168-79

of the health-promoting benefits of fruit and vegetable consumption comes from the unique plant-based chemicals—phytochemicals—contained therein. For example, while in the past we might have thought of the benefits of eating apples as being derived from the vitamin C content, we now know that vitamin C only provides 0.4% of the antioxidant action contained within a whole apple—obviously the other components of the apple, namely the phenolic compounds are responsible for most of an apple's antioxidant activity.[116] Recent research has shown that cranberries, apples, red grapes, and strawberries have the most antioxidant power of the fruits[117], while red peppers, broccoli, carrots, and spinach are the best antioxidant vegetables[118]; see the tables that follow. This is a very important concept to appreciate and remember: **the benefits derived from fruits and vegetables are _not_ derived principally from the vitamins and therefore can never be obtained from the use of multivitamin pills as a substitute for whole foods. Multivitamin and multimineral supplements are valuable and worthwhile _supplements_ to a whole-foods diet but should not be used as _substitutes_ for a whole-foods diet. Fruits and vegetables contain more than 8,000 phytochemicals, most of which have anti-inflammatory, anti-proliferative, and anti-cancer benefits**[119]—**the best and only way to benefit from these chemicals is to change the diet in favor of relying principally on fruits and vegetables as the major component of the diet**, and the easiest way to do this is to eliminate carbohydrate-rich antioxidant-poor foods such as bread, pasta, rice, sweets, crackers, chips and "junk foods."

Phenolic content and antioxidant capacity of common vegetables and fruits[120,121]

Vegetables		Fruits	
Phenolic content	**Antioxidant capacity**	**Phenolic content**	**Antioxidant capacity**
1. Broccoli	1. Red pepper	1. Cranberry	1. Cranberry
2. Spinach	2. Broccoli	2. Apple	2. Apple
3. Yellow onion	3. Carrot	3. Red grape	3. Red grape
4. Red pepper	4. Spinach	4. Strawberry	4. Strawberry
5. Carrot	5. Cabbage	5. Pineapple	5. Peach
6. Cabbage	6. Yellow onion	6. Banana	6. Lemon
7. Potato	7. Celery	7. Peach	7. Pear
8. Lettuce	8. Potato	8. Lemon	8. Banana
9. Celery	9. Lettuce	9. Orange	9. Orange
10. Cucumber	10. Cucumber	10. Pear	10. Grapefruit
		11. Grapefruit	11. Pineapple

Different fruits and vegetables contain different types, quantities, and ratios of vitamins, minerals, and phytochemicals; therefore, **_dietary diversity_ will therefore help patients obtain a broad spectrum of and maximum benefit from these different nutrients**. Taking appropriate action with the data that a fruit/vegetable-based diet has powerful health-promoting benefits means that we as doctors and patients have to change our lifestyles with regard to how we plan our meals, what we buy, what we prepare, and what we eat. Behavior modification is a tremendous challenge for people, especially those who lack sufficient motivation or insight. This text is providing the _insight_—the data, references, and concepts. But without _motivation_—from doctors to help their patients attain the highest levels of health, and from patients to change their lifestyles to become as healthy as possible—the research itself does little to promote health.

Many people (most Americans especially) need to increase potassium intake: The physiologic effect of potassium is influenced by the potassium:sodium ratio (sodium reduces effectiveness and retention of potassium),

---

[116] "We propose that the additive and synergistic effects of phytochemicals in fruit and vegetables are responsible for their potent antioxidant and anticancer activities, and that the benefit of a diet rich in fruit and vegetables is attributed to the complex mixture of phytochemicals present in whole foods." Liu RH. Health benefits of fruit and vegetables are from additive and synergistic combinations of phytochemicals. _Am J Clin Nutr_. 2003 Sep;78(3 Suppl):517S-520S
[117] "Cranberry had the highest total antioxidant activity (177.0 +/- 4.3 micromol of vitamin C equiv/g of fruit), followed by apple, red grape, strawberry, peach, lemon, pear, banana, orange, grapefruit, and pineapple." Sun et al. Antioxidant and antiproliferative activities of common fruits. _J Agric Food Chem_. 2002 Dec 4;50(25):7449-54
[118] "Red pepper had the highest total antioxidant activity, followed by broccoli, carrot, spinach, cabbage, yellow onion, celery, potato, lettuce, and cucumber." Chu YF, Sun J, Wu X, Liu RH. Antioxidant and antiproliferative activities of common vegetables. _J Agric Food Chem_. 2002 Nov 6;50(23):6910-6
[119] Liu RH. Health benefits of fruit and vegetables are from additive and synergistic combinations of phytochemicals. _Am J Clin Nutr_. 2003 Sep;78(3 Suppl):517S-520S
[120] Chu YF, Sun J, Wu X, Liu RH. Antioxidant and antiproliferative activities of common vegetables. _J Agric Food Chem_. 2002;50:6910-6
[121] Sun J, Chu YF, Wu X, Liu RH. Antioxidant and antiproliferative activities of common fruits. _J Agric Food Chem_. 2002;50:7449-54

potassium:chloride ratio (chloride reduces effectiveness and retention of potassium), and the overall pH/acid-base balance of the human host (i.e., metabolic acidosis reduces effectiveness and retention of potassium, while an alkaline state improves retention and effectiveness of potassium). Importantly, magnesium status is an important positive-direct determinant of potassium status, particularly in patients with recalcitrant hypokalemia and/or hyperaldosteronism.[122] Respective amounts of potassium per serving of food or juice (1 cup = 8 fluid ounces =240 milliliters) are provided in the table below; renal insufficiency and potassium-sparing drugs/diuretics promote hyperkalemia, generally contraindicate high intake of potassium, and mandate periodic assessment of serum potassium.

Potassium content of common foods

Food serving	Potassium in mg (Na as available)
One papaya	780
One cup of mixed vegetable juice	740 (35-630 mg Na)
One cup of prune juice	700
One cup of carrot juice	520 (160 mg Na)
One cup plain low-fat yogurt	510 (150 mg Na)
One cup of cantaloupe	490
One cup of orange juice	470
One small banana	465
One cup of honeydew melon	460
One-third cup of raisins	365
One cup of carrot-orange juice	360 (35 mg Na)
One medium mango	320
One medium kiwi	250
One small orange	240
One medium pear	210

The importance of potassium

"**Adults should consume at least 4.7 grams of potassium per day to lower blood pressure**, blunt the effects of salt, and reduce the risk of kidney stones and bone loss. However, most American women 31 to 50 years old consume no more than half of the recommended amount of potassium, and men's intake is only moderately higher."

Food and Nutrition Board of the Institute of Medicine of the National Academies. "Dietary Reference Intakes: Water, Potassium, Sodium, Chloride, and Sulfate." Released: February 11, 2004
iom.edu/Reports/2004/Dietary-Reference-Intakes-Water-Potassium-Sodium-Chloride-and-Sulfate.aspx

Antihypertensive mechanisms of potassium include vasodilator activity, diuretic and naturietic effects, and suppression of renin, angiotensin, and adrenergic tone.[123] In February 2004, the Institute of Medicine (IOM) set the Adequate Intake of potassium for adults at 4.7 grams a day—more than double previous recommendations; more than 90% of American adults do not meet these recommendations. If 90% of the population is not meeting recommended intakes of potassium, and these recommendations from the IOM come after an extensive review of the scientific literature, then potassium assessment and supplementation should be routine components of patient care; furthermore, this shows to the inadequacy of current laboratory assessments for evaluating potassium status and potassium balance.

- Randomized trial with 1-year follow-up and a title that says it all: Increasing the dietary potassium intake reduces the need for antihypertensive medication (*Annals of Internal Med* 1991 Nov): Forty-seven patients with medication-controlled hypertension completed one year of dietary treatment (or control nonintervention); dietary intervention focused on potassium-rich foods, with compliance monitored by 3-day food records and 24-hour urinary potassium excretion. Results showed: "After 1 year, the average drug consumption (number of pills per day) relative to that at baseline was 24% in group 1 (potassium-rich diet) and 60% in group 2 (control diet). By the end of the study, blood pressure could be controlled using less than 50% of the initial [drug] therapy in 81% of the patients in group 1 compared with 29% of the patients in group 2. ... CONCLUSION: Increasing the dietary potassium intake from natural foods is a feasible and effective measure to reduce antihypertensive drug treatment."

---

[122] "Magnesium deficiency is frequently associated with hypokalemia. Concomitant magnesium deficiency aggravates hypokalemia and renders it refractory to treatment by potassium. Herein is reviewed literature suggesting that magnesium deficiency exacerbates potassium wasting by increasing distal potassium secretion. A decrease in intracellular magnesium, caused by magnesium deficiency, releases the magnesium-mediated inhibition of ROMK channels and increases potassium secretion. Magnesium deficiency alone, however, does not necessarily cause hypokalemia. An increase in distal sodium delivery or elevated aldosterone levels may be required for exacerbating potassium wasting in magnesium deficiency." Huang CL, Kuo E. Mechanism of hypokalemia in magnesium deficiency. *J Am Soc Nephrol*. 2007 Oct;18(10):2649-52
[123] Patki et al. Efficacy of potassium and magnesium in essential hypertension: a double-blind, placebo controlled, crossover study. *BMJ*. 1990 Sep 15;301(6751):521-3

Eat "complex carbohydrates"—emphasizing whole foods and avoiding grains and sugars—to stabilize blood sugar, mood, and energy: Choose items with a "low glycemic index"[124] to stabilize blood sugar and—for many people—to lower triglycerides and cholesterol levels. Foods with a low Glycemic Index (GI < 55)[125] include yogurt, apple (36), whole orange (43), peach (28), legumes, lentils (28), and soybeans (18), cherries, dried apricots, nuts, most meats, and most vegetables. Foods that have both a low *glycemic index* as well as a low *glycemic load* include: apples, carrots, chick peas, grapes, green peas, kidney beans, oranges, peaches, peanuts, pears, pinto beans, red lentils, and strawberries.[126]

Reduce or eliminate simple sugars from the diet (as necessary): Nearly everyone should minimize intake of table sugar (sucrose), fructose and high-fructose corn syrup, and all artificial sweeteners. Of important and recent note, high-fructose corn syrup has been shown to be contaminated by mercury due to the manufacturing process[127], and fructose has been shown to induce hypertension and the metabolic syndrome in humans.[128] Chronic overconsumption of refined carbohydrates promotes disease by 1) increasing urinary excretion of magnesium and calcium, 2) inducing oxidative stress, 3) promoting fat deposition and obesity, which then generally leads to insulin resistance and hyperinsulinemia with an increase in production of cholesterol, triglycerides, and proinflammatory adipokines[129], and 4) reducing function of leukocytes.[130] Among sweeteners, honey is the best choice since it is the only natural sweetener available with a wide range of health-promoting benefits including anti-inflammatory, antibacterial, antioxidant and anti-allergy effects.[131] Also consider the herb stevia as a non-caloric and nutritive sweetener. Occasional intake of sweets is likely to be of little consequence for people who are generally healthy and who are willing to sustain relatively short-term endothelial dysfunction[132], oxidative stress[133], increased LDL oxidation[134], and activation of NF-kappaB[135] as a result of their self-induced hyperglycemia. Postexertional hyperglycemia can be used to enhance athletic performance by sustaining and inducing glycogen storage following and during exercise (i.e., carbohydrate loading for glycogen "supercompensation"[136,137]). Similarly, consumption of "simple" carbohydrate without protein can be used to promote entry of tryptophan across the blood-brain barrier and into the brain to promote serotonin synthesis.[138] In summary, *habitual overconsumption* of simple carbohydrates promotes disease by numerous oxidative and pro-inflammatory mechanisms, while conversely *periodic consumption* of simple carbohydrates can be used to promote athletic performance and to increase brain tryptophan uptake and thus serotonin synthesis for the promotion of enhanced mood and cognitive performance and for the regulation of food intake.

---

[124] For more information on glycemic index, consult a nutrition book or website such as stanford.edu/~dep/gilists.htm
[125] Janette Brand-Miller, Kaye Foster-Powell. Diets with a low glycemic index. *Nutr Today* 1999 Mar findarticles.com/cf_dls/m0841/2_34/54654508/p1/article.jhtml
[126] Mendosa D. Glycemic Values of Common American Foods mendosa.com/common_foods.htm Accessed on August 4, 2004
[127] "Average daily consumption of high fructose corn syrup is about 50 grams per person in the United States. With respect to total mercury exposure, it may be necessary to account for this source of mercury in the diet of children and sensitive populations." Dufault et al. Mercury from chlor-alkali plants. *Environ Health*. 2009 Jan 26;8:2. See also: "High fructose corn syrup has been shown to contain trace amounts of mercury as a result of some manufacturing processes, and its consumption can also lead to zinc loss." Dufault et al. Mercury exposure, nutritional deficiencies and metabolic disruptions may affect learning in children. *Behav Brain Funct*. 2009 Oct 27;5:44.
[128] News release from American Heart Association's 63rd High Blood Pressure Research Conference. High-sugar diet increases men's blood pressure; gout drug protective. Abstract P127. Sept. 23, 2009. americanheart.mediaroom.com/index.php?s=43&item=829 Accessed December 19, 2009
[129] "Because visceral and subcutaneous adipose tissues are the major sources of cytokines (adipokines), increased adipose tissue mass is associated with alteration in adipokine production (eg, overexpression of tumor necrosis factor-a, interleukin-6, plasminogen activator inhibitor-1, and underexpression of adiponectin in adipose tissue)." Aldhahi W, Hamdy O. Adipokines, inflammation, and the endothelium in diabetes. *Curr Diab Rep*. 2003 Aug;3(4):293-8
[130] Sanchez A, et al. Role of sugars in human neutrophilic phagocytosis. *Am J Clin Nutr*. 1973 Nov;26(11):1180-4
[131] Al-Waili NS. Effects of daily consumption of honey solution on hematological indices and blood levels of minerals and enzymes. *J Med Food*. 2003 Summer;6(2):135-4
[132] "Modest hyperinsulinemia, mimicking fasting hyperinsulinemia of insulin-resistant states, abrogates endothelium-dependent vasodilation in large conduit arteries, probably by increasing oxidant stress. These data may provide a novel pathophysiological basis to the epidemiological link between hyperinsulinemia/insulin-resistance and atherosclerosis in humans." Arcaro G, et al. Insulin causes endothelial dysfunction in humans: sites and mechanisms. *Circulation*. 2002 Feb 5;105(5):576-82
[133] "Hyperglycemia increased plasma MDA concentrations, but the activities of GSH-Px and SOD were significantly higher after a larger dose of glucose only. Plasma catecholamines were unchanged. These results indicate that the transient increase of plasma catecholamine and insulin concentrations did not induce oxidative damage, while glucose already in the low dose was an important triggering factor for oxidative stress." Koska J, Blazicek P, Marko M, Grna JD, Kvetnansky R, Vigas M. Insulin, catecholamines, glucose and antioxidant enzymes in oxidative damage during different loads in healthy humans. *Physiol Res*. 2000;49 Suppl 1:S95-100
[134] "In conclusion, insulin at physiological doses is associated with increased LDL peroxidation independent of the presence of hyperglycemia." Quinones-Galvan et al. Evidence that acute insulin administration enhances LDL cholesterol susceptibility to oxidation in healthy humans. *Arterioscler Thromb Vasc Biol*. 1999 Dec;19(12):2928-32
[135] "These data show that the intake of a mixed meal results in significant inflammatory changes characterized by a decrease in IkappaBalpha and an increase in NF-kappaB binding, plasma CRP, and the expression of IKKalpha, IKKbeta, and p47(phox) subunit." Aljada A, Mohanty P, Ghanim H, Abdo T, Tripathy D, Chaudhuri A, Dandona P. Increase in intranuclear nuclear factor kappaB and decrease in inhibitor kappaB in mononuclear cells after a mixed meal. *Am J Clin Nutr*. 2004 Apr;79(4):682-90
[136] "A significant glycogen sparing, as well as supercompensation within 24 h of recovery, was observed after [carbohydrate] supplementation." Brouns F, Saris WH, Beckers E, Adlercreutz H, et al. Metabolic changes induced by sustained exhaustive cycling and diet manipulation. *Int J Sports Med*. 1989 May;10 Suppl 1:S49-62
[137] "The accepted method of increasing muscle glycogen stores is by "glycogen loading," which classically involves depletion of muscle glycogen, usually by exercise, followed by consumption of a high-CHO diet for several days (e.g., 3, 39). ...increase muscle glycogen concentrations ([glycogen]) to between 150 and 200% of normal resting levels." Robinson et al. Role of submaximal exercise in promoting creatine and glycogen accumulation in human skeletal muscle. *J Appl Physiol*. 1999 Aug;87(2):598-604
[138] "Our results suggest that high-carbohydrate meals have an influence on serotonin synthesis. We predict that carbohydrates with a high glycemic index would have a greater serotoninergic effect than carbohydrates with a low glycemic index." Lyons PM, Truswell AS. Serotonin precursor influenced by type of carbohydrate meal in healthy adults. *Am J Clin Nutr*. 1988 Mar;47(3):433-9

Avoid artificial sweeteners, colors and other additives: Absolutely never use **aspartame**—this is a synthetic chemical that is easily converted to the toxin formaldehyde.[139] Aspartame causes cancer in animals and is strongly linked to brain tumors in humans.[140,141] **Sodium benzoate** is a food preservative that can cause asthma[142] and skin rashes[143] in sensitive individuals. **Tartrazine (yellow dye #5)** is a food/drug coloring agent that can cause asthma and skin rashes in sensitive individuals.[144] **Carrageenan** is a naturally-occurring carbohydrate extracted from red seaweed. Common sources of carrageenan are certain brands of "rice milk" and "soy milk." In addition to suppressing immune function[145], carrageenan causes intestinal ulcers and inflammatory bowel disease in animals[146] and some research indicates that carrageenan consumption is associated with an increased risk for cancer in humans.[147,148]

Consume sufficient daily water in the form of water and health-promoting teas and juices: Daily "water" intake should be approximately 30 ml/kg; thus, for a 150-lb (70-kg) person, fluid intake should be at least 2.1 liters, and for a person who weighs 220 lbs (100 kg) the daily intake should be approximately 3 liters. More fluids may be used during times of exercise, heat exposure, illness, or detoxification, while fluid restriction can be indicated in patients with heart failure, renal failure, anasarca (generalized edema), and hyponatremia.

Consider reducing or eliminating caffeine: This is especially important for people with reactive hypoglycemia, insomnia, anxiety, hypertension, low-back pain, and for women with fibrocystic breast disease. Caffeine ingestion also leads to the activation of brain noradrenergic receptors; activation of noradrenergic receptors can cause inhibition of dopaminergic neurotransmission.[149] For people who are in good health, 1-3 servings of caffeine per day are not harmful. Herbal teas in general and green tea in particular have significant health-promoting effects due to their phytonutrient components and antioxidant, anti-inflammatory, and anticancer properties.

To the extent possible, eat "organic" foods rather than industrially-produced foods: Organic foods (i.e., foods which are *naturally grown* rather than being treated with insect poisons, synthetic fertilizers, and chemicals to enhance shelf-life) tend to cost more than chemically-produced foods; but the increased phytonutrient content justifies the cost. Organic foods contain more nutrients than do chemically-produced foods.[150] More importantly, recent research has also indicated that organic foods are better able to prevent the genetic damage that can lead to cancer than are foods that have been grown in an environment of artificial fertilizers and pesticides.[151]

- Reduction in urinary organophosphate pesticide metabolites in adults after a week-long organic diet. (*Environ Res* 2014 Jul[152]): Industrial/corporate food production commonly uses organophosphate (OP) pesticides; this prospective, randomised, crossover study was conducted to determine if an organic food diet reduces organophosphate exposure in adults. "Thirteen participants were randomly allocated to consume a diet of at least 80% organic or conventional food for 7 days and then crossed over to the opposite diet. Urinary levels of six dialkylphosphate (DAP) metabolites were analysed in first-morning voids collected on day 8 of each phase using GC-MS/MS with detection limits of 0.11-0.51µg/L. RESULTS: The mean total DAP results in the organic phase were 89% lower than in the conventional phase. For total

---

[139] Trocho C, et al. Formaldehyde derived from dietary aspartame binds to tissue components in vivo. *Life Sci*. 1998;63(5):337-4949
[140] Compared to other environmental factors putatively linked to brain tumors, the artificial sweetener aspartame is a promising candidate to explain the recent increase in incidence and degree of malignancy of brain tumors. ...exceedingly high incidence of brain tumors in aspartame-fed rats compared to no brain tumors in concurrent controls..." Olney JW, Farber NB, Spitznagel E, Robins LN. Increasing brain tumor rates: is there a link to aspartame? *J Neuropathol Exp Neurol* 1996;55(11):1115-23
[141] Russell Blaylock MD. *Excitotoxins*. Health Press; December 1996 [ISBN: 0929173252] Pages 211-214
[142] "Adverse reactions to benzoate in this patient required avoidance of some drugs, some of those classically prescribed under the form of syrups in asthma." Petrus M, Bonaz S, Causse E, Rhabbour M, Moulie N, Netter JC, Bildstein G. [Asthma and intolerance to benzoates] [Article in French] *Arch Pediatr*. 1996;3(10):984-7
[143] Munoz FJ, et al. Perioral contact urticaria from sodium benzoate in a toothpaste. *Contact Dermatitis*. 1996 Jul;35(1):51
[144] "Tartrazine sensitivity is most frequently manifested by urticaria and asthma... Vasculitis, purpura and contact dermatitis infrequently occur as manifestations of tartrazine sensitivity." Dipalma JR. Tartrazine sensitivity. *Am Fam Physician*. 1990 Nov;42(5):1347-50
[145] "Impairment of complement activity and humoral responses to T-dependent antigens, depression of cell-mediated immunity, prolongation of graft survival and potentiation of tumour growth by carrageenans have been reported." Thomson AW, Fowler EF. Carrageenan: a review of its effects on the immune system. *Agents Actions*. 1981;11:265-73
[146] Watt J, Marcus R. Experimental ulcerative disease of the colon. *Methods Achiev Exp Pathol*. 1975;7:56-71
[147] Tobacman JK. Review of harmful gastrointestinal effects of carrageenan in animal experiments. *Environ Health Perspect*. 2001 Oct;109(10):983-94
[148] "However, the gum carrageenan which is comprised of linked, sulfated galactose residues has potent biological activity and undergoes acid hydrolysis to poligeenan, an acknowledged carcinogen." Tobacman JK, Wallace RB, Zimmerman MB. Consumption of carrageenan and other water-soluble polymers used as food additives and incidence of mammary carcinoma. *Med Hypotheses*. 2001 May;56(5):589-98
[149] "The results suggest that noradrenergic innervation of dopamine cells can directly inhibit the activity of dopamine cells." Paladini CA, Williams JT. Noradrenergic inhibition of midbrain dopamine neurons. *J Neurosci*. 2004 May 12;24(19):4568-75
[150] Smith B. Organic Foods versus Supermarket Foods: element levels. *Journal of Applied Nutrition* 1993; 45(1), p35-9
[151] "Against BaP, three species of OC vegetables showed 30-57% antimutagenecity, while GC ones did only 5-30%." Ren H, Endo H, Hayashi T. The superiority of organically cultivated vegetables to general ones regarding antimutagenic activities. *Mutat Res*. 2001 Sep 20;496(1-2):83-8
[152] Oates L, Cohen M, Braun L, et al. Reduction in urinary organophosphate pesticide metabolites in adults after a week-long organic diet. *Environ Res*. 2014 Jul;132:105-11

dimethyl DAPs there was a 96% reduction. Mean total diethyl DAP levels in the organic phase were half [-50% reduction] those of the conventional phase, yet the wide variability and small sample size meant the difference was not statistically significant. CONCLUSIONS: The consumption of an organic diet for one week significantly reduced organophosphate pesticide exposure in adults. Larger scale studies in different populations are required to confirm these findings and investigate their clinical relevance."

Recognize the importance of avoiding food allergens: Biomedical research has established that adverse food reactions, regardless of the underlying mechanisms or classification of allergy, intolerance, or sensitivity, can exacerbate a wide range of human illnesses, including thyroid disease[153], mental depression[154,155], asthma, rhinitis,[156] recurrent otitis media[157], migraine[158,159,160], attention deficit and hyperactivity disorders[161], epilepsy[162,163,164], gastrointestinal inflammation[165], hypertension[166], joint pain and inflammation[167,168,169,170,171,172,173,174] and a wide range of other health problems. Any program of health promotion and health maintenance must include consideration of food allergies, food intolerances, and food sensitivities. The elimination-and-challenge technique is the most cost-effective and it also teaches patients how to identify their own food allergies and intolerances, which may change for the better or worse over time; when the patient is empowered with this technique, he/she can take an active and on-going role in his/her own healthcare. Patients may be allergic to foods that are generally considered healthy, including whole organic foods. The more common food allergens—exemplified here by a list of offending foods identified in a study of patients with migraine[175]—are wheat (78%), orange (65%), eggs (45%), tea and coffee (40% each), chocolate and milk (37%) each), beef (35%), and corn, cane sugar, and yeast (33% each).

Avoid microwave heating/cooking: Microwave ovens have been noted to exude electromagnetic radiation and may also structurally change native amino acids, forming racemic derivatives that might have no nutritional value (e.g., when converted from the natural L isomer to the abnormal R isomer) and/or toxic effects. In his extensive and clinically-experienced review of the nutrition literature, Gaby[176] writes, "Microwaving of infant formulas caused racemization of some amino acids that did not occur with conventional heating. One of these racemized amino acids, D-proline, has been shown to be neurotoxic, nephrotoxic, and hepatotoxic."

Supplement the health-promoting whole-foods diet with specific vitamins, minerals, fatty acids, and probiotics: Despite the fact that America is one of the richest nations on earth, and that we produce more than enough food to feed ourselves and many other nations with a healthy diet, Americans tend to have poor dietary habits and

---

[153] Sategna-Guidetti et al. Prevalence of thyroid disorders in untreated adult celiac disease patients and effect of gluten withdrawal. *Am J Gastroenterol*. 2001 Mar;96(3):751-7
[154] "The detection and treatment of psychological dysfunction related to food intolerance with particular reference to the problem of objective evaluation is discussed... Long-term follow-up revealed maintenance of marked improvements in psychological and physical functioning." Mills N. Depression and food intolerance: a single case study. *Hum Nutr Appl Nutr*. 1986 Apr;40(2):141-5
[155] "OBJECTIVE: To describe a patient with food intolerance probably contributing to depressive symptoms, intolerance to psychotropic medication and treatment resistance... RESULTS: The patient's course improved considerably with an elimination diet." Parker G, Watkins T. Treatment-resistant depression: when antidepressant drug intolerance may indicate food intolerance. *Aust N Z J Psychiatry*. 2002 Apr;36(2):263-5
[156] Speer F. The allergic child. *Am Fam Physician*. 1975 Feb;11(2):88-94
[157] Juntti H, Tikkanen S, Kokkonen J, Alho OP, Niinimaki A. Cow's milk allergy is associated with recurrent otitis media during childhood. *Acta Otolaryngol*. 1999;119:867-73
[158] "Foods which provoked migraine in 9 patients with severe migraine refractory to drug therapy were identified... These observations confirm that a food-allergic reaction is the cause of migraine in this group of patients." Monro J, Carini C, Brostoff J. Migraine is a food-allergic disease. *Lancet*. 1984 Sep 29;2(8405):719-21
[159] Egger J, Carter CM, Wilson J, et al. Is migraine food allergy? A double-blind controlled trial of oligoantigenic diet treatment. *Lancet*. 1983 Oct 15;2(8355):865-9
[160] Monro J, Brostoff J, Carini C, Zilkha K. Food allergy in migraine. Study of dietary exclusion and RAST. *Lancet*. 1980 Jul 5;2(8184):1-4
[161] Boris M, Mandel FS. Foods and additives are common causes of the attention deficit hyperactive disorder in children. *Ann Allergy*. 1994 May;72(5):462-8
[162] Egger J, Carter CM, Soothill JF, Wilson J. Oligoantigenic diet treatment of children with epilepsy and migraine. *J Pediatr*. 1989;114(1):51-8
[163] Pelliccia et al. Partial cryptogenetic epilepsy and food allergy/intolerance. Reflections on three clinical cases. *Minerva Pediatr*. 1999 May;51(5):153-7
[164] Frediani T, Lucarelli S, Pelliccia A, Vagnucci B, et al. Allergy and childhood epilepsy: a close relationship? *Acta Neurol Scand*. 2001;104(6):349-52
[165] Marr HY, Chen WC, Lin LH. Food protein-induced enterocolitis syndrome: report of one case. *Acta Paediatr Taiwan*. 2001;42(1):49-52
[166] Grant EC. Food allergies and migraine. *Lancet*. 1979 May 5;1(8123):966-9
[167] "Food allergy appeared to be responsible for the joint symptoms in three patients and in one it was possible to precipitate swelling of a knee due to synovitis with effusion by drinking milk a few hours beforehand, the synovial fluid having mildly inflammatory features and a relatively high eosinophil count." Golding DN. Is there an allergic synovitis? *J R Soc Med*. 1990 May;83(5):312-4
[168] Panush RS. Food induced ("allergic") arthritis: clinical and serologic studies. *J Rheumatol*. 1990 Mar;17(3):291-4
[169] Pacor ML, Lunardi C, Di Lorenzo G, Biasi D, Corrocher R. Food allergy and seronegative arthritis: report of two cases. *Clin Rheumatol*. 2001;20(4):279-81
[170] Schrander JJ, Marcelis C, de Vries MP, van Santen-Hoeufft HM. Does food intolerance play a role in juvenile chronic arthritis? *Br J Rheumatol*. 1997 Aug;36(8):905-8
[171] van de Laar MA, van der Korst JK. Food intolerance in rheumatoid arthritis. I. A double blind, controlled trial of the clinical effects of elimination of milk allergens and azo dyes. *Ann Rheum Dis*. 1992 Mar;51(3):298-302
[172] Haugen MA, Kjeldsen-Kragh J, Forre O. A pilot study of the effect of an elemental diet in the management of rheumatoid arthritis. *Clin Exp Rheumatol*. 1994;12(3):275-9
[173] van de Laar MA, Aalbers M, Bruins FG, et al. Food intolerance in rheumatoid arthritis. II. Clinical and histological aspects. *Ann Rheum Dis*. 1992;51(3):303-6
[174] Panush RS, Stroud RM, Webster EM. Food-induced (allergic) arthritis. Inflammatory arthritis exacerbated by milk. *Arthritis Rheum* 1986; 29(2): 220-6
[175] Grant EC. Food allergies and migraine. *Lancet*. 1979 May 5;1(8123):966-9
[176] Gaby AR. *Nutritional Medicine*. 2011

inadequate levels of nutritional intake that do not meet the minimal standards, such as the Recommended Daily Allowance (RDA, now Daily Reference Intake (DRI)).[177] Many people are under the misperception that if they appear healthy or are even overweight then they could not possibly have nutritional deficiencies. The truths of this matter are that 1) gross/obvious nutritional deficiencies are common among "apparently healthy" individuals, 2) common situations like stress, poor diets, and use of medications predispose people to nutritional deficiencies, 3) hereditary/genetic disorders affect a large portion of the population and lead to an increased need for nutritional intake which can generally only be met with supplementation in addition to a healthy whole-foods diet. Taking a "one-a-day" multivitamin is insufficient for people who truly desire significant benefit from supplementation. These one-a-day preparations generally only provide the minimum daily allowance—this dose is not large enough to provide truly preventive medicine results; also, such one-a-day products tend to contain low-quality nutrients, such as ergocalciferol rather than cholecalciferol[178], cyanocobalamin rather than the hydroxyl-, methyl-, or adenosyl- forms[179], and DL-tocopherol or exclusively L-alpha-tocopherol rather than a mix of tocopherols with a high concentration (generally approximately 40%) of gamma tocopherol.[180] Additional rationale for the routine and case-specific use of nutritional supplements is provided in later sections of this book and in the clinical protocols published in following volumes; the points below serve to introduce a few basic concepts:

- Many people think that eating a "healthy diet" will supply them with the nutrients that they need and that they do not need to take a vitamin supplement. This may have been true 2000 years ago, but today's industrially produced "foods" are generally stripped of much of their nutritional value long before they leave the factory. Industrially-produced fruits and vegetables contain lower quantities of nutrients than does naturally raised "organic" produce.[181]
- The reason that people can be of normal weight or can even be overweight and obese and still have nutrient deficiencies is that the body lowers the metabolic rate when the intake of vitamins and minerals is low. This is referred to as the "physiologic adaptation to marginal malnutrition." Even though people may eat enough calories and protein, they can still suffer from growth retardation and behavioral problems as a result of micronutrient malnutrition, even though they *appear* nourished.[182]
- Most nutrition-oriented doctors will agree that magnesium is one of the most important nutrients, especially for helping prevent heart attack and stroke. **Magnesium deficiency is an epidemic in so-called "developed" nations, with 20-40% of different populations showing objective laboratory evidence of magnesium deficiency.**[183,184,185,186]
- Add to the above that every day we are confronted with more chronic emotional stress and toxic chemicals than has ever before existed on the planet, and it becomes easy to see that basic nutritional support and an organic whole foods diet is just the start of attaining improved health.

<u>**General Guidelines for the Safe Use of Nutritional Supplements**</u>: Supplementation with vitamins and minerals is generally safe, especially if the following guidelines are followed:

- <u>Vitamins and minerals should generally be taken with food in order to eliminate the possibility of nausea and to increase absorption</u>: Most vitamins and other supplements should be taken with food so that nausea is avoided.

---

[177] "Most people do not consume an optimal amount of all vitamins by diet alone. Pending strong evidence of effectiveness from randomized trials, it appears prudent for all adults to take vitamin supplements." Fletcher RH, Fairfield KM. Vitamins for chronic disease prevention in adults: clinical applications. *JAMA* 2002 Jun 19;287(23):3127-9
[178] "Vitamin D(2) potency is less than one third that of vitamin D(3). Physicians resorting to use of vitamin D(2) should be aware of its markedly lower potency and shorter duration of action relative to vitamin D(3)." Armas et al. Vitamin D2 is much less effective than vitamin D3 in humans. *J Clin Endocrinol Metab*. 2004 Nov;89(11):5387-91
[179] Freeman AG. Cyanocobalamin--a case for withdrawal: discussion paper. *J R Soc Med*. 1992 Nov;85(11):686–687
[180] "gamma-tocopherol is the major form of vitamin E in many plant seeds and in the US diet, but has drawn little attention compared with alpha-tocopherol, the predominant form of vitamin E in tissues and the primary form in supplements. However, recent studies indicate that gamma-tocopherol may be important to human health and that it possesses unique features that distinguish it from alpha-tocopherol." Jiang Q, Christen S, Shigenaga MK, Ames BN. gamma-tocopherol, the major form of vitamin E in the US diet, deserves more attention. *Am J Clin Nutr*. 2001 Dec;74(6):714-22 ajcn.org/content/74/6/714.full.pdf
[181] Smith B. Organic Foods versus Supermarket Foods: element levels. *Journal of Applied Nutrition* 1993; 45(1), p35-9
[182] Allen LH. The nutrition CRSP: what is marginal malnutrition, and does it affect human function? *Nutr Rev* 1993 Sep;51(9):255-67
[183] "The American diet is low in magnesium, and with modern water systems, very little is ingested in the drinking water." Innerarity S. Hypomagnesemia in acute and chronic illness. *Crit Care Nurs Q*. 2000 Aug;23(2):1-19
[184] "Altogether 43% of 113 trauma patients had low magnesium levels compared to 30% of noninjured cohorts." Frankel et al. Hypomagnesemia in trauma patients. *World J Surg*. 1999 Sep;23(9):966-9
[185] "There was a 20% overall prevalence of hypomagnesemia among this predominantly female, African American population." Fox et al. An investigation of hypomagnesemia among ambulatory urban African Americans. *J Fam Pract*. 1999 Aug;48(8):636-9
[186] "Suboptimal levels were detected in 33.7 per cent of the population under study. These data clearly demonstrate that the Mg supply of the German population needs increased attention." Schimatschek HF, Rempis R. Prevalence of hypomagnesemia in an unselected German population of 16,000 individuals. *Magnes Res*. 2001 Dec;14(4):283-90

- Iron is potentially harmful: Iron promotes the formation of reactive oxygen species ("free radicals") and is thus implicated in several diseases, such as infections, cancer, liver disease, diabetes, and cardiovascular disease. Iron supplements should not be consumed except by people who have been definitively diagnosed with iron deficiency by measurement of serum ferritin. Iron supplementation without documentation of iron deficiency by measurement of serum ferritin is inappropriate. [187]
- Vitamin A is one of the only vitamins with the potential for serious toxicity even at low doses: Attention should be given to vitamin A intake so that toxicity is avoided. Total intake of vitamin A must account for all sources—foods, fish oils, and vitamin supplements. Manifestations of vitamin A toxicity include: skin problems (dry skin, flaking skin, chapped or split lips, red skin rash, hair loss), joint pain, bone pain, headaches, anorexia (loss of appetite), edema (water retention, weight gain, swollen ankles, difficulty breathing), fatigue, and/or liver damage. Whenever vitamin A is used in high doses, it must be used for a defined period of time in order to avoid the toxicity that will result from high-dose long-term vitamin A supplementation.
    - Adults: Women who are pregnant or might become pregnant and who are planning to carry the baby to full term delivery should not ingest more than 10,000 IU of vitamin A per day. Vitamin A toxicity is seen with chronic ingestion of therapeutic doses (for example: 25,000 IU per day for 6 years, or 100,000 IU per day for 2.5 years[188]). Most patients should not consume more than 25,000 IU of vitamin A per day for more than 2 months without express supervision by a healthcare provider. Vitamin A is present in some multivitamins, in animal liver and products such as fish liver oil, and in other supplements—read labels to ensure that the total daily intake is not greater than 25,000 IU per day.
    - Infants and Children: Different studies have used either daily or monthly schedules of vitamin A supplementation. In a study with extremely low-birth weight infants, 5,000 IU of vitamin A per day for 28 days was safely used.[189] In another study conducted in sick children, those aged less than 12 months received 100,000 IU on two consecutive days, while children between ages 12-60 months received a larger dose of 200,000 IU on two consecutive days.[190]
- Preexisting kidney problems (such as renal insufficiency) increase the risks associated with nutritional supplementation: Supplementation with vitamins and minerals does not cause kidney damage. However, if a patient already has kidney problems, then nutritional supplementation may become hazardous; this is particularly true with magnesium and potassium and perhaps also with vitamin C. Assessment of renal function with serum or urine tests is encouraged before beginning an aggressive plan of supplementation. Conditions which cause kidney damage include use of specific drugs (e.g., acetaminophen, aspirin, contrast and chemotherapy agents, cocaine), acute or chronic high blood pressure, diabetes mellitus and other diseases such as lupus (SLE), polycystic kidney disease, and scleroderma.
- Pre-existing medical conditions may make supplementation unsafe: A few rare medical conditions may cause nutritional supplementation to be unsafe, including severe liver disease, renal failure, electrolyte imbalances, hyperparathyroidism and other vitamin D hypersensitivity syndromes.
- Several drugs/medications may adversely interact with vitamin/mineral supplements and with botanical medicines: Vitamins/minerals may reduce the effectiveness of some prescription medications. For example, taking certain antibiotics such as ciprofloxacin or tetracycline with calcium reduces absorption of the drugs, therefore rendering the drugs much less effective. Taking botanical medicines with medications may make the drugs dangerously less effective (such as when St. John's Wort is combined with protease inhibitor drugs[191]) or may make the drug dangerously more effective (such when Kava is combined with the anti-

---

[187] Hollán S, Johansen KS. Adequate iron stores and the 'Nil nocere' principle. *Haematologia* (Budap). 1993;25(2):69-84

[188] "The smallest continuous daily consumption leading to cirrhosis was 25,000 IU during 6 years, whereas higher daily doses (greater than or equal to 100,000 IU) taken during 2 1/2 years resulted in similar histological lesions. ... The data also indicate that prolonged and continuous consumption of doses in the low "therapeutic" range can result in life-threatening liver damage." Geubel et al. Liver damage caused by therapeutic vitamin A administration: estimate dose-related toxicity in 41 cases. *Gastroenterol* 1991 Jun:1701-9

[189] "Infants with birth weight < 1000 g were randomised at birth to receive oral vitamin A supplementation (5000 IU/day) or placebo for 28 days." Wardle SP, Hughes A, Chen S, Shaw NJ. Randomised controlled trial of oral vitamin A supplementation in preterm infants to prevent chronic lung disease. *Arch Dis Child Fetal Neonatal Ed.* 2001 Jan;84(1):F9-F13 Available on-line at adc.bmjjournals.com/cgi/content/full/fetalneonatal%3b84/1/F9

[190] "Children were assigned to oral doses of 200 000 IU vitamin A (half that dose if <12 months) or placebo on the day of admission, a second dose on the following day, and third and fourth doses at 4 and 8 months after discharge from the hospital, respectively." Villamor E, Mbise R, Spiegelman D, Hertzmark E, Fataki M, Peterson KE, Ndossi G, Fawzi WW. Vitamin A supplements ameliorate the adverse effect of HIV-1, malaria, and diarrheal infections on child growth. *Pediatrics*. 2002 Jan;109(1):E6

[191] Piscitelli SC, Burstein AH, Chaitt D, Alfaro RM, Falloon J. Indinavir concentrations and St John's wort. *Lancet*. 2000 Feb 12;355(9203):547-8

anxiety drug alprazolam[192]). If vitamin D is used in doses greater than 1,000 IU/d in patients taking hydrochlorothiazide or other calcium-retaining drugs, serum calcium should be monitored at least monthly until safety (i.e., lack of hypercalcemia) has been established per patient.[193] Patients should not combine nutritional or botanical medicines with chemical/synthetic drugs without specific advice from a knowledgeable doctor. Do not increase vitamin K consumption from supplements or dietary improvements in patients taking coumadin/warfarin. A reasonable recommendation is that nutritional supplements be taken 2 hours away from pharmaceutical medications to avoid complications such as intraintestinal drug-nutrient binding.

Advanced concepts in nutrition—an introduction

Biochemical Individuality and Orthomolecular Medicine:

"Biochemical individuality" was the term coined by biochemist Dr. Roger Williams of the University of Texas[194] to describe the genetic and physiologic variations in human beings that produced different nutritional needs among individuals. Some enzymes essential for proper cellular function are adversely affected by defects in their construction (i.e., amino acid sequence) that reduce their efficiency. Dr. Linus Pauling, who discovered the molecular basis for the hemoglobinopathy of sickle cell anemia, noted that single amino acid substitutions could produce dramatic alterations in protein function.[195] Pauling discovered that sickle cell disease was caused by a single amino acid substitution in the hemoglobin molecule, and for this discovery he won the Nobel Prize in Chemistry in 1954.[196] With recognition of the importance of individual molecules in determining health or disease, Pauling coined the phrase "orthomolecular medicine" based on his thesis that many diseases could be effectively prevented and treated if we used the "right molecules" to correct abnormal physiologic function. Pauling contrasted the clinical use of nutrients for the improvement of physiologic function (orthomolecular medicine) with the use of chemical drugs, which generally work by interfering with normal physiology (toximolecular medicine). Since nutrients are the fundamental elements of the human body from which all enzymes, chemicals, and cellular structures are formed, Pauling advocated that the use of customized nutrition and nutritional supplements could promote optimal health by optimizing cellular function and efficiency. More recently, Dr. Bruce Ames has thoroughly documented the science of the orthomolecular precepts[197] and has advocated optimal diets along with nutritional supplementation as a highly efficient and cost-effective method for preventing disease and optimizing health.[198,199] In sum, we see that 1) the foundational diet must be formed from whole foods such as fruits, nuts, seeds, vegetables, and lean meats, 2) processed and artificial foods should be avoided, and 3) the use of nutritional supplements is necessary to provide sufficiently high levels of nutrition to overcome defects in enzymatic activity.

Orthomolecular precepts

- The functions of the body are dependent upon thousands of enzymes. Because of genetic defects that are common in the general population, some of these enzymes are commonly defective – even if only slightly – in large portions of the human population.
- Enzyme defects reduce the function and efficiency of important chemical reactions. Because enzymes are so important for normal function and the prevention of disease, defects in enzyme function can result in disruptions in physiology and the creation of what later manifests as "disease."
- Rather than treating these diseases with synthetic chemical drugs, it is commonly possible to prevent and treat disease with high-doses of vitamins, minerals, and other nutrients to compensate for or bypass metabolic dysfunctions, thus allowing for the promotion of optimal health by promoting optimal physiologic function.

Ames BN, et al. High-dose vitamin therapy stimulates variant enzymes with decreased coenzyme binding affinity (increased K(m)). *Am J Clin Nutr.* 2002 Apr

---

[192] Almeida JC, Grimsley EW. Coma from the health food store: interaction between kava and alprazolam. *Ann Intern Med.* 1996 Dec 1;125(11):940-1
[193] Vasquez A, Manso G, Cannell J. The clinical importance of vitamin D (cholecalciferol): a paradigm shift. *Altern Ther Health Med.* 2004 Sep-Oct;10(5):28-36
[194] "Every individual organism that has a distinctive genetic background has distinctive nutritional needs which must be met for optimal well-being. ...[N]utrition applied with due concern for individual genetic variations...offers the solution to many baffling health problems." Williams RJ. *Biochemical Individuality*. University of Texas, 1956. Page x
[195] "...the concentration of coenzyme [vitamins and minerals] needed to produce the amount of active enzyme required for optimum health may well be somewhat different for different individuals. ...many individuals may require a considerably higher concentration of one or more coenzymes than other people do for optimum health..." Pauling L. On the Orthomolecular Environment of the Mind: Orthomolecular Theory. In: Williams RJ, Kalita DK. *A Physician's Handbook on Orthomolecular Medicine*. Keats Publ: 1977, p76
[196] nobel.se/chemistry/laureates/1954/pauling-bio.html on April 4, 2004
[197] "About 50 human genetic dis-eases due to defective enzymes can be remedied or ameliorated by the administration of high doses of the vitamin component of the corresponding coenzyme, which at least partially restores enzymatic activity." Ames BN, Elson-Schwab I, Silver EA. High-dose vitamin therapy stimulates variant enzymes with decreased coenzyme binding affinity (increased K(m)): relevance to genetic disease and polymorphisms. *Am J Clin Nutr.* 2002 Apr;75(4):616-58
[198] "An optimum intake of micronutrients and metabolites, which varies with age and genetic constitution, would tune up metabolism and give a marked increase in health, particularly for the poor and elderly, at little cost." Ames BN. The metabolic tune-up: metabolic harmony and disease prevention. *J Nutr.* 2003 May;133(5 Suppl 1):1544S-8S
[199] "Optimizing micronutrient intake [through better diets, fortification of foods, or multivitamin-mineral pills] can have a major impact on public health at low cost." Ames BN. Cancer prevention and diet: help from single nucleotide polymorphisms. *Proc Natl Acad Sci* U S A. 1999 Oct 26;96(22):12216-8

Molecular rationale for high-dose nutrient supplementation
"As many as **one-third of mutations** in a gene result in the corresponding enzyme having an increased Michaelis constant, or Km, (decreased binding affinity) for a coenzyme, resulting in a lower rate of reaction. **About 50 human genetic diseases due to defective enzymes can be remedied or ameliorated by the administration of high doses of the vitamin component of the corresponding coenzyme**, which at least partially restores enzymatic activity."
"**High doses of vitamins are used to treat many inheritable human diseases**. The molecular basis of disease arising from as many as one-third of the mutations in a gene is an increased Michaelis constant, or Km, (decreased binding affinity) of an enzyme for the vitamin-derived coenzyme or substrate, which in turn lowers the rate of the reaction."
Ames BN, et al. High-dose vitamin therapy stimulates variant enzymes. *Am J Clin Nutr.* 2002 Apr;75:616-58

Nutrigenomics—Nutritional Genomics: "Genome" refers to all of the genetic material in an organism, and "genomics" is the field of study of this information. The field of nutritional genomics—nutrigenomics—refers to the clinical synthesis of 1) research on the human genome, and 2) the advancing science of clinical nutrition, including research on nutraceuticals (nutritional medicines) and phytomedicinals (botanical medicines). Nutrigenomics represents a major advance in our understanding of the underlying biochemical and physiologic mechanisms of the effects of nutrition.

Nutrition is far more than "fuel" for our biophysiologic machine; we know now that nutrition—the consumption of specific proteins, amino acids, vitamins, minerals, fatty acids, and phytochemicals—can alter genetic expression and can thus either promote health or disease at the very fundamental level of genetic expression. The commonly employed excuse that many patients use—"I just have bad genes"—now takes on a whole new meaning; it may be that these patients suffer from the expression of "bad genes" *because of the food that they eat.*

The concept and phenomenon of nutrigenomics can be described by saying that each of us has the genes for health, as well as the genes for disease; what largely determines our level of health is how we treat our genes with environmental inputs, especially nutrition. We appear able, to a large extent, to "turn on" disease-promoting genes with poor nutrition and a pro-inflammatory lifestyle[200,201], while, to a lesser extent, we are able to activate or "turn on" health-promoting genes with a healthy diet[202] and with proper nutritional supplementation.[203]

Putting it all together with "the supplemented Paleo-Mediterranean diet": The health-promoting diet of choice for the majority of people is a diet based on abundant consumption of fruits, vegetables, seeds, nuts, omega-3 and monounsaturated fatty acids, and lean sources of protein such as lean meats, fatty cold-water fish, soy and whey proteins. This diet prohibits and obviates overconsumption of chemical preservatives, artificial sweeteners, and carbohydrate-dominant foods such as candies, pastries, breads, potatoes, grains, and other foods with a high glycemic load and high glycemic index. This "Paleo-Mediterranean Diet" is a combination of the "Paleolithic" or "Paleo diet" and the well-known "Mediterranean diet", both of which are well described in peer-reviewed journals and the lay press. The Mediterranean diet is characterized by increased proportions of legumes, nuts, seeds, whole grain products, fruits, vegetables (including potatoes), fish and lean meats, and monounsaturated and n-3 fatty acids.[204] Consumption of the Mediterranean diet is associated with improvements in insulin sensitivity and reductions in cardiovascular disease, diabetes, cancer, and all-cause mortality when contrasted to the effects of *ad libitum* eating, particularly in the standard American diet (SAD) eating pattern.[205] The Paleolithic diet detailed by collaborators Eaton[206], O'Keefe[207], and Cordain[208] is similar to the Mediterranean diet except for stronger emphasis on fruits and vegetables (preferably raw or minimally cooked), omega-3-rich lean meats, and reduced consumption of starchy foods such as potatoes and grains, the latter of which were not staples in the human diet until the last few thousand years. Emphasizing the olive oil and red wine of the Mediterranean diet and the absence of grains and potatoes per the Paleo diet appears to be the way to get the best of both dietary worlds; the remaining diet is characterized by fresh whole fruits, vegetables, nuts (especially almonds), seeds, berries, olive oil, lean meats rich

---

[200] Rusyn et al. Corn oil rapidly activates nuclear factor-kappaB in hepatic Kupffer cells by oxidant-dependent mechanisms. *Carcinogenesis.* 1999 Nov;20(11):2095-100
[201] Aljada et al. Increase in intranuclear nuclear factor kappaB and decrease in inhibitor kappaB in mononuclear cells after a mixed meal. *Am J Clin Nutr.* 2004 Apr;79(4):682-90
[202] OKeefe JH Jr,Cordain L.Cardiovascular disease resulting from a diet and lifestyle at odds with our Paleolithic genome.*Mayo Clin Proc.*2004;79:101-8
[203] Kaput J, Rodriguez LR. Nutritional genomics: the next frontier in the postgenomic era. *Physiol Genomics* 16: 166–177
[204] Curtis BM, O'Keefe JH Jr. Understanding the Mediterranean diet. Could this be the new "gold standard" for heart disease prevention? *Postgrad Med.* 2002;112:35-8,41-5
[205] Knoops KT, et al. Mediterranean diet, lifestyle factors, and 10-year mortality in elderly European men and women: the HALE project. *JAMA.* 2004 Sep 22;292(12):1433-9
[206] Eaton SB, Shostak M, Konner M. *The Paleolithic Prescription: A program of diet & exercise and a design for living*, New York: Harper & Row, 1988
[207] O'Keefe JH Jr, Cordain L. Cardiovascular disease resulting from a diet and lifestyle at odds with our Paleolithic genome. *Mayo Clin Proc.* 2004 Jan;79(1):101-8
[208] Cordain L. *The Paleo Diet.* Indianapolis; John Wiley and Sons, 2002

in n-3 fatty acids, and red wine in moderation. In sum, this dietary plan along with the inclusion of garlic and dark chocolate (a rich source of cardioprotective, antioxidative, antihypertensive, and anti-inflammatory polyphenolic flavonoids[209,210]) is expected to reduce adverse cardiovascular events by more than 76%.[211] Biochemical justification for this type of diet is ample and is well supported by numerous long-term studies in humans wherein both Mediterranean and Paleolithic diets result in statistically significant and clinically meaningful reductions in disease-specific and all-cause mortality.[212,213,214,215] Diets rich in fruits and vegetables are sources of more than 8,000 phytochemicals, many of which have antioxidant, anti-inflammatory, and anti-cancer properties.[216] Oleic acid, squalene, and phenolics in olive oil and phenolics and resveratrol in red wine have antioxidant, anti-inflammatory, and anti-cancer properties and also protect against cardiovascular disease.[217] N-3 fatty acids have numerous health benefits via multiple mechanisms as described in the sections that follow. Increased intake of dietary fiber from fruits and vegetable favorably modifies gut flora, promotes xenobiotic elimination (via flora modification, laxation, and overall reductions in enterohepatic recirculation), and is associated with reductions in morbidity and mortality. Such a "Paleolithic diet" can also lead to urinary alkalinization (average urine pH of ≥ 7.5 according to Sebastian et al[218]) which increases renal *retention of minerals* for improved musculoskeletal health[219,220,221] and which increases *urinary elimination of many toxicants and xenobiotics* for a tremendous reduction in serum levels and thus adverse effects from chemical exposure or drug overdose.[222] Furthermore, therapeutic alkalinization was recently shown in an open trial with 82 patients to reduce symptoms and disability associated with low-back pain and to increase intracellular magnesium concentrations by 11%.[223] **Ample intake of amino acids via dietary proteins supports phase-2 detoxification** (amino acid and sulfate conjugation) for proper xenobiotic elimination[224,225], **provides amino acid precursors for neurotransmitter synthesis** and maintenance of mood, memory, and cognitive performance[226,227,228,229], **and prevents the immunosuppression and decrements in musculoskeletal status caused by low-protein diets**.[230] Described originally by this author[231], the "supplemented Paleo-Mediterranean diet" provides patients the best of current knowledge in nutrition by relying on a foundational diet plan of fresh fruits, vegetables, nuts, seeds, berries, fish, and lean meats which is adorned with olive oil for its squalene, phenolic antioxidant/anti-inflammatory and monounsaturated fatty acid content. Inclusive of medical foods such as red wine, garlic, and dark chocolate which may synergize to effect at least a 76% reduction in cardiovascular disease[232], this diet also reduces the risk for cancer[233] and can be an integral component of a health-promoting lifestyle.[234] Competitive athletes are allowed increased carbohydrate consumption before and after training and competition to promote glycogen storage supercompensation.[235,236]

---

[209] Schramm et al. Chocolate procyanidins decrease the leukotriene-prostacyclin ratio in humans and human aortic endothelial cells. *Am J Clin Nutr*. 2001;73(1):36-40
[210] Engler et al. Flavonoid-rich dark chocolate improves endothelial function and increases plasma epicatechin concentrations in healthy adults. *J Am Coll Nutr* 2004;23:197-204
[211] Franco et al. The Polymeal: a more natural, safer, and probably tastier (than the Polypill) strategy to reduce cardiovascular disease by more than 75%. *BMJ*. 2004:1447-50
[212] de Lorgeril M, et al. Mediterranean dietary pattern in a randomized trial: prolonged survival and possible reduced cancer rate. *Arch Intern Med*. 1998 Jun 8;158(11):1181-7
[213] Knoops KT, et al. Mediterranean diet, lifestyle factors, and 10-year mortality in elderly European men and women: the HALE project. *JAMA*. 2004 Sep 22;292(12):1433-9
[214] Lindeberg S, Cordain L, and Eaton SB. Biological and clinical potential of a Paleolithic diet. *J Nutri Environ Med* 2003; 13:149-160
[215] O'Keefe JH Jr, Cordain L, et al. Optimal low-density lipoprotein is 50 to 70 mg/dl: lower is better and physiologically normal. *J Am Coll Cardiol*. 2004 Jun 2;43(11):2142-6
[216] Liu RH. Health benefits of fruit and vegetables are from additive and synergistic combinations of phytochemicals. *Am J Clin Nutr*. 2003;78(3 Sup):517S-520S
[217] Alarcon de la Lastra C, Barranco MD, Motilva V, Herrerias JM. Mediterranean diet and health: biological importance of olive oil.*Curr Pharm Des*. 2001;7:933-50
[218] Sebastian, Frassetto et al. Estimation of the net acid load of the diet of ancestral preagricultural Homo sapiens and their hominid ancestors. *Am J Clin Nutr*. 2002;76:1308-16
[219] Sebastian A, et al. Improved mineral balance and skeletal metabolism in postmenopausal women treated with potassium bicarbonate. *N Engl J Med*. 1994;330(25):1776-81
[220] Tucker et al. Potassium, magnesium, fruit and vegetable intakes are associated with greater bone mineral density in elderly men and women. *Am J Clin Nutr*. 1999;69:727-36
[221] Whiting et al. Dietary protein, phosphorus, potassium are beneficial to bone mineral density in men consuming adequate dietary calcium. *J Am Coll Nutr*. 2002;21:402-9
[222] Proudfoot AT, Krenzelok EP, Vale JA. Position Paper on urine alkalinization. *J Toxicol Clin Toxicol*. 2004;42(1):1-26
[223] "The results show that a disturbed acid-base balance may contribute to the symptoms of low back pain. The simple and safe addition of an alkaline multimineral preparate was able to reduce the pain symptoms in these patients with chronic low back pain." Vormann J, et al. Supplementation with alkaline minerals reduces symptoms in patients with chronic low back pain. *J Trace Elem Med Biol*. 2001;15:179-83
[224] Liska DJ. The detoxification enzyme systems. *Altern Med Rev*. 1998;3:187-9
[225] Anderson KE, Kappas A. Dietary regulation of cytochrome P450. *Annu Rev Nutr*. 1991;11:141-67
[226] Rogers et al. Tryptophan depletion alters the decision-making of healthy volunteers through altered processing of reward cues. *Neuropsychopharmacology*. 2003;28:153-62
[227] Arnulf I, et al. Mid-morning tryptophan depletion delays REM sleep onset in healthy subjects. *Neuropsychopharmacology*. 2002;27(5):843-51
[228] Thomas JR,Lockwood PA,Singh A, Deuster PA.Tyrosine improves working memory in a multitasking environment.*Pharmacol Biochem Behav*.1999;64:495-500
[229] Markus CR, et al. The bovine protein alpha-lactalbumin increases the plasma ratio of tryptophan to the other large neutral amino acids, and in vulnerable subjects raises brain serotonin activity, reduces cortisol concentration, and improves mood under stress. *Am J Clin Nutr*. 2000;71:1536-44
[230] Castaneda C, et al. Elderly women accommodate to a low-protein diet with losses of body cell mass, muscle function, and immune response. *Am J Clin Nutr*. 1995;62:30-9
[231] Vasquez A. Five-Part Nutritional Protocol that Produces Consistently Positive Results. *Nutr Wellness* 2005 Sept. InflammationMastery.com/reprints and updated in Chapter 4.
[232] Franco et al. The Polymeal: a more natural, safer, and probably tastier (than the Polypill) strategy to reduce cardiovascular disease by more than 75%.*BMJ* 2004;329:1447-50
[233] "The combination of 4 low risk factors lowered the all-cause mortality rate to 0.35 (95% CI, 0.28-0.44). In total, lack of adherence to this low-risk pattern was associated with a population attributable risk of 60% of all deaths, 64% of deaths from coronary heart disease, 61% from cardiovascular diseases, and 60% from cancer." Knoops KT, de Groot LC, Kromhout D, et al. Mediterranean diet, lifestyle factors, and 10-year mortality in elderly European men and women: the HALE project. *JAMA*. 2004 Sep 22;292(12):1433-9
[234] Orme-Johnson DW, Herron RE. An innovative approach to reducing medical care utilization and expenditures. *Am J Manag Care*. 1997;3(1):135-44
[235] "A significant glycogen sparing, as well as supercompensation within 24 h of recovery, was observed after [carbohydrate] supplementation." Brouns F, Saris WH, Beckers E, Adlercreutz H, et al. Metabolic changes induced by sustained exhaustive cycling and diet manipulation. *Int J Sports Med*. 1989 May;10 Suppl 1:S49-62
[236] "The accepted method of increasing muscle glycogen stores is by "glycogen loading," which classically involves depletion of muscle glycogen, usually by exercise, followed by consumption of a high-CHO diet for several days (e.g., 3, 39). …increase muscle glycogen concentrations ([glycogen]) to between 150 and 200% of normal resting levels." Robinson TM, et al. Role of submaximal exercise in promoting creatine and glycogen accumulation in human skeletal muscle. *J Appl Physiol*. 1999 Aug;87(2):598-604

Profile of the Supplemented Paleo-Mediterranean Diet (Vasquez 2005, 2011)[237]

Foods to consume:	Foods to avoid:
☺ **Everything organic**: to enhance nutrition, avoid pesticides/herbicides, and to avoid GMO as much as possible (detailed and cited later) ☺ **Lean sources of protein** • Fish (avoiding tuna which is commonly loaded with mercury) • Chicken and turkey • Lean cuts of free-range grass-fed meats: beef, buffalo, lamb are occasionally acceptable • Soy protein[238] and whey protein isolate[239,240] ☺ **Fruits and fruit juices** ☺ **Vegetables and vegetable juices** ☺ **Nuts, seeds, berries** ☺ **Generous use of olive oil**: On sautéed vegetables and fresh salads ☺ **Daily vitamin/mineral supplementation**: With a high-potency broad-spectrum multivitamin and multimineral supplement[241] ☺ **Sun exposure or vitamin D3 supplementation**: To ensure provision of 2,000-5,000 IU of vitamin D3 per day for adults[242] ☺ **Balanced broad-spectrum fatty acid supplementation**: With ALA, GLA, EPA, and DHA[243] ☺ **Water, tea, home-made fruit/vegetable juices**: Commercial vegetable juices are commonly loaded with sodium chloride; choose appropriately. Fruit juices can be loaded with natural and superfluous sugars. Herbal teas can be selected based on the medicinal properties of the plant that is used.	☒ **Avoid as much as possible fat-laden arachidonate-rich meats** like beef, liver, pork, and lamb, as well as high-fat cream and other dairy products with emulsified, readily absorbed saturated fats and arachidonic acid ☒ **High-sugar pseudofoods**: • Corn syrup • Cola and soda • Donuts, candy, etc…."junk food" ☒ **Grains such as wheat, rye, barley**: These have only existed in the human diet for less than 10,000 years and are consistently associated with increased prevalence of degenerative diseases due to the allergic response they invoke and because of their high glycemic load and high glycemic index. ☒ **Potatoes and rice**: High in sugar, low in phytonutrients ☒ **Avoid allergens**: Determined per individual ☒ **Chemicals to avoid**: • Pesticides, Herbicides, Fungicides • Carcinogenic sweeteners: aspartame[244] • Artificial flavors • Artificial colors: tartrazine • Preservatives: benzoate • Flavor enhancers: carrageenan and monosodium glutamate • GMO: avoid genetically manipulated corporate products and do not contribute to unethical profiteering businesses; rather support local and sustainable farmers as much as possible for a wide range of ethical, nutritional, and environmental reasons

---

[237] Vasquez A. Five-Part Nutritional Protocol. *Nutritional Wellness* 2005 Sept. and Vasquez A. The Supplemented Paleo-Mediterranean Diet. *Nutritional Perspectives* 2011 Jan
[238] "These results indicate that for healthy adults, the isolated soy protein is of high nutritional quality, comparable to that of animal protein sources, and that the methionine content is not limiting for adult protein maintenance." Young et al. Evaluation of the protein quality of an isolated soy protein in young men. *Am J Clin Nutr*. 1984 Jan;39:16-24
[239] Bounous G. Whey protein concentrate (WPC) and glutathione modulation in cancer treatment. *Anticancer Res*. 2000 Nov-Dec;20(6C):4785-92
[240] Markus CR, et al. The bovine protein alpha-lactalbumin increases the plasma ratio of tryptophan to the other large neutral amino acids, and in vulnerable subjects raises brain serotonin activity, reduces cortisol concentration, and improves mood under stress. *Am J Clin Nutr*. 2000 Jun;71(6):1536-44
[241] "Most people do not consume an optimal amount of all vitamins by diet alone. …it appears prudent for all adults to take vitamin supplements." Fletcher RH, Fairfield KM. Vitamins for chronic disease prevention in adults: clinical applications. *JAMA*. 2002;287:3127-9
[242] Vasquez A, et al. The clinical importance of vitamin D (cholecalciferol). *Altern Ther Health Med*. 2004 Sep 10:28-36
[243] Vasquez A. New Insights into Fatty Acid Supplementation and Its Effect on Eicosanoid Production and Genetic Expression. *Nutr Perspectives* 2005; Jan: 5-16
[244] "In the past two decades brain tumor rates have risen in several industrialized countries, including the United States... Compared to other environmental factors putatively linked to brain tumors, the artificial sweetener aspartame is a promising candidate to explain the recent increase in incidence and degree of malignancy of brain tumors." Olney JW, Farber NB, Spitznagel E, Robins LN. Increasing brain tumor rates: is there a link to aspartame? *J Neuropathol Exp Neurol* 1996 Nov;55(11):1115-23

Local Mediterranean market fare: Plants provide fiber, antioxidants, numerous functional phytochemicals with anti-inflammatory properties, and prebiotic and antimicrobial constituents that favorably modulate human gastrointestinal flora to provide anti-inflammatory immunomodulation; seafood generally provides low-fat high-quality protein with favorable fatty acid profiles. Supporting local farmers, fishers, and personal store owners helps promote environmental and community sustainability.

Emotional, Mental, and Social Health

Stress management and authentic living: Mental, emotional, and physical "stress" describes any unpleasant living condition which can lead to negative effects on health, such as increased blood pressure, depression, apathy, increased muscle tension, and, according to some research, increased risk of serious health problems such as early death from cardiovascular disease and cancer. Many people find that their modern lives are characterized by excess amounts of multitasking, job responsibilities, family responsibilities, commuter traffic, financial pressures in combination with an insufficient amount of relaxation, sleep, community support, exercise, time in nature, healthy nutrition, and time to simply *be* rather than *do*. Stress comes in many different forms and includes malnutrition, trauma, insufficient exercise (epidemic), excess exercise (rare), sleep deprivation, emotional turmoil, and exposure to chemicals and radiation. When most people talk about "stress" they are referring to either chronic anxiety (such as with high-pressure work situations or dysfunctional interpersonal relationships) or the acute stress reaction that is typical of unpredictable rapid-onset events such as an injury, accident, or other physically threatening situation. **These "different types of stress" are not separate from each other; rather, they are interconnected:**

- Emotional stress causes nutritional depletion, particularly of vitamin A[245], magnesium, tryptophan, and vitamin C—most mammals (other than those that lost L-gulonolactone oxidase function such as humans/primates, guinea pigs, most bats, some birds and fish[246]) can internally produce ascorbate and greatly increase endogenous production during times of stress,
- Sleep deprivation alters immune response and mental functioning,[247]
- Emotional stress triggers increased microbial virulence, growth, and mucosal adhesion; the sensing of the neuroendocrine stress response by microorganisms, many of which have receptors for catecholamines, is termed "microbial endocrinology",[248]
- Chemical exposure can disrupt endocrine function.[249]

Therefore, **any type of [emotional] stress can cause other types of [physiologic] stress**. Avoiding stressful situations is, of course, an effective way to avoid being bothered or harmed by them. If work-related stress is the problem, then finding a new position or occupation is certainly an option worth considering and implementing. High-stress jobs are often high-paying jobs; but if in the process of making money, a person ruins her health and loses years from her life, then no one would ever say, "It was worth it." **Money, success, and freedom only have value for the person alive and healthy to enjoy them.** Toxic relationships, whether at home or work, are relationships that cause more harm than good by re-injuring old emotional wounds and by creating new emotional injuries. We can all benefit from affirming our right to a happy and healthy life by minimizing/eliminating contact with people who cause emotional harm to us—this requires conscious effort.[250] Engel[251] provides a clear articulation and description of abusive relationships, along with checklists for their recognition and exercises for their remediation. Healthy relationships are difficult to create and maintain these days, and probably a few basic components contribute to this phenomenon. ❶ With the society-wide disintegration of the extended family, most people in our society have never even seen a healthy family unit and therefore have no model and no available mentors to help them recreate a lasting family structure. ❷ Due specifically to the structure of our educational systems and (pseudo)culture of entertainment, most people have very short attention spans and are accustomed to inattention, distraction, and externally derived entertainment and gratification. ❸ Modern schools and fragmented families both fail to teach conflict resolution and relationship skills. ❹ Poor nutritional status—very common in the general population—promotes impulsivity, irritability, depression, and mood instability.

> **How to test relationship quality at home/work**
> "Good relationships make you feel loved, wanted, and cared for."
> Malcolm. *Health Style*. 2001,133

---

[245] Ingenbleek Y, Bernstein L. The stressful condition as a nutritionally dependent adaptive dichotomy. *Nutrition* 1999 Apr;15(4):305-20
[246] Drouin et al. The genetics of vitamin C loss in vertebrates. *Curr Genomics*. 2011 Aug;12(5):371-8 and "...bats lost the ability to biosynthesize vitamin C recently by exhibiting stepwise mutation patterns during GULO evolution..." Cui et al. Recent Loss of Vitamin C Biosynthesis Ability in Bats. *PLoS ONE* 2011;6(11):e27114
[247] Heiser P, e. Alterations of host defense system after sleep deprivation are followed by impaired mood and psychosocial functioning. *World J Biol Psychiatry* 2001 Apr;2:89-94
[248] Freestone et al. Microbial endocrinology: how stress influences susceptibility to infection. *Trends Microbiol*. 2008 Feb;16(2):55-64
[249] "Evidence suggests that environmental exposure to some anthropogenic chemicals may result in disruption of endocrine systems in human and wildlife populations." epa.gov/endocrine on March 7, 2004
[250] Collins BC. *How to Recognize Emotional Unavailability and Make Healthier Relationship Choices*. [Mjf Books; ISBN: 1567313442]
[251] Engel B. *The Emotionally Abusive Relationship: How to Stop Being Abused and How to Stop Abusing*. Wiley Publishers: 2003

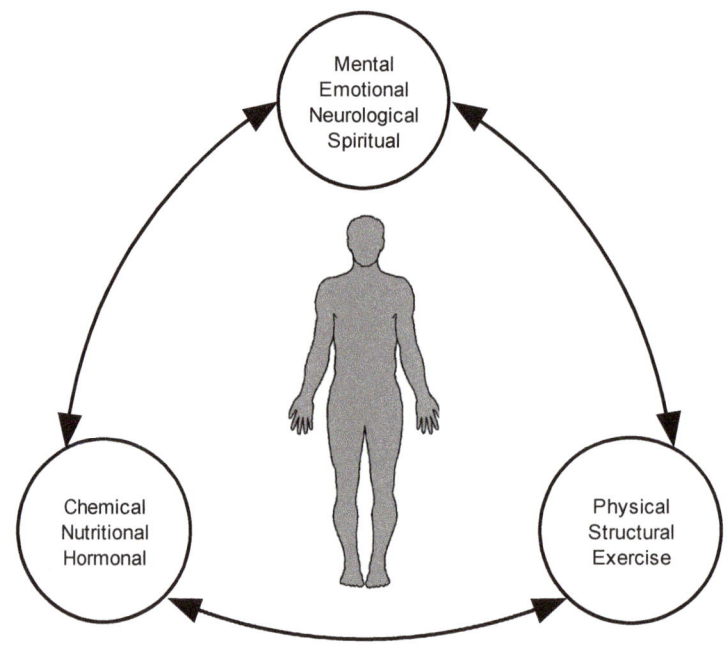

Stress affects the whole body.

Therefore, a complete stress management program must address the whole body:

Physical Structural

Biochemical Hormonal Nutritional

Mental Emotional Spiritual

An important concept is that <mark>psychoemotional stress is a "whole body" phenomenon</mark>: affecting the mind, the brain, emotional state, the physical body (including musculoskeletal, immune, and cardiovascular systems), as well as the nutritional status of the individual. The adverse effects of stress can be reduced with an integrated combination of therapeutics that addresses each of the major body systems affected by stress, which are 1) mental/emotional, 2) physical, and 3) nutritional/biochemical.

Approaching stress management from a tripartite perspective

	Mental/emotional	**Physical**	**Nutritional/biochemical**
Therapeutic considerations	• Social support • Re-parenting • Conversational style[252] • Meditation, prayer • Healthy boundaries • Books, tapes, groups • REST—reduced environmental stimulation therapy[253] • Expressive writing[254] • Time to simply rest and relax	• Yoga • Massage • Exercise • Stretching • Swimming • Resting • Biking • Hiking • Physical touch and affection	• Vitamins, especially vitamin C[255] • Fish oil[256] • Hormones, cytokines, neurotransmitters, and eicosanoids • Tryptophan, pyridoxine, whey protein • Botanical medicines such as *kava*[257], *Ashwaganda,* and *Eleutherococcus*

---

[252] Rick Brinkman ND and Rick Kirschner ND. *How to Deal With Difficult People* [Audio Cassette. Career Track, 1995]
[253] For more information on REST and its use in weight loss and alcohol consumption: Borrie et al. Restricted environmental stimulation therapy in a weight reduction program. *J Behav Med*. 1980 Jun;3(2):147-61. Cooper et al. Reduced Environmental Stimulation Therapy (REST) and reduced alcohol consumption. *J Subst Abuse Treat*. 1988;5(2):61-8
[254] Smyth et al. Effects of writing about stressful experiences on symptom reduction in patients with asthma or rheumatoid arthritis. *JAMA*. 1999 Apr 14;281(14):1304-9
[255] Brody S, Preut R, Schommer K, Schurmeyer TH. A randomized controlled trial of high dose ascorbic acid for reduction of blood pressure, cortisol, and subjective responses to psychological stress. *Psychopharmacology* (Berl). 2002 Jan;159(3):319-24
[256] Hamazaki T, Itomura M, Sawazaki S, Nagao Y. Anti-stress effects of DHA. *Biofactors*. 2000;13(1-4):41-5
[257] Cagnacci A, et al. Kava-Kava administration reduces anxiety in perimenopausal women. *Maturitas*. 2003 Feb 25;44(2):103-9

The body functions as a whole—not as independent, autonomous organ systems: Problems with one aspect of health create problems in other aspects of health. **Treatment of disease and promotion of wellness must therefore improve overall health and functioning while simultaneously addressing the disease or presenting complaint.**

The influences on "functional phenotype" can originate from psychosocial health or dysfunction or "toxic" emotional exposures and the resulting physiologic and microbial responses: The model presented here is a simple one, but it serves to demonstrate how psychological health status can affect the entirety of all body systems, either directly or indirectly. Due to the interconnected nature of each component/system, problems can become synergistic and reinforced and thus self-perpetuating. For example, psychological stress increases microbial virulence (e.g., microbial endocrinology) and total microbial load while reducing mucosal immunity (e.g., reduced secretory IgA) and immunomodulating hormones (e.g., DHEA and testosterone are reduced with severe stress); complicating these are the facts that people tend to make poor dietary choices when they are stressed (e.g., "stress eaters") and that xenobiotic accumulation can only follow xenobiotic exposure and that most xenobiotic exposure results from corporate irresponsibility, government complicity, and population-wide sociopolitical ineffectiveness.

Stress always has a biochemical/physiologic component: Regardless of its origins, stress invariably takes a toll on the body—*the whole body*. Well-documented effects of stress include:
1. Increased levels of cortisol—higher levels are associated with osteoporosis, memory loss, slow healing, and insulin resistance.
2. Reduced function of thyroid hormones[258] (i.e., induction of peripheral/metabolic hypothyroidism)
3. Reduced levels of testosterone (in men)
4. Increased intestinal permeability and "leaky gut"[259]
5. Increased excretion of minerals in the urine
6. Increased need for vitamins, minerals, and amino acids
7. Suppression of immune function and of natural killer cells that fight viral infections and tumors
8. Decreased production of sIgA—main defense of the lungs, gastrointestinal tract, and genitourinary tract
9. Increased populations of harmful bacteria in the intestines and an associated increased rate of lung and upper respiratory tract infections
10. Increased incidence of food allergies[260]
11. Sleep disturbance

---
[258] Ingenbleek Y, Bernstein L. The stressful condition as a nutritionally dependent adaptive dichotomy. *Nutrition* 1999 Apr;15(4):305-20
[259] Hart A, Kamm MA. Review article: mechanisms of initiation and perpetuation of gut inflammation by stress. *Aliment Pharmacol Ther* 2002;16(12):2017-28
[260] Anderzen et al. Stress and sensitization: controlled prospective psychophysiological study of children exposed to international relocation. *J Psychosom Res* 1997;43:259-69

Sometimes a stressful situation can be modified into one that is less stressful or dysfunctional, so that the benefits are retained, yet the negative aspects are reduced. Of course, the best example of this is interpersonal relationships, which easily lend themselves to improvement with the application of conscious effort. Many audiotapes, books, and seminars are available for people interested in having improved interpersonal relationships. Selected resources are listed here:
- Men and Women: Talking Together by Deborah Tannen and Robert Bly [Sound Horizons, 1992. ISBN: 1879323095] A lively discussion of the different communication and relationship styles of men and women by two respected experts in their fields.
- How to Deal with Difficult People by Drs. Rick Brinkman and Rick Kirschner. [Audio Cassette. Career Track, 1995] An entertaining format with solutions to common workplace and situational difficulties. Authored and performed by two naturopathic physicians.
- Men are From Mars, Women are From Venus by John Gray. [Audio Cassette and Books]. Phenomenally popular concepts in understanding, accepting, and effectively integrating the differences between men and women.
- The ManKind Project (ManKindProject.org). An international organization hosting events for men and women. The men's events, formats, and groups are authentic, clear, and healthy. The ManKind Project has an organization for women called The WomanWithin (womanwithin.org). No book or tape can substitute for the dynamics and personal attention that can be experienced by a conscious, empowered, and well-intended group.

When "the problem" cannot be avoided, and the interaction/relationship with the problem cannot be improved, a remaining option is to supplement the internal environment so that it is somewhat "strengthened" to deal with the stress of the bothersome event or situation. For example, when dealing with emotional stress, we can use counseling, support groups, or various relaxation techniques.[261] If we determine that the emotional stress has a biochemical component, then we can use specific botanical and nutritional supplementation to safely and naturally support and restore normal function. Moving deeper into the issue of "stress management" requires that we ask why a person is in a stressful situation to begin with. Of course, with *random acts of chaos* like car accidents, we cannot always ascribe the problem to the person, unless the accident resulted from their own negligence. But **when people are chronically stressed and unhappy about their jobs and/or relationships, then we need to employ more than stress reduction techniques**, and as clinicians we need to offer more than the latest adaptogen. **We have to ask why a person would subject himself/herself to such a situation, and what fears or limitations (self-imposed and/or externally applied) keep him/her from breaking free into a life that works.**[262,263,264,265,266,267]

Six fundamental components of Self-esteem
1. Living consciously
2. Self-acceptance
3. Self-responsibility
4. Self-assertiveness
5. Living purposefully
6. Personal integrity
Branden N. *Six Pillars of Self-Esteem*. Bantam: 1995

Autonomization, intradependence, emotional literacy, corrective experience:

"None of us are completely developed people when we reach adulthood.
We are each incomplete in our own way." *Merle Fossum*[268]

Consciousness-raising is a keystone gift that holistic physicians can impart to their patients and one which may be necessary for true healing to be manifested and maintained. Healthcare providers are quick to enlighten their patients to the details of diet, exercise, nutrition, medications, surgeries, and other *biomechanical* and *biochemical* aspects of health, but are routinely negligent when it comes to sharing with patients the emotional tools that may be necessary to repair or construct the "self" which is supposed to implement the treatment plan that the doctor has designed. Passivity and ignorance are not hindrances to the success of the *medical paradigm*, which requires that

---

[261] Martha Davis PhD, Matthew McKay MSW, Elizabeth Robbins Eshelman PhD. *The Relaxation & Stress Reduction Workbook 5th edition*. New Harbinger Publishers; 2000
[262] Rick Jarow. *Creating the Work You Love: Courage, Commitment and Career*; Inner Traditions Intl Ltd; 1995 [ISBN: 0892815426]
[263] Breton D, Largent C. *The Paradigm Conspiracy: Why Our Social Systems Violate Human Potential-And How We Can Change Them*. Hazelden: 1998
[264] Dominguez JR. *Transforming Your Relationship with Money*. Sounds True; Book and Cassette edition: 2001 Audio tape.
[265] Miller A. *The truth will set you free: overcoming emotional blindness and finding your true adult self*. New York: Basic Books; 2001
[266] Bradshaw J. *Healing the Shame that Binds You* [Audio Cassette (April 1990) Health Communications Audio; ISBN: 1558740430]
[267] Miller A. *The Drama of the Gifted Child: The Search for the True Self*. Basic Books: 1981
[268] Fossum M. *Catching Fire: Men Coming Alive in Recovery*. New York; Harper/Hazelden: 1989, 4-7

patients are "compliant" rather than self-directed; however, for *authentic, holistic healthcare* to be successful, it must empower the patient sufficiently such that he/she attains/regains appropriate *autonomy*—an "internal locus of control"—sufficient for lifelong internally-driven health maintenance. Health implications of autonomy (or its absence) are obvious and intuitive. Patients with an underdeveloped internal locus of control appear to experience greater degrees of social stress which can lead to hypercortisolemia and hippocampal atrophy.[269] A developed internal locus of control correlates strongly with the success of weight-loss programs, and for nonautonomous patients it is necessary to encourage the development of autonomous self-care behavior in addition to the provision of information about diet and exercise.[270]

Primary, secondary, and tertiary means for developing an autonomous, authentic self: Ideally, positive childhood experiences (A) merge into adolescent and adult experiences of confidence and maturity (B) for the development of a true adult (C). If A or B is lacking or insufficient, the result is an incomplete self often incapable of *effective* and *appropriate* action. Corrective experiences must then be pursued to re-establish the foundation from which an authentic self can arise.

Completely formed internal identities are the natural result of the *continuum* of positive childhood experiences (inclusive of stability, "unconditional love", healthy parenting, and active, conscious intergenerational social contact) which are ideally merged into adolescent and adulthood experiences of success, acceptance, inclusion,

---

[269] "Cumulative exposure to high levels of cortisol over the lifetime is known to be related to hippocampal atrophy... Self-esteem and internal locus of control were significantly correlated with hippocampal volume in both young and elderly subjects." Pruessner JC, Baldwin MW, Dedovic K, Renwick R, Mahani NK, Lord C, Meaney M, Lupien S. Self-esteem, locus of control, hippocampal volume, and cortisol regulation in young and old adulthood. *Neuroimage*. 2005 Dec;28(4):815-26

[270] "Their weight loss was significant and associated with an internal locus of control orientation (P < 0.05)... Participants with an internal orientation could be offered a standard weight reduction programme. Others, with a more external locus of control orientation, could be offered an adapted programme, which also focused on and encouraged the participants' internal orientation." Adolfsson B, Andersson I, Elofsson S, Rossner S, Unden AL. Locus of control and weight reduction. *Patient Educ Couns*. 2005 Jan;56:55-61

independence, interdependence, and intradependence with the end result being a socially-conscious adult with an internal locus of control. Where the patient has experienced a relative absence of these natural and expected prerequisites, a truncated—wounded, reactive, shame-based, dissatisfied—self is likely to result. The failure to develop self-esteem and an internal locus of control largely explains why so many adult patients feign that they are incapable of action, "can't exercise", and "can't leave" their abusive jobs and relationships, and "can't resist" the dietary habits which daily contribute to their physical and psychoemotional decline. Thus, for more than a few patients, a therapeutic path must be explored which helps to re-create the foundation from which an autonomous adult and authentic self can grow—it is a *process* (not an event) of **emotional recovery**.[271] To this extent, interventional or therapeutic *autonomization* resembles a *recovery program* that can include various forms of conscious action, including goal-setting, positive reinforcement, developing emotional literacy[272] and emotional intelligence[273], and consciousness-raising experiences such as therapy and group work—all of which serve to intentionally (re)create and maintain the necessary climate for authentic selfhood. Therewith, the patient can accept challenges to further develop an *empowered self* by participating in exercises in which the ability to decide, choose, and act responsibly and appropriately are reinforced to eventually become second nature, replacing passivity, inaction, and ineffectiveness.[274]

"Empowerment" can only be authentic if it is built on the foundation of a developed self. While *emotional recovery* and *personal empowerment* are separate spheres of activity and attention, they are not mutually exclusive and indeed are synergistic. However, emotional recovery—that process of recounting one's own history, delving into the depths of one's own psyche, and integrating what is found into a cohesive, functional and healthy whole— must occur before the program of personal development emphasizes empowerment. *Empowerment* cannot succeed without *recovery* because otherwise the so-called "empowerment" is likely to add to the defense mechanisms that protect against pain and thereby block the development of an authentic self. Stated concisely by Janov[275], "**Anything that builds a stronger defense system deepens the neurosis.**"

Patients lacking an internal locus of control are much more likely to succumb to the tantalizing barrage of direct-to-consumer drug advertising[276] which infantilizes patients by 1) oversimplifying diseases, their causes, and treatments, 2) exonerating patients from responsibility and reinforcing the illusion of victimization and helplessness, and 3) encouraging a dependent, passively receptive role by telling patients that they have no proactive role other than to "ask your doctor if a prescription is right for you." **Americans have traditionally consumed more prescription and OTC medications per capita than people in any other country**[277,278], **and this trend continues to worsen per new data in 2013 showing** "More than 4 billion prescriptions were written in 2011. That is the most ever. Everything from sleeping pills to drugs for anxiety and depression—you name it." "Something changed in the 1990s, when it became legal for drug makers to advertise. … Demand for drugs skyrocketed."[279] With the combined and synergistic effects of 1) the dissolution of first the extended family and now the nuclear family[280], 2) a society-wide famine of mentors, elders, and community[281,282,283], 3) a dearth of autonomous, genuine exploration from childhood to adulthood, and 4) primary and secondary "educational" institutions designed to squelch independence and autonomy in favor of the more efficient, predictable, and controllable conformity and "standardization"[284,285], **industrialized societies have raised generations of people who lack completely formed internal identities**. Lacking an internal locus of control and identity from which to think independently and critically, these "adults" are easy prey for slick and flashy drug advertisements that promise the illusion of perfect health in exchange for passivity, abdication, and lifelong medicalization. That the typical American watches four

---

[271] Bradshaw J. *Healing the Shame that Binds You* [Audio Cassette (April 1990) Health Communications Audio; ISBN: 1558740430]
[272] Dayton T. *Trauma and Addiction: Ending the Cycle of Pain through Emotional Literacy*. Deerfield Beach; Health Communications, 2000
[273] Goleman D. *Emotional Intelligence*. New York; Bantam Books: 1995. Although the book as a whole was considered pioneering for its time, and the book continues to make a valuable contribution, a few of the concepts and author's personal stories are embarrassingly simplistic.
[274] Gatto JT. *A Schooling Is Not An Education: interview by Barbara Dunlop*. johntaylorgatto.com/bookstore/index.htm
[275] Janov A. *The Primal Scream*. New York; GP Putnam's Sons: 1970, page 20
[276] Aronson E. *The Social Animal*. San Fransisco; WH Freeman and company: 1972: 21-22, 53
[277] America the medicated. cbsnews.com/stories/2005/04/21/health/printable689997.shtml, msnbc.msn.com/id/7503122/, usgovinfo.about.com/od/healthcare/a/usmedicated.htm.
[278] Kivel P. *You Call This a Democracy*? Apex Press (August, 2004). ISBN: 1891843265 paulkivel.com/
[279] Costello T. Pill Nation: are we too reliant on prescription meds? 2013 Apr today.com/video/today/51490407/#51490407
[280] Bly R. *Iron John*. Reading, Mass.: Addison Wesley, 1990
[281] Bly R. *The Sibling Society*. Vintage Books USA; Reprint edition (June 1, 1997) ISBN: 0679781285 (Abridged audio edition (May 1, 1996), ASIN: 0679451269)
[282] Bly R. *Where have all the parents gone? A talk on the Sibling Society*. New York: Sound Horizons, 1996 Highly recommended.
[283] Bly R, Hillman J, Meade M. *Men and the Life of Desire*. Oral Tradition Archives. ISBN: 1880155001. Audio Cassette
[284] Gatto JT. *Dumbing Us Down: the Hidden Curriculum of Compulsory Education*. Gabriola Island, Canada; New Society Publishers: 2005
[285] Gatto JT. *The Paradox of Extended Childhood*. [From a presentation in Cambridge, Mass. October 2000] johntaylorgatto.com/bookstore/index.htm

hours of television per day[286] is bad enough, what makes this worse is that "Americans who watch average amounts of television may be exposed to more than 30 hours of direct-to-consumer drug advertisements each year, far surpassing their exposure to other forms of health communication."[287] If we are to wean our suckling culture from undue dependence on the pharmaceutical industry, we have to address our patient population directly and transform them from *passive, nonautonomous, and ignorant about health and disease* to pro-active, autonomous, and well-informed about health and the means required to obtain and sustain it.

Health ⇔ Healing
"The object of healing is… to move closer to wholeness." Kreinheder A. *Body and soul*, 1991, p 38

Insight into a patient's internal dynamic can provide the clinician with an understanding that explains the phenomena of *non-compliance* and *disease identification*. Rather than seeing non-compliance as "weakness of will", non-compliance as a form of "disobedience" may be a reflection of the patient's unconscious need to wrestle with and resolve parental introjects. For example, if a patient had a rejecting, nonaffirming parent, he/she may need to find another rejecting authority figure in order to continue playing the role of the child; by assuming this role and "setting the stage", the patient is unconsciously attempting to create a situation wherein the primary relationship can be healed.[288] Complicating this is *disease identification*—in which patients use their disease as a source of identity and secondary gain for martyrdom, social support, group participation, acceptance, admiration, purpose, excitement, and—perhaps and at times—the drama of victimization, usually by the universe/life/world, thus confirming one's importance in that sense. Maxwell Maltz MD provided an alternate approach in his classic *PsychoCybernetics*, 1960 (page 121): "Stop dramatizing yourself as an object of pity and injustice."

Spiritual strength: "How much truth can a spirit bear, how much truth can a spirit dare? ... That became for me more and more the real measure of value." "For a tree to become great, it seeks to twine hard roots around hard rocks." Nietzsche FW. *Ecce homo*, Introduction, sect. #3, and *Thus spoke Zarathustra*, *Diminishing virtue*, sect. #3; photo by DrV, Oregon coast near Astoria 2013 Aug.

---

[286] "American children view over 23 hours of television per week. Teenagers view an average of 21 to 22 hours of television per week. By the time today's children reach age 70, they will have spent 7 to 10 years of their lives watching television." Am. Acad.Pediatrics aapca1.org/aapca1/tv.html
[287] Brownfield ED, et al. Direct-to-consumer drug advertisements on network television. *J Health Commun*. 2004 Nov-Dec;9(6):491-7
[288] Miller A. *The Drama of the Gifted Child: The Search for the True Self*. Basic Books: 1981, page 88

Helping patients create and maintain authentic selves

An absent or underdeveloped locus of control is the key problem that underlies many anxiety disorders, addictive behavioral traits such as overeating, overworking, codependency, as well as chronic ineffectiveness in the pursuit of one's goals. The solutions to this problem are logical, practical, and accessible to everyone; the major costs associated with each are open-mindedness, attentiveness, discipline and persistence. There is scant mention of this concept and its intervention in the biomedical literature; however, it is well described in the psychological literature, particularly that which focuses on various types of "recovery" such as that from addiction, co-dependence, and low self-esteem, the latter two of which are virtually synonymous with an insufficient internal locus of control.

There is no single path here. There are many paths. The goal is not to choose the right path; rather the goal is to travel several paths to the degree necessary, implement what has been learned, travel other paths, and return to the same path again to retrace one's steps in new ways. The process is similar to that of *ceremonial initiation*, the purpose of which is to formally mark the *beginning* of a process that is *ongoing* and *infinite*.[1] Each path and each process has its gifts, significance, and limitations. However, the ultimate goal of each must be a tangible and positive change in the ways which the patient feels and/or behaves in and interacts with the world on a day-to-day basis.

In no particular order (since the proper sequence will have to be customized to the situation and willingness of the patient), the following are some of the more commonly cited exercises, processes, and sources of additional information:

Apprenticeship and Mentoring: books, tapes, and lectures: Children and non-autonomous adults are pulled into authentic adulthood by mentors, elders, and true adults. The therapeutic encounters thus provided—whether interpersonal or vicarious in the form of lectures, books, or audiotapes— serve as sources of information from which new possibilities can be gleaned, and these therefore serve as infinitely valuable resources for expanding the narrow horizons that characterize an underdeveloped internal locus of control. In essence, books, tapes, and lectures allow the patient to become a student and to choose a vicarious mentor. _Advantages_: Books and tapes allow access to many of the best minds in psychology; books and tapes are inexpensive; allow patients to explore and benefit from many different perspectives; books and tapes are always available and are therefore amenable to various schedules of work and responsibility. _Disadvantages_: Books and tapes do not re-create the interpersonal bridge which is essential for authentic recovery; do not provide a direct and objective means of accountably, thus potentially allowing patients to delude themselves about the effectiveness (or lack thereof) of their recovery process. Examples of better-known books, tapes and recorded lectures on the *process* of emotional recovery:

- **_The Six Pillars of Self-Esteem_** by Nathaniel Branden PhD. This is a very accessible yet very structured work in which Dr Branden brilliantly elucidates key concepts in psychology relevant to self-efficacy and self-esteem; also available as an audiobook excellently narrated by Dr Branden.
- **_Healing the Shame that Binds You_** by John Bradshaw [Audio Cassette (April 1990) Health Communications Audio; ISBN: 1558740430] Available as book and cassette with identical titles and different content.
- **_A Little Book on the Human Shadow_** by Robert Bly. Certainly among the most concise, accessible, and complete books ever written on the processes involved in losing and recovering the self; also available as an audio presentation.
- **_The Drama of the Gifted Child_** by Alice Miller. This internationally acclaimed book is considered a true classic among therapists and patients alike. Available as book and a brilliantly performed audio cassette.
- **_You Can Heal Your Life_** by Louise Hay. Another standard for recovery; very "new age."
- **_Codependent No More: How to Stop Controlling Others and Start Caring for Yourself_** by Melody Beattie. Pioneering for its time.
- **_The Artist's Date Book_** by Julia Cameron. Each page has a new creative idea for creative expression and "creative recovery."
- **_The Psychology of Self-Esteem_** by Nathaniel Branden PhD. More advanced and perhaps less widely relevant than his "six pillars" work, this is also an excellent encapsulation of important concepts in personal psychology.

Helping patients create and maintain authentic selves—*continued*
<u>*Therapy*</u>: *"Therapy is a conversation that matters."* Therapy in this context specifically means face-to-face, active interaction, either one-on-one or in a group setting, with the specific intention to give and/or provide support for personal growth. Whether 12-step groups such as Codependents Anonymous qualify as a form of therapy depends entirely upon the level of engagement of the participant; sitting in a room while *other people* do *their* work provides slow or no benefit for the passive observer. **Recovery is an *active* process, which is why it is antithetical to depression, which is a *passive* state of being.** Patients should go in knowing that this is a *process* and to not expect to be "fixed" after the first hour or even the first month. **Advantages**: Therapists can provide crucial support and insight while the client wrestles with undecipherable and convoluted emotional and psychic data. Therapists can help the client set goals ("stretches" and "homework") by which the client reaches beyond his/her comfort zone to attain the next expansion in being and experience. Therapists must create a safe space or "container" in which ideas and feelings can be brought forth to intermingle and be consciously appreciated. **Disadvantages**: Requires a flexible and disciplined schedule; costs money; bad therapists can do more harm than good if they misdirect their clients away from volatile and core issues and authentic expression. Therapy can be disempowering if the patient continues to project his/her locus of control onto the therapist. Some of the more commonly used tools of the psychotherapeutic trade include: • **Active listening** • **Insight, explanation of events**: their origins, reasons, and significance • **Reminders** of previous conclusions and stories • **Challenge old ideas and habits**: Therapy that generally or completely lacks confrontation and accountability is ineffective. • **Encourage exploration and new modes of being and interacting** • **Creating a safe container wherein the client can review the details, significance, and feelings associated with past events** • **Modeling the expression of feeling** • **Defining goals and helping the client focus on what is significant** • **Correcting distortions of reality** • **Asking patients to get in touch with and then express their feelings** • **Support and encourage clients to take calculated risks for the sake of self-expansion** • **Pointing out errors in logic** • **Coaching patients in the proper and responsible use of emotional language** • **Discouraging evasiveness; requiring accountability**[1] <u>*Creativity*</u>: All types of self-expression reinforce and validate the patient's sense of self. Creative self-expression, such as writing about thoughts and feelings about significant experiences, can reduce symptomatology in patients with rheumatoid arthritis and asthma.[1] <u>*Experiential*</u>: Corrective experiences can be obtained in therapy, with friends and family, in integration groups, and during "experiential" retreats. **Advantages**: Experiential events orchestrated by therapists and various groups such as ManKind Project (mkp.org) and WomanWithin.org can rapidly facilitate personal growth while also providing an ongoing container and support system that encourages self-development rather than the ego-inflation that accompanies short-term events. **Disadvantages**: "Adventures" like driving across the nation or climbing a mountain are unconscious and largely impotent attempts at self-initiation; authentic initiation has always been supervised by community elders. However, once a well-founded initiation has taken place, preferably with an on-going community that facilitates continued refinement and self-exploration, then "adventures" can be undertaken consciously to maintain and reinforce the experience of autonomy and competent selfhood. Eventually, transformative and sustenative experiences can be integrated and created in the daily life experience so that dramatic adventures become unnecessary for the continued renewal and "recharging" of the self.

Creating and Re-Creating the Self: An on-going process that involves various types of "therapy" such as healthy formal/informal interpersonal and group relationships, creative expression and exploration, the periodic infusion of new ideas from teachers and mentors, attendance in workshops and seminars (and other forms of on-going consciousness-raising), reflection, and the integration of transformative and sustentative significance into everyday life, in such a way that daily life itself becomes *therapeutic* and *affirmative*.

Become your own source of transformation

"However you may be, be your own source of experience! Throw off your discontent about your nature; forgive yourself *your own self*, for you have in your life experience a ladder with a hundred rungs, on which you can climb to knowledge. ... You have it in your power to merge everything you have lived through—attempts, false starts, errors, delusions, passions, your love and your hope—into your future self and goal, with nothing left over."

Nietzsche FW. Human, All Too Human: A Book for Free Spirits. #292

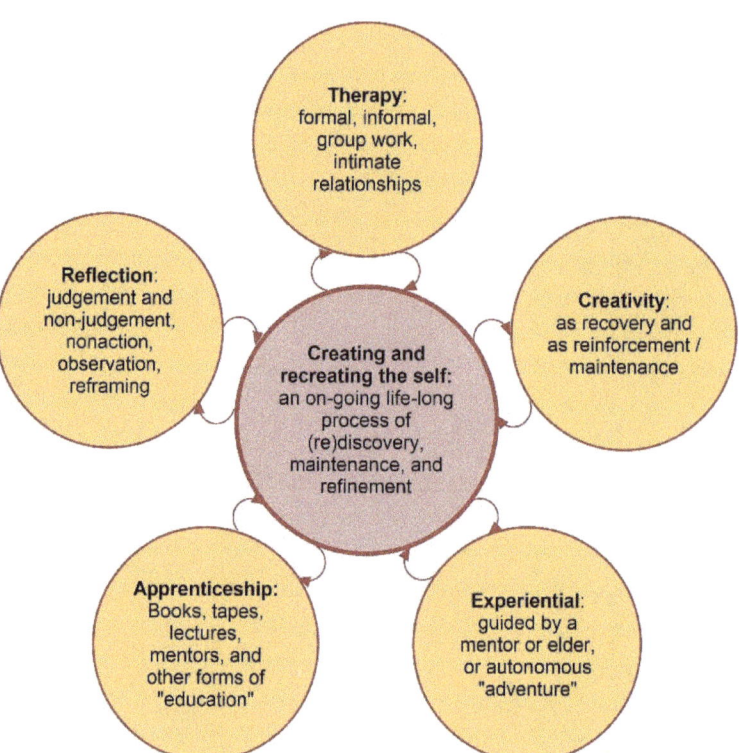

One possible sequence of events for effective, lasting, and authentic autonomization: The caterpillar does not blossom into a butterfly without spending time in its cocoon. The airborne seed descends into the earth for its nourishment before it sprouts and searches for the sun. Similarly, gratification of our ascentionist and impatient ego must be deferred for the sake of allowing the time and descent that provide "grounding" and developing of a solid foundation from which authentic growth can arise. The Western view of "personal development" idealizes a life course of constant ascension that is generally inconsistent with living in a real world fraught with imperfections; two of the major complications arising from such a perfectionistic paradigm are 1) that it causes people to feel anxious and ashamed when confronted with otherwise normal delays and failures, and 2) that it biases people into believing that improvement comes only from advancement rather than also from the return and short-term regression that are characteristic of most historically-proven societal traditions. With modification of the stepwise model proposed by Bradshaw[289], here I propose the following sequence:

1. **Short-term behavior modification**: For people whose behavior is acutely dysfunctional or harmful to themselves or others, they must stop the "acting out" that is the symptom of the underlying emotional injury or schism. Accepting abuse—at work or home—is a form of **acting out** that perpetuates old wounds and saps the strength required for recovery. Enacting addictive behavior is injurious to the psyche because self-injurious behavior reinforces the image of oneself as an object of contempt while also reinforcing the image of psychological dependency and emotional helplessness.

2. **Emotional recovery**: Complete healing is only possible when consciously pursued, and conscious healing can only be pursued after one has become conscious of the wounds, injuries, absences, dynamics, and events that lead to the current state. This process of recovery is referred to mythologically as the "descent" or the time of "eating ashes" that is a recurrent theme in various fairy tales ("Cinderella" literally means "ash girl") and cultural-religious histories (such as Jesus' *descent* into the tomb).[290] The biggest blockades to this process are 1) the ego, which prefers to ascend and to deny intrapersonal "negativity"[291], and 2) the challenge in finding elders and mentors in a society that constantly perpetuates and encourages immaturity, materialism, and superficiality.[292] In the words of famed psychologist Carl Jung, "One does not become enlightened by imagining figures of light, but by making the darkness *conscious*. The latter procedure, however, is disagreeable, and

---

[289] Bradshaw J. *Healing the Shame that Binds You* [Audio Cassette (April 1990) Health Communications Audio; ISBN: 1558740430]
[290] Bly R, Hillman J, Meade M. *Men and the Life of Desire*. Oral Tradition Archives. ISBN: 1880155001
[291] Robert Bly. *The Human Shadow*. Sound Horizons, New York 1991 [ISBN: 1879323001] and Bly R. *A Little Book on the Human Shadow*.[ISBN: 0062548476]
[292] Bly R. *Where have all the parents gone? A talk on the Sibling Society*. New York: Sound Horizons, 1996

therefore unpopular." People often have tremendous resistances to the process of self-exploration and internal learning; as Jeffrey Kottler[293] wrote of his own experience in *The Compleat Therapist*, "…like most prospective consumers of therapy, I made up a bunch of excuses for why I could handle this on my own… I was smiling like an idiot…"

3. **Long-term behavior modification and integration**: Insight allows for an illumination of the internal mental-emotional landscape, and effective insight must then be manifested externally by changes/modifications in behavior, habits, and interaction in the world. **Externalized behaviors simultaneously reflect and reinforce thoughts and feelings.** According to Grieneeks[294], patients (and their healthcare providers) can "*think* their way into new ways of *acting*" and "*act* their way into new ways of *thinking*." Eventually, a consciously designed life can be created so that actions, interactions, thoughts, and feelings are melded together in such ways that everyday life itself becomes simultaneously *therapeutic*, *affirmative*, *sustentative*, and *empowering*. In this way, the person and his/her life are unified in such ways as to become self-perpetuating and self-sustaining cycles of ascents and descents, thought-feeling and action, reflection and courage, independence and interdependence—in sum: "a wheel rolling from its own center."[295] At this point the self is established, though it must be maintained and developed with the continuous application of consciousness, reflection, and action.

4. **Metapersonal involvement in community, religion, spirituality, and the world**: Many people are tempted to move from a state of woundedness, relative incompleteness and the feelings of shame and disempowerment to a state of illusory *perfection*, *enlightenmeir* and *omnipotence* without doing the requisite hard work that makes authentic personal growth possible. People with unhealed emotional wounds often seek to camouflage those deficiencies by becoming pious and projecting an image of completeness and of "having it all figured out" and "having it all together"; religion and the acquisition of power are often misused for this purpose. Many people are successful in wearing this mask for many years; but its crumbling—often manifested as the "midlife crisis"—heralds an opportunity for personal growth if not medicated with anti-depressants, vacations, affairs, gambling, new cars and other distractions common in the American "midlife crisis." The temptation to bypass Stages 2 [emotional recovery] and 3 [integration] and leapfrog from Stage 1 [woundedness] to Stage 4 [spirituality] should be resisted because the religion or spirituality is then used as a shield *against authenticity* and as a tool for illusory control. Religion can be misused in this way by providing an "identity" and sense of redemption for people with incompletely formed identities and for those with incompletely reconciled shadows and unresolved childhood-parental introjects.[296,297,298] Nietzsche's[299] response to this problem was to encourage self-knowledge and self-reconciliation as prerequisites to religious devotion, hence his admonition, "By all means love your neighbor as yourself – but *first* be such that you love yourself." Historical and recent events remind us of how religion can be misused for misanthropic ends.[300] What is commonly referred to as "spiritual development"—a level of resolution, reconciliation, and autonomy that allows for compassionate interdependence with people, the planet and the larger "world"—is synergistic with and can be supported by religion; but the latter is not a substitute for the former.[301,302] Religion and other forms of metapersonal involvement (e.g., community participation and social generosity) are *important* and *necessary* extensions of self-development. In order for personal development to blossom from the germ of necessary narcissism into its flower of functional completeness, it must eventually manifest in the larger community and the world.

---

[293] Kottler JA. *The Compleat Therapist*. San Francisco; Jossey-Bass publishers; 1991, pages 2-3
[294] Keith Grieneeks PhD. "Psychological Assessment" taught in 1998 at Bastyr University.
[295] Friedrich Wilhelm Nietzsche, Walter Kaufmann (Translator). *Thus Spoke Zarathustra*. Penguin USA; 1978, page 27
[296] Bradshaw J. *Healing the Shame that Binds You* [Audio Cassette (April 1990) Health Communications Audio; ISBN: 1558740430]
[297] Miller A. *The Drama of the Gifted Child: The Search for the True Self*. Basic Books: 1981
[298] Miller A. *The truth will set you free: overcoming emotional blindness and finding your true adult self*. New York: Basic Books; 2001
[299] Nietzsche N. *Thus spoke Zarathustra*. Read by Jon Cartwright and Alex Jennings and published by Naxos AudioBooks. I think this is among the more brilliant achievements in human history. naxosaudiobooks.com/nabusa/pages/432512.htm
[300] *Bonhoeffer*, movie documentary by director/writer Martin Doblmeier described online bonhoeffer.com
[301] Lozoff B. *It's a Meaningful Life: It Just Takes Practice*. March 1, 2001. ISBN: 0140196242
[302] Bradshaw J. *Healing the Shame that Binds You* [Audio Cassette Version (April 1990) Health Communications Audio; ISBN: 1558740430]

5. *Acceptance of mortality and death*: No individual person or any system of thought, whether scientific or religious, can feign completeness without accounting for the end of life and incorporating this account into its overarching paradigm. The event is too significant, and the fear and concerns it provokes are too weighty to not be addressed directly and held in consciousness on a periodic—if not frequent—basis. This topic is of practical importance, too, not only in our own lives and those of our friends and family, but also to the national healthcare system, which currently spends the bulk of its money and resources vainly attempting to preserve life in the last few years and months after which disease or age call unrelentingly for the end of life. Perhaps if we as individuals and as participants in the healthcare system could accept and deal with our own deaths, then we would not have to panic and participate in such superfluous expenditures of time, energy, emotion, and money when death seeks to arrive, either for our patients, our friends and family, or ourselves. Proximal to the panic and aversion that characterizes the West's relationship to death is the "subclinical" panic and aversion that infiltrate the lives, practices, and policies that we experience every day. Surely, many unconscious events and subconscious influences contribute to the "lives of quiet desperation"[303] and "universal anxiety"[304] that subtly yet powerfully afflict most people; surely, lack of reconciliation with death is a major contributor. Especially in western cultures, death is commonly seen as some type of failure or shortcoming, either on behalf of the patient or his/her doctors, and the most common questions asked on the topic of death are "*how can this be avoided*?" before the event and "*who is to blame*?" after the event. Other cultures accept death as a natural part of life, and indeed, people are seen to have an obligation to die so that the next generations can have their turn in the cycle of life. Alternatives to western hysteria are founded on acceptance of death, and the prerequisites for the acceptance of death are 1) the dedication of sufficient time for its consideration (most people would rather watch a bad movie or attend spectator sports), 2) reframing the event in terms of its being a natural part of our lives, certainly nothing to be ashamed of (discussed below), 3) making necessary logistical preparations (e.g., writing of wills, providing for dependents, and other obvious technicalities), and 4) living as completely, consciously, compassionately, effectively, and authentically as possible so that remorse can be minimized, perhaps completely mitigated. Reframing the event of death begins with its description in general terms so that its enigma, from which its power over the hearts and minds of humanity is derived, can be deciphered and thus deflated. The main characteristics of death which precipitate its fear are 1) the unpredictability of its arrival, 2) the duration of the dying process, and 3) the quality of that process, for example whether it is painful or associated with or precipitated by severe illness or injury. The first characteristic of *timeliness*—the unpredictability of its arrival—stresses people because of their inadequate preparation and the feeling that they have only recently begun to live or have not quite yet begun to live their authentic lives. These concerns are allayed by preparation, both logistical and intrapersonal. Each of us has the responsibility to "become authentically whole" so that we do not inflict our incompleteness onto others, either directly through various forms of transference or deprivation or indirectly though the more subtle means of politics and cultural mores.[305,306] If a person can live with vitality, authenticity, compassion and effectiveness then little is left to want, and fears of death and its untimely arrival are diminished. The remaining variables are both controllable and uncontrollable; they are uncontrollable to the extent that we are all subject to chaos and accidents, whether in cars, planes, or bathtubs. *Duration* and *quality*

> **Failure to accept aging and death can only create a fragmented and neurotic society**
> "The event of death is not a tragedy—to rabbit, fox or man. But **the *concept* of death *is* a tragedy**, for man, and *indirectly* for poor fox, rabbit, bush, bird, just anything and everything in man's path."
> Pearce JC, *Exploring the Crack in the Cosmic Egg*. Washington Square Press; 1974, page 59

> **Failure to accept aging and death can only create a fragmented and neurotic society**
> "Once accepted, death is an integral component of every event, as the left hand to the right. The cultural death concept could only be instilled in a mind split from its own life flow."
> Pearce JC, *Exploring the Crack in the Cosmic Egg*.1974, p59

---

[303] Throeau HD, (Thomas O, ed). *Walden and Civil Disobedience*. New York: WW Norton and Company; 1966, page 5
[304] Becker E. *The Denial of Death*. New York: Free Press; 1973, pages 11 and 21
[305] Miller A. *The Drama of the Gifted Child: The Search for the True Self*. Basic Books: 1981
[306] Robert Bly. *The Human Shadow*. Sound Horizons, New York 1991 [ISBN: 1879323001] and Bly R. *A Little Book on the Human Shadow* [ISBN: 0062548476

are both controllable on an inpatient setting to the extent that palliative care and autonomous decision-making is made available.[307,308]

Life can only be authentically and completely experienced after one has created an authentic self and has thereafter accepted life *as it is*. Since death is part of life, the full engagement of life requires *acceptance of* and *reconciliation with* death. Acceptance of death does not necessarily entail that life becomes permeated with nihilistic resignation; on the contrary, it infuses daily events with significance and makes all experiences unique and worthy of appreciation.

> **Growth, integration, and acceptance**: Starting at the top, the progression of personal growth, emotional recovery, integration and daily practice is followed by the more advanced integration of one's chosen purpose, mission, and life work with one's chosen spiritual/religious practice, family and community involvement, and acceptance of and preparation for the end of life and the continuity of society and the environment.

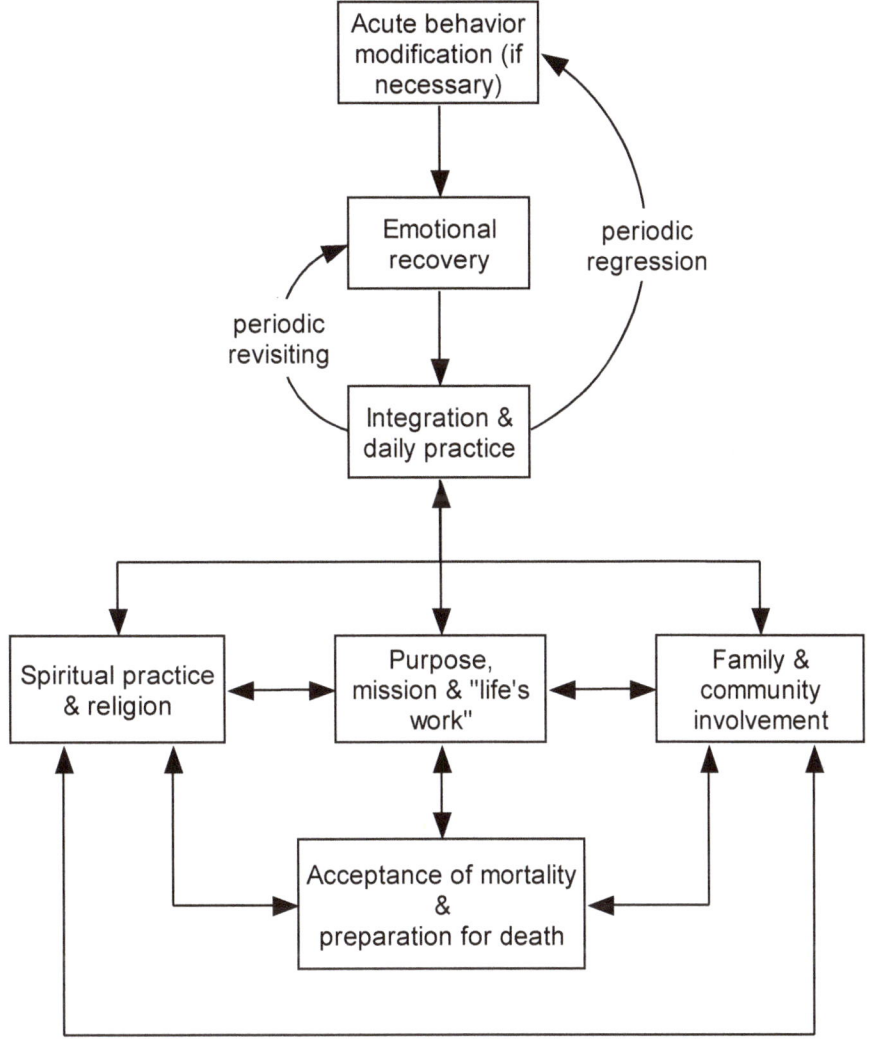

> "They say there's no future for us. They're right, which is fine with us." *Rumi*[309]

---

[307] Steinbrook R. Medical marijuana, physician-assisted suicide, and the Controlled Substances Act. *N Engl J Med.* 2004 Sep 30;351(14):1380-3
[308] "Failure to give an effective therapy to seriously ill patients, either adults or children, violates the core principles of both medicine and ethics… Therefore, in the patient's best interest, patients and parents/surrogates, have the right to request medical marijuana under certain circumstances and physicians have the duty to disclose medical marijuana as an option and prescribe it when appropriate." Clark PA. Medical marijuana: should minors have the same rights as adults? *Med Sci Monit*.2003;9:ET1-9
[309] Rumi in Barks C (translator). *The Essential Rumi*. HarperSanFransisco: 1995, page 2

Town Lake in Austin, Texas just as a light rain began, circa 2004: Photo by Dr V

Environmental Health, Toxicity, and Detoxification

> *"Man's attitude toward nature is today critically important simply because we have now acquired a fateful power to alter and destroy nature. But man is a part of nature, and his war against nature is inevitably a war against himself."* Rachel Carson[310]

Environmental exposures to chemicals and toxic substances: Studies using blood tests and tissue samples from Americans across the nation have consistently shown that all Americans have toxic chemical accumulation whether or not they work in chemical factories or are obviously exposed at home or work.[311,312] **The recent report from the CDC found toxic chemicals such as pesticides in all Americans, especially minorities, women, and children.**[313] Nearly all of these chemicals are known to contribute to health problems in humans—problems such as cancer, fatigue, poor memory, endocrinopathy, subfertility/infertility, Parkinson's disease, autoimmune diseases like lupus, and many other serious conditions. Therefore, *detoxification programs are a necessity—not a luxury*.

Examples of toxicants commonly found in Americans

Environmental pollutant (population frequency)	Biologic effects as quoted from HSDB: Hazardous Substances Data Bank. National Library of Medicine, NIH[314] or other reference as noted
DDE (found in 99% of Americans): DDE is the main metabolite of DDT, a pesticide that was presumably banned in the US in 1972	<ul><li>DDT is known to be immunosuppressive in animals.</li><li>A study published in 2004 showed that increasing levels of DDE in African-American male farmers in North Carolina correlated with a higher prevalence of antinuclear antibodies and up to 50% reductions in serum IgG.[315]</li><li>Other studies in humans have suggested an estrogenic or anti-androgenic effect.[316]</li><li>Virtually all US women have evidence of DDT/DDE accumulation. Women with higher levels of DDT and/or its metabolites show pregnancy and childbirth complications and have higher rates of infant mortality.[317]</li></ul>

---

[310] Rachel Carson. *Silent Spring*. Boston, Houghton Mifflin Company (2002). ISBN: 0395683297. See also Rachel Carson Dies of Cancer; 'Silent Spring' Author Was 56. New York Times 1956. rachelcarson.org/ on August 1, 2004
[311] "The average concentration of 2,3,7,8-tetrachlorodibenzo-p-dioxin in the adipose tissue of the US population was 5.38 pg/g, increasing from 1.98 pg/g in children under 14 years of age to 9.40 pg/g in adults over 45." Orban JE, Stanley JS, Schwemberger JG, Remmers JC. Dioxins and dibenzofurans in adipose tissue of the general US population and selected subpopulations. *Am J Public Health* 1994 Mar;84(3):439-45
[312] "Although the use of HCB as a fungicide has virtually been eliminated, detectable levels of HCB are still found in nearly all people in the USA." Robinson PE, Leczynski BA, Kutz FW, Remmers JC. An evaluation of hexachlorobenzene body-burden levels in the general population of the USA. *IARC Sci Publ* 1986;77:183-92
[313] "Many of the pesticides found in the test subjects have been linked to serious short- and long-term health effects including infertility, birth defects and childhood and adult cancers." panna.org/campaigns/docsTrespass/chemicalTrespass2004.dv.html July 25, 2004
[314] Primary source for this data is the Hazardous Substances Data Bank. National Library of Medicine, National Institutes of Health: toxnet.nlm.nih.gov/cgi-bin/sis/htmlgen?HSDB accessed on August 1, 2004
[315] Cooper GS, Martin SA, Longnecker MP, Sandler DP, Germolec DR. Associations between plasma DDE levels and immunologic measures in African-American farmers in North Carolina. *Environ Health Perspect.* 2004 Jul;112(10):1080-4
[316] Dalvie MA, Myers JE, Lou Thompson M, Dyer S, Robins TG, Omar S, Riebow J, Molekwa J, Kruger P, Millar R. The hormonal effects of long-term DDT exposure on malaria vector-control workers in Limpopo Province, South Africa. *Environ Res.* 2004 Sep;96(1):9-19
[317] "The findings strongly suggest that DDT use increases preterm births, which is a major contributor to infant mortality. If this association is causal, it should be included in any assessment of the costs and benefits of vector control with DDT." Longnecker MP, Klebanoff MA, Zhou H, Brock JW. Association between maternal serum concentration of the DDT metabolite DDE and preterm and small-for-gestational-age babies at birth. *Lancet.* 2001 Jul 14;358(9276):110-4

Examples of toxicants commonly found in Americans—*continued*

Environmental pollutant (population frequency)	Biologic effects as quoted from HSDB: Hazardous Substances Data Bank. National Library of Medicine, NIH[318] or other reference
2,5-dichlorophenol (88% nationally and up to 96% in select children populations): Dichlorophenols can occur in tap water as a result of standard chlorination treatment. General population may be exposed to 2,5-dichlorophenol through oral consumption or dermal contact with chlorinated tap water. 2,5-Dichlorophenol was identified in 96% of the urine samples of children residing in Arkansas near an herbicide plant at concentrations of 4-1,200 ppb. The sole manufacturer for herbicide use is Sandoz (Clariant Corporation).	- Human Toxicity Excerpts: 1. Burning pain in mouth and throat. White necrotic lesions in mouth, esophagus, and stomach. Abdominal pain, vomiting ... and bloody diarrhea. 2. Pallor, sweating, weakness, headache, dizziness, tinnitus. 3. Shock: Weak irregular pulse, hypotension, shallow respirations, cyanosis, pallor, and a profound fall in body temperature. 4. Possibly fleeting excitement and confusion, followed by unconsciousness. ... 5. Stentorous breathing, mucous rales, rhonchi, frothing at nose and mouth and other signs of pulmonary edema are sometimes seen. Characteristic odor of phenol on the breath. 6. Scanty, dark-colored ... urine ... moderately severe renal insufficiency may appear. 7. Methemoglobinemia, Heinz body hemolytic anemia and hyperbilirubinemia have been reported. ... 8. Death from respiratory, circulatory or cardiac failure. 9. If spilled on skin, pain is followed promptly by numbness. The skin becomes blanched, and a dry opaque eschar forms over the burn. When the eschar sloughs off, a brown stain remains.
Chlorpyrifos (found in 93% of Americans): Insecticide used on corn and cotton and for termite control. Conservative estimates hold that 80% of the chlorpyrifos in the US was produced directly or indirectly by Dow Chemical Corporation.[319] **This pesticide is routinely used in schools and is thus found in blood and tissue samples of nearly all American children.**	- Toxic if inhaled, in contact with skin, and if swallowed. - All the organophosphorus insecticides have a cumulative effect by progressive inhibition of cholinesterase. - The symptoms of chronic poisoning due to organophosphorus pesticides include headache, weakness, feeling of heaviness in head, decline of memory, quick onset of **fatigue, disturbed sleep**, loss of appetite, and loss of orientation. Other manifestations of accumulation include **tension, anxiety, restlessness, insomnia, headache, emotional instability, fatigue**... - Chlorpyrifos is a suspected endocrine disruptor.[320] - **Higher chlorpyrifos levels in children correlate with higher incidences attention problems, attention-deficit/hyperactivity disorder, and pervasive developmental disorder.**[321]

---

[318] Primary source for this data is the Hazardous Substances Data Bank, National Institutes of Health: toxnet.nlm.nih.gov/cgi-bin/sis/htmlgen?HSDB accessed on August 1, 2004
[319] Kristin S. Schafer, Margaret Reeves, Skip Spitzer, Susan E. Kegley. Chemical Trespass: Pesticides in Our Bodies and Corporate Accountability. Pesticide Action Network North America. May 2004 Available at panna.org/campaigns/docsTrespass/chemicalTrespass2004.dv.html on August 1, 2004
[320] panna.org/resources/documents/factsChlorpyrifos.dv.html accessed August 1, 2004
[321] "Highly exposed children (chlorpyrifos levels of >6.17 pg/g plasma) scored, on average, 6.5 points lower on the Bayley Psychomotor Development Index and 3.3 points lower on the Bayley Mental Development Index at 3 years of age compared with those with lower levels of exposure. Children exposed to higher, compared with lower, chlorpyrifos levels were also significantly more likely to experience Psychomotor Development Index and Mental Development Index delays, attention problems, attention-deficit/hyperactivity disorder problems, and pervasive developmental disorder problems at 3 years of age." Rauh VA, Garfinkel R, Perera FP, Andrews HF, Hoepner L, Barr DB, Whitehead R, Tang D, Whyatt RW. Impact of prenatal chlorpyrifos exposure on neurodevelopment in the first 3 years of life among inner-city children. *Pediatrics*. 2006 Dec;118(6):e1845-59

Examples of toxicants commonly found in Americans—*continued*

Environmental pollutant (population frequency)	Biologic effects as quoted from **HSDB**: Hazardous Substances Data Bank. National Library of Medicine, NIH[322] or other reference as noted
Mercury (8% of American women of reproductive age have mercury levels high enough to cause adverse health effects)	- Mercury is a well-known neurotoxin, immunotoxin, and nephrotoxin. Mercury toxicity is also a known cause of hypertension in humans. - A recent study published in *JAMA—Journal of the American Medical Association*[323] noted that **"**Humans are exposed to methylmercury, a well-established neurotoxin, through fish consumption. The fetus is most sensitive to the adverse effects of exposure. … **approximately 8% of women had concentrations higher than the US EPA's recommended reference dose (5.8 microg/L),** below which exposures are considered to be without adverse effects." **The most obvious interpretation of this data published in *JAMA* is that 8% of American women have chronic mercury poisoning—poisoning in this case refers specifically to elevated blood levels of a known toxicant that consistently demonstrates adverse effects on human health.** Logical deduction holds that such a high prevalence of human poisoning should be unacceptable and should lead directly to legislative restrictions on corporate emissions to protect and salvage the health of the public.
2,4-dichlorophenol (found in 87% of Americans): Pesticide	- Human Toxicity Excerpts: same as for 2,5-dichlorophenol - In males, significant increases in relative risk ratios for lung cancer, rectal cancer, and soft tissue sarcomas were reported; in females, there were increases in the relative risk of cervical cancer.

Toxicity and detoxification—basics: The physiologic processes by which toxins—whether chemicals or metals—are referred to generally as "detoxification." Clinically, doctors can implement treatment interventions to promote and facilitate the removal of chemical and metal toxins; this, too, is generally referred to as detoxification or clinical/therapeutic detoxification programs. Detoxification programs are popular with patients and some doctors and are most often misused and misapplied. The recent findings that mercury poisoning can result from once-weekly consumption of tuna[324] and that the average American has 13 pesticides in his/her body[325] should be seen as an indication of how dangerously toxic our environment has become, largely due to irresponsible corporate and government policies that value profitability over sustainability.

Detoxification procedures: Though a detailed clinical explanation of detoxification procedures will not be included here (see Chapter 4 of *Integrative Rheumatology*[326]), the general concepts for detoxification are as follows:
1. *Avoidance*: reduced exposure = reduced problem
    a. If there were less chemical pollution, then our environment would be less toxic and therefore we would not have such problems with environmental poisoning.
    b. Limit or eliminate exposure to paint fumes, car exhaust, new carpet, solvents, adhesives, artificial foods, synthetic chemical drugs, copier fumes, pesticides, herbicides, chemical fertilizers, etc.

---

[322] Primary source for this data is the Hazardous Substances Data Bank, National Institutes of Health: toxnet.nlm.nih.gov/cgi-bin/sis/htmlgen?HSDB Accessed Aug 1, 2004
[323] Schober SE, Sinks TH, Jones RL, Bolger PM, McDowell M, Osterloh J, Garrett ES, Canady RA, Dillon CF, Sun Y, Joseph CB, Mahaffey KR. Blood mercury levels in US children and women of childbearing age, 1999-2000. *JAMA*. 2003 Apr 2;289(13):1667-74
[324] "The neurobehavioral performance of subjects who consumed tuna fish regularly was significantly worse on color word reaction time, digit symbol reaction time and finger tapping speed (FT)." Carta P, Flore C, Alinovi R, Ibba A, Tocco MG, Aru G, Carta R, Girei E, Mutti A, Lucchini R, Randaccio FS. Sub-clinical neurobehavioral abnormalities associated with low level of mercury exposure through fish consumption. *Neurotoxicology*. 2003 Aug;24(4-5):617-23
[325] "A comprehensive survey of more than 1,300 Americans has found traces of weed- and bug-killers in the bodies of everyone tested, …. The survey, conducted by the U.S. Centers for Disease Control and Prevention, found that the body of the wellness average American contained 13 of these chemicals." Martin Millelstaedt. 13 pesticides in body of average American. *The Globe and Mail*. Friday, May 21, 2004 - Page A17 theglobeandmail.com/servlet/ArticleNews/TPStory/LAC/20040521/HPEST21/TPEnvironment/ 2004 Aug
[326] Vasquez A. *Integrative Rheumatology*. InflammationMastery.com

3. *Depuration*: "The act or process of freeing from foreign or impure matter"[327]
    a. Exercise and sauna
    b. Bowel cleansing, fiber, probiotics, antibiotics, laxatives
    c. Liver and bile stimulators
    d. Cofactors for phase 1 oxidation and phase 2 conjugation
    e. Chelation for heavy metals
    f. Urine alkalinization
4. *Damage control*: managing the consequences of chemical and heavy metal toxicity
    a. Hormone replacement
    b. Antioxidant therapy
    c. Occupational and rehabilitative training
    d. Management of resultant diseases, particularly autoimmune diseases
5. *Political and social action*: Due in large part to corporate influence and government deregulation, environmental contamination with pesticides from American corporations has increased to such an extent over the past few decades that now all Americans show evidence of pesticide accumulation in their bodies. Failure to hold corporations to tight regulatory standards has jeopardized the future of humanity. Voter passivity combined with collusion between multinational corporations and government officials is the underlying problem. Political action is the solution. The past and recent history on this topic is clear and well documented for those who wish to access the facts.[328,329,330,331,332,333,334,335,336]

> **"The only thing necessary for the triumph of evil is for good men to do nothing."**
> **Edmond Burke (1729 – 1797)**
>
> "Your lack of interest in the past, your lack of involvement, your unwillingness to develop coherent strategies, your unwillingness to challenge authority - these have created a vacuum in decision-making, that has been filled by professional groups with close relationships with the chemical industries…"   Samuel Epstein, M.D.[337]

---

[327] Webster's 1913 Dictionary
[328] Van den Bosch R. *The pesticide conspiracy*. Garden City, NY: Doubleday, 1978. ISBN: 0385133847
[329] "Monsanto Corporation is widely known for its production of the herbicide Roundup and genetically engineered Roundup-ready crops… altered to survive a dousing of the toxic herbicide. …glyphosate, is known to cause eye soreness, headaches, diarrhea, and other flu-like symptoms, and has been linked to non-Hodgkin's lymphoma." Bush Names Former Monsanto Executive as EPA Deputy Administrator. Daily News Archive From March 29, 2001 beyondpesticides.org/NEWS/daily_news_archive/2001/03_29_01.htm accessed on August 1, 2004
[330] "They pointed to budgets cuts for research and enforcement, to steep declines in the number of cases filed against polluters, to efforts to relax portions of the Clean Air Act, to an acceleration of federal approvals for the spraying of restricted pesticides and more." Patricia Sullivan. Anne Gorsuch Burford, 62, Dies; Reagan EPA Director. *Washington Post*. Thursday, July 22, 2004; Page B06 washingtonpost.com/wp-dyn/articles/A3418-2004Jul21.html on August 2, 2004
[331] "In fact, amongst the crimes of Reagan and Bush which will go down in history are their emasculation of Federal regulatory apparatus… But in 1988, under the Bush administration, the EPA - illegally, in our view - revoked the Dellaney Law…" Samuel Epstein MD, 1993. Professor of Occupational and Environmental Medicine at the School of Public Health, University of Illinois Medical Center Chicago. converge.org.nz/pirm/pestican.htm accessed August 1, 2004
[332] "The Environmental Protection Agency will be free to approve pesticides without consulting wildlife agencies to determine if the chemical might harm plants and animals protected by the Endangered Species Act, according to new Bush administration rules…. It also is intended to head off future lawsuits, the officials said." Associated Press. Bush Eases Pesticide Laws cbsnews.com/stories/2004/07/29/tech/main633009.shtml accessed August 1, 2004
[333] "The new policy also could bolster pesticide makers' contention that federal labeling insulates them from suits alleging that their products cause illness or environmental damage, Olson says. 'It . . . could really be disastrous for public health.'" Bush Exempts Pesticide Companies from Lawsuits. Law on Pesticides Reinterpreted: Government Alters Policy in Effort to Protect Manufacturers. Peter Eisler. *USA TODAY*. October 6, 2003 organicconsumers.org/foodsafety/bushpesticides100703.cfm Accessed Aug 2004
[334] "The Environmental Protection Agency will be free to approve pesticides without consulting wildlife agencies to determine if the chemical might harm plants and animals protected by the Endangered Species Act, according to new Bush administration rules." Bush eases pesticide reviews for endangered species. usatoday.com/news/washington/2004-07-29-epa-pesticides_x.htm?csp=34 Accessed August 2004
[335] "It is simply intolerable that the EPA, instead of providing an example for open scientific discussion, has continuously violated key environmental legislation, stifling legitimate dissent. The failure of EPA to properly encourage and protect whistleblowing has undermined the ability of the EPA and state environmental agencies to enforce environmental laws." Letter to Carol Browner, Administrator U.S. Environmental Protection Agency from Stephen Kohn, Chair National Whistleblower Center Board of Directors dated March 23, 1999. Availble at whistleblowers.org/statements.htm on October 10, 2004
[336] "The Bush administration has imposed a gag order on the U.S. Environmental Protection Agency from publicly discussing perchlorate pollution, even as two new studies reveal high levels of the rocket-fuel component may be contaminating the nation's lettuce supply." Peter Waldman. Rocket Fuel Residues Found in Lettuce: Bush administration issues gag order on EPA discussions of possible rocket fuel tainted lettuce. *THE WALL STREET JOURNAL*. See organicconsumers.org/toxic/lettuce042903.cfm rhinoed.com/epa's_gag_order.htm peer.org/press/508.html yubanet.com/artman/publish/article_13637.shtml
[337] Excerpted from lecture by Samuel Epstein MD, 1993. Professor of Occupational and Environmental Medicine at the School of Public Health, University of Illinois Medical Center Chicago. converge.org.nz/pirm/pestican.htm Accessed 2004 Sep and reviewed again 2014 Jun

Chapter 2: Wellness Promotion, Re-establishing the Foundation for Health

Overview of toxicant exposure and detoxification/depuration: Details are discussed later in this text.

Integrative/functional/naturopathic healthcare empowers patients with the ability to understand and effectively participate in the course of their life and health

Drug/surgery-based medicine	*Paradigm*	Holistic natural healthcare
• Doctor as "savior" and indifferent "objective" observer	*Role of the doctor*	• Doctor as "teacher" and active caring partner and co-participant in the process
• Helpless victim, disempowered, dependent	*Role of the patient*	• Active participant, empowered, responsible
• Illness is impossibly complex, and treating this with natural means is generally impossible • Treatment is simple: you have this disease, and you need to take one or more drugs for every problem • Diet and lifestyle modifications are generally viewed as secondary to drugs • The disease is more important than the patient	*Nature of illness*	• Multifactorial: involving many different aspects of lifestyle, diet, exercise, genetic inheritance, psychology, and environment • Many causes allows for many different treatment approaches and different ways of attaining health • Illness can be modified via selective dietary and lifestyle changes and a custom-tailored treatment plan • The patient is more important than the disease
• Disease-centered, drug-centered	*Viewpoint*	• Patient-centered, wellness-centered
• Drugs, including chemotherapy • Surgery • Radiation • Electroconvulsive treatment • Vaccinations	*Treatment and options*	• Diet and lifestyle improvement • Relationship/emotional work • Botanical and nutritional medicines • Physical medicine, chiropractic, exercise • Acupuncture • *Selective* rather than *first-line* use of pharmaceuticals and medical procedures
• Symptom suppression • Drug side-effects are a significant cause of death in the US • Only *treats disease*, does not *promote health*; cannot reach optimal health by only reactively treating established health problems • Enormous expense, often subsidized by private or public "insurance"	*Long-term outcome*	• Improved health • Potential for successful prevention, treatment or eradication of chronic disease • Potential to become optimally healthy • Proven cost-reduction
• Heightened risk, since drugs are foreign chemicals that have action in the body by interfering with the way that the body normally works • Every drug has side-effects, some of which can be life-threatening • Surgery causes irreparable changes to the body, often for the worse. • Radiation and chemotherapy can cause a secondary cancer to develop	*Risks*	• Reduced risk, since most of the botanical treatments and all of the nutritional medicines have been a major part of the human diet for centuries/millennia and have proven safety • Delayed onset of action: most treatments are not fast-acting enough to be of value in traumatic or acutely life-threatening situations • Patients must be willing to adopt healthier lifestyles
• Allows a doctor to see many patients within a short amount of time, thus increasing profitability • Since drugs do not cure problems, patients must return for lifelong prescription renewals • Therapeutic passivity: minimal action or effort required by patient and doctor • The doctor holds all the power, and the patient is completely dependent on the doctor for treatment	*Benefits*	• Improved short-term and long-term health • Empowerment • Understanding of body processes as well as healthcare directions and goals • Options

Chapter 2: Wellness Promotion, Re-establishing the Foundation for Health

Health-promoting:
- Frequent exercise and physical activity
- Plenty of sleep
- Maintaining ideal body weight
- Avoiding exposure to chemicals, drugs, pollution, exhaust, tobacco smoke
- Daily consumption of fruits and vegetables
- Ideal protein intake for body size, physical activity, and health status
- Diet high in fiber and complex carbohydrates
- Use of health-promoting beverages such as green tea, fruit/vegetable juices, water, and light consumption of beer or red wine
- Increased intake of ALA, EPA, DHA, GLA, and oleic acid
- Multi-vitamin and multi-mineral supplementation
- Optimal vitamin D and iron status
- Beneficial gastrointestinal flora
- Natural and phytonutraceutical interventions to promote optimal health
- Pro-active healthcare
- Healthy and supportive relationships that foster responsibility, independence, interdependence, health and feelings of being wanted and cared for
- Work environments that promote collaboration and creativity and which appreciate personal time and allow for schedule flexibility

Disease-promoting:
- Physical inactivity and sedentary lifestyle
- Insufficient sleep
- Obesity
- Frequent exposure to chemicals, drugs, pollution, exhaust, tobacco smoke
- Daily consumption of processed and artificial foods
- Insufficient (common) or excessive (rare) protein
- Diet high in simple carbohydrates and sugars
- Use of disease-promoting beverages such as cola, artificially colored/flavored/sweetened drinks, and hard liquor
- Increased intake of linoleic acid (vegetable oils) and arachidonic acid (beef, liver, pork, lamb and most farm-raised land animals)
- Low intake of vitamins and minerals
- Excess iron and insufficient vitamin D
- Dysbiosis: intestinal overgrowth of yeast, parasites, and harmful bacteria
- Use of synthetic chemical drugs to suppress symptoms of poor health
- Reactive healthcare that only responds to problems after they have developed
- Dysfunctional relationships that enable and foster illness, dependency and isolation
- Work environments that promote isolation, pressure, perfectionism and which disapprove of creativity, personal time, and flexibility

Maximize factors that promote health ☯ Minimize factors that promote disease

<u>Opposite influences of health promotion vs. disease promotion: Lifestyle concept</u>: Improved clinical outcomes will be attained when doctors and patients attend to both **prescription of health-promoting activities** and **proscription of disease-promoting activities**. Indeed, attention needs to be given to the **ratio** of these disparate and opposing forces, which ultimately influence genetic expression and physiologic function of many organ systems.

Optimize the influences on the health-disease continuum

""The work of the naturopathic physician is to elicit healing by helping patients to create or recreate conditions for health to exist within them. Health will occur where the conditions for health exist. Disease is the product of conditions which allow for it."

Jared Zeff, N.D. *Journal of Naturopathic Medicine* 1997

The experience and celebration of health and physicality: Playa Barceloneta 2013, photo by Dr Vasquez.

Chapter 3:
Basic Concepts and Therapeutics in (Nondrug) Musculoskeletal Care and Integrative Pain Management

> **Introduction**
> *Nonpharmacologic* management of musculoskeletal problems is preferred over pharmacologic (e.g., NSAID, Coxib, steroid, opioid) management because of the collateral benefits, safety, and cost-effectiveness associated with manual, dietary, botanical, and physiologic/physiotherapeutic treatments. A brief discussion of **the current "crisis in musculoskeletal medicine"** is provided for contextualization and emphasis of the importance of expanding clinicians' knowledge of effective nondrug treatments; the image below graphically demonstrates the *b.e.n.d. s.t.e.m.s.* acronym of treatments for pain and inflammation outlined later in this chapter.

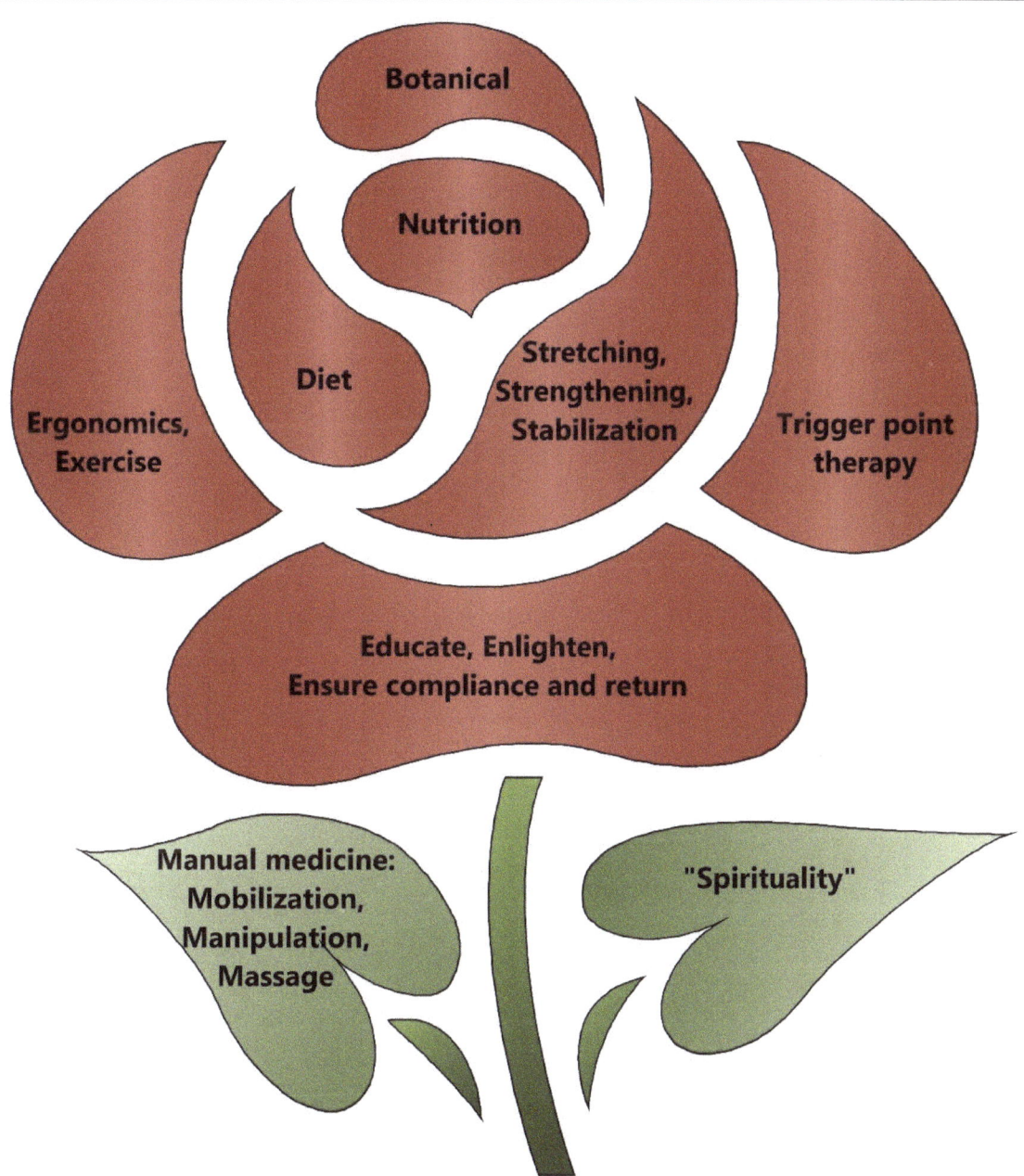

Topics:
- **Introduction**
- **Pervasive and persistent inadequacies in musculoskeletal education and training among physicians**
- **Adverse effects of nonsteroidal anti-inflammatory drugs (NSAIDs) and COX-2 inhibitors (coxibs)**
- **Nonpharmacologic Musculoskeletal Care & Integrative Pain Management**
    - Protect, prevent re-injury
    - Relative rest
    - Ice/heat, individualize treatment
    - Compression
    - Elevation, establish treatment program
    - Anti-inflammatory & analgesic treatments
    - Treat with physical/manual medicine
    - Uncover the underlying problem
    - Re-educate, rehabilitate, resourcefulness, return to active life, refer to specialist
    - Nutrition, diet, and supplements
- **Myofascial trigger points (MFTP): diagnosis and treatment**
- **Musculoskeletal Manipulation and Manual Medicine: Brief Introduction and Sample Techniques**
    - Carpal Tunnel Syndrome as an example of a neuromusculoskeletal problem that responds very well to the combination of nutritional and manual manipulative interventions
- **Proprioceptive retraining/rehabilitation**
- **Introduction to Injection Therapies: Trigger Points, Anesthetics, Viscous Agents, Prolotherapy**
- **Additional clinical tool: the B.E.N.D.S.T.E.M.S. treatment acronym**

Core Competencies:
- Provide one example from each letter of the *p.r.i.c.e. a. t.u.r.n.* and/or *b.e.n.d. s.t.e.m.s.* mnemonic acronyms for integrative care for musculoskeletal injuries.
- List at least 6 of the 10 mechanisms of action of spinal manipulative therapy.
- List the two most common clinical findings associated with myofascial trigger points and describe appropriate physical/manual and nutritional treatments.
- Describe plans for low-back and ankle proprioceptive retraining/rehabilitation for a patient who has no exercise equipment.
- Describe the effects of stereotypic NSAIDs on chondrocyte metabolism and the long-term effects on joint structure.
- Name four biochemical/physiologic mechanisms by which COX-2 inhibiting drugs predispose to cardiovascular death.
- Demonstrate the proper clinical use of the following non-drug therapeutics for pain:
    - Fish oil: Eicosapentaenoic acid (EPA), Docosahexaenoic acid (DHA)
    - Gamma-linolenic acid (GLA)
    - Vitamin D3: Cholecalciferol
    - Vitamin E: Alpha-tocopherol, beta-tocopherol, delta-tocopherol, gamma-tocopherol
    - Niacinamide
    - Glucosamine sulfate and Chondroitin Sulfate
    - Pancreatin, bromelain, papain, trypsin and alpha-chymotrypsin: "proteolytic enzymes" and "pancreatic enzymes"
    - *Zingiber officinale*, Ginger
    - *Uncaria tomentosa*, *Uncaria guianensis*, "Cat's claw", "una de gato"
    - *Salix alba*, Willow Bark
    - *Capsicum annuum*, *Capsicum frutescens*, Cayenne pepper, hot chili pepper
    - *Boswellia serrata*, Frankincense, Salai guggal
    - *Harpagophytum procumbens*, Devil's claw

Introduction to Basic Musculoskeletal Care and Integrative Nonpharmacologic Pain Management: Whether dealing with a *recent and acutely painful injury* or an *exacerbation of a chronic injury or musculoskeletal disease*, all integrative clinicians are wise to have at their disposal a comprehensive protocol for the management of acute and subacute pain and exacerbations of joint inflammation. Undertraining and incompetence in musculoskeletal medicine are very common among healthcare providers[1,2,3,4,5], leaving doctors to overuse simplistic and dangerous treatments (i.e., pharmaceutical drugs) because they are unaware of better options.[6] Failure to understand how to arrive at an accurate diagnosis and subsequent failure to know how to manage musculoskeletal pain leaves doctors *and thus their patients* with "no other option" than the overuse of so-called anti-inflammatory drugs such as non-steroidal anti-inflammatory drugs (NSAIDs, such as aspirin), which kill at least 17,000 patients per year[7], and the cyclooxygenase-2 inhibiting drugs (COX-2 inhibitors, coxibs, such as Vioxx and Celebrex) which have killed tens of thousands of patients.[8,9,10,11]

- Opioid epidemic in the United States (*Pain Physician.* 2012 Jul[12]): "Over the past two decades, as the prevalence of chronic pain and health care costs have exploded, an opioid epidemic with adverse consequences has escalated. ...dramatic increases in opioid use... ...aggressive marketing by the pharmaceutical industry. These positions are based on unsound science and blatant misinformation, and accompanied by the dangerous assumptions that opioids are highly effective and safe, and devoid of adverse events when prescribed by physicians. ... The escalating use of therapeutic opioids shows hydrocodone topping all prescriptions with 136.7 million prescriptions in 2011, with all narcotic analgesics exceeding 238 million prescriptions. It has also been illustrated that opioid analgesics are now responsible for more deaths than the number of deaths from both suicide and motor vehicle crashes, or deaths from cocaine and heroin combined. ... The majority of [opioid-induced] deaths (60%) occur in patients when they are given prescriptions based on prescribing guidelines by medical boards, with 20% of deaths in low dose opioid therapy of 100 mg of morphine equivalent dose or less per day and 40% in those receiving morphine of over 100 mg per day. In comparison, 40% of deaths occur in individuals abusing the drugs obtained through multiple prescriptions, doctor shopping, and drug diversion. ... The obstacles that must be surmounted are primarily inappropriate prescribing patterns, which are largely based on a lack of knowledge, perceived safety, and inaccurate belief of undertreatment of pain."
- Influence of profiteering public and private interests in drug regulation (*The Nation* 2014 July[13]): "Prescription opioids…are the most dangerous drugs abused in America, with more than 16,000 deaths annually linked to opioid addiction and overdose. The Centers for Disease Control and Prevention report that more Americans now die from painkillers than from heroin and cocaine combined. ... People in the United States, a country in which painkillers are routinely overprescribed, now consume more than 84 percent of the entire worldwide supply of oxycodone and almost 100 percent of hydrocodone opioids. In Kentucky, to take just one example, about one in fourteen people is misusing prescription painkillers...."

The crisis in pain medicine and rheumatology: The epidemic of opioid overuse, the paucity of musculoskeletal training among medical physicians, the spike in analgesic and anti-inflammatory drug-related deaths, and the heightened costs of treating musculoskeletal conditions compared with other conditions[14] are summatively

---

[1] Joy EA, Hala SV. Musculoskeletal Curricula in Medical Education: Filling In the Missing Pieces. *The Physician and Sportsmedicine*. 2004; 32: 42-45
[2] Freedman KB, Bernstein J. The adequacy of medical school education in musculoskeletal medicine. *J Bone Joint Surg Am*. 1998;80(10):1421-7
[3] Freedman KB, Bernstein J. Educational deficiencies in musculoskeletal medicine. *J Bone Joint Surg Am*. 2002;84-A(4):604-8
[4] Matzkin E, Smith ME, Freccero CD, Richardson AB. Adequacy of education in musculoskeletal medicine. *J Bone Joint Surg Am*. 2005 Feb;87-A(2):310-4
[5] Schmale GA. More evidence of educational inadequacies in musculoskeletal medicine. *Clin Orthop Relat Res*. 2005 Aug;(437):251-9
[6] See Vasquez A. *Integrative Orthopedics, Third Edition* (2012), *Fibromyalgia in a Nutshell* (2012), *Inflammation Mastery and Integrative Rheumatology, Third Edition* (2014)
[7] Singh G. Recent considerations in nonsteroidal anti-inflammatory drug gastropathy. *Am J Med*. 1998;105(1B):31S-38S
[8] "The results from VIGOR showed that the relative risk of developing a confirmed adjudicated thrombotic cardiovascular event (myocardial infarction, unstable angina, cardiac thrombus, resuscitated cardiac arrest, sudden or unexplained death, ischemic stroke, and transient ischemic attacks) with rofecoxib treatment compared with naproxen was 2.38." Mukherjee D, Nissen SE, Topol EJ. Risk of cardiovascular events associated with selective COX-2 inhibitors. *JAMA*. 2001 Aug 22-29;286(8):954-9
[9] Topol EJ. Failing the public health--rofecoxib, Merck, and the FDA. *N Engl J Med*. 2004 Oct 21;351(17):1707-9
[10] Ray WA, Griffin MR, Stein CM. Cardiovascular toxicity of valdecoxib. *N Engl J Med*. 2004;351(26):2767
[11] "Patients in the clinical trial taking 400 mg. of Celebrex twice daily had a 3.4 times greater risk of CV events compared to placebo. For patients in the trial taking 200 mg. of Celebrex twice daily, the risk was 2.5 times greater. The average duration of treatment in the trial was 33 months." FDA Statement on the Halting of a Clinical Trial of the cox-2 Inhibitor Celebrex. fda.gov/bbs/topics/news/2004/NEW01144.html Available on January 4, 2005
[12] Manchikanti L, Helm S 2nd, Fellows B, Janata JW, Pampati V, Grider JS, Boswell MV. Opioid epidemic in the United States. *Pain Physician*. 2012 Jul;15(3 Suppl):ES9-38
[13] Fang L. The Real Reason Pot Is Still Illegal. *The Nation* 2014 July 21-28 thenation.com/article/180493/anti-pot-lobbys-big-bankroll. For additional social context see JF. What civil-asset forfeiture means. *The Economist* 2014 Apr 14 economist.com/blogs/economist-explains/2014/04/economist-explains-7
[14] European League Against Rheumatism. Higher health care cost burden of musculoskeletal conditions. eurekalert.org/pub_releases/2014-06/elar-hhc061114.php. 2014 Jun

contributing to what is now called a crisis in pain medicine[15] and rheumatology[16]. For these reasons—and the humanitarian need to alleviate human suffering—this chapter provides an important review of nondrug treatments for musculoskeletal pain.

Previously, any medical treatment that was non-surgical was commonly described as "conservative" simply because it was *non-invasive/non-surgical*. However, many so-called "conservative" drug treatments are dangerously lethal and expensive, as the coxibs (cyclooxygenase-2 inhibitors), with their lethality and high costs, have demonstrated. Further, "conservative" has become such a confusing term in modern politics that even people who identify themselves as such are often at a loss for an accurate definition of the term. This updated version of this chapter will provide an expedient review of clinically relevant considerations in the management of pain and should be used in conjunction with the information in other chapters and volumes of this work.

The audience for this book—health science students and healthcare providers—should already be familiar with the components of basic care for injuries and the popular—yet overly simplistic—*r.i.c.e.* acronym, which stands for *rest, ice, compression, elevation* and is an easy and convenient approach to managing minor injuries, such as occurs during sports/athletics, e.g., the classic sprained ankle. When I taught Orthopedics at Bastyr University in 2000, I expanded this list to include protect, prevent re-injury, relative rest, ice, individualize treatment, compression, elevation, establish treatment program, anti-inflammatory and analgesic treatments, treat with physical/manual medicine,

> **Higher cost burden of musculoskeletal conditions compared to other diseases— Press Release from European League against Rheumatism (EULAR) 2014**
>
> In a new study released at the European League Against Rheumatism Annual Congress (EULAR 2014), **health care costs associated with musculoskeletal conditions were noted to be almost 50% higher for people with a musculoskeletal condition compared to any other singly occurring condition**.
> - Musculoskeletal conditions have a larger impact on healthcare costs than any other disease category, whether occurring alone or as co-morbidity.
> - "It is clear that the cost of delivering care to those patients with musculoskeletal conditions is considerably higher than those with other diseases."
> - More than 150 conditions affect the muscles, bones, and joints, and these are collectively described as musculoskeletal conditions, and their prevalence increases considerably with age making them **the main cause of disability among the elderly**.
> - Healthcare costs increase steeply as the number of diseases in an individual increased, but the presence of musculoskeletal conditions has a larger impact on the total cost than any other condition.
>
> European League Against Rheumatism (EULAR), 2014 Jun eurekalert.org/pub_releases/2014-06/elar-hhc061114.php

uncover the underlying problem, re-educate, rehabilitate, retrain, resourcefulness, return to active life, and nutrition including diet and nutritional and botanical supplements. The mnemonic acronym spells *p.r.i.c.e. a. t.u.r.n.* which is cumbersome but perhaps easy to remember and therefore useful; the major point is to think outside of the *r.i.c.e.* box. As integrative doctorate and multidoctorate clinicians, we certainly have much more to offer our patients than rest, ice, compression, and elevation; this chapter reviews some of these options using an outline based on the previous *p.r.i.c.e. a. t.u.r.n.* acronym and then concludes with the more pleasant *b.e.n.d. s.t.e.m.s.* acronym which was graphically demonstrated on the first page of this chapter.

Whereas the allopathic/drug-based approach stops with minimal pain/injury treatment and provides essentially nothing in terms of prevention or comprehensive patient management—let alone promotion of optimal health—the holistic and integrative approach is centered on the *patient* and seeks to help him/her attain optimal health while being treated for the musculoskeletal disorder. We can and must help our patients attain optimal health while effectively managing their acute and chronic musculoskeletal problems.[17,18,19] **Indeed, since for many patients their only interaction with the healthcare system is when they are injured or in pain, we must seize upon this opportunity to enroll patients in preventive and pro-active healthcare**; the alternative to *proactive* healthcare (maintaining/optimizing health and addressing health problems *before* they start or are still small) is *reactive* healthcare (managing problems *after* they have fully developed), which is now proven to be a colossal failure in terms of finances, health outcomes, resource utilization and other ethical considerations.

---

[15] "The main causes of this crisis are: 1) the high prevalence of chronic pain, reaching levels of 17% in the adult population;2) the lack of appropriate training of primary care physicians in the field of chronic pain management; and 3) the paucity of consultation services in the field of chronic pain." Minerbi et al. Pain Medicine in Crisis—A Possible Model toward a Solution: Empowering Community Medicine to Treat Chronic Pain. Rambam Maimonides Med J. Oct 2013; 4(4): e0027
[16] Morris AJ. The approaching crisis in rheumatologic care. *J Rheumatol* 2003; 30: 1890
[17] Vasquez A. New Insights into Fatty Acid Supplementation and Its Effect on Eicosanoid Production and Genetic Expression. *Nutritional Perspectives* 2005; January: 5-16
[18] Vasquez A. Improving overall health while safely and effectively treating musculoskeletal pain. *Nutritional Perspectives* 2005; 28: 34-38, 40-42
[19] Vasquez A. The Importance of Integrative Chiropractic Health Care in Treating Musculoskeletal Pain and Reducing the Nationwide Burden of Medical Expenses and Iatrogenic Injury and Death: A Concise Review of Current Research and Implications for Clinical Practice and Healthcare Policy. *The Original Internist* 2005; 12(4): 159-182

Pervasive and persistent inadequacies in musculoskeletal education and training among physicians—the obvious need to enhance and advance clinicians' knowledge musculoskeletal care and pain management

Question: What would be the expected clinical outcome if physicians are inadequately trained in musculoskeletal medicine and then given prescriptive rights for potent NSAIDs, coxibs, steroids, DMARDs, etc and placed in a position of ethical and professional responsibility for managing patients' pain?

Answer: We would logically expect the profession to overuse potentially lethal drugs, to diagnose conditions incompletely and inaccurately, to overuse expensive (and with regard to computed tomography, dangerous) imaging technology to compensate for poor diagnostic skills, and to overuse procedures and surgery in an attempt to provide (the appearance of) competence in the clinical management of musculoskeletal problems. That is, in fact exactly what occurs; this is an accurate description of medical practice with regard to musculoskeletal problems.

- Medical student musculoskeletal education (*J Bone Joint Surg Am* 2012 Oct[20]): "The survey contained a validated orthopedic examination of musculoskeletal competency (passing grade, 70% ... The mean score was 51.1%; only sixty-seven (19.3%) of the students passed. Fourth-year students scored significantly higher (59.0% [which is still an average grade of failure]) compared with first-year students (37.3%), but 65% of students in both groups failed. Only 34.2% of the graduating students had completed a musculoskeletal elective. Students who participated in elective musculoskeletal education had a higher pass rate (67.5%) than those who did not (43.9%)."
- Musculoskeletal education in US medical schools (*Curr Rev Musculoskelet Med* 2011 Sep[21]): "Despite the prevalence of musculoskeletal disorders in the United States, physicians have received inadequate training during medical school on how to examine, diagnose, and manage these conditions."
- Assessment of the musculoskeletal medicine attitudes and knowledge of medical students at Harvard Medical School (*Acad Med* 2007 May[22]): "Participants were asked to fill out a 30-question survey and a nationally validated basic competency exam in musculoskeletal medicine. ... Medical students rated musculoskeletal education to be of major importance (3.8/5) but rated the amount of curriculum time spent on musculoskeletal medicine as poor (2.1/5). Third-year students felt a low to adequate level of confidence in performing a musculoskeletal physical examination (2.7/5) and failed to demonstrate cognitive mastery in musculoskeletal medicine (passing rate on competency exam: 7%), whereas fourth-year students reported a similar level of confidence (2.7/5) and exhibited a higher passing rate (26%). ... These findings, which are consistent with those from other schools, suggest that medical students do not feel adequately prepared in musculoskeletal medicine and lack both clinical confidence and cognitive mastery in the field."
- Musculoskeletal cognitive competency in chiropractic interns (*J Manipulative Physiol Ther* 2007 Jan[23]): 123 fourth-year chiropractic students at a single school (Canadian Memorial Chiropractic College) were given a standardized musculoskeletal examination (basic competency examination [BCE], originally developed by Freedman and Bernstein, cited below, 1998 and 2002); very tellingly, these chiropractic researchers decided that twenty percent (5 questions) of the standardized musculoskeletal examination were not relevant to or were outside of the scope of chiropractic practice, i.e., that chiropractic practice scope is narrower than that of primary care and medical training. "Interns achieved a 51.2% passing rate (mean score, 73.2%) for the 25-item BCE,... For the modified 20-item BCE [narrowed for chiropractic education and practice scope], the interns' mean score was 80.8%..." This study is interesting in that, while chiropractic students performed better (51.5% for >73% passing grade; 64.7% for >70% passing grade) than their allopathic counterparts as would be expected for a four-year training program that focuses with near exclusively on musculoskeletal diagnosis and management, nearly half of them failed the exam if 73% accuracy is the standard; further, the researchers' modification of the exam appears to be an admission that chiropractic education/training scope is not on par with that of medical students and clinicians as they noted that 20% of questions "fell outside the scope of chiropractic practice." *What were the topics of these questions that were excluded?*: Congenital hip dislocation, knee dislocation following motor vehicle accident, skin laceration and metacarpal fracture of the hand following minor trauma, appropriate indications for

---

[20] Skelley NW, Tanaka MJ, Skelley LM, LaPorte DM. Medical student musculoskeletal education: an institutional survey. *J Bone Joint Surg Am*. 2012 Oct 3;94(19):e146(1-7)
[21] Monrad SU, et al. Musculoskeletal education in US medical schools: lessons from the past and suggestions for the future. *Curr Rev Musculoskelet Med*. 2011 Sep;4(3):91-8
[22] Day CS, et al. Musculoskeletal medicine: an assessment of the attitudes and knowledge of medical students at Harvard Medical School. *Acad Med*. 2007 May;82(5):452-7
[23] Humphreys et al. An examination of musculoskeletal cognitive competency in chiropractic interns. *J Manipulative Physiol Ther*. 2007 Jan;30(1):44-9

radiographs in patients with low-back pain, and simple clinical anatomy of the femoral neck and head. Thus, the admission by these researchers/clinicians that chiropractic students/clinicians are not prepared to deal with these issues is also a clear statement from them that they perceive that the profession is not prepared to deal with routine musculoskeletal issues at the primary care level.

- Insufficient musculoskeletal knowledge among academic primary care physicians (*J Bone Joint Surg Am* 2006 Jul[24]): "RESULTS: ... Fifty-nine (64%) of the ninety-two physicians scored < 70% [on an examination of basic musculoskeletal knowledge]. Higher examination scores were associated with male gender (p = 0.01) and participation in a musculoskeletal course (p = 0.009). Practitioners who took elective courses demonstrated higher scores compared with those who took required courses (p = 0.014). Greater musculoskeletal confidence was associated with the number of years in clinical practice (p = 0.045), male gender (p = 0.01), residency training in family practice (p < 0.00001), and prior participation in a musculoskeletal course (p = 0.0004). ... CONCLUSIONS: Although a large proportion of primary care visits are for musculoskeletal symptoms, the majority of primary care providers tested at a large, regional, academic primary care institution failed to demonstrate adequate musculoskeletal knowledge..."

- More evidence of educational inadequacies in musculoskeletal medicine (*Clin Orthop Relat Res* 2005 Aug[25]): "In their study, Freedman and Bernstein suggested that 80% of a group of graduates from many of the best medical schools in the United States were deficient in their knowledge of basic facts and concepts in musculoskeletal medicine. ... Despite generally improved levels of competency with each year at medical school, less than 50% of fourth-year students showed competency."

- Educational deficiencies in musculoskeletal medicine (*J Bone Joint Surg Am* 2002 Apr[26]): "Two hundred and forty (58%) of the 417 program directors of internal medicine residency departments responded. They suggested a mean passing score (and standard deviation) of 70.0% +/- 9.9%. As reported previously, the mean test score of the eighty-five examinees was 59.6%. Sixty-six (78%) of them failed to demonstrate basic competency on the examination according to the criterion set by the internal medicine program directors. ... According to the standard suggested by the program directors of internal medicine residency departments, a large majority of the examinees once again failed to demonstrate basic competency in musculoskeletal medicine on the examination. It is therefore reasonable to conclude that medical school preparation in musculoskeletal medicine is inadequate."

- Inadequacy of medical school education in musculoskeletal medicine (*J Bone Joint Surg Am* 1998 Oct[27]): "Seventy (82 per cent) of the eighty-five residents failed to demonstrate basic competency on the examination according to the chairpersons' criterion. In summary, seventy (82 per cent) of eighty-five medical school graduates failed a valid musculoskeletal competency examination. We therefore believe that medical school preparation in musculoskeletal medicine is inadequate."

- Training and clinical competency in musculoskeletal medicine (*Sports Med* 1993 May[28]): "Injuries and diseases of the musculoskeletal system account for more than 20% of patient visits to primary care and emergency medical practitioners. However, less than 3% of the pre-clinical medical school curriculum is devoted to teaching all aspects of musculoskeletal disease... Available elective training in musculoskeletal injuries and diseases is commonly taught by hospital-affiliated physicians and surgeons, with the result that this teaching case load is typically skewed towards serious and/or surgical problems."

In sum: The data and conclusions consistently report the fact that health professional education and training are both inadequate to ensure competence among (American) physicians in the understanding, diagnosis, and management of musculoskeletal disorders based on a verified and standardized *yet very basic* examination of musculoskeletal competence. The anticipated implications and consequences—inadequate care with overuse of invasive, expensive, and dangerous drugs, procedures, and surgeries—is well borne-out.

> **What purpose education?**
> "Education is a system of imposed ignorance."
> Chomsky N. *Manufacturing Consent*, 1992 documentary film

---

[24] Lynch et al. Important demographic variables impact musculoskeletal knowledge and confidence of academic primary care physicians. *J Bone Joint Surg Am* 2006;88:1589-95
[25] Schmale GA. More evidence of educational inadequacies in musculoskeletal medicine. *Clin Orthop Relat Res*. 2005 Aug;(437):251-9
[26] Freedman KB, Bernstein J. Educational deficiencies in musculoskeletal medicine. *J Bone Joint Surg Am*. 2002 Apr;84-A(4):604-8
[27] Freedman KB, Bernstein J. The adequacy of medical school education in musculoskeletal medicine. *J Bone Joint Surg Am*. 1998 Oct;80(10):1421-7
[28] Craton N, Matheson GO. Training and clinical competency in musculoskeletal medicine. Identifying the problem. *Sports Med*. 1993 May;15(5):328-37

Pervasive and persistent inadequacies in nutrition education and training among physicians

Introduction: Despite the acknowledged importance of diet in the prevention of obesity, diabetes, hypertension and other components of cardiometabolic syndrome/disease, physicians are consistently and systematically untrained in nutrition. A few exemplary citations are summarized per the following:

- What do resident physicians know about nutrition? (*J Am Coll Nutr* 2008 Apr[29]): "OBJECTIVE: Despite the increased emphasis on obesity and diet-related diseases, nutrition education remains lacking in many internal medicine training programs. We evaluated the attitudes, self-perceived proficiency, and knowledge related to clinical nutrition among a cohort of internal medicine interns. METHODS: Nutrition attitudes and self-perceived proficiency were measured using previously validated questionnaires. Knowledge was assessed with a multiple-choice quiz. ... RESULTS: Of the 114 participants, 61 (54%) completed the survey. Although 77% agreed that nutrition assessment should be included in routine primary care visits, and 94% agreed that it was their obligation to discuss nutrition with patients, only 14% felt physicians were adequately trained to provide nutrition counseling. ... CONCLUSIONS: Internal medicine interns' perceive nutrition counseling as a priority, but lack the confidence and knowledge to effectively provide adequate nutrition education." These are impressive results showing that internal medicine doctors—specialists who commonly deal with diabetes, hypertension, obesity, and metabolic syndrome—do not have competence in nutrition, even by weak and basic standards.

- Relevance of clinical nutrition education and role models to the practice of medicine (*Eur J Clin Nutr*. 1999 May[30]): "Yet, despite the prevalence of nutritional disorders in clinical medicine and increasing scientific evidence on the significance of dietary modification to disease prevention, present day practitioners of medicine are typically untrained in the relationship of diet to health and disease."

- How much do gastroenterology fellows know about nutrition? (*J Clin Gastroenterol*. 2009 Jul[31]): "The mean total test score was 50.04%. ...CONCLUSIONS: Gastroenterology fellows think their knowledge of nutrition is suboptimal; objective evaluation of nutrition knowledge in this cohort confirmed this belief. A formal component of nutrition education could be developed in the context of GI fellowship education and continuing medical education as necessary."

In sum: The data consistently demonstrate that healthcare providers at the doctorate level are untrained in nutrition when assessed by rather simple standards; their knowledge of functional nutrition at the level of clinical intervention in the treatment of serious disease would reasonably be expected to be approximately zero. Thus, given that doctors are trained neither in musculoskeletal management (despite the fact that all patients have musculoskeletal systems and that related disorders represent no less than 20% of general practice) nor nutrition (despite the fact that all patients eat food and that such dietary habits (and/or the use of nutritional interventions) impact nearly all known diseases in the known universe), one might wonder as to the cause and perpetuation of this systematically imposed ignorance on such topics of major importance.

> **Dumbing Us Down: The Hidden Curriculum of Systematized Educational Systems**
>
> "Look again at the seven lessons of school teaching: confusion, class position, indifference, emotional and intellectual dependency, conditional self-esteem, and surveillance. All of these lessons are prime training for permanent underclasses, people deprived forever of finding the center of their own special genius."
>
> Such a curriculum produces physical, moral, and intellectual paralysis, and no curriculum of content will be sufficient to reverse its hideous effects. ... Schools teach exactly what they are intended to teach and they do it well."
>
> Gatto JT. *Dumbing Us Down: The Hidden Curriculum of Compulsory Schooling*, p. 16.

Adverse effects of nonsteroidal anti-inflammatory drugs (NSAIDs) and COX-2 inhibitors (coxibs)

Introduction: Nonsteroidal anti-inflammatory drugs (NSAIDs) have many common and serious adverse effects, including the promotion of joint destruction. Paradoxically, these drugs *cause* or *exacerbate* the very symptoms and disease they are supposed to treat: joint pain and destruction. In a tragic exemplification of Orwellian newspeak[32],

---

[29] Vetter et al. What do resident physicians know about nutrition? An evaluation of attitudes, self-perceived proficiency and knowledge. *J Am Coll Nutr*. 2008 Apr;27(2):287-98
[30] Halsted CH. The relevance of clinical nutrition education and role models to the practice of medicine. *Eur J Clin Nutr*. 1999 May;53 Suppl 2:S29-34
[31] Raman M, Violato C, Coderre S. How much do gastroenterology fellows know about nutrition? *J Clin Gastroenterol*. 2009 Jul;43(6):559-64
[32] Orwell G. *1984*. Harcourt Brace Jovanovich: 1949. "Newspeak" is defined by the Merriam-Webster Dictionary (m-w.com) as "propagandistic language marked by euphemism, circumlocution, and the inversion of customary meanings" and as "a language designed to diminish the range of thought," in the novel *1984* (1949) by George Orwell.

the habitual utilization and long-term prescription of NSAIDs for joint pain and inflammation as advocated by the pharmaceutical industry[33] and medical textbooks[34] is not described as *malpractice*; rather it is described as the "*standard of care*" and "*first-line therapy.*" Adverse effects include:

- Promotion of bone necrosis and cartilage destruction: Several NSAIDs cause osteonecrosis[35] and many of these drugs interfere with chondrocyte function and cartilage formation and thus promote the destruction of joints.[36] As noted by Newman and Ling[37], "**...femoral head collapse and acceleration of osteoarthritis have been well documented in association with the NSAIDs...**" The subchondral osteonecrosis induced by many NSAIDs may both necessitate and complicate arthroplasty (joint replacement with prosthesis) because of extensive joint damage and because the underlying bone that must hold the new implant is too weak to provide a stable foundation.[38] *In vivo* studies have shown that salicylate, acetylsalicylic acid, fenoprofen, isoxicam, tolmetin, and ibuprofen reduce glycosaminoglycan synthesis.[39] COX-2 inhibition impairs anabolic bone activity that is necessary for the preservation of bone strength.[40,41]

- Gastric ulceration and gastrointestinal bleeding: Nearly all NSAIDs promote gastric ulceration and gastrointestinal bleeding. Among patients who chronically use NSAIDs 65% will develop intestinal inflammation[42] and up to 30% will develop gastroduodenal ulceration.[43] Drugs differ greatly in their propensity to damage the gastrointestinal mucosa and cause bleeding, and aspirin appears to be the most problematic.[44] NSAIDs can also promote and exacerbate colitis and inflammation of the large intestine.[45]

- Increased intestinal permeability: NSAIDs damage the mucosa of the small intestine and promote macromolecular absorption and paracellular permeability—"leaky gut." As described in greater detail later in this text, increased intestinal permeability most certainly contributes to the exacerbation and perpetuation of many rheumatic and musculoskeletal disorders by inducing inflammation via immune activation and by promoting the formation of immune complexes that are then deposited into synovial tissues for the induction of a local inflammatory response inside the joint.[46]

- Promotion of hepatic and renal injury and failure: Chronic use of NSAIDs is an important risk factor for the development of renal failure.[47] Hepatic injury is less common than NSAID-induced renal failure but can be achieved with higher drug doses (especially with the non-NSAID analgesic acetaminophen), coadministration of drugs, and concomitant consumption of alcohol.

- Death: NSAIDs have been an impressively significant cause of death in countries wherein they are used and overused. According to the 1998 review by Singh in *American Journal of Medicine*[48], "**Conservative calculations estimate that approximately 107,000 patients are hospitalized annually for nonsteroidal anti-inflammatory drug (NSAID)-related gastrointestinal (GI) complications and at least 16,500 NSAID-related deaths occur each year among arthritis patients alone. The figures for all NSAID users would be overwhelming, yet the scope of this problem is generally under-appreciated.**" The profile of NSAID-

---

[33] "Congratulations: you've joined the 20 million people who have taken CELEBREX, the #1 doctor-prescribed brand of arthritis medication." celebrex.com 2004 Jan
[34] "The first drug to treat rheumatoid arthritis is an NSAID." Tierney et al (eds). *Current Medical Diagnosis and Treatment 2002, 41st Edition*. Lange Medical; 2002. Page 856
[35] "The case of a young healthy man, who developed avascular necrosis of head of femur after prolonged administration of indomethacin, is reported here." Prathapkumar KR, Smith I, Attara GA. Indomethacin induced avascular necrosis of head of femur. *Postgrad Med J*. 2000 Sep; 76(899): 574-5
[36] "At...concentrations comparable to those... in the synovial fluid of patients treated with the drug, several NSAIDs suppress proteoglycan synthesis... These NSAID-related effects on chondrocyte metabolism ... are much more profound in osteoarthritic cartilage than in normal cartilage, due to enhanced uptake of NSAIDs by the osteoarthritic cartilage." Brandt KD. Effects of nonsteroidal anti-inflammatory drugs on chondrocyte metabolism in vitro and in vivo. *Am J Med*. 1987 Nov 20; 83(5A): 29-34
[37] Newman NM, Ling RS. Acetabular bone destruction related to non-steroidal anti-inflammatory drugs. *Lancet*. 1985 Jul 6; 2(8445): 11-4
[38] "This highly significant association between NSAID use and acetabular destruction gives cause for concern, not least because of the difficulty in achieving satisfactory hip replacements in patients with severely damaged acetabula." Newman et al. Acetabular bone destruction related to non-steroidal anti-inflammatory drugs. *Lancet*. 1985; 2: 11-4
[39] Brandt KD. Effects of nonsteroidal anti-inflammatory drugs on chondrocyte metabolism in vitro and in vivo. *Am J Med*. 1987 Nov 20; 83(5A): 29-34
[40] "Histological observations suggest that cox-2 is required for normal endochondral ossification during fracture healing. Because mice lacking Cox2 form normal skeletons, our observations indicate that fetal bone development and fracture healing are different and that cox-2 function is specifically essential for fracture healing." Simon AM, Manigrasso MB, O'Connor JP. Cyclo-oxygenase 2 function is essential for bone fracture healing. *J Bone Miner Res*. 2002 Jun;17(6):963-76
[41] "The results indicate that cox-2 and constitutive NOS are important signaling molecules in the anabolic responses of neonatal tibial bone to the micromechanical load in vitro." Kunnel JG, Igarashi K, Gilbert JL, Stern PH. Bone anabolic responses to mechanical load in vitro involve cox-2 and constitutive NOS. *Connect Tissue Res*. 2004;45(1):40-9
[42] "NSAIDs cause small intestinal inflammation in 65% of patients receiving the drugs long-term." Bjarnason I, Macpherson AJ. Intestinal toxicity of non-steroidal anti-inflammatory drugs. *Pharmacol Ther*. 1994 Apr-May;62(1-2):145-57
[43] "Endoscopic studies indicate that up to 30% of chronic NSAID users will develop gastroduodenal ulceration." Blower AL. Considerations for nonsteroidal anti-inflammatory drug therapy: safety. *Scand J Rheumatol Suppl*. 1996;105:13-24
[44] "ASA (1,500 mg/day for 5 days) caused about a 6-fold increase in blood loss. Four days after withdrawal of ASA, faecal blood was still about twice as high as in faeces of subjects given ibuprofen and indoprofen." Porro GB, et al. Gastro-intestinal blood loss during administration of indoprofen, aspirin and ibuprofen. *J Int Med Res* 1977;5(3):155-60
[45] "Non-steroidal anti-inflammatory drugs (NSAIDs) may adversely affect the colon, either by causing a non-specific colitis or by exacerbating a preexisting colonic disease. ... Local and/or systemic effects of NSAIDs on mucosal cells might lead to an increased intestinal permeability, which is a prerequisite for colitis." Faucheron JL, Parc R. Non-steroidal anti-inflammatory drug-induced colitis. *Int J Colorectal Dis*. 1996;11(2):99-101
[46] Inman RD. Antigens, the gastrointestinal tract, and arthritis. *Rheum Dis Clin North Am*. 1991 May; 17(2): 309-21
[47] "Patients with chronic arthritis who consume excessive amount of NSAIDs are at risk of developing renal papillary necrosis and chronic renal impairment." Segasothy M, Chin GL, Sia KK, Zulfiqar A, Samad SA. Chronic nephrotoxicity of anti-inflammatory drugs used in the treatment of arthritis. *Br J Rheumatol*. 1995 Feb; 34(2): 162-5
[48] Singh G. Recent considerations in nonsteroidal anti-inflammatory drug gastropathy. *Am J Med*. 1998 Jul 27; 105(1B): 31S-38S

induced death is likely very different from country to country, and would be expected to change over time as new drugs are introduced; however, one should—ultimately—look at the aggregate of, in this example, not only NSAIDs but also their modern replacements, particularly the Coxibs, which cause *fewer gastrohemorrhagic deaths* but *more cardiovascular deaths*.

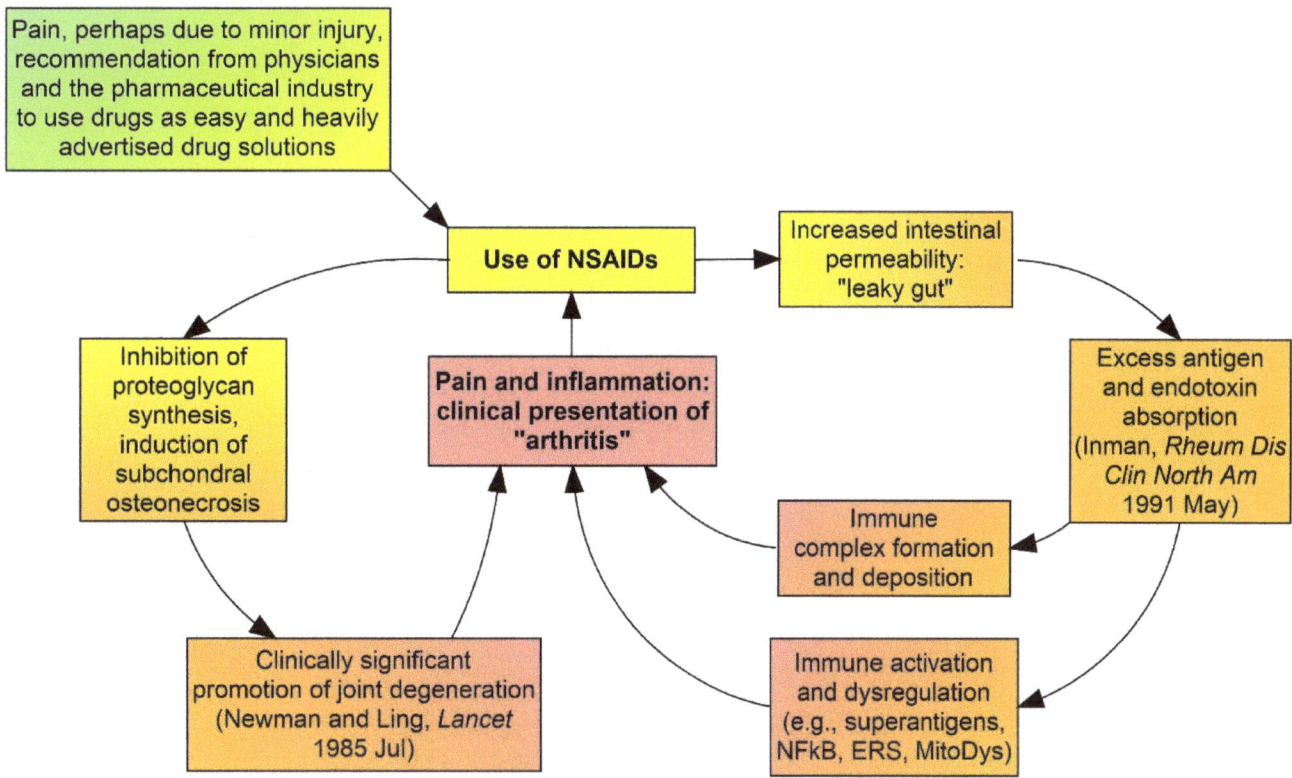

The vicious cycle of NSAID use: Pain prompts use of NSAIDS, which promote joint destruction and increased intestinal permeability, promoting systemic inflammation which then contribute(s) to the perpetuation of joint pain.

- Adverse effects specific to Coxibs: Drugs specifically designed to inhibit the isoform of cyclooxygenase known as cyclooxygenase-2 (coxibs) carry their own list of adverse effects, namely membranous glomerulopathy and acute interstitial nephritis[49], acute cholestatic hepatitis[50], toxic epidermal necrolysis[51,52], and—perhaps most importantly—increased risk for cardiovascular disease (e.g., stroke, hypertension, myocardial infarction) and cardiovascular death. Immediately following the withdrawal of the arthritis drug rofecoxib (Vioxx) in late September 2004, Topol[53] extrapolated that as many as 160,000 adverse cardiovascular events (including stroke, myocardial infarction, and death) may have resulted from the overuse of Vioxx/rofecoxib due to the collusion of Merck's intentional failure to withdraw what was known for years to be a dangerous drug, the FDA's failure to enforce regulatory standards to protect the public, and the overutilization of Vioxx by the medical profession, which was well informed of the lethality of Vioxx for several years[54] before Merck's confessionary and belated withdrawal of the drug. Soon thereafter, several other so-called "anti-inflammatory drugs" such as valdecoxib (Bextra)[55], celecoxib (Celebrex)[56], and

---

[49] Markowitz GS, et al. Membranous glomerulopathy and acute interstitial nephritis following treatment with celecoxib. *Clin Nephrol*. 2003;59(2):137-42
[50] Grieco A, Miele L, Giorgi A, Civello IM, Gasbarrini G. Acute cholestatic hepatitis associated with celecoxib. *Ann Pharmacother*. 2002;36(12):1887-9
[51] Berger P, Dwyer D, Corallo CE. Toxic epidermal necrolysis after celecoxib therapy. *Pharmacotherapy*. 2002 Sep;22(9):1193-5.
[52] Friedman B, Orlet HK, Still JM, Law E. Toxic epidermal necrolysis due to administration of celecoxib (Celebrex). *South Med J*. 2002;95(10):1213-4
[53] Topol EJ. Failing the public health--rofecoxib, Merck, and the FDA. *N Engl J Med*. 2004 Oct 21;351(17):1707-9
[54] Mukherjee D, Nissen SE, Topol EJ. Risk of cardiovascular events associated with selective cox-2 inhibitors. *JAMA* 2001; 286(8):954-9
[55] Ray WA, Griffin MR, Stein CM. Cardiovascular toxicity of valdecoxib. *N Engl J Med*. 2004;351(26):2767
[56] "Patients in the clinical trial taking 400 mg. of Celebrex twice daily had a 3.4 times greater risk of CV events compared to placebo. For patients in the trial taking 200 mg. of Celebrex twice daily, the risk was 2.5 times greater. The average duration of treatment in the trial was 33 months." FDA Statement on the Halting of a Clinical Trial of the cox-2 Inhibitor Celebrex. fda.gov/bbs/topics/news/2004/NEW01144.html Available on January 4, 2005

naproxen (Aleve)[57] were likewise associated with excess cardiovascular injury and death. Although the advertising-induced feeding frenzy on Celebrex made it the most "successful" drug launch in US history with more than 7.4 million prescriptions written within its first 6 months[58], major adverse effects due to the drug were noted within 2 years of its release onto the medical market[59]; current guidelines hold that patients must be informed of the excess cardiovascular risk associated with this drug and that its use should be limited to the lowest dose for the shortest time possible (weeks).[60] When compared with placebo in cardiac surgery patients, Bextra/valdecoxib is associated with a 3-fold to 4-fold increased risk of heart attack, stroke, and death[61], and recently 7 million arthritis patients, many of whom were already at high risk for cardiovascular disease, were being treated with this drug.[62] Use of Bextra was also strongly associated with toxic epidermal necrolysis, a potentially fatal condition.[63] Due primarily to the adverse cardiovascular effects[64], in the interest of protecting the public from additional adverse effects and unnecessary deaths, in April 2005 the FDA ordered that Bextra/valdecoxib be taken off the market in the US[65], and Health Canada followed suit by removing the drug from Canadian markets.[66] **It is inexcusable that these drugs were so highly utilized despite evidence of relative analgesic inefficacy** (not better than earlier NSAIDs like aspirin), **exorbitant costs** (US $90-180 per month[67]) and **clear evidence of danger** (e.g., cardiovascular death) by two well-identified biochemical/physiologic mechanisms, namely: 1) inhibiting the formation of vasodilating and anti-aggregatory prostacyclin, which is formed by COX-2, and 2) shunting arachidonate toward formation of pro-atherosclerotic leukotrienes[68] by blocking cyclooxygenase. Inhibition of prostacyclin formation promotes thrombosis and hypertension. Of recent interest is the finding that celecoxib induces endoplasmic reticulum stress (detailed later in Chapter 4 of Volume 1) and—ironically—cox2 expression; thus, per the research cited below presented in 2013, this drug actually induces/promotes expression of the same enzyme it is designed to inhibit. In order to foreshadow the discussion on endoplasmic reticulum stress (ERS) and the unfolded protein response (UPR) and to help readers begin to develop a more profound understanding of the subtle *pro-inflammatory effects of anti-inflammatory drugs*, the following sample quotes and citations are offered:

- Celecoxib induces apoptosis, ER stress, and cyclooxygenase-2 expression on lung cancer cells (*J Immunol* 2013 May[69]): "Paradoxically, celecoxib stimulated COX-2 mRNA and protein on A549, but indomethacin, inhibitor of COX-1 and COX-2 did not induce COX-2 expression. Taken together, we suggest that celecoxib induces apoptosis and ER stress on lung cancer cell line."
- Drug-induced perturbation of ER stress and the unfolded protein response (*Toxicol Pathol* 2013 Feb[70]): "Marketed pharmaceuticals developed for various diseases can also cause ER stress by either on- or off-target mechanisms for which they were developed including bortezomib, nelfinavir, atazanavir, ritonavir, lopinavir, sorafenib, indomethacin, and celecoxib."

---

[57] "Preliminary information from the study showed some evidence of increased risk of cardiovascular events, when compared to placebo, to patients taking naproxen." FDA Statement on Naproxen. fda.gov/bbs/topics/news/2004/NEW01148.html Available on January 4, 2005
[58] Monsanto, Pfizer celebrate Celebrex. *St. Louis Business Journal*. July 20, 1999 bizjournals.com/stlouis/stories/1999/07/19/daily5.html Accessed on January 5, 2005
[59] Mukherjee D, Nissen SE, Topol EJ. Risk of cardiovascular events associated with selective cox-2 inhibitors. *JAMA*. 2001 Aug 22-29;286(8):954-9
[60] "Celecoxib should be used in the lowest effective doses for short periods (weeks) only. A risk–benefit discussion is necessary for those requiring the drug for a longer period." Cotter J, Wooltorton E. New restrictions on celecoxib (Celebrex) use and the withdrawal of valdecoxib (Bextra). *CMAJ*. 2005 May 10;172(10):1299
[61] Lenzer J. Pfizer criticised over delay in admitting drug's problems. *BMJ*. 2004;329(7472):935
[62] Ray WA, Griffin MR, Stein CM. Cardiovascular toxicity of valdecoxib. *N Engl J Med*. 2004;351(26):2767
[63] "There is a strong association between Stevens-Johnson syndrome/toxic epidermal necrolysis and the use of the sulfonamide cox-2 inhibitors, particularly valdecoxib." La Grenade et al. Comparison of Reporting of Stevens-Johnson Syndrome and Toxic Epidermal Necrolysis in Association with Selective cox-2 Inhibitors. *Drug Saf*. 2005;28:917-24
[64] Nussmeier NA, et al. Complications of the cox-2 inhibitors parecoxib and valdecoxib after cardiac surgery. *N Engl J Med*. 2005 Mar 17;352(11):1081-91
[65] "On April 7, the Food and Drug Administration requested that Pfizer suspend sales of BEXTRA in the United States. As a result, BEXTRA will no longer be available to patients in the United States... In light of the FDA's position that there is an increased cardiovascular risk for all prescription non-steroidal anti-inflammatory arthritis medicines, as well as the increased rate of rare, serious skin reactions with BEXTRA, the FDA has requested that sales of BEXTRA be suspended." bextra.com/ September 28, 2005
[66] Sibbald B. Pfizer withdraw valdecoxib (Bextra) at Health Canada's request. *CMAJ*. 2005 May 10;172(10):e1298. Epub 2005 Apr 7 cmaj.ca/cgi/reprint/172/10/e1298
[67] walgreens.com/library/finddrug/druginfo1.jsp?particularDrug=Celebrex&id=15102 Accessed September 29, 2005
[68] "CONCLUSIONS: Variant 5-lipoxygenase genotypes identify a subpopulation with increased atherosclerosis. The observed diet-gene interactions further suggest that dietary n-6 polyunsaturated fatty acids promote, whereas marine n-3 fatty acids inhibit, leukotriene-mediated inflammation that leads to atherosclerosis in this subpopulation." Dwyer JH, et al. Arachidonate 5-lipoxygenase promoter genotype, dietary arachidonic acid, and atherosclerosis. *N Engl J Med*. 2004 Jan 1;350(1):29-37
[69] Kim et al. Celecoxib induces apoptosis, ER stress, and cyclooxygenase-2 expression on lung cancer cells (P2090). *J Immunol* 2013 May; 190 (Meeting Abstract) 132.35
[70] Lafleur MA et al. Xenobiotic perturbation of ER stress and the unfolded protein response. *Toxicol Pathol*. 2013 Feb;41(2):235-6

Perspective: If we summarize that at least 17,000 people die each year from NSAIDs, that other "medication errors" kill over 7,000 people in America[71] and that an additional 180,000 Americans die due to hospital errors[72], then we have a situation where at least 200,000 Americans die each year due to drug effects and hospital/physician errors. Furthermore, according to estimates by David Graham, MD, MPH, (Associate Director for Science, Office of Drug Safety, US FDA), more than 139,000 Americans who took Vioxx suffered serious side effects and between 26,000 and 55,000 people died from using the drug.[73] This aggregate is significantly greater than the annual deaths due to diabetes (71,000), suicide (30,000), homicide (20,000)[74], and—as a most dramatic example—the September 11, 2001 American terrorist attack (up to 3,000) *combined*.[75] Data suggests that nondrug treatments such as spinal manipulation[76], glucosamine sulfate[77], *Harpagophytum*[78] and capsicum are safer and/or more effective than pharmaceutical drugs for the relief of many types of pain. The increased utilization of these and other nonpharmacologic treatments would result in reductions in morbidity, mortality, and overall healthcare expenses when compared to our current overutilization of NSAIDs and other medical/allopathic pharmacosurgical treatments.[79]

> **In the US, 493 patients die each day —3,452 deaths per week— due to adverse events in hospitals**
>
> "Recent estimates suggest that each year more than 1 million patients are injured while in the hospital and approximately 180,000 die because of these injuries. Furthermore, drug-related morbidity and mortality are common and are estimated to cost more than $136 billion a year."
>
> Holland, Degruy. *Am Fam Physician*, 1997

Basic Concepts and Commonly Employed Therapeutics in Integrative Pain Management

The following pages summarize the basic therapeutics most commonly employed by integrative physicians in the treatment of acute and chronic musculoskeletal conditions. Knowledge of some of the clinical skills relied upon in orthopedics[80] is necessary when treating rheumatic musculoskeletal problems[81] because an acutely inflamed joint associated with a *chronic* and *systemic* disorder may need to be treated as if it were a *recent* and *focal* injury. Although *rheumatology* is generally concerned with the treatment of *non-traumatic* disorders of an inflammatory or autoimmune nature, knowledge of orthopedics is necessary during the course of evaluating and treating patients with autoimmunity because differential diagnosis, qualification/quantification, and comanagement of joint disorders *within the same patient* are commonly necessary. For example, a patient with rheumatoid arthritis (long-term autoimmune disease) affecting the knees and hips may also develop carpal tunnel syndrome (orthopedic problem) and later present with neck pain and leg spasticity secondary to atlantoaxial instability (neuro-orthopedic emergency).

Orthopedics generally centers on the clinical management of 1) **acute injuries** (e.g., whiplash), 2) **chronic repetitive strain injuries** (tendonitis and myofasciitis/myofascitis), and 3) **congenital/developmental anomalies**, (odontoid hypoplasia and scoliosis). For most clinicians, management of congenital anomalies centers on accurate diagnosis and then either observation or appropriate referral. For the treatment of common acute and chronic injuries encountered in general practice, integrative clinical care can include the facets described in the following section, modified for the clinical situation and individual patient.

---

[71] "In 1983, 2876 people died from medication errors. ... By 1993, this number had risen to 7,391 - a 2.57-fold increase." Phillips DP, Christenfeld N, Glynn LM. Increase in US medication-error deaths between 1983 and 1993. *Lancet*. 1998 Feb 28;351(9103):643-4
[72] "Recent estimates suggest that each year more than 1 million patients are injured while in the hospital and approximately 180,000 die because of these injuries. Furthermore, drug-related morbidity and mortality are common and are estimated to cost more than $136 billion a year." Holland EG, Degruy FV. Drug-induced disorders. *Am Fam Physician*. 1997;56(7):1781-8, 1791-2
[73] commondreams.org/views05/0223-35.htm and fda.gov/cder/drug/infopage/vioxx/vioxxgraham.pdf Accessed July 26, 2006
[74] Centers for Disease Control and Prevention (CDC), National Center for Health Statistics. Deaths: Final Data for 2001. 116 pp. (PHS) 2003-1120. Available at cdc.gov/nchs/releases/03facts/mortalitytrends.htm on January 18, 2004
[75] "On September 11, 2001, four U.S. planes hijacked by terrorists crashed into the World Trade Center, the Pentagon and a field in Pennsylvania killing nearly 3,000 people in a matter of hours." From cnn.com/SPECIALS/2001/memorial/ on January 26, 2004
[76] "CONCLUSION: The best evidence indicates that cervical manipulation for neck pain is much safer than the use of NSAIDs, by as much as a factor of several hundred times. There is no evidence that indicates NSAID use is any more effective than cervical manipulation for neck pain." Dabbs V, Lauretti WJ. A risk assessment of cervical manipulation vs. NSAIDs for the treatment of neck pain. *J Manipulative Physiol Ther*. 1995 Oct;18(8):530-6
[77] Muller-Fassbender H, et al. Glucosamine sulfate compared to ibuprofen in osteoarthritis of the knee. *Osteoarthritis Cartilage*. 1994 Mar;2(1):61-9
[78] Chrubasik S, et al. A randomized double-blind pilot study comparing Doloteffin and Vioxx in the treatment of low back pain. *Rheumatology* (Oxford). 2003 Jan;42(1):141-8
[79] Orme-Johnson DW, Herron RE. An innovative approach to reducing medical care utilization and expenditures. *Am J Manag Care*. 1997 Jan;3:135-44
[80] Vasquez A. *Integrative Orthopedics*. Third Edition (2012) or later. InflammationMastery.com
[81] Vasquez A. *Integrative Rheumatology*. Third Edition (2014) or later. InflammationMastery.com

Generally, different types and locations of injuries can be treated from a common framework of interventions that are then customized for the three following primary considerations:
1) <u>Location</u>: The specific location and associated functional considerations, e.g., lower extremity injuries may require crutches while upper extremity injuries may benefit from a brace or sling; ergonomic modifications,
2) <u>Tissue</u>: The type of tissue that is injured—i.e., muscle, cartilage, tendons, or ligaments—may respond to a customized nutritional and rehabilitative protocol,
3) <u>Patient</u>: The specific goals, needs, comorbidities, medications, occupation, recreational activities, age, and other characteristics of the individual patient. Also included here is consideration/correction of the patient's *internal inflammatory tendency* and *inflammatory balance/imbalance*, e.g. pro-inflammatory diet, acid-base balance, mitochondrial function, AGE and allergen consumption, etc.

<u>Protect & prevent re-injury</u>:
- **Avoid motions and activities that cause significant pain, as pain indicates that damaged/inflamed tissues are being stressed.** The goals are 1) to allow healing of injured tissues, and 2) to promote maximal physical restoration and functional ability. An excess of rest promotes functional disability, muscle atrophy, and psychological dysfunction (e.g., iatrogenic neurosis, inaccurate perception of patient being permanently damaged or defective, loss of confidence, loss of social contact [especially for children, and adults for whom physical activity is important]). Returning to activities and work too quickly may not allow time for sufficient healing and may thus promote re-injury, temporary exacerbation, progression from mild to severe injury, and/or progression to repetitive strain injury.
- **Use bracing, taping, bandages, wrapping, canes, crutches, and walkers as needed.**[82,83]

<u>Relative rest</u>:
- **"Relative rest" simply means to take time away from the activities that either promote additional injury or that unnecessarily drain energies which could otherwise be used for healing and recuperation.** For some patients, this means avoiding certain exercises during a workout, while for other patients this may mean using a crutch or taking days off from work.
- "Bed rest" is generally to be avoided since it promotes muscle atrophy, intraarticular adhesions, loss of neuromuscular coordination, constipation, and patients' assumption of the sick role.[84]

<u>Ice/heat</u>:
- **First 48-72 hours after injury: Apply ice or cold pack for 10 minutes each 30-60 minutes for reduction in pain and inflammation.** The best protocol appears to be interrupted application of ice to maximize deep cooling of tissues while minimizing cold-induced damage to the skin.[85] Ice massage is more effective than stationary application of ice or an ice bag.[86] Intraarticular temperatures can be lowered with topical application of ice[87], and immersion into ice water appears to be the best method for reducing intraarticular temperature according to an animal study.[88] Greater skin thickness due to subcutaneous adipose increases the amount of time needed to achieve clinically significant cooling of deep tissues.[89] Avoid frostbite and cold injuries to skin and superficial nerves. Use caution in patients with decreased skin sensitivity, circulatory insufficiency, and/or suboptimal ability to follow directions and employ good judgment.
- **After 48-72 hours post-injury: Apply gentle heat as needed for the relief of pain and reduction in muscle spasm and to promote healing by increasing circulation.** Avoid heat injuries to skin. Use caution in patients with decreased skin sensitivity (e.g., diabetics and the elderly) or suboptimal ability to follow directions and employ good judgment.

---

[82] Van Hook FW, Demonbreun D, Weiss BD. Ambulatory devices for chronic gait disorders in the elderly. *Am Fam Physician*. 2003 Apr 15;67(8):1717-24
[83] Joyce BM, Kirby RL. Canes, crutches and walkers. *Am Fam Physician*. 1991 Feb;43(2):535-42
[84] "Glucose intolerance, anorexia, constipation, and pressure sores might develop. Central nervous system changes could affect balance and coordination and lead to increasing dependence on caregivers." Teasell R, Dittmer DK. Complications of immobilization and bed rest. Part 2: Other complications. *Can Fam Physician*. 1993 Jun;39:1440-2, 1445-6
[85] "... melting iced water applied through a wet towel for repeated periods of 10 minutes is most effective." MacAuley DC. Ice therapy. *Int J Sports Med*. 2001 Jul;22(5):379-84
[86] Zemke JE, et al. Intramuscular temperature responses in the human leg to two forms of cryotherapy: ice massage and ice bag. *J Orthop Sports Phys Ther*. 1998 Apr;27(4):301-7
[87] Martin SS, et al. Cryotherapy: an effective modality for decreasing intraarticular temperature after knee arthroscopy. *Am J Sports Med*. 2001 May-Jun;29(3):288-91
[88] Bocobo C, Fast A, Kingery W, Kaplan M. The effect of ice on intra-articular temperature in the knee of the dog. *Am J Phys Med Rehabil*. 1991 Aug;70(4):181-5
[89] Otte JW, et al. Subcutaneous adipose tissue thickness alters cooling time during cryotherapy. *Arch Phys Med Rehabil*. 2002 Nov;83(11):1501-5

Individualize treatment:
- **The cornerstone of effective holistic and integrative treatment is to design treatment plans that simultaneously 1) address "the problem" while also 2) improving the patient's overall health.** Often, serious and so-called "untreatable" diseases can be ameliorated or eradicated simply with general, non-specific, overall health improvement even when these conditions repeatedly fail to respond to specific "disease-targeting" medical treatments.

Compression:
- Snug bandages/wraps may help to reduce swelling and can provide support for injured tissues and weakened joints. Care must be utilized to avoid arterial, venous, or lymphatic obstruction. Overuse of bandages/wraps/braces limits motion and thereby promotes neuromuscular discoordination, which can promote local instability and re-injury.

Educate, establish treatment program, elevation:
- Educate patient about the injury. Educate patient about the need for appropriate follow-up office visits for reexamination, reassessment, and treatment.
- Estimate the amount of time during which most recovery will take place. Estimate the extent of return to previous status.
- Elevate the injured part to minimize swelling and edema.

Anti-inflammatory & analgesic treatments:
- Avoidance of pro-inflammatory foods: **Arachidonic acid** (high in cow's milk, beef, liver, pork, and lamb) is the direct precursor to pro-inflammatory prostaglandins and leukotrienes[90] and pain-promoting isoprostanes.[91] **Saturated fats** promote inflammation by activating/enabling pro-inflammatory Toll-like receptors, which are otherwise "specific" for inducing pro-inflammatory responses to microorganisms.[92] Consumption of saturated fat in the form of **cream** creates marked oxidative stress and lipid peroxidation that lasts for at least 3 hours postprandially.[93] **Corn oil** rapidly activates NFkB (in hepatic Kupffer cells) for a pro-inflammatory effect[94]; similarly, consumption of **linoleic acid** promotes intracellular antioxidant depletion and may thus promote oxidation-mediated inflammation via activation of NFkB. **Linoleic acid** causes intracellular oxidative stress and calcium influx and results in increased NFkB-stimulated transcription of pro-inflammatory genes.[95] **High glycemic foods** cause oxidative stress[96,97] and inflammation via activation of NFkB and other mechanisms—e.g., *white bread causes inflammation*[98] as does *a high-fat high-carbohydrate fast-food breakfast.*[99] **High glycemic foods** suppress immune function[100,101] and thus promote the development of infection/dysbiosis.[102] Delivery of a **high carbohydrate load** to the gastrointestinal lumen promotes bacterial overgrowth[103,104], which is inherently pro-inflammatory[105,106] and

---

[90] Vasquez A. New Insights into Fatty Acid Supplementation and Its Effect on Eicosanoid Production and Genetic Expression. *Nutritional Perspectives* 2005; January: 5-16
[91] Evans AR, et al. Isoprostanes, novel eicosanoids that produce nociception and sensitize rat sensory neurons. *J Pharmacol Exp Ther*. 2000 Jun;293(3):912-20
[92] Lee et al. Saturated fatty acids but not unsaturated fatty acids induce expression of cyclooxygenase-2 mediated through Toll-like receptor 4. *J Biol Chem* 2001 May;276:16683-9
[93] "CONCLUSIONS: Both fat and protein intakes stimulate ROS generation. The increase in ROS generation lasted 3 h after cream intake and 1 h after protein intake. Cream intake also caused a significant and prolonged increase in lipid peroxidation." Mohanty P, Ghanim H, Hamouda W, Aljada A, Garg R, Dandona P. Both lipid and protein intakes stimulate increased generation of reactive oxygen species by polymorphonuclear leukocytes and mononuclear cells. *Am J Clin Nutr*. 2002 Apr;75(4):767-72
[94] Rusyn I, et al. Corn oil rapidly activates nuclear factor-kappaB in hepatic Kupffer cells by oxidant-dependent mechanisms. *Carcinogenesis*. 1999 Nov;20(11):2095-100
[95] "Exposing endothelial cells to 90 micromol linoleic acid/L for 6 h resulted in a significant increase in lipid hydroperoxides that coincided wih an increase in intracellular calcium concentrations." Hennig B, Toborek M, Joshi-Barve S, Barger SW, Barve S, Mattson MP, McClain CJ. Linoleic acid activates nuclear transcription factor-kappa B (NF-kappa B) and induces NF-kappa B-dependent transcription in cultured endothelial cells. *Am J Clin Nutr*. 1996 Mar;63(3):322-8 ajcn.org/cgi/reprint/63/3/322
[96] Mohanty et al. Glucose challenge stimulates reactive oxygen species (ROS) generation by leucocytes. *J Clin Endocrinol Metab*. 2000 Aug;85(8):2970-3
[97] Koska J, et al. Insulin, catecholamines, glucose and antioxidant enzymes in oxidative damage during different loads in healthy humans. *Physiol Res*. 2000;49 Suppl 1:S95-100
[98] "Conclusion - The present study shows that high GI carbohydrate, but not low GI carbohydrate, mediates an acute proinflammatory process as measured by NF-kappaB activity." Dickinson S, et al. High glycemic index carbohydrate mediates acute proinflammatory process measured by NF-kappaB activation. *Asia Pac J Clin Nutr*. 2005;14:S120
[99] Aljada A, et al. Increase in intranuclear nuclear factor kappaB and decrease in inhibitor kappaB in mononuclear cells after a mixed meal. *Am J Clin Nutr*. 2004 Apr;79(4):682-90
[100] Sanchez A, Reeser JL, Lau HS, et al. Role of sugars in human neutrophilic phagocytosis. *Am J Clin Nutr*. 1973 Nov;26(11):1180-4
[101] "Postoperative infusion of carbohydrate solution leads to moderate fall in the serum concentration of inorganic phosphate. ... The hypophosphatemia was associated with significant reduction of neutrophil phagocytosis, intracellular killing, consumption of oxygen and generation of superoxide during phagocytosis." Rasmussen A, Segel E, Hessov I, Borregaard N. Reduced function of neutrophils during routine postoperative glucose infusion. *Acta Chir Scand*. 1988 Jul-Aug;154(7-8):429-33
[102] Vasquez A. Part 6: Nutritional and Botanical Treatments against "Silent Infections" and Gastrointestinal Dysbiosis. *Nutritional Perspectives* 2006; January
[103] Ramakrishnan et al. Beneficial effects of fasting and low carbohydrate diet in D-lactic acidosis with short-bowel syndrome. *JPEN J Parenter Enteral Nutr* 1985;9:361-3
[104] Gottschall E. *Breaking the Vicious Cycle: Intestinal Health through Diet*. Kirkton Press; Rev edition (August 1, 1994)
[105] Lin HC. Small intestinal bacterial overgrowth: a framework for understanding irritable bowel syndrome. *JAMA*. 2004 Aug 18;292(7):852-8
[106] Lichtman SN, et al. Reactivation of arthritis induced by small bowel bacterial overgrowth in rats. *Infect Immun*. 1995 Jun;63(6):2295-301

which appears to be myalgenic in humans[107] at least in part due to the ability of endotoxin to impair muscle function.[108] Overconsumption of high-carbohydrate low-phytonutrient **grains, potatoes, and manufactured foods** displaces phytonutrient-dense foods such as fruits, vegetables, nuts, seeds, and berries which contain more than 8,000 phytonutrients, many of which have antioxidant and thus anti-inflammatory actions.[109,110]

- Anti-inflammation versus hemostasis: Anti-inflammatory/analgesic medications that impair coagulation (e.g., aspirin) are contraindicated in patients with possible internal bleeding such as severe hematoma, hemarthrosis, spleen injury, intracranial hemorrhage (i.e., subdural hematoma following a whiplash injury) and in patients about to undergo surgery. Theoretically, some caution might also be used with nutritional/botanical supplements that have anti-coagulant effects, such as *Ginkgo biloba*[111] and garlic.[112]

- Anti-inflammatory diet, the "supplemented Paleo-Mediterranean diet": The health-promoting diet of choice for the majority of people is a diet based on **abundant consumption of fruits, vegetables, nuts, seeds, berries, omega-3 and monounsaturated fatty acids, and lean sources of protein such as lean (e.g., grass-fed or game) meats, fatty cold-water fish, soy and whey protein isolate.** This diet obviates overconsumption of chemical preservatives, artificial sweeteners, and carbohydrate-dominant foods such as candies, pastries, breads, potatoes, grains, and other foods with a high glycemic load and high glycemic index. This "Paleo-Mediterranean Diet" is a combination of the "Paleolithic" or "Paleo diet" and the well-known "Mediterranean diet", both of which are well described in peer-reviewed journals and the lay press, particularly by Eaton[113], O'Keefe[114], and Cordain[115] — see Chapter 2 and my other reviews[116,117,118] (included in Chapter 4 of *Inflammation Mastery: Volume 1* series starting in 2014) for details. This diet is the most nutrient-dense diet available, and its benefits are further enhanced by supplementation with vitamins, minerals, probiotics, and the health-promoting polyunsaturated fatty acids: ALA, GLA, EPA, and DHA.

- Anti-inflammatory nutrients and botanicals: Nutritional and botanical therapeutics are prescribed *per patient* and *per condition*. Doses listed are for adults and can be reduced when numerous interventions are simultaneously applied.

Importance of removing/counteracting the common pro-inflammatory diet

"RESULTS: The typical American diet is deficient in fruits and vegetables and contains excessive amounts of meat, refined grain products, and dessert foods. **Such a diet can have numerous adverse biochemical effects, all of which create a proinflammatory state and predispose the body to degenerative diseases**. It appears that an inadequate intake of fruits and vegetables can result in a suboptimal intake of antioxidants and phytochemicals and an imbalanced intake of essential fatty acids. Through different mechanisms, **each nutritional alteration can promote inflammation and disease**. CONCLUSION: We can no longer view different diseases as distinct biochemical entities. Nearly all degenerative diseases have the same underlying biochemical etiology, that is, a **diet-induced proinflammatory state**. Although specific diseases may require specific treatments, such as adjustments for hypomobile joints, beta-blockers for hypertension, and chemotherapy for cancer, **the treatment program must also include nutritional protocols to reduce the proinflammatory state**."

Seaman DR. The diet-induced proinflammatory state. *J Manipulative Physiol Ther* 2002 Mar

---

[107] Pimentel M, et al. A link between irritable bowel syndrome and fibromyalgia may be related to findings on lactulose breath testing. *Ann Rheum Dis*. 2004 Apr;63(4):450-2
[108] Bundgaard H, et al. Endotoxemia stimulates skeletal muscle Na+-K+-ATPase and raises blood lactate. *Am J Physiol Heart Circ Physiol*. 2003 Mar;284(3):H1028-34
[109] "We propose that the additive and synergistic effects of phytochemicals in fruit and vegetables are responsible for their potent antioxidant and anticancer activities, and that the benefit of a diet rich in fruit and vegetables is attributed to the complex mixture of phytochemicals present in whole foods." Liu RH. Health benefits of fruit and vegetables are from additive and synergistic combinations of phytochemicals. *Am J Clin Nutr*. 2003 Sep;78(3 Suppl):517S-520S
[110] Seaman DR. The diet-induced proinflammatory state: a cause of chronic pain and other degenerative diseases? *J Manipulative Physiol Ther*. 2002;25(3):168-79
[111] "A structured assessment of published case reports suggests a possible causal association between using ginkgo and bleeding events... Patients using ginkgo, particularly those with known bleeding risks, should be counseled about a possible increase in bleeding risk." Bent S, Goldberg H, Padula A, Avins AL. Spontaneous bleeding associated with ginkgo biloba: a case report and systematic review of the literature: a case report and systematic review of the literature. *J Gen Intern Med*. 2005 Jul;20(7):657-61
[112] "The authors report a case of spontaneous spinal epidural hematoma causing paraplegia secondary to a qualitative platelet disorder from excessive garlic ingestion." Rose KD, et al. Spontaneous spinal epidural hematoma with associated platelet dysfunction from excessive garlic ingestion: a case report. *Neurosurgery*. 1990 May;26(5):880-2
[113] Eaton SB, Shostak M, Konner M. *The Paleolithic Prescription*, New York: Harper & Row, 1988
[114] O'Keefe JH Jr, Cordain L. Cardiovascular disease resulting from a diet and lifestyle at odds with our Paleolithic genome. *Mayo Clin Proc*. 2004 Jan;79(1):101-8
[115] Cordain L. *The Paleo Diet*. Indianapolis; John Wiley and Sons, 2002
[116] Vasquez A. A Five-Part Nutritional Protocol that Produces Consistently Positive Results. *Nutritional Wellness* 2005 Sep
[117] Vasquez A. Implementing the Five-Part Nutritional Wellness Protocol for the Treatment of Various Health Problems. *Nutritional Wellness* 2005 Nov
[118] Vasquez A. Revisiting the five-part nutritional wellness protocol: the supplemented Paleo-Mediterranean diet. *Nutritional Perspectives* 2011 Jan

- Fish oil: EPA with DHA: Three grams per day (3,000 mg/d) of combined EPA and DHA is a reasonable therapeutic dose[119] and is generally supplied in one tablespoon of liquid fish oil. Encapsulated fish oil supplements vary tremendously in their concentration of EPA and DHA and may require consumption of as few as five and as many as 21 capsules per day to achieve the same dosage and of EPA+DHA found in one tablespoon of liquid fish oil; encapsulated fish oil supplements also generally cost significantly more than do liquid fish oil supplements. The routine use of eicosapentaenoic acid (EPA) and docosahexaenoic acid (DHA) supplements is justified based on the following data: ❶ Most modern diets are profoundly deficient in omega-3 fatty acids[120], ❷ Dietary/supplemental intake of omega-3 fatty acids is a necessary prerequisite to reducing the pro-inflammatory effects of omega-6 fatty acids[121], ❸ Supplementation with EPA+DHA is safe and reduces all-cause mortality[122], ❹ Supplementation with EPA+DHA consistently provides clinically significant benefits in the treatment of a wide range of painful/inflammatory conditions.[123,124]

  > **Clinical review of fatty acid metabolism**
  > Chapter 4 of *Inflammation Mastery: Volume 1* (2014) includes an update of previous reviews published on clinical applications of CFAT—combination fatty acid therapy.

  - Clinical trial—Omega-3 fatty acids (fish oil) as an anti-inflammatory alternative to NSAIDs for discogenic back pain (*Surg Neurol* 2006 Apr[125]): The authors note that the use of NSAID medications is a well-established effective therapy for both acute and chronic nonspecific neck and back pain and yet can carry "extreme complications, including gastric ulcers, bleeding, myocardial infarction, and even deaths." 250 patients who had been seen by a neurosurgeon and were found to have nonsurgical neck or back pain were asked to take a total of 1200 mg per day of omega-3 EFAs (eicosapentaenoic acid and docosahexaenoic acid) found in fish oil supplements. ... Seventy-eight percent were taking 1200 mg and 22% were taking 2400 mg of EFAs. Fifty-nine percent discontinued to take their prescription NSAID medications for pain. Sixty percent stated that their overall pain was improved, and 60% stated that their joint pain had improved. Eighty percent stated they were satisfied with their improvement, and 88% stated they would continue to take the fish oil. There were no significant side effects reported. ... omega-3 EFA fish oil supplements appear to be a safer alternative to NSAIDs for treatment of nonsurgical neck or back pain in this selective group."

- GLA, Gamma-linolenic acid: Approximately 500 mg per day is the common anti-inflammatory dose[126] although higher doses of 2.8 grams per day have been safely used in patients with rheumatoid arthritis.[127] Except in the rarest circumstances (perhaps including temporal lobe epilepsy[128]), **GLA (most concentrated in borage oil) should always be co-administered with EPA and DHA (from fish oil) in order to obtain maximal benefit and avoid the increased formation of arachidonic acid that occurs when GLA is administered alone and the reduction in GLA/DGLA that occurs when fish oil is administered alone.**

---

[119] "…clinical benefits of the n-3 fatty acids were not apparent until they were consumed for > or =12 wk. It appears that a minimum daily dose of 3 g eicosapentaenoic and docosahexaenoic acids is necessary to derive the expected benefits [in patients with rheumatoid arthritis]." Kremer JM. n-3 fatty acid supplements in rheumatoid arthritis. *Am J Clin Nutr*.2000;71(1Suppl):349S-51S

[120] Simopoulos AP. Essential fatty acids in health and chronic disease. *Am J Clin Nutr*. 1999 Sep;70(3 Suppl):560S-569S

[121] Rubin D, Laposata M. Cellular interactions between n-6 and n-3 fatty acids: a mass analysis of fatty acid elongation/desaturation, distribution among complex lipids, and conversion to eicosanoids. *J Lipid Res*. 1992 Oct;33(10):1431-40.

[122] "The recent GISSI (Gruppo Italiano per lo Studio della Sopravvivenza nell'Infarto miocardico)-Prevention study of 11,324 patients showed a 45% decrease in risk of sudden cardiac death and a 20% reduction in all-cause mortality in the group taking 850 mg/d of omega-3 fatty acids. These fatty acids have potent anti-inflammatory effects and may also be antiatherogenic." O'Keefe JH Jr, Harris WS. From Inuit to implementation: omega-3 fatty acids come of age. *Mayo Clin Proc*. 2000 Jun;75(6):607-14

[123] "Many of the placebo-controlled trials of fish oil in chronic inflammatory diseases reveal significant benefit, including decreased disease activity and a lowered use of anti-inflammatory drugs." Simopoulos AP. Omega-3 fatty acids in inflammation and autoimmune diseases. *J Am Coll Nutr*. 2002 Dec;21(6):495-505

[124] Vasquez A. New Insights into Fatty Acid Supplementation and Its Effect on Eicosanoid Production and Genetic Expression. *Nutritional Perspectives* 2005; January: 5-16

[125] Maroon et al. Omega-3 fatty acids (fish oil) as an anti-inflammatory: alternative to nonsteroidal anti-inflammatory drugs for discogenic pain. *Surg Neurol*. 2006 Apr;65:326-31

[126] "Forty patients with rheumatoid arthritis and upper gastrointestinal lesions due to non-steroidal anti-inflammatory drugs entered a prospective 6-month double-blind placebo controlled study of dietary supplementation with gamma-linolenic acid 540 mg/day..." Brzeski M, Madhok R, Capell HA. Evening primrose oil in patients with rheumatoid arthritis and side-effects of non-steroidal anti-inflammatory drugs. *Br J Rheumatol*. 1991 Oct;30(5):370-2

[127] Zurier RB, Rossetti RG, Jacobson EW, DeMarco DM, Liu NY, Temming JE, White BM, Laposata M. gamma-Linolenic acid treatment of rheumatoid arthritis. A randomized, placebo-controlled trial. *Arthritis Rheum*. 1996 Nov;39(11):1808-17

[128] "Three long-stay, hospitalised schizophrenics who had failed to respond adequately to conventional drug therapy were treated with gamma-linolenic acid and linoleic acid in the form of evening primrose oil. They became substantially worse and electroencephalographic features of temporal lobe epilepsy became apparent." Vaddadi KS. The use of gamma-linolenic acid and linoleic acid to differentiate between temporal lobe epilepsy and schizophrenia. *Prostaglandins Med*. 1981 Apr;6(4):375-9

- Clinical trial—Alpha-lipoic acid (ALA), gamma linolenic acid (GLA) and rehabilitation in the treatment of back pain (*Int J Immunopathol Pharmacol* 2009 Jul-Sep[129]): This is a very interesting study which applied a partial nutritional protocol for the treatment of neuropathy as adjunct to usual rehabilitation in the treatment of neuropathic pain associated with disc herniation/degeneration and associated nerve root compression. The treatment group (n=101) received oral alpha-lipoic acid (ALA) 600 mg/d and gamma-linolenic acid (GLA) 360 mg/d and a physical rehabilitation program for six weeks, the second (n = 102) treated with only rehabilitation program. The authors noted and concluded, "Significant improvements was noted in the ALA and GLA group for paresthesia, stabbing and burning pain, as showed by VAS (Visual Analogue Scale), Oswestry Low Back Pain Disability Questionnaire, Aberdeen Low Back Pain Scale; also, improvements of quality of life has been noted, in the same group, as showed by SF-36, LDQ (Revised Leeds Disability Questionnaire), Roland and Morris disability questionnaire. All these outcome measure showed statistically significant decreases. Oral treatment with alpha-lipoic acid (ALA) and gamma-linolenic acid (GLA) for six weeks in synergy with rehabilitation therapy improved neuropathic symptoms and deficits in patients with radicular neuropathy."

- *Zingiber officinale* (Ginger): Ginger is a well-known spice and food with a long history of use as an anti-inflammatory, anti-nausea, and gastroprotective agent[130], and components of ginger have been shown to reduce production of the leukotriene LTB4 by inhibiting 5-lipoxygenase and to reduce production of the prostaglandin PGE2 by inhibiting cyclooxygenase.[131,132] With its dual reduction in the formation of pro-inflammatory prostaglandins and leukotrienes, ginger has been shown to safely reduce nonspecific musculoskeletal pain[133,134] and to provide relief from osteoarthritis of the knees[135] and migraine headaches.[136] Ginger can be consumed liberally as a supplement or as whole food, and it is safe for use in pregnancy up to one gram per day.[137]

- Willow bark (*Salix* spp): In a double-blind placebo-controlled clinical trial in 210 patients with moderate/severe low-back pain (20% of patients had positive straight-leg raising test), willow bark extract showed a dose-dependent analgesic effect with benefits beginning in the first week of treatment.[138] In a head-to-head study of 228 patients comparing willow bark (standardized for 240 mg salicin) with Vioxx (rofecoxib), treatments were equally effective yet willow bark was safer and 40% less expensive.[139] Because willow bark's salicylates were the original source for the chemical manufacture of acetylsalicylic acid (aspirin), researchers and clinicians have erroneously mistaken willow bark to be synonymous with aspirin; this is certainly inaccurate and therefore clarification of willow's mechanism of action will be provided here. Aspirin has two primary effects via three primary mechanisms of action: 1) anticoagulant effects mediated by the acetylation and permanent inactivation of thromboxane-A synthase, which is the enzyme that makes the powerfully proaggregatory thromboxane-A2; 2) antiprostaglandin action via acetylation of both isoforms of cyclooxygenase (COX-1 inhibition 25-166x more than COX-2) with widespread inhibition of prostaglandin formation, and 3) antiprostaglandin formation via retroconversion of acetylsalicylate into salicylic acid which then inhibits cyclooxygenase-2 gene transcription.[140] Notice that the acetylation reactions are specific to aspirin and thus actions #1 and #2 are not seen with willow bark; whereas #3—inhibition of COX-2 transcription by salicylates—appears to be the

---

[129] Ranieri et al. Use of alpha-lipoic acid (ALA), gamma linolenic acid (GLA) and rehabilitation in treatment of back pain. *Int J Immunopathol Pharmacol*. 2009 Jul-Sep;22:45-50
[130] Langner E, Greifenberg S, Gruenwald J. Ginger: history and use. *Adv Ther* 1998 Jan-Feb;15(1):25-44
[131] Kiuchi F, et al. Inhibition of prostaglandin and leukotriene biosynthesis by gingerols and diarylheptanoids. *Chem Pharm Bull* (Tokyo) 1992 Feb;40(2):387-91
[132] Tjendraputra E, et al. Effect of ginger constituents and synthetic analogues on cyclooxygenase-2 enzyme in intact cells. *Bioorg Chem* 2001 Jun;29(3):156-63
[133] Srivastava KC, Mustafa T. Ginger (Zingiber officinale) in rheumatism and musculoskeletal disorders. *Med Hypotheses*. 1992 Dec;39(4):342-8
[134] Srivastava KC, Mustafa T. Ginger (Zingiber officinale) and rheumatic disorders. *Med Hypotheses*. 1989 May;29(1):25-8
[135] Altman RD, Marcussen KC. Effects of a ginger extract on knee pain in patients with osteoarthritis. *Arthritis Rheum*. 2001 Nov;44(11):2531-8
[136] Mustafa T, Srivastava KC. Ginger (Zingiber officinale) in migraine headache. *J Ethnopharmacol*. 1990 Jul;29(3):267-73
[137] "...oral ginger 1 g per day... No adverse effect of ginger on pregnancy outcome was detected." Vutyavanich T, Kraisarin T, Ruangsri R. Ginger for nausea and vomiting in pregnancy: randomized, double-masked, placebo-controlled trial. *Obstet Gynecol* 2001 Apr;97(4):577-82.
[138] Chrubasik S, et al. Treatment of low-back pain exacerbations with willow bark extract: a randomized double-blind study. *Am J Med*. 2000;109:9-14
[139] Chrubasik S, et al. Treatment of low-back pain with a herbal or synthetic anti-rheumatic: a randomized controlled study. *Rheumatology* (Oxford). 2001;40:1388-93
[140] Hare LG, Woodside JV, Young IS. Dietary salicylates. *J Clin Pathol* 2003 Sep;56(9):649-50 jcp.bmj.com/cgi/content/full/56/9/649

major mechanism of action of willow bark extract. Proof of this principle is supported by the lack of adverse effects associated with willow bark in the research literature. If willow bark were pharmacodynamically synonymous with aspirin, then we would expect case reports of gastric ulceration, hemorrhage, and Reye's syndrome to permeate the research literature; this is not the case and therefore—**with the exception of possible allergic reactions in patients previously allergic/anaphylactic to aspirin and salicylates—extensive "warnings" on willow bark products**[141] **are unnecessary.**[142] Salicylates are widely present in fruits, vegetables, herbs and spices and are partly responsible for the anti-cancer, anti-inflammatory, and health-promoting benefits of fruit and vegetable consumption.[143,144] With willow bark products, the daily dose should not exceed 240 mg of salicin, and products should include other components of the whole plant. **Except for rare allergy in patients previously sensitized to aspirin or salicylates, no adverse effects are known**; to be on the medicolegal safe side, use is discouraged during pregnancy, before surgery, or when anti-coagulant medications are being used.

- *Uncaria guianensis* and *Uncaria tomentosa* ("cat's claw", "una de gato"): A double-blind placebo-controlled study using 100 mg daily of highly-concentrated freeze-dried aqueous extract of *Uncaria tomentosa* found significant pain relief (reduction by 36%) and minimal adverse effects after 4 weeks of treatment in 30 male patients with osteoarthritis of the knees, a benefit mediated via antioxidant activities and inhibition of NF-kappaB, TNFα, COX-2, and PGE-2 production.[145] Inhibition of NFkB and iNOS are of primary importance in the treatment of inflammatory conditions.[146] A year-long study of patients with active rheumatoid arthritis (RA) treated with sulfasalazine or hydroxychloroquine showed "relative safety and modest benefit" of coadministration of *Uncaria tomentosa*.[147] Other studies with *Uncaria tomentosa* have shown enhancement of post-vaccination immunity[148] and enhancement of DNA repair in humans.[149] Traditional uses have included the use of the herb as a contraceptive and as treatment for gastrointestinal ulcers.

- *Boswellia serrata*: *Boswellia* inhibits 5-lipoxygenase[150] with no apparent effect on cyclooxygenase[151] and has been shown effective in the treatment of osteoarthritis of the knees[152] as well as asthma[153] and ulcerative colitis.[154] When used as monotherapy, the target dose is approximately 150 mg of boswellic acids TID.

- *Harpagophytum procumbens* (Devil's claw): The safety and effectiveness of *Harpagophytum* has been established in patients with hip pain, low-back pain, and knee pain.[155,156,157] The mechanisms of action include weak anti-inflammatory effects and a stronger analgesic effect.[158,159] Research

---

[141] Clauson KA, et al. Evaluation of Presence of Aspirin-Related Warnings with Willow Bark (July/August). *Ann Pharmacother*. 2005 Jul-Aug;39(7-8):1234-7 The article by Clauson et al contained/s numerous inaccuracies and should either be withdrawn or read only in conjunction with my refutation: Vasquez A, Muanza D. Evaluation of Presence of Aspirin-Related Warnings with Willow Bark: Comment on the Article by Clauson et al. *Ann Pharmacotherapy* 2005 Oct;39(10):1763
[142] Vasquez et al. Evaluation of Presence of Aspirin-Related Warnings with Willow Bark: Comment on the Article by Clauson et al. *Ann Pharmacotherapy* 2005 Oct;39(10):1763
[143] Lawrence JR, et al. Urinary excretion of salicyluric and salicylic acids by non-vegetarians, vegetarians, and patients taking low dose aspirin. *J Clin Pathol*. 2003 Sep;56:651-3
[144] Paterson JR, Lawrence JR. Salicylic acid: a link between aspirin, diet and the prevention of colorectal cancer. *QJM*. 2001 Aug;94(8):445-8
[145] Piscoya J, et al. Efficacy and safety of freeze-dried cat's claw in osteoarthritis of the knee. *Inflamm Res*. 2001 Sep;50(9):442-8
[146] Sandoval-Chacon M, et al. Antiinflammatory actions of cat's claw: the role of NF-kappaB. *Aliment Pharmacol Ther*. 1998 Dec;12(12):1279-89
[147] "This small preliminary study demonstrates relative safety and modest benefit to the tender joint count of a highly purified extract from the pentacyclic chemotype of UT in patients with active RA taking sulfasalazine or hydroxychloroquine." Mur E, Hartig F, Eibl G, Schirmer M. Randomized double blind trial of an extract from the pentacyclic alkaloid-chemotype of uncaria tomentosa for the treatment of rheumatoid arthritis. *J Rheumatol*. 2002 Apr;29(4):678-81
[148] "...Uncaria tomentosa or Cat's Claw which is known to possess immune enhancing and antiinflammatory properties in animals. There were no toxic side effects observed as judged by medical examination, clinical chemistry and blood cell analysis. However, statistically significant immune enhancement for the individuals on C-Med-100 supplement was observed..." Lamm S, Sheng Y, Pero RW. Persistent response to pneumococcal vaccine in individuals supplemented with a novel water soluble extract of Uncaria tomentosa, C-Med-100. *Phytomedicine*. 2001;8(4):267-74
[149] Sheng Y, Li L, Holmgren K, Pero RW. DNA repair enhancement of aqueous extracts of Uncaria tomentosa in a human volunteer study. *Phytomedicine*. 2001 Jul;8(4):275-82
[150] Wildfeuer A, Neu IS, Safayhi H, Metzger G, Wehrmann M, Vogel U, Ammon HP. Effects of boswellic acids extracted from a herbal medicine on the biosynthesis of leukotrienes and the course of experimental autoimmune encephalomyelitis. *Arzneimittelforschung* 1998 Jun;48(6):668-74
[151] Safayhi H, et al. Boswellic acids: novel, specific, nonredox inhibitors of 5-lipoxygenase. *J Pharmacol Exp Ther* 1992 Jun;261(3):1143-6
[152] Kimmatkar N, et al. Efficacy and tolerability of Boswellia serrata extract in treatment of osteoarthritis of knee. *Phytomedicine*. 2003 Jan;10(1):3-7
[153] Gupta I, et al. Effects of Boswellia serrata gum resin in patients with bronchial asthma. *Eur J Med Res*. 1998 Nov 17;3(11):511-4
[154] Gupta I, et al. Effects of Boswellia serrata gum resin in patients with ulcerative colitis. *Eur J Med Res*. 1997 Jan;2(1):37-43
[155] Chrubasik S, et al. Comparison of outcome measures during treatment with the proprietary Harpagophytum extract doloteffin in patients with pain in the lower back, knee or hip. *Phytomedicine* 2002 Apr;9(3):181-94
[156] Chantre P, et al. Efficacy and tolerance of Harpagophytum procumbens versus diacerhein in treatment of osteoarthritis. *Phytomedicine* 2000 Jun;7(3):177-83
[157] Leblan D, Chantre P, Fournie B. Harpagophytum procumbens in the treatment of knee and hip osteoarthritis. *Joint Bone Spine* 2000;67(5):462-7
[158] Whitehouse et al. Devil's Claw (Harpagophytum procumbens): no evidence for anti-inflammatory activity in treatment of arthritic disease. *Can Med Assoc J* 1983;129:249-51
[159] Moussard C, Alber D, Toubin MM, Thevenon N, Henry JC. A drug used in traditional medicine, harpagophytum procumbens: no evidence for NSAID-like effect on whole blood eicosanoid production in human. *Prostaglandins Leukot Essent Fatty Acids* 1992 Aug;46(4):283-6

suggests that *Harpagophytum* is an effective analgesic for low back pain[160], including low back pain with radiculitis and radiculopathy.[161] The common dose is 60 mg harpagoside per day.[162]

- <u>Topical application of *Capsicum annuum, Capsicum frutescens* (Cayenne pepper, hot chili pepper)</u>: Capsaicin reduces pain perception by depleting sensory fibers of substance P—blocking transport as well as de-novo synthesis of substance P. Topical capsaicin alleviates diabetic neuropathy[163], low back pain[164], chronic neck pain[165], osteoarthritis[166], rheumatoid arthritis[167], notalgia paresthetica[168], reflex sympathetic dystrophy[169], and cluster headache (intranasal application).[170,171,172] Notable with capsaicin are the absence of adverse effects (other than local burning sensation, which abates), high efficacy, and lower cost—all of which are often superior to prescription drug analgesics; an outline of notable studies is provided below:

  - <u>Topical capsaicin versus oral amitriptyline for diabetic neuropathy</u>: An 8-week, double-blind, multicenter parallel study compared the safety and efficacy of topical capsaicin and oral amitriptyline in 235 patients with painful diabetic neuropathy involving the feet; pain relief and reduction in disability were comparable, but topical capsaicin was much safer and avoided the costs and adverse effects of amitriptyline (somnolence [46%], neuromuscular [23%] and cardiovascular [9%] effects). The authors concluded, "Topically applied capsaicin is an equally effective but considerably safer alternative to amitriptyline for relief of the pain of diabetic neuropathy."[173]

  - <u>High-potency topical capsaicin 5-10% for severe intractable pain</u>: A very assertive intervention study by Robbins et al[174] used high-concentration (5%–10%) capsaicin administered with regional anesthesia in patients with intractable pain, complex regional pain syndromes and neuropathic pain; the effectiveness of this approach lead the authors to conclude, "The intermittent application of large-dose topical capsaicin may provide significant pain relief, decrease chronic analgesic dependence, and decrease aggregate health care expenditures."

  - <u>Topical capsaicin for pediatric hernia repair analgesia</u>: A double-blind, placebo-controlled study among 108 children undergoing pediatric hernia repair showed that acupoint capsaicin application provided pain relief and allowed for reduced dependence on meperidine (opioid analgesic).[175]

  - <u>Topical capsaicin for hysterectomy analgesia</u>: A double-blind, placebo-controlled study among 90 women undergoing abdominal hysterectomy showed that topical capsaicin reduced the need for morphine and postoperative antiemetics.[176]

---

[160] Chrubasik S, et al. A randomized double-blind pilot study comparing Doloteffin and Vioxx in the treatment of low back pain. *Rheumatology* (Oxford). 2003 Jan;42(1):141-8
[161] "The majority of responders were patients who had suffered less than 42 days of pain, and subgroup analyses suggested that the effect was confined to patients with more severe and radiating pain accompanied by neurological deficit... There was no evidence for Harpagophytum-related side-effects, except possibly for mild and infrequent gastrointestinal symptoms." Chrubasik S, Junck H, Breitschwerdt H, Conradt C, Zappe H. Effectiveness of Harpagophytum extract WS 1531 in the treatment of exacerbation of low back pain: a randomized, placebo-controlled, double-blind study. *Eur J Anaesthesiol* 1999 Feb;16(2):118-29
[162] "They took an 8-week course of Doloteffin at a dose providing 60 mg harpagoside per day... Doloteffin is well worth considering for osteoarthritic knee and hip pain and nonspecific low back pain." Chrubasik S, Thanner J, Kunzel O, Conradt C, Black A, Pollak S. Comparison of outcome measures during treatment with the proprietary Harpagophytum extract doloteffin in patients with pain in the lower back, knee or hip. *Phytomedicine* 2002 Apr;9(3):181-94
[163] "Study results suggest that topical capsaicin cream is safe and effective in treating painful diabetic neuropathy. "[No authors listed] Treatment of painful diabetic neuropathy with topical capsaicin. A multicenter, double-blind, vehicle-controlled study. The Capsaicin Study Group. *Arch Intern Med*. 1991 Nov;151(11):2225-9
[164] Keitel W, et al. Capsicum pain plaster in chronic non-specific low back pain. *Arzneimittelforschung*. 2001 Nov;51(11):896-903
[165] Mathias BJ, Dillingham TR, Zeigler DN, Chang AS, Belandres PV. Topical capsaicin for chronic neck pain. A pilot study. *Am J Phys Med Rehabil* 1995 Jan-Feb;74(1):39-44
[166] McCarthy GM, McCarty DJ. Effect of topical capsaicin in the therapy of painful osteoarthritis of the hands. *J Rheumatol*. 1992;19(4):604-7
[167] Deal CL, et al. Treatment of arthritis with topical capsaicin: a double-blind trial. *Clin Ther*. 1991 May-Jun;13(3):383-95
[168] Leibsohn E. Treatment of notalgia paresthetica with capsaicin. *Cutis* 1992 May;49(5):335-6
[169] "Capsaicin is effective for psoriasis, pruritus, and cluster headache; it is often helpful for itching and pain of postmastectomy pain syndrome, oral mucositis, cutaneous allergy, loin pain/hematuria syndrome, neck pain, amputation stump pain, and skin tumor; and it may be beneficial for neural dysfunction (detrusor hyperreflexia, reflex sympathetic dystrophy, and rhinopathy)." Hautkappe et al. Review of effectiveness of capsaicin for painful cutaneous disorders and neural dysfunction. *Clin J Pain* 1998;14:97-106
[170] "Capsaicin application to human nasal mucosa was found to induce painful sensation, sneezing, and nasal secretion. All of these factors exhibit desensitization upon repeated applications." Sicuteri F, et al. Beneficial effect of capsaicin application to the nasal mucosa in cluster headache. *Clin J Pain*. 1989;5(1):49-53
[171] "The efficacy of repeated nasal applications of capsaicin in cluster headache is congruent with previous reports on the therapeutic effect of capsaicin in other pain syndromes (post-herpetic neuralgia, diabetic neuropathy, trigeminal neuralgia) and supports the use of the drug to produce a selective analgesia." Fusco BM, Marabini S, Maggi CA, Fiore G, Geppetti P. Preventative effect of repeated nasal applications of capsaicin in cluster headache. *Pain*. 1994 Dec;59(3):321-5
[172] "These results indicate that intranasal capsaicin may provide a new therapeutic option for the treatment of this disease." Marks DR, Rapoport A, Padla D, Weeks R, Rosum R, Sheftell F, Arrowsmith F. A double-blind placebo-controlled trial of intranasal capsaicin for cluster headache. *Cephalalgia*. 1993 Apr;13(2):114-6
[173] Biesbroeck et al. A double-blind comparison of topical capsaicin and oral amitriptyline in painful diabetic neuropathy. *Adv Ther*. 1995 Mar-Apr;12(2):111-20
[174] Robbins WR, et al. Treatment of intractable pain with topical large-dose capsaicin: preliminary report. *Anesth Analg*. 1998 Mar;86(3):579-83
[175] Kim KS, Kim DW, Yu YK. The effect of capsicum plaster in pain after inguinal hernia repair in children. *Paediatr Anaesth*. 2006 Oct;16(10):1036-41
[176] Kim KS, Nam YM. The analgesic effects of capsicum plaster at the Zusanli point after abdominal hysterectomy. *Anesth Analg*. 2006;103(3):709-13

- Topical capsaicin for low-back pain: A double-blind, randomized, placebo-controlled, multicenter parallel study with 320 patients with chronic low back pain" used topical capsicum to safely obtain clinically relevant reductions in pain and disability.[177]
- Intranasal capsaicin for cluster headache: Treatment of active cluster headache with intranasal capsaicin (compared with placebo) reduced severity after 7 days of treatment.[178]
- Intranasal capsaicin for migraine headache: In a small controlled trial, patients stated that intranasal application of capsaicin alleviated migraine suffering by 50% to 80%.[179]

Capsaicin is applied externally and therefore has no internal adverse effects; delivery is typically via inexpensive OTC cream or patch with strengths ranging from 0.025, 0.075, 0.1%; more potent and expensive physician-authorized and physician-applied patches are also available. Capsaicin products are applied topically per product instructions and patient tolerance; the medically benign burning sensation abates with continued use. Doctors should experiment on themselves with this treatment before administering to patients in order to gain understanding by experience; care must always be used to avoid contact with eyes or genitals, especially at the same time, because that would really hurt, and would be socially awkward (contorted body posturing, facial grimacing, futile cries for help, etc—especially at a medical conference with colleagues or fine dining events with friends and family), and would make washing/rinsing difficult for technical (reduced vision due to excess lacrimation) and psychoepistimological (how to prioritize?) reasons.

o *Cannabis sativa* and related variants (Cannabis): Cannabis is an inexpensive and impressively safe botanical providing therapeutic efficacy against a wide range of debilitating medical disorders (notably chronic pain), and it is readily cultivable by individual citizens/patients and increasingly available through decriminalized commercial channels. Clinicians and "premedical healers" have used Cannabis for its medicinal benefits for more than five thousand years; the world's oldest surviving medical text, the Chinese *Shen-nung Pen-tshao Ching* (*Divine Farmer's Materia Medica*), recommends Cannabis to reduce the pain of rheumatism and to address digestive disorders.[180] The plant has been used medically for thousands of years with an objectively favorable risk:benefit ratio with the added benefit of low cost and notably easy cultivation. The plant was later made illegal for purposes of social divisiveness/targeting (e.g., independent thinkers, and because of its low cost and numerous medical uses, it was preferentially used by poor sections of the population, particularly minorities) and for market protection (i.e., because the medical and social uses of the drug dissuaded people from using patentable high-profit pharmaceutical drugs, taxable high-profit corporate-produced alcoholic beverages and tobacco products); currently, the criminalization of Cannabis is financially supported by police unions, privatized prison corporations in America, alcoholic beverage companies, prescription drug companies, and prison guard unions; see compilation footnote for citations.

> **The Responsibility of Intellectuals**
>
> "It is the responsibility of intellectuals to speak the truth and to expose lies."
>
> Chomsky N. *New York Review of Books* 1967 nybooks.com

> **Private interests supporting criminalization of Cannabis and therefore penalization/incarceration of citizens**
>
> 1. Prescription drug makers: **Purdue Pharma** makes OxyContin, **Abbott Laboratories** makes Vicodin, **Alkermes** makes Zohydrol ("reportedly ten times stronger than OxyContin"), **Janssen Pharmaceutical** is a **Johnson & Johnson** subsidiary that makes Nucynta, and **Pfizer** makes several opioid drugs
> 2. Alcohol and beer companies
> 3. Privatized prison corporations
> 4. Police unions and (privatized) prison guard unions: recipients of federal funding; police departments, as authorized by the Reagan administration, gained the ability to financially profit via the seizure and sale of personal property ("asset forfeiture") called "policing for profit"
> 5. Community nonprofit groups: recipients of federal funding connected to the "War on Drugs"
> 6. Drug rehabilitation centers: benefit from court-ordered rehabilitation sentences
> 7. Partnership for Drug-Free Kids, formerly Partnership for a Drug-Free America: paid by opioid manufacturers and other pharmaceutical companies.
>
> Fang L, *Nation* 2014 Jul and JF, *The Economist* 2014 Apr. See compilation footnote.

---

[177] Frerick H, Keitel W, Kuhn U, Schmidt S, Bredehorst A, Kuhlmann M. Topical treatment of chronic low back pain with a capsicum plaster. *Pain*. 2003 Nov;106(1-2):59-64
[178] Marks et al. A double-blind placebo-controlled trial of intranasal capsaicin for cluster headache. *Cephalalgia*. 1993 Apr;13(2):114-6
[179] Fusco BM, Barzoi G, Agrò F. Repeated intranasal capsaicin applications to treat chronic migraine. *Br J Anaesth*. 2003 Jun;90(6):812
[180] Thomas J. The Past, Present, and Future of Medical Marijuana in the United States. *Psychiatric Times* 2010 Jan psychiatrictimes.com/articles/

The criminalization of Cannabis use has no legitimate medical or social basis especially when contrasted against costlier, riskier, less effective, and readily available ethanol/alcohol, tobacco, and innumerable government-approved pharmaceutical drugs, particularly analgesic, opioid, antispasmodic, antidepressant and antianxiety drugs. Recently and only after spending trillions of dollars and wasting innumerable *tens-hundreds of thousands* of human lives, laws regarding Cannabis are being relaxed internationally. Oral consumption of Cannabis products obviates concern regarding adverse effects from inhalation of smoked (and therefore chemically altered) plant material. See compilation footnote for citations/information.[181]

- Pharmacologic and clinical effects of medical cannabis (*Pharmacotherapy* 2013 Feb[182]): "Pain and muscle spasms are the most common reasons that medical cannabis is being recommended. Studies of medical cannabis show significant improvement in various types of pain and muscle spasticity. Reported adverse effects are typically not serious, with the most common being dizziness."

- Cannabis as an adjunct to or substitute for opiates in the treatment of chronic pain (*J Psychoactive Drugs* 2012 Apr[183]): "There is a growing body of evidence to support the use of medical cannabis as an adjunct to or substitute for prescription opiates in the treatment of chronic pain. When used in conjunction with opiates, cannabinoids lead to a greater cumulative relief of pain, resulting in a reduction in the use of opiates (and associated side-effects) by patients in a clinical setting. Additionally, cannabinoids can prevent the development of tolerance to and withdrawal from opiates, and can even rekindle opiate analgesia after a prior dosage has become ineffective."

> **Cannabis: Current medical uses**
> "Various well-designed, randomized, placebo-controlled trials have shown that smoked cannabis can relieve peripheral, posttraumatic, and HIV-induced neuropathic pain."
>
> Evidence from Clinical Studies:
> - Tourette syndrome
> - Glaucoma
> - Post-operative pain
> - Refractory neuropathic pain
> - Nausea due to many causes
> - HIV anorexia, weight loss
> - Multiple sclerosis spasticity, central pain, bladder dysfunction
> - Opioid synergism
>
> Safety: "much less dangerous than opiates, amphetamines, and barbiturates and also less dangerous than alcohol."
>
> Leung, *Journal of the American Board Family Medicine* 2011 Jul

- Medical uses of Cannabis (*J Am Board Family Med* 2011 Jul[184]): Accepted applications of Cannabis per Canadian regulations: "end-of-life care; seizures from epilepsy; severe pain and/or persistent muscle spasms caused by multiple sclerosis, spinal cord diseases, or spinal cord injury; severe pain; cachexia; anorexia; weight loss and/or severe nausea from cancer or HIV/AIDS infection."

- Modulation of amygdala-cortical connectivity contributes to the dissociative effect of cannabis on pain perception (*Pain* 2013 Jan[185]): Functional magnetic resonance imaging was used to investigate the effects of delta-9-tetrahydrocannabinol (THC), a naturally occurring cannabinoid, on brain activity related to cutaneous ongoing pain and hyperalgesia that were temporarily induced by capsaicin in healthy volunteers. THC reduced reported unpleasantness but not intensity of ongoing pain and hyperalgesia. … THC significantly reduced primary sensorimotor functional connectivity between the right amygdala and the primary sensorimotor cortex during the ongoing pain state."

- Low-dose vaporized cannabis significantly improves neuropathic pain (*J Pain* 2013 Feb[186]): "The analgesia obtained from a low dose of delta-9-tetrahydrocannabinol (1.29%) in patients, most of whom were experiencing neuropathic pain despite conventional treatments, is a clinically significant outcome. …As a result, one might not anticipate a significant impact on daily functioning."

- Medical cannabis reduces opioid analgesic overdose mortality (*JAMA Intern Med* 2014 Aug[187]): "States with medical cannabis laws had a 24.8% lower mean annual opioid overdose mortality rate (95% CI, -37.5% to -9.5%; P = .003) compared with states without medical cannabis laws. … Medical cannabis laws are associated with significantly lower state-level opioid overdose mortality rates."

---

[181] Compilation footnote: Brecher EM. *Licit and Illicit Drugs: The Consumers Union Report on Narcotics, Stimulants, Depressants, Inhalants, Hallucinogens, and Marijuana.* 1972. Fang L. The Real Reason Pot Is Still Illegal. *The Nation* 2014 July 21-28. JF. What civil-asset forfeiture means. *Economist* 2014 Apr
[182] Borgelt et al. The pharmacologic and clinical effects of medical cannabis. *Pharmacotherapy.* 2013 Feb;33(2):195-209
[183] Lucas P. Cannabis as an adjunct to or substitute for opiates in the treatment of chronic pain. *J Psychoactive Drugs.* 2012 Apr-Jun;44(2):125-33
[184] Leung L. Cannabis and its derivatives: review of medical use. *J Am Board Fam Med.* 2011 Jul-Aug;24(4):452-62
[185] Lee et al. Amygdala activity contributes to the dissociative effect of cannabis on pain perception. *Pain.* 2013 Jan;154(1):124-34
[186] Wilsey et al. Low-dose vaporized cannabis significantly improves neuropathic pain. *J Pain.* 2013 Feb;14(2):136-48
[187] Bachhuber et al. Medical Cannabis Laws and Opioid Analgesic Overdose Mortality in the United States, 1999-2010. *JAMA Intern Med.* 2014 Aug 25. doi: 10.1001/jamainternmed.2014.4005. [Epub ahead of print]

Treat with physical/manual medicine:
- Massage: Gentle massage provides comfort, increases circulation, reduces edema, and promotes healing. After the acute phase, deeper massage may help restore range of motion by breaking adhesions and reducing the feeling of vulnerability that may occur after injury. Research indicates that massage can reduce adolescent aggression[188], improve outcome in preterm infants[189], alleviate premenstrual syndrome[190], improve flexibility, reduce pain, increase serotonin and dopamine in patients with low back pain[191], and improve function and alleviate depression in patients with Parkinson's disease (Alexander technique).[192]
- Joint mobilization and manipulation: Applied as appropriate (after contraindications have been excluded) and to the level of patient comfort. Mechanisms of action and sample techniques are listed later in this section.
- Treatment of associated muscle spasm and myofascial trigger points (MFTP): Such treatment can increase range of motion and decrease pain. See notes on the diagnosis and treatment of MFTP in the following section in this chapter.

Uncover the underlying problem:
- In the case of most acute injuries, the underlying problem is often the injury itself. However, the physician must not be overly naïve and must conduct a thorough history and examination to assess for possible underlying pathologies that cause or contribute to the problem that "appears" to be injury related. Congenital anomalies, underlying pathology, previous injury, and psychoemotional disorders may have been present before the "injury."
    - **In children and young adults, 5% of "sports-related" injuries are associated with preexisting infection, anomalies, or other conditions.**
    - In adult women: "In three cases of carcinoma, the breast mass was not noticed until after the [auto accident] and was initially thought by the patient to have been caused by the trauma. **Indeed between 9% and 20% of women with breast cancer attribute their symptoms to previous trauma to the breast.**"[193]
- Look for leg length inequalities and biomechanical faults such as hyperpronation and pelvic torque.
- Assess and correct poor posture, poor ergonomics, lack of flexibility, muscle strength imbalances, and proprioceptive/coordination deficits.
- Patients may experience a reduction in pain—particularly low-back pain and osteoarthritis pain—when they eliminate coffee/caffeine, food allergens, and/or specific foods to which they are sensitive, most notably the *Solanaceae*/nightshade family—eggplant, tobacco, tomatoes, potatoes, and bell peppers. Foods in the *Solanaceae* family contain anti-acetylcholinesterases[194] that may effect increased synaptic transmission of afferent pain sensations.
- Correction of **diet-induced chronic metabolic acidosis**[195] with the use of alkalinizing diets/supplements can alleviate musculoskeletal pain, at least in part by raising/normalizing intracellular magnesium levels and by reducing intracellular calcium levels. Additional benefits of alkalinization include increased mineral retention, reduced bone resorption[196] and enhanced clearance of toxic xenobiotics and toxins (per the excellent internationally endorsed position paper by Proudfoot et al[197]). Generally speaking and after renal

---

[188] Diego MA, et al. Aggressive adolescents benefit from massage therapy. *Adolescence* 2002 Fall;37(147):597-607
[189] Mainous RO. Infant massage as a component of developmental care: past, present, and future. *Holist Nurs Pract* 2002 Oct;16(5):1-7
[190] Hernandez-Reif M, et al. Premenstrual symptoms are relieved by massage therapy. *J Psychosom Obstet Gynaecol* 2000 Mar;21(1):9-15
[191] "RESULTS: By the end of the study, the massage therapy group, as compared to the relaxation group, reported experiencing less pain, depression, anxiety and improved sleep. They also showed improved trunk and pain flexion performance, and their serotonin and dopamine levels were higher." Hernandez-Reif M, Field T, Krasnegor J, Theakston H. Lower back pain is reduced and range of motion increased after massage therapy. *Int J Neurosci* 2001;106(3-4):131-45
[192] Stallibrass C, Sissons P, Chalmers C. Randomized controlled trial of the Alexander technique for idiopathic Parkinson's disease. *Clin Rehabil* 2002 Nov;16(7):695-708
[193] Seifert S. Medical Illness Simulating Trauma (MIST) syndrome: case reports and discussion of syndrome. *Fam Med* 1993 Apr;25(4):273-6
[194] Krasowski MD, McGehee DS, Moss J. Natural inhibitors of cholinesterases: implications for adverse drug reactions. *Can J Anaesth*. 1997 May;44(5 Pt 1):525-34
[195] "Results of recent observational studies confirm an association between insulin resistance and metabolic acidosis markers, including low serum bicarbonate, high serum anion gap, hypocitraturia, and low urine pH." Adeva MM, Souto G. Diet-induced metabolic acidosis. *Clin Nutr*. 2011 Aug;30(4):416-21
[196] "In postmenopausal women, the oral administration of potassium bicarbonate at a dose sufficient to neutralize endogenous acid improves calcium and phosphorus balance, reduces bone resorption, and increases the rate of bone formation." Sebastian A, Harris ST, Ottaway JH, Todd KM, Morris RC Jr. Improved mineral balance and skeletal metabolism in postmenopausal women treated with potassium bicarbonate. *N Engl J Med*. 1994 Jun 23;330(25):1776-81 content.nejm.org/cgi/content/abstract/330/25/1776
[197] "Urine alkalinization is a treatment regimen that increases poison elimination by the administration of intravenous sodium bicarbonate to produce urine with a pH > or = 7.5." Proudfoot AT, et al. Position Paper on urine alkalinization. *J Toxicol Clin Toxicol*. 2004;42:1-26 eapcct.org/publicfile.php?folder=congress&file=PS_UrineAlkalinization.pdf

and electrolyte disorders have been excluded, the goal is to achieve and maintain a urine pH of 7.5 or slightly higher.

- o Clinical trial—Alkaline mineral supplementation decreases pain in rheumatoid arthritis patients (*Open Nutrition Journal* 2008[198]): Thirty-seven patients with active RA of at least two years duration receiving drug treatment participated in this 12-week study. "All patients were randomly allocated to a supplemented group (30g of an alkaline mineral supplement daily) or to an unsupplemented group. … DAS 28 and VAS decreased in the supplemented group, whereas there was no change in these parameters during the trial in the control group. The functions (HAQ) of the supplemented patients improved. The immunoreactive **endorphin levels increased** in both groups but to a higher degree in the supplemented group. During the trial, **medication (NSAIDs and steroids) could be reduced** in the supplemented group only. Conclusion: This study suggests that an alkaline supplement may improve function and pain in rheumatoid arthritis and may represent an easy and safe addition to the usual treatment of RA patients."

> **Correcting the common diet-induced metabolic acidosis: the importance of maintaining urinary alkalinization**
>
> Benefits of alkalinization correlating with urine pH 7.5 – 8, reasonably up to 8.5:
> - **Elevated endorphins** improves mood and alleviates pain (thereby alleviating depression, addiction, and need for analgesic/anti-inflammatory drugs)
> - **Reduced cortisol** (thereby lessening insulin resistance and hippocampal atrophy)
> - **Enhanced retention of minerals** (improved nutritional status)
> - **Enhanced excretion of poisons** (reduced xenobiotic load)
>
> For patients who do not achieve alkalinization with diet alone, oral administration of potassium/magnesium citrate/bicarbonate should be used.
>
> Proudfoot et al. *J Toxicol Clin Toxicol*. 2004
> Vormann et al. *J Trace Elem Med Biol*. 2001
> Maurer et al. *Am J Physiol Renal Physiol*. 2003

- o Clinical trial—Supplementation with alkaline minerals alleviates low back pain (*J Trace Elem Med Biol* 2001[199]): "The results show that a disturbed acid-base balance may contribute to the symptoms of low back pain. The simple and safe addition of an alkaline multimineral preparate was able to reduce the pain symptoms in these patients with chronic low back pain."

Re-educate, rehabilitate, resourcefulness, return to active life, reassure, referral:
- Educate patient on ways to avoid re-injury and to decrease likelihood of recurrence.
- Pre-rehabilitation assessment has three main goals: 1) identification of the type of injury, 2) quantification of the severity of the injury, and 3) determining the appropriate interventions.[200] Rehabilitative exercises **emphasizing strength, coordination, proprioception, range of motion, and functional utility** (appropriate per occupation and hobbies) should be employed.
- **Isometric exercises** can be used to maintain/increase muscle strength in patients for whom range-of-motion exercises are painful or contraindicated.
- **Work hardening** has been defined by the American Physical Therapy Association as "a highly structured goal-oriented, individualized treatment program designed to return a person to work. Work Hardening programs…use real or simulated work activities designed to restore physical, behavioral, and vocational functions."[201] Teperman[202] defined the specific goals of work hardening as:
    1. Improved lifting strength (loading and unloading) to/from different heights, including overhead,
    2. Improved carrying capacity (various objects, different distances, unilateral and bilateral),
    3. Improved functional tolerance (coordination and manipulation) at different levels,
    4. Improved cardiovascular endurance,
    5. Improved dexterity tasks (counting, weighing, sorting, packaging/unpacking),
    6. Improved biomechanics in any setting (work/leisure).
- **Work conditioning** has been defined as "a work-related, intensive, and goal-oriented treatment program specifically designed to restore an individual's systemic, neuromuscular (strength, endurance, flexibility,

---

[198] Cseuz et al. Alkaline mineral supplementation decreases pain in rheumatoid arthritis patients: a pilot study. *Open Nutrition Journal* 2008:10;2
[199] Vormann J, et al. Supplementation with alkaline minerals reduces symptoms in patients with chronic low back pain. *J Trace Elem Med Biol*. 2001;15(2-3):179-83
[200] Geffen SJ. 3: Rehabilitation principles for treating chronic musculoskeletal injuries. *Med J Aust*. 2003 Mar 3;178(5):238-42
[201] American Physical Therapy Association, "Guidelines for Programs for Injured Workers" 1995. Quoted by Washington State Department of Labor and Industries. lni.wa.gov/Main/MostAskedQuestions/ClaimsIns/WorkHardFaq.asp. Accessed July 23, 2006
[202] Teperman LJ. Active functional restoration and work hardening program returns patient with 2½-year-old elbow fracture-dislocation to work after 6 months: a case report. *J Can Chiropr Assoc* 2002; 46(1): 22-30 jcca-online.org/client/cca/JCCA.nsf/objects/Active+functional+restoration+elbow+fracture-dislocation/$file/5-Teperman.pdf

etc.) and cardiopulmonary function."[203] While overlaps exist between work hardening and work conditioning, and both are generally designed to "return the patient to work", work hardening is focused more on the performance of work-related tasks (task-oriented) while work conditioning tends to focus more on the cardiopulmonary and neuromuscular fitness of the patient (fitness-oriented).

- **Rehabilitation can become more than *restorative*; if the plan is comprehensive and it effects long-term improvements in overall health, then such a program can become *transformative*.** For example, while the oversimplified medical model as commonly practiced in HMO and PPO systems might describe a patient's problem as "low-back pain, refer for physiotherapy and begin Vioxx 25 mg b.i.d.", a more comprehensive assessment and treatment of the same patient's problem might be described as "low-back pain secondary to sedentary lifestyle, obesity, mild systemic inflammation, hypovitaminosis D, and proprioceptive deficits. Begin program of daily general exercise along with specific exercises for low-back region, low-carbohydrate diet to promote weight loss, balance training twice daily, begin supplementation with cholecalciferol 4,000 IU/d and fish oil 3 g/d." Notice that the typical allopathic plan *requires* and *thus ensures* patient passivity and does nothing to promote overall health, whereas the comprehensive natural/integrative plan is more in accord with current biomedical literature, requires active patient participation, offers the probability of improved overall health, and will reduce the severity and risk of present and future diseases, respectively.
- Patients should be supported in the tolerance of minor discomfort to avoid overuse of analgesics, to avoid an excessive reduction in activities, and to avoid playing the "sick role." While validating the patient's concerns, physicians should not encourage dysfunctional behavior or contribute to "iatrogenic neurosis."
- **Symptomatic treatment that provides no lasting benefit can foster psychological dependency and therapeutic passivity**. "Therapeutic dependency" describes the situation wherein the patient becomes dependent on treatment sessions for secondary gain of attention, physical contact, and time off from work (etc.) rather than focusing on the goal of getting as healthy as possible as quickly as possible. Therapeutic dependency is fostered by doctors who fail to educate patients to take an active role in their own care and by doctors who take on the role of "savior" rather than empowering patients to take effective action in improving their health. **Therapeutic passivity** is related to **therapeutic dependency** since patients who fail to take responsible action tend to become dependent on healthcare providers to "cure me", "fix me" and "rescue me."
- Modify home and occupational workstations to minimize strain and stress on injured tissues. Educate patients to use tools, machines, props, and stepstools to work efficiently and to reduce unnecessary lifting and straining motions.
- Physical activities can be fully resumed when symptoms have decreased and when physical examination findings (e.g., reflexes, strength, range of motion, spinal segmental function, and trigger points) are within normal limits. Note that in many situations returning the patient to their previous duration, frequency, and intensity of activity may predispose to re-injury since the patient is re-entering the situation wherein the original injury occurred; therefore at least one of these lifestyle/occupational/recreational variables must change in order to reduce the likeliness of re-injury.
- Books, websites, and national/local support groups and organizations may be available for emotional, physical, psychological-emotional, and legal assistance.
- While detailed individual descriptions of therapeutic exercise and rehabilitative programs are not the subject of this book, we can readily appreciate the many options that are available to us for the rehabilitation of injuries:
    - <u>Weight optimization</u>: For the majority of patients living in our society where obesity is pandemic, weight reduction is important not only to improve overall health and to reduce mechanical stresses on joints, but perhaps even more importantly to reduce the production of proinflammatory chemicals made in adipose tissue (adipokines) which promote an overall internal climate of pain and inflammation. Some patients may need to gain muscle strength to promote healing and avoid

---

[203] Howar JM. *Keys to Effective Work Hardening and Limited Duty Programs.* eh.doe.gov/feosh/contacts/LimitedDutyPrograms.pdf Accessed July 23, 2006. Ironically, even though the third page of this presentation clearly shows the use of spinal manipulation, chiropractic doctors are notably absent from the list of "Industrial Rehab Specialists."

re-injury; this can generally be achieved with resistance training and increased protein consumption.
- Therapeutic exercise: Includes strength training, stretching, improving endurance, and functional training specific to the patient's occupational or athletic activities. These can be tailored to great detail to the patient's condition and goals.[204]
- Proprioceptive retraining/rehabilitation: As discussed later in this chapter, restoration and optimization of proprioceptive function and balance control is especially important for the long-term functional improvement of patients with proprioceptive deficits, commonly seen in patients with chronic low-back pain[205], neck pain[206], knee arthritis[207], and ankle instability.[208]
- Treatment of myofascial trigger points: Since joint injuries and chronic pain—*especially in the neck, back and shoulder*—are commonly associated with trigger points[209], addressing this secondary and occult cause of pain is important to maximize pain relief and functional restoration.
- Analgesic and anti-inflammatory botanicals and nutraceuticals: Safe and effective natural means for achieving a timely reduction in pain include topical capsaicin, *Harpagophytum*, *Uncaria*, acupuncture, willow, and spinal manipulation. Fish oil, GLA, vitamin E, *Boswellia*, willow bark, *Harpagophytum*, and *Zingiber* are just a few of the effective natural anti-inflammatory treatments available.
- Manipulation, mobilization, and massage: Joint manipulation has numerous physiologic and anatomic effects, most of which are relevant for the alleviation of pain and improvement of joint function. These mechanisms include:
    1. Releasing entrapped intraarticular menisci and synovial folds,
    2. Acutely reducing intradiscal pressure, thus promoting replacement of decentralized disc material,
    3. Stretching of deep periarticular muscles to break the cycle of chronic autonomous muscle contraction by lengthening the muscles and thereby releasing excessive actin-myosin binding,
    4. Promoting restoration of proper kinesthesia and proprioception,
    5. Promoting relaxation of paraspinal muscles by stretching facet joint capsules,
    6. Promoting relaxation of paraspinal muscles via "postactivation depression", which is the temporary depletion of contractile neurotransmitters,
    7. Temporarily elevating plasma beta-endorphin,
    8. Temporarily enhancing phagocytic ability of neutrophils and monocytes,
    9. Activating the diffuse descending pain inhibitory system located in the periaqueductal gray matter—this is an important aspect of nociceptive inhibition by intense sensory/mechanoreceptor stimulation, and
    10. Improving neurotransmitter balance and reducing pain (soft-tissue manipulation).[210]

Additional details are provided in numerous published reviews and primary research[211,212,213,214,215,216,217] and by Leach[218], whose extensive description of the mechanisms of action of spinal manipulative therapy is unsurpassed. Given such a wide base of experimental and clinical

---

[204] Basmajian JV (ed). *Therapeutic Exercise. Fourth Edition*. Baltimore: Williams and Wilkins. 1984
[205] Newcomer KL, et al. Muscle activation patterns in subjects with and without low back pain. *Arch Phys Med Rehabil*. 2002;83(6):816-21
[206] McPartland JM, et al. Chronic neck pain, standing balance, and suboccipital muscle atrophy--a pilot study. *J Manipulative Physiol Ther*. 1997 Jan;20(1):24-9
[207] Callaghan MJ, et al. The Effects of Patellar Taping on Knee Joint Proprioception. *J Athl Train*. 2002 Mar;37(1):19-24
[208] Olmsted LC, et al. Efficacy of the Star Excursion Balance Tests in Detecting Reach Deficits in Subjects With Chronic Ankle Instability. *J Athl Train*. 2002 Dec;37(4):501-506
[209] "The mean number of TrPs present on each neck pain patient was 4.3, of which 2.5 were latent and 1.8 were active TrPs. Control subjects also exhibited TrPs (mean: 2; SD: 0.8). All were latent TrPs." Fernandez-de-Las-Penas C, et al. Myofascial trigger points in subjects presenting with mechanical neck pain. *Man Ther*. 2006 Jun 10
[210] "RESULTS: By the end of the study, the massage therapy group, as compared to the relaxation group, reported experiencing less pain, depression, anxiety and improved sleep. They also showed improved trunk and pain flexion performance, and their serotonin and dopamine levels were higher." Hernandez-Reif M, Field T, Krasnegor J, Theakston H. Lower back pain is reduced and range of motion increased after massage therapy. *Int J Neurosci* 2001;106(3-4):131-45
[211] Maigne JY, Vautravers P. Mechanism of action of spinal manipulative therapy. *Joint Bone Spine*. 2003;70(5):336-41
[212] Brennan PC, et al. Enhanced neutrophil respiratory burst as a biological marker for manipulation forces. *J Manipulative Physiol Ther*. 1992 Feb;15(2):83-9
[213] Brennan PC, et al. Enhanced phagocytic cell respiratory burst induced by spinal manipulation: potential role of substance P. *J Manipulative Physiol Ther*. 1991;14(7):399-408
[214] Heikkila et al. Effects of acupuncture, cervical manipulation, NSAID therapy on dizziness and impaired head repositioning of suspected cervical origin. *Man Ther* 2000;5:151-7
[215] Rogers RG. The effects of spinal manipulation on cervical kinesthesia in patients with chronic neck pain: a pilot study. *J Manipulative Physiol Ther*. 1997;20(2):80-5
[216] Bergman, Peterson, Lawrence. *Chiropractic Technique*. New York: Churchill Livingstone 1993. An updated edition is now availabe published by Mosby.
[217] Herzog WH. Mechanical and physiological responses to spinal manipulative treatments. *JNMS: J Neuromusculoskeltal System* 1995; 3: 1-9
[218] Leach RA. (ed). *The Chiropractic Theories: A Textbook of Scientific Research, Fourth Edition*. Baltimore: Lippincott, Williams & Wilkins, 2004

support published in peer-reviewed journals and widely-available textbooks, denigrations directed toward spinal manipulation on the grounds that it is "unscientific" or "unsupported by research" are unfounded and are indicative of selective ignorance.[219]

- Eicosanoid modulation: Historically, the balance of omega-3 to omega-6 fatty acids in the human diet has been approximately 1:1 or 1:2.[220] Since omega-3 fatty acids are generally *anti-inflammatory* while omega-6 fatty acids are generally proinflammatory (with the exception of GLA/DGLA), the former *quantitative* dietary balance translated to a *qualitative* balance with regard to the body's inherent inflammatory tendency. Modern diets today, however, provide a ratio of 1:30, with anti-inflammatory omega-3 fatty acids greatly outnumbered by the proinflammatory omega-6 fatty acids. Thus, human physiology has been altered by the widespread consumption of a *pro-inflammatory acidogenic diet*.[221,222] **Correction of these problems at the level of dietary intake rather than by the use of** and dependence upon by both doctors and patients **anti-inflammatory medications is essential for the attainment of health and the long-term relief of pain and inflammation**.[223,224]
- Reassurance: Education, explanation, reassurance, and support help to address the mental and emotional aspects of injury.
- Alkalinization: The American/Western style of eating results in subclinical diet-induced pathogenic chronic metabolic acidosis[225] which can be corrected with a Paleo-Mediterranean diet[226] or alkalinizing supplements[227] (including potassium citrate and magnesium bicarbonate) for the alleviation of musculoskeletal pain in general and low-back pain in particular.[228]
- **Referral: Patients with severe pain, serious conditions/complications, or documented noncompliance are excellent candidates for co-management or unidirectional referral.**

Nutrition:

- Supplementation with a high-potency broad-spectrum multivitamin and multimineral product: This will help correct common nutritional deficiencies and support optimal healing. Certain nutrients such as vitamin C, zinc, and copper are commonly considered "specific" for promoting optimal repair of connective tissue.
- Dietary protein for tissue repair: In otherwise healthy patients with no liver, renal, or other metabolic disorders, ensure adequate intake of 0.5-0.9 gram of protein per pound of body weight.[229] Vegetarians may heal more slowly after injury than do omnivores; vegetarians and lacto-vegetarians undergoing cosmetic surgery reportedly have more complications and slower healing than do people eating a diet containing meat.[230] Additionally, low-protein diets have shown to reduce muscle mass and suppress immune function.[231] See the table below for protein intake recommendations:

---

[219] Vasquez A. The Science of Chiropractic and Spinal Manipulation, Part 2. mercola.com/2005/mar/12/chiropractic_spine.htm
[220] Simopoulos AP. Essential fatty acids in health and chronic disease. *Am J Clin Nutr*. 1999 Sep;70(3 Suppl):560S-569S
[221] Seaman DR. The diet-induced proinflammatory state: a cause of chronic pain and other degenerative diseases? *J Manipulative Physiol Ther*. 2002;25(3):168-79
[222] Adeva MM1, Souto G. Diet-induced metabolic acidosis. *Clin Nutr*. 2011 Aug;30(4):416-21
[223] Vasquez A. A Five-Part Nutritional Protocol that Produces Consistently Positive Results. *Nutritional Wellness* 2005 September
[224] Vasquez A. Dietary, Nutritional and Botanical Interventions to Reduce Pain and Inflammation. *Naturopathy Digest* 2006, March *Nutritional Wellness* 2006, March
[225] "As a result, healthy adults consuming the standard US diet sustain a chronic, low-grade pathogenic metabolic acidosis that worsens with age as kidney function declines." Cordain L, Eaton SB, Sebastian A, Mann N, Lindeberg S, Watkins BA, O'Keefe JH, Brand-Miller J. Origins and evolution of the Western diet: health implications for the 21st century. *Am J Clin Nutr*. 2005 Feb;81(2):341-54 ajcn.org/cgi/content/full/81/2/341
[226] Cordain L. *The Paleo Diet*. John Wiley and Sons, 2002
[227] "An acidogenic Western diet results in mild metabolic acidosis in association with a state of cortisol excess, altered divalent ion metabolism, and increased bone resorptive indices." Maurer et al. Neutralization of Western diet inhibits bone resorption independently of K intake and reduces cortisol secretion in humans. *Am J Physiol Renal Physiol*. 2003 Jan;284(1):F32-40
[228] "The results show that a disturbed acid-base balance may contribute to the symptoms of low back pain. The simple and safe addition of an alkaline multimineral preparate was able to reduce the pain symptoms in these patients with chronic low back pain." Vormann J, Worlitschek M, Goedecke T, Silver B. Supplementation with alkaline minerals reduces symptoms in patients with chronic low back pain. *J Trace Elem Med Biol*. 2001;15(2-3):179-83
[229] Nancy Clark, MS, RD. The Power of Protein. *The Physician and Sportsmedicine* 1996, volume 24, number 4. physsportsmed.com/issues/1996/04_96/protein.htm
[230] Vegetarians and healing. *JAMA* 1995; 273: 910
[231] Castaneda C, et al. Elderly women accommodate to a low-protein diet with losses of body cell mass, muscle function, and immune response. *Am J Clin Nutr* 1995 Jul;62:30-9

Recommended Grams of Protein per Patient Profile and Body Weight Per Day		
Patient Profile	Per **pound** of weight[232]	Per **kilogram** of weight
RDA for sedentary adult and children ages 6-18 years[233]	0.4	0.88
Adult recreational exerciser—average for adults	**0.5-0.75**	**1.1-1.65**
Adult competitive athlete	0.6-0.9	1.32-1.98
Adult building muscle mass	0.7-0.9	1.54-1.98
Dieting athlete	0.7-1.0	1.54-2.2
Growing teenage athlete	0.9-1.0	1.98-2.2

- Vegetables, fruit, and fiber: Whole foods provide micronutrients, natural anti-inflammatory components, and immune modulators; the fiber/phytonutrient content provides positive effects on gut flora while maintaining proper waste elimination and reducing straining (e.g., reduced need for the Valsalva maneuver).
- Carbohydrates: Carbohydrate intake should be adequate to supply energy-expenditure needs and to support healing but should not be excessive such as to unfavorably increase body weight during times of decreased physical activity. Preferred sources of carbohydrates are fruits and vegetables.
- Water: Adequate intake of water is important to flush out wastes, toxins, and to prevent constipation. Eight glasses per day is the classic recommendation; however increased fluid intake is appropriate during exercise, heat exposure, stress, and to promote clearance of nitrogenous wastes and xenobiotics. Fluid restriction may be appropriate for persons with adrenal insufficiency to avoid hyponatremia and those with cardiovascular failure, fluid overload, or edema.
- Identification and elimination of adverse food reactions: Adverse food reactions—regardless of the underlying mechanism(s) or classification of allergy, intolerance, or sensitivity—can precipitate joint pain and inflammation[234,235,236,237,238,239,240] and a wide range of other health problems.
- Vitamin D3: The data is very clear that 1) vitamin D deficiency causes pain—both axial and peripheral, 2) the pain of vitamin D deficiency is difficult-to-treat or unresponsive to NSAIDs and opioids, thus forcing pharmacocentric physicians to use higher and thus more dangerous doses of drugs, 3) replacement with vitamin D3 quickly and effectively alleviates the pain of vitamin D deficiency, 4) all "pain patients" should have their vitamin D levels tested and optimized per the data in this book. For adults without existing or predisposition toward hypercalcemia, the appropriate dose of vitamin D3 is typically 4,000-10,000 IU/d; serum calcium is periodically monitored for safety while serum 25-hydroxy-vitamin D is optimize per the graphic that follows.[241] Given the quantity and consistency of the data substantiating the causative connection between vitamin D3 deficiency and pain, the high frequency of this problem in clinical practice, the consequences of nontreatment, and the dependable success of treatment, failure to assess and treat vitamin D deficiency in patients with persistent major pain is not consistent with quality contemporary clinical care.
    - Exemplary case report—A woman who left her wheelchair (*Lancet* 1999 Mar[242]): 32yo patient with progressive muscular weakness of her legs and diffuse skeletal pain and required used of crutches or wheelchair. She had waddling gait, proximal hip-muscle weakness and hypotonia, and from the age of 21 she had been treated with steroids for ileal Crohn's disease, for which she had one small-bowel resection. She was given parenteral 1,25-dihydroxyvitaminD3 (1 microg/d) and

---

[232] Slightly modified from Nancy Clark, MS, RD. Protein Power. *The Physician and Sportsmedicine* 1996, volume 24, number 4
[233] 0.83 g.kg-1.d-1 (equivalent to 0.37 grams per pound of body weight) Pellet PL. Protein requirements in humans. *Am J Clin Nutr* 1990 May;51:723-37
[234] Golding DN. Is there an allergic synovitis? *J R Soc Med*. 1990 May;83(5):312-4
[235] Panush RS. Food induced ("allergic") arthritis: clinical and serologic studies. *J Rheumatol*. 1990 Mar;17(3):291-4
[236] Pacor ML, Lunardi C, Di Lorenzo G, Biasi D, Corrocher R. Food allergy and seronegative arthritis: report of two cases. *Clin Rheumatol*. 2001;20(4):279-81
[237] Schrander JJ, Marcelis C, de Vries MP, van Santen-Hoeufft HM. Does food intolerance play a role in juvenile chronic arthritis? *Br J Rheumatol*. 1997 Aug;36(8):905-8
[238] van de Laar et al. Food intolerance in rheumatoid arthritis. *Ann Rheum Dis*. 1992;51:298-302
[239] Haugen et al. A pilot study of the effect of an elemental diet in the management of rheumatoid arthritis. *Clin Exp Rheumatol*. 1994 May-Jun;12(3):275-9
[240] van de Laar et al. Food intolerance in rheumatoid arthritis. II. *Ann Rheum Dis*. 1992 Mar;51(3):303-6
[241] **Vasquez A, Manso G, Cannell J. The clinical importance of vitamin D (cholecalciferol): a paradigm shift with implications for all healthcare providers.** *Altern Ther Health Med.* 2004 Sep-Oct;10(5):28-36 Full-text available at ICHNFM.org/pdf
[242] Mingrone G et al. A woman who left her wheelchair. *Lancet*. 1999 Mar 6;353(9155):806

enhanced oral intake of calcium and phosphate-rich food (meat, fish, liver, and root vegetables), and "after 3 weeks she could walk again, and her muscle weakness and bone pain disappeared."

- Severe hypovitaminosis D in patients with persistent, nonspecific musculoskeletal pain (*Mayo Clin Proc* 2003 Dec[243]): "All patients with persistent, nonspecific musculoskeletal pain are at high risk for the consequences of unrecognized and untreated severe hypovitaminosis D. ... Because osteomalacia is a known cause of persistent, nonspecific musculoskeletal pain, screening all outpatients with such pain for hypovitaminosis D should be standard practice in clinical care."
- Clinical trial—Vitamin D deficiency and chronic low back pain (*Spine* 2003 Jan[244]): "Findings showed that 83% of the study patients (n = 299) had an abnormally low level of vitamin D before treatment with vitamin D supplements. After treatment, clinical improvement in symptoms was seen in all the groups that had a low level of vitamin D, and in 95% of all the patients (n = 341). Vitamin D deficiency is a major contributor to chronic low back pain in areas where vitamin D deficiency is endemic. Screening for vitamin D deficiency and treatment with supplements should be mandatory in this setting."
- Clinical trial—Vitamin D supplementation for diffuse musculoskeletal pain (*Eur J Gen Pract* 2014 Mar[245]): Patients 18-50yo with pain or unexplained asthenia/fatigue with hypovitaminosis D (average 25[OH]D level 23.7 nmol/l). After vitamin D supplementation, the adjusted mean serum 25ohD level increased to 118.8 nmol/l, the quality of life score increased and the pain evaluation score decreased. In this study, vitamin D supplementation decreased pain scores in adult patients with diffuse musculoskeletal pain and vitamin D deficiency.
- Review of 450 cases—Low vitamin D as a risk factor for the development of myalgia in patients taking high-dose simvastatin (*Clin Ther* 2014 May[246]): "This was a retrospective medical record review of 450 patients who were prescribed simvastatin 80 mg at the Veterans Affairs Western New York Healthcare System between August 1, 2006, and July 31, 2011. ... The mean vitamin D level in patients experiencing myalgia was 26.2 versus 36.3 ng/mL. The 25-hydroxyvitamin D level in those who reported myalgia was approximately 10 ng/mL lower compared with those who tolerated simvastatin 80 mg. Vitamin D insufficiency appears to be a risk factor for the development of [statin-induced] myalgia." Comment by DrV: Several studies have documented the correlation between statin-induced myalgia and vitamin D deficiency; sadly, both the vitamin D deficiency and the overuse of statin drugs would be avoided if clinicians and physicians had a better knowledge of nutrition.
- Case series—Improvement of chronic back pain or failed back surgery with vitamin D repletion (*J Am Board Fam Med* 2009 Jan-Feb[247]): "Chronic low back pain and failed back surgery may improve with repletion of vitamin D from a state of deficiency/insufficiency to sufficiency. Vitamin D insufficiency is common; repletion of vitamin D to normal levels in patients who have chronic low back pain or have had failed back surgery may improve quality of life or, in some cases, result in complete resolution of symptoms."
- Severity of vitamin D deficiency correlates with opioid drug need (dose and duration) for pain control (*Pain Med* 2008 Nov[248]): Among 267 chronic pain patients, the prevalence of vitamin D inadequacy was 26%. "Among patients using opioids, the mean morphine equivalent dose for the inadequate vitamin D group was 133.5 mg/day compared with 70.0 mg/day for the adequate group. The mean duration of opioid use for the inadequate and adequate groups were 71.1 months and 43.8 months, respectively. Opioid users with inadequate [vitamin D] levels reported worse physical functioning and health perception than opioid users with adequate levels."

---

[243] Plotnikoff GA, Quigley JM. Prevalence of severe hypovitaminosis D in patients with persistent, nonspecific musculoskeletal pain. *Mayo Clin Proc*. 2003 Dec;78(12):1463-70
[244] Al Faraj S, Al Mutairi K. Vitamin D deficiency and chronic low back pain in Saudi Arabia. *Spine* 2003 Jan 15;28(2):177-9
[245] Le Goaziou MF et al. Vitamin D supplementation for diffuse musculoskeletal pain: results of a before-and-after study. *Eur J Gen Pract*. 2014 Mar;20(1):3-9
[246] Mergenhagen K et al. Low vitamin d as a risk factor for the development of myalgia in patients taking high-dose simvastatin. *Clin Ther*. 2014 May 1;36(5):770-7
[247] Schwalfenberg G. Improvement of chronic back pain or failed back surgery with vitamin D repletion: a case series. *J Am Board Fam Med*. 2009 Jan-Feb;22(1):69-74
[248] Turner et al. Prevalence and clinical correlates of vitamin D inadequacy among patients with chronic pain. *Pain Med*. 2008 Nov;9(8):979-84

Excess vitamin D
> 100 ng/mL (250 nmol/L) with hypercalcemia

Optimal range
50 - 100 ng/mL (125 - 250 nmol/L)

Insufficiency range
< 20- 40 ng/mL (50 - 100 nmol/L)

Deficiency
< 20 ng/mL (50 nmol/L)

<u>Serum 25(OH) vitamin D levels</u>: Modified from earlier peer-reviewed versions published in Vasquez et al, *Alternative Therapies in Health and Medicine* 2004)

The vitamin D "clinical paradigm shift" consolidated by Vasquez et al in 2004

"Given the depth and breadth of the peer-reviewed research documenting the frequency and consequences of hypovitaminosis D, failure to diagnose and treat this disorder is ethically questionable and is inconsistent with the delivery of quality, science-based healthcare. ... Until proven otherwise, the balance of the research clearly indicates that oral supplementation in the range of 1,000 IU/day for infants, 2,000 IU/day for children, and 4,000 IU/day for adults is safe and reasonable to meet physiologic requirements, to promote optimal health, and to reduce the risk of several serious diseases. Safety and effectiveness of supplementation are assured by periodic monitoring of serum 25(OH)D and serum calcium."

Vasquez A et al. The clinical importance of vitamin D (cholecalciferol): a paradigm shift with implications for all healthcare providers. *Altern Ther Health Med* 2004 Sep ICHNFM.org/pdf

---

- <u>Other specific supplements/botanicals</u>: Supplementation is tailored to the type of tissue that has been injured, such as calcium, magnesium, and vitamins D and K for bone fractures, glucosamine sulfate and niacinamide for cartilage injuries, and proteolytic enzymes for muscle strains.
    - <u>Niacinamide</u>: The niacinamide form of vitamin B3 was proven effective against osteoarthritis by Kaufman more than 50 years ago.[249] Furthermore, Kaufman's documentation of an "anti-aging" effect of vitamin supplementation in general and niacinamide therapy in particular[250] is consistent with recent experimental data demonstrating rapid reversion of aging phenotypes by niacinamide through modulation of histone acetylation.[251] A recent double-blind placebo-controlled repeat study found that niacinamide therapy improved joint mobility, reduced objective inflammation as assessed by ESR, reduced the impact of the arthritis on the activities of daily living, and allowed a reduction in analgesic/anti-inflammatory medication use.[252] While the mechanism of action is probably multifaceted, inhibition of joint-destroying nitric oxide appears to be an important benefit.[253] The standard dose of 500 mg given orally 6 times per day is more effective than 1,000 mg 3 times per day. Hepatic dysfunction is rare when daily doses are kept below 3,000 mg per day, yet Gaby[254] suggests measurement of liver enzymes after 3 months of treatment and yearly thereafter. Antirheumatic benefit is generally significant following 2-6 weeks of treatment, and patients may also notice an anxiolytic benefit, possibly mediated by the binding of niacinamide to GABA/benzodiazepine receptors.[255]
    - <u>Glucosamine sulfate and chondroitin sulfate</u>: Glucosamine and chondroitin are the "building blocks" from which cartilage is built and oral supplementation is intended to enhance cartilage anabolism and to thus counteract the enhanced cartilage catabolism seen in destructive arthritic processes.[256] Clinical trials with glucosamine and chondroitin sulfates have shown consistently positive results in clinical trials involving patients with osteoarthritis of the hands, hips, knees,

---

[249] Kaufman W. Niacinamide therapy for joint mobility. Therapeutic reversal of a common clinical manifestation of the normal aging process. *Conn State Med J* 1953;17:584-591
[250] Kaufman W. The use of vitamin therapy to reverse certain concomitants of aging. *J Am Geriatr Soc* 1955;3:927-936
[251] Matuoka K, et al. Rapid reversion of aging phenotypes by nicotinamide through possible modulation of histone acetylation. *Cell Mol Life Sci*. 2001;58(14):2108-16
[252] Jonas WB, Rapoza CP, Blair WF. The effect of niacinamide on osteoarthritis: a pilot study. *Inflamm Res* 1996 Jul;45(7):330-4
[253] McCarty et al. Niacinamide therapy for osteoarthritis--does it inhibit nitric oxide synthase induction by interleukin 1 in chondrocytes? *Med Hypotheses*. 1999;53(4):350-60
[254] Gaby AR. Literature review and commentary: Niacinamide for osteoarthritis. *Townsend Letter for Doctors and Patients*. 2002: May; 32
[255] Mohler H, Polc P, Cumin R, Pieri L, Kettler R. Nicotinamide is a brain constituent with benzodiazepine-like actions. *Nature*. 1979; 278(5704): 563-5
[256] Vidal y Plana et al. Articular cartilage pharmacology: I. In vitro studies on glucosamine and non steroidal antiinflammatory drugs. *Pharmacol Res Commun* 1978;10:557-69

temporomandibular joint, and low-back.[257,258,259,260,261,262,263] For example, glucosamine sulfate was superior to placebo for pain reduction and preservation of joint space in a 3-year clinical trial in patients with knee osteoarthritis.[264] Arguments against the use of glucosamine due to inflated concern about inefficacy or exacerbation of diabetes[265] are without scientific merit[266,267] as evidenced by a 90-day trial of diabetic patients consuming 1500 mg of glucosamine hydrochloride with 1200 mg of chondroitin sulfate which showed no significant alterations in serum glucose or hemoglobin A1c[268] and by the previously cited 3-year study which found significant clinical benefit and no adverse effects on glucose homeostasis.[269] The adult dose of glucosamine sulfate is generally 1500-2000 mg per day in divided doses, and the dose of chondroitin sulfate is approximately 1000 mg daily; these treatments can be used singly, in combination, and with other treatments. Both treatments are safe for multiyear use, and rare adverse effects include allergy and nonpathologic gastrointestinal upset. Clinical benefit is generally significant following 4-6 weeks of treatment and is maintained for the duration of treatment. In contrast to coxib and other mislabeled "anti-inflammatory" drugs that consistently elevate the incidence of cardiovascular disease, death, and other adverse effects[270,271,272,273,274], supplementation with chondroitin sulfate appears to safely reduce the pain and disability associated with osteoarthritis while simultaneously reducing incidence of cardiovascular morbidity and mortality.[275,276] In a study with animals that spontaneously develop atherosclerosis[277], administration of chondroitin sulfate induced regression of existing atherosclerosis. In a six-year study with 120 patients with established cardiovascular disease, 60 chondroitin-treated patients suffered 6 coronary events and 4 deaths compared to 42 events and 14 deaths in a comparable group of 60 patients receiving "conventional" therapy; chondroitin-treated patients reported enhancement of well-being while no adverse clinical or laboratory effects were noted during the 6 years of treatment.[278] Glucosamine sulfate is strongly preferred over glucosamine hydrochloride due to higher efficacy of the former. The negative study by Clegg et al[279] in *New England Journal of Medicine* 2006 was not a scientific study, but rather it was a pseudostudy designed with the intention to make "glucosamine and chondroitin sulfate" appear inefficacious so that drug sales of coxibs would remain high—this study is so ridiculously corrupt that 1) it should have never been published, 2) it should be withdrawn, and 3) it exemplifies the extent to which the *New England Journal of Medicine* panders to the pharmaceutical industry at the expense of quality patient care and good science.

---

[257] "…patients taking GS had a significantly greater decrease in TMJ pain with function, effect of pain, and acetaminophen used between Day 90 and 120 compared with patients taking ibuprofen." Thie et al. Evaluation of glucosamine sulfate compared to ibuprofen for the treatment of temporomandibular joint osteoarthritis. *J Rheumatol* 2001;28:1347-55
[258] Braham R, Dawson B, Goodman C. The effect of glucosamine supplementation on people experiencing regular knee pain. *Br J Sports Med*. 2003;37(1):45-9
[259] "…oral glucosamine therapy achieved a significantly greater improvement in articular pain score than ibuprofen, and the investigators rated treatment efficacy as 'good' in a significantly greater proportion of glucosamine than ibuprofen recipients. In comparison with piroxicam, glucosamine significantly improved arthritic symptoms after 12 weeks of therapy…" Matheson AJ, Perry CM. Glucosamine: a review of its use in the management of osteoarthritis. *Drugs Aging*. 2003; 20(14): 1041-60
[260] Uebelhart D, Malaise M, Marcolongo R, DeVathaire F, Piperno M, Mailleux E, Fioravanti A, Matoso L, Vignon E. Intermittent treatment of knee osteoarthritis with oral chondroitin sulfate: a one-year, randomized, double-blind, multicenter study versus placebo. *Osteoarthritis Cartilage*. 2004;12:269-76
[261] van Blitterswijk WJ, et al. Glucosamine and chondroitin sulfate supplementation to treat symptomatic disc degeneration. *BMC Complement Altern Med*. 2003;3(1):2
[262] Morreale P, et al. Comparison of the antiinflammatory efficacy of chondroitin sulfate and diclofenac sodium in patients with knee osteoarthritis. *J Rheumatol*. 1996;23:1385-91
[263] Mazieres B, et al. Chondroitin sulfate in osteoarthritis of the knee: a prospective, double blind, placebo controlled multicenter clinical study. *J Rheumatol*. 2001;28(1):173-81
[264] Reginster JY et al. Long-term effects of glucosamine sulphate on osteoarthritis progression: a randomised, placebo-controlled clinical trial. *Lancet*. 2001;357(9252):251-6
[265] Adams ME. Hype about glucosamine. *Lancet*. 1999;354(9176):353-4
[266] Cumming A. Glucosamine in osteoarthritis. *Lancet*. 1999;354(9190):1640-1
[267] Rovati LC, Annefeld M, Giacovelli G, Schmid K, Setnikar I. *Glucosamine in osteoarthritis*. Lancet. 1999;354(9190):1640
[268] Scroggie et al. Effect of glucosamine-chondroitin supplementation on glycosylated hemoglobin in patients with type 2 diabetes mellitus. *Arch Intern Med* 2003;163:1587-9
[269] Reginster JY, et al. Long-term effects of glucosamine sulphate on osteoarthritis progression: a randomised, placebo-controlled clinical trial. *Lancet*. 2001;357(9252):251-6
[270] Topol EJ. Failing the public health--rofecoxib, Merck, and the FDA. *N Engl J Med*. 2004 Oct 21;351(17):1707-9
[271] Mukherjee D, Nissen SE, Topol EJ. Risk of cardiovascular events associated with selective cox-2 inhibitors. *JAMA* 2001; 286(8):954-9
[272] Ray WA, Griffin MR, Stein CM. Cardiovascular toxicity of valdecoxib. *N Engl J Med*. 2004;351(26):2767
[273] "Patients in the clinical trial taking 400 mg. of Celebrex twice daily had a 3.4 times greater risk of CV events compared to placebo. For patients in the trial taking 200 mg. of Celebrex twice daily, the risk was 2.5 times greater. The average duration of treatment in the trial was 33 months." FDA Statement on the Halting of a Clinical Trial of the cox-2 Inhibitor Celebrex. fda.gov/bbs/topics/news/2004/NEW01144.html Available on January 4, 2005
[274] "Preliminary information from the study showed some evidence of increased risk of cardiovascular events, when compared to placebo, to patients taking naproxen." FDA Statement on Naproxen. fda.gov/bbs/topics/news/2004/NEW01148.html Available on January 4, 2005
[275] Morrison LM. Treatment of coronary arteriosclerotic heart disease with chondroitin sulfate-A: preliminary report. *J Am Geriatr Soc*. 1968;16(7):779-85
[276] Morrison LM, et al. The prevention of coronary arteriosclerotic heart disease with chondroitin sulfate A: preliminary report. *Exp Med Surg*. 1969;27(3):278-89
[277] Morrison et al. Absence of naturally occurring coronary atherosclerosis in squirrel monkeys (Saimiri sciurea) treated with chondroitin sulfate A. *Experientia* 1972 ;28:1410-1
[278] Morrison LM, Enrick N. Coronary heart disease: reduction of death rate by chondroitin sulfate A. *Angiology*. 1973 May;24(5):269-87
[279] Clegg DO, Reda DJ, Harris CL, et al. Glucosamine, chondroitin sulfate, and the two in combination for painful knee osteoarthritis. *N Engl J Med*. 2006;354:795-808

> **Characteristics of the (pseudo)study by Clegg et al published and widely cited from *New England J Med* 2006**
> - **Misleading title**: The term "glucosamine and chondroitin sulfate" gives the impression that—if a distinction is being made—glucosamine sulfate is being used in the study, rather than glucosamine hydrochloride. Given that glucosamine sulfate is more popular among consumers and more clinically efficacious, one would reasonably assume that this is the form being used; in fact, the opposite is true: the authors used glucosamine hydrochloride, which is notably less effective than glucosamine sulfate (GS). This suggests that the authors were either ignorant or intentionally designing the study to produce negative results.
> - **Misleading title**: The title makes no mention of the use of Celebrex/celecoxib in the study, while in fact the study was designed as a competition between these two interventions.
> - **Unequal study design—duration**: GS typically takes several months to be effective, with optimal results not appreciated until treatment has been continued up to 3 years. In contrast, celecoxib is known to be much faster acting. By using a shorter term trial duration, the researchers gave the advantage to celecoxib.
> - **Unequal study design—dose**: The dosing of celecoxib was more assertive than the dosing of GS and chondroitin.
> - **Misleading conclusions published versus the authors' data**: According to Figure 2 of the article, glucosamine and chondroitin—alone or in combination—was equal to or generally better than placebo in every measure. Yet, the published conclusion and popular headlines in the lay press conclude that the nondrug treatments were inefficacious; this study has also been cited in otherwise reputable medical textbooks, such as *Cecil's Essentials of Medicine*, a medical textbook widely read by medical students and allopathic clinicians.
> - Several of the authors had received payment from Pfizer, the drug company that makes Celebrex/celecoxib: Drs. Brandt, Moskowitz, Schnitzer, and Schumacher report having received consulting fees or having served on advisory boards for Pfizer. Dr. Brandt reports having equity interests in Pfizer. Drs. Moskowitz and Weisman report having received lecture fees from Pfizer. Drs. Bingham, Clegg, Hooper, Jackson, Molitor, Sawitzke, and Schnitzer, grant support from Pfizer. Dr. Moskowitz reports having served as an expert consultant for Pfizer.
>
> Clegg DO, Reda DJ, Harris CL, Klein MA, O'Dell JR, Hooper MM, Bradley JD, Bingham CO 3rd, Weisman MH, Jackson CG, Lane NE, Cush JJ, Moreland LW, Schumacher HR Jr, Oddis CV, Wolfe F, Molitor JA, Yocum DE, Schnitzer TJ, Furst DE, Sawitzke AD, Shi H, Brandt KD, Moskowitz RW, Williams HJ. Glucosamine, chondroitin sulfate, and the two in combination for painful knee osteoarthritis. *N Engl J Med*. 2006;354:795-808. This article is an embarrassment to science; note the long list of agreeable authors.

- Vitamin E, with an emphasis on gamma-tocopherol: The *gamma* form of tocopherol inhibits cyclooxygenase and has anti-inflammatory activity.[280] Clinical trials and case reports have demonstrated benefit of vitamin E supplementation in patients with rheumatoid arthritis[281,282], spondylosis[283] and osteoarthritis[284], and autoimmune diseases including scleroderma, discoid lupus erythematosus, porphyria cutanea tarda, vasculitis, and polymyositis.[285,286,287] In 2013, we as clinicians gained valuable insight into the mechanism of action of vitamin E thanks to the work of Salinthone et al[288] who showed that, rather than functioning simply/solely as an antioxidant, vitamin E significantly raises cyclic adenosine monophosphate (cAMP) levels and thereby has an anti-inflammatory effect; they showed that "vitamin E resulted in a greater than 2-fold increase in cAMP level (29.19 pmol/mg protein) compared to baseline. Lipoic acid was used as a positive control, which generated 45.49 pmol/mg protein of cAMP." Elevation of cAMP—such as by alpha-tocopherol and lipoic acid—results in a dose-dependent inhibition of inflammatory IL-2 and IL-17 cytokine generation and by this mechanism—additive/synergistic with the antioxidant and mitochondrial-supportive effects—reduces inflammation. Generally, cAMP-elevating agents

---

[280] Jiang Q, Christen S, Shigenaga MK, Ames BN. gamma-tocopherol, the major form of vitamin E in the US diet, deserves more attention. *Am J Clin Nutr* 2001 Dec;74(6):714-22
[281] Helmy M, Shohayeb M, Helmy MH, el-Bassiouni EA. Antioxidants as adjuvant therapy in rheumatoid disease. A preliminary study. *Arzneimittelforschung*. 2001;51(4):293-8
[282] Edmonds SE, et al. Putative analgesic activity of repeated oral doses of vitamin E in the treatment of rheumatoid arthritis. *Ann Rheum Dis*. 1997 Nov;56(11):649-55
[283] "Vitamin E administration at a dose of 100 mg daily for three weeks resulted in a significant increase in serum vitamin E level accompanied by complete relief of pain... The results therefore strongly indicate that vitamin E is effective in curing spondylosis and most probably due to its antioxidant activity." Mahmud Z, Ali SM. Role of vitamin A and E in spondylosis. *Bangladesh Med Res Counc Bull*. 1992 Apr;18(1):47-59. See also "The results of this double-blind controlled clinical trial showed that vitamin E was superior to placebo with respect to the relief of pain (pain at rest, pain during movement, pressure-induced pain) and the necessity of additional analgetic treatment. Improvement of mobility was better in the group treated with vitamin E." Blankenhorn G. [Clinical effectiveness of Spondyvit (vitamin E) in activated arthroses. A multicenter placebo-controlled double-blind study] [Article in German—information from abstract] *Z Orthop Ihre Grenzgeb* 1986;124:340-3. See also This is a very interesting study because the clinical response to vitamin E was proportional to the increase in plasma levels of vitamin E, thus confirming the dose-response relationship that implies causality as well as indicating that the failure of such treatment in some patients may be due to malabsorption or unquenchable systemic oxidative stress rather than the inefficacy of vitamin E supplementation, per se. "There were no significant differences in the efficacy of the two drugs, although one patient of the V-group refused further treatment after 8 days because of inefficacy. V reduced or abolished the pain at rest in 77% (D in 85%), the pain on pressure in 67% (D in 50%), and the pain on movement in 62% (D in 63%). Both treatments appeared to be equally effective in reducing the circumference of the knee joints (p = 0.001) and the walking time (p less than 0.001) and in increasing the joint mobility (p less than 0.002)." Scherak O, et al. [High dosage vitamin E therapy in patients with activated arthrosis] [Article in German—information from abstract] *Z Rheumatol*. 1990 Nov-Dec;49(6):369-73
[284] Machtey I, Ouaknine L. Tocopherol in Osteoarthritis: a controlled pilot study. *J Am Geriatr Soc*. 1978 Jul;26(7):328-30
[285] Killeen RN, Ayres S Jr, Mihan R. Polymyositis: response to vitamin E. *South Med J*. 1976 Oct;69(10):1372-4
[286] Ayres S Jr, Mihan R. Lupus erythematosus and vitamin E: an effective and nontoxic therapy. *Cutis*. 1979 Jan;23(1):49-52, 54
[287] Ayres S Jr, Mihan R. Is vitamin E involved in the autoimmune mechanism? *Cutis*. 1978 Mar;21(3):321-5
[288] Salinthone et al. α-Tocopherol stimulates cyclic AMP production in human peripheral mononuclear cells and alters immune function. *Mol Immunol*. 2013 Mar;53(3):173-8

demonstrate anti-inflammatory actions by increasing production of anti-inflammatory IL-10 and reducing production of pro-inflammatory TNF-alpha.[289]
- Vitamin C: Doses of 1-2 grams per day have been suggested to reduce pain and the need for surgery in patients with low-back pain by improving disc integrity.[290] Vitamin C reduces production of isoprostanes, which promote inflammation and pain. Ascorbate is also necessary for the production of the anti-inflammatory prostaglandin E-1. Supplemental vitamin C may also reduce the severity and progression of osteoarthritis.[291]
- Pancreatic/proteolytic enzymes: Orally-administered pancreatic and proteolytic enzymes are absorbed from the gastrointestinal tract into the systemic circulation[292,293] to exert analgesic, anti-inflammatory, anti-edematous benefits with therapeutic relevance for acute and chronic musculoskeletal disorders.[294,295,296,297]

---

[289] Eigler et al. Anti-inflammatory activities of cAMP-elevating agents: enhancement of IL-10 synthesis and suppression of TNF production. *J Leukoc Biol*. 1998 Jan;63(1):101-7
[290] Greenwood J. Optimum vitamin C intake as a factor in the preservation of disc integrity. *Med Ann Dist Columbia*. 1964 Jun;33:274-6
[291] "A 3-fold reduction in risk of OA progression was found for both the middle tertile and highest tertile of vitamin C intake. This related predominantly to a reduced risk of cartilage loss. Those with high vitamin C intake also had a reduced risk of developing knee pain." McAlindon TE, et al. Do antioxidant micronutrients protect against the development and progression of knee osteoarthritis? *Arthritis Rheum*. 1996 Apr;39(4):648-56
[292] Gotze H, Rothman SS. Enteropancreatic circulation of digestive enzymes as a conservative mechanism. *Nature* 1975; 257(5527): 607-609
[293] Liebow C, Rothman SS. Enteropancreatic Circulation of Digestive Enzymes. *Science* 1975; 189(4201): 472-474
[294] Trickett P. Proteolytic enzymes in treatment of athletic injuries. *Appl Ther*. 1964;30:647-52
[295] Walker JA, Cerny FJ, Cotter JR, Burton HW. Attenuation of contraction-induced skeletal muscle injury by bromelain. *Med Sci Sports Exerc*. 1992 Jan;24(1):20-5
[296] Walker et al. Bromelain reduces mild acute knee pain and improves well-being in a dose-dependent fashion in an open study of healthy adults. *Phytomedicine*. 2002;9:681-6
[297] Brien S, et al. Bromelain as a Treatment for Osteoarthritis: a Review of Clinical Studies. *Evidence-based Complementary and Alternative Medicine*. 2004;1(3)251–257

Myofascial trigger points (MFTP)

Description/pathophysiology:
- Many patients suffer from chronic pain that originates from myofascial trigger points—localized areas within muscle tissue that produce chronic pain, promote muscle contraction and tightness, and which mediate autonomous autonomic responses. Physicians who take the time to locate and treat MFTP and educate patients about effective home care can often rapidly and permanently reduce their patients' pain in a safe and highly cost-effective manner.
- MFTP have been defined as "a highly localized and hyperirritable spot in a palpable taut band of skeletal muscle fibers"[298] characterized by the following:
    1. Referred pain with compression: Digital compression of the MFTP causes local pain and most often causes referred pain in a distribution similar or identical to the patient's presenting complaint. The distribution of pain may appear radicular and may thus be described as "pseudoradicular."
    2. Twitch response: When digital pressure is applied perpendicularly to the direction of muscle fibers at the location of the MFTP and the muscle is "plucked" or allowed to "snap" as if one were plucking a taut rubber band or the string of a guitar, the muscle being assessed undergoes a rapid contraction.
    3. Muscle tightness: The muscle involved is tighter than usual, and it is resistant to stretch.
    4. Associated autonomic phenomena: Regions of the body near a localized MFTP may display associated autonomic dysregulation such as vasoconstriction, sweating, pilomotor response, and the patient may experience nausea, dizziness, light-headedness[299] or atrial fibrillation.[300]
    5. MFTP may be "active" or "latent": Active MFTP are those which cause spontaneous pain with joint motion or muscle contraction, whereas latent MFTP cause pain only when provoked by an examiner's deep palpation and physical compression.[301]
    6. Normal muscle strength: Muscle weakness and atrophy are not associated with MFTP unless the weakness or atrophy is secondary to pain.
- The initiation and perpetuation of MFTP is complex and commonly associated with previous injury or chronic static posturing (such as sitting in front of a computer for 8-14 hours per day) and also with emotional stress. Since **intrafusal fibers of muscle spindles receive direct sympathetic innervation**, and since adrenaline/epinephrine directly increases the contractile tone and tension of muscles, it is reasonable to conclude that attention to emotional stress and stress management techniques should be part of the comprehensive treatment plan for MFTP. A significant reduction in emotional tension and work-related repetitive strain injuries may follow a comprehensive and "body-based" approach to healthy living and appropriate career choices.[302]
- The pathogenesis and physiology-based treatment of MFTP follow this route are as follows:
    Pathogenesis[303]
    1. Excess calcium is released from the sarcoplasmic reticulum, leading to local muscle fiber contraction.
    2. Intense and chronic muscle contractions cause relative local ischemia.
    3. The reduction in local blood supply limits energy replacement and leads to the depletion of adenosine triphosphate (ATP).
    4. The muscle cell now has insufficient ATP for the active return of calcium from the contractile elements to the sarcoplasmic reticulum, thus maintaining the muscle fibers in a contracted state.
    Physiology-based treatment:
    5. Stretching the muscle fibers reduces the overlap between actin and myosin, which then leads to a reduction in energy demand of the cell and thus helps to "break the cycle" of **contraction** *leading to* **energy depletion** *leading to* **contraction** *leading to* **energy depletion**...

---

[298] Hong CZ, Simons DG. Pathophysiologic and electrophysiologic mechanisms of myofascial trigger points. *Arch Phys Med Rehabil*. 1998;79(7):863-72
[299] Hubbard DR, Berkoff GM. Myofascial trigger points show spontaneous needle EMG activity. *Spine*. 1993 Oct 1;18(13):1803-7
[300] Simons DG. Cardiology and myofascial trigger points: Janet G. Travell's contribution. *Tex Heart Inst J*. 2003;30(1):3-7
[301] Hubbard DR, Berkoff GM. Myofascial trigger points show spontaneous needle EMG activity. *Spine*. 1993 Oct 1;18(13):1803-7
[302] Jarrow R. *Creating the Work You Love: Courage, Commitment and Career*. Inner Traditions Intl Ltd; December 1995) [ISBN: 0892815426]
[303] Simons DG. Cardiology and myofascial trigger points: Janet G. Travell's contribution. *Tex Heart Inst J*. 2003;30(1):3-7

6. Application of ice (or other benign, intense afferent stimuli such as capsaicin or spinal manipulation) floods the dorsal horn and thus blocks transmission of nociceptive stimuli via the hypothesized "gate control" mechanism of pain reception.
7. Magnesium supplementation is appropriate for many patients with MFTP since many patients do not consume sufficient dietary magnesium and since magnesium inhibits calcium release from the sarcoplasmic reticulum[304] and thereby has a muscle relaxing effect. **Magnesium deficiency is an epidemic** in so-called "developed" nations, with 20-40% of different populations showing objective serologic/cytologic evidence of magnesium deficiency.[305,306,307,308]

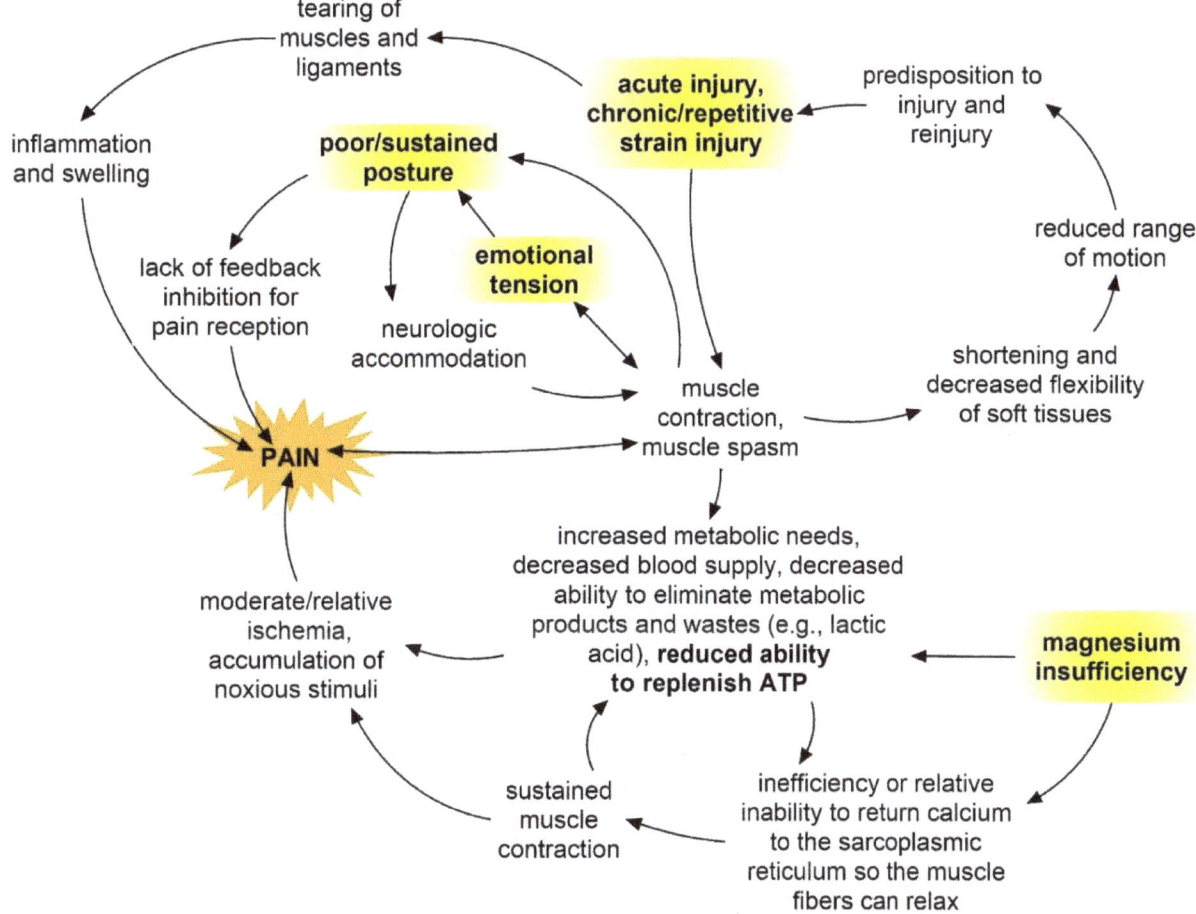

Hypothesized model for the initiation and promotion of myofascial trigger points with self-perpetuating cycles: Emotional tension, sustained posturing, and magnesium deficiency are a few of the "entry points" to neuromuscular pain.

Clinical presentations:
- The pain pattern from MFTP is varied and is dependent on the muscle(s) involved. Each muscle has a unique pattern of pain referral; e.g., a MFTP in the deltoid or supraspinatus may cause shoulder pain and arm pain that can mimic cervical radiculitis. MFTP in the sternocleidomastoid commonly causes "headache" and pain over the side of the face and TMJ; MFTP in the psoas can cause low back and leg pain. Patients may also report subjective numbness or tingling in addition to pain. Differentiation of MFTP pain from radiculitis and radiculopathy should be pursued clinically and documented in the patient chart.

---

[304] "Mg2+ inhibits Ca2+ release from the sarcoplasmic reticulum." Mathew R, Altura BM. The role of magnesium in lung diseases: asthma, allergy and pulmonary hypertension. *Magnes Trace Elem*. 1991-92;10(2-4):220-8
[305] "The American diet is low in magnesium, and with modern water systems, very little is ingested in the drinking water." Innerarity S. Hypomagnesemia in acute and chronic illness. *Crit Care Nurs Q*. 2000 Aug;23(2):1-19
[306] "43% of 113 trauma patients had low magnesium levels compared to 30% of noninjured cohorts." Frankel et al. Hypomagnesemia in trauma patients. *World J Surg* 1999;23:966-9
[307] "There was a 20% overall prevalence of hypomagnesemia among this predominantly female, African American population." Fox CH, Ramsoomair D, Mahoney MC, Carter C, Young B, Graham R. An investigation of hypomagnesemia among ambulatory urban African Americans. *J Fam Pract*. 1999 Aug;48(8):636-9
[308] "Suboptimal levels were detected in 33.7 per cent of the population under study. These data clearly demonstrate that the Mg supply of the German population needs increased attention." Schimatschek HF, Rempis R. Prevalence of hypomagnesemia in an unselected German population of 16,000 individuals. *Magnes Res*. 2001 Dec;14(4):283-90

<u>Major differential diagnoses</u>:
- <u>Arthropathy and arthritis</u>: Passive joint provocation tests are negative with MFTP; no laboratory abnormalities (such as elevated CRP) are seen with MFTP.
- <u>Acute muscle injury, strain</u>: History of *recent* injury is often negative; history of *chronic* strain and *previous* injury are common with MFTP
- <u>Radiculitis</u>: The pain associated with MFTP is not dermatomal and is reproduced with local muscle compression, whereas the pain of radiculitis is dermatomal and reproduced with nerve tension tests.
- <u>Radiculopathy</u>: Radiculopathy is associated with muscle weakness, which is not a characteristic of MFTP.

<u>Clinical assessments</u>:
- <u>History/subjective</u>: Pain is always present (although it may be mild or latent).
- <u>Physical examination/objective</u>: The most reliable physical signs of MFTP are **1) spot tenderness within a taut band of muscle, 2) reproduction of pain and referred pain with palpation and provocation**, and 3) local twitch response with palpation and provocation.
- <u>Imaging & laboratory assessments</u>: Lab tests and imaging assessments are normal. Myofascial trigger points show spontaneous electromyographic activity.[309]

<u>Establishing the diagnosis</u>:
- Reasonable clinical exclusion of acute strain, radiculopathy and radiculitis combined with characteristic clinical findings mentioned above, including at least **1) spot tenderness within a taut band of muscle, 2) reproduction of pain and referred pain with palpation/provocation.**

<u>Complications</u>:
- Many patients with MFTP suffer from pain for years before being properly diagnosed. Many patients are prescribed hazardous and inappropriate medications to treat the pain and symptoms of MFTP, and surgical interventions are periodically used inappropriately in patents who have not been accurately diagnosed. For example when a patient with low back pain due to MFTP is found to have an incidental disc herniation, the patient may undergo surgery on the intervertebral disc only to have pain continue postoperatively until it is treated with simple techniques directed at the MFTP.[310]

<u>Clinical management</u>:
- Simple nutritional and physical treatments as described below.
- Patients should be advised that deep massage of the area is often necessary and that pain may be temporarily exacerbated.

<u>Treatments</u>:
- <u>Post-isometric stretching</u>: Lewit and Simons described this simple and highly effective treatment succinctly in a highly recommended article[311], "The post-isometric relaxation technique begins by placing the muscle in a stretched position. Then an isometric contraction is exerted against minimal resistance. Relaxation and then gentle stretch follow as the muscle releases." In a large study involving 244 patients, post-isometric stretching "produced **immediate pain relief in 94%, lasting pain relief in 63%**, as well as lasting relief of point tenderness in 23% of the sites treated. Patients who practiced autotherapy on a home program were more likely to realize lasting relief." Clinically the technique is simultaneously performed, explained, and taught by the clinician: 1) stretch the target muscle, 2) weakly contract the target muscle against resistance for 10 seconds, 3) stretch the target muscle to a greater length than before for at least 20 seconds, 4) repeat this procedure 2-3 times. Pretreatment heating or exercising of the target muscles along with post-treatment application of ice helps to increase treatment efficacy and minimize post-treatment soreness, respectively.

---

[309] Hubbard DR, Berkoff GM. Myofascial trigger points show spontaneous needle EMG activity. *Spine*. 1993 Oct 1;18(13):1803-7
[310] Rubin D. Myofascial trigger point syndromes: an approach to management. *Arch Phys Med Rehabil*. 1981 Mar;62(3):107-10
[311] Lewit K, Simons DG. Myofascial pain: relief by post-isometric relaxation. *Arch Phys Med Rehabil*. 1984 Aug;65(8):452-6

- Cold and stretch: The application of cold and the simultaneous stretching of the muscle is an effective treatment for MFTP.[312] Cold can be applied with ice. The previously popular "spray and stretch" technique that used a vapocoolant spray such as Fluori-Methane is unnecessary and is environmentally irresponsible.
- Dry needling or injection of local anesthetic or saline: While local injection of anesthetic or saline may appear more complex and therefore more effective, dry needling (rapid insertion and withdrawal of a needle) directly into the MFTP is just as effective, safer, and is less complicated than using anesthetic or saline solution. Increased efficacy of this technique is associated with the elicitation of a local twitch response immediately upon insertion and withdrawal of the needle. The accuracy of the needle insertion directly into the "sensitive locus" of the MFTP is essential for the effectiveness of this approach. Common locations for MFTP correlate with commonly used acupuncture points, and the technique of acupuncture is analogous to the dry needling technique except that dry needling is performed more quickly and with highly localized precision into the MFTP sensitive locus. [313]
- Topical application: Capsaicin helps to relieve neuromuscular pain, too, and may help break the cycle of pain and spasm by 1) providing afferent stimuli to block nociceptive stimuli, and 2) by depleting local tissues of substance P, which not only serves as a transmitter of pain sensations, but may also perpetuate muscle contraction and spasm. Another mechanism by which capsaicin can alleviate trigger points is by desensitizing the vanilloid receptor (VR-1) to ultimately decrease local neurotransmitter release.[314]
- Adjunctive nutritional support: Supplementation with **magnesium** (600 mg per day or to bowel tolerance[315]) and **calcium** are often helpful, particularly when used with an **alkalinizing Paleo-Mediterranean diet** (as discussed in Chapter 2), which—at the very least—promotes renal retention of calcium and magnesium to thus facilitate mineral retention. Other treatments to reduce intracellular calcium levels (intracellular hypercalcinosis[316]) include supplementation with **physiologic doses of vitamin D3** and **fish oil for EPA**[317] along with avoidance/reduction of factors which promote renal loss of calcium and magnesium such as caffeine, sugar, alcohol/ethanol, and psychoemotional stress.

---

[312] Rubin D. Myofascial trigger point syndromes: an approach to management. *Arch Phys Med Rehabil*. 1981 Mar;62(3):107-10

[313] Hong CZ, Simons DG. Pathophysiologic and electrophysiologic mechanisms of myofascial trigger points. *Arch Phys Med Rehabil*. 1998 Jul;79(7):863-72

[314] "Massage with capsaicin cream (0.075%, available over the counter) is useful for treating TrPs located in surgical scars,36 which are particularly refractory to treatment." McPartland JM. Travell trigger points—molecular and osteopathic perspectives. *J Am Osteopath Assoc*. 2004 Jun;104(6):244-9 jaoa.org/cgi/content/full/104/6/244

[315] "When the practitioner has been convinced to start Mg on the basis of his diagnosis or through insistence of the patient, the often recommended dose of 300 mg per day is insufficient. Experience of successful therapy indicates that no less than 600 mg per day is required." Liebscher DH, Liebscher DE. About the misdiagnosis of magnesium deficiency. *J Am Coll Nutr*. 2004 Dec;23(6):730S-1S coldcure.com/html/misdiagnosis-magnesium-deficiency.pdf

[316] naturopathydigest.com/archives/2006/sep/vasquez.php for additional discussion

[317] "This is a consequence of the ability of EPA to release Ca2+ from intracellular stores while inhibiting their refilling via capacitative Ca2+ influx that results in partial emptying of intracellular Ca2+ stores and thereby activation of protein kinase R." Palakurthi SS, Fluckiger R, Aktas H, Changolkar AK, Shahsafaei A, Harneit S, Kilic E, Halperin JA. Inhibition of translation initiation mediates the anticancer effect of the n-3 polyunsaturated fatty acid eicosapentaenoic acid. *Cancer Res*. 2000 Jun 1;60(11):2919-25

Musculoskeletal Manipulation and Manual Medicine: Brief Introduction and Sample Techniques

Manual medicine in general and spinal manipulation in particular are mentioned in nearly every section of *Integrative Orthopedics*, and select techniques are described with accompanying text and photographs. Manipulative techniques are included in this textbook to remind practitioners of a few of the more useful and commonly applied maneuvers and to provide descriptions and citations for refinement of their application. However, the level of detail provided here is insufficient unless the reader has received hands-on professionally-supervised training in an accredited institution wherein other important concepts have been taught and implemented under experienced guidance. Competence and proficiency in the art and skill of manipulation cannot be learned from a textbook; these can only be approached with personal mentoring and in-person coursework amply provided in colleges and post-graduate trainings specializing in manipulative technique. **Manipulative medicine** is a *time-space* objective-subjective-intuitive **kinesthetic phenomenon** which might be described as occurring in four dimensions—*anteroposterior, transverse/horizontal, vertical,* and *chronological* due to variations in speed and power; all the while, the doctor is monitoring subjective and objective responses of the what might be considered the fifth dimension—the doctor's dynamic *perception of, influence upon,* and *interaction with* the patient's affect, posture, muscle tension, dynamic joint positioning, tissue response, and compressive tension. As the doctor assesses and provides force, the patient's response changes the target, and so the doctor must adapt to a constantly moving target—the lesion being treated.

These sections presume professional training by the reader has already been begun or completed and that the reader is familiar with manipulative concepts, technique, terminology, and commonly used abbreviations. Again, the intention here is to remind clinicians of manipulation in general and these specific techniques in particular; only a few *subjectively chosen* techniques are included from the several hundred vertebral, myofascial, visceral, and extravertebral/extremity maneuvers that are available.

General Layout and Description of Manipulative Techniques	
Patient position:	• Patient position may be prone, supine, lateral recumbent or "side-posture", standing, or seated
Doctor position:	• Usually standing, either *upright, forward flexed,* or using an oblique *fencer's stance*; knees are almost always bent in order to bring doctor's torso near treatment area to increase mechanical force from the upper limbs
Assessment:	• <u>Subjective</u>: Patient's experience, sensations, and effect on daily living • <u>Motion palpation</u>: Intersegmental motion analysis generally used for assessing the presence of vertebral motion restrictions or aberrant motion. The patient is relaxed and passive while the doctor takes the joint that is being assessed through its normal range of motion in various directions while palpating near adjacent joint surfaces for nuance of pattern and end-feel. Motion lesions are generally described as **restrictions** and/or **hypermobility** • <u>Static palpation</u>: Boney and other landmarks are compared symmetrically and to the practitioner's experience for the detection of abnormality consistent with subjective, motion, and soft tissue findings; static palpations are usually described in terms of prominence or relative superiority/inferiority when compared symmetrically • <u>Soft tissue palpation</u>: Subcutaneous tissues, tendons, ligaments, muscles, and joint spaces can be palpated to assess myofascial status and function. Soft tissue findings commonly include edema, joint swelling, bogginess, "ropiness" of muscles, tenderness, restricted motion of soft tissues, hypertonicity, spasm, and adhesions
Treatment contact, directive hand:	• Generally the doctor provides therapeutic contact with one of the contact surfaces of the hands—digital, hypothenar, pisiform, index, thumb, thenar, or "calcaneal" when using the heel of the hand[318]; other contacts such as the elbow or chest might be used for deep myofascial or compressive manipulative procedures, respectively. The *treatment contact* is provided by the *directive hand*—the hand that is delivering the therapeutic *thrust* or *direction*;

---

[318] Kirk CR, et al. *States Manual of Spinal, Pelvic, and Extravertebral Technics. Second Edition*. Lombard, Il: National College of Chiropractic; 1985, page 20

	the treatment contact of the directive hand works in cooperation with the *supporting contact* of the *supporting hand*
Supporting contact:	This generally refers to the supportive hand, the one that is either holding or stabilizing the patient in contrast to the hand that is delivering the manipulative force. The indirect hand can provide at least three different types of support • <u>Neutral/stabilizing support</u>: The supportive hand plays a relatively neutral role with regard to the manipulative force • <u>Synergistic/cooperative/assistive support</u>: In this situation, the supportive hand moves with the therapeutic force in the same direction. An example of this would be the head-holding hand moving in the same direction as the directive/treatment hand when performing manipulation of the upper cervical spine • <u>Counterthrust/resistive support</u>: In this situation, the supportive hand moves counter/against the direction of the directive force. A common example is the force applied to the upper torso when performing a side-posture manipulation of the lumbar spine or pelvis. Another important example is the counterthrust by the supportive hand when performing a more forceful manipulation of the cervical spine; in this case the supportive hand is serving to limit the motion that would otherwise be imposed by forceful motion by the directive hand; more forceful manipulations such as used to increase afferent input to joint proprioceptors should *not* result in more motion; rather the increased speed and force of the directive hand is countered rather than assisted by the supportive hand
Pretreatment positioning:	• Joints are generally—but not always—taken to the end range of motion before the manipulative thrust is applied because the general purpose of high-velocity low-amplitude manipulation is to break myofascial restrictions and/or forcefully activate joint proprioceptors. In chiropractic terms, this is described as taking the joint into the **paraphysiologic space** because the physiologic range of motion is temporarily though safely exceeded[319]; in osteopathic terms, this part of the range of motion is described as being within the range of **passive motion** but still within the **anatomic barrier**[320]
Therapeutic action:	• For joint manipulation, this is usually the **chiropractic adjustment** or the **osteopathic HVLA** (high-velocity low-amplitude thrust); <u>thrust vectors</u> can be *straight*, *curvilinear*, or *rotary* into **segmental directions** of *rotation, extension, flexion, side-bending, traction*, and combinations of those directions • Other common manual techniques include stretching, post-isometric stretching, massage, compression, percussion, joint springing, mobilization, articulation, traction
Image:	• Photographs will be provided when relevant and available
Resources:	Textbook and article citations for additional information will be provided in this last row when relevant and available; the most commonly cited works include: • *States Manual, Second Edition*[321] by Constance Kirk DC, Dana Lawrence DC, Nila Valvo DC • *Kimberly Manual, 2006 Edition*[322] by Paul Kimberly DO • *Chiropractic Technique*[323] by Thomas Bergmann DC, David Peterson DC, Dana Lawrence DC • *Chiropractic Management of Spine-Related Disorders*[324] edited by Meridel Gatterman DC

Examples of manipulative medicine techniques

The following samples are an obvious underrepresentation of the diversity of manipulative techniques available, which easily numbers into the hundreds. Various techniques are—of course—described with greater range and depth in textbooks wholly dedicated to the topic of manipulation, which by itself is not the subject of this text. Rather, **use these samples as reminders to include or at least consider manipulative therapy** when composing your treatment plan; oftentimes, the manipulative therapy is the fastest and shortest route between *pain* and *relief from pain*.

---

[319] Leach RA. (ed). *The Chiropractic Theories: A Textbook of Scientific Research, Fourth Edition*. Baltimore: Lippincott, Williams & Wilkins, 2004, page 32-33
[320] Kimberly PE. *Outline of Osteopathic Manipulative Procedures. The Kimberly Manual 2006*. Kirksville College of Osteopathic Medicine. Walsworth Publishing, page 7
[321] Kirk CR, et al. *States Manual of Spinal, Pelvic, and Extravertebral Technics. Second Edition*. Lombard, Illinois: National College of Chiropractic; 1985
[322] Kimberly PE. *Outline of Osteopathic Manipulative Procedures. The Kimberly Manual 2006*. Kirksville College of Osteopathic Medicine. Walsworth Publishing
[323] Bergmann TF, Peterson DH, Lawrence DJ. *Chiropractic Technique*. New York; Churchill Livingstone: 1993
[324] Gatterman MI. *Chiropractic Management of Spine Related Disorders*. Baltimore; Williams and Wilkins: 1990

Cervical Spine: Rotation Emphasis

Patient position:
- Supine, neck slightly flexed

Doctor position:
- At 45° angle from head of table; may also be in a more lateral position aside the patient's head and neck; while it is acceptable to assess and set-up with straight legs, at the time of impulse, doctor's legs should be bent to provide the doctor with greater power, stability, and biomechanical safety

Assessment:
- Subjective: neck pain, headaches
- Motion palpation: rotation restriction; primary or compensatory hypermobile segments may be detected above or below the restricted segment
- Static palpation: vertebra may feel relatively posterior on the side opposite the rotational restriction, e.g., a right rotational restriction may present with a relative left rotational malposition that brings the vertebral lamina and articular pillars posterior on the left
- Soft tissue: tenderness, may also have muscle spasm

Treatment contact:
- Doctor uses either an index or proximal phalange contact on the posterior aspect of the transverse process and/or articular pillar
- The doctor's vector and hence the positioning of the forearm of the contact hand must change depending on the level of the cervical spine that is being treated
- Notice in this photograph that the thumb of the doctor's contact hand is placed on the angle of the mandible, this is more to help anchor the contact and stabilize the doctor's wrist than to assist with the manipulation; very little pressure and zero thrust are applied to the mandible

Supporting contact:
- Head is held into rotation and slight flexion; as with all techniques, nuanced adjustments in flexion-extension, rotation, and side-bending are made until the premanipulative tension is localized to the specific direction/tissue of restriction

Pretreatment positioning:
- Slight flexion and extension may be used below and above the treatment contact to create motion restriction at the adjacent motion segments; this helps to focus the motion and therapeutic force at the specific; importantly the support hand is largely responsible for proper positioning with the correct amount of nuanced flexion-extension and side-bending so that the rotational force is accurately delivered

Thrust:
- Rotational thrust with contact hand; support hand keeps head off table allowing rotation

Image:

Cervical Spine: Lateral Flexion (Side-Bending) Emphasis; Treatment of Lateral Malposition

Patient position:
- Supine, head is neutrally placed—neither flexed nor extended; slight flexion is allowed; this technique can also be adapted for use in a seated position

Doctor position:
- At 45° angle from head of table; may also be in a more lateral position aside the patient's head and neck

Assessment:
- Subjective: neck pain, headaches
- Motion palpation: lateral flexion restriction
- Static palpation: vertebra may feel laterally displaced
- Soft tissue: tenderness, may also have muscle spasm

Treatment contact:
- Using an index (metacarpal-phalangeal) contact at the tip of the transverse process or slightly posterior to the transverse process; an index phalangeal contact can also be used on the articular pillars as long as doctor is careful not to thrust in a rotational direction; notice in this picture how Dr Harris has the forearm of his contact hand perfectly aligned in the treatment vector, which is almost purely in the patient's transverse/horizontal plane; notice also that Dr Harris has his knees bent and is forward flexed to bring his torso closer to his contact and thereby minimize stress and strain on his own shoulders; with slight modifications in vector direction, this technique can be applied throughout the cervical spine from C0-C7

Supporting contact:
- Lateral aspect of head, opposite contact; generally the supporting hand is neutral, however it can supply some traction and can help induce lateral flexion at impulse; with more aggressive adjustments, the supporting hand can supply a counterforce to minimize motion following the application of a faster and more powerful thrust

Pretreatment positioning:
- Lateral flexion at the targeted segment; the slightest amount of contralateral rotation is applied

Therapeutic action:
- Establish minimal premanipulative tension once the end range of motion has been reached, then use quick and very shallow trust to induce lateral flexion

Image:

Posterior Ribs: Manipulation of the Costovertebral Junction

Patient position:
- Supine on table; to facilitate positioning, patient's leg opposite doctor may be flexed at hip and knee with foot flat on table. Patient's arms are crossed over the front of their body; my preference is that the arm closest to the doctor (the arm opposite to the side of the thorax being treated) is atop.

Doctor position:
- Modified fencer's stance facing cephalad

Assessment:
- <u>Subjective</u>: mechanical paraspinal pain; often discomfort with inhalation.
- <u>Motion palpation</u>: stiffness at the affected costotransverse junction.
- <u>Static palpation</u>: prominence in the posterior direction of the rib near the costotransverse junction.
- <u>Soft tissue</u>: local tenderness to palpation is very common

Treatment contact:
- Contact on the specific rib immediately lateral to the costotransverse junction is made with the doctor's thenar eminence with the doctor's hand in a firm, pursed position. Initial contact is made superior and lateral to the final location of manipulative contact in order to attain proper premanipulative tissue tension

Supporting contact:
- The doctor's supporting (noncontact) hand along with the doctor's torso deliver the manipulative thrust through the patient's arm atop the patient's thorax

Pretreatment positioning:
- Patient is supine; after positioning the contact hand posteriorly, the doctor grasps the patient's upper arm, then pulls downward and then applies progressively compressive force (body weight, not muscular force) while raising the supporting contact and rolling the patient over atop the contact hand

Thrust:
- Body-drop thrust generally superiorly and laterally in the direction of the patient's opposite shoulder; the angle of the thrust changes depending on the spinal-costal level being treated, with more superior segments requiring a more superiorly directed thrust, while lower segments require a progressively laterally-yet-sagittally directed thrust. Notably, the manipulative thrust is applied to the anterior thorax via contact with the patient's upper arm, yet the true manipulative force is from posterior to anterior via the doctor's thenar eminence positioned posteriorly.

Image:

Thoracic Spine: Supine Thoracic Flexion, "Anterior Thoracic"

Patient position:
- Supine on table; to facilitate positioning, patient's leg opposite doctor may be flexed at hip and knee with foot flat on table
- Patient is instructed to place right hand on right trapezius and left hand on left trapezius; the patient is instructed, "Do not place your hands behind your neck and do not interlace your fingers."

Doctor position:
- Facing table at 45° angle in fencer stance with feet apart and knees bent
- Doctor must be midline and balanced at time of impulse in order to provide symmetric force

Assessment:
- Subjective: mechanical midback pain
- Motion palpation: flexion restriction
- Static palpation: extension malposition; focal loss of thoracic kyphosis; focal approximation of spinous processes consistent with extension malposition; vertebra may feel anteriorly displaced
- Soft tissue: local paravertebral myohypertonicity is common; local paresthesia is very common, and patients are often exquisitely sensitive to the lightest touch

Treatment contact:
- Closed fist contact with spinous processes between doctor's distal interphalangeal joints and thenar eminence; the trust is delivered from the doctor's chest through the patient's arms which compress the patient's chest; Dr Harris (pictured as patient) prefers to use a forearm contact to reduce wear-and-tear on his hands and wrists

Supporting contact:
- The supporting contact is the hand-arm that supports the patient's upper torso; the supporting contact pulls toward the doctor and superiorly at time of impulse

Pretreatment positioning:
- Patient lifts head from table; doctor uses supporting hand and arm to lift patient off table to allow placement of contact hand and to facilitate spinal flexion

Therapeutic action:
- Doctor uses **body drop thrust** technique at 45° toward ground and toward the head of the table; the trust should simultaneously generate compression and long-axis traction; the contact hand remains tense to provide solid leverage *inferior* to the targeted motion segment; the supporting hand and arm pull toward doctor at time of impulse to accentuate traction and spinal flexion; patient is instructed to breathe deeply then relax and exhale; upon exhalation, the doctor establishes and maintains premanipulative tension to achieve joint flexion, then applies HVLA thrust; the thrust must be fast and shallow; slow and deep impulses can sprain the interspinous ligaments

Lumbar Side-Posture Rotational Manipulation/Mobilization, "Lumbar Roll"

Patient position:
- Side-posture, lateral recumbent; lower leg is straight; upper leg is flexed at hip and knee with foot behind calf of the leg that is straight on the table

Doctor position:
- Facing table at 45° angle in fencer stance with feet apart and knees bent
- Notice in the photograph how Dr Harris approximates his center of gravity and biomechanical leverage directly over his therapeutic contact

Assessment:
- <u>Subjective</u>: asymptomatic or with lumbar pain; lumbar disc herniation[325], use a cautious and gentle technique if the patient has radicular symptoms, and as a rule of thumb the patient should be positioned with the symptomatic leg down on the table (e.g., "good leg *up*, bad leg *down*")
- <u>Motion palpation</u>: focal restrictions with focal pain are perhaps better treated with a lesion-specific technique such as the "push-pull" maneuver; this is an excellent technique if the patient has general discomfort without localization, or has pain and will benefit from rotational manipulation for its muscle stretching and afferent-stimulating analgesic benefits
- <u>Static palpation</u>: minor displacements and malpositions may be noted; if specific biomechanical lesions are found, use a more specific technique such as the "push-pull" maneuver
- <u>Soft tissue</u>: palpate for hypertonicity/spasm with or without relative muscle atrophy; patients with chronic low-back pain tend to have weaker extensor muscles than the general population; however, during an acutely painful episode, their otherwise weakened muscles will be hypertonic thus leading to a paradoxical **atrophic hypertonicity**

Treatment contact:
- Doctor uses a palmar/calcaneal ("heel of the hand") contact over the lumbar facet joints
- Rotation and traction are provided at the time of impulse with the doctor's thigh which is compressed and providing long-axis traction against the patient's upper leg, which is flexed at the hip and knee

Support:
- Doctor's cephalad hand applies rotational resistance to patient's shoulder as shown

Pretreatment positioning:
- Premanipulative tension is attained and maintained prior to **body drop impulse**
- The premanipulative tension and the therapeutic impulse are established and delivered through the contact hand and the doctor's caudad leg which has compressive contact with the patient's flexed leg

Therapeutic action:
- Body drop thrust impulse with rotational emphasis; notice how the forearm of his contact hand perpendicular to the patient's coronal plane to direct his impulse in a posterior-to-anterior direction

[325] Quon JA, et al. Lumbar intervertebral disc herniation: treatment by rotational manipulation. *J Manipulative Physiol Ther*. 1989 Jun;12(3):220-7

Lumbar Spine: Side-Posture Segmental Rotation (Lumbar "Push-Pull")

Patient position:
- Lateral recumbent (side-posture) with no/minimal lateral flexion and minimal thoracic rotation; upper leg is flexed at hip and knee, with foot placed/locked behind the calf that is on the table; the patient grasps his/her own forearms and maintains modest tension to provide anchoring for the doctor's caudad arm, which is placed under the patient's superior arm; the patient's lower leg is straight

Doctor position:
- Doctor is facing the table standing on the cephalad leg while the caudad leg is flexed at the hip and knee and placed atop the patient's flexed upper leg to provide additional leverage at the time of manipulative thrust. Regarding the doctor's cephalad arm, the humerus is directed toward the patient's shoulder, and the elbow is bent allowing the forearm to push into the sulcus formed by the pectoralis major and deltoid; doctors forearm emerges under patient's elbow, so that fingertips are on the superior/lateral aspect of the lumbar spinous process of the superior vertebra of the targeted motion segment. Regarding the doctor's caudad arm, the elbow is flexed and the forearm is placed along the posterior aspect of the patient's superior ilium; fingers hook the inferior/lateral aspect of the lumbar spinous process of the inferior vertebra of the targeted motion segment

Assessment:
- <u>Subjective</u>: asymptomatic or lumbar pain, which may not be at the affected segment
- <u>Motion palpation</u>: rotational restriction
- <u>Static palpation</u>: may have rotational malposition
- <u>Soft tissue</u>: may have muscle spasm at nearby area of hypermobility

Treatment contact:
- The doctor's cephalad contacts are at the patient's deltopectoral sulcus and directly on the superior/lateral aspect of the lumbar spinous process of the superior vertebra of the targeted motion segment. This maneuver has three caudad contacts: 1) doctor's fingertips pull directly on the inferior/lateral aspect of the lumbar spinous process of the inferior vertebra of the targeted motion segment; 2) doctor's forearm on patient's ilium; 3) doctors caudad lower leg is atop patient's flexed leg

Support:
- All contacts are active

Pretreatment positioning:
- Rotational tension is applied and focused at the lumbar spinal segment being treated
- Thoracic rotation and lateral flexion are minimized to the extent possible
- Modest lumbar lateral flexion toward the table helps to gap the inferior articular process of the superior segment from the superior articular process of the inferior segment

Therapeutic action:
- 1) Doctor's cephalad elbow thrusts toward patient's shoulder to create simultaneous rotation and long-axis traction; 2) cephalad fingertips push toward the ground while atop the superior/lateral aspect of the lumbar spinous process of the superior vertebra of the targeted motion segment; 3) doctor's caudad fingertips hook and pull the inferior vertebra; 4) forearm pushes patient's ilium into rotation; 5) extension "kick" of doctor's knee quickly creates rotational force. All five actions occur simultaneously

Image:

Carpal tunnel syndrome, CTS

Description/pathophysiology:
- Symptoms resultant from compression of the median nerve in the osteofibrous tunnel bordered by the carpal bones and the transverse carpal ligament. This compression may be due to:
    o Inflammatory edema of the finger flexor tendons and their associated synovial sheaths as they traverse the carpal tunnel; inflammation/edema may be due to overuse, injury, systemic edema (e.g., secondary to estrogen excess, pregnancy), hypothyroidism, or inflammatory process such as RA
    o May be exacerbated by external compression due to poor ergonomics, posture, or habits, such as sleeping prone on wrists, working with wrist on edge of desk/table, working with wrists in extreme flexion or extension
    o Rarely caused by congenital stenosis of the carpal tunnel
    o Specific nutritional deficiencies responsive to nutritional supplementation in many patients[326]
    o The median nerve can be compressed anywhere from its origin at the nerve roots all the way to the carpal tunnel. The concept of the "double crush" holds that two or more areas of minor compression to a nerve can result in a functional lesion similar to what would be expected with a single major compression; these compressive locations and their clinical assessment will be reviewed later in this section on CTS.

> **Carpal tunnel syndrome is an example of a neuromusculoskeletal problem that responds very well to the combination of nutritional and manual manipulative interventions**
>
> Nutritional and manipulative interventions for CTS have proven safety and efficacy and should be used by expert practitioners before surgical intervention for CTS is even considered. Correctly placing manipulative and nutritional nondrug interventions into CTS care protocols would likely save healthcare dollars and help patients improve overall health and therefore reduce the medical/personal/financial burdens of surgical care.

Complications:
- Loss of strength, muscle atrophy (intrinsic thenar muscles), and compromise of function of the hand; in severe cases, patients lose function of one or both hands and may be largely unable to work and function in their daily lives.
- Pain, paresthesia in the distribution of the median nerve

Clinical presentations:
- Pain-numbness-tingling in the thumb, index and middle fingers, and radial surface of the palm
- Symptoms are often worse at night
- May also have weakness of grip strength and loss of coordination of fine motor skills of the hand

Major differential diagnoses and contributing conditions:
- Double crush syndrome[327]
- Hypothyroidism
- Diabetes mellitus
- Acromegaly
- Amyloidosis
- Estrogen excess
- Pregnancy
- Nutritional deficiency or nutritional dependency, especially pyridoxine and riboflavin

Clinical assessments:
- History:
    o Pain, numbness, tingling in the median nerve distribution
    o Symptoms are worse at night.
    o May also have weakness of grip strength

---

[326] Folkers K, et al. Enzymology of the response of carpal tunnel syndrome to riboflavin and to combined riboflavin and pyridoxine. *Proc Natl Acad Sci* 1984 Nov;81(22):7076-8
[327] "Results supported the DSC hypothesis. DCS evaluation requires both structural and functional diagnosis of peripheral neurones ...." Flak et al. Double crush syndrome evaluation in the median nerve in clinical, radiological and electrophysiological examination. *Stud Health Technol Inform*. 2006;123:435-41

- **Physical examination**:
  - Intrinsic thumb muscles may be weak
  - Assess for atrophy of the thenar eminence by observation and bilateral comparison
  - Positive neuro-orthopedic assessment:
    - Phalen's test
    - Reverse Phalen's test
    - Tinel's test
    - Direct pressure at the carpal tunnel reproduces symptoms, i.e., numbness or tingling of the thenar palm
  - Assessment for compression of the median nerve and its contributory nerve roots:

Location	Screening assessments	Therapeutic considerations
Intervertebral disc of any level from C5-T1	- Cervical compression tests - MRI if clinically warranted	- Consider traction for disc decompression
Intervertebral foramina on the affected side	- Provocative positioning to exacerbate hand paresthesia: combinations of ipsilateral side-bending and extension to exacerbate foraminal compression of nerve root - Cervical oblique radiographs to assess IVFs	- Osseous and soft-tissue manipulation as indicated per patient to cervical and shoulder region - Improve spinal health and posture - Ergonomic and workstation improvements
Compression of brachial plexus due to thoracic outlet compression at anterior-middle scalenes, costoclavicular space, or secondary to tight pectoralis major	- Tests for TOS (see Chapter on shoulder)	- Stretch scalenes and pectoralis minor to relieve chronic compression of neurovascular bundle - Improve posture - Ergonomic and workstation improvements
Compression of median nerve at pronator teres	- Palpation and provocation at dual origin of pronator teres: proximal medial ulna and medial epicondyle	- Osseous and soft-tissue manipulation as indicated per patient to elbow region and pronator teres

Imaging & laboratory assessments:
- Assessment for hypothyroidism with TSH, free T4, free T3, and anti-TPO antibodies: **Hypothyroidism is relatively common among patients with CTS.**[328] **Musculoskeletal complaints are common in patients with thyroid problems, particularly hypothyroidism.**[329] With a suggestive or compelling clinical presentation, treatment of overt or subclinical hypothyroidism with thyroid hormone replacement is justified unless specifically contraindicated when the TSH value is greater than 2 µIU/mL[330], greater than 3 µIU/mL[331], or when antithyroid antibodies are present.[332] For most patients, treatment of hypothyroidism is best accomplished with a natural glandular source of thyroid hormone (such as a "nutritional" glandular product or Armour thyroid) or a hypoallergenic synthetic bioidentical combination of both T3 and T4[333] (such as Liotrix/Thyrolar) and should also be accompanied by general nutritional supplementation with a high-

---

[328] Palumbo CF, et al. The effects of hypothyroidism and thyroid replacement on the development of carpal tunnel syndrome. *J Hand Surg* [Am]. 2000 Jul;25(4):734-9
[329] Cakir M, Samanci N, Balci N, Balci MK. Musculoskeletal manifestations in patients with thyroid disease. *Clin Endocrinol* (Oxf). 2003 Aug;59(2):162-7
[330] Weetman AP. Hypothyroidism: screening and subclinical disease. *BMJ*. 1997 Apr 19;314(7088):1175-8 bmj.com/cgi/content/full/314/7088/1175
[331] "Now American Association of Clinical Endocrinologists encourages doctors to consider treatment for patients who test outside the boundaries of a narrower margin based on a target TSH level of 0.3 to 3.04. AACE believes the new range will result in proper diagnosis for millions of Americans who suffer from a mild thyroid disorder, but have gone untreated until now." aace.com/pub/tam2003/press.php 2004 Jan
[332] Beers MH, Berkow R (eds). *The Merck Manual of Diagnosis and Therapy, 17th Edition*. Whitehouse Station; Merck Research Laboratories 1999 page 96
[333] Bunevicius R, et al. Effects of thyroxine as compared with thyroxine plus triiodothyronine in patients with hypothyroidism. *N Engl J Med*. 1999 Feb 11;340(6):424-9

potency broad-spectrum multivitamin/multimineral supplement that contains 200-600 mcg of selenium[334,335] and 15-25 mg of zinc.[336] Zinc, selenium, and iron are required for peripheral conversion and function of thyroid hormones; corresponding mineral deficiencies can precipitate a mild functional hypothyroidism.

- <u>Basic routine laboratory assessment with CBC, CRP, CCP, and chemistry/metabolic panel</u>: This approach is sufficient to screen for diabetes and rheumatoid arthritis, both of which are more common in patients with CTS.[337,338]
- <u>Assessment of vitamin levels and functional enzyme status</u>: This is generally not necessary; consider assessment of vitamin B6 status with erythrocyte glutamic oxaloacetic transaminase (EGOT) and/or serum P5P levels.
- <u>Electromyography</u>: EMG can be used to objectively quantify impaired nerve conduction
- <u>Serum ferritin</u>: Assess for iron overload or iron deficiency.

<u>Clinical management</u>: Referral if clinical outcome is unsatisfactory.

<u>Treatments</u>:
- **<u>Pyridoxine (vitamin B-6; concomitant administration with magnesium)</u>:** Many patients with CTS have serum and biochemical evidence of pyridoxine deficiency[339] which remit along with the CTS following supplementation with pyridoxine, thus helping to obviate the need for surgery.[340,341,342,343,344,345] *The Merck Manual of Diagnosis and Therapy, 17th Edition* advocates a trial of 50 mg twice daily[346] while others have recommended a dose of 200 mg per day.[347] A recent clinical trial[348] showed that enzyme saturation proceeds from 83% with 30 mg of pyridoxine to 93% with 200 mg of pyridoxine, thus proving again that dose-responsiveness is not maximized until higher *supranutritional* doses are used; this precept was previously reviewed in a brilliant *required reading* article by Bruce Ames et al.[349] In my practice I commonly use at least 250 mg daily with breakfast for a *loading dose* trial period of 2-12 weeks before tapering down to a maintenance dose of 50 mg/day. Long-term ultrahigh-dose administration of pyridoxine HCL can be neurotoxic, producing a peripheral neuropathy that is not unlike the presentation of carpal tunnel syndrome. One of the problems with supplementation with vitamin B-6 in the form of pyridoxine HCL is that this particular synthetic form of vitamin B-6 appears to be mildly neurotoxic and must be converted to the active form(s) of the vitamin before becoming harmless and physiologically functional. The phosphorylation of pyridoxine HCL into its active phosphorylated forms (e.g., pyridoxal-5-phosphate, P5P) requires the presence of magnesium. Many people are deficient in magnesium and therefore may not respond to supplementation with pyridoxine HCL because of deficiency-induced biochemical inability to convert the vitamin to its active form in sufficient quantities to achieve a therapeutic effect. Obviously, either using an activated form of pyridoxine such as the commercially available pyridoxal-5-phosphate would obviate this problem; gastrointestinal absorption of P5P appears to be limited. Coadministration of magnesium is advised with the use of pyridoxine HCL, and generally long-term high-dose (i.e., bowel tolerance) supplementation is necessary to replenish body magnesium levels. If necessary, assessment of magnesium status is performed by measuring either RBC or WBC intracellular magnesium levels; serum levels of magnesium are generally

---

[334] Duntas LH, et al. Effects of a six month treatment with selenomethionine in patients with autoimmune thyroiditis. *Eur J Endocrinol*. 2003 Apr;148(4):389-93
[335] Olivieri et al. Selenium, zinc, and thyroid hormones in healthy subjects: low T3/T4 ratio in elderly is related to impaired selenium status. *Biol Trace Elem Res* 1996;51:31-41
[336] Nishiyama S, et al. Zinc supplementation alters thyroid hormone metabolism in disabled patients with zinc deficiency. *J Am Coll Nutr*. 1994 Feb;13(1):62-7
[337] Van Dijk MA, et al. Indications for requesting laboratory tests for concurrent diseases in patients with carpal tunnel syndrome:. *Clin Chem*. 2003 Sep;49(9):1437-44
[338] Solomon DH, Katz JN, Bohn R, Mogun H, Avorn J. Nonoccupational risk factors for carpal tunnel syndrome. *J Gen Intern Med*. 1999 May;14(5):310-4
[339] Fuhr JE, Farrow A, Nelson HS Jr. Vitamin B6 levels in patients with carpal tunnel syndrome. *Arch Surg*. 1989 Nov;124(11):1329-30
[340] Ellis et al, Folkers K. Vitamin B6 deficiency in patients with clinical syndrome including the carpal tunnel defect. *Res Commun Chem Pathol Pharmacol* 1976 Apr;13:743-57
[341] Ellis J, Folkers K, et al. Clinical results of a cross-over treatment with pyridoxine and placebo of the carpal tunnel syndrome. *Am J Clin Nutr*. 1979 Oct;32(10):2040-6
[342] Ellis J, Folkers K, Levy M, Takemura K, Shizukuishi S, Ulrich R, Harrison P. Therapy with vitamin B6 with and without surgery for treatment of patients having the idiopathic carpal tunnel syndrome. *Res Commun Chem Pathol Pharmacol*. 1981 Aug;33(2):331-44
[343] Ellis JM, Folkers K, et al. Response of vitamin B-6 deficiency and the carpal tunnel syndrome to pyridoxine. *Proc Natl Acad Sci* U S A. 1982 Dec;79(23):7494-8
[344] Kasdan ML, Janes C. Carpal tunnel syndrome and vitamin B6. *Plast Reconstr Surg*. 1987 Mar;79(3):456-62
[345] Ellis JM. Treatment of carpal tunnel syndrome with vitamin B6. *South Med J*. 1987 Jul;80(7):882-4
[346] Beers MH, Berkow R (eds). <u>*The Merck Manual of Diagnosis and Therapy, 17th Edition*</u>. Whitehouse Station; Merck Research Laboratories 1999 Page 492
[347] "Current treatment for carpal tunnel syndrome should include NSAIDs, nighttime splinting, ergonomic workstation review, and vitamin B6 200 mg per day." Holm G, Moody LE. Carpal tunnel syndrome: current theory, treatment, and the use of B6. *J Am Acad Nurse Pract*. 2003 Jan;15(1):18-22
[348] "The in vivo study showed increasing aspartate aminotransferase saturation with increasing pyridoxine doses. 83% saturation was reached with 30 mg daily, 88% with 100 mg, and 93% with 200 mg after 20 days of oral supplementation." Oshiro M, Nonoyama K, Oliveira RA, Barretto OC. Red cell aspartate aminotransferase saturation with oral pyridoxine intake. *Sao Paulo Med J*. 2005 Mar 2;123(2):54-7 scielo.br/scielo.php?script=sci_arttext&pid=S1516-31802005000200004&tlng=es&lng=en&nrm=iso
[349] Ames BN, Elson-Schwab I, Silver EA. High-dose vitamin therapy stimulates variant enzymes with decreased coenzyme binding affinity (increased K(m)): relevance to genetic disease and polymorphisms. *Am J Clin Nutr*. 2002 Apr;75(4):616-58 ajcn.org/cgi/content/full/75/4/616

meaningless from a nutritional standpoint. Furthermore, magnesium supplementation should occur along with concomitant urinary alkalinization so that supplemented magnesium will be retained. Failure to alkalinize the urine with either diet[350] or alkalinization therapy such as sodium bicarbonate and/or potassium citrate[351], or alkaline minerals[352] allows for facilitated excretion of magnesium and subsequent "failure" of pyridoxine therapy due to insufficient magnesium-dependent phosphorylation and activation of the vitamin. Vitamin B6 probably exerts its beneficial effects in the treatment of CTS via several mechanisms, including:
- o Facilitating biosynthesis of pain-relieving serotonin
- o Reducing excitatory glutamate levels
- o Diuretic effect: perhaps via inhibition of anti-diuretic hormone (ADH) secretion
- o Diuretic effect via estrogen-lowering[353]: probably effected via upregulation of hepatic transaminases but possibly also via a direct pituitary effect[354]

Likewise, magnesium supplementation appears to provide some analgesic benefit which is at least partially due to its role in inhibiting activation of NMDA receptors and reducing/normalizing neuronal transmission. Magnesium is a required co-factor for tissue alkaline phosphatase, the enzyme required for pyridoxine dephosphorylation prior to tissue uptake of pyridoxal-5-phosphate; thus, magnesium deficiency appears to cause tissue/cellular deficiency of vitamin B6 by reducing cellular uptake of the vitamin.[355]

- o **Drug-nutrient interactions**: High doses of **vitamin B6** can reduce blood levels and effectiveness of **barbiturate drugs** such as pentobarbital [Nembutal], phenobarbital [Phenobarbitone], secobarbital [Seconal], and thiopental [Pentothal]
- o **Drug-nutrient interactions**: High doses of **magnesium** may decrease the absorption or effectiveness of several drugs, including: Azithromycin (Zithromax), Cimetidine (Tagamet), Ciprofloxacin (Ciloxan, Cipro), Doxycycline (Atridox, Doryx, Doxy, Monodox, Periostat, Vibramycin), Famotidine (Mylanta-AR, Pepcid, Pepcid AC), Hydroxychloroquine (Plaquenil), Levofloxacin (Levaquin), Nitrofurantoin (Furadantin, Macrobid, Macrodantin), Nizatidine (Axid, Axid AR), Ofloxacin (Floxin, Ocuflox), Tetracycline (Achromycin, Sumycin, Helidac), Warfarin (Coumadin). Misoprostol (Cytotec, Arthrotec) with magnesium may result in diarrhea. Spironolactone (Aldactone, Aldactazide) or Amiloride (Midamor, Moduretic) may cause dangerously high levels of magnesium

Before moving on to the next section readers should have crystalline clarity with regard to the following:
- o Most patients consuming an American/Western-style diet have subtle chronic metabolic acidosis, which results in many adverse effects, one of which is increased urinary excretion of magnesium and reduced tissue/intracellular levels of magnesium.
- o This acidotic predisposition toward magnesium deficiency is exacerbated by low dietary intake of magnesium, as well as other factors such as overconsumption of caffeine, sugar, and also by chronic mental/emotional stress.
- o The resultant magnesium deficiency thus impairs activation/phosphorylation of pyridoxine HCL into the active form pyridoxal-5-phosphate via magnesium-dependent pyridoxal kinase; this results in a simultaneous diminution of effectiveness and enhancement of pyridoxine HCL-mediated neurotoxicity. Cofactors for various tissue-specific isoforms of pyridoxal kinase include magnesium, zinc, cobalt, and manganese; of these, zinc appears most important, particularly in the liver and brain. The final production of active P5P requires a (ribo)flavin-dependent oxidase; thus, *B2 insufficiency precipitates B6 insufficiency.*[356]

---

[350] Cordain L. *The Paleo Diet*. Indianapolis; John Wiley and Sons, 2002
[351] Maurer et al. Neutralization of Western diet inhibits bone resorption independently of K intake, reduces cortisol secretion in humans. *Am J Physiol Renal Physiol* 2003;284:F32-40
[352] Vormann J, et al. Supplementation with alkaline minerals reduces symptoms in patients with chronic low back pain. *J Trace Elem Med Biol*. 2001;15(2-3):179-83
[353] "Administration of vitamin B6 at doses of 200-800 mg/day reduces blood estrogen, increases progesterone and results in improved symptoms under double-blind conditions." Abraham GE. Nutritional factors in the etiology of the premenstrual tension syndromes. *J Reprod Med*. 1983 Jul;28(7):446-64
[354] "These results indicate that pharmacological doses of PLP inhibit pituitary cell proliferation and hormone secretion, in part mediated through PLP-induced cell-cycle arrest and apoptosis. Pyridoxine may therefore be appropriate for testing as a relatively safe drug for adjuvant treatment of hormone-secreting pituitary adenomas." Ren SG, Melmed S. Pyridoxal phosphate inhibits pituitary cell proliferation and hormone secretion. *Endocrinology*. 2006 Aug;147(8):3936-42
[355] "Mg deficiency impairs vitamin B6 status by depleting intracellular Mg and thus inhibits the activity of alkaline phosphatase, a metalloenzyme required for the uptake of pyridoxal phosphate by tissues." Planells E, et al. Effect of magnesium deficiency on vitamin B2 and B6 status in the rat. *J Am Coll Nutr*. 1997 Aug;16(4):352-6
[356] Holman P. Pyridoxine - Vitamin B6. *Journal of the Australasian College of Nutritional & Environmental Medicine*, Vol. 14, No. 1, July 1995, pages 5-16 acnem.org/journal/14-1_july_1995/pyridoxine-vitamin_b6.htm Congratulations to Mr. Holman for his excellent summation of pyridoxine metabolism.

- o Furthermore, magnesium deficiency impairs alkaline phosphatase, the enzyme required for cellular uptake of pyridoxal-5-phosphate; in this way, magnesium deficiency causes tissue insufficiency of pyridoxine.
- o Additionally, chronic metabolic acidosis further impairs intracellular accumulation of magnesium, apparently because the elevated intracellular concentration of hydrogen ions creates an electrochemically repulsive force, given that both hydrogen and magnesium are positively-charged cations.
- o In this situation, if a patient is supplemented with pyridoxine HCL *without magnesium* and *without systemic alkalinization*, we should not expect that optimal clinical responsiveness will be observed even if the patient is functionally vitamin B6 deficient and if the condition is pyridoxine responsive. Thus, the *correct treatment* in the *correct patient* **fails** not because of failure of the treatment *per se*, but rather due failure to create an internal milieu wherein vitamin B6 can function optimally.
    - ▪ Readers should now understand the inherent bias of the medical studies that have "proved" the "ineffectiveness" of vitamin B6 supplementation. Why did so many of these studies fail to show positive benefit? *The supplementation failed because the doctors had no training in nutrition and thus implemented a treatment that had little hope for optimal success because the researchers failed to* ❶ *improve the diet,* ❷ *correct the diet-induced metabolic acidosis, and* ❸ *provide co-factors necessary for B6 function.*
    - ▪ Readers should now understand how to reduce B6 toxicity while increasing its effectiveness. *Alkalinization followed by supplementation with zinc, magnesium, and riboflavin.*
    - ▪ Readers should now understand why an alkalinizing Paleo-Mediterranean diet is *primarily* essential for creating an internal environment wherein the *secondary* addition of high-dose nutritional supplements can function.
- Riboflavin (vitamin B2): Patients with CTS may respond to riboflavin therapy alone, and the combination of riboflavin 50 mg with pyridoxine 500 mg appears more efficacious than the use of either B2 or B6 alone.[357] Per data that migraine headaches are alleviated with riboflavin 400 mg/d[358], in patients with CTS we may safely proceed with riboflavin 400 mg, preferably administered with breakfast.
- Yoga: Yoga postures and relaxation showed superior results compared to use of a night splint in the treatment of CTS.[359] In contrast to surgical lesion of the transverse carpal ligament, yoga is fun, feels good, and can improve aspects of overall health[360] and socioemotional wellbeing.
- Mobilization and manipulation of the carpal bones, myofascial release: Symptoms of CTS may be effectively reduced simply by a mobilization technique of squeezing the metacarpal heads together and also stretching the third and fourth digits into extension.[361] Osteopathic-type manipulation (similar to chiropractic manipulation) of the wrist has shown clinical, electromyographic, and MRI evidence of efficacy[362,363], and the technique is intuitive and commonly known among clinicians with training in manipulation. Additional effectiveness can be obtained when patients are taught to regularly perform stretching maneuvers with the forearm in supination, wrist in forced extension, and the thumb brought firmly back toward the body with the use of the contralateral hand.
- Trial of anti-inflammatory botanicals: Particularly bromelain and proteolytic enzymes.
- Reduce intake of dietary salt: Excess sodium ingestion promotes water retention and magnesium excretion (among many other adverse effects).
- Deep tissue massage to the muscles of the forearm: The median nerve can be compressed proximal to the carpal tunnel at its relationships to the flexor digitorum superficialis, pronator teres[364], and/or the lacertus

---

[357] Folkers et al. Enzymology of the response of the carpal tunnel syndrome to riboflavin and to combined riboflavin and pyridoxine. *Proc Natl Acad Sci* 1984 Nov;81(22):7076-8
[358] Schoenen J, Jacquy J, Lenaerts M. Effectiveness of high-dose riboflavin in migraine prophylaxis. A randomized controlled trial. *Neurology* 1998 Feb;50(2):466-70
[359] Garfinkel MS, Singhal A, Katz WA, et al. Yoga-based intervention for carpal tunnel syndrome: a randomized trial. *JAMA*. 1998 Nov 11;280:1601-3
[360] "It is likely that the yoga practices of controlling body, mind, and spirit combine to provide useful psychophysiological effects for healthy people and for people compromised by musculoskeletal and cardiopulmonary disease." Raub JA. Psychophysiologic effects of Hatha Yoga on musculoskeletal and cardiopulmonary function: a literature review. *J Altern Complement Med*. 2002 Dec;8(6):797-812
[361] Manente G, Torrieri F, Pineto F, Uncini A. A relief maneuver in carpal tunnel syndrome. *Muscle Nerve*. 1999 Nov;22(11):1587-9
[362] "All participants who were treated improved clinically, with decrease in both symptoms and palpatory restriction." Sucher BM. Palpatory diagnosis and manipulative management of carpal tunnel syndrome. *J Am Osteopath Assoc*. 1994 Aug;94(8):647-63
[363] Sucher BM. Myofascial manipulative release of carpal tunnel syndrome: documentation with magnetic resonance imaging. *J Am Osteopath Assoc*. 1993 Dec;93(12):1273-8
[364] Olehnik WK, Manske PR, Szerzinski J. Median nerve compression in the proximal forearm. *J Hand Surg* [Am]. 1994 Jan;19(1):121-6

fibrosus extension from the biceps tendon.[365] Soft-tissue manipulative treatments should be used as part of the comprehensive treatment plan for CTS before any patient is considered a surgical candidate.
- Behavioral and occupational ergonomic modifications: Improve work station functionality, avoid overuse of the hands and wrists, and particularly avoid direct compression of the wrist while working.
- Treatment of endocrine abnormalities and concomitant disease: Diabetes mellitus, thyroid disease, rheumatoid arthritis, in women: assess for high estrogen/ low progesterone, or the use of estrogen supplementation.[366]
- Weight loss: If the patient is overweight, the patient should lose weight.
- Use of a wrist splint at night: A commonly advocated treatment in allopathic textbooks.
- Surgery: For non-responsive cases only as a last resort after nutrition, diet, weight loss, ergonomics, and competent manipulation, mobilization, and massage have been utilized *in combination* along with assessment for and treatment of endocrinologic contributions.

---

[365] Wertsch JJ, Melvin J. Median nerve anatomy and entrapment syndromes: a review. *Arch Phys Med Rehabil*. 1982 Dec;63(12):623-7
[366] "Recent weight gain and use of estrogen replacement therapy were identified as possible risk factors; this provides some support for the theory that fluid retention in the soft tissues of the carpal tunnel is etiologically involved, although these results are preliminary and further research must be carried out to refute or support these findings." Dieck GS, Kelsey JL. An epidemiologic study of the carpal tunnel syndrome in an adult female population. *Prev Med*. 1985 Jan;14(1):63-9

Myofascial Release Techniques for the Treatment of Carpal Tunnel Syndrome: Respectfully attributed to and adapted from the work of Benjamin Sucher, D.O.[367,368,369]

In this demonstration, the doctor is working on the patient's right wrist. In the doctor's right hand, the patient's pisiform, triquetral, and hamate bones are grasped and rolled externally, in a clockwise direction. In the doctor's left hand, the patient's scaphoid and trapezium bones are grasped and rolled externally from midline, in a counterclockwise direction. The combination of these two motions generates strong tension in the transverse carpal ligament (flexor retinaculum) that eventually leads to relaxation of the ligament and allows for increased cross-sectional area within the carpal tunnel, thus relieving pressure on its contents, particularly the median nerve. This maneuver is generally referred to as the *opponens roll*, and the following techniques are variations of same.

In this maneuver, the doctor's contacts and motions are the same as above, except that in this case the doctor's fingers are interposed between those of the patient. This positioning provides for greater control of the patient's distal palm, allowing the doctor to force the patient's wrist into extension while applying tension to the transverse carpal ligament. The addition of wrist extension appears to increase the clinical efficacy of the maneuver.

In this positioning, the actions are the same as above, but the doctor is using his fingers rather than thumbs to apply the mobilizing force. In the doctor's right hand, the patient's scaphoid and trapezium bones are grasped and rolled externally from the palmar surface, in a counterclockwise direction. In the doctor's left hand, the patient's pisiform, triquetral, and hamate bones are grasped and rolled externally from the palmar surface, in a clockwise direction. The action and concept are to "open" the carpal tunnel by tractioning the transverse carpal ligament.

---

[367] Sucher BM. Palpatory diagnosis and manipulative management of carpal tunnel syndrome. *J Am Osteopath Assoc.* 1994 Aug;94(8):647-63
[368] Sucher BM. Myofascial manipulative release of carpal tunnel syndrome: documentation with magnetic resonance imaging. *J Am Osteopath Assoc.* 1993 Dec;93(12):1273-8
[369] Sucher BM, et al. Manipulative treatment of carpal tunnel syndrome: biomechanical and osteopathic intervention to increase the length of the transverse carpal ligament: part 2. Effect of sex differences and manipulative "priming". *J Am Osteopath Assoc.* 2005 Mar;105(3):135-43 jaoa.org/cgi/content/full/105/3/135

> **Proprioceptive Rehabilitation: Essential in the Management of Chronic/Back Pain and Knee/Ankle Injuries**

The central nervous system plays a silent and often underappreciated role in the maintenance of joint integrity and the prevention of joint injuries. Finely coordinated, minute alterations in muscle tension and joint position are essential for proper musculoskeletal biomechanics. Impaired coordination of this delicate neuromuscular system—either by injury or more commonly by disuse—predisposes to subtle and gross injuries and the perpetuation of chronic pain. **Muscle spasm, myofascial trigger points, and neuromuscular uncoupling must be viewed within a context that appreciates how the Western diet and lifestyle contribute to the genesis and perpetuation of painful musculoskeletal problems.**

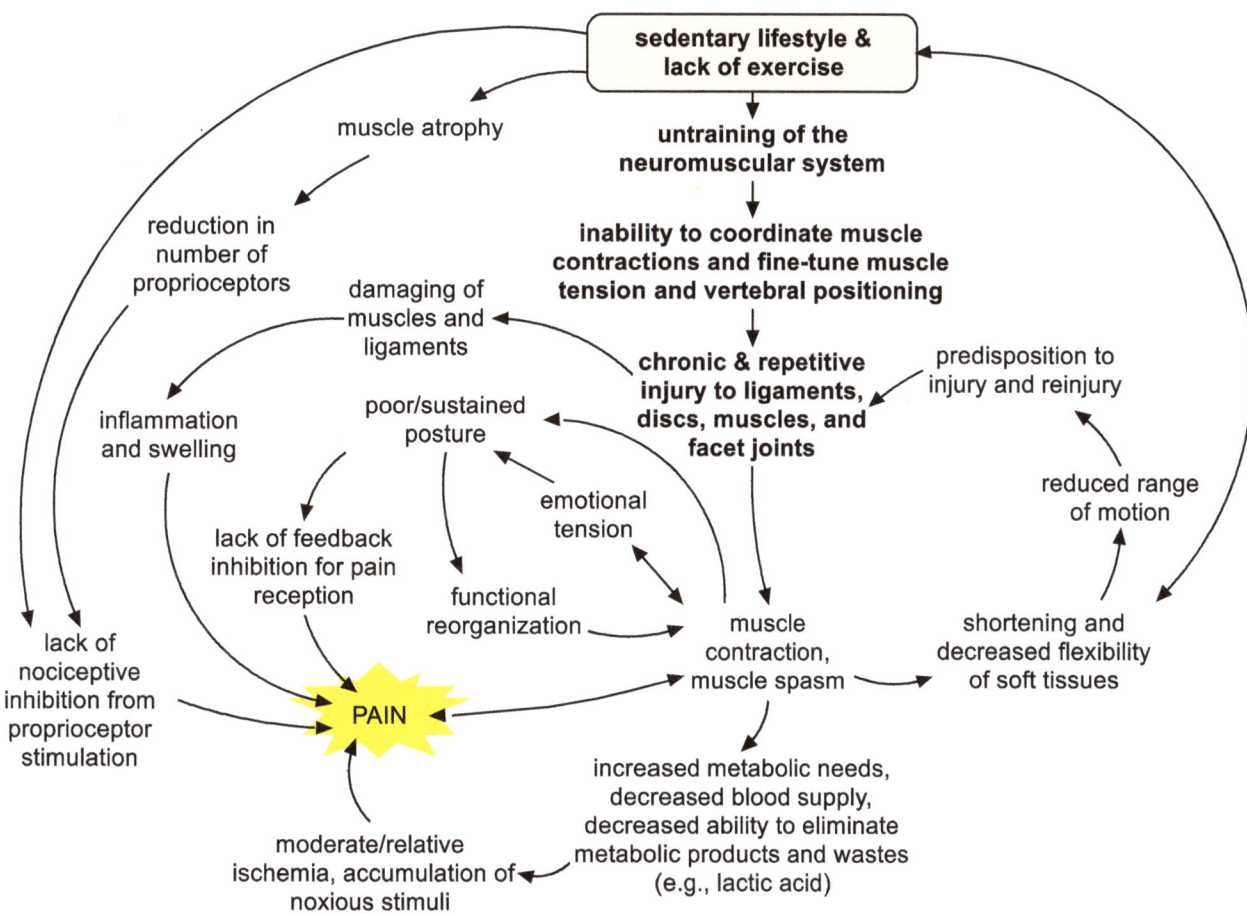

Processed pro-inflammatory nutrient-poor diet and sedentary lifestyle contribute to the genesis and perpetuation of painful musculoskeletal problems: Many people have undernourished (nutritional deficiencies promote pain) overfed (carbohydrates promote inflammation) bodies with weak muscles (lack of exercise) and an untrained (lack of coordination due to sitting nearly motionless most of the day) nervous system.

Proprioceptive deficits are common in patients with chronic low-back pain[370], neck pain[371], knee pain and arthritis[372], and ankle instability.[373] Not only does poor proprioception leave joints vulnerable to recurrent microtrauma, but also lack of proprioceptive inhibition of nociceptors negates the proposed "gate-control" mechanism of pain inhibition and thus opens the door to the perception of chronic pain.[374] Thus, **proprioceptive deficits both increase**

---

[370] Newcomer KL, et al. Muscle activation patterns in subjects with and without low back pain. *Arch Phys Med Rehabil*. 2002;83(6):816-21
[371] McPartland JM, Brodeur RR, Hallgren RC. Chronic neck pain, standing balance, and suboccipital muscle atrophy. *J Manipulative Physiol Ther*. 1997 Jan;20(1):24-9
[372] Callaghan MJ, Selfe J, Bagley PJ, Oldham JA. The Effects of Patellar Taping on Knee Joint Proprioception. *J Athl Train*. 2002 Mar;37(1):19-24
[373] Olmsted LC, et al. Efficacy of the Star Excursion Balance Tests in Detecting Reach Deficits in Subjects with Chronic Ankle Instability. *J Athl Train*. 2002 Dec;37(4):501-506
[374] "The lack of proprioceptive inhibition of nociceptors at the dorsal horn of the spinal cord would result in chronic pain and a loss of standing balance." McPartland JM, Brodeur RR, Hallgren RC. Chronic neck pain, standing balance, and suboccipital muscle atrophy--a pilot study. *J Manipulative Physiol Ther*. 1997 Jan;20(1):24-9

joint injury and increase pain perception. Chronic pain may lead to functional reorganization in the central nervous system and self-perpetuate pain as "pain memories"[375]—rewiring of the nervous system to maintain pain.

An important component to injury rehabilitation and prevention is proprioceptive retraining.[376] Proprioceptive retraining programs have been shown to reduce the severity of pain and the occurrence and recurrence of injuries. With the simple investment of a few minutes per day, patients and athletes can retrain their nervous systems to respond more quickly and to increase the accuracy of proprioception. Muscle-strengthening rehabilitative programs that fail to address proprioceptive retraining do not result in improved neuromuscular coordination as evaluated by electromyography.[377] Furthermore, muscle-strengthening programs may actually lead to a reduction in postural stability when compared to balance training.[378] The **physical medicine portion** of musculoskeletal rehabilitative programs should generally include:

- Correction of faulty movement patterns: Addressing each of the three major components: 1) initial posture, 2) quality of somatosensory input, and 3) CNS motor programs,
- Promotion of spinal stability: Addressing both the *active* and the *passive* components,
- Proprioceptive/sensorimotor training: Target the neck, torso, lumbar spine, pelvis, and lower extremity,
- Strengthening exercises: Strengthen the neck, shoulders, back, legs, and abdominal and oblique muscles,
- Myofascial and spinal manipulative therapy: Use manual medicine to alleviate pain, facilitate and effect proprioceptive/sensorimotor restoration, and promote optimal joint biomechanics.

A very comprehensive and dense review of this topic was published by Murphy[379] in 2000, and this article is highly recommended for practitioners specializing in rehabilitation.

Clinical techniques for proprioceptive/sensorimotor retraining and rehabilitation:
- Wobble board, balance shoes, standing foam, exercise ball, or other labile support surface: At the very least, patients should be advised to use a wobble board, balance board, balance shoes or exercise sandals for *at least* 5 minutes 2 times per day every day of the week. Exercise sandals appear to be highly efficient for increasing muscular activity in the lower leg and ankle.[380] Sedentary patients can easily integrate proprioceptive training into their lives—they can use the wobble board or balance shoes while they are watching television. This easy treatment has been shown to facilitate rapid subconscious neuromuscular coordination of the gluteal muscles, thus enhancing pelvic and low-back stability.[381] Other techniques include standing on thick foam or walking in thick sand, which are labile surfaces that require increased neuromuscular control. Standing on one leg and performing gentle motions while blindfolded or with closed eyes further challenges *and therefore improves* the coordination of proprioceptive input with neuromuscular responsiveness.[382,383,384]
    - Reflex activation of gluteal muscles in walking (*Spine* 1993 May[385]): In this very important and notably brief report, the authors note that gluteal activation and pelvic stability often are decreased in chronic low-back pain

> **Neuromuscular faults in low back pain**
> ❶ Weak spinal extensors,
> ❷ Weak abdominal muscles,
> ❸ Delayed activation of deep stability muscles especially multifidus and transversus abdominis
>
> "The biggest problem of low back pain is lumbar instability. Unbalanced mobilization order among stability muscles and mobility muscles, as well as muscle length, causes low back pain. ... For lumbar region stability, strengthening and co-contraction of the multifidus and transversus abdominis (TA), which are deep stability muscles, and the erector spinae (ES) and abdominal muscles, which are superficial stabilizer muscles, is required."
>
> Lee et al. *J Phys Ther Sci*. 2014 Jan

---

[375] "Functional reorganisation in both the somatosensory and motor system... In patients with chronic low back pain and fibromyalgia... reorganisational change increases with chronicity; ...cortical reorganisation is correlated with the amount of pain... central alterations may be viewed as pain memories ... influence the processing of both painful and nonpainful input..." Flor H. Cortical reorganisation and chronic pain: implications for rehabilitation. *J Rehabil Med*. 2003 May;(41 Suppl):66-72
[376] Murphy DR. Chiropractic rehabilitation of the cervical spine. *J Manipulative Physiol Ther*. 2000 Jul-Aug; 23(6): 404-8
[377] "Unbalanced electromyographic patterns found in patients with LBP given symmetrical tasks were not affected by rehabilitation treatment." Lu WW, et al. Back muscle contraction patterns of patients with low back pain before and after rehabilitation treatment: an electromyographic evaluation. *J Spinal Disord*. 2001 Aug;14(4):277-82
[378] "RESULTS: After 1 month, back extensor strengthening led to decreased postural stability on hard surface... Balance skill training, however, increased postural stability as indicated by a decreased low-frequency component." Kollmitzer J, Ebenbichler GR, Sabo A, Kerschan K, Bochdansky T. Effects of back extensor strength training versus balance training on postural control. *Med Sci Sports Exerc*. 2000 Oct;32(10):1770-6
[379] Murphy DR. Chiropractic rehabilitation of the cervical spine. *J Manipulative Physiol Ther*. 2000 Jul-Aug;23(6):404-8
[380] Troy Blackburn J, et al. Exercise Sandals Increase Lower Extremity Electromyographic Activity during Functional Activities. *J Athl Train*. 2003 Sep;38(3):198-203
[381] Bullock-Saxton JE, Janda V, Bullock MI. Reflex activation of gluteal muscles in walking. *Spine* 1993 May;18(6):704-8
[382] Olmsted LC, et al. Efficacy of the Star Excursion Balance Tests in Detecting Reach Deficits in Subjects with Chronic Ankle Instability. *J Athl Train*. 2002 Dec;37(4):501-506
[383] Troy Blackburn et al. Exercise Sandals Increase Lower Extremity Electromyographic Activity during Functional Activities. *J Athl Train*. 2003 Sep;38(3):198-203
[384] Willems T, et al. Proprioception and Muscle Strength in Subjects with a History of Ankle Sprains and Chronic Instability. *J Athl Train*. 2002 Dec;37(4):487-493
[385] Bullock-Saxton JE, Janda V, Bullock MI. Reflex activation of gluteal muscles in walking. *Spine* 1993 May;18(6):704-8

sufferers. "Labile support, through wearing "balance shoes," offered facilitation of cerebellovestibular circuits." With one week of treatment the authors note "Significant increases in gluteal activity and significant decreases in time to 75% maximum contraction, demonstrated the value of sensorimotor elicitation of subconscious and automatic responses in muscles often weakened in back pain sufferers."

- o Combination patterns of proprioceptive neuromuscular facilitation and ball exercise on pain and muscle activity of chronic low back pain patients (*J Phys Ther Sci* 2014 Jan[386]): This study shows that pain measured by the validated visual analog scale (VAS) and muscle electromyographic activity (EMG) were both improved to a greater extent in patients using proprioceptive neuromuscular facilitation (PNF). The alleviation of low back pain with proprioceptive training proves the causative relationship between proprioceptive loss and low back pain and—perhaps even more importantly—the therapeutic value of proprioceptive rehabilitation for alleviation of back pain. "VAS and EMG activity were significantly reduced in the PNF combination pattern group and the ball exercise group. A comparison of the groups showed significant differences. In VAS and EMG activity; in particular, the combination pattern group using PNF increased EMG activity more than the ball exercise group did after six weeks of intervention.

Wobble board (and other labile surface) variations

Foot variations:
- Two feet wide, two feet narrow
- One foot centered, other leg for balance *pictured*
- One food centered, other leg moving in controlled pattern in all directions, e.g., star pattern
- One foot centered, other leg moving somewhat randomly, i.e., dancing to music

Arm variations:
- Arms for balance
- Arms moving in symmetry
- Arms moving differently, randomly, e.g., dance
- Arms lifting weights: biceps curl, lateral raises for deltoids and shoulders (single-sided *pictured* and double-sided)

Eye variations:
- Open or closed; closed eyes forces greater/exclusive reliance on proprioceptive input

Posture:
- As perfect as possible while retraining the nervous system to improved posture *not pictured*

Proprioceptive rehabilitation—demonstration of use of wobble-board for single-leg empty-arm exercise and double-leg weight-lifting (single-side lateral raises for deltoids and shoulders): These pictured examples show the simple implementation of proprioceptive retraining, which is generally the simple implementation of proprioceptive/cerebellar challenge to enhance neuromuscular coordination. The effect (enhanced neuromuscular coordination) is rapid (occurring within 3 sessions of 5 minutes each) and the results (alleviation of pain) are clinically significant. For most purposes, wobble boards and other labile surfaces can be made from items purchased locally or found in-house. The brief original video is available online: vimeo.com/drvasquez/proprioceptive1

- Spinal manipulation: Spinal manipulation appears to improve proprioceptive function.[387]
- Barefoot exercise: Barefoot exercise increases proprioceptive input and helps alleviate back pain.[388]
- Vigorous full-body exercise of any and all types, especially those that are relatively fast and require high-frequency complex neuromuscular responses, such as:

---

[386] Lee CW et al. The effects of combination patterns of proprioceptive neuromuscular facilitation and ball exercise on pain and muscle activity of chronic low back pain patients. *J Phys Ther Sci.* 2014 Jan;26(1):93-6
[387] "RESULTS: Subjects receiving manipulation demonstrated a mean reduction in visual analogue scores of 44%, along with a 41% improvement in mean scores for the head repositioning skill." Rogers RG. The effects of spinal manipulation on cervical kinesthesia in patients with chronic neck pain. *J Manipulative Physiol Ther* 1997 Feb;20(2):80-5
[388] Bullock-Saxton JE, Janda V, Bullock MI. Reflex activation of gluteal muscles in walking. *Spine* 1993 May;18(6):704-8

- o Swimming: Excellent for promoting fitness in a way that is generally easy on joints and muscles and is without impact; requires and thus promotes coordination and timing
- o Indoor aerobics: Excellent for cardiovascular fitness and weight loss, requires and thus promotes coordination and timing
- o Outdoor cycling (road): Excellent for cardiovascular fitness and weight loss, easy on the joints; requires and promotes coordination and balance.
- o Outdoor cycling (mountain and trail): Same as above; requires more balance and coordination than road cycling due to unpredictability of surface; rough surfaces provide flood of afferent stimuli through feet and hands.
- o Hiking: Excellent combination of lower extremity strengthening and aerobics; random and uneven trails provide proprioceptive challenge; helps people get in touch with nature.
- o Yoga, Pilates, Calisthenics: Yoga and calisthenics are ways convenient, can be done alone or with others, do not require expensive equipment, and can be tailored for low-back rehabilitation.[389,390,391]

Relaxing, convenient, yoga/calisthenics for improved strength and neuromuscular control: The yoga/calisthenics exercise demonstrated above promotes strengthening of gluteal muscles and spinal extensors; the crossed pattern of (right) arm and (left) leg raising requires much more neuromuscular control than would be required if both hands were being used for stabilization. Repetitions should be repeated until muscular failure is achieved.

- Skin taping to increase afferent stimuli: Applying tape to the skin can increase sensory input from cutaneous mechanoreceptors and can improve sensorimotor coordination.[392,393,394,395]
- Vitamin D3: Identification and correction of vitamin D deficiency has been shown to improve muscular strength, alleviate pain, improve neuromuscular coordination, and—in several studies—reduce the incidence of falling and osteoporotic fractures. The increasingly

Correction of vitamin D deficiency improves muscle strength and neuromuscular coordination

"Vitamin D supplementation, in fallers with vitamin D insufficiency, has a **significant beneficial effect on functional performance, reaction time and balance**... This suggests that **vitamin D supplementation improves neuromuscular or neuroprotective function**, which may in part explain the mechanism whereby vitamin D reduces falls and fractures."

Dhesi et al. *Age Ageing*. 2004 Nov

---

[389] Shiple B. Relieving Low-Back Pain with Exercise. *Physician and Sportsmedicine* 1997; 25: physsportsmed.com/issues/1997/08aug/shiplepa.htm
[390] Drezner JA. Exercises in the Treatment of Low- Back Pain. *Physician and Sportsmedicine* 2001; 29: physsportsmed.com/issues/2001/08_01/pa_drezner.htm
[391] Kuritzky L, White J. Extend Yourself for Low-Back Pain Relief. *Physician and Sportsmedicine* 1997; 25: physsportsmed.com/issues/1997/01jan/back_pa.htm
[392] "This suggests that ankle taping partly corrects impaired proprioception caused by modern athletic footwear and exercise." Robbins S, Waked E, Rappel R. Ankle taping improves proprioception before and after exercise in young men. *Br J Sports Med*. 1995 Dec;29(4):242-7
[393] "We concluded that increased cutaneous sensory feedback provided by strips of athletic tape applied across the ankle joint of healthy individuals can help improve ankle joint position perception in nonweightbearing, especially for a midrange plantar-flexed ankle position." Simoneau GG, Degner RM, Kramper CA, Kittleson KH. Changes in Ankle Joint Proprioception Resulting From Strips of Athletic Tape Applied Over the Skin. *J Athl Train*. 1997 Apr;32(2):141-147 pubmedcentral.nih.gov
[394] Callaghan MJ, Selfe J, Bagley PJ, Oldham JA. The Effects of Patellar Taping on Knee Joint Proprioception. *J Athl Train*. 2002 Mar;37(1):19-24 pubmedcentral.nih.gov/
[395] "Application of stretch to the skin over VMO via the tape can increase VMO activity, suggesting that cutaneous stimulation may be one mechanism by which patella taping produces a clinical effect." Macgregor et al. Cutaneous stimulation from patella tape causes differential increase in vasti muscle activity in people with patellofemoral pain. *J Orthop Res* 2005;23:351-8

widespread realization that patients with chronic joint pain and recurrent injuries have proprioceptive defects is a paradigm shift of its own right, and it obviously sheds new light on therapy and prevention of musculoskeletal pain and recurrent injuries. **Spinal manipulation, skin taping,** and **specific exercises** have all been shown to improve sensorimotor coordination. Very interestingly, **vitamin D supplementation** also improves sensorimotor coordination and thereby helps prevent falls and subsequent musculoskeletal injuries, particularly in the elderly.[396] Vitamin D3 supplementation helps prevent fractures (especially in elderly patients) by at least three different mechanisms: ❶ Vitamin D3 increases calcium absorption in the gut and helps preserve bone strength, ❷ it improves balance and coordination so that falls are avoided, and ❸ vitamin D further protects bone and defends against osteoporosis via a systemic anti-inflammatory effect that reduces the catabolic effect of inflammation on bone.

- o The clinical importance of vitamin D: a paradigm shift with implications for all healthcare providers (*Altern Ther Health Med* 2004 Sep[397]): "Given the depth and breadth of the peer-reviewed research documenting the frequency and consequences of hypovitaminosis D, failure to diagnose and treat this disorder is ethically questionable and is inconsistent with the delivery of quality, science-based healthcare. ... Until proven otherwise, the balance of the research clearly indicates that oral supplementation in the range of 1,000 IU/day for infants, 2,000 IU/day for children, and 4,000 IU/day for adults is safe and reasonable to meet physiologic requirements, to promote optimal health, and to reduce the risk of several serious diseases. Safety and effectiveness of supplementation are assured by periodic monitoring of serum 25(OH)D and serum calcium."
- o Effects of vitamin D on the musculoskeletal system and the prevention of falls (*J Am Osteopath Assoc* 2012 Jan[398]): "Vitamin D supplementation helps prevent falls not only because of its effect on bone density and the regulation of calcium and phosphate metabolism, but also because of its effect on muscle and nervous system function. ... One study demonstrated that vitamin D supplementation improves muscle strength and postural equilibrium, which may in turn reduce the risk of falling."

---

[396] Dhesi JK, et al. Vitamin D supplementation improves neuromuscular function in older people who fall. *Age Ageing*. 2004 Nov;33(6):589-95
[397] Vasquez A, et al. Clinical importance of vitamin D: paradigm shift with implications for all healthcare providers. *Altern Ther Health Med* 2004 Sep ICHNFM.org/pdf
[398] Fraix M. Role of the musculoskeletal system and the prevention of falls. *J Am Osteopath Assoc*. 2012 Jan;112(1):17-21

Introduction to Injection Therapies: Trigger Points, Anesthetics, Viscous Agents, Prolotherapy

Injection therapies will be detailed and demonstrated in much greater detail in the next edition of *Integrative Orthopedics* (i.e., 4th Edition) and are overviewed here for the sake of introduction; their clinical application requires relevant review of anatomy, pharmacology, and clinical procedures is thus best contextualized in chapters that focus on musculoskeletal regions and specific disorders.

- <u>Trigger point and tender point injections</u>: Muscles can be injected with anesthetic such as lidocaine for pain relief; interestingly, many patients achieve lasting pain relief that extends far beyond the time anticipated by the drug's half-life. Injected normal saline and vitamin B-12 are also used frequently for muscular pain relief.
- <u>Intraarticular injection of anesthetics and viscous agents</u>: This is a particularly gratifying in-office procedure that often provides pain relieve and improved functional status in patients not sufficiently helped by oral and topical pain relievers; while anesthetics and steroids can be injected into any joint (or ligament or muscle for that matter), viscous agents are most specifically used in the knee.
- <u>Prolotherapy (*proliferative therapy*)</u>: "Finally, in 1939, I arrived at the conclusion that relaxation of the articular ligaments was responsible for a considerable number of low back disabilities. I decided to attempt strengthening the ligaments by the injection of a proliferating solution within the fibrous bands to stimulate the production of fibrous tissue. The treatment proved to be satisfactory almost from the beginning, and it was cautiously extended until now articular ligaments of the entire spine and pelvis and some other joints are treated with great satisfaction both to the patient and to me. ... A joint is only as strong as its weakest ligament."[399] Due to its ability to promote proliferation of connective tissue, dextrose prolotherapy may provide benefit for patients with ligamentous laxity and disc degeneration, as demonstrated in studies of patients with back pain, knee pain, and hand osteoarthritis.[400,401,402,403,404]

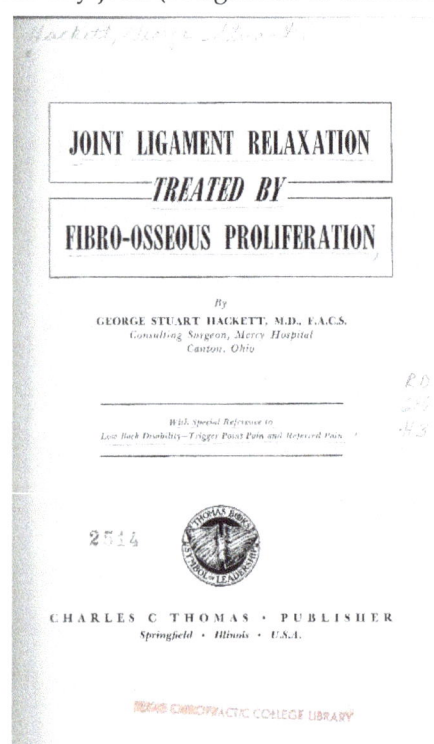

- <u>Intravenous colchicine</u>: Michael Rask MD has been the strongest advocate of the use of intravenous colchicine for the treatment of herniated spinal discs, and his monograph "*Colchicine use in 6,000 patients with disk disease and other related resistantly-painful spinal disorders*"[405] is required reading for any physician interested in using this technique clinically—the details of his protocol are much too extensive to review here, and clinicians will be better served by reading the original article. Notably, as part of the protocol for patients with disc herniation, in addition to intravenous colchicine, Rask advocates 1) treatment of myofascial trigger points, 2) weight loss, 3) cessation of alcohol, tobacco, and caffeine, 4) avoidance of *Solanaceae* plants such as eggplant, potato, tomato, and green and red peppers, 5) avoidance of sugars and junk foods, and 6) a strict vegan diet, especially for patients who are overweight. Although Rask (op cit 1989) notes that colchicine is "extremely effective" and "an exceedingly safe medication", other authors[406] have been less optimistic noting that the benefit was "often of short duration." Given that intravenous colchicine has been

---

[399] Hackett GS. *Joint Ligament Relaxation Treated by Fibro-Osseous Proliferation*. Springfield Illinois, Charles C Thomas Publishers, 1956
[400] "Prolotherapy injection with 10% dextrose resulted in clinically and statistically significant improvements in knee osteoarthritis. Preliminary blinded radiographic readings (1-year films, with 3-year total follow-up period planned) demonstrated improvement in several measures of osteoarthritis severity. ACL laxity, when present in these osteoarthritic patients, improved." Reeves KD, Hassanein K. Randomized prospective double-blind placebo-controlled study of dextrose prolotherapy for knee osteoarthritis with or without ACL laxity. *Altern Ther Health Med* 2000 Mar;6(2):68-74, 77-80
[401] Mooney V. Prolotherapy at the fringe of medical care, or is it the frontier? *Spine J.* 2003 Jul-Aug;3(4):253-4
[402] This study used intradiscal injection therapy with glucosamine, chondroitin sulfate, hypertonic dextrose and DMSO. "Although the results were statistically significant for the 30 patients as a whole, 17 of the 30 patients (57%) improved markedly with an average of 72% improvement in disability scores and 76% in visual analogue scores. The other 13 patients (43%) had little or no improvement." Klein RG, et al. Biochemical injection treatment for discogenic low back pain: a pilot study. *Spine J.* 2003 May-Jun;3(3):220-6
[403] "Dextrose prolotherapy was clinically effective and safe in the treatment of pain with joint movement and range limitation in osteoarthritic finger joints." Reeves KD, Hassanein K. Randomized, prospective, placebo-controlled double-blind study of dextrose prolotherapy for osteoarthritic thumb and finger (DIP, PIP, and trapeziometacarpal) joints: evidence of clinical efficacy. *J Altern Complement Med.* 2000 Aug;6(4):311-20
[404] "RESULTS: Each patient was injected an average of 3.5 times. Overall, 43.4% of patients fell into the sustained improvement group with an average improvement in numeric pain scores of 71%, comparing pretreatment and 18 month measurements." Miller MR, Mathews RS, Reeves KD. Treatment of painful advanced internal lumbar disc derangement with intradiscal injection of hypertonic dextrose. *Pain Physician.* 2006 Apr;9(2):115-21 painphysicianjournal.com/linkout_vw.php?issn=1533-3159&vol=9&page=115
[405] Rask MR. Colchicine use in 6,000 patients with disk disease and other related resistantly-painful spinal disorders. *J Neurological Orthopaedic Med Surgery* 1989; 10: 291-298
[406] "Results indicate a significant difference between the two groups, the intravenous colchicine group showing improvement in symptoms for a few hours or days over a 3-week course of treatment. However, the relief was often of short duration." Simmons et al. Intravenous colchicine for low back pain: a double-blind study. *Spine.* 1990 Jul;15(7):716-7

associated with complications such as pancytopenia, organ failure, and death[407], it is not a treatment to be taken lightly nor should inexperienced physicians administer it. Colchicine can be administered orally, but its low therapeutic efficacy in relation to its moderate gastrointestinal toxicity limits its applicability. In a poorly designed study by Schnebel and Simmons[408], orally administered colchicine was no better yet was more toxic than placebo; this study appears to have been designed specifically to show inefficacy and toxicity of colchicine since the patients were either given *no treatment* alternating with a *gastroirritative toxic dose* of colchicine.

Statue of Silvius Brabo, a mythical Roman soldier who is said to have killed a giant and thrown his hand into the river, hence the name of the city Antwerp, which translates to "hand throwing." Photo at Antwerp City Hall, Belgium 2012 by DrV.

---

[407] "Bone marrow depression has been reported, primarily in cases of acute colchicine intoxication, and intravenous administration of the drug has been associated with severe pancytopenia and death." Levy M, Spino M, Read SE. Colchicine: a state-of-the-art review. *Pharmacotherapy*. 1991;11(3):196-211
[408] Schnebel BE, Simmons JW. The use of oral colchicine for low back pain. A double-blind study. *Spine*. 1988 Mar;13(3):354-7 Use of colchicine in this study varied from abstinence for 3 days followed by a toxic dose on day 4; therefore patients in the treatment group were subjected to no treatment for 75% of the time, followed by a dose that caused gastrointestinal toxicity—vomiting and diarrhea—the other 25% of the time. At neither phase of the study were patients exposed to a treatment that had any possibility of being effective in relation to the potential toxicity. This study was so poorly designed that its publication brings into question the editorial quality of *Spine* during this era.

Another Clinically Useful Mnemonic Acronym: "B.e.n.d. S.t.e.m.s."

As an alternative to the "p.r.i.c.e. a. t.u.r.n." acronym as previously described and which is admittedly cumbersome, clinicians may use the following alternate, either additively or substitutionally. "B.e.n.d. s.t.e.m.s." is aesthetically more appealing, though it is less complete than *price a turn*. The goal, of course, is to have a useful memory key available when the clinician is formulating the treatment plan. Just as all doctors are familiar with the *s.o.a.p.* format for writing chart notes to ensure their inclusion of *subjective, objective, assessment*, and *plan* for each visit, when arriving to the "p" portion of the note, integrative clinicians can use *price a turn* and/or *bend stems* to help remember key components to integrative and holistic care.

B   <u>Botanical</u>: Numerous botanical medicines are available for a wide range of indications. Among the botanical medicines with the best research support for the treatment of musculoskeletal pain and inflammation are willow bark, *Boswellia, Harpagophytum, Uncaria*, ginger, and *Capsicum*.

E   <u>Ergonomics/posture and Exercise</u>: Patients can improve their ergonomics at home, at work, and (occasionally) in the car. Likewise, attention to posture—the "style" with which one holds one's body—is important in the prevention of repetitive strain injuries, particularly to the shoulders and neck region. Most patients are overweight, out of shape, weak, and neuromuscularly uncoordinated; problems correctible with exercise.

N   <u>Nutrition</u>: Nutritional supplements are extremely valuable in the treatment and prevention of a wide range of mild and serious health problems. Use of high-dose "supranutritional" levels of vitamins can be used to help patients overcome their enzyme and receptor defects to facilitate improved physiological function and improved overall health.[409]

D   <u>Diet</u>: In order to remain consistent with the time-proven wisdom of the *Hierarchy of Therapeutics* (discussed in Chapter 2) and to avoid becoming an aimless horde of drug-pushing symptom-suppressors, holistic integrative clinicians must always attend to the basics—the foundational influences which powerfully affect metabolism and thus overall health. Clearly, diet is one of those basics, along with emotions and lifestyle—exercise, work, stress management, outlook, and relationships.

S   <u>Stretching, strengthening, and stabilization</u>: Tight muscles can be stretched in the office, where the doctor is able to teach the patient proper methods and is able to refine the diagnosis and specificity of the stretch to ensure that targeted muscles are effectively addressed. Thereafter, the patient *must* continue these stretches at home—both physically and mentally. ***Physical stretching*** involves the therapeutic lengthening of muscles and fascia to maintain or restore ease of myofascial motion and to alleviate adhesions or restrictions that impair function. ***Mental stretching*** involves the patient's active use of reframing and discipline in order to attain a higher level of functioning and effectiveness in his/her relationships, lifestyle, work situation, mental outlook, habits and other phenomena in order to overcome the external or internal *adhesions* or *restrictions* that are impairing and preventing optimal function *of the patient as a whole*. Exercise and proproceptive rehabilitation for spinal and peripheral joint stabilization are essential requirements for neuromusculoskeletal health.

T   <u>Trigger points</u>: Always remember to address the trigger point component (discussed previously in this chapter) when working with musculoskeletal pain. Seek and ye shall find; treat and the patient will improve. Think outside the region. A trigger point in the low-back or gluteal region may cause the patient to assume an antalgic posture that results in altered biomechanics and leads to a clinical presentation of shoulder or neck pain with chronic tension headaches; direct treatment of the painful shoulders or neck will provide improvement, but cure will not be effected until the cause—often distant from the region of complaint—is effectively addressed.[410]

E   <u>Educate and Ensure return</u>: Educate the patient about the condition, its cause and solutions. Educate about PAR-B—procedures, risks, alternatives, and benefits of treatment. Also, educate the patient *in writing* about the importance of follow-up visits and time limitations on treatments; failure to ensure that the patient was educated to return for follow-up visits is grounds for malpractice if the patient's condition changes or deteriorates due to complications associated with the presenting complaint at the last office visit.

M   <u>Manual medicine—mobilization, manipulation, massage</u>: Treat the problem effectively and directly with the skilled use of your hands. Practice produces proficiency.

S   <u>Spirituality (emotions, psychology)</u>: Perceptions create our emotional and mental realities, and from these subjective realities do we engage the world. Inaccurate perceptions skew and misshape one's interactions with the world. Creating more accurate perceptions—a process that requires intentionality and hard work—enhances *effectiveness* and ultimately *enjoyment* of one's life experience.

---

[409] Ames BN, Elson-Schwab I, Silver EA. High-dose vitamin therapy stimulates variant enzymes. *Am J Clin Nutr*. 2002 Apr;75(4):616-58 ajcn.org/cgi/content/full/75/4/616
[410] "This patient seemed to respond favorably to conservative care that included regions of spine not traditionally associated with headache pain." Stude DE, Sweere JJ. A holistic approach to severe headache symptoms in a patient unresponsive to regional manual therapy. *J Manipulative Physiol Ther*. 1996 Mar-Apr;19(3):202-7

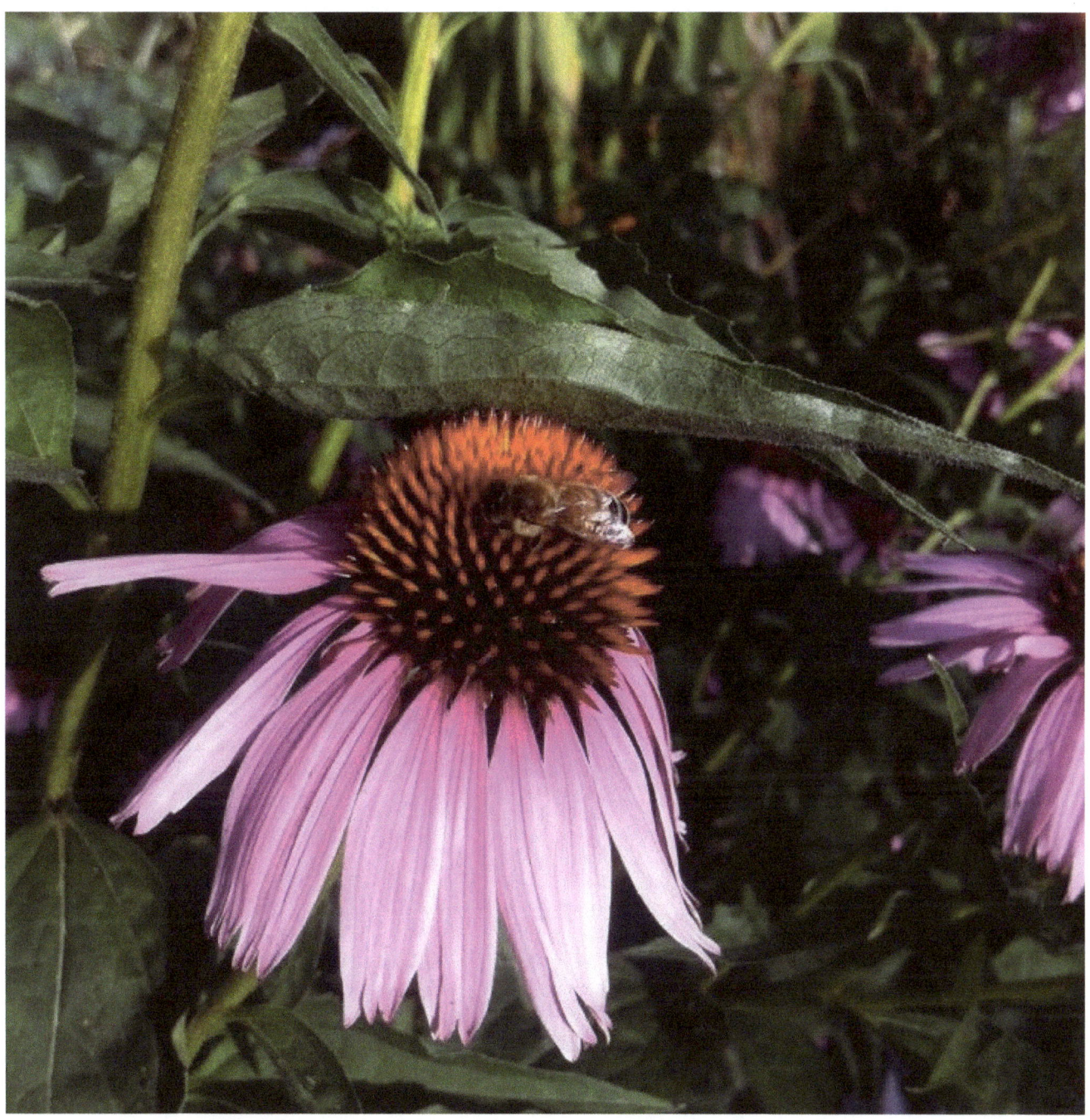

Purple coneflower (*Echinacea purpurea*) with honey bee (*Apis* genus): Portland Oregon 2011, photo by DrV

Progressive awakening
"Only that day dawns to which we are awake." Henry David Thoreau, *Walden*[411] "In virtually all of the great spiritual and philosophical traditions of the world there appears some form of the idea that most human beings are sleepwalking through their own existence. **Enlightenment is identified with waking up.** Evolution and progress are identified with an expansion of consciousness." Nathaniel Branden, *Six Pillars of Self-Esteem*[412] "And once you are awake, then shall you ever remain awake." Friedrich Nietzsche, *Thus Spoke Zarathustra*[413]

---

[411] Thoreau HD. (Owen Thomas, Ed). *Walden and Civil Disobedience*. New York; WW Norton and Company: 1966, page 221
[412] Nathaniel Branden *The Six Pillars of Self-Esteem*, p. 67
[413] Nietzsche FW. *Thus Spoke Zarathustra*.

Columbia River Gorge: Wahkeena Falls, Oregon *above*, Dog Mountain, Washington *below*.

Chapter 4:
Introduction to DrV's Functional Inflammology Protocol: The Seven Major Modifiable Factors in Systemic Inflammation, Allergy, and Autoimmunity

Major Modifiable Influences on Immune and Inflammatory Balance

This section reviews clinically-relevant information related to the pathogenesis and etiology of inflammatory/allergic/autoimmune conditions. Following extensive reviews of the research literature in conjunction with the author's impressively successful clinical experience with patients with "idiopathic" and inflammatory/autoimmune disorders, the original version of this information was published in the first edition of *Integrative Rheumatology* (2006). This section is a distillation of thousands of research articles, abstracts, seminar notes, conversations with colleagues, one-on-one patient encounters and the author's own considerations and reflections.

Following my review and perusal of thousands of research articles in addition to the attentive application of my interest in these conditions throughout three doctoral programs, I have come to appreciate seven major modifiable factors that are chiefly relevant for the initial and long-term management of patients with inflammatory conditions and rheumatic diseases. These 7 factors are:

1. <u>Food intake and nutritional status</u>: The pro/anti-inflammatory effects of diet, including food allergies and intolerances, nutrient deficiencies and dependencies,
2. <u>Infections and dysbiosis</u>: Chronic exposure to microbial effectors/effects,
3. <u>Nutritional modulation of the immune system</u>: Nutrigenomic modification of immunocyte phenotype,
4. <u>Dysmetabolism and Dysfunctional organelles, most notably mitochondria</u>: Especially the pro-inflammatory, pro-oxidant, and anti-apoptotic consequences of dysfunctional mitochondria (DysMito or MitoDys); more recently the conversation has extended beyond mitochondrial dysfunction to include endoplasmic reticulum stress/dysfunction (ERS) and resultant unfolded protein response (UPR),
5. <u>Stress, sleep deprivation vs sleep sufficiency, spinal health, social and psychological considerations</u>: Included in this section is a collection of important considerations which—in the first draft of this acronym—started with stress management, sleep hygiene, and pSychological and social factors. Later versions have included spinal health (chiropractic model), somatic dysfunction (osteopathic model), surgery, specialized supplementation, and "stamp your passport"—sometimes we all just need to vacate for a while and implement some *geographic cure* for the sake of inspiration, life enhancement, exposure to new ideas and lifestyles, and the breaking of (dysfunctional) thought patterns and routines,
6. <u>Endocrine imbalances</u>: Hormones can promote or retard the genesis and perpetuation of inflammation/allergy/autoimmunity; therapeutic correction with prescription or nonprescription interventions can have a profound anti-inflammatory benefit.
7. <u>Xenobiotic immunotoxicity</u>: Exposure to and accumulation of toxic chemicals and/or toxic metals can alter immune responses toward allergy and autoimmunity and away from immunosurveillance against infections and cancer.

Common diseases such as psoriasis and rheumatoid arthritis are greater public health concerns and are more commonly encountered in clinical practice than are the more rare conditions; proportionate mention is made in the following section. Importantly, readers should appreciate that the information in various sections likely applies either conceptually or specifically to conditions described in other sections and that therefore the best way to understand inflammatory/allergic/autoimmune disorders in their totality is to appreciate the nuances of each and the common themes among all.

I am quite pleased to see that the original five variables that I defined in the first two editions of *Integrative Rheumatology* (2006, 2007) have stood the tests of time, science, and clinical practice: in fact, all have been strengthened in the intervening years.

Affirmation and consistency of common themes in an interconnected reality; the importance of transitioning from reception to comprehension to conception to behavior

"The fact that today I still stand by these ideas, **that in the intervening time they themselves have constantly become more strongly associated with one another, even to the point of growing into each other, intertwining, and becoming *one***, that has reinforced in me the joyful confidence that they may not have originally developed in me as single, random, or sporadic ideas, but up out of common roots, from some fundamental *will for knowledge* ruling from deep within, always speaking with greater clarity, always demanding greater clarity.

In fact, this is the only thing appropriate and proper for a philosopher. **We have no right to be isolated in any way: we are not permitted to make isolated mistakes or to run into isolated truths**. Our ideas, our values, our affirmations and denials, our *if*s and *but*s—these rather grow out of us from the same necessity which makes a tree bear its fruit—totally related and interlinked amongst each other: witnesses of one will, one health, one soil, one sun."

Nietzsche FW. *On the Genealogy of Morals*, 1887, Preface essay #2

"In order for a particular species to maintain itself and increase its power, **its conception of reality must comprehend enough of the calculable and constant** for it to **base a scheme of behavior on it**."

Nietzsche FW. *Will to Power*, 1901, #480

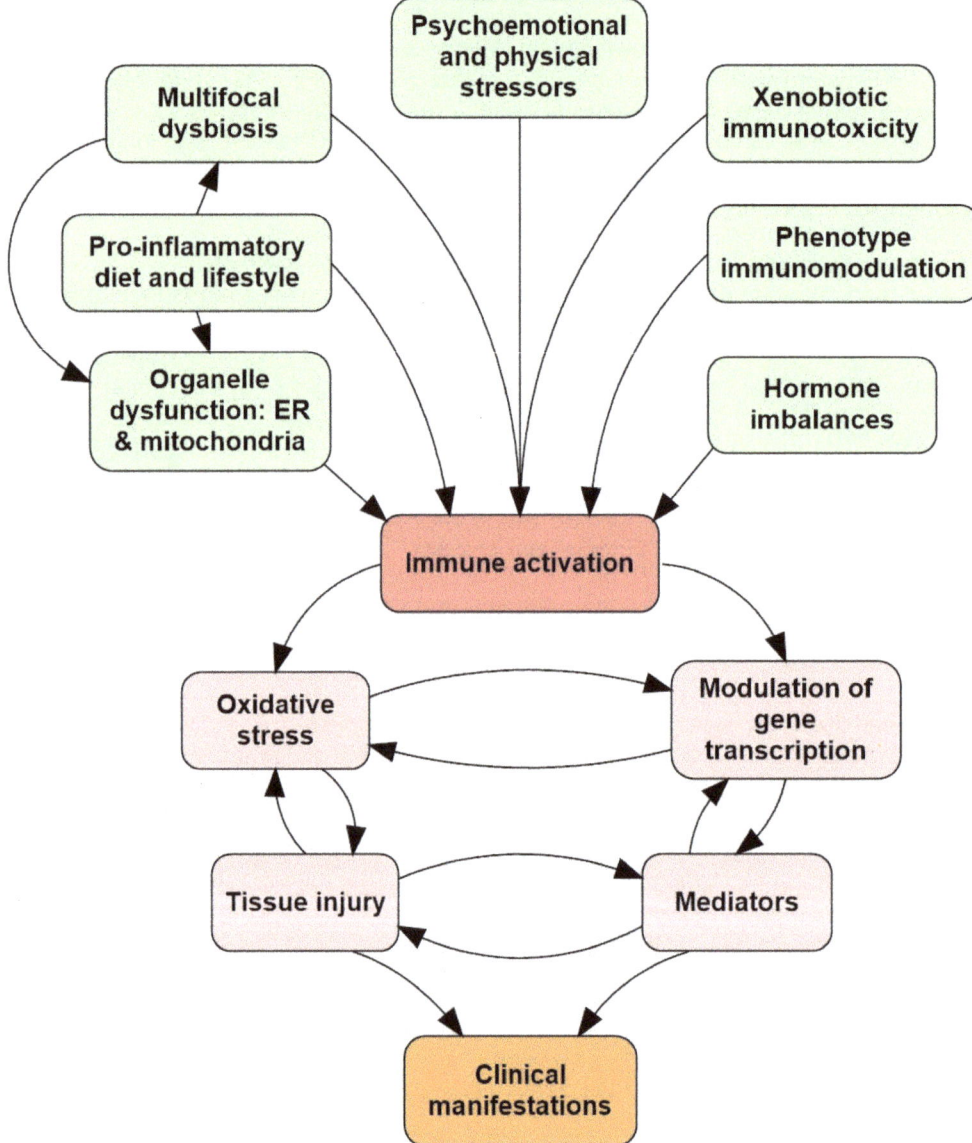

Inflammation in a simple cause-and-effect diagram: The major causative factors amenable to clinical implementation are represented, along with the pathophysiologic consequences and clinical effects. Molecular details, clinical assessments, and therapeutic interventions are introduced/reviewed in this chapter; in later volumes of this work, clinical protocols detail the drugs and doses, etc.

Chapter 4: Major Modifiable Factors in Systemic Inflammation

Nutrition & FxMed for chronic immune-inflammatory disorders

Causes of Inflammation-Immune-Metabolic Imbalance:

1. Food, Lifestyle
2. Infection, Dysbiosis
3. Nutritional Immunomodulation
4. Dysfunctional mitochondria
5. Stress, Emotions, Psychology, Sociology, Lifestyle
6. Endocrine, Hormones
7. Xenobiotics, Toxins

Notice that these 7 factors can be remembered by the acronym: **F.I.N.D.S.E.X.**
♥ First presented in Paris in 2012 ♥

The "Functional Inflammology Protocol" and FINDSEX® acronym: As the clinical protocol expanded from five components (diet, dysbiosis, xenobiotics, hormones, and stress) published in 2006 and 2007 to seven components (adding nutritional immunomodulation and mitochondrial dysfunction) in 2012, I realized that the time had come to attempt an acronym in order to facilitate student memorization and clinician application. I applied some priority to the sequence of the categories, and then experimented with a few acronyms. The rest, as is said, is history. This occurred just before a series of presentations in France (starting in Paris), Holland, and Belgium in March of 2012. The FINDSEX acronym is a registered trademark (e.g., ® and ™) in association with *Functional Immunology and Nutritional Immunomodulation*[1], *F.I.N.D.S.E.X. The Easily Remembered Acronym for the Functional Inflammology Protocol*[2], *Integrative Rheumatology and Inflammation Mastery, Third Edition*[3], and other books, videos[4], audios[5], and presentations by Dr Vasquez since 2012. One of the more recent introductions to this protocol was delivered at the International Conference on Human Nutrition and Functional Medicine in Portland Oregon in September 2013 and is posted here vimeo.com/ichnfm/drv-functional-inflammology-intro2013 and accessed with the password "DrVprotocol"; any changes to passwords, as well as access to new videos, book updates, and articles are periodically distributed by email newsletter inflammationmastery.com/join_email.html. Purchasers of this book can attend several hours of video introduction/review of this protocol via the access provided in the links below.[6]

---

[1] Published Jun 2012, ISBN-10: 1477603859, ISBN-13: 978-1477603857
[2] Published Apr 2013, ISBN-10: 1484046765, ISBN-13: 978-1484046760
[3] Published Jan 2014, ISBN-10: 1495272621, ISBN-13: 978-1495272622
[4] vimeo.com/drvasquez and vimeo.com/ichnfm
[5] itunes.apple.com/us/artist/dr-alex-vasquez/id475526413 and cdbaby.com/Artist/DrAlexVasquez
[6] Vasquez A. "Introduction to Functional Inflammology Protocol" presented at International Conference on Human Nutrition and Functional Medicine in Portland, Oregon September 25-29, 2013. More than eight hours of video introducing the functional inflammology protocol—to be used with the printed slides in the final section of this book—is available online: vimeo.com/album/2943155. Password: **DrVprotocol_volume1**

❶ **Food** ❷ Infections ❸ Nutri-immunomod ❹ Dysmetab ❺ Stress/Sleep/Socio/Surg/Sup ❻ Endo ❼ Xeno

❶ Food: Diet and Basic Nutritional Supplementation

Major Concepts in this Section

"Food" is the first part of the protocol and the foundation of the overall plan, not simply for improving nutritional status, but for setting the biochemical stage for more profound improvements in immune balance, mitochondrial function, et al. Patients can and should appreciate that they have near complete control over what they consume; unfortunately and conversely, however, in countries such as the United States where much of the food supply is contaminated with pesticide residues and genetically manipulated food-type (GMO) products, consuming a health-promoting diet can present unique challenges.

Contents of this section:
1. Introduction to Nutrigenomics: Gene-Expression Effects of Foods and Nutrients
2. Basic Concepts and Practical Applications via Previously Published Articles
    a. A Five-Part Nutritional Wellness Protocol That Produces Consistently Positive Results: Brief Review of Scientific Rationale
    b. Implementing the Five-Part Nutritional Wellness Protocol for the Treatment of Various Health Problems
    c. Common Oversights and Shortcomings in the Study and Implementation of Nutritional Supplementation
    d. Revisiting the Five-Part Nutritional Wellness Protocol: The Supplemented Paleo-Mediterranean Diet
3. Diet Details, Biochemical Concepts, and Clinical Pearls
    a. Macronutrients and "The Big Picture": Protein, Carbohydrates, Lipids, Fiber, pH Balance
    b. Micronutrients and Nutritional Supplementation—Overview and Concepts: Vitamins, Minerals, Combination Fatty Acids, Probiotics
    c. Additional Considerations: GMO (Genetically Manipulated Organisms/Foods) and related toxins, Gluten, Fructose, TLR, AGE/RAGE, food-induced hypothalamic inflammation, GPR-120
4. Additional Details and Mini-Monographs:
    a. The Major Fatty Acids and End-products of Clinical Significance
    b. NFkB and Its Phytonutritional Modulation
    c. Food Allergy and Adverse Food Reactions: A few considerations and perspectives

Introduction to Nutrigenomics: Pro-Inflammatory and Anti-Inflammatory Effects of Foods and Nutrients

We must look beyond the nutritional properties of foods to appreciate that dietary patterns and the consumption of specific foods can influence genetic expression and either promote or retard the development of inflammation and related clinical disorders. The purpose of this section is to help clinicians attain a more profound understanding of the value of nutrition and its critical role as a foundational component in the treatment plan of patients with inflammatory disorders. The "correct" diet for the vast majority of patients with inflammatory disorders is the "supplemented Paleo-Mediterranean diet" which I have described in several other publications. The diet is modified for the specific exclusion of allergenic foods; it is implemented on a rotation basis, and it allows for periodic fasting and vegetarianism/veganism. The implementation of health-promoting dietary modifications is an *absolutely mandatory* component of the treatment plan, upon which other treatments depend for their success. The study of how dietary components and nutritional supplements influence genetic expression is referred to as *nutrigenomics* or *nutritional genomics* and has been described as "the next frontier in the postgenomic era."[7] Various nutrients have been shown to modulate genetic expression and thus alter phenotypic manifestations of disease by upregulating or downregulating specific genes, interacting with nuclear receptors, altering hormone receptors, and modifying the influence of transcription factors, such as pro-inflammatory NFkB (NFkB) and the anti-inflammatory peroxisome-proliferator activated receptors (PPARs).[8,9,10,11] **The previous view that nutrients only interact with human physiology at the metabolic/post-transcriptional level must be updated in light of current research showing that nutrients can, in fact, modify human physiology and phenotype at the genetic/pre-transcriptional level.** Fatty acids and their *eicosanoid*, *leukotriene*, and *isoprostane* intermediates and end-products modulate genetic expression in several ways. In general, n-3 fatty acids decrease inflammation and promote health while n-6 fatty acids (except for GLA, which is generally health-promoting) increase inflammation, oxidative stress, and the manifestation of disease. Corn oil, probably as a result of its high n-6 LA (linoleic acid) content, rapidly activates NFkB and thus promotes tumor development, atherosclerosis, and elaboration of proinflammatory mediators such as TNFa.[12,13,14] Similarly n-6 arachidonic acid increases production of the free radical *superoxide* approximately 4-fold when added to isolated Kupffer cells *in vitro*. Prostaglandin-E2 is produced from arachidonic acid by cyclooxygenase and increases genetic expression of cyclooxygenase and IL-6; thus, an increase in PG-E2 leads to additive expression of cyclooxygenase, which further increases inflammation and elevates C-reactive protein.[15] Some of the unique health-promoting effects of GLA are nutrigenomically mediated via activation of PPAR-gamma, resultant inhibition of NFkB, and impairment of estrogen receptor function.[16,17] Supplementation with ALA leads to a dramatic reduction of prostaglandin formation in humans[18], and this effect is probably mediated by downregulation of proinflammatory gene transcription, as evidenced by reductions in CRP, IL-6, and serum amyloid A.[19] EPA appears to exert much of its anti-inflammatory benefit by suppressing NFkB activation and thus reducing elaboration of proinflammatory mediators.[20,21] EPA also indirectly modifies gene expression and cell growth by reducing intracellular calcium levels and thus activating protein kinase R which impairs eukaryotic initiation factor-2alpha and inhibits protein synthesis at the level of translation

> **Ayurvedic proverb**
> "When the diet is wrong, medicine is of no use. When the diet is correct, medicine is of no need."

---

[7] Kaput J, Rodriguez RL. Nutritional genomics: the next frontier in the postgenomic era. *Physiol Genomics*. 2004 Jan 15;16(2):166-77. Very important article.
[8] Vamecq J, Latruffe N. Medical significance of peroxisome proliferator-activated receptors. *Lancet*. 1999;354:141-8
[9] Ehrmann J Jr, Vavrusova N, Collan Y, Kolar Z. Peroxisome proliferator-activated receptors (PPARs) in health and disease. *Biomed Pap Med Fac Univ Palacky Olomouc Czech Repub*. 2002 Dec;146(2):11-4 publib.upol.cz/~obd/fulltext/Biomed/2002/2/11.pdf
[10] Kliewer SA, Xu HE, Lambert MH, Willson TM. Peroxisome proliferator-activated receptors: from genes to physiology. *Recent Prog Horm Res*. 2001;56:239-63
[11] Delerive P, Fruchart JC, Staels B. Peroxisome proliferator-activated receptors in inflammation control. *J Endocrinol*. 2001;169(3):453-9
[12] Rusyn I, et al. Corn oil rapidly activates nuclear factor-kappaB in hepatic Kupffer cells by oxidant-dependent mechanisms. *Carcinogenesis*. 1999 Nov;20(11):2095-100
[13] Rose DP, et al. Effect of diets containing different levels of linoleic acid on human breast cancer growth and lung metastasis in nude mice. *Cancer Res* 1993;53:4686-90
[14] Dichtl et al. Linoleic acid-stimulated vascular adhesion molecule-1 expression in endothelial cells depends on nuclear factor-kappaB. *Metabolism* 2002;51:327-33
[15] Bagga D, Wang L, Farias-Eisner R, Glaspy JA, Reddy ST. Differential effects of prostaglandin derived from omega-6 and omega-3 polyunsaturated fatty acids on COX-2 expression and IL-6 secretion. *Proc Natl Acad Sci* U S A. 2003 Feb 18;100(4):1751-6. pnas.org/cgi/reprint/100/4/1751.pdf
[16] Menendez JA, Colomer R, Lupu R. Omega-6 polyunsaturated fatty acid gamma-linolenic acid (18:3n-6) is a selective estrogen-response modulator in human breast cancer cells: gamma-linolenic acid antagonizes estrogen receptor-dependent transcriptional activity, transcriptionally represses estrogen receptor expression and synergistically enhances tamoxifen and ICI 182,780 (Faslodex) efficacy in human breast cancer cells. *Int J Cancer*. 2004 May 10;109(6):949-54
[17] Jiang WG, Redfern A, Bryce RP, Mansel RE. Peroxisome proliferator activated receptor-gamma (PPAR-gamma) mediates the action of gamma linolenic acid in breast cancer cells. *Prostaglandins Leukot Essent Fatty Acids*. 2000 Feb;62(2):119-27
[18] Adam O, et al. Effect of alpha-linolenic acid in the human diet on linoleic acid metabolism and prostaglandin biosynthesis. *J Lipid Res*. 1986 Apr;27(4):421-6
[19] Rallidis et al. Dietary alpha-linolenic acid decreases C-reactive protein, serum amyloid A and interleukin-6 in dyslipidaemic patients. *Atherosclerosis*. 2003;167:237-42
[20] Zhao Y, et al. Eicosapentaenoic acid prevents LPS-induced TNF-alpha expression by preventing NFkB activation. *J Am Coll Nutr*. 2004 Feb;23(1):71-8
[21] Mishra A, et al. Oxidized omega-3 fatty acids inhibit NFkB activation via a PPARalpha-dependent pathway. *Arterioscler Thromb Vasc Biol*. 2004 Sep;24:1621-7

initiation, thereby mediating an anti-cancer benefit.[22] DHA is the precursor to docosatrienes and resolvins which downregulate gene expression for IL-1, inhibit TNFa, and reduce neutrophil entry to sites of inflammation.[23] Oxidized EPA activates PPAR-alpha and thereby suppresses NFkB.[24,25] Other nutrients that inhibit the activation of NFkB include vitamin D[26,27], lipoic acid[28], green tea[29], rosemary[30], grape seed extract[31], resveratrol[32,33], caffeic acid phenethyl ester (CAPE) from bee propolis[34], indole-3-carbinol[35], N-acetyl-L-cysteine[36], selenium[37], and zinc.[38] **Therefore, we see that fatty acids and nutrients directly affect gene expression by complex and multiple mechanisms, as graphically illustrated in the accompanying diagram, and the synergism and potency of these anti-inflammatory nutraceuticals supports the rationale for the use of nutrition and select botanicals for the safe and effective treatment of inflammatory disorders.**

---

[22] Palakurthi et al. Inhibition of translation initiation mediates the anti-cancer effect of the n-3 polyunsaturated fatty acid EPA. *Cancer Res.* 2000 Jun 1;60(11):2919-25

[23] "These results indicate that DHA is the precursor to potent protective mediators generated via enzymatic oxygenations to novel docosatrienes and 17S series resolvins that each regulate events of interest in inflammation and resolution." Hong S, Gronert K, Devchand PR, Moussignac RL, Serhan CN. Novel docosatrienes and 17S-resolvins generated from docosahexaenoic acid in murine brain, human blood, and glial cells. Autacoids in anti-inflammation. *J Biol Chem.* 2003 Apr 25;278(17):14677-87

[24] Mishra A, et al. Oxidized omega-3 fatty acids inhibit NFkB activation via a PPARalpha-dependent pathway. *Arterioscler Thromb Vasc Biol.* 2004 Sep;24:1621-7

[25] Delerive P, Fruchart JC, Staels B. Peroxisome proliferator-activated receptors in inflammation control. J Endocrinol. 2001;169(3):453-9

[26] "1Alpha,25-dihydroxyvitamin D3 (1,25-(OH)2-D3), the active metabolite of vitamin D, can inhibit NFkB activity in human MRC-5 fibroblasts, targeting DNA binding of NFkB but not translocation of its subunits p50 and p65." Harant H, Wolff B, Lindley IJ. 1Alpha,25-dihydroxyvitamin D3 decreases DNA binding of nuclear factor-kappaB in human fibroblasts. *FEBS Lett.* 1998 Oct 9;436(3):329-34

[27] "Thus, 1,25(OH)2D3 may negatively regulate IL-12 production by downregulation of NF-kB activation and binding to the p40-kB sequence." D'Ambrosio D, et al. Inhibition of IL-12 production by 1,25-dihydroxyvitamin D3. Involvement of NFkB downregulation. *J Clin Invest.* 1998 Jan 1;101(1):252-62

[28] "ALA reduced the TNF-alpha-stimulated ICAM-1 expression in a dose-dependent manner, to levels observed in unstimulated cells. Alpha-lipoic acid also reduced NFkB activity in these cells in a dose-dependent manner." Lee HA, Hughes DA.Alpha-lipoic acid modulates NFkB activity in human monocytic cells by direct interaction with DNA. *Exp Gerontol.* 2002 Jan-Mar;37(2-3):401-10

[29] "In conclusion, EGCG is an effective inhibitor of IKK activity. This may explain, at least in part, some of the reported anti-inflammatory and anti-cancer effects of green tea." Yang F, et al. The green tea polyphenol (-)-epigallocatechin-3-gallate blocks nuclear factor-kappa B activation by inhibiting I kappa B kinase activity in the intestinal epithelial cell line IEC-6. *Mol Pharmacol.* 2001 Sep;60(3):528-33

[30] "These results suggest that carnosol suppresses the NO production and iNOS gene expression by inhibiting NFkB activation, and provide possible mechanisms for its anti-inflammatory and chemopreventive action." Lo AH, Liang YC, Lin-Shiau SY, Ho CT, Lin JK. Carnosol, an antioxidant in rosemary, suppresses inducible nitric oxide synthase through down-regulating nuclear factor-kappaB in mouse macrophages. *Carcinogenesis.* 2002 Jun;23(6):983-91

[31] "Constitutive and TNFalpha-induced NFkB DNA binding activity was inhibited by GSE at doses > or =50 microg/ml and treatments for > or =12 h." Dhanalakshmi S, et al. Inhibition of NFkB pathway in grape seed extract-induced apoptotic death of human prostate carcinoma DU145 cells. *Int J Oncol.* 2003 Sep;23(3):721-7

[32] "Resveratrol's anticarcinogenic, anti-inflammatory, and growth-modulatory effects may thus be partially ascribed to the inhibition of activation of NFkB and AP-1 and the associated kinases." Manna SK, Mukhopadhyay A, Aggarwal BB. Resveratrol suppresses TNF-induced activation of nuclear transcription factors NF-kappa B, activator protein-1, and apoptosis: potential role of reactive oxygen intermediates and lipid peroxidation. *J Immunol.* 2000 Jun 15;164(12):6509-19

[33] "Both resveratrol and quercetin inhibited NFkB-, AP-1- and CREB-dependent transcription to a greater extent than the glucocorticosteroid, dexamethasone." Donnelly LE, et al. Anti-inflammatory Effects of Resveratrol in Lung Epithelial Cells. *Am J Physiol Lung Cell Mol Physiol.* 2004 Oct;287(4):L774-83

[34] "Caffeic acid phenethyl ester (CAPE) is an anti-inflammatory component of propolis (honeybee resin). CAPE is reportedly a specific inhibitor of nuclear factor-kappaB (NFkB)." Fitzpatrick LR, Wang J, Le T. Caffeic acid phenethyl ester, an inhibitor of nuclear factor-kappaB, attenuates bacterial peptidoglycan polysaccharide-induced colitis in rats. *J Pharmacol Exp Ther.* 2001 Dec;299(3):915-20

[35] Takada Y, Andreeff M, Aggarwal BB. Indole-3-carbinol suppresses NF-{kappa}B and I{kappa}B{alpha} kinase activation causing inhibition of expression of NF-{kappa}B-regulated antiapoptotic and metastatic gene products and enhancement of apoptosis in myeloid and leukemia cells. *Blood.* 2005 Apr 5; [Epub ahead of print]

[36] Paterson RL, Galley HF, Webster NR. The effect of N-acetylcysteine on nuclear factor-kappa B activation, interleukin-6, interleukin-8, and intercellular adhesion molecule-1 expression in patients with sepsis. *Crit Care Med.* 2003 Nov;31(11):2574-8

[37] Faure P, Ramon O, Favier A, Halimi S. Selenium supplementation decreases nuclear factor-kappa B activity in peripheral blood mononuclear cells from type 2 diabetic patients. *Eur J Clin Invest.* 2004;34(7):475-81

[38] Uzzo RG, et al. Zinc inhibits nuclear factor-kappa B activation and sensitizes prostate cancer cells to cytotoxic agents. *Clin Cancer Res.* 2002;8(11):3579-83

Chapter 4: Major Modifiable Factors in Systemic Inflammation

Schematic Representation of Simultaneous Nutrigenomic and Metabolic Effects of Nutrients: Although conceptually accurate, this diagram is highly simplified and not all-inclusive; rather, this diagram focuses exclusively on nutrients that affect the NFkB pathway. Updated from Vasquez 2005.[39,40]

---

[39] Vasquez A. New Insights into Fatty Acid Supplementation and Its Effect on Eicosanoid Production and Genetic Expression. *Nutritional Perspectives* 2005; Jan: 5-16
[40] Vasquez A. Nutritional and Botanical Inhibition of NFkB, the Major Intracellular Amplifier of the Inflammatory Cascade. A Practical Clinical Strategy Exemplifying Anti-Inflammatory Nutrigenomics. *Nutritional Perspectives* 2005;July: 5-12

A Five-Part Nutritional Wellness Protocol That Produces Consistently Positive Results: Brief Review of Scientific Rationale

This article was originally published in *Nutritional Wellness*
nutritionalwellness.com/archives/2005/sep/09_vasquez.php

Introduction: When I am lecturing here in the U.S., as well as in Europe, doctors often ask if I will share the details of my protocols with them. Thus, in 2004, I published a 486-page textbook for doctors that includes several protocols and important concepts for the promotion of wellness and treatment of musculoskeletal disorders.[41] In this article, I will share with you what I consider a basic protocol for wellness promotion. I've implemented this protocol as part of the treatment plan for a wide range of clinical problems. In my next column, I will provide several case reports of patients from my office to exemplify the effectiveness of this program and show how it can be the foundation upon which additional treatments can be added as necessary.

Nutrients are required in the proper amounts, forms, and approximate ratios for essential physiologic function; if nutrients are lacking, the body cannot function normally, let alone optimally. Impaired function results in subjective and objective manifestations of what is commonly labeled as "disease." Thus, a powerful and effective alternative to treating diseases with drugs is to re-establish normal/optimal physiologic function by replenishing the body with essential nutrients.

Of course, many diseases are multifactorial and therefore require multicomponent treatment plans, and some diseases actually require the use of drugs. However, while only a relatively small portion of patients actually need drugs for their problems, I am sure we all agree that everyone needs a foundational nutrition plan, as outlined and substantiated below.

1. <u>Health-promoting diet</u>: Following an extensive review of the research literature, I developed what I call the "supplemented Paleo-Mediterranean diet," which I have described in greater detail elsewhere.[42] In essence, this diet plan combines the best of the Mediterranean diet with the best of the Paleolithic diet, the latter of which has been detailed and popularized by Dr. Loren Cordain in his book, *The Paleo Diet*, and his numerous scientific articles.[43] This diet places emphasis on fruits, vegetables, nuts, seeds, and berries that meet the body's needs for fiber, carbohydrates, and most importantly, the 8,000+ phytonutrients that have additive and synergistic health benefits.[44] Preferred protein sources are lean meats such as fish and poultry. In contrast to Cordain's Paleo diet, I also advocate soy and whey for their high-quality protein and anticancer, cardioprotective, and mood-enhancing benefits. Rice and potatoes are discouraged due to their relatively high glycemic indexes and high glycemic loads, and their lack of fiber and phytonutrients (compared to other fruits and vegetables). Generally speaking, grains such as barley, rye, and wheat (e.g., the "toxic triad" of inflammatory gluten) are discouraged due to the high glycemic loads/indexes of most breads and pastries, as well as the allergenicity/immunogenicity of gluten, a protein that appears to help trigger disorders such as migraine, celiac disease, psoriasis, epilepsy, and autoimmunity. Sources of simple sugars such as high-fructose corn syrup (e.g., cola, soda) and processed foods (e.g., "TV dinners" and other manufactured snacks and convenience foods) are strictly forbidden. Chemical preservatives, colorants, sweeteners and carrageenan are likewise prohibited. In summary, this diet plan provides plenty of variety, as most dishes comprised of poultry, fish, soy, fruits, vegetables, nuts, berries, and seeds are allowed. The diet also provides plenty of fiber, phytonutrients, carbohydrates, potassium, and protein, while simultaneously being low in fat, sodium, arachidonic acid, and "simple sugars." The diet must be customized with regard to total protein and calorie intake, as determined by the size, status, and activity level of the patient, and individual food allergens should be avoided. Regular consumption of this diet has shown the ability to reduce hypertension, alleviate diabetes, ameliorate migraine headaches, and result in improvement of overall health and a lessening of the severity of many common "diseases." This diet is supplemented with vitamins, minerals, and fatty acids as described below.

2. <u>Multivitamin and multimineral supplementation</u>: Vitamin and mineral supplementation finally received endorsement from "mainstream" medicine when researchers from Harvard Medical School published a review

---

[41] Vasquez A. *Integrative Orthopedics: The Art of Creating Wellness While Managing Acute and Chronic Musculoskeletal Disorders*. 2004, 2007, 2012
[42] Vasquez A. The Importance of Integrative Chiropractic Health Care in Treating Musculoskeletal Pain and Reducing the Nationwide Burden of Medical Expenses and Iatrogenic Injury and Death: Concise Review of Current Research and Implications for Clinical Practice and Healthcare Policy. *The Original Internist* 2005; 12(4): 159-182
[43] Cordain L. *The Paleo Diet*. (John Wiley and Sons, 2002). Also: Cordain L. Cereal grains: humanity's double edged sword. *World Rev Nutr Diet* 1999;84:19-73 Access to most of Dr Cordain's articles is available at thepaleodiet.com/
[44] Liu RH. Health benefits of fruit and vegetables are from additive and synergistic combinations of phytochemicals. *Am J Clin Nutr* 2003;78(3 Suppl):517S-520S

article in *Journal of the American Medical Association* that concluded, "Most people do not consume an optimal amount of all vitamins by diet alone. ...It appears prudent for all adults to take vitamin supplements."[45] Long-term nutritional insufficiencies experienced by the majority of the population promote the development of "long-latency deficiency diseases" such as cancer, neuroemotional deterioration, and cardiovascular disease.[46] Impressively, the benefits of multivitamin/multimineral supplementation have been demonstrated in numerous clinical trials. Multivitamin/multimineral supplementation has been shown to improve nutritional status and reduce the risk for chronic diseases[47], improve mood[48], potentiate antidepressant drug treatment[49], alleviate migraine headaches (when used with diet improvement and fatty acids[50]), improve immune function and infectious disease outcomes in the elderly[51] (especially diabetics[52]), reduce morbidity and mortality in patients with HIV infection[53,54] alleviate premenstrual syndrome[55,56] and bipolar disorder[57], reduce violence and antisocial behavior in children[58] and incarcerated young adults (when used with essential fatty acids[59]), and improve scores of intelligence in children.[60] Vitamin supplementation has anti-inflammatory benefits, as evidenced by significant reduction in C-reactive protein, (CRP) in a double-blind, placebo-controlled trial.[61] The ability to safely and affordably deliver these benefits makes multimineral-multivitamin supplementation and essential component of any and all health-promoting and disease-prevention strategies. Vitamin A can result in liver damage with chronic consumption of 25,000 IU or more, and intake should generally not exceed 10,000 IU per day in women of childbearing age. Iron should not be supplemented except in patients diagnosed with iron deficiency by the blood test ferritin. Additional vitamin D should be used, as described in the next section.

3. <u>Physiologic doses of vitamin D3</u>: The prevalence of vitamin D deficiency varies from 40 percent (general population) to almost 100 percent (patients with musculoskeletal pain) in the American population. I described the many benefits of vitamin D3 supplementation in the previous issue of *Nutritional Wellness* and in the major monograph published in 2004.[62] In summary, vitamin D deficiency causes or contributes to depression, hypertension, seizures, migraine, polycystic ovary syndrome, inflammation, autoimmunity, and musculoskeletal pain such as low-back pain. Clinical trials using vitamin D supplementation have proven the cause-and-effect relationship between vitamin D deficiency and these conditions by showing that each of these could be cured or alleviated with vitamin D supplementation. In our review of the literature, we concluded that daily vitamin D doses should be 1,000 IU for infants, 2,000 IU for children, and 4,000 IU for adults. Cautions and contraindications include the use of thiazide diuretics (e.g., hydrochlorothiazide) or any other medications that can promote hypercalcemia, as well as granulomatous diseases such as sarcoidosis, tuberculosis, and certain types of cancer, especially lymphoma. Effectiveness is monitored by measuring serum 25-OH-vitamin D, and safety is monitored by measuring serum calcium.

4. <u>Balanced and complete fatty acid supplementation</u>: A detailed survey of the literature reveals five major health-promoting anti-inflammatory fatty acids found in the human diet.[63] These are alpha-linolenic acid (ALA; omega-3, from flaxseed oil), eicosapentaenoic acid (EPA; omega-3, from fish oil), docosahexaenoic acid (DHA; omega-3, from fish oil and algae), gamma-linolenic acid (GLA; omega-6, most concentrated in borage oil), and oleic acid (omega-9, mainly from olive oil, also found in flaxseed and borage oils). Each of these fatty acids has health benefits that cannot be fully attained from supplementing a different fatty acid. The benefits of GLA

---

[45] Fletcher RH, Fairfield KM. Vitamins for chronic disease prevention in adults: clinical applications. *JAMA* 2002;287:3127-9
[46] Heaney RP. Long-latency deficiency disease: insights from calcium and vitamin D. *Am J Clin Nutr* 2003;78:912-9
[47] McKay DL, Perrone G, Rasmussen H, Dallal G, Hartman W, Cao G, Prior RL, Roubenoff R, Blumberg JB. The effects of a multivitamin/mineral supplement on micronutrient status, antioxidant capacity and cytokine production in healthy older adults consuming a fortified diet. *J Am Coll Nutr* 2000;19(5):613-21
[48] Benton D, Haller J, Fordy J. Vitamin supplementation for 1 year improves mood. *Neuropsychobiology* 1995;32(2):98-105
[49] Coppen A, Bailey J. Enhancement of the antidepressant action of fluoxetine by folic acid: a randomised, placebo controlled trial. *J Affect Disord* 2000;60:121-30
[50] Wagner W, Nootbaar-Wagner U. Prophylactic treatment of migraine with gamma-linolenic and alpha-linolenic acids. *Cephalalgia* 1997;17:127-30
[51] Langkamp-Henken et al. Nutritional formula enhanced immune function and reduced days of symptoms of URI in seniors. *J Am Geriatr Soc* 2004;52:3-12
[52] Barringer TA, et al. Effect of a multivitamin and mineral supplement on infection and quality of life. *Ann Intern Med* 2003;138:365-71
[53] Fawzi WW, Msamanga GI, et al. A randomized trial of multivitamin supplements and HIV disease progression and mortality. *N Engl J Med* 2004;351:23-32
[54] Burbano X, et al. Impact of a selenium chemoprevention clinical trial on hospital admissions of HIV-infected participants. *HIV Clin Trials* 2002;3:483-91
[55] Abraham GE. Nutritional factors in the etiology of the premenstrual tension syndromes. *J Reprod Med* 1983;28(7):446-64
[56] Stewart A. Clinical and biochemical effects of nutritional supplementation on the premenstrual syndrome. *J Reprod Med* 1987;32:435-41
[57] Kaplan BJ, et al. Effective mood stabilization with a chelated mineral supplement: an open-label trial in bipolar disorder. *J Clin Psychiatry* 2001;62:936-44
[58] Kaplan BJ, et al. Treatment of mood lability and explosive rage with minerals and vitamins: two case studies. *J Child Adolesc Psychopharmacol* 2002;12(3):205-19
[59] Gesch et al. Influence of supplementary vitamins, minerals and essential fatty acids on the antisocial behaviour of young adult prisoners. *Br J Psychiatry* 2002;181:22-8
[60] Benton D. Micro-nutrient supplementation and the intelligence of children. *Neurosci Biobehav Rev* 2001;25:297-309
[61] Church TS, Earnest CP, Wood KA, Kampert JB. Reduction of C-reactive protein levels through use of a multivitamin. *Am J Med* 2003;115:702-7
[62] Vasquez A, Manso G, Cannell J. The clinical importance of vitamin D (cholecalciferol): a paradigm shift. *Alternative Therapies in Health and Medicine* 2004;10:28-37
[63] Vasquez A. New Insights into Fatty Acid Supplementation and Its Effect on Eicosanoid Production and Genetic Expression. *Nutritional Perspectives* 2005; Jan: 5-16

(borage oil) are not attained by consumption of EPA and DHA (fish oil); in fact, consumption of fish oil can actually promote a deficiency of GLA.[64] Likewise, consumption of GLA alone can reduce EPA levels while increasing levels of proinflammatory arachidonic acid; both of these problems are avoided with co-administration of fish oil any time borage oil is used. Using ALA (flaxseed oil) alone only slightly increases EPA but generally leads to no improvement in DHA status and can lead to a reduction of oleic acid; thus, fish oil, olive oil (and borage oil) should be supplemented when flaxseed oil is used.[65] Obviously, the goal here is a balanced intake of all of the health-promoting fatty acids; using only one or two sources of fatty acids is not balanced and results in suboptimal improvement, at best. In clinical practice, I routinely use combination fatty acid therapy comprised of ALA, EPA, DHA, and GLA for essentially all patients. The product also contains a modest amount of oleic acid, and I encourage use of olive oil for salads and cooking. This approach results in complete and balanced fatty acid intake, and the clinical benefits are impressive.

5. Probiotics /gut flora modification: Proper levels of good bacteria promote intestinal health, proper immune function, and support overall health. Excess bacteria or yeast, or the presence of harmful bacteria, yeast, or "parasites" such as amoebas and protozoans, can cause "leaky gut," systemic inflammation, and a wide range of clinical problems. Intestinal flora can become imbalanced by poor diets, excess stress, immunosuppressive drugs, antibiotics, or exposure to contaminated food or water, all of which are common among American patients. Thus, as a rule, I reinstate the good bacteria by the use of probiotics (good bacteria and yeast), prebiotics (fiber, arabinogalactan, and inulin), and the use of fermented foods such as kefir (in patients not allergic to milk). Harmful yeast, bacteria, and other "parasites" can be eradicated with the combination of dietary change, drugs, and/or herbal extracts. For example, oregano oil in an emulsified, time-released form has proven safe and effective for the elimination of various parasites encountered in clinical practice.[66] Likewise, the herb *Artemisia annua* (sweet wormwood) commonly is used to eradicate specific bacteria and has been used for thousands of years in Asia for the treatment and prevention of infectious diseases, including malaria.[67]

Conclusion: In this brief review, I have outlined and scientifically substantiated a fundamental protocol that can serve as effective therapy for patients with a wide range of "diseases." Customizing the Paleo-Mediterranean diet to avoid food allergens, using vitamin-mineral supplements along with physiologic doses of vitamin D and broad-spectrum balanced fatty acid supplementation, and ensuring gastrointestinal health with the skillful use of probiotics, prebiotics, and antimicrobial treatments provides an excellent health-promoting and disease-eliminating foundation and lifestyle for many patients. Often, this simple protocol is all that is needed for the effective treatment of a wide range of clinical problems. For other patients with more complex illnesses, of course, additional interventions and laboratory assessments can be used to customize the treatment plan. However, we must always remember that the attainment and preservation of health requires that we meet the body's basic nutritional needs. This five-step protocol begins the process of meeting those needs. In my next article, I'll give you some examples from my clinical practice and additional references to show this protocol's safety and effectiveness.

Implementing the Five-Part Nutritional Wellness Protocol for the Treatment of Various Health Problems

This article was originally published in *Nutritional Wellness*
nutritionalwellness.com/archives/2005/nov/11_vasquez.php

Introduction: In my last article in *Nutritional Wellness* I described a 5-part nutritional protocol that can be used in the vast majority of patients without adverse effects and with major benefits. For many patients, the basic protocol consisting of 1) the Paleo-Mediterranean diet, 2) multivitamin/multimineral supplementation, 3) additional vitamin D3, 4) combination fatty acid therapy with an optimal balance of ALA, GLA, EPA, DHA, and oleic acid, and 5) probiotics (including the identification and eradication of harmful yeast, bacteria, and other "parasites") is all the treatment that they need. For patients who need additional treatment, this foundational plan still serves as the core of the biochemical aspect of their intervention. Of course, in some cases, we have to use other lifestyle modifications

---

[64] Cleland LG, Gibson RA, Neumann M, French JK. The effect of dietary fish oil supplement upon the content of dihomo-gammalinolenic acid in human plasma phospholipids. *Prostaglandins Leukot Essent Fatty Acids* 1990 May;40(1):9-12
[65] Jantti J, Nikkari T, Solakivi T, et al. Evening primrose oil in rheumatoid arthritis: changes in serum lipids and fatty acids. *Ann Rheum Dis* 1989;48(2):124-7
[66] Force M, Sparks WS, Ronzio RA. Inhibition of enteric parasites by emulsified oil of oregano in vivo. *Phytother Res* 2000;14:213-4
[67] Schuster BG. Demonstrating the validity of natural products as anti-infective drugs. *J Altern Complement Med* 2001;7 Suppl 1:S73-82

(such as exercise), additional supplements (such as policosanol or antimicrobial herbs), manual treatments (including spinal manipulation) and occasionally select medications (such has hormone modulators) to obtain our goal of maximum improvement.

The following examples show how the 5-part protocol serves to benefit patients with a wide range of conditions. For the sake of saving space, I will use only highly specific citations to the research literature, since I have provided the other references in the previous issue of *Nutritional Wellness* and elsewhere.[68]

- A Man with High Cholesterol: This patient is a 41-year-old slightly overweight man with very high cholesterol. His total cholesterol was 290 (normal < 200), LDL cholesterol was 212 (normal <130), and his triglycerides were 148 (optimal <100). I am quite certain that nearly every medical doctor would have put this man on cholesterol-lowering statin drugs for life. *Treatment*: In contrast, I advised a low-carb Paleo-Mediterranean diet because such diets have been shown to reduce cardiovascular mortality more powerfully that "statin" cholesterol-lowing drugs in older patients.[69] Likewise, fatty acid supplementation is more effective than statin drugs for reducing cardiac and all-cause mortality.[70] We added probiotics, because supplementation with *Lactobacillus* and *Bifidobacterium* has been shown to lower cholesterol levels in humans with high cholesterol.[71] Finally, I also prescribed 20 mg of policosanol for its well-known ability to favorably modify cholesterol levels.[72] *Results*: Within *one month* the patient had lost weight, felt better, and his total cholesterol had dropped to normal at 196 (from 290!), LDL was reduced to 141, and triglycerides were reduced to 80. Basically, this treatment plan was "the protocol + policosanol." Drug treatment of this patient would have been more expensive, more risky, and would not have resulted in global health improvements.

- A Child with Intractable Seizures: This is a 4-year-old nonverbal boy with 3-5 seizures per day despite being on two anti-seizure medications and having previously had several other "last resort" medical and surgical procedures. He also had a history of food allergies. *Treatment*: Obviously, there was no room for error in this case. We implemented a moderately low-carb hypoallergenic diet since both carbohydrate restriction[73] and allergy avoidance[74] can reduce the frequency and severity of seizures. Since many "anti-seizure" medications actually cause seizures by causing vitamin D deficiency[75], I added 800 IU per day of emulsified vitamin D3 for its antiseizure benefit.[76] We used 1 tsp per day of a combination fatty acid supplement that provides balanced amounts of ALA, GLA, EPA, and DHA, since fatty acids appear to have potential antiseizure benefits.[77] Vitamin B-6 (250 mg of P5P) and magnesium (bowel tolerance) were also added to reduce brain hyperexcitability.[78] Stool testing showed an absence of *Bifidobacteria* and *Lactobacillus*; probiotics were added for their anti-allergy benefits.[79] *Results*: Within about 2 months seizure frequency reduced from 3-5 per day to one seizure every other day: *an 87% reduction in seizure frequency*. Patient was able to discontinue one of the anti-seizure medications. His parents also noted several global improvements: the boy started making eye contact with people, he was learning again, and intellectually he was "making gains every day." His parents considered this an "amazing difference." Going from 30 seizures per week to 4 seizures per week while reducing medication use by 50% is a major achievement. Notice that we simply used the basic wellness protocol with some additional B6 and magnesium. It is highly unlikely that B6 and magnesium alone would have produced such a favorable response.

- A Young Woman with Full-Body Psoriasis Unresponsive to Drug Treatment: This is a 17-year-old woman with head-to-toe psoriasis since childhood. She wears long pants and long-sleeved shirts year-round, and the psoriasis is a major interference to her social life. Medications have ceased to help. *Treatment*: The Paleo-Mediterranean diet was implemented with an emphasis on food allergy identification.[1] We used a multivitamin-

---

[68] Vasquez A. *Integrative Orthopedics*. By now of course, this book has been surpassed in content of nutritional information, particularly in books printed past 2009.
[69] Knoops KT, et al. Mediterranean diet, lifestyle factors, and 10-year mortality in elderly European men and women. *JAMA*. 2004 Sep 22;292(12):1433-9
[70] Studer M, et al. Effect of different antilipidemic agents and diets on mortality: a systematic review. *Arch Intern Med*. 2005;165:725-30
[71] Xiao JZ, et al. Effects of milk products fermented by Bifidobacterium longum on blood lipids in rats and healthy adult male volunteers. *J Dairy Sci*. 2003;86:2452-61
[72] Cholesterol-lowering action of policosanol compares well to that of pravastatin and lovastatin. *Cardiovasc J S Afr*. 2003;14(3):161
[73] Freeman JM, et al. The efficacy of the ketogenic diet-1998: a prospective evaluation of intervention in 150 children. *Pediatrics*. 1998;102:1358-63
[74] Egger J, Carter CM, Soothill JF, Wilson J. Oligoantigenic diet treatment of children with epilepsy and migraine. *J Pediatr*. 1989;114:51-8
[75] Ali FE, Al-Bustan MA, Al-Busairi WA, Al-Mulla FA. Loss of seizure control due to anticonvulsant-induced hypocalcemia. *Ann Pharmacother*. 2004;38:1002-5
[76] Christiansen C, Rodbro P, Sjo O."Anticonvulsant action" of vitamin D in epileptic patients? A controlled pilot study. *Br Med J*. 1974 May 4;2(913):258-9
[77] Yuen AW, et al. Omega-3 fatty acid supplementation in patients with chronic epilepsy: A randomized trial. *Epilepsy Behav*. 2005 Sep;7(2):253-8
[78] Mousain-Bosc M, et al. Magnesium VitB6 intake reduces central nervous system hyperexcitability in children. *J Am Coll Nutr*. 2004;23(5):545S-548S
[79] Majamaa H, Isolauri E.Probiotics: a novel approach in the management of food allergy. *J Allergy Clin Immunol*. 1997 Feb;99(2):179-85

mineral supplement with 200 mcg selenium to compensate for the nutritional insufficiencies and selenium deficiency that are common in patients with psoriasis; likewise 10 mg of folic acid was added to address the relative vitamin deficiencies and elevated homocysteine that are common in these patients.[80] Combination fatty acid therapy with EPA and DHA from fish oil and GLA from borage oil was used for the anti-inflammatory and skin-healing benefits.[81] Vitamin E (1200 IU of mixed tocopherols) and lipoic acid (1,000 mg per day) were added for their anti-inflammatory benefits and to combat the oxidative stress that is characteristic of psoriasis.[82] Of course, probiotics were used to modify gut flora, which is commonly deranged in patients with psoriasis.[83] ***Results***: Within a few weeks, this patient's "lifelong psoriasis" was essentially gone. Food allergy identification and avoidance played a major role in the success of this case. When I saw the patient again 9 months later for her second visit, she had no visible evidence of psoriasis. Her "medically untreatable" condition was essentially cured by the use of my basic protocol, with the addition of a few extra nutrients.

- A Man with Fatigue and Recurrent Numbness in Hands and Feet. This 40-year-old man had seen numerous neurologists and had spent tens of thousands of dollars on MRIs, CT scans, lumbar punctures, and other diagnostic procedures. No diagnosis had been found, and no effective treatment had been rendered by medical specialists. ***Assessments***: We performed a modest battery of lab tests which revealed elevations of fibrinogen and C-reactive protein (CRP), two markers of acute inflammation. Assessment of intestinal permeability with the lactulose-mannitol assay showed major intestinal damage ("leaky gut"). Follow-up parasite testing on different occasions showed dysbiosis caused by *Proteus*, *Enterobacter*, *Klebsiella*, *Citrobacter*, and *Pseudomonas aeruginosa*—of course, these are gram-negative bacteria that can induce immune dysfunction and autoimmunity, as described elsewhere.[1] Specifically, *Pseudomonas aeruginosa* has been linked to the development of nervous system autoimmunity, such as multiple sclerosis.[84] ***Treatment***: We implemented a plan of diet modification, vitamins, minerals, fatty acids, and probiotics. The dysbiosis was further addressed with specific antimicrobial herbs (including caprylic acid and emulsified oregano oil[85]) and drugs (such as tetracycline, Bactrim, and Augmentin). The antibiotic drugs proved to be ineffective based on repeat stool testing. ***Results***: Within one month we witnessed impressive improvements, both subjectively and objectively. Subjectively, the patient reported that the numbness and tingling almost completely resolved. Fatigue was reduced, and energy was improved. Objectively, the patient's elevated CRP plummeted from abnormally high at 11 down to completely normal at 1. Eighteen months later, the patient's CRP had dropped to less than 1 and fatigue and numbness were no longer problematic. Notice that this treatment plan was basically "the protocol" with additional attention to eradicating the dysbiosis we found with specialized stool testing.
- A 50-year-old Man with Rheumatoid Arthritis. This patient presented with a 3-year history of rheumatoid arthritis that had been treated unsuccessfully with drugs (methotrexate and intravenous Remicade). The first time I tested his hsCRP level, it was astronomically high at 124 mg/L (normal is <3). Because of the severe inflammation and other risk factors for sudden cardiac death, I referred this patient to an osteopathic internist for immune-suppressing drugs; the patient refused, stating that he was no longer willing to rely on immune-suppressing chemical medications. His treatment was entirely up to me. ***Assessments and Treatments***: We implemented the Paleo-Mediterranean diet and a program of vitamins, minerals, optimal combination fatty acid therapy (providing ALA, GLA, EPA, DHA, and oleic acid), and 4000 IU of vitamin D in emulsified form to overcome defects in absorption that are seen in older patients and those with gastrointestinal problems.[86] Hormone testing showed abnormally low DHEA, low testosterone, and slightly elevated estrogen; these problems were corrected with DHEA supplementation and the use of a hormone-modulating drug (Arimidex) that lowers estrogen and raises testosterone. Specialized stool testing showed absence of *Lactobacillus* and *Bifidobacteria* and intestinal overgrowth of *Citrobacter* and *Enterobacter* which was corrected with probiotics and antimicrobial treatments including undecylenic acid and emulsified oregano oil. Importantly, I also decided to inhibit NFkB (the primary transcription factor that upregulates the pro-inflammatory response[87]) by using a

---

[80] Vanizor Kural B, et al. Plasma homocysteine and its relationships with atherothrombotic markers in psoriatic patients. *Clin Chim Acta*. 2003 Jun;332(1-2):23-3
[81] Vasquez A. New Insights into Fatty Acid Supplementation and Its Effect on Eicosanoid Production and Genetic Expression. *Nutritional Perspectives* 2005; January: 5-16
[82] Kokcam I, Naziroglu M. Antioxidants and lipid peroxidation status in the blood of patients with psoriasis. *Clin Chim Acta*. 1999 Nov;289(1-2):23-31
[83] Waldman A, et al. Incidence of Candida in psoriasis--a study on the fungal flora of psoriatic patients. *Mycoses*. 2001 May;44(3-4):77-81
[84] Hughes LE, et al. Antibody responses to Acinetobacter spp. and Pseudomonas aeruginosa in multiple sclerosis. *Clin Diagn Lab Immunol.* 2001;8(6):1181-8
[85] Force M, Sparks WS, Ronzio RA. Inhibition of enteric parasites by emulsified oil of oregano in vivo. *Phytother Res*. 2000 May;14(3):213-4
[86] Vasquez A. Subphysiologic Doses of Vitamin D are Subtherapeutic: Comment on the Study by The Record Trial Group. *TheLancet.com* Accessed June 16, 2005
[87] Tak PP, Firestein GS. NFkB: a key role in inflammatory diseases. *J Clin Invest*. 2001 Jan;107(1):7-11

combination botanical formula that contains curcumin, piperine, lipoic acid, green tea extract, propolis, rosemary, resveratrol, ginger, and Phytolens™ (an antioxidant extract from lentils that may inhibit autoimmunity[88])—all of these herbs and nutrients have been shown to inhibit NFkB and to thus downregulate inflammatory responses.[89] **Results**: Within 6 weeks, this patient had happily lost 10 lbs of excess weight and was able to work without pain for the first time in years. **Follow-up testing showed that his hsCRP had dropped from 124 to 7 mg/L—a drop of 114 points—95%!—in less than one month: better than had ever been achieved even with the use of intravenous immune-suppressing drugs!** This patient continues to make significant progress. Obviously this case was complex, and we needed to do more than the basic protocol. Nonetheless, the basic protocol still served as the foundation for the treatment plan. Note that vitamin D has significant anti-inflammatory benefits and can cause major reductions in inflammation measured by CRP.[90] The correction of the hormonal abnormalities and the dysbiosis, and downregulating NFkB with several botanical extracts were also critical components of this successful treatment plan.

Summary and Conclusions: These examples show how the nutritional wellness protocol that I described in the September issue of *Nutritional Wellness* can be used as the foundational treatment for a wide range of health problems. In many cases, implementation of the basic protocol is all that is needed. In more complex situations, we use the basic protocol and then add more specific treatments to address dysbiosis and hormonal problems, and we can add additional nutrients as needed. However, nothing will ever replace a healthy diet, sufficiencies of vitamin D and all five of the health-promoting fatty acids (i.e., ALA, GLA, EPA, DHA, and oleic acid), and normalization of gastrointestinal flora. Without these basics, survival and the appearance of health are possible, but true health and recovery from "untreatable" illnesses is not possible. In order to attain optimal health, we have to create the conditions that allow for health to be attained, and we start this process by supplying the body with the nutrients that it needs to function optimally. In the words of naturopathic physician Jared Zeff from the *Journal of Naturopathic Medicine*, "The work of the naturopathic physician is to elicit healing by helping patients to create or recreate the conditions for health to exist within them. Health will occur where the conditions for health exist. Disease is the product of the conditions which allow for it."[91]

Common Oversights and Shortcomings in the Study and Implementation of Nutritional Supplementation

This article was originally published in *Naturopathy Digest*
naturopathydigest.com/archives/2007/jun/vasquez.php

Introduction: An impressive discrepancy often exists between the low efficacy of nutritional interventions reported in the research literature and the higher efficacy achieved in the clinical practices of clinicians trained in the use of interventional nutrition (i.e., naturopathic physicians). This discrepancy is dangerous for at least two reasons. First, it results in an undervaluation of the efficacy of nutritional supplementation, which ultimately leaves otherwise treatable patients untreated. Second, such untreated and undertreated patients are often then forced to use dangerous and expensive pharmaceutical drugs and surgical interventions to treat conditions that could have otherwise been easily and safely treated with nutritional supplementation and diet modification. Consequently, the burden of suffering, disease, and healthcare expense in the US is higher than it would be if nutritionally-trained clinicians were more fully integrated into the healthcare system.

Obstacles to Efficacy in the Use of Nutritional Supplementation: Below are listed some of the most common causes for the underachievement of nutritional supplementation in practice and in published research. While this list is not all-inclusive, it will serve as a review for clinicians and an introduction for chiropractic/naturopathic students.

---

[88] Sandoval M, et al. Peroxynitrite-induced apoptosis in epithelial (T84) and macrophage (RAW 264.7) cell lines: effect of legume-derived polyphenols (phytolens). *Nitric Oxide*. 1997;1(6):476-83
[89] Vasquez A. Nutritional and Botanical Inhibition of NFkB, the Major Intracellular Amplifier of the Inflammatory Cascade. A Practical Clinical Strategy Exemplifying Anti-Inflammatory Nutrigenomics. *Nutritional Perspectives* 2005;July: 5-12
[90] Timms PM, et al. Circulating MMP9, vitamin D and variation in the TIMP-1 response with VDR genotype. *QJM*. 2002 Dec;95(12):787-96
[91] Zeff JL. The process of healing: a unifying theory of naturopathic medicine. *Journal of Naturopathic Medicine* 1997; 7: 122-5

In both practice and research, the problems listed below often overlap and function synergistically to reduce the efficacy of nutritional supplementation.

1. <u>Inadequate dosing (quantity)</u>: Many clinical trials published in major journals and many doctors in clinical practice have used inadequate doses of vitamins (and other natural therapeutics) and have thus failed to achieve the results that would have easily been obtained had they implemented their protocol with the proper physiologic or supraphysiologic dose of intervention. The best example in my experience centers on vitamin D, where so many of the studies are performed with doses of 400-800 IU per day only to conclude that vitamin supplementation is ineffective for the condition being treated. The problem here is that the researchers failed to appreciate that the physiologic requirement for vitamin D3 in adults is approximately 3,000-5,000 IU per day[92] and that therefore their supplemental dose of 400-800 IU is only 10-20% of what is required. Subphysiologic doses are generally subtherapeutic. In this regard, I have had to correct journals such as *The Lancet*[93], *JAMA*[94], and *British Medical Journal*[95] from misleading their readers (many of whom are major policymakers) from concluding that nutritional supplementation is impotent; rather, their researchers and editors were not sufficiently educated in the design and review of studies using nutritional interventions. These journals should hire chiropractic and naturopathic physicians so that they have staff trained in natural treatments and who can thus provide an educated review of studies on these topics.[96]

2. <u>Inadequate dosing (duration)</u>: Often the effects of long-term nutritional deficiency are not fully reversible and/or may require a treatment period of months or years to achieve maximal clinical response. For example, full replacement of fatty acids in human brain phospholipids is an ongoing process that occurs over a period of several years; thus studies using fatty acid supplements for a period of weeks or 2-3 months generally underestimate the enhanced effectiveness that can be obtained with administration over many months or several years of treatment. Relatedly, recovery from vitamin D deficiency takes several weeks of high-dose supplementation in order to achieve tissue saturation and subsequent cellular replenishment; studies of short duration are destined to underestimate the results that could have been achieved with supplementation carried out over several months.[97]

3. <u>Failure to use proper forms of nutrients (quality)</u>: Nutrients are often available in different forms, not the least of which are "active" versus "inactive" and "natural" versus "unnatural." Most vitamin supplements, particularly high-potency B vitamins, are manufactured synthetically and are not from "natural sources" despite the marketing hype promulgated by companies that, for example, mix their synthetic vitamins with a vegetable powder and then call their vitamin supplements "natural." The simple fact is that production of high-potency supplements from purely natural sources would be prohibitively wasteful, inefficient, and expensive. Thus, while it is not necessary for vitamins to be "natural" in order to be useful, it is necessary that the vitamins are useable and preferably not "unnatural." The best example of the use of unnatural supplements is the use of synthetic DL-tocopherol in the so-called "vitamin E" studies; DL-tocopherol is 50% comprised of the L-isomer of tocopherol which is not only unusable by the human body but is actually harmful in that it interferes with normal metabolism and can exacerbate hypertension and cause symptomatic complications (e.g., headaches). Further, tocopherols exist within the body in relationship with the individual forms of the vitamin, such that supplementation with one form (e.g., alpha-tocopherol) can result in a relative deficiency of another form (e.g., gamma-tocopherol). One final example of the failure to use proper forms of nutrients is in the use of pyridoxine HCl as a form of vitamin B6; while this practice itself is not harmful, clinicians need to remember that pyridoxine HCl is ineffective until converted to the more active forms of the vitamin including pyridoxal-5-phosphate. Since this conversion requires co-nutrients such as magnesium and zinc, we can easily see that the reputed failure of B6 supplementation when administered in the form of pyridoxine HCl might actually be due to untreated insufficiencies of required co-nutrients, as discussed in the following section.

4. <u>Failure to ensure adequacy of co-nutrients</u>: Vitamins, minerals, amino acids, and fatty acids work together in an intricately choreographed and delicately orchestrated dance that culminates in the successful completion of

---

[92] Heaney RP, et al. Human serum 25-hydroxycholecalciferol response to extended oral dosing with cholecalciferol. *Am J Clin Nutr*. 2003 Jan;77(1):204-10
[93] Vasquez A. Subphysiologic Doses of Vitamin D are Subtherapeutic: Comment on the Study by The Record Trial Group. *The Lancet* 2005 Published on-line May 6
[94] Muanza DN, Vasquez A, Cannell J, Grant WB. Isoflavones and Postmenopausal Women. [letter] *JAMA* 2004; 292: 2337
[95] Vasquez A, Cannell J. Calcium and vitamin D in preventing fractures: data are not sufficient to show inefficacy. [letter] *BMJ: British Medical Journal* 2005;331:108-9
[96] Vasquez A. Allopathic Usurpation of Natural Medicine. *Naturopathy Digest* 2006 Feb naturopathydigest.com/archives/2006/feb/vasquez.php
[97] Vasquez A, Manso G, Cannell J. The clinical importance of vitamin D (cholecalciferol): a paradigm shift. *Altern Ther Health Med*. 2004 Sep-Oct;10(5):28-36

interconnected physiologic functions. If any of the performers in this event are missing (i.e., nutritional deficiency) or if successive interconversions are impaired due to lack of enzyme function, then the show cannot go on, or—if it does go on—impaired metabolism and defective function will result. So, if we take a patient with "vitamin B6 deficiency" and give him vitamin B6 in the absence of other co-nutrients needed for the proper activation and metabolic utilization of vitamin B6, we cannot honestly expect the "nutritional supplementation" to work in this case; rather, we might see a marginal benefit or perhaps even a negative outcome as an imbalanced system is pushed into a different state of imbalance despite supplementation with the "correct" vitamin. In the case of vitamin B6, necessary co-nutrients include zinc, magnesium, and riboflavin; deficiency of any of these will result in a relative "failure" of B6 supplementation even if a patient has a B6-responsive condition. Notably, overt magnesium deficiency is alarmingly common among patients and citizens in industrialized nations[98,99,100], and this epidemic of magnesium deficiency is due not only to insufficient intake but also to excessive excretion caused by consumption of high-glycemic foods, caffeine, and a diet that promotes chronic metabolic acidosis with resultant urinary acidification.

5. <u>Failure to achieve urinary alkalinization</u>: Western/American-style diets typified by overconsumption of grains, dairy, sugar, and salt result in a state of subclinical chronic metabolic acidosis which results in urinary acidification, relative hypercortisolemia, and consequent hyperexcretion of minerals such as calcium and magnesium.[101][102] Thus, the common conundrum of magnesium replenishment requires not only magnesium supplementation but also dietary interventions to change the internal climate to one that is conducive to bodily retention and cellular uptake of magnesium.[103]

6. <u>Use of mislabeled supplements</u>: Even in the professional arena of nutritional supplement manufacturers, some companies habitually underdose their products either in an attempt to spend less in the manufacture of their products or as a consequence of poor quality control. If a product is labeled to contain 1,000 IU of vitamin D but only contains 836 IU of the nutrient, then obviously full clinical efficacy will not be achieved; this was a problem in a recent clinical trial involving vitamin D.[104] The problem for clinicians is in trusting the companies that supply nutritional supplements; some companies do "in house" testing which lacks independent review, while other companies use questionable "independent testing" which is not infrequently performed by a laboratory that is a wholly owned subsidiary of the parent nutritional company. Manufacturing regulations that are sweeping through the industry will cleanse the nutritional supplement world of poorly made products, and these same regulations will sweep some unprepared companies right out the door when they are unable to meet the regulatory requirements.

7. <u>Failure to ensure/assess bioavailability and optimal serum/cellular levels</u>: Clinical trials with nutritional therapies need to monitor serum or cellular levels to ensure absorption, product bioavailability, and the attainment of optimal serum levels. This is particularly relevant in the treatment of chronic disorders such as the autoimmune diseases, wherein so many of these patients have gastrointestinal dysbiosis and often have concomitant nutrient malabsorption.[105] Simply dosing these patients with supplements is not always efficacious; often the gut must be cleared of dysbiosis so that the mucosal lining can be repaired and optimal nutrient absorption can be reestablished.

8. <u>Coadministration of food with nutritional supplements (sometimes right, sometimes wrong)</u>: Food can help or hinder the absorption of nutritional supplements. Phytate and tannins in grains and teas, respectively, are notorious for inhibiting mineral absorption. Some supplements, like coenzyme Q10, should be administered with fatty food to enhance absorption. Other supplements, like amino acids, should be administered away from

---

[98] "Altogether 43% of 113 trauma patients had low magnesium levels compared to 30% of noninjured cohorts." Frankel H, Haskell R, Lee SY, Miller D, Rotondo M, Schwab CW. Hypomagnesemia in trauma patients. *World J Surg*. 1999 Sep;23(9):966-9
[99] "There was a 20% overall prevalence of hypomagnesemia among this predominantly female, African American population." Fox CH, Ramsoomair D, Mahoney MC, Carter C, Young B, Graham R. An investigation of hypomagnesemia among ambulatory urban African Americans. *J Fam Pract*. 1999 Aug;48(8):636-9
[100] "Suboptimal levels were detected in 33.7 per cent of the population under study. These data clearly demonstrate that the Mg supply of the German population needs increased attention." Schimatschek et al. Prevalence of hypomagnesemia in an unselected German population of 16,000 individuals. *Magnes Res*. 2001 Dec;14(4):283-90
[101] Cordain L, et al. Origins and evolution of the Western diet: health implications for the 21st century. *Am J Clin Nutr*. 2005 Feb;81(2):341-54
[102] Maurer M, Riesen W, Muser J, Hulter HN, Krapf R. Neutralization of Western diet inhibits bone resorption independently of K intake and reduces cortisol secretion in humans. *Am J Physiol Renal Physiol*. 2003 Jan;284(1):F32-40
[103] Vormann J, et al. Supplementation with alkaline minerals reduces symptoms in patients with chronic low back pain. *J Trace Elem Med Biol*. 2001;15(2-3):179-83
[104] Heaney RP, et al. Human serum 25-hydroxycholecalciferol response to extended oral dosing with cholecalciferol. *Am J Clin Nutr*. 2003 Jan;77(1):204-10
[105] Vasquez A. Nutritional and Botanical Treatments Against "Silent Infections" and Gastrointestinal Dysbiosis. *Nutritional Perspectives* 2006; January

protein-rich foods and are often better administered with simple carbohydrate to enhance cellular uptake; this is especially true with tryptophan.

9. <u>Correction of gross dietary imbalances enhances supplement effectiveness</u>: If the diet is grossly imbalanced, then nutritional supplementation is less likely to be effective. The best example of this is in the use of fatty acid supplements, particularly in the treatment of inflammatory disorders. If the diet is laden with dairy, beef, and other sources of arachidonate, then fatty acid supplementation with EPA, DHA, and GLA is much less likely to be effective, or much higher doses of the supplements will need to be used in order to help restore fatty acid balance. Generally speaking, the diet needs to be optimized to enhance the efficacy of nutritional supplementation.

Conclusion: In this brief review, I have listed and discussed some of the most common impediments to the success of nutritional supplementation. I hope that naturopathic students, clinicians, and researchers will find these points helpful in their design of clinical treatment protocols.

Revisiting the Five-Part Nutritional Wellness Protocol: The Supplemented Paleo-Mediterranean Diet

This article was originally published in the January 2011 issue of *Nutritional Perspectives*

Abstract: This article reviews the five-part nutritional protocol that incorporates a health-promoting nutrient-dense diet and essential supplementation with vitamins/minerals, specific fatty acids, probiotics, and physiologic doses of vitamin D3. This foundational nutritional protocol has proven benefits for disease treatment, disease prevention, and health maintenance and restoration. Additional treatments such as botanical medicines, additional nutritional supplements, and pharmaceutical drugs can be used atop this foundational protocol to further optimize clinical effectiveness. The rationale for this five-part protocol is presented, and consideration is given to adding iodine-iodide as the sixth component of the protocol.

Introduction: In 2004 and 2005 I first published a "five-part nutrition protocol"[106,107] that provides the foundational treatment plan for a wide range of health disorders. This protocol served and continues to serve as the foundation upon which other treatments are commonly added, and without which those other treatments are likely to fail, or attain suboptimal results at best.[108] Now as then, I will share with you what I consider a basic foundational protocol for wellness promotion and disease treatment. I have used this protocol in my own self-care for many years and have used it in the treatment of a wide range of health-disease conditions in clinical practice.

This nutritional protocol is validated by biochemistry, physiology, experimental research, peer-reviewed human trials, and the clinical application of common sense. It is the most nutrient-dense diet available, satisfying nutritional needs and thereby optimizing metabolic processes while promoting satiety and weight loss/optimization. Nutrients are required in the proper amounts, forms, and approximate ratios for critical and innumerable physiologic functions; if nutrients are lacking, the body cannot function *normally*, let alone *optimally*. Impaired function results in subjective and objective manifestations of what is eventually labeled as "disease." Thus, a powerful and effective alternative to treating diseases with drugs is to re-establish normal/optimal physiologic function by replenishing the body with essential nutrients, reestablishing hormonal balance ("orthoendocrinology"), promoting detoxification of environmental toxins, and by reestablishing the optimal microbial milieu, especially the eradication of (multifocal) dysbiosis; this multifaceted approach can be applied to several diseases, especially those of the inflammatory and autoimmune varieties.[109]

Of course, most diseases are multifactorial and therefore require multicomponent treatment plans, and some diseases actually require the use of drugs in conjunction with assertive interventional nutrition. However, while only a smaller portion of patients actually need drugs for the long-term management their problems, all clinicians should agree that everyone needs a foundational nutrition plan because nutrients—not drugs—are universally required for life and health. This five-part nutrition protocol is briefly outlined below; a much more

---

[106] Vasquez A. *Integrative Orthopedics: The Art of Creating Wellness While Managing Acute and Chronic Musculoskeletal Disorders*. 2004, 2007, 2012
[107] Vasquez A. Five-Part Nutritional Protocol that Produces Consistently Positive Results. *NutrWellness* 2005Sep nutritionalwellness.com/archives/2005/sep/09_vasquez.php
[108] Vasquez A. Common Oversights and Shortcomings in the Study and Implementation of Nutritional Supplementation. *Naturopathy Digest* 2007 June.
[109] Vasquez A. Integrative Rheumatology. IBMRC: 2006, 2009.

detailed substantiation of the underlying science and clinical application of this protocol was recently published in a review of more than 650 pages and approximately 3,500 citations.[110]

1. <u>Health-promoting Paleo-Mediterranean diet</u>: Following an extensive review of the research literature, I developed what I call the "supplemented Paleo-Mediterranean diet." In essence, this diet plan combines the best of the Mediterranean diet with the best of the Paleolithic diet, the latter of which has been best distilled by Dr. Loren Cordain in his book "The Paleo Diet"[111] and his numerous scientific articles.[112,113,114] The Paleolithic diet is superior to the Mediterranean diet in nutrient density for promoting satiety, weight loss, and improvements/normalization in overall metabolic function.[115,116] This diet places emphasis on fruits, vegetables, nuts, seeds, and berries that meet the body's needs for fiber, carbohydrates, and most importantly, the 8,000+ phytonutrients that have additive and synergistic health effects[117]—including immunomodulating, antioxidant, anti-inflammatory, and anti-cancer benefits. High-quality protein sources such as fish, poultry, eggs, and grass-fed meats are emphasized. Slightly modifying Cordain's Paleo diet, I also advocate soy and whey protein isolates for their high-quality protein and their anticancer, cardioprotective, and mood-enhancing (due to the high tryptophan content) benefits. Potatoes and other starchy vegetables, wheat and other grains including rice are discouraged due to their high glycemic indexes and high glycemic loads, and their relative insufficiency of fiber and phytonutrients compared to fruits and vegetables. Grains such as wheat, barley, and rye are discouraged due to the high glycemic loads/indexes of most breads, pastries, and other grain-derived products, as well as due to the immunogenicity of constituents such as gluten, a protein composite (consisting of a prolamin and a glutelin) that can contribute to disorders such as migraine, epilepsy, eczema, arthritis, celiac disease, psoriasis and other types of autoimmunity. Sources of simple sugars and foreign chemicals such as colas/sodas (which contain artificial colors, flavors, and high-fructose corn syrup, which contains mercury[118] and which can cause the hypertensive-diabetic metabolic syndrome[119]) and processed foods (e.g., "TV dinners" and other manufactured snacks and convenience foods) are strictly forbidden. Chemical preservatives, colorants, sweeteners, flavor-enhancers such as monosodium glutamate and carrageenan are likewise avoided. In summary, this diet plan provides plenty of variety, as most dishes comprised of poultry, fish, lean meats, soy, eggs, fruits, vegetables, nuts, berries, and seeds are allowed. The diet provides an abundance of fiber, phytonutrients, carbohydrates, potassium, and protein, while simultaneously being low in fat, sodium, arachidonic acid, and "simple sugars." The diet must be customized with regard to total protein and calorie intake, as determined by the size, status, and activity level of the patient; individual per-patient food allergens should be avoided. Regular consumption of this diet has shown the ability to reduce hypertension, alleviate diabetes, ameliorate migraine headaches, and result in improvement of overall health and a lessening of the severity of many common "diseases", particularly those with an autoimmune or inflammatory component. This Paleo-Mediterranean diet is supplemented with vitamins, minerals, fatty acids, and probiotics—making it the "supplemented Paleo-Mediterranean diet" as described below.

2. <u>Multivitamin and multimineral supplementation</u>: Vitamin and mineral supplementation has been advocated for decades by the chiropractic/naturopathic professions while being scorned by so-called "mainstream

---

[110] Vasquez A. *Chiropractic and Naturopathic Mastery of Common Clinical Disorders*. IBMRC: 2009
[111] Cordain L. *The Paleo Diet*. John Wiley and Sons, 2002
[112] O'Keefe JH Jr, Cordain L. Cardiovascular disease resulting from a diet and lifestyle at odds with our Paleolithic genome. *Mayo Clin Proc*. 2004 Jan;79(1):101-8
[113] Cordain L. Cereal grains: humanity's double edged sword. *World Rev Nutr Diet* 1999;84:19-73
[114] Cordain L, et al. Origins and evolution of the Western diet: health implications for the 21st century. *Am J Clin Nutr*. 2005 Feb;81(2):341-54
[115] "A high micronutrient density diet mitigates the unpleasant aspects of the experience of hunger even though it is lower in calories. Hunger is one of the major impediments to successful weight loss. Our findings suggest that it is not simply the caloric content, but more importantly, the micronutrient density of a diet that influences the experience of hunger. It appears that a high nutrient density diet, after an initial phase of adjustment during which a person experiences "toxic hunger" due to withdrawal from pro-inflammatory foods, can result in a sustainable eating pattern that leads to weight loss and improved health." Fuhrman J, Sarter B, Glaser D, Acocella S. Changing perceptions of hunger on a high nutrient density diet. *Nutr J*. 2010 Nov 7;9:51 nutritionj.com/content/9/1/51
[116] "The Paleolithic group were as satiated as the Mediterranean group but consumed less energy per day (5.8 MJ/day vs. 7.6 MJ/day, Paleolithic vs. Mediterranean, p=0.04). Consequently, the quotients of mean change in satiety during meal and mean consumed energy from food and drink were higher in the Paleolithic group (p=0.03). Also, there was a strong trend for greater Satiety Quotient for energy in the Paleolithic group (p=0.057). Leptin decreased by 31% in the Paleolithic group and by 18% in the Mediterranean group with a trend for greater relative decrease of leptin in the Paleolithic group." Jonsson T, Granfeldt Y, Erlanson-Albertsson C, Ahren B, Lindeberg S. A Paleolithic diet is more satiating per calorie than a Mediterranean-like diet in individuals with ischemic heart disease. *Nutr Metab (Lond)*. 2010 Nov 30;7(1):85.
[117] Liu RH. Health benefits of fruit and vegetables are from additive and synergistic combinations of phytochemicals. *Am J Clin Nutr* 2003;78(3 Suppl):517S-520S
[118] "With daily per capita consumption of HFCS in the US averaging about 50 grams and daily mercury intakes from HFCS ranging up to 28 µg, this potential source of mercury may exceed other major sources of mercury especially in high-end consumers of beverages sweetened with HFCS." Dufault R, et al. Mercury from chlor-alkali plants: measured concentrations in food product sugar. *Environ Health*. 2009 Jan 26;8:2 ehjournal.net/content/8/1/2
[119] Vasquez A. *Integrative Medicine and Functional Medicine for Chronic Hypertension: An Evidence-based Patient-Centered Monograph for Advanced Clinicians*. IBMRC; 2011. See also: Reungjui S, et al. Thiazide diuretics exacerbate fructose-induced metabolic syndrome. *J Am Soc Nephrol*. 2007 Oct;18(10):2724-31

medicine." Vitamin and mineral supplementation finally received bipartisan endorsement when researchers from Harvard Medical School published a review article in *Journal of the American Medical Association* that concluded, "Most people do not consume an optimal amount of all vitamins by diet alone. ...it appears prudent for all adults to take vitamin supplements."[120] Long-term nutritional insufficiencies experienced by "most people" promote the development of "long-latency deficiency diseases"[121] such as cancer, neuroemotional deterioration, and cardiovascular disease. Impressively, the benefits of multivitamin/multimineral supplementation have been demonstrated in numerous clinical trials. Multivitamin/multimineral supplementation has been shown to improve nutritional status and reduce the risk for chronic diseases[122], improve mood[123], potentiate antidepressant drug treatment[124], alleviate migraine headaches (when used with diet improvement and fatty acids[125]), improve immune function and infectious disease outcomes in the elderly[126] (especially diabetics[127]), reduce morbidity and mortality in patients with HIV infection[128,129], alleviate premenstrual syndrome[130,131] and bipolar disorder[132], reduce violence and antisocial behavior in children[133] and incarcerated young adults (when used with essential fatty acids[134]), and improve scores of intelligence in children.[135] Multivitamin and multimineral supplementation provides anti-inflammatory benefits, as evidenced by significant reduction in C-reactive protein (CRP) in a double-blind, placebo-controlled trial.[136] The ability to safely and affordably deliver these benefits makes multimineral-multivitamin supplementation an essential component of any and all health-promoting and disease-prevention strategies. A few cautions need to be observed; for example, vitamin A can (rarely) result in liver damage with chronic consumption of 25,000 IU or more, and intake should generally not exceed 10,000 IU per day in women of childbearing age. Also, iron should not be supplemented except in patients diagnosed with iron deficiency by a blood test (serum ferritin).

3. <u>Physiologic doses of vitamin D3</u>: The prevalence of vitamin D deficiency varies from 40-80 percent (general population) to almost 100 percent (patients with musculoskeletal pain) among Americans and Europeans. Vasquez, Manso, and Cannell described the many benefits of vitamin D3 supplementation in a "paradigm-shifting" review published in 2004.[137]

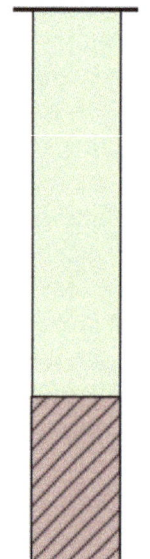

Excess vitamin D
> 100 ng/mL (250 nmol/L) with hypercalcemia

Optimal range
50 - 100 ng/mL (125 - 250 nmol/L)

Insufficiency range
< 20- 40 ng/mL (50 - 100 nmol/L)

Deficiency
< 20 ng/mL (50 nmol/L)

<u>Image right: Interpretation of serum 25(OH) vitamin D levels:</u> Updated from Vasquez et al, *Alternative Therapies in Health and Medicine* 2004 Sep

---

[120] Fletcher RH, Fairfield KM. Vitamins for chronic disease prevention in adults: clinical applications. *JAMA* 2002;287:3127-9
[121] Heaney RP. Long-latency deficiency disease: insights from calcium and vitamin D. *Am J Clin Nutr* 2003;78:912-9
[122] McKay et al. The effects of a multivitamin/mineral supplement on micronutrient status, antioxidant capacity and cytokine production in healthy older adults consuming a fortified diet. *J Am Coll Nutr* 2000;19(5):613-21
[123] Benton D, Haller J, Fordy J. Vitamin supplementation for 1 year improves mood. *Neuropsychobiology* 1995;32(2):98-105
[124] Coppen A, Bailey J. Enhancement of the antidepressant action of fluoxetine by folic acid: a randomised, placebo controlled trial. *J Affect Disord* 2000;60:121-30
[125] Wagner W, Nootbaar-Wagner U. Prophylactic treatment of migraine with gamma-linolenic and alpha-linolenic acids. *Cephalalgia* 1997;17:127-30
[126] Langkamp-Henken et al. Nutritional formula enhanced immune function and reduced days of symptoms upper respiratory tract infection in seniors. *J Am Geriatr Soc* 2004:3-12
[127] Barringer TA, et al. Effect of a multivitamin and mineral supplement on infection and quality of life. *Ann Intern Med* 2003;138:365-71
[128] Fawzi WW, Msamanga GI, et al. A randomized trial of multivitamin supplements and HIV disease progression and mortality. *N Engl J Med* 2004;351:23-32
[129] Burbano X, et al. Impact of a selenium chemoprevention clinical trial on hospital admissions of HIV-infected participants. *HIV Clin Trials* 2002;3:483-91
[130] Abraham GE. Nutritional factors in the etiology of the premenstrual tension syndromes. *J Reprod Med* 1983;28(7):446-64
[131] Stewart A. Clinical and biochemical effects of nutritional supplementation on the premenstrual syndrome. *J Reprod Med* 1987;32:435-41
[132] Kaplan BJ, et al. Effective mood stabilization with a chelated mineral supplement: an open-label trial in bipolar disorder. *J Clin Psychiatry* 2001;62:936-44
[133] Kaplan et al. Treatment of mood lability and explosive rage with minerals and vitamins: two case studies in children. *J Child Adolesc Psychopharmacol* 2002;12(3):205-19
[134] Gesch et al. Influence of supplementary vitamins, minerals and essential fatty acids on the antisocial behaviour of young adult prisoners. *Br J Psychiatry* 2002;181:22-8
[135] Benton D. Micro-nutrient supplementation and the intelligence of children. *Neurosci Biobehav Rev* 2001;25:297-309
[136] Church TS, Earnest CP, Wood KA, Kampert JB. Reduction of C-reactive protein levels through use of a multivitamin. *Am J Med* 2003;115:702-7
[137] Vasquez A, Manso G, Cannell J. The clinical importance of vitamin D (cholecalciferol). *Alternative Therapies in Health and Medicine* 2004;10:28-37

Our review showed that vitamin D deficiency causes or contributes to depression, hypertension, seizures, migraine, polycystic ovary syndrome, inflammation, autoimmunity, and musculoskeletal pain, particularly low-back pain. Clinical trials using vitamin D supplementation have proven the cause-and-effect relationship between vitamin D deficiency and most of these conditions by showing that each could be cured or alleviated with vitamin D supplementation. Per our review, daily vitamin D doses should be 1,000 IU for infants, 2,000 IU for children, and 4,000 IU for adults, although some adults respond better to higher doses of 10,000 IU per day. Cautions/contraindications include the use of thiazide diuretics (e.g., hydrochlorothiazide) or any other medications that promote hypercalcemia, as well as granulomatous diseases such as sarcoidosis, tuberculosis, and certain types of cancer, especially lymphoma. Effectiveness is monitored by measuring serum 25-OH-vitamin D, and safety is monitored by measuring serum calcium. Dosing should be tailored for the attainment of optimal serum levels of 25-hydroxy-vitamin D3, generally 50-100 ng/ml (125-250 nmol/l) as illustrated.

4. Balanced and complete fatty acid supplementation: A detailed survey of the literature shows that five fatty acids have major health-promoting disease-preventing benefits and should therefore be incorporated into the daily diet and/or regularly consumed as dietary supplements.[138] These are alpha-linolenic acid (ALA; omega-3, from flaxseed oil), eicosapentaenoic acid (EPA; omega-3, from fish oil), docosahexaenoic acid (DHA; omega-3, from fish oil and algae), gamma-linolenic acid (GLA; omega-6, most concentrated in borage oil but also present in evening primrose oil, hemp seed oil, black currant seed oil), and oleic acid (omega-9, most concentrated in olive oil, which contains in addition to oleic acid many anti-inflammatory, antioxidant, and anticancer phytonutrients). Supplementing with one fatty acid can exacerbate an insufficiency of other fatty acids; hence the importance of balanced combination supplementation. Each of these fatty acids has health benefits that cannot be fully attained from supplementing a different fatty acid; hence, again, the importance of balanced combination supplementation. The benefits of GLA are not attained by consumption of EPA and DHA; in fact, consumption of fish oil can actually promote a deficiency of GLA.[139] Likewise, consumption of GLA alone can reduce EPA levels while increasing levels of proinflammatory arachidonic acid; both of these problems are avoided with co-administration of EPA any time GLA is used because EPA inhibits delta-5-desaturase, which converts dihomo-GLA into arachidonic acid. Using ALA alone only slightly increases EPA but generally leads to no improvement in DHA status and can lead to a reduction of oleic acid; thus, DHA and oleic acid should be supplemented when flaxseed oil is used.[140] Obviously, the goal here is physiologically-optimal (i.e., "balanced") intake of all of the health-promoting fatty acids; using only one or two sources of fatty acids is not balanced and results in suboptimal improvement. In clinical practice, I routinely use combination fatty acid therapy comprised of ALA, EPA, DHA, and GLA for essentially all patients; when one appreciates that the average daily Paleolithic intake of n-3 fatty acids was 7 grams per day contrasted to the average daily American intake of 1 gram per day, we can see that—by using combination fatty acid therapy emphasizing n-3 fatty acids—we are simply meeting physiologic expectations via supplementation, rather than performing an act of recklessness or heroism. The product I use also contains a modest amount of oleic acid that occurs naturally in flax and borage seed oils, and I encourage use of olive oil for salads and cooking. This approach results in complete and balanced fatty acid intake, and the clinical benefits are impressive. Benefits are to be expected in the treatment of premenstrual syndrome, diabetic neuropathy, respiratory distress syndrome, Crohn's disease, lupus, rheumatoid arthritis, cardiovascular disease, hypertension, psoriasis, eczema, migraine headaches, bipolar disorder, borderline personality disorder, mental depression, schizophrenia, osteoporosis, polycystic ovary syndrome, multiple sclerosis, and musculoskeletal pain. The discovery in September 2010 that the G protein-coupled receptor 120 (GPR120) functions as an n-3 fatty acid receptor that, when stimulated with EPA or DHA, exerts broad anti-inflammatory effects (in cell experiments) and enhances systemic insulin sensitivity (in animal study) confirms a new mechanism of action of fatty acid supplementation and shows that we as clinician-researchers are still learning the details of the beneficial effects of commonly used treatments.[141]

---

[138] Vasquez A. New Insights into Fatty Acid Biochemistry and the Influence of Diet. *Nutritional Perspectives* 2004; October: 5, 7-10, 12, 14
[139] Cleland LG, Gibson RA, Neumann M, French JK. The effect of dietary fish oil supplement upon the content of dihomo-gammalinolenic acid in human plasma phospholipids. *Prostaglandins Leukot Essent Fatty Acids* 1990 May;40(1):9-12
[140] Jantti J, Nikkari T, Solakivi T, et al. Evening primrose oil in rheumatoid arthritis: changes in serum lipids and fatty acids. *Ann Rheum Dis* 1989;48(2):124-7
[141] Oh da Y, et al. GPR120 is an omega-3 fatty acid receptor mediating potent anti-inflammatory and insulin-sensitizing effects. Cell. 2010 Sep 3;142(5):687-98

5. <u>Probiotics /gut flora modification</u>: Proper levels of good bacteria promote intestinal health, support proper immune function, and encourage overall health. Excess bacteria or yeast, or the presence of harmful bacteria, yeast, or "parasites" such as amoebas and protozoans, can cause "leaky gut," systemic inflammation, and a wide range of clinical problems, especially autoimmunity. Intestinal flora can become imbalanced by poor diets, excess stress, immunosuppressive drugs, and antibiotics, and all of these factors are common among American patients. Thus, as a rule, I reinstate the good bacteria by the use of probiotics (good bacteria and yeast), prebiotics (fiber, arabinogalactan, and inulin), and the use of fermented foods such as kefir and yogurt for patients not allergic to milk. Harmful yeast, bacteria, and other "parasites" can be eradicated with the combination of dietary change, antimicrobial drugs, and/or herbal extracts. For example, oregano oil in an emulsified, time-released form has proven safe and effective for the elimination of various parasites encountered in clinical practice.[142] Likewise, the herb *Artemisia annua* (sweet wormwood) commonly is used to eradicate specific bacteria and has been used for thousands of years in Asia for the treatment and prevention of infectious diseases, including drug-resistant malaria.[143] Restoring microbial balance by providing probiotics, restoring immune function (immunorestoration) and eliminating sources of dysbiosis, especially in the gastrointestinal tract, genitourinary tract, and oropharynx, is a very important component in the treatment plan of autoimmunity and systemic inflammation.[144]

Should combinations of iodine and iodide be the sixth component of the Protocol?*: Both iodine and iodide have biological activity in humans. An increasing number of clinicians are using combination iodine-iodide products to provide approximately 3-6 mg/d [changed/corrected*]. Collectively, iodine and iodide provide antioxidant, antimicrobial, mucolytic, immunosupportive, antiestrogen, and anticancer benefits that extend far beyond the mere incorporation of iodine into thyroid hormones.[5] Benefits of iodine/iodide in the treatment of asthma[145,146] and systemic fungal infections[147,148] have been documented, and many clinicians use combination iodine/iodide supplementation for the treatment of estrogen-driven conditions such as fibrocystic breast disease.[149] While additional research is needed and already underway to further establish the role of iodine-iodide as a routine component of clinical care, clinicians can reasonably begin incorporating this nutrient into their protocols based on the above-mentioned physiologic roles and clinical benefits. **See update/addendum following this reprint.*

Summary and Conclusions: In this brief review, I have described and substantiated a fundamental protocol that can serve as effective therapy for patients with a wide range of diseases and health disorders. Customizing the Paleo-Mediterranean diet to avoid patient-specific food allergens, using vitamin-mineral supplements along with physiologic doses of vitamin D and broad-spectrum balanced fatty acid supplementation, and ensuring "immunomicrobial" health with the skillful use of probiotics, prebiotics, immunorestoration, and antimicrobial treatments provides an excellent health-promoting and disease-eliminating foundation and lifestyle for many patients. Often, this simple protocol is all that is needed for the effective treatment of a wide range of clinical problems, even those that have been "medical failures" for many years. For other patients with more complex illnesses, of course, additional interventions and laboratory assessments can be used to optimize and further customize the treatment plan. Clinicians should avoid seeking "silver bullet" treatments that ignore overall metabolism, immune function, and inflammatory balance, and we must always remember that the attainment and preservation of health requires that we first meet the body's basic nutritional and physiologic needs. This five-step protocol begins the process of meeting those needs. With it, health can be restored and the need for disease-specific treatment is obviated or reduced; without it, fundamental physiologic needs are not met, and health cannot be obtained and maintained. Addressing core physiologic needs empowers doctors to deliver the most effective healthcare possible, and it allows patients to benefit from such treatment.

---

[142] Force M, Sparks WS, Ronzio RA. Inhibition of enteric parasites by emulsified oil of oregano in vivo. *Phytother Res* 2000;14:213-4
[143] Schuster BG. Demonstrating the validity of natural products as anti-infective drugs. *J Altern Complement Med* 2001;7 Suppl 1:S73-82
[144] Vasquez A. Integrative Rheumatology. IBMRC: 2006, 2009.
[145] Tuft L. Iodides in bronchial asthma. *J Allergy Clin Immunol*. 1981 Jun;67(6):497
[146] Falliers CJ, McCann WP, Chai H, Ellis EF, Yazdi N. Controlled study of iodotherapy for childhood asthma. *J Allergy*. 1966 Sep;38(3):183-92
[147] Tripathy S, et al. Rhinofacial zygomycosis successfully treated with oral saturated solution of potassium iodide. *J Eur Acad Dermatol Venereol*. 2007 Jan;21(1):117-9
[148] Bonifaz A, et al. Sporotrichosis in childhood: clinical and therapeutic experience in 25 patients. *Pediatr Dermatol*. 2007 Jul-Aug;24(4):369-72
[149] Ghent WR, Eskin BA, Low DA, Hill LP. Iodine replacement in fibrocystic disease of the breast. *Can J Surg*. 1993 Oct;36(5):453-60

*Update and addendum to information on iodine and iodide:
- Authoritative enthusiasm for high-dose iodine-iodide: Several authoritative articles/authors stated that an advisable level of intake for iodine-iodide for the prevention and treatment of various conditions is approximately 12 mg/d. Because of these well-referenced and apparently authoritative publications, many clinicians and nutrition professionals began using higher doses iodine-iodide with patients and clients, quite often with benefit and nearly always with the absence of serious adverse effects. Several popular nutritional supplements used by clinicians and nutritionists contain both iodi*ne* (the *n*atural, diatomic form) and iodi*de* (the *d*ivided/ionic form most commonly consumed in *d*ietary supplements, such as potassium iodi*de*); both forms of this volatile metal have biologic properties in humans. Benefits of iodine-iodide supplementation focus mostly on the mucolytic, antimicrobial, and anti-estrogen effects.
    - Dr Jonathan V Wright (*Nutrition and Healing* 2002 Nov and 2005 May): In *Nutrition and Healing* (2002 Nov), well-respected nutrition expert, pioneer, and clinician Jonathan V. Wright MD advocated high-dose iodine-iodide for a wide range of conditions, particularly those related to inflammation, excess estrogen, and microbial infections. In another issue of *Nutrition and Healing* (2005 May) Dr Wright wrote "12.5 milligrams (that's 12,500 micrograms) is the optimal daily amount of iodine, not only for your thyroid but for the rest of your body, too." In that same article, Dr Wright stated, "The Japanese have traditionally consumed more iodine, mostly from seaweed, than any other population. The average daily intake of iodine in Japan [is] 13.8 milligrams…", and throughout the article Dr Wright advocates that 12.5 mg/d is "the optimal daily dose" of combined iodine-iodine.
    - Extrathyroidal benefits of iodine (*Journal of American Physicians and Surgeons* 2006 Winter): Independently and in a peer-reviewed publication, Donald Miller MD (Professor of Surgery, Division of Cardiothoracic Surgery, University of Washington School of Medicine) supported the daily intake of 12.5 mg/d in *Journal of American Physicians and Surgeons* and even supported higher doses with the statement "More than 4,000 patients in this project [Iodine Project] take iodine in daily doses ranging from 12.5 to 50 mg, and those with diabetes can take up to 100 mg /day." Miller also noted that dermatologists "treat inflammatory dermatoses, like nodular vasculitis and pyoderma gangrenosum, with SSKI (supersaturated potassium iodide), beginning with an iodine dose of 900 mg/day, followed by weekly increases of up to 6 g/day as tolerated. Fungal eruptions, like sporotrichosis, are treated initially in gram amounts with great effect."
    - Iodine deficiency and therapeutic considerations (*Alternative Medicine Review* 2008 Jun): In 2008, Patrick wrote "Estimates of the average daily Japanese iodine consumption vary from 5,280 mcg to 13,800 mcg…" and this again supported and reinforced enthusiasm for doses of approximately 12 mg/d of iodine-iodine. However, in this article, Patrick did not advocate any specific daily dosage, citing 3-6 mg/d as beneficial and without adverse effect.
- Review, reanalysis, and caution: Soon after these enthusiastic publications, Alan Gaby MD published in several magazines, presented in post-graduate educational events, and discussed in his book *Nutritional Medicine* a review and reanalysis of the original data and concluded that the estimated average daily intake of iodine-iodine in Japan had been *overestimated* by a mathematical error (mistakenly interchanging wet and dry weights of seaweed and thus overestimating the daily Japanese intake of iodine-iodine). Per Gaby (*Nutritional Medicine*, page 175), the true intake of iodine-iodide in Japan averages 330-500 mcg/d, which is 25-fold lower than the estimate of 13.8 mg/d, upon which rested much of the rationale for implementing high-dose iodine-iodide supplementation empirically and routinely.
- Benefits, perspectives, and additional research: Many clinicians including the current author have used high-dose iodine-iodide ranging from approximately 12-48 mg/d for variable periods of time without personally experiencing or clinically observing apparent adverse effects; that statement does not imply endorsement of routine universal high-dose iodine-iodide supplementation. Some degree of caution is advised in consideration of the risks of inducing thyroid dysfunction (hyperthyroidism, hypothyroidism), intestinal hemorrhage[150], and

---

[150] Kinoshita et al. Severe duodenal hemorrhage induced by Lugol's solution administered for thyroid crisis treatment. *Intern Med.* 2010;49(8):759-61

anaphylaxis-like reactions.[151] Topical and systemic antimicrobial benefits of iodine-iodide are well known and well documented; oral high-dose iodine-iodide has been used to treat drug-resistant fungal infections (cited below). When applied for sufficient concentrations and durations, both diatomic iodine and ionic iodide possess potent broad-spectrum antimicrobial properties; essentially no "drug resistance" against iodine-iodide exists for bacteria, fungi, viruses, and protozoans. Iodine also has documented molecular and clinical anti-estrogen effects, thus providing scientific explanation for its ability to treat and prevent estrogen-related disorders ranging from fibrocystic breast disease to cancer. Indeed, iodine treatment of breast cancer cells has been shown to increase the mRNA levels of several genes involved in estrogen metabolism and "detoxification" such as cytochrome p450-1A1 while also decreasing the levels of estrogen responsive genes such as TFF1 and WISP2; also noted following iodine treatment is upregulation of gene expression for the enzyme glutathione peroxidase, an important selenium-dependent component of antioxidant defense mechanisms.[152]

- Ultra-high dose iodide for sporotrichosis in childhood (*Pediatric Dermatology* 2007 Jul-Aug): Nineteen pediatric patients with proven sporotrichosis were successfully treated with potassium iodide per the following quoted protocol: "All patients were initially treated with potassium iodide (KI), and only those who were unresponsive or who developed side effects were given itraconazole. The dose of KI used was 1–3 g/day, starting at 1 g/day and increasing until the dose of 3 g/day was reached. … Treatments were sustained until remission was reached, which ranged from 3 to 6 months."[153] Per the review by Miller[154] cited previously, KI 1g (1,000 mg) contains 770 mg of iodide. Thus, the pediatric patients in this case series were treated with 770-2,310 mg/d of iodide for successful antimycotic treatment. Two patients from the original group of 23 patients experienced nausea and vomiting from the KI and were switched to itraconazole; two other patients were lost to follow-up. The authors note that, "Side effects occur in 5% to 10% of patients, mainly presenting as gastrointestinal symptoms as well as headache and rhinorrhea to a lesser extent."

- Ultra-high dose iodide for rhinofacial zygomycosis—case report (*Journal of European Academy of Dermatology and Venereology* 2007 Jan): A 19-year-old male "was put on oral SSKI at an initial dose of 0.5 mL three times daily. This was gradually increased by 0.1 mL/dose/day until a dose of 5 mL three times daily was reached."[155] Generic formulation of "saturated solution of potassium iodide" (SSKI) contains 1000 mg of KI per mL of solution, which provides roughly 750 mg iodide; thus, SSKI dosed at 5 mL thrice daily = 15 mL/d = 11,250 mg/d (slightly more than 11 grams per day) of iodide for this adult patient with rhinofacial zygomycosis. Treatment was continued for at least 12 months without report of adverse effect.

- Modest dose iodine replacement in fibrocystic disease of the breast (*Canadian Journal of Surgery* 1993 Oct): Ghent and colleagues[156] sought to determine the response of patients with fibrocystic breast disease to "iodine replacement therapy" and reviewed three clinical studies of different design containing 233, 145 (later up to 1365), and 23 subjects; overall, subjective alleviation of pain and objective alleviation of breast fibrosis was seen in approximately 70% of patients. Consistent with other reports and impressions, the authors noted that, "Molecular iodine is nonthyrotropic and was the most beneficial." The dose of molecular iodine averaged 0.08 mg/kg body weight, which for an average 140-lb (63-kg) patient equates to approximately 5 mg/d.

- Modest dose iodine in patients with cyclic mastalgia (*Breast Journal* 2004 Jul-Aug): Kessler[157] reports a randomized, double-blind, placebo-controlled, multicenter clinical trial was conducted with 111 otherwise healthy euthyroid women with a history of breast pain and fibrosis; subjects received molecular iodine for 6 months. Physicians assessed breast pain, tenderness, and nodularity each cycle; patients assessed breast pain and tenderness with the Lewin breast pain scale at 3-month intervals and with a VAS at each cycle. All iodine-treated subjects improved compared to no improvement seen in

---

[151] Indraccolo et al. Anaphylactic-like reaction to Lugol solution during colposcopy. *South Med J* 2009 Jan;102(1):96-7
[152] "Quantitative RT-PCR confirmed the array data demonstrating that iodine/iodide treatment increased the mRNA levels of several genes involved in estrogen metabolism (CYP1A1, CYP1B1, and AKR1C1) while decreasing the levels of the estrogen responsive genes TFF1 and WISP2." Stoddard FR 2nd, et al. Iodine alters gene expression in the MCF7 breast cancer cell line: evidence for an anti-estrogen effect of iodine. *Int J Med Sci*. 2008 Jul 8;5(4):189-96
[153] Bonifaz A, et al. Sporotrichosis in childhood: clinical and therapeutic experience in 25 patients. *Pediatr Dermatol*. 2007 Jul-Aug;24(4):369-72
[154] Said of KI, "The standard dose was 1g, which contains 770 mg of iodine." Miller DW. Extrathyroidal benefits of iodine. *J Am Physicians Surgeons* 2006;Winter,106-10
[155] Tripathy et al. Rhinofacial zygomycosis successfully treated with oral saturated solution of potassium iodide. *J Eur Acad Dermatol Venereol*. 2007;21:117-9
[156] Ghent et al. Iodine replacement in fibrocystic disease of the breast. *Can J Surg*. 1993 Oct;36(5):453-60
[157] Kessler JH. The effect of supraphysiologic levels of iodine on patients with cyclic mastalgia. *Breast J*. 2004 Jul-Aug;10(4):328-36

the placebo group. "Reductions in all three physician assessments were observed in patients after 5 months of therapy in the 3.0 mg/day (7/28; 25%) and 6.0 mg/day (15/27; 18.5%) treatment groups, but not the 1.5 mg/day or placebo group. Patients recorded statistically significant decreases in pain by month 3 in the 3.0 and 6.0 mg/day treatment groups, but not the 1.5 mg/day or placebo group; more than 50% of the 6.0 mg/day treatment group recorded a clinically significant reduction in overall pain. All doses were associated with an acceptable safety profile. No dose-related increase in any adverse event was observed." Notably, the failure of the 1.5 mg/day dose implies that this dose is inadequate and thereby justifies higher routine dosing.

- Clinical implementation and the author's perspective: Iodide has a stronger effect on thyroid function and provides tissue-penetrating antimicrobial benefits from oral administration. Molecular iodine has anti-estrogen effects that correlate with the clinical alleviation of cyclic breast pain and fibrocystic breast disease; other anti-estrogen benefits such as an anti-cancer benefit are reasonably anticipated from supplemental iodine. Products with combined iodine and iodide are available and reasonable for clinical use, and a daily dose range of 3-6 mg does not appear unreasonable and has been shown to be beneficial in human studies. Iodine and iodide are impressively well tolerated. Nicely summarized in a personal email from Michael Gonzalez DSc PhD in November 2012, an overview of iodine-iodide's clinical applications may be stated as follows:

   "Different tissues of the body respond to different forms of iodine. The Iodide form is believed to be particularly useful for the thyroid. But the supplement of choice for the breast is "iodine" not "iodide." Lugol's formula is Iodine 5% + Potassium iodide (KI) 10% in distilled water. Because different tissues concentrate different forms of iodine, using a supplement that contains both iodine and iodide is preferable to using a supplement that contains only one form. With different tissues responding to different forms of iodine, it would make common sense that a greater therapeutic benefit from iodine will be achieved by using a combination of iodide and iodine. ... The most frequent adverse reactions to potassium iodide are stomach upset, diarrhea, nausea, vomiting, stomach pain, salivary gland swelling/tenderness, acne and skin rash."

Antioxidant support in general and supplementation with selenium in particular are recommended always, and particularly when iodine-iodide doses greater than 1-3 mg/d are used. Selenium 200 mcg/d has been shown in several studies to have an ameliorating effect on thyroid autoimmunity and a supportive effect on peripheral thyroid hormone metabolism. Although iodi*n*e is generally considered *n*onthyrotropic, periodic assessment of thyroid function and for thyroid autoimmunity is reasonable for patients taking long-term high-dose treatment. Clinicians should take advantage of iodine-iodide's safe and effective mucolytic, antimicrobial, and anti-estrogen benefits.

Distinguishing iodiNe from iodiDe

IodiNe
- **Natural** elemental form—diatomic.
- **Nonthyrotropic**—no immediate adverse effects on thyroid function.
- **Nuclear**—affects gene expression, for example by promoting estrogen detoxification and reducing estrogen responsiveness.
- **Nixes microbes**, antimicrobial—very broad spectrum; povidone iodine is one of the most widely used topical antimicrobials in the history of microbiology and medicine.

IodiDe
- **Divided**—ionic, nondiatomic.
- **Dietary** form, such as in iodized salt which typically contains potassium iodate, potassium iodide, sodium iodate, or sodium iodide.
- **Dissolves mucus**—mucolytic benefits advantageous in the treatment of asthma, bronchitis and respiratory tract infections. Potassium iodide is thought to act as an expectorant by increasing respiratory tract secretions and thereby decreasing the viscosity of mucus; iodide levels increase in respiratory secretions within approximately 15 minutes after oral administration.
- **Directly thyrotropic**—necessary for thyroid hormone production; high doses can cause thyroid dysfunction, which may be problematic (exacerbation of thyroid autoimmunity, hypothyroidism, or hyperthyroidism) or therapeutic (inhibition of thyroid hormone production during hyperthyroidism).
- **Deals death to microbes**, antimicrobial—very broad spectrum, used in the form of potassium iodide (KI, SSKI) for the treatment of microbial infections such as zygomycosis and sporotrichosis.

Reply to "Role of Western Diet in Inflammatory Autoimmune Diseases" by Manzel et al. in *Current Allergy and Asthma Reports*, Volume 14, Issue 1, 2014 January

The short version of this letter was originally published in digital/online and printed formats in *Current Allergy and Asthma Reports* 2014 Aug[158]

Interested readers should access ICHNFM.org/publications/ to see if the full version of this letter has been published in digital/online open-access format in *International Journal of Human Nutrition and Functional Medicine*[159]

I think the original article by Manzel et al[160] is/was a disservice to science, to clinicians, and to the *Journal* that published their intellectually impoverished 8-page 100-citation review. The full version of my original reply—as short as I could make it consistent with most *Letters to the Editor*—was approximately 1,500 words and 21 citations; the version accepted and published by the *Journal* was approximately 450 words and 4 citations, and it notably excluded my five main concluding statements, which I have included here:

"In sum, the review by Manzel et al is characterized by:
1) Questionable and/or erroneous statements presented as matter of fact without any citation,
2) Failure to include important research showing significant and replicated clinical data in humans,
3) Inappropriate promotion of drug treatments over nutritional treatments,
4) Apparent failure to disclose financial relationships with drug companies[161], and
5) Inaccurate, denigrating, and sweeping generalizations misrepresenting the (in)efficacy of nutritional supplements."

Out of respect and appreciation for the (new) editorial team at the *Journal*, and because of this book's space limitation (printing limit of 630 pages) and my own overscheduled schedule, I have chosen to not make the full version of my reply public yet, but may do so later in *International Journal of Human Nutrition and Functional Medicine* available at ICHNFM.org/publications/. While I honestly think the original article by Manzel et al is a horrid (mis)representation of the current state of the science, I do appreciate the modest-yet-significant show of integrity by the *Journal* editors in their acceptance and publication of my *Reply*; anything less would have warranted a potent response in defense of science, intellectual integrity, and the clinicians and patients dependent on the integrity of science for pain-alleviating and life-saving decisions.

---

[158] Vasquez A. Reply to "role of Western diet in inflammatory autoimmune diseases" by Manzel et Al. In *Current Allergy and Asthma Reports* (volume 14, issue 1, January 2014). *Curr Allergy Asthma Rep*. 2014 Aug;14(8):454. Published online 20 Jun 2014 link.springer.com/journal/11882
[159] Vasquez A. Rebuttal to "Role of Western Diet in Inflammatory Autoimmune Diseases" by Manzel et al in Current Allergy Asthma Reports 2014 January. *International Journal of Human Nutrition and Functional Medicine* ® 2014:2(2);2 ICHNFM.org/publications/
[160] Manzel A, Muller DN, Hafler DA, et al. Role of "Western diet" in inflammatory autoimmune diseases. *Curr Allergy Asthma Rep*. 2014 Jan;14(1):404
[161] "Dr. Linker has received personal compensation for activities with BayerVital, Biogen Idec, NovartisPharma, Merck Serono, and TEVA Pharma. Dr. Linker has received research support from BayerVital, Biogen Idec, NovartisPharma, Merck Serono, and TEVA Pharma. Dr. Kleinewietfeld has received royalty payments from Stemcell-Technologies. Dr. Hafler has received personal compensation for activities with Wyeth, Beckman Coulter, and Novartis." S50 Multiple Sclerosis: Novel Mechanisms of Action High Dietary Salt Aggravates Experimental Neuroinflammation in Mice via Induction of Th17 Cells. *Neurology* February 12, 2013 neurology.org/cgi/content/meeting_abstract/80/1_MeetingAbstracts/S50.003

Reply to "Role of Western Diet in Inflammatory Autoimmune Diseases" by Manzel et al. in *Current Allergy and Asthma Reports* (Volume 14, Issue 1, January 2014)

Alex Vasquez

© Springer Science+Business Media New York 2014

To the Editor,

Regarding the recent review "Role of Western Diet in Inflammatory Autoimmune Diseases" [1], while I appreciate the importance of this topic and the authors' review, I noted several shortcomings in this review and have questions about the omission of certain information. The authors failed to include relevant and important human data while instead relying on animal studies (their Table 1). The authors also include erroneous information, without appropriate citation.

The authors state that "a high-fat diet is a prominent factor in promoting obesity" but failed to provide citation for this. Importantly, other researchers have shown that high-fat ketogenic diets promote weight loss rather than obesity.

I found the reliance on animal data (especially their Table 1) and the exclusion of human data inappropriate for a review article of this nature and at this time in biomedical history. Several clinical trials have already documented the effectiveness of dietary intervention in human autoimmune diseases. For example, diets which emphasize increased consumption of plant foods (excluding gluten-containing grains) and dietary alteration of gastrointestinal flora have already shown clinical benefits [2]. Exclusion of gluten is of critical importance for some patients, and well established is gluten's role in inflammation, alteration of gastrointestinal flora, increasing intestinal permeability, and direct stimulation of inflammatory pathways. The authors mentioned hypertension four times in their review but failed to mention the remarkable efficacy of therapeutic fasting for this condition [3]. Clinical trials showing the safety and efficacy of dietary fatty acid supplementation were also excluded from the review, despite showing remarkable clinical safety and antirheumatic efficacy [4]. Antiinflammatory mechanisms of dietary intervention not mentioned in their review include alleviation of oxidative stress, alleviation of dysbiosis, reduced reactivity to dietary antigens, normalization of intestinal hyperpermeability, and alleviation of proinflammatory mitochondrial dysfunction [5].

This article is part of the Topical Collection on *Autoimmunity*

A. Vasquez
International College of Human Nutrition and Functional Medicine in Barcelona, Barcelona, Spain
e-mail: ichnfm@gmail.com

A. Vasquez
Biotics Research Corporation in Rosenberg, Rosenberg, TX, USA

Published online: 20 June 2014

References

1. Manzel A, Muller DN, Hafler DA, Erdman SE, Linker RA, Kleinewietfeld M. Role of "Western diet" in inflammatory autoimmune diseases. Curr Allergy Asthma Rep. 2014;14(1):404.
2. Peltonen R, Nenonen M, Helve T, et al. Faecal microbial flora and disease activity in rheumatoid arthritis during a vegan diet. Br J Rheumatol. 1997;36(1):64–8.
3. Goldhamer A, Lisle D, Parpia B, Anderson SV, Campbell TC. Medically supervised water-only fasting in the treatment of hypertension. J Manip Physiol Ther. 2001;24(5):335–9.
4. Belch JJ, Ansell D, Madhok R, O'Dowd A, Sturrock RD. Effects of altering dietary essential fatty acids on requirements for non-steroidal anti-inflammatory drugs in patients with rheumatoid arthritis: a double blind placebo controlled study. Ann Rheum Dis. 1988;47(2):96–104.
5. Vasquez A. Integrative rheumatology and inflammation mastery, Third Edition. Create Space Publishers; 2014.

Mechanisms of diet in autoimmunity—partial representation: Vasquez A. Reply to "role of Western diet in inflammatory autoimmune diseases" by Manzel et Al. In *Current Allergy and Asthma Reports* (volume 14, issue 1, January 2014). *Curr Allergy Asthma Rep.* 2014 Aug;14(8):454. **Copyright Statement from Publisher**: The final publication is available at Springer via dx.doi.org/10.1007/s11882-014-0454-4. Author retains the right to use his/her article for his/her further scientific career by including the final published journal article in other publications such as dissertations and postdoctoral qualifications provided acknowledgement is given to the original source of publication.

Diet—Details, Biochemical Concepts, and Clinical Pearls
- **Macronutrients and "The Big Picture"**: The following section balances details with practicality to review necessary "real world" information for clinicians who aspire to efficacy en route to excellence in the realm of nutritional medicine.

  > **Nutritional Biochemistry: Words of Wisdom**
  >
  > "You can do no better than the food that you eat, but you can do a whole lot worse."
  >
  > Jeffrey Bland PhD, *Nutritional Biochemistry* lecture series, circa 1985

  - Protein: As with all nutrients, we can begin the conversation by breaking-down a large topic into its components, the main two of which are consumption and utilization, with the former obviously preceding the latter; realistically, those are preceded by availability, affordability, and selection.
    - Protein acquisition: Challenges to dietary protein acquisition include: availability, cost, knowledge of need, social/political norms, and frequency of utilization. In famished countries and regions, carbohydrate-sufficient protein malnutrition (*kwashiorkor*) is noted, while a milder form of "subclinical protein malnutrition" is impressively common among vegetarians, vegans, and persons who simply do not consume sufficient dietary protein due to habit or ignorance. As my teacher Dr Jeffrey Bland wisely said in his lecture series on *Nutritional Biochemistry* several decades ago, "You can do no better than the food that you eat, but you can do a whole lot worse." As such, the minimum requirement for proper protein nutriture begins with consumption of the proper amount of high-quality dietary protein per age, size/weight, activity and physiologic needs; the following table provides excellent objective guidance:

Recommended <u>Grams of Protein</u> per <u>Patient Profile</u> and <u>Body Weight</u> Per Day		
Patient Profile	*Per* **pound** *of weight*[162]	*Per* **kilogram** *of weight*
Adult recreational exerciser	0.5-0.75	1.1-1.65
Adult competitive athlete	0.6-0.9	1.32-1.98
Adult building muscle mass	0.7-0.9	1.54-1.98
Dieting athlete	0.7-1.0	1.54-2.2
Growing teenage athlete	0.9-1.0	1.98-2.2

Sufficient dietary protein is essential for patients with musculoskeletal injuries because tissue healing relies on the constant availability of amino acids and micronutrients[163], which should be supplied by a healthy, balanced, whole-foods diet that may be supplemented with specific vitamins, minerals, and phytonutrients. Increased protein intake does not adversely affect bone health as long as dietary calcium intake is adequate[164]; acid-base balance, and intakes of vitamin D3, magnesium, anti-inflammatory fatty acids, and other nutrients such as vitamin K and phytonutrients are also clinically important. Per the excellent review by Lemon[165], "Those involved in strength training might need to consume as much as …1.7 g protein x kg(-1) x day(-1)…while those undergoing endurance training might need about 1.2 to 1.6 g x kg(-1) x day(-1)… **…there is no evidence that protein intakes in the range suggested will have adverse effects in healthy individuals.**" To calculate protein requirements for patients who are completely sedentary, multiply body weight in pounds by 0.4 and this will give the number of grams of protein that should be eaten each day.[166] For patients who are very active (frequent weight lifting, or competitive athlete), multiply body weight in pounds by 0.7-0.9 and this will give the number of grams of protein that should be eaten each day. Again, compared with *sedentary* people, those who are **sick, injured, and athletic need more dietary protein** to maintain weight, fight infections, repair injuries, and build and maintain muscle mass. Low-

---

[162] Slightly modified from Nancy Clark, MS, RD. Protein Power. *The Physician and Sportsmedicine* 1996, volume 24, number 4
[163] "Supplementation with protein and vitamins, specifically arginine and vitamins A, B, and C, provides optimum nutrient support of the healing wound." Meyer NA, Muller MJ, Herndon DN. Nutrient support of the healing wound. *New Horiz* 1994 May;2(2):202-14
[164] Heaney RP. Excess dietary protein may not adversely affect bone. *J Nutr* 1998 Jun;128(6):1054-7
[165] Lemon PW. Effects of exercise on dietary protein requirements. *Int J Sport Nutr* 1998 Dec;8(4):426-47
[166] Pellet PL. Protein requirements in humans. *Am J Clin Nutr* 1990 May;51(5):723-37

protein diets suppress immune function, reduce muscle mass, and impair healing[167,168] whereas intakes of higher amounts of protein safely facilitate healing and the maintenance of muscle mass.

- Carbohydrates, CHO: Carbohydrate intake should be sufficient but otherwise minimal because carbohydrates—much more so than proteins and lipids and in many cases exclusively—promote dyslipidemia, immunosuppression, mitochondrial impairment, hunger, tumorigenesis, inflammation, oxidative stress and antioxidant depletion. Importantly, carbohydrate intake is the most important macronutrient *inverse* determinant of endogenous bHB production; excessive carbohydrate intake suppresses bHB production and therefore leads to direct/relative mitochondrial impairment, oxidative stress, and an aging (rather than rejuvenative) phenotype. Excess carbohydrate intake—notably fermentable carbohydrates such as from wheat and potatoes—is also the most important dietary cause of small intestinal bacterial overgrowth (SIBO), which is the primary cause the majority of cases of fibromyalgia (FM)[169], gastroesophageal reflux[170], irritable bowel syndrome (IBS)[171], and restless leg syndrome (RLS)[172], especially when accompanied by IBS or FM. Benefits of carbohydrate intake include maintenance of glucose/glycogen stores and relative elevation of serum tryptophan (depression of other amino acid levels) for enhanced serotonergic cerebral neurotransmission. Although patients and doctors alike have been conditioned to believe that carbohydrate intake is necessary at every meal and via snacks and sugared beverages throughout the day, the more profound truths are that ❶ carbohydrate-rich foods are better avoided, ❷ carbohydrate intake should be minimized to meet physiologic requirements (e.g., recovery from exercise, maintenance of desired weight), and ❸ constant intake of carbohydrates produces what I term *carbohydrate-mediated carbohydrate dependence*—excessive physiologic dependence on carbohydrates via adaptation to this fuel source (for example in part via dietary modification of

Adverse effects of dietary carbohydrates (general) and processed fructose (specific)
- Adipogenesis
- Hyperphagia (absolute or relative)
- Immunosuppression
- Oxidative stress
- Antioxidant nutrient depletion
- Endogenous antimetabolites: Promotion of palmitate and ceramide production, with resultant insulin resistance.
- Hyperinsulinemia: Stimulation of sodium retention (promoting HTN) and HMG-CoA reductase (promoting hypercholesterolemia).
- Loss of endogenous bHB: Inhibition of bHB (beta-hydroxy-butyrate) production; loss of bHB causes a relative increase in oxidant stress and loss of mitochondrial function.
- GI microbial overgrowth: Residual and fermentable carbohydrates in the gastrointestinal tract directly promote microbial overgrowth in gut, promoting systemic inflammation (e.g., via LPS, increased intestinal permeability, and immune complexes), fibromyalgia, GERD, RLS.
- Problems specific to fructose: Induction of bacterial dysbiosis and increased intestinal permeability leading to endotoxinemia; induction of AGE / Maillard reaction / glycosylation glycation; rapid influx of processed/acellular fructose causes ATP depletion at fructokinase, activates inflammatory pathways, leads to increase in serum urate which causes endothelial dysfunction and insulin resistance—proof of this comes from inhibition of fructose-induced metabolic syndrome via allopurinol and avoidance of fructose-induced metabolic syndrome and weight gain when fructose is consumed with antioxidant/anti-inflammatory phytochemicals and citrate, the latter of which promotes urinary alkalinization for efficient urate excretion and thereby avoidance of problems induced by relative/absolute hyperuricaemia.

---

[167] Castaneda et al. Elderly women accommodate to a low-protein diet with losses of body cell mass, muscle function, and immune response. *Am J Clin Nutr* 1995;62:30-9
[168] [No author listed]. Vegetarians and healing. *JAMA* 1995; 273: 910
[169] Pimentel M, Wallace D, Hallegua D, Chow E, Kong Y, Park S, Lin HC. A link between irritable bowel syndrome and fibromyalgia may be related to findings on lactulose breath testing. *Ann Rheum Dis*. 2004 Apr;63(4):450-2. For much greater detail and explanation, see my later works/books/chapters on fibromyalgia which integrate this research with the secondary problems such as microbial mitochondriopathy; my most recent update to the fibromyalgia model was published in *Integrative Rheumatology and Inflammation Mastery* (2014); visit InflammationMastery.com for additional publications and updated publications and videos.
[170] Austin GL, Thiny MT, Westman EC, Yancy WS Jr, Shaheen NJ. A very low-carbohydrate diet improves gastroesophageal reflux and its symptoms. *Dig Dis Sci*. 2006 Aug;51(8):1307-12. Yancy WS Jr, Provenzale D, Westman EC. Improvement of gastroesophageal reflux disease after initiation of a low-carbohydrate diet: five brief case reports. *Altern Ther Health Med*. 2001 Nov-Dec;7(6):120, 116-9. Piche T, des Varannes SB, Sacher-Huvelin S, Holst JJ, Cuber JC, Galmiche JP. Colonic fermentation influences lower esophageal sphincter function in gastroesophageal reflux disease. *Gastroenterology*. 2003 Apr;124(4):894-902
[171] Lin HC. Small intestinal bacterial overgrowth: a framework for understanding irritable bowel syndrome. *JAMA*. 2004 Aug 18;292(7):852-8
[172] Weinstock et al. Restless legs syndrome in patients with irritable bowel syndrome: response to SIBO therapy. *Dig Dis Sci*. 2008 May;53(5):1252-6

electron transport chain supercomplex assembly[173]). Dietary carbohydrate sources can be selected based on their ability to promote or inhibit intestinal microbial growth; this is the basis for the specific carbohydrate diet (SCD)[174] and variations on that theme to prevent microbial overgrowth in the intestines and its complications such as autobrewery syndrome.[175, 176]

- Fats, lipids: Average Paleolithic intake of n3 fatty acids was approximately 7 grams per day; and modern (American diet) intake is 1 gram per day; therefore, relatively speaking and contrasting physiologic expectations with modern dietary intakes, persons/patients can be considered n3-deficient unless they are consuming n3 supplementation or what would be considered today "special" (or by the allopathic paradigm: "faddish") diets. What is commonly called fatty acid *supplementation* should more appropriately be called fatty acid *replacement* since generally all that is being done is *normalizing* intake of fatty acids, rather than doing anything heroic or unnatural. All of the main dietary n3 fatty acids (FA)—ALA, EPA, DHA—have clinically significant anti-inflammatory benefits; n6FA linolenic and arachidonic acids are both clearly pro-inflammatory and tumorigenic, while n6FA GLA is clearly anti-inflammatory and anti-tumorigenic. In the gastrointestinal tract, dietary long-chain saturated fats promote LPS absorption from the gastrointestinal tract via chylomicron formation; in this way "saturated fat promotes inflammation" *via a mechanism completely independent from the metabolic and adipogenic effects of fat*: by serving as a carrier/container for pro-inflammatory bacterial LPS.

- Fiber: Basically—from the perspective of clinicians, "fibers" and indigestible carbohydrate from plants can be considered in three different ways: ❶ Soluble—think "absorbing", bulking, and fermentable: Best example is oat bran, absorbs and reduces absorption of cholesterol, serves as fermentable food source for bacteria and in this manner increases fecal bulk (along with water retention), not necessarily a good idea for patients with SIBO, ❷ Insoluble—think "binding", bulking, and mostly nonfermentable: Best example is wheat bran, but rice bran is also commercially available and avoids the problems of wheat's toxic gluten; vegetable fibers are mostly insoluble fiber; more likely to bind minerals such as zinc and iron, generally/relatively nonfermentable and thus increases fecal bulk via mass and some water retention (rather than promoting growth of bacteria); reasonable for patients with SIBO; vegetable matter in general and brown rice in particular have favorable effects on human gastrointestinal flora, promoting eubiosis; in regard to the latter, carrots are notable for their antimicrobial/eubiosis effect for which carrots have been used for the treatment of infectious diarrhea (and SIBO); ❸ Fermentable carbohydrates lacking physical bulking action: Best examples are inulin and fructooligosaccharides (FOS) which generally promote growth of beneficial bacteria excepting *Klebsiella pneumoniae* growth on FOS; no physical bulking action except via bacterial proliferation; no absorbing/binding action of clinical significance.

- pH and acid-base balance: Given the body's inherent acid-forming tendency, alkalinizing measures must be available to prevent what would otherwise be inevitable metabolic acidosis resulting specifically from cellular metabolism and its attendant production of organic acids, carbon dioxide, ketoacids, and sulfuric acid, the last in this list from sulfur-containing amino acid catabolism. Both acute and long-term acid-base balance are *grossly* regulated by respiration and urination, while the more subtle fine-tuning occurs via dietary input. In accord with the concept of biochemical individuality and the truism that treatment must always be individualized, some people tend to be more or less *acidic* or *basic* than others as measured by urine pH, which is a reasonable measure of systemic acid-base status provided adequate renal function and which allows direct measurement of urine pH, which—per the position paper by Proudfoot et al—should be at least 7.5 to promote

---

[173] Lapuente-Brun et al. Supercomplex assembly determines electron flux in the mitochondrial electron transport chain. *Science*. 2013 Jun 28;340(6140):1567-70
[174] Gottschall EG. *Breaking the Vicious Cycle: Intestinal Health Through Diet*, 1994
[175] Dahshan et al. Auto-brewery syndrome in a child with short gut syndrome: case report and review of the literature. *J Pediatr Gastroenterol Nutr*. 2001 Aug;33(2):214-5
[176] Cordell et al. Case Study of Gut Fermentation Syndrome (Auto-Brewery) with Saccharomyces cerevisiae as the Causative Organism. *Int J Clin Med* 2013, 4, 309-312

xenobiotic excretion. However, generally speaking for most of the population consuming a Western diet characterized by *gross* insufficiency of plants (thus lack of [potassium] citrate as an immediate precursor for alkalinizing bicarbonate) and a *relative* excess of animal/dairy/grain protein (thereby promoting endogenous formation of sulfuric acid); in this manner, the Western diet is said to promote **diet-induced metabolic acidosis**, which promotes many long-term (not acute) health problems such as osteoporosis, insulin resistance, hypertension, and possibly malignant disease.[177] Urinary alkalinization can be maintained via *a personalized combination of* plant-based diets, regular deep-breathing and exercise to promote respiratory alkalosis, and supplemental potassium/magnesium citrate/bicarbonate (rarely sodium bicarbonate, which has the disadvantage of sodium but the advantage of greater public availability); benefits of alkalinization include enhanced detoxification/clearance of xenobiotics, thereby contributing to alleviation of current disease and reduced risk of future disease[178], ◐ increased endorphin production for alleviation of pain[179] and depression, possible lessening of (tobacco) addiction[180], ◉ reduced serum cortisol and bone loss[181] and likely reductions in hippocampal atrophy and insulin resistance also via reductions in serum cortisol, ◓ enhanced intracellular retention of magnesium by 11%[182], ◒ enhanced xenobiotic excretion (generally).[183]

Net acid and base production from common foods
Acid-producing foods: Notice that these foods represent the majority of food intake for many people, thereby promoting population-wide diet-induced metabolic acidosis: • Fish, shellfish, meat, poultry, eggs, • Cheese, milk • Cereal grains • Chloride ion (added in the form of sodium chloride, table salt)
Base-producing foods: • Fruit, vegetables, tubers, roots, and nuts
Neutral: • Legumes • Fats • Refined sugars
Cordain et al. Origins and evolution of Western diet. *Am J Clin Nutr*. 2005

o **Micronutrients and nutritional supplementation with vitamins, minerals, combination fatty acids, and probiotics**: Space, time, and scope do not allow an exhaustive review of all vitamins and minerals in this volume; my last outline of all major vitamins and minerals was printed in *Chiropractic and Naturopathic Mastery of Common Clinical Disorders* (2009) and the next version of such will be published in an upcoming volume in this *Inflammation Mastery* series and/or in an open-access review published in *International Journal of Human Nutrition and Functional Medicine*. Here, I will only discuss a few classic must-know topics while the nutrients relevant for the **functional inflammology protocol** are discussed within contexts of clinical application; the subject of routine nutritional supplementation is also addressed in my accompanying presentation from ICHNFM 2013.[184] **Combination fatty acid therapy (CFAT)** is discussed in the minimonograph in this chapter; additional applications are mentioned in the description of the protocol and in additional volumes detailing clinical applications for specific conditions. **Probiotics** should be pretty well known to most of my readers; additional details are provided elsewhere in the book and are not replicated here; my clinical approach to probiotic therapy emphasizes 1) dietary optimization since diet is the most important determinant of intestinal microbial ecology, 2) daily consumption of fermented/probiotic foods such as yogurt, kefir, miso, real sauerkraut, etc, 3) stress reduction and nutrient supplementation (e.g., vitamins A and D, along with zinc and glutamine) to improve intestinal immunity and thereby reduce dysbiosis and promote eubiosis, 4) use

---

[177] "Even a very mild degree of metabolic acidosis induces skeletal muscle resistance to the insulin action and dietary acid load may be an important variable in predicting the metabolic abnormalities and the cardiovascular risk of the general population, the overweight and obese persons, and other patient populations including diabetes and chronic kidney failure. High dietary acid load is more likely to result in diabetes and systemic hypertension and may increase the cardiovascular risk." Adeva MM, Souto G. Diet-induced metabolic acidosis. *Clin Nutr*. 2011 Aug;30(4):416-21
[178] Minich DM, Bland JS. Acid-alkaline balance: role in chronic disease and detoxification. *Altern Ther Health Med*. 2007 Jul-Aug;13(4):62-5
[179] Vormann J, et al. Supplementation with alkaline minerals reduces symptoms in patients with chronic low back pain. *J Trace Elem Med Biol*. 2001;15(2-3):179-83
[180] This study showed a small initial trend toward less tobacco smoke use/inhalation following urinary alkalinization with sodium bicarbonate. Cherek DR, Mauroner RF, Brauchi JT. Effects of increasing urinary pH on cigarette smoking. *Clin Pharmacol Ther*. 1982 Aug;32(2):253-60
[181] Maurer M, Riesen W, Muser J, Hulter HN, Krapf R. Neutralization of Western diet inhibits bone resorption independently of K intake and reduces cortisol secretion in humans. *Am J Physiol Renal Physiol*. 2003 Jan;284(1):F32-40
[182] Vormann J, et al. Supplementation with alkaline minerals reduces symptoms in patients with chronic low back pain. *J Trace Elem Med Biol*. 2001;15(2-3):179-83
[183] Proudfoot AT, Krenzelok EP, Vale JA. Position Paper on urine alkalinization. *J Toxicol Clin Toxicol*. 2004;42(1):1-26
[184] Vasquez A. "Introduction to Functional Inflammology Protocol" presented at International Conference on Human Nutrition and Functional Medicine in Portland, Oregon September 25-29, 2013. More than eight hours of video introducing the functional inflammology protocol—to be used with the printed slides in the final section of this book—is available online: vimeo.com/album/2943155. Password: **DrVprotocol_volume1**

of probiotic and synbiotic supplements to further ensure intake of beneficial microbes. The subsections that follow detail some of the most important general concepts and specific *must know* information about vitamins and minerals—again see the accompanying presentation from the 2013 International Conference on Human Nutrition and Functional Medicine (vimeo.com/ICHNFM) for additional details, rationale, and citations. Before reviewing the important articles summarized and cited immediately following, I'd like to offer one additional consideration: Per standard definitions, our whole idea of "nutritional deficiency" and therefore the need/rightness/wrongness of nutritional supplementation is wrong. Nutritional deficiency should be defined as "insufficient amount relative to individual need" – not absolute amount. We have two intellectually defensible options: 1) scientific but impractical: test all levels and functional parameters to determine month-by-month/year-by-year nutritional needs which change per diet, illness, medication, lifestyle, age, or 2) reasonable and practical: provide a reasonable dose of nutrients to "cover the bases" and meet biochemical needs to safely, inexpensively, and effectively avoid the problems caused by common and occult micronutrient deficiency. The third option which requires zero thought is to 3) deny reality to the detriment of the patient: ignore this data and pretend everything will work out fine on its own.

- General rationale for routine nutritional supplementation #1—Vitamins for chronic disease prevention in adults (*JAMA* 2002 Jun[185]): "However, suboptimal intake of some vitamins, above levels causing classic vitamin deficiency, is a risk factor for chronic diseases and common in the general population, especially the elderly. ...low levels of the antioxidant vitamins (vitamins A, E, and C) may increase risk for several chronic diseases. Most people do not consume an optimal amount of all vitamins by diet alone. Pending strong evidence of effectiveness from randomized trials, it appears prudent for all adults to take vitamin supplements. ... Physicians should make specific efforts to learn about their patients' use of vitamins to ensure that they are taking vitamins they should...."
- General rationale for routine nutritional supplementation #2—Prevention of long-latency deficiency disease: insights from calcium and vitamin D (*Am J Clin Nutr* 2003 Nov[186]): "Nutrient intake recommendations and national nutritional policies have focused primarily on prevention of short-latency deficiency diseases. Most nutrient intake recommendations today are based on prevention of the index disease only. However, inadequate intakes of many nutrients are now recognized as contributing to several of the major chronic diseases that affect the populations of the industrialized nations. Often taking many years to manifest themselves, these disease outcomes should be thought of as long-latency deficiency diseases."
- General rationale for routine nutritional supplementation #3—Promotion of optimal metabolism in lieu of the expense and unavailability of extensive laboratory testing for each patient (*Am J Clin Nutr* 2002 Apr[187]): "As many as one-third of mutations in a gene result in the corresponding enzyme having an increased Michaelis constant, or K(m), (decreased binding affinity) for a coenzyme, resulting in a lower rate of reaction. About 50 human genetic dis-eases due to defective enzymes can be remedied or ameliorated by the administration of high doses of the vitamin component of the corresponding coenzyme, which at least partially restores enzymatic activity. Several single-nucleotide polymorphisms, in which the variant amino acid reduces coenzyme binding and thus enzymatic activity, are likely to be remediable by raising cellular concentrations of the cofactor through high-dose vitamin therapy."
- General rationale for routine nutritional supplementation #4—Vitamin D deficiency is the most common and most clinically significant nutrient deficiency seen regularly in the practice of primary care medicine (*Altern Ther Health Med* 2004 Sep[188]): Beyond vitamin and mineral supplementation in general is the clinicians' need to focus on vitamin D3 supplementation, especially given that most multivitamin formulations do not meet the physiologic requirement

---

[185] Fletcher RH, Fairfield KM. Vitamins for chronic disease prevention in adults: clinical applications. *JAMA*. 2002 Jun 19;287(23):3127-9
[186] Heaney RP. Long-latency deficiency disease: insights from calcium and vitamin D. *Am J Clin Nutr*. 2003 Nov;78(5):912-9
[187] Ames BN, et al. High-dose vitamin therapy stimulates variant enzymes with decreased coenzyme binding affinity (increased Km). *Am J Clin Nutr* 2002 Apr;75:616-58
[188] Vasquez A, Manso G, Cannell J. The clinical importance of vitamin D (cholecalciferol): a paradigm shift. *Altern Ther Health Med.* 2004 Sep-Oct;10(5):28-36

in adults of approximately 4,000 IU/d; per my 2004 "paradigm shift with implications for all healthcare providers" all readers should know that vitamin D deficiency causes—in large percentages of patients per diagnosis—hypertension, migraine headaches, widespread body pain identical to fibromyalgia, local pain consistent with low-back pain, insulin resistance, systemic inflammation and autoimmunity.

- General rationale for routine nutritional supplementation #5—DNA damage from micronutrient deficiencies is likely to be a major cause of cancer (*Mutat Res.* 2001 Apr[189]): " A deficiency of any of the micronutrients: folic acid, Vitamin B12, Vitamin B6, niacin, Vitamin C, Vitamin E, iron, or zinc, mimics radiation in damaging DNA by causing single- and double-strand breaks, oxidative lesions, or both. For example, the percentage of the US population that has a low intake (<50% of the RDA) for each of these eight micronutrients ranges from 2 to >20%. ... Some evidence, and mechanistic considerations, suggest that Vitamin B12 (14% US elderly) and B6 (10% of US) deficiencies also cause high uracil and chromosome breaks. ...Common micronutrient deficiencies are likely to damage DNA by the same mechanism as radiation and many chemicals, appear to be orders of magnitude more important, and should be compared for perspective. Remedying micronutrient deficiencies should lead to a major improvement in health and an increase in longevity at low cost."

- Additional clinical details on iron: Necessary for formation of hemoglobin and dopamine, iron—when accumulated "too much and in the wrong location"—promotes ROS-mediated cellular toxicity, leading to cardiomyopathy, hypogonadism, hepatopathy, and diabetes mellitus; an insufficiency of iron causes immune impairment, mitochondrial dysfunction, anemia, and depression/fatigue/anhedonia due to insufficient CNS dopamine and norepinephrine.
    - Excess absorption and altered storage: Hereditary iron-accumulation disorders such as genetic hemochromatosis are among the most common hereditary diseases in the human population, occurring in all races, both genders, with a clinical presentation occurring at any age but typically in adulthood. Among Caucasians and Hispanics, genetic hemochromatosis has a homozygote frequency of approximately 1 per 200-250 and a heterozygote frequency of 1 per 7; among Africans and African Americans, the clinical phenotype of severe iron overload has been reported as high as 1 per 80 in hospital populations. Genotropic iron-accumulation disorders are quantitative (i.e., excess intestinal absorption of iron) and qualitative (i.e., parenchymal storage which is abnormal and more cytotoxic than the normal deposition of iron in the mononuclear phagocyte system (MPS, previously termed the reticuloendothelial system).
    - Defective/deficient blood-brain transport: A subset of the population has a defect in transport of iron from the blood into the brain can thus develop "brain-specific iron deficiency" with anticipated deficiencies in dopamine, norepinephrine, and mitochondrial function. Clinical consequences of "cerebral iron deficiency" would therefore be expected to include deficits in attention, hedonia/pleasure/mood, motor control, and migraine precipitated by mitochondrial dysfunction. In 2005 Mizuno et al[190] showed low brain iron concentrations in patients with restless leg syndrome (RLS) was due to "dysfunction of iron transportation from serum to CNS in patients with idiopathic RLS" while a more detailed study performed in 2011 by Connor et al[191] confirmed "alterations in the iron management protein profile in RLS compared with controls at the site of blood-brain interface" and also noted a consistent "decrease in transferrin receptor expression in the microvasculature in the presence of relative brain iron deficiency."

---

[189] Ames BN. DNA damage from micronutrient deficiencies is likely to be a major cause of cancer. *Mutat Res.* 2001 Apr 18;475(1-2):7-20
[190] "These results indicate low brain iron concentration caused by the dysfunction of iron transportation from serum to CNS in patients with idiopathic RLS." Mizuno S, Mihara T, Miyaoka T, Inagaki T, Horiguchi J. CSF iron, ferritin and transferrin levels in restless legs syndrome. *J Sleep Res.* 2005 Mar;14(1):43-7
[191] Connor JR, et al. Profile of altered brain iron acquisition in restless legs syndrome. *Brain.* 2011 Apr;134(Pt 4):959-68

- Food consumption: Reviewed here are some clinically important facts about food preparation, consumption, digestion, and metabolism. Advancements in technology and our molecular biology understanding make a conversation about digestion and mastication seem comparatively primitive. But we all need to pause and reflect on the importance of basic digestion, mastication, salvation etc for proper digestion. Regardless of advances in technology, certain physiologic truths remain inviolable.
  - Preparation: Many people lack basic cooking skills, and are thus dependent on processed/packaged/industrial food products; indeed, one of the most important medical consequences of the dissolution of social and familial structure is the pervasive loss of essential life skills—one of the most important of which is food selection and preparation. Fundamental courses in food preparation should be required for all healthcare professionals, who have the responsibility to educate their patients and model good health practices. Most protein-dense animal-based foods can be consumed raw if fresh and sourced from noninfected animals; social customs and concern about microbial contamination commonly prompt cooking, which—despite denaturing dietary proteins—often increases digestibility, palatability, and ease of mastication, thereby increasing total protein intake. The most notable concern with diet-induced parasitosis is cysticercosis and neurocysticercosis caused from consumption of pork which is both undercooked and infected, classically with the pork tapeworm *Taenia solium*.[192] Food-transmitted prion-induced spongiform encephalopathies have been very rarely reported in humans following consumption of deer, boar, elk, and—classically in the case of *kuru*—cultural cannibalism of human brain.
  - Consumption: Desire is psychoepistimological, a translation of intellectual and emotional presuppositions into emotional/visceral/emotive responses and actions. Acquisition is motivated by desire, and either facilitate or restrained by social, cultural, and financial realities. Proper protein nutriture requires adequate protein consumption. Psychosocial stress, depression, zinc deficiency, and certain medications (especially stimulants) commonly contribute to anorexia (inadequate appetite and food consumption). Zinc deficiency causes anorexia (reduced appetite/intake), hypogeusia (reduced sense of taste), and hyposmia (reduced sense of smell): all of which contribute to reduced food consumption.
  - Mastication: Generally and simplistically speaking, digestion is the break-down of food from animal and plant tissue/material to its component proteins and constituent amino acids and peptides for absorption and cellular uptake; the enzymatic/biochemical breakdown of foods is facilitated by mechanical degradation, allowing greater surface area and thus more enzyme-protein contact, resulting in better "digestion." ==Teeth (dentition) and time (patience) are needed for proper mastication==; an insufficiency of either via dental disease or lack of time allowance/prioritization, respectively, will compromise mastication and thus digestion and thus protein nutriture.

The biggest dietary deficiencies are those of time, information, and prioritization
• Most people do not have/make time to relax, consider, prepare and masticate a health-promoting diet. Without time and the prioritization of that time for self-care, parasympathetic-mediated and rejuvenative activities, health will always have to be pursued artificially.
• Consider the alternate: overeating fast food (pesticides, GMO toxins; excess fat, carbohydrates, salt; absence of phytonutrients) in a hurry and relying on drugs for resultant problems—in America, approximately 15-21% of food consumed by young adults 20-40y is "fast food" while a much larger proportion is processed and unhealthy food; thus, most of the food eaten promotes disease, not health.

  - Digestion—gastric: An adequacy of gastric hydrochloric acid (HCl) is necessary, especially for digestion of proteins, ionization of minerals for enhanced absorption, and microbicidal actions. Production/function of HCl is compromised by antacid substances (e.g., bicarbonate, histamine-2 receptor antagonists, proton-pump antagonists), *Helicobacter pylori* infection/colonization, zinc deficiency, hypocortisolemia, hypothyroidism, hypogonadism, and various types of psychoemotional stress. Inadequate HCl production is noted with

---

[192] See cdc.gov/parasites/cysticercosis/ and cdc.gov/parasites/taeniasis/ for discussion and images. Accessed April 2014

atrophic gastritis (such as due to alcoholism) and pernicious anemia; incidence of these is increased in patients with autoimmune thyroiditis and/or vitiligo. HCL replacement with capsules/tablets of betaine HCl can be helpful, and may only need to be maintained for a limited period of time (e.g., 6-12 months), after which endogenous production may return. HCl production can be assessed clinically, via response to HCl supplementation, or by Heidelberg radiotelemetry.
- Digestion—pancreatic: Production and function of pancreatic enzymes is notably zinc-dependent. With pancreatic insufficiency—as especially noted in patients with cystic fibrosis, postpancreatitis pancreatic insufficiency, or acne rosacea—oral supplementation with pancreatic/proteolytic enzymes from porcine/botanical sources can be highly beneficial.
- Digestion—mucosal: Mucosal proteases and peptidases contribute to protein digestion and peptide and amino acid absorption; these enzymes can be damaged/reduced by intestinal disorders such as celiac, Crohn's, and by degradation of mucosal enzymes by bacterial proteases as seen in SIBO—small intestine bacterial overgrowth.
- Absorption: Efficient nutrient absorption is dependent on mucosal/villous integrity, vascular and lymphatic integrity (e.g., impaired in congestive heart failure, which leads to bowel wall edema and reduced intestinal absorption), and all of the above previous steps. Mucosal integrity and absorption can be objectively and practically assessed by measuring urine levels of orally administered Lactulose (increased with a Leaky gut and increased paracellular absorption) and Mannitol (decreased with Malabsorption and reduced transcellular absorption); 24-hour fecal fat can also be measured, as steatorrhea can be seen with both pancreatic insufficiency (maldigestion) and mucosal injury (malabsorption). Mucosal injury is always an active and current problem, since the intestinal mucosa is otherwise and generally rapidly replicative and reparative; as expected, mucosal replication and repair is nutrient-dependent (especially zinc, vitamin A, and glutamine), and malnutrition and malabsorption can become a vicious cycle.
- Transport, cellular uptake, reception: Classic and clinically important considerations with nutrient transport, uptake, reception are as follows:
  - All/many nutrients: To promote the essential catalytic functions of enzymes to sustain organismal life, vitamins and minerals serve as coenzymes and cofactors, respectively. When genotropic amino acid substitutions, an example of single nucleotide polymorphisms (SNPs or "snips"), occur in enzyme structure, the result is a generally a subtle or gross alteration in enzyme function, generally reduced enzyme function, commonly due to reduced affinity for binding with the required coenzyme or cofactor. When enzymes are "slow" or "defective" due to alterations in structure due to altered amino acid composition due to SNPs, the provision of supradietary amounts of cofactors and coenzymes—vitamin and mineral supplementation—can be used to partly/completely restore enzymatic function and thus the biochemical reactions necessary for life and health. As this model is scientifically established, clinically proven, and generally irrefutable, these facts establish the scientific and intellectual basis for vitamin and mineral supplementation among "apparently healthy" and ill patients alike, which has been referred to as "orthomolecular medicine" (per Pauling[193], "use the right molecules") and "mega-nutrient" therapy.[194]
    - Review: High-dose vitamin therapy stimulates variant enzymes with decreased coenzyme binding affinity (*Am J Clin Nutr* 2002 Apr[195])—quite likely the most authoritative article ever written on this topic: "As many as one-third of mutations in a gene result in the corresponding enzyme having an increased

---

[193] Pauling L. Orthomolecular psychiatry. *Science*. 1968 Apr 19;160(3825):265-71
[194] Newbold HL. *Mega-nutrients for your nerves*. P. H. Wyden; First Edition edition 1975
[195] Ames BN, et al. High-dose vitamin therapy stimulates variant enzymes with decreased coenzyme binding affinity (increased Km). *Am J Clin Nutr* 2002 Apr;75:616-58

Michaelis constant, or K(m), (decreased binding affinity) for a coenzyme, resulting in a lower rate of reaction. ==About 50 human genetic dis-eases due to defective enzymes can be remedied or ameliorated by the administration of high doses of the vitamin component of the corresponding coenzyme, which at least partially restores enzymatic activity.== Several single-nucleotide polymorphisms, in which the variant amino acid reduces coenzyme binding and thus enzymatic activity, are likely to be remediable by raising cellular concentrations of the cofactor through ==high-dose vitamin therapy==."

- <u>Processed foods and the Western/American diet—general description and bioclinical considerations</u>: The general pattern eating described as the Western diet or the American diet (the latter with a higher specific emphasis on consumption of genetically manipulated organisms [GMO]) includes overconsumption of carbohydrates in general and sucrose, high-fructose corn syrup, wheat, potatoes, dairy in particular; insufficiency of fiber and phytonutrient-dense foods such as fruits and vegetables; overconsumption of chemicals such as colorants and preservatives and "flavor enhancers" such as MSG (excitoneurotoxic) and carrageenan (immunosuppressive, inflammatory, carcinogenic); overconsumption of sodium and chloride and underconsumption of potassium, magnesium, citrate, and bicarbonate; rampant vitamin and mineral deficiencies despite the outward appearance of obesity/overweight; diet-induced hunger, metabolic impairment, endoplasmic reticulum stress, mitochondrial dysfunction, and hypothalamic inflammation.
    - <u>GMO (genetically manipulated organisms and related toxins): introduction and survey of literature</u>: GMO foods were released onto the commercial food market in America in 1996 without adequate safety testing on animals, humans, and the environment. Genetic "*modification*" is a euphemism for interspecies **manipulation** of gene sequence and content; "modification" is far too benign a term, considering the *manipulation* (of politics, science, public opinion), *mistreatment* (of people, including what has been described as a *suicide belt* and *GM genocide* resulting from farmers bankrupted after using GMO crops and the imposition of profiteering corporate policies[196]), *maleficence* (harming people, animals, environment) that actually occurs, and the *metastatic* nature of GMO plants which have now contaminated previously nonGMO crops internationally, even in countries that have banned GMO crops, thus suggesting that airborne cross-pollination/contamination is inevitable, threatening global food security.[197] Because (multi)gene manipulation is used in tandem with high-dose pesticides and herbicides (therefore, in the real world, these are always used in complex synergistic combinations) and to reduce/avoid the ongoing problems that occur in science when these items are studied in isolation (note that doing so does *not* reflect the real world application and therefore such science is itself *unscientific* insofar as it is *unrealistic*), I use the term "GMO toxins" to include all genetic changes such as Bt and Ht and GMO-associated chemicals especially pesticides, herbicides, and the other falsely labeled "inert" chemicals in these formations; indeed, my use of the term GMO toxins is appropriate since virtually all of these gene changes and chemicals are designed to directly/indirectly kill life forms, in this case insects and plants, some of which are necessary for the cycle of life, parts of which include pollination of crops and the consumption/degradation of plant material for recovery of nutrients for reuse. I find the term "GMO toxins" less cumbersome than the alternative proposed elsewhere of "pesticides associated to genetically modified foods" (PAGMF), which is both longer and less inclusive. Human safety studies have not been performed on GMO foods and toxins despite the fact that in

---

[196] "Imagine a storm blows across your property – and that now, without your knowledge or consent, genetically manipulated seeds are present in the garden you have tended for years. A few days later, representatives of a multi-national corporation pay you a visit, demand that you surrender your produce - and simultaneously file a criminal complaint against you for the illegal use of patented, genetically-manipulated seeds. Around the world, this story represents the bitter truth. It's the real-life experience of Canadians Percy und Louise Schmeiser, who have been fighting chemical and seed manufacturer Monsanto since 1996. Today, nearly three-fourths of genetically manipulated plants harvested worldwide originated in Monsanto labs." Percy Schmeiser - David versus Monsanto, film by Bertram Verhaag. denkmalfilm.tv/index.php?l=en&page=percy-schmeiser-4 and amazon.com/David-vs-Monsanto-Percy-Schmeiser/dp/B004R14BZ8/. "So Shankara became one of an estimated 125,000 farmers to take their own life as a result of the ruthless drive to use India as a testing ground for genetically modified crops. The crisis, branded the 'GM Genocide' by campaigners, was highlighted recently when Prince Charles claimed that the issue of GM had become a 'global moral question' - and the time had come to end its unstoppable march." dailymail.co.uk/news/article-1082559/The-GM-genocide-Thousands-Indian-farmers-committing-suicide-using-genetically-modified-crops.html. "The highest acreage of Bt cotton is in Maharashtra and this is also where the highest farmer suicides are. Suicides increased after Bt cotton was introduced — Monsanto's royalty extraction, and the high costs of seed and chemicals have created a debt trap. According to Government of India data, nearly 75 per cent rural debt is due to purchase inputs. As Monsanto's profits grow, farmers' debt grows. It is in this systemic sense that Monsanto's seeds are seeds of suicide." globalresearch.ca/the-seeds-of-suicide-how-monsanto-destroys-farming/5329947.
[197] Quist D, Chapela IH. Transgenic DNA introgressed into traditional maize landraces in Oaxaca, Mexico. *Nature*. 2001 Nov 29;414(6863):541-3

America (the country that produces and consumes the most GM food) citizens eat more than their weight in GM foods per year.[198]

> **GMO toxins: all genes and chemicals related to GMO crops designed to kill insects, plants, and promote use of higher levels of other pesticides and herbicides**
> - **3-MPPA**: 3-methylphosphinicopropionic acid, metabolite of gluphosinate herbicide
> - **AMPA: aminomethyl phosphoric acid**, metabolite of glyphosate herbicide
> - **Bt**: bacterial toxin bacillus thuringiensis
> - **Cry1Ab protein**: one of the Bt toxins
> - **GLUF**: gluphosinate herbicide
> - **GLYP**: glyphosate herbicide
> - **Ht**: Herbicide tolerant, plants genetically altered to tolerate otherwise poisonous levels of herbicides
> - **"Inert" ingredients**: Several of these have been found harmful at real-life levels, promoting direct or indirect toxicity
> - **PAGMF**: pesticides associated to genetically modified foods
> - **"Stacked GMO"**: single plants with multiple genetic manipulations, such as combinations of Bt and Ht. For example, DK 42-88RRYGPL corn is a "triple stack of NK603, MON863 and MON810 genes" while Pannar 4E-705RR/Bt corn is a "double stack" of NK603 and MON810.

- Bt toxin—insecticidal via intestinal cell toxicity; reported link to intestinal toxicity in animals: *Bacillus thuringiensis* (or Bt) is a Gram-positive, soil-dwelling bacterium that produces crystal proteins called δ-endotoxins (Delta endotoxins, pore-forming toxins, also called Cry and Cyt toxins), which have insecticide action via binding of the delta-endotoxin to gut epithelium, causing cell lysis and insect death; this has led to the commercialized and patented insertion of Bt genes into plant crops to produce one common type of "genetically modified food" that, as a plant, provides its own endogenously-produced pesticide, theoretically leading to crop protection but possibly harming nontarget insects, including those necessary for pollination and other important functions in the web of life. Variants of the Bt gene can be inserted into plants to target specific insects; again, this basically converts what was previously a food (e.g., corn) into an unnatural hybrid of food-producing-a-bacterial-toxin-to-kill-intestinal-epithelial-cells. The question as to whether GMO/Bt causes biochemical/functional intestinal injury in animals and humans has not been answered; gross visualization (used in the study by Carman et al described below) is likely too insensitive and should be superseded by histologic or biochemical assessments such as the well-established sucrose/lactulose/mannitol absorption tests that are clinically and commercially available.
    - Long-term toxicology study on pigs fed a combined genetically modified (GM) soy and GM maize diet (*Journal of Organic Systems* 2013[199]): "The GM diet was associated with gastric and uterine differences in pigs. GM-fed pigs had uteri that were 25% heavier than non-GM fed pigs. GM-fed pigs had a higher rate of severe stomach inflammation with a rate of 32% of GM-fed pigs compared to 12% of non-GM-fed pigs. The severe stomach inflammation was worse in GM-fed males compared to non-GM fed males by a factor of 4.0, and GM-fed females compared to non-GM fed females by a factor of 2.2." Publicized reviews of this article followed professional or business interests. Coverage by the news service Reuters[200] reported the research as accurate and quoted commentary from the industry group CropLife International, a global federation representing the plant science industry, stating "more than 150 scientific studies have been done on animals fed biotech crops and to date, there is no scientific evidence of any detrimental impact"; this statement by CropLife International—whose website in 2014 Jun reads that the private-interest group "promotes agricultural technologies such as pesticides and plant biotechnology" and whose members include Dow, Monsanto, Syngenta and other multinational chemical corporations—is

---

[198] "Americans are eating their weight and more in genetically engineered food every year, a new Environmental Working Group analysis shows. On average, people eat an estimated 193 pounds of genetically engineered food in a 12-month period. The typical American adult weighs 179 pounds. ... Shockingly, virtually no long-term health studies have been done on consumption of genetically engineered food." Sharp R. Americans Eat Their Weight In Genetically Engineered Food. *Environmental Working Group's AgMag* 2012 Oct ewg.org/agmag/2012/10/americans-eat-their-weight-genetically-engineered-food

[199] Carman et al. A long-term toxicology study on pigs fed a combined genetically modified (GM) soy and GM maize diet. *Journal of Organic Systems* 2013; 8(1),38-54

[200] Gillam C. Scientists say new study shows pig health hurt by GMO feed. *Reuters* 2013 reuters.com/article/2013/06/11/us-gmo-pigs-study-idUSBRE95A14K20130611

obviously a lie, given the multiple studies demonstrating abnormalities in GMO-fed animals, only a small sample of which is presented in these pages. Criticism of the original research published by *Business Insider*[201] described the research as "misleading and flawed" and thereafter barraged the article with innuendo, *argumentum ad hominem*, accurate criticism (an example of which is the lack of major differences between groups in the combination of moderate and severe stomach inflammation), and illogic (e.g., "The enlarged uterus finding, while statistically significant, is not likely to be clinically relevant."). My (DrV) personal reading of the article finds the uterine abnormalities more significant/reliable than the stomach abnormalities.

- Glyphosate—the widely used herbicide produced by Monsanto: Glyphosate (gly-FO-SATE) is a broad-spectrum systemic herbicide used to kill plants, especially annual broadleaf weeds and grasses known to compete with commercial crops; it was brought to market in the 1970s by the biotechnology company Monsanto under the trade name "Roundup®." Glyphosate-based herbicides are currently the most commonly used herbicides in the world despite evidence of toxicity; glyphosate-based herbicide mixtures are applied internationally to food, air, and water without demonstration of safety and increasing evidence of harm. Glyphosate's *designated but not solitary* mode of action is to inhibit an enzyme involved in the synthesis of the aromatic amino acids tyrosine, tryptophan and phenylalanine. Some patented crops have been genetically engineered to be resistant to glyphosate (i.e., "Roundup Ready", also created by Monsanto Company); soy was the first "Roundup Ready" crop, and in the United States 94% of soy is GMO[202]—some have suggested that this is evidence of a market monopoly. Many articles in the scientific literature note problems with the population-wide and world-wide application of this chemical mixture and the financial and political policies that commonly accompany. The most consistent and painful theme in the research

> **GMO foods (e.g., soy, corn, cotton, canola, sugar beet, alfalfa, papaya [Chinese and Hawaiian], zucchini, and yellow squash*): imposed on an unconsenting population, without their knowledge, and without proper safety testing**
>
> "Americans are eating their weight and more in genetically engineered food every year, a new Environmental Working Group analysis shows. On average, people eat an estimated 193 pounds of genetically engineered food in a 12-month period. The typical American adult weighs 179 pounds. ... Shockingly, virtually no long-term health studies have been done on consumption of genetically engineered food."**
>
> The whole situation is complicated by the fact that these patented food such as soy, corn, and alfalfa are used as major feed sources for farm-raised fish, cows, pigs, and poultry. This has three major implications:
> 1) People are eating GMO-sourced food and related proteins and chemicals even when they think they are eating fish, beef, milk, cheese, yogurt, pork, chicken, turkey, and eggs,
> 2) These toxins and chemicals can be expected to bioconcentrate in animal tissues as do other nutrients and chemicals,
> 3) **Whoever controls these patented plants controls the entire grown food supply beyond the GMO foods themselves.**
>
> *Jeffrey M. Smith, personal communication, 2014 Jul. **Sharp R, Environmental Working Group. *AgMag* 2012

literature is the combination of data showing that GMO toxins have been imposed on entire large populations of the world (e.g., the entire country of the United States, with a population of more than 318 million people who eat the largest portion of GMO foods in the world) without any reasonable safety data and very clear evidence of biological harm; adding salt to this wound is the fact that major health organizations such as the American Medical Association, which claims "To promote the art and science of medicine and the betterment of public health" and promises "Together, we can shape a better, healthier future – not just for patients and physicians, but for the country as a whole"[203] have been completely quiescent,

---

[201] Welsh J. Scientists Shred Study That Says Genetically Modified Food Makes Pigs Sick. *BusinessInsider.com* 2013 Jun businessinsider.com/gm-pig-study-is-deeply-flawed-2013-6#ixzz36bYn2igT
[202] Carman et al. A long-term toxicology study on pigs fed a combined genetically modified (GM) soy and GM maize diet. *Journal of Organic Systems* 2013; 8(1),38-54
[203] ama-assn.org/ama/pub/about-ama/our-mission.page 2014 Jul

allowing this uncontrolled experiment on the American population. Some people have suggested that this is a human rights offense, an almost-certain health hazard, and worldwide environmental threat; yet most Americans are eating GMO foods+chemicals every day.

- Exposure to glyphosate-based herbicide alters aromatase levels in rat testis and sperm nuclear quality (*Environ Toxicol Pharmacol* 2014 May[204]): The authors of this report write, "Roundup is the major pesticide used in agriculture worldwide; it is a glyphosate-based herbicide. Its molecular effects are studied following an acute exposure (0.5%) of fifteen 60-day-old male rats during an 8-day period. ...The major disruption is an increase of aromatase mRNA levels at least by 50% in treated rats at all times, as well as the aromatase protein. ... A rise of abnormal sperm morphology and a decrease of the expression of protamine 1 and histone 1 testicular in epididymal sperm are observed despite a normal sperm concentration and motility."

- Toxicity of a glyphosate-based herbicide on the Neotropical fish Prochilodus lineatus (*Comp Biochem Physiol C Toxicol Pharmacol* 2008 Mar[205]): The authors note, "However, toxic effects of Roundup at sub-lethal concentrations have now been demonstrated in fish. Sub-lethal concentrations of glyphosate, corresponding to less than 2% of the LC50, caused ultrastructural damage in the liver of *C. carpio*. Histological alterations were also observed in liver, gills and kidneys of Nile tilapia (*Oreochromis niloticus*) after acute and chronic exposure to sub-lethal concentrations of Roundup. Despite the fact that Roundup is widely used in Brazil, only a limited amount of information is available on its toxic effects to native freshwater fishes." This data on glyphosate/Roundup-induced fish toxicity is increasingly important given the impending *death of the oceans*[206] and extinction of salt-water fish as a food source.[207]

> **GMO documentaries, social context, health effects**
> Genetic Roulette
> seedsofdeception.com
> David versus Monsanto
> youtube.com and
> rclvideolibrary.com
> Scientists under Attack
> scientistsunderattack.com
> GMO Food, Dr. Russell Blaylock
> youtube.com
> Seeds of Death: Unveiling The Lies of GMO youtube.com
> Confessions of an Economic Hitman youtube.com
> Hoodwinked: An Economic Hit Man Reveals Why the Global Economy Imploded—and How to Fix It economichitman.com
> GMO OMG gmofilm.com

- Glyphosate and gluten intolerance (*Interdiscip Toxicol* 2013 Dec[208]): The authors propose that glyphosate, the active ingredient in the herbicide Roundup is the most important causal factor in the epidemics of celiac disease and gluten intolerance. "Glyphosate residues in wheat and other crops are likely increasing recently due to the growing practice of crop desiccation just prior to the harvest. We argue that the practice of "ripening" sugar cane with glyphosate may explain the recent surge in kidney failure among agricultural workers in Central America. We conclude with a plea to governments to reconsider policies regarding ... glyphosate residues in foods."

- Glyphosate's suppression of cytochrome P450 enzymes and other pathways to modern diseases (*Entropy* 2013 Apr[209]): These researchers report that glyphosate/Roundup chemical residues are found in the main foods of the Western diet, comprised primarily of sugar, corn, soy and wheat. Glyphosate's inhibition of cytochrome P450 (CYP) enzymes is an overlooked component of its toxicity to mammals because CYP enzymes play crucial roles in biology, one of which is to detoxify xenobiotics. The researchers further note that glyphosate enhances the damaging effects of other chemical residues and environmental toxins. ... "Consequences are most of the diseases and conditions associated with a Western diet, which include gastrointestinal disorders, obesity, diabetes, heart disease, depression, autism, infertility, cancer and Alzheimer's disease."

- **Additive and synergistic toxicities of mislabeled "inert" chemicals—reproductive toxicity:** Extremely low dilutions of chemical combinations show additive/synergistic toxicities—

---

[204] Cassault-Meyer et al. Acute exposure to glyphosate-based herbicide alters aromatase levels in testis, sperm nuclear quality. *Environ Toxicol Pharmacol* 2014;38:131-40
[205] Langiano Vdo et al. Toxicity of glyphosate-based herbicide on Neotropical fish Prochilodus lineatus. *Comp Biochem Physiol C Toxicol Pharmacol* 2008 Mar:222-31
[206] Renton A. The Death of the Oceans. *Newsweek* 2014 Jul newsweek.com/2014/07/11/disaster-weve-wrought-worlds-oceans-may-be-irrevocable-256962.html
[207] DeNoon D. Salt-Water Fish Extinction Seen By 2048. *CBS News* 2006 Nov 2 cbsnews.com/news/salt-water-fish-extinction-seen-by-2048/
[208] Samsel et al. Glyphosate, pathways to modern diseases II: Celiac sprue and gluten intolerance. *Interdiscip Toxicol*. 2013 Dec;6(4):159-84
[209] Samsel et al. Glyphosate's Suppression of Cytochrome P450 Enzymes and Amino Acid Biosynthesis by the Gut Microbiome. *Entropy* 2013 Apr, 15(4), 1416-1463

specifically affecting cells of the reproductive system; this is a very concerning finding given that GMO-related toxins have been detected in pregnant human women and human fetal tissue, giving us every reason to believe that the cytotoxicity induced by pesticide formulations is affecting human lives in real time.

> > ▫ Human cytotoxicity of pesticide additives (*Scientific American* 2009 Jun[210]): "One specific inert ingredient, polyethoxylated tallowamine, or POEA, was more deadly to human embryonic, placental and umbilical cord cells than the herbicide itself – a finding the researchers call "astonishing." "This clearly confirms that the [inert ingredients] in Roundup formulations are not inert," wrote the study authors from France's University of Caen. "Moreover, the proprietary mixtures available on the market could cause cell damage and even death [at the] residual levels" found on Roundup-treated crops, such as soybeans, alfalfa and corn, or lawns and gardens. The research team suspects that Roundup might cause pregnancy problems by interfering with hormone production, possibly leading to abnormal fetal development, low birth weights or miscarriages."
> > ▫ Ethoxylated adjuvants of glyphosate-based herbicides are active principles of human cell toxicity (*Toxicology* 2013 Nov[211]): "Pesticides are always used in formulations as mixtures of an active principle with adjuvants. ... Here we demonstrate that all formulations are more toxic than glyphosate [alone], ... POE-15 [polyethoxylated tallowamine] clearly appears to be the most toxic principle against human cells, even if others are not excluded. It begins to be active with negative dose-dependent effects on cellular respiration and membrane integrity between 1 and 3ppm, at environmental/occupational doses. We demonstrate in addition that POE-15 induces necrosis when its first micellization process occurs, by contrast to glyphosate which is known to promote endocrine disrupting effects after entering cells. Altogether, these results challenge the establishment of guidance values such as the acceptable daily intake of glyphosate, when these are mostly based on a long term in vivo test of glyphosate alone. Since pesticides are always used with adjuvants that could change their toxicity, the necessity to assess their whole formulations as mixtures becomes obvious. This challenges the concept of active principle of pesticides for non-target species."
>
> ▪ GMO toxins absorbed by humans: One of the main arguments espoused by the chemical industry is that GMO toxins and pesticides do not reach human consumers because such chemicals are said to decompose with time, cooking (assuming that the foods are cooked rather than eaten raw as many foods are), digestion; data in humans with analysis of human tissue samples has proven this argument to be a lie: humans *indeed* accumulate GMO toxins—Bt toxin and associated pesticide chemicals.
> > ▫ Maternal and fetal exposure to pesticides associated to genetically modified foods (*Reprod Toxicol* 2011 May[212]): "Pesticides associated to genetically modified foods (PAGMF), are engineered to tolerate herbicides such as glyphosate (GLYP) and gluphosinate (GLUF) or insecticides such as the bacterial toxin bacillus thuringiensis (Bt). ... Blood of thirty pregnant women (PW) and thirty-nine nonpregnant women (NPW) were studied. Serum GLYP and GLUF were detected in nonpregnant women and not detected in pregnant women. Serum 3-MPPA and CryAb1 toxin were detected in pregnant women, their fetuses and nonpregnant women. This is the first study to reveal the presence of circulating pesticides associated to genetically modified foods in women with and without pregnancy, ..."

"Inert" can be cytotoxic

A chemical that is "inert" against insects and plants can be harmful for humans.

A chemical that is "inert in isolation" can be devastating when combined with other toxic chemicals and/or other "inert" chemicals.

---

[210] Gammon C et al. Weed-Whacking Herbicide Proves Deadly to Human Cells. *Scientific American* 2009 Jun scientificamerican.com/article/weed-whacking-herbicide-p/
[211] Mesnage et al. Ethoxylated adjuvants of glyphosate-based herbicides are active principles of human cell toxicity. *Toxicology*. 2013 Nov 16;313(2-3):122-8
[212] Aris et al. Maternal and fetal exposure to pesticides associated to genetically modified foods in Eastern Townships of Quebec, Canada. *Reprod Toxicol*. 2011;31:528-33

- Glyphosate in humans correlates with disease (*J Environ Anal Toxicol* 2014 Jan[213]): "Glyphosate excretion in German dairy cows was significantly lower than Danish cows. Cows kept in genetically modified free area had significantly lower glyphosate concentrations in urine than conventional husbandry cows. Also glyphosate was detected in different organs of slaughtered cows as intestine, liver, muscles, spleen and kidney. Fattening rabbits showed significantly higher glyphosate residues in urine than hares. Moreover, glyphosate was significantly higher in urine of humans with conventional feeding [non-organic foods]. Furthermore, chronically ill humans showed significantly higher glyphosate residues in urine than healthy population. The presence of glyphosate residues in both humans and animals could haul the entire population towards numerous health hazards, studying the impact of glyphosate residues on health is warranted and the global regulations for the use of glyphosate may have to be re-evaluated. ... Glyphosate residues can remain stable in foods for a year or more, even if the foods are frozen, dried or processed. ... Exposure of mammals to glyphosate may cause loss of mitochondrial transmembrane potential and result in oxidative stress to liver and brain. Both apoptosis and autophagy are involved in glyphosate toxicity mechanisms."

- **Commercial influence of science and politics**: One of the most damning research articles documenting adverse effects of GMO foods and toxins was published by Séralini et al[214] in *Food Chem Toxicol* 2012 Nov; in this paper, the authors show massive tumorigenesis and multiple organ abnormalities in animals fed GMO foods and related GMO toxins, e.g., genetically manipulated proteins and –*cidal* chemicals. The original research was deemed properly conducted, and the original manuscript was accepted by the journal with minimal editorial input; in other words: this was deemed by the editors to be good research. Following publication of the article, a deluge of letters refuting the article was published, and many of these denigrations and refutations were written by authors affiliated with Monsanto, the agrichemical multinational corporation that sells and massively profits from GMO. In 2014 Jan, the Séralini article was retracted by the journal after it created a new editorial position and filled that position with a researcher who worked for Monsanto. This unprecedented retraction violates scientific publication standards by well-established bioethics criteria; if biomedical journals and their publishers are going to pander to corporate interests, then the entirety of science—of truth, of medicine and healthcare, of reality itself—is at risk. GMO foods and toxins will be seen as "safe" if corporate-funded studies are published and independently/academically-funded articles are blocked or retracted; at this rate, if we as educated healthcare professionals and policymakers responsible for public welfare are going to allow the disgrace of reality, then we are resigning our integrity, courage, and our intellects

> **We must maintain our integrity and intellect lest we become pawns in the service of evil**
>
> "Must the citizen ever for a moment, or in the least degree, resign his conscience to the legislator? Why has every man a conscience, then? I think that we should be men first, and subjects afterward. ... Law never made men a whit more just; and, by means of their respect for it, **even the well-disposed are daily made the agents of injustice**. ... Now, what are they? Men at all? Or small movable forts and magazines, at the service of some unscrupulous man in power? — **a mere shadow and reminiscence of humanity**, a man laid out alive and standing, and already, as one may say, buried under arms with funeral accompaniments...
>
> I saw yet more distinctly the State in which I lived. I saw to what extent the people among whom I lived could be trusted as good neighbors and friends; that their friendship was for summer weather only; that they did not greatly propose to do right; that they were a distinct race from me ... that in their sacrifices to humanity, they ran no risks, not even to their property."
>
> Thoreau HD. *Civil Disobedience*, 1849

---

[213] Krüger et al. Detection of Glyphosate Residues in Animals and Humans. *J Environ Anal Toxicol* 2014 Jan 4:2. This article is open-access: omicsonline.org
[214] Séralini et al. Long term toxicity of a Roundup herbicide and a Roundup-tolerant genetically modified maize. *Food Chem Toxicol*. 2012 Nov;50(11):4221-31

in favor of passive idiocy and might as well therefore agree that ketchup is a vegetable[215] and therefore that frozen pizza is a vegetable[216], that climate change and global warming and ocean acidification are not occurring and that the icecaps aren't melting[217], and that 2 + 2 = 5.[218] If doctors, medical societies/associations, and public health groups do not stand for the truth and for the health of the public, if their only (conveniently self-chosen) professional tasks are **patient-by-patient micromanagement of public health** and the protection of their own professional niche, then they are no better than other private interest groups seeking their own aggrandizement and profitability.

> **The Responsibility of Intellectuals**
> "It is the responsibility of intellectuals to speak the truth and to expose lies."
> Noam Chomsky PhD. *New York Review of Books*, 1967 Feb 23

- Betrayal of science by Elsevier and its journal *Food and Chemical Toxicology* (*Bioethics Forum* 2014 Jan[219]): "11 of the [13] authors of letters to the editor slamming Séralini's study had undisclosed financial relationships with Monsanto. In 2013, Paul Christou, the editor of *Transgenic Research*, coauthored an attack on Séralini and the FCT editors in his own journal, calling for a retraction of the study. Christou did not disclose his multiple conflicts of interest, including being an inventor on patents on GM crop technology, many of which Monsanto owns. Meanwhile, back at *Food and Chemical Toxicology*, a new position for an associate editor was filled by Richard E. Goodman, a University of Nebraska professor who previously worked for Monsanto, and who has a longstanding association with the industry-funded International Life Sciences Institute (ILSI). Months later, Elsevier, FCT's publisher, announced the retraction. ... The retraction of the Séralini study is a black mark on medical publishing, a blow to science, and a win for corporate bullies."

- The Goodman Affair: Monsanto Targets the Heart of Science (*Independent Science News* 2013 May[220]): "But just a few months later, in early 2013 the *FCT* editorial board acquired a new "Associate Editor for biotechnology", Richard E. Goodman. This was a new position, seemingly established especially for Goodman in the wake of the "Séralini affair". Richard E. Goodman is...a former Monsanto employee, who worked for the company between 1997 and 2004. While at Monsanto he assessed the allergenicity of the company's GM crops and published papers on its behalf on allergenicity and safety issues relating to GM food (Goodman and Leach 2004). Goodman had no documented connection to the journal until February 2013. His fast-tracked appointment, directly onto the upper editorial board raises urgent questions. Does Monsanto now effectively decide which papers on biotechnology are published in FCT? And is this part of an attempt by Monsanto and the life science industry to seize control of science? ... FCT took on Goodman, a former Monsanto employee and well-known supporter of industry viewpoints, immediately following the publication of a controversial paper that was critical of Monsanto's principal products."

- Article by former Assistant Secretary of the US Treasury Dr Paul Craig Roberts—2013 Feb[221]): As a former Assistant Secretary of the US Treasury working with Ronald

---

[215] "The New York Times (9-28-81) noted that "Democrats are still chortling at what they hail as 'the Emperor's New Condiments' -- the attempt to declare ketchup a school-lunch vegetable." Nestle M. Ketchup Is a Vegetable? Again? The Atlantic 2011 Nov theatlantic.com/health/archive/2011/11/ketchup-is-a-vegetable-again/248538/
[216] "If there were any lingering doubts as to whom our elected representatives really work for, they were put to rest Tuesday when Congress announced that frozen pizza was a vegetable. The United States Congress voted to rebuke new USDA guidelines for school lunches that would have increased the amount of fresh fruit and vegetables in school cafeterias and instead declared that the tomato paste on frozen pizza qualified it as a vegetable. For this we can thank large food companies -- in this case ConAgra and Schwan -- which pressured Congress to comply with their financial interests. It simply doesn't suit the makers of frozen pizza, chicken nuggets and tater tots for schools to offer real food in the form of fresh fruits and vegetables." Wartman K. Pizza Is a Vegetable? Congress Defies Logic, Betrays Our Children. *Huffington Post* 2011 Nov huffingtonpost.com/kristin-wartman/pizza-is-a-vegetable_b_1101433.html. "As long as a serving of pizza contains at least 2 tablespoons of tomato sauce, this allows it to squeak in as a vegetable under the current rules." Petri A. Move over, ketchup! Pizza is a vegetable. 2011 Nov *Washington Post* washingtonpost.com/blogs/compost/post/move-over-ketchup-pizza-is-a-vegetable/2011/11/16/gIQAk1okRN_blog.html
[217] Cohen N. Climate change deniers have won. *The Guardian* 2014 Mar theguardian.com/commentisfree/2014/mar/22/climate-change-deniers-have-won-global-warming
[218] Orwell G. *1984*. Also: Moustaki N (Author), Podehl N (Narrator). *CliffsNotes 1984*, cliffsnotes.com/literature/n/1984/book-summary amazon.com/1984-CliffsNotes/dp/B004S8NFZ2/. Also: Video SparkNotes: Orwell's 1984 video summary. youtube.com/watch?v=pTqIVvUPAjw
[219] Fugh-Berman A, Sherman TG. Rounding Up Scientific Journals. *Bioethics Forum* 2014 Jan thehastingscenter.org/Bioethicsforum/Post.aspx?id=6684
[220] Robinson C, Latham J. The Goodman Affair: Monsanto Targets the Heart of Science. *Independent Science News* 2013 May independentsciencenews.org/science-media/the-goodman-affair-monsanto-targets-the-heart-of-science/
[221] Roberts PC. America the Polluted: One Nation, Under Monsanto. *CounterPunch.com* 2013 Feb counterpunch.org/2013/02/26/one-nation-under-monsanto/

Reagan, and as former Associate Editor of the *Wall Street Journal*, Dr Roberts (PhD, Economics) can speak very authoritatively from experience on government politics; his 2013 article "America the Polluted: One Nation, Under Monsanto" is publicly available online and describes how Monsanto holds powerful influence in American politics and is able to influence political outcomes through key positions; examples of such influence and conflict of interest are as follows:

> **Years of falsity have blinded people to accurate perception**
>
> "We have been poisoned on so much [falsity and lies] for so many years, when the truth comes along and it's right in your face, you don't know what to do with it... You wake up one morning with a footprint on your face... You have to look the lie right in the eye and not be afraid to see too clearly."
>
> Rollins H. *One from None*, 1991, p106-144

- **Tom Vilsack, appointed US Secretary of Agriculture** in 2009, is former "Biotech Governor (Iowa 2001) of the Year", an award bestowed by the Biotechnology Industry Organization, "the world's largest trade association representing biotechnology companies", a proGMO/pesticide/herbicide trade group supported by multinationals such as AstraZeneca, Genentech/Roche, DuPont, and Monsanto[222]
- **Michael Taylor, appointed to the newly created position of Deputy Commissioner for Foods and Veterinary Medicine** (aka, "US Food Czar"), is former outside attorney Monsanto, then Deputy Commissioner of Policy at the US Food and Drug Administration, then VP of Government Affairs for Monsanto[223]
- **Clarence Thomas, US Supreme Court Justice**, is a former employed attorney of Monsanto[224]

Dr Roberts argues that the infiltration of US political positions by people intimately connected with the business interests of private corporations is powerfully influencing the quality and availability of biomedical research, legislative changes, legal decisions, and voters' perceptions of issues related to GMO and biotechnology. Dr Roberts concludes, "Monsanto is not only sufficiently powerful to prevent any research other than that which it purchases with its funding, but also Monsanto succeeded last year in blocking with money and propaganda the GMO labeling law in California. I would tell you to be careful what you eat as it can make you ill and infertile, but you can't even find out what you are eating."

- <u>Allergenicity, immunogenicity, inflammatory effects</u>: The article cited below carries devastating implications for connecting GMO foods with autism, allergy, autoimmunity, obesity, and other inflammatory disorders. The finding that GMO corn—but not natural corn—lead to increases in IL-6 (which promotes Th-17 cell development, as well as cardiometabolic disease) and gamma-delta T cells is sufficient to mechanistically connect GMO foods with inflammatory and dysmetabolic disease in humans.
    - <u>Intestinal and peripheral immune response to MON810 maize ingestion in weaning and old mice (*J Agric Food Chem* 2008 Dec[225])</u>: The authors' abstract understates the importance of their findings, noting immune system abnormalities and an increase in the pro-inflammatory cytokine IL-6 following consumption of GMO corn compared with natural corn. The increase in IL-6 is by itself significant, given the role of inflammation in essentially all human diseases and the ability of IL-6 to induce Th-17 phenotype characteristic of more severe allergic and autoimmune diseases. However,

---

[222] "September 20, 2001: The Biotechnology Industry Organization (BIO) today named Iowa Gov. Tom Vilsack as Governor of the Year for his support of the industry's economic growth and agricultural biotechnology research." bio.org/media/press-release/iowas-vilsack-named-bio-governor-year 2014 Jul. "Tom Vilsack serves as the Nation's 30th Secretary of Agriculture. As leader of the U.S. Department of Agriculture (USDA), Vilsack is working hard to strengthen the American agricultural economy,... USDA is promoting American agriculture by conducting cutting-edge research and expanding markets at home and abroad." usda.gov/wps/portal/usda/usdahome?contentidonly=true&contentid=bios_vilsack.xml 2014 Jul

[223] "Michael R. Taylor was named deputy commissioner for foods at the Food and Drug Administration (FDA) in January 2010. He is the first individual to hold the position, which was created along with a new Office of Foods in August 2009. Other positions held by Mr. Taylor include senior fellow, Resources for the Future; professor, School of Medicine, University of Maryland; partner, King & Spalding law firm; and vice president for public policy, Monsanto Company. fda.gov/aboutfda/centersoffices/officeoffoods/ucm196721.htm 2014 Jul. Michael R. Taylor, J.D. (1991-1994), Deputy Commissioner for Policy. fda.gov/AboutFDA/WhatWeDo/History/Leaders/DeputyCommissioners/default.htm 2014 Jul

[224] "Clarence Thomas, Associate Justice... an attorney with the Monsanto Company from 1977–1979" supremecourt.gov/about/biographies.aspx 2014 Jul

[225] Finamore et al. Intestinal and peripheral immune response to MON810 maize ingestion in weaning and old mice. *J Agric Food Chem*. 2008 Dec 10;56(23):11533-9

per my reading of the full text of the article, I find this article to sound the alarm on GMO foods per the authors' report, "One of the more recurrent alterations in lymphocyte phenotypes observed in this study was an increase in the TCRγδ+ (gamma-delta T-cells) population. A high percentage of these lymphocytes are localized in the gut and ... γδT cells seem to be important regulatory elements of the immune system, being capable of modulating inflammatory response associated with infectious agents and autoantigens. Higher numbers of γδT cells have been observed in humans with asthma, in intraepithelial lymphocytes (IELs) of children with untreated food allergy, and in the duodenum of children with juvenile idiopathic arthritis or connective tissue disease with gastrointestinal symptoms." Further, gamma-delta T-cells are known to secrete IL-17, the cytokine responsible for the massive tissue damage seen in autoimmune diseases such as multiple sclerosis, rheumatoid arthritis, and psoriasis, and which is also elevated in autism.[226]

GMO-induced increase in IL-6 and gamma-delta Tcells + induction of mitochondrial dysfunction by GMO toxins: possible (synergistic) explanation to GMO connection to a wide range of human health problems
1. GMO-induced gamma-delta T cells: Rats fed GMO corn showed important increases in IL-6 (pro-inflammatory cytokine associated with many and perhaps nearly all human diseases) and in gamma-delta T cells (known to contribute to human allergic and autoimmune disease and to promote inflammatory damage and induction of pathogenic Th-17 cells). If GMO toxins cause the same inflammatory changes in humans, then this would be sufficient to explain the dramatic increases in autoimmunity, autism, and inflammatory and allergic diseases.
2. Induction of mitochondrial dysfunction by GMO toxins, especially glyphosate and associated (pseudo)inert chemicals: Mitochondrial dysfunction is known to contribute to inflammatory diseases, allergy, autoimmunity, Alzheimer's disease, Parkinson's disease, hypertension, diabetes mellitus type-2, and many other diseases; additionally, mitochondrial dysfunction promotes increased secretion of and sensitivity to inflammatory cytokines. If GMO toxins cause mitochondrial dysfunction in humans, then this would be sufficient to explain the marked increases in inflammatory diseases, allergy, autoimmunity, Alzheimer's disease, Parkinson's disease, hypertension, diabetes mellitus type-2, and many other diseases.
3. Potential additive and synergistic effects: Researchers should look for evidence of additive and synergistic effects of IL-6, IL-17, Th-17 cells, gamma-delta T-cells, and mitochondrial dysfunction in human patients, especially those with inflammatory disorders ranging from obesity to autoimmunity.

- Grains with "toxic gluten"—barley, wheat, rye: Many grains including corn and rice contain variants of "gluten", but from a clinical and immunologic standpoint our main consideration is on "toxic gluten" (differentiated by its adverse immunologic/histologic/clinical effect rather than its general categorization); the most immunogenic forms of gluten are found in wheat, rye, barley and their related processed products ranging from bread to beer. Thus, when we talk about "gluten" from a clinical standpoint, the implication is that we are talking about "toxic gluten" found in barley, wheat, rye.
    - Specificity of tissue transglutaminase explains cereal toxicity in celiac disease (*J Exp Med*. 2002 Mar[227]): In this important article, the authors note that celiac disease is caused immunogenic inflammation triggered by gluten, a complex mixture of storage proteins found in wheat, and that tissue transglutaminase (tTG) is involved in the generation of T-cell stimulatory gluten peptides through deamidation of glutamine. "Only particular glutamine residues, however, are modified by tTG. Here we provide evidence that the spacing between glutamine and proline, the second most abundant amino acid in gluten, plays an essential role in the specificity of deamidation. ... Strikingly, these algorithms [developed in this study] identified many similar peptides in the gluten-like hordeins from barley and secalins from rye but not in the avenins from oats. The avenins contain significantly lower percentages of proline residues, which offers a likely explanation for the lack of toxicity of oats. Thus, the unique amino acid composition of gluten and related proteins in barley and rye favors the generation of toxic T cell stimulatory gluten peptides by tTG."
  Beyond acute/subacute prevention of starvation, no medical need exists for the consumption of wheat (nor rye, nor barley); the few nutrients available in wheat are better acquired in other foods that have

---

[226] Al-Ayadhi LY, Mostafa GA. Elevated serum levels of interleukin-17A in children with autism. *J Neuroinflammation*. 2012 Jul 2;9:158
[227] Vader et al. Specificity of tissue transglutaminase explains cereal toxicity in celiac disease. *J Exp Med*. 2002 Mar 4;195(5):643-9

less carbohydrate, more protein (e.g., meat) or phytonutrients (egg, fruits and vegetables). Wheat contains indigestible polysaccharides and therefore promotes small intestinal bacterial/microbial overgrowth (SIBO), especially when overconsumed; many people have wheat with breakfast (e.g., bread, toast, cereal, pancakes/waffles, donuts), lunch (sandwich, pizza), dinner (pasta in its various forms, bread as the international side-dish) and dessert (cake, pie). The proper term for the allergy, sensitivity, and intolerance associated with wheat and gluten is "gluten-related disorders." My judgment is that most organizations advocating "whole grains" and "whole wheat" as healthy food have basically sold their souls and resigned their consciousness to grain industry propaganda and "research" showing that whole grains are a healthier option than fiber-free hyperprocessed grain products which are essentially the nutritional equivalent of table sugar; whole oats, brown rice, and the inclusion of a few other relatively rare/primitive/nonGMO/organic grains is reasonable, again in contrast to blanket endorsements of "whole grains" which allows patients to eventually feel good about eating bread, pastries, and other sugar-laden, AGE-loaded, phytonutrient-depleted, carbohydrate-rich and SIBO-promoting foods. In concise summation, reasons to avoid wheat include the following:

1. Nutrient-poor: Wheat is very low in nutrients compared with fruits and especially vegetables. When wheat is consumed, the opportunity is lost to have consumed a food with greater nutritional quantity and quality and (generally) of lower immunogenicity.
2. Phytonutrient-poor: Wheat is very low in health-promoting phytonutrients when compared to fruits (e.g., antioxidant flavonoids) and vegetables (I3C/DIM).
3. High fermentation: As demonstrated in three clinical trials in humans, wheat promotes microbial overgrowth of the small bowel due to its content of indigestible polysaccharides. The resulting microbial overgrowth promotes increased intestinal permeability and a pro-inflammatory state via low-grade endotoxinemia, which also promotes the development of chronic pain via inflammatory/immunogenic mechanisms and peripheral and central sensitization.[228]
4. Increased intestinal permeability: Recent research has shown that wheat/gluten triggers increased intestinal permeability—leaky gut—in essentially everyone; this finding is consistent with the finding that wheat triggers immune complex formation in apparently healthy patients (i.e., those considered to be without wheat allergy, celiac disease, or other gluten-related disorder).
5. Wheat/gluten/gliadin promotes formation of circulating immune complexes (CIC): These are formed even in health people; pathogenically, CIC contribute to vasculitis, nephritis, arthritis, and dermatitis.
   - Gliadin IgG antibodies and circulating immune complexes (*Scand J Gastroenterol* 2009 Jan[229]): "Circulating immune complexes (CICs) in blood are associated with autoimmune-diseases such as systemic lupus erythematosus, immune complex glomerulonephritis, rheumatoid arthritis and vasculitis. … 352 (265 F, 87 M), so far, healthy individuals were tested for CICs containing C1q and immunoglobulin G (IgG) as well as for gliadin IgG antibodies using the ELISA technique. … In our study, 15.3% (54/352) of the patients presented with elevated CIC concentrations (above 50 microg/ml) and 6.5% (23/352) of the study population were positive for gliadin IgG antibodies (above 20 U/ml). CIC concentration levels were significantly higher in the group with elevated gliadin IgG antibodies (CIC median: 49.0 microg/ml) compared with the group with normal levels of gliadin IgG antibodies (CIC median: 30.0 microg/ml). … The results of this study indicate that certain food antigens (e.g. gluten) could play a role in the formation of CICs."
6. Celiac disease is common: 1 per 141 people in USA (per *Am J Gastroenterol* 2012 Oct). Factors proposed to enhance the development of celiac disease are *Candida albicans* and glyphosate.

---

[228] Yamaguchi et al. Low rather than high dose lipopolysaccharide 'priming' of muscle provides an animal model of persistent elevated mechanical sensitivity for study of chronic pain. *Eur J Pain*. 2011Aug;724-31. Amaral et al. Commensal microbiota is fundamental for development of inflammatory pain. *Proc Natl Acad Sci* 2008 Feb:2193-7
[229] Eisenmann et al. Gliadin IgG antibodies and circulating immune complexes. *Scand J Gastroenterol*. 2009 Jan;44(2):168-71

7. <u>Inherently proinflammatory</u>: In vitro, gliadin stimulates human monocytes to produce of IL-8 and TNF-alpha through a mechanism involving NF-kappaB (per *FEBS Lett* 2004 Jul); in this manner, wheat proteins can be said to be directly pro-inflammatory *independently from any allergy/intolerance/sensitivity*.

8. <u>Wheat/gluten can trigger an assortment of health problems which "necessitate" medical/drug treatment if the underling dietary cause is not addressed</u>: Gluten-induced disorders can include gluten ataxia, dermatitis herpetiformis, acne, skin rashes, migraine headache, somatic pain, Meniere's disease, infertility, IgA nephropathy, thyroid disease; these are commonly (mis)diagnosed as other problems and are "medically managed" with drugs—skin creams, analgesics, anti-inflammatory drugs, steroid pills and creams, etc—while the dietary origin under the guise of a "healthy whole grain" remains in place for years or the patient's lifetime. Avoidance of the "toxic glutens" in wheat, rye, barley along with a program of intestinal healing (discussed elsewhere in this book) and nutritional immunomodulation (detailed in this book with complete protocol) should be used in all patients with gluten-related disorders.
    - <u>Gluten sensitivity masquerading as systemic lupus erythematosus</u> (*Ann Rheum Dis* 2004 Nov[230]): "Three patients are described whose original presentation and immunological profile led to the erroneous diagnosis of systemic lupus erythematosus (SLE). The correct diagnosis of gluten sensitivity was made after years of treatment with steroids and other immunosuppressive drugs."
    - <u>Celiac disease (CD) increases risk of SLE</u> (*J Rheumatol.* 2012 Oct[231]): "Individuals with CD were at a 3-fold increased risk of SLE compared to the general population."
    - <u>Remission without insulin therapy on gluten-free diet in type 1 diabetes mellitus</u> (*BMJ Case Rep.* 2012 Jun[232]): "A 5-year and 10-month old boy was diagnosed with classical type 1 diabetes mellitus (T1DM) without celiac disease. ... At 16 months after diagnosis the fasting blood glucose was 4.1 mmol/l and after 20 months he is still without daily insulin therapy. ...The authors propose that the gluten-free diet has prolonged remission in this patient with T1DM and that further trials are indicated."

9. <u>Chronic pain and cognitive dysfunction</u>: Two contemporary studies showed that wheat consumption contributes to cognitive impairment in patients *with* celiac disease[233] and pain and fatigue in IBS patients *without* celiac disease—this second study is summarized below:
    - <u>Gluten causes gastrointestinal symptoms in subjects without celiac disease</u> (*Am J Gastroenterol* 2011 Mar[234]): This is a double-blind, randomized, placebo-controlled rechallenge trial undertaken in patients with IBS in whom celiac disease was excluded and who were symptomatically controlled on a gluten-free diet. "Participants received either gluten or placebo in the form of two bread slices plus one muffin per day with a gluten-free diet for up to 6 weeks. ... On a visual analog scale, patients were significantly worse with gluten within 1 week for overall symptoms, pain, bloating, satisfaction with stool consistency, and tiredness." Noteworthy is the fact that all of these adverse clinical manifestations are directly attributable to wheat-induced SIBO regardless of any antigenicity of or immunosensitivity to wheat or gluten.

10. <u>Net acid load</u>: As noted previously, "fish, meat, poultry, eggs, shellfish, cheese, milk, and cereal grains are net acid producing, whereas fresh fruit, vegetables, tubers, roots, and nuts are net base producing."[235] Given the space limitations of the stomach and time and financial limitations of most humans, consuming wheat and other acid-forming foods by definition means that fewer base-forming foods will be consumed; this imbalance promotes/perpetuates diet-induced/maintained low-grade metabolic acidosis.

---

[230] Hadjivassiliou et al. Gluten sensitivity masquerading as systemic lupus erythematosus. *Ann Rheum Dis.* 2004 Nov;63(11):1501-3
[231] Ludvigsson et al. Increased risk of systemic lupus erythematosus in 29,000 patients with biopsy-verified celiac disease. *J Rheumatol.* 2012 Oct;39(10):1964-70
[232] Sildorf et al. Remission without insulin therapy on gluten-free diet in a 6-year old boy with type 1 diabetes mellitus. *BMJ Case Rep.* 2012 Jun 21;2012. pii: bcr0220125878
[233] Biesiekierski et al. Gluten causes gastrointestinal symptoms in subjects without celiac disease. *Am J Gastroenterol.* 2011 Mar;106(3):508-14
[234] "In newly diagnosed coeliac disease, cognitive performance improves with adherence to the gluten-free diet in parallel to mucosal healing." Lichtwark et al. Cognitive impairment in celiac disease improves on a gluten-free diet and correlates with histological and serological indices of disease severity. *Aliment Pharmacol Ther* 2014 Jul;40:160-70
[235] Cordain et al. Origins and evolution of the Western diet. *Am J Clin Nutr.* 2005 Feb;81(2):341-54. Thanks, Pedro Bastos, for reminding me of this.

- High fructose corn syrup (HFCS)—nonnutritive calories, ATP depletion, mercury: In the United States, much/most HFCS is sourced from GMO corn; the process of producing this nonphysiologic unnatural nutrient-depleted carbohydrate source introduces mercury—a toxic metal famous for its causation of hypertension and psychosis/neurotoxicity—in clinically meaningful amounts.[236] Initial metabolic processing of fructose occurs via fructokinase and causes ATP depletion leading to activation of inflammatory pathways and resultant production of uric acid which causes insulin resistance and clinical manifestations of weight gain, hypertension, and dyslipidemia and dysglycemia—the metabolic syndrome.[237] Fructose promotes urate formation, and urate formation stimulates fructokinase activity; in this manner a vicious cycle is established promoting the development of fructose-induced urate-mediated diseases such as fatty liver.[238] Fructose consumption from whole foods such as fruits does not cause the same problems noted with HFCS because 1) *cellular* carbohydrates—sugars within the context of fibers and other (phyto)nutrients—do not cause the same adverse physiologic affects noted with *acellular* carbohydrate sources, 2) lower carbohydrate:fiber ratio, 3) fruits contain ant inflammatory and antioxidant phytonutrients that offset and physiologically "balance" the adverse effects of the sugars, 4) plants generally have an alkalinizing effect via their content of citrates such as potassium citrate—this promotes urinary excretion of the fructose-induced urate via urinary alkalinization—in contrast to the acidifying effect of many "soft drinks" and "sodas" which are acidic due to the carbonation process that introduces carbon dioxide and subsequently carbonic acid—systemic/urinary acidification promotes retention of uric acid and thereby promotes exacerbation of fructose-induced and urate-mediated insulin resistance.
- Pasteurization, Maillard reaction, polyol pathway, advanced glycation end-products (AGE) and their receptor (RAGE): The nonenzymatic reaction wherein sugars such as glucose/fructose/lactose are bound to proteins in general and the amino acid lysine (also tryptophan and arginine) in particular to form amino sugars; this process is called glycation, glycosylation, or the Maillard reaction, and as with most nonenzymatic reactions, it occurs slowly over time, is dose/substrate-dependent, and is expedited by heat. The sequence below is slightly modified from Gaby[239]; in this diagram AGE = advanced glycation end product, which—as discussed below, interacts with its receptor, RAGE.

Reducing Sugar + Amino Acid + Heat/time ➔ N-Glycosylamine ➔ Amadori rearrangement ➔ AGE/RAGE

Other pathways and several other AGEs and RAGE ligands exist. Methylglyoxal, also called pyruvaldehyde or 2-oxopropanal, is formed by the nonenzymatic degradation of the glycolytic intermediates, including dihydoxyacetone phosphate and glyceraldehyde-3-phosphate; its production is increased during sustained hyperglycemia, and methylglyoxal can be converted into AGE via reaction with free amino groups of lysine and arginine and with thiol groups of cysteine. Methylglyoxal is degraded/detoxified by the enzyme glyoxalase-1 (Glo1); however, GLo1 is downregulated by RAGE, and in this manner RAGE activation leads to additional RAGE activation via increased ligand availability.

Excess glycolytic intermediates ➔ Methylglyoxal + lysine/arginine/cysteine ➔ AGE ➔ RAGE activation

Fructose is the most reactive of the reducing sugars, promoting hemoglobin glycosylation, protein cross-linking, and (lipid) peroxidation much more rapidly than does glucose. Glycosylated proteins can be further modified ultimately to advanced glycation end-products (AGE), which bind to DNA

---

[236] "Mercury contamination of food products as a result of the use of mercury contaminated HFCS seems like a very real possibility. With daily per capita consumption of HFCS in the US averaging about 50 grams and daily mercury intakes from HFCS ranging up to 28 µg, this potential source of mercury may exceed other major sources of mercury especially in high-end consumers of beverages sweetened with HFCS." Dufault et al. Mercury from chlor-alkali plants: measured concentrations in food product sugar. *Environ Health*. 2009 Jan 26;8:2

[237] "High doses of fructose raise the BP and cause the features of metabolic syndrome. Lowering the uric acid level prevents the increase in mean arterial blood pressure. Excessive intake of fructose may have a role in the current epidemics of obesity and diabetes." Perez-Pozo et al. Excessive fructose intake induces the features of metabolic syndrome in healthy adult men: role of uric acid in the hypertensive response. *Int J Obes* 2010 Mar;34(3):454-61

[238] "In conclusion, present study shows that metabolism of fructose by fructokinase results in the intracellular production of uric acid that feeds back to up-regulate fructokinase and increase sensitivity of the cell to the triglyceride-raising effects of fructose. Of interest, blockade of intracellular uric acid with allopurinol could inhibit the effect of fructose to increase fat accumulation." Lanaspa et al. Uric acid stimulates fructokinase and accelerates fructose metabolism in the development of fatty liver. *PLoS One*. 2012;7(10):e47948

[239] Gaby AR. Adverse effects of dietary fructose. *Altern Med Rev*. 2005 Dec;10(4):294-306

and also promote chronic pain and inflammation at least in part via interaction with the receptor for AGE (RAGE) which, as part of the innate immune system, is a pattern-recognition receptor predominantly involved in the recognition of endogenous molecules released in the context of infection, physiological stress or chronic/sustained inflammation.[240] AGE levels are increased in patients who are diabetic, fibromyalgic, elderly, and those with renal insufficiency; readers should appreciate that AGE levels reflect endogenous production (obviously exacerbated by hyperglycemia) and exogenous consumption (consumption of a diet high in processed foods, especially aged/cooked milk products and baked items such as pastries). As expected, the use of heat to reduce the bacterial load of cow's milk greatly increases the quantity of amino sugars in comparison with non-heated milk; in this manner, pasteurization changes the way these milk proteins are digested and thereafter perceived/processed by the intestinal immune system in a manner that promotes allergic sensitization.[241] The clinical significance of RAGE activation is its vicious contribution to inflammation, as perfectly summarized by Lee and Parker[242], "Interestingly, unlike other receptors, expression of RAGE is positively regulated by its ligand stimulation, which means that increasing concentration of ligands leads to up-regulation of RAGE. So, RAGE signals are accelerated more and more by the accumulation of signal stimulants. RAGE is found on the cell surface of various immune cells, and most of its ligands are mainly secreted by immune cells, including macrophages and dendritic cells; therefore one of the major roles of RAGE is involved in inflammation. Stimulation of RAGE by its ligands activates the proinflammatory transcription factor nuclear factor kappa B (NFkB)..." AGEs are excreted by the kidneys, which are also damaged by AGEs; thus a vicious cycle of AGE exposure, intrarenal AGE retention, renal injury, upregulation of RAGE receptors can culminate in renal failure, particularly due to diabetic nephropathy.

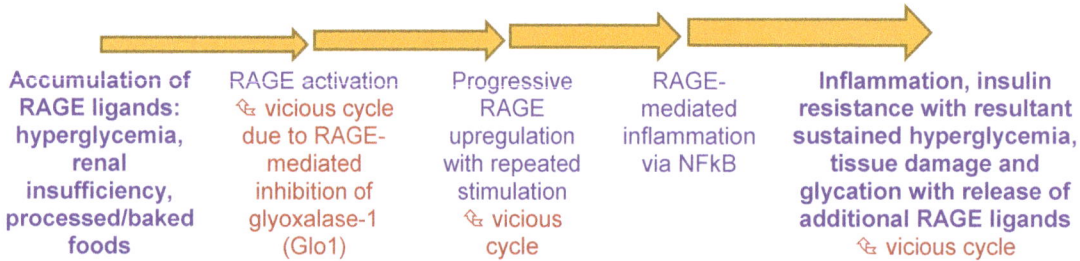

The polyol pathway, also called the sorbitol-aldose reductase pathway, is implicated in diabetic complications, especially in microvascular damage to the retina, kidney, and nerves. From a clinical perspective, the conversion of glucose to sorbitol via aldose reductase is important due to the resulting osmotic and oxidative stresses (and possible AGE production via sorbitol-amino binding), while the formation of fructose from sorbitol via sorbitol dehydrogenase is less consequential. Because the retina, kidney, and nervous tissues are insulin-independent, glucose enters in a dose-dependent manner per serum glucose levels, which reflect the balance between glucose intake (i.e., diet) and peripheral glucose uptake. In a hyperglycemic state, the affinity of aldose reductase for glucose rises, causing an escalating/disproportionate accumulation of sorbitol while also causing an escalating/disproportionate depletion of NADPH, resulting in tissue-specific glucose-induced oxidative stress. In these ways (osmotic stress, oxidative stress, AGE formation, inhibition nitric oxide and thus vasodilation and mitochondrial biogenesis), the polyol pathway is a major contributor to hyperglycemia-induced cellular/tissue damage and oxidative stress seen with sustained hyperglycemia, leading to the classic complications of diabetes: cataract, renal injury, neuropathy[243], and -more rarely and to a lesser extent- diabetic cerebral edema.

---

[240] Ibrahim et al. RAGE and TLRs: relatives, friends or neighbours? *Mol Immunol*. 2013 Dec;56(4):739-44
[241] Roth-Walter et al. Pasteurization of milk proteins promotes allergic sensitization by enhancing uptake through Peyer's patches. *Allergy*. 2008 Jul;63(7):882-90
[242] Lee EJ, Park JH. Receptor for Advanced Glycation Endproducts (RAGE), Its Ligands, and Soluble RAGE. *Genomics Inform*. 2013 Dec;11(4):224-9
[243] Chung et al. Contribution of polyol pathway to diabetes-induced oxidative stress. *J Am Soc Nephrol*. 2003 Aug;14(8 Suppl 3):S233-6

Glucose excess → **Sorbitol formation via aldose reductase and depletion of NADPH: consequences are ❶ intracellular osmotic stress (e.g., diabetic cataractogenesis), ❷ reduced ability to reduce/regenerate glutathione (GSH), ❸ reduced ability to produce nitric oxide, ❹ formation of AGEs** → **Limited formation of fructose of via sorbitol dehydrogenase; fructose contributes to AGE formation and thus RAGE activation**

- Dietary activation and modulation of Toll-like receptors (TLR): Toll-like receptors (TLR), especially TLR-2 and TLR-4, are part of the innate immune system activated by microbial motifs (pathogen-associated molecular patterns, PAMPs) and saturated fatty acids (SFA) to induce inflammation generally via NFkB-mediated pathways. As components of the innate immune system, TLR and RAGE can be seen as pro-inflammatory receptors with somewhat of an *outward* and *inward* focus, respectively, and for which some overlap in activation is likely to exist; TLR-2/4 are sensitive to PAMPS (hence an *outward* focus on external invaders) and saturated fatty acids while RAGE are predominantly sensitive to endogenous physiological/metabolic insults (e.g., resulting from hyperglycemia) or inflammation (hence an *inward* focus on homeodynamic balance). TLR activation by microbes and saturated fatty acids is of particular relevance for the development of insulin resistance and diabetes mellitus type-2 and the associated problems of obesity, hypertension, and appetite insatiation. The most simple model for understanding the sequence of events is as follows; this model of "metabolic inflammation" will be developed further in a following section in this book:

Overeating of sugars, especially without phytonutrients and exercise → **Hyperglycemia + Hyperinsulinemia** → **Endogenous SFA production (e.g., palmitate)** → **TLR activation and TLR-mediated inflammation** → **Insulin resistance with resultant sustained hyperglycemia, hyperinsulinemia, hyperphagia, hypercholesterolemia**; ↻ vicious cycle

TLR activation is *primarily* abrogated by treatment of causative dysglycemia/diabetes, dysbiosis, and dietary recklessness, *secondarily* mitigated via olive oil and fish oil which modulate intracellular TLR signaling, and *tertiarily* modulated by phytonutritional NFkB inhibitors.

- Processed food/fuel overload (PFO)—excess carbohydrates, excess (saturated and n6) fatty acids: Quantitative and persistent excess of calories in the form of dietary sugars and fats (dietary fat in the Western diet is typically unprecedentedly high in n6 fatty acids [notably linoleic acid and arachidonic acid, both of which are notably inflammatory], long-chain saturated fatty acids, and hydrogenated oils); the general and obvious descriptive term for this caloric excess is "fuel overload." The metabolic consequence of diet-induced hyperglycemia is hyperinsulinemia, which promotes increased production of ceramide, which is itself a mediator of insulin resistance; one of the most logical explanation for this glucose-induced insulin resistance via insulin-induced ceramide production is that it is a self-regulatory and self-protective mechanism whereby cells are able to protect themselves from fuel overload. Notably, the medical/pharmacologic/allopathic interpretation of this phenomenon is that the insulin resistance is a problem that needs to be "cured" with drugs that override this self-regulatory mechanism to enhance insulin sensitivity; in the end, this overriding of physiologic insulin resistance leads to exacerbation of pathologic intracellular fuel overload. The consequences of intracellular fuel overload due to excess dietary carbohydrates and fats include ❶ excess intracellular lipid (e.g., palmitate, ceramide) accumulation, which leads to ER stress, mitochondrial dysfunction, and the activation of oxidant and inflammatory pathways, ❷ suppression of mitochondrial ATP production at the level of ETC oxidative phosphorylation, ❸ intracellular accumulation of lipids that have physiologic consequences, notably palmitate and ceramide and their ability to mediate insulin resistance, ❹ intracellular accumulation of lipids that are biochemically altered (e.g., modified by LOX-mediated hydroperoxidation), ❺ fuel-induced activation of pro-inflammatory enzymes such as lipoxygenase (LOX) which promotes inflammatory macrophage recruitment, hydroperoxidation of unsaturated fatty acids, insulin resistance, mitochondrial dysfunction, ER stress and the subsequent UPR, ❻ hyperglycemia caused by dietary excess of carbohydrates and the above-mentioned complications leads to oxidative stress, activation of inflammatory pathways such as NFkB, and results in formation of endogenous AGEs which promote biological aging, inflammation, and pain perception/sensitization, ❼ the activation of inflammatory pathways causes suppression of endothelial nitric oxide synthase (eNOS), and the resultant decrease in nitric oxide (NO) production impairs vasodilation (promoting hypertension and erectile dysfunction) and mitochondrial biogenesis (promoting mitopenia which results in overwork and excess ROS production from remaining mitochondria, while also reducing ATP production and fatty acid oxidation/clearance). An efficient quote from the 2013 article by Mabalirajan and Ghosh[244] provides an excellent summary of many of these concepts: "It is a surprising paradox that high nutrient [carbohydrate and lipid] intake can lead to decreased oxidative phosphorylation. The imbalance between nutrient intake and its utilization leads to store abnormal lipid in adipocytes and obesity. This accumulated lipid induces various stress pathways and activates various lipid oxidative enzymes. It has been demonstrated that mice which were fed either high fat or western diet had shown the increased expression of 12/15-lipoxygenase (12/15-LOX), a nonheme iron dioxygenase, which catalyzes the hydroperoxidation of polyunsaturated fatty acids, in adipocytes." Mabalirajan and Ghosh should have specified overconsumption of *lipids* and *carbohydrates* since this is the real problem—not "high nutrient intake" since this is misleading.

o Food-induced hypothalamic inflammation, dietary activation of Toll-like receptors: As described in an excellent article by Milanski et al[245], ❶ long-chain saturated fatty acids produce an inflammatory response predominantly through the activation of TLR4 in hypothalamus with resultant local release of cytokines, and ❷ the physiologic consequences of diet-induced hypothalamic inflammation include local endoplasmic reticulum stress, systemic inflammation, adiposity, insulin resistance, and enhanced hunger, the latter via inhibited reception/function of anorexigenic (hunger-suppressing; the roots *orexi-*, *orex-*, *-orexia* are Greek with the denotation of hunger, desire, searching) hormones insulin and leptin. Inflammation in the hypothalamic region of the brain, which can occur following TLR activation secondary to glucose, saturated long-chain fatty acids, or exposure to microbial motifs (e.g., bacterial or viral). In the CNS, TLR4 are found in the microglia. Of additional note regarding brain inflammation, "…recent studies in the brain provide in vivo evidence supporting the model that both ER stress and inflammation are able to activate each other and to inhibit normal cellular metabolism."[246] Toll-like receptors (TLR, e.g., TLR2 and TLR4) are upregulated and activated by microbial motifs such as bacterial endotoxin/LPS as well as by glucose (hyperglycemia), long-chain saturated fatty acids, free fatty acids and "vegetable oil" (term used but undefined by Milanski et al, presumably n6 PUFA especially linoleic acid, known for its proinflammatory effects). The endoplasmic reticulum (ER) functions to synthesize and process proteins, whether used intracellularly, within the cell membrane, or secreted from the cell. In certain adverse situations—notably exposure to viruses, bacteria, hyperglycemia and hyper(long-chain saturated)lipidosis, disruption of ER function leads to accumulation of unfolded/misfolded proteins within the ER

> **Saturated fatty acids produce an inflammatory response through the activation of TLR4 in the hypothalamus, promoting obesity**
>
> "… the activation of an inflammatory response in the hypothalamus leads to the molecular and functional resistance to the adipostatic hormones, leptin and insulin, resulting in a defective control of food intake and energy expenditure. … In conclusion, saturated fatty acids activate TLR2 and TLR4 signaling and ER stress in hypothalamus. … TLR4, which determines ER stress induction. The presence of a functional TLR4 signaling is required for the development of hyperlipidic dietary obesity."
>
> Milanski et al. *J Neurosci*. 2009 Jan

---

[244] Mabalirajan U, Ghosh B. Mitochondrial dysfunction in metabolic syndrome and asthma. *J Allergy* (Cairo). 2013;2013:340476
[245] Milanski et al. Saturated fatty acids produce an inflammatory response predominantly through activation of TLR4 signaling in hypothalamus. *J Neurosci*. 2009 Jan;29:359-70
[246] Hotamisligil GS. Endoplasmic reticulum stress and the inflammatory basis of metabolic disease. *Cell*. 2010 Mar 19;140(6):900-17

lumen; this *ER stress* (ERS) leads to a complex adaptive cellular response termed the *unfolded protein response* (UPR), which increases production and release of proteins and cytokines needed for immune surveillance. Induction of ERS-UPR occurs following stimulation of TLR2 or TRL4, leading to activation of the NFkB pathway; the linear flow can be depicted as follows:

Long-chain saturated fatty acids ➔ TLR4 ➔ NFkB ➔ ERS+UPR ➔ orexia, insulin resistance

ERS is obviously an adaptive mechanism, which most likely developed for sensing microbes, and which becomes maladaptive when chronically stimulated by overconsumption of carbohydrates and saturated fats; the sequel UPR is notably appropriate for response to microbes, and notably harmful when activated by habitual dietary excess. When ERS-UPR activation is sustained, the result is excess inflammation and immune system hypervigilance (e.g., pathophysiologic priming for disorders of metabolic/allergic/autoimmune inflammation); more intense activation of ERS may result in apoptosis.

Endoplasmic reticulum stress is somewhat analogous to a "traffic jam" inside the ER, and the unfolded protein response is a pro-inflammatory "traffic alert" in response; another more creative analogy would be that of an origami artist forced to fold and produce more than possible, with the resultant emotional breakdown/outrage analogous to the inflammatory UPR. Without the metabolic insults of excess glucose and excess saturated fatty acids—both of which are overpresent in Americanized/Westernized diets but which would have been absent for the vast majority of human history—the main expected stressors for induction of ERS would have been of microbial origin, and thus the resultant "alarms" and amplification of immune responses would have clearly been a positive and meaningful response; now that industrialized societies have essentially codified hyperglycemia and higher intakes of saturated fat, this ERS-UPR pathway is maintained in a higher state (quantitatively more) of sustained activation (longer duration).

Dysnutrition/dysmetabolism causes TLR4-mediated ERS and proinflammatory UPR: Dietary and metabolic insults cause endoplasmic reticulum stress (largely but not entirely) mediated by TLR4 and lead to the UPR, which primes the immune system and leads to enhanced pro-inflammatory cytokine release.

Saturated long-chain fatty acids activate TLR4 and induce NFkB-mediated inflammation via ERS-UPR and routes that are independent from ERS-UPR. While the ERS-UPR pathway effects elaboration of pro-inflammatory cytokines in an NFkB-dependent manner, the opposite is also true: NFkB activation causes ERS-UPR. Therefore, one would reasonably expect that inhibitors/modulators of the NFkB pathway (detailed elsewhere in this chapter) would be of therapeutic value in conditions of ERS-UPR; however, the clinical focus should always remain on identifying and eliminating the *origin* of the ERS-UPR/NFkB activation.

o   Conveniently and consistently overlooked social causes and medical consequences of obesity, insulin resistance, and medical management thereof: I wish to make an extra effort to point out a few items here to underscore their importance; in this paragraph, I will restate and reframe a few ideas to ensure that readers fully grasp the realization I am trying to impart. Readers, of course, have the option to bypass these particular perspectives, but let's at least consider them *before* making that decision. ❶ The medical-pharmaceutical goal of using drugs to "enhance insulin sensitivity" is simple-minded, noncurative, and self-serving: Pharmacologic enhancement of insulin sensitivity *in lieu* of actually correcting the causes (mostly dietary, microbial, xenobiotic, and lifestyle) of insulin resistance increasingly occurs to me as a stupid idea (i.e., a forced pharmacologic override of normal physiology), leveraged by drug companies via drug-promotional journal articles and advertisements upon uninformed doctors and patients, who are purposefully kept ignorant by medical school and public education, respectively. The drug treatments for long-term management of insulin resistance offer no chance for curing the disease and simply keep patients in a state of perpetual drug dependency while medical doctors have basically become enslaved to the pharmaceutical industry. Many of these facts also apply to the long-term management of so-called chronic hypertension, which is likewise nearly always readily curable (not merely treatable) with nonpharmacologic means; some of this data was reviewed in my earlier books and articles covering diabetes and hypertension and will be revisited and expanded in Volume 2 of the *Inflammation Mastery* series. ❷ Insulin resistance is cytoprotective: The idea that the human body could be an infinite repository for glucose and other high-energy fuel substrates—storing these reactive molecules endlessly and without consequence—is among the feeblest ideas to permeate and be absorbed into the clinical practice of medicine in general and the treatment of diabetes mellitus type-2 in particular. Fuel overload—caused solely by an excess of glucose+fructose with variable amounts of lipid and sodium and an insufficiency of nutrients and physical exercise—causes numerous consequential intracellular and organism-damaging events including oxidative damage, immune impairment, antioxidant depletion, mitochondrial dysfunction, endoplasmic reticulum dysfunction, and systemic inflammation; faced with an excess intake of glucose+fructose and fatty acids sourced from processed and nutrient-depleted foods, the body's only way of blocking these intracellular events is by blocking cellular uptake of fuel in general and glucose in particular, and by this innate self-protective wisdom of the body do we have "insulin resistance" formerly called by a more accurate name of "glucose intolerance." Very importantly, note that the term "glucose intolerance" implies a problem with glucose (consumption) and therefore suggests a low-cost low-carbohydrate dietary remedy, while the term "insulin resistance" is much more ambiguous and suggests a problem with insulin and the "need" for "insulin-sensitizing drugs", or simply more insulin (pharmaceutical grade, via injection). ❸ Insulin resistance is the predictable outcome of an unnatural diet and physically-constrained lifestyle: The overconsumption of processed foods is the primary cause of insulin resistance via nutrient deficiencies (e.g., chromium, cholecalciferol, magnesium, fiber and phytonutrients), substrate overload (e.g., glucose, n6 fatty acids, fructose, and pro-inflammatory sodium), and accumulation of dysmetabolic intermediates such as palmitate and ceramide; adding dysbiotic microbial exposures (natural) and xenobiotic exposures (artifactual from corporate-government irresponsibility) synergizes with modern malnutrition (fuel overload with nutrient deficiency) to create the perfect storm for insulin resistance, obesity, metabolic syndrome and hypertension. ❹ Insulin resistance and related inflammatory and cardiometabolic consequences can be produced on a population-wide basis: Making nutrient-poor fuel-rich foods less expensive than health-promoting foods, excising nutrition education and physical education (formerly "P.E." from when I was a grade-school student) from public and private schools, allowing xenobiotics to be distributed among the population at levels severe enough to cause endocrinologic (e.g., metabolic and reproductive) impairment, limiting opportunities and incentives for public recreation and exercise (e.g., making car-ownership mandatory in many communities while blocking access to parks, bikeways, etc) is a perfect way to make an entire population obese and diabetic—witness the trends in the United States (images below). ❺ **Obesity and related inflammatory and cardiometabolic consequences are expensive (to the benefit of pharmaceutical-medical interests) and are unequally distributed among social/racial/economic groups**: According to the US CDC[247] in 2014, "More than one-third of U.S. adults (34.9%) are obese and obesity-related conditions include heart disease, stroke, type 2 diabetes and certain types of cancer, some of the leading causes of preventable death. The estimated annual medical cost of obesity in the U.S. was $147 billion in 2008 U.S. dollars; the medical costs for people who are obese were $1,429 higher than those of normal weight. Obesity affects some groups more than others: Non-Hispanic blacks have the highest age-adjusted rates of obesity (47.8%) followed by Hispanics (42.5%), non-Hispanic whites (32.6%), and non-Hispanic Asians." ❻ **Obesity trends (in America) follow very clear changes in governmental, social and economic policy—when people are insecure/scared about their personal finances and the stability of their society, they eat more**: In a brilliant Op-Ed article titled "The Political Roots of American Obesity", Kihn describes what he calls "the American syndrome" as having started most clearly with changes in America's political climate in 1980; before this time, obesity trends had been both low and consistent for decades. Starting in 1980, economic insecurity started to skyrocket in the United States, and the obesity epidemic was initiated on a population-wide level.

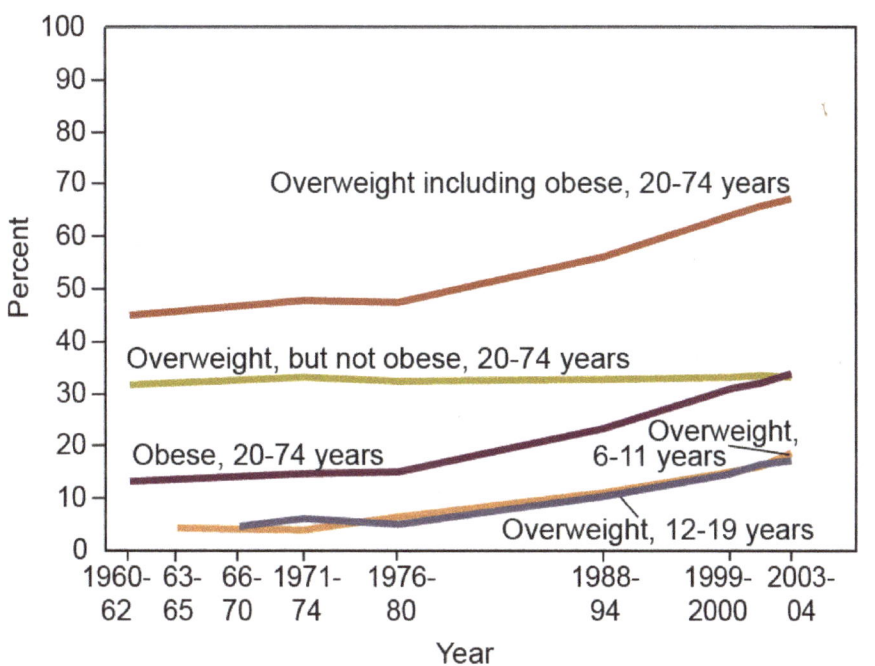

Who benefits from the obesity epidemic? What forces contribute to its perpetuation?

"The obesity epidemic helps American capitalism in two ways. On one side of the coin, **it creates a population that is more compliant, tired, sick,** self-hating and resigned to its misery. The last thing those sitting at the top want to see is a lean, clean and mean population. On the other side of the coin, **obese and overweight Americans bring in enormous profits for many vital industries** - agribusiness, food processing and transportation, food stores, restaurants, the medical industry, the diet industry and the pharmaceutical industry."

Kihn, Political Roots of American Obesity. *Truthout* 2013

Obesity trends in the United States: Rapid obesification of Americans cannot be attributed to genetic causes; however it follows economic and political trends. "Obesity is the toxic consequence of economic insecurity and a failing economic environment." Image from cdc.gov/nchs/data/hus/hus06.pdf; quote from Drewnowski, *Nutr Rev* 2009.

---

[247] cdc.gov/obesity/data/adult.html 2014 Jul

According to Kihn, starting in 1980, new government policies acted quickly to dismantle unionized worker protections *and thus quality of work life—where people spend much or most of their adult lives, job security, worker safety, and quality pay with living wages*; the most obvious single event (which had a ripple effect throughout the country and clearly indicated the change in America's social contract) was the President-authorized firing of more than 11,000 unionized air traffic controllers which was followed by nation-wide "union busting", the marked declines in job/income security, and the now famous processes of "out-sourcing" jobs to temporary and part-time workers and "off-shoring" jobs to low-paying countries with no worker protections and no sustainable environmental policies. Kihn argues very cogently that while obesity may result from overeating fats and sugars, ==the drive to overeat has an emotional basis== in survival and resource insecurity; this trend of society-wide insecurity and anxiety has its origins in national policies that make people fearful for their survival—namely, job and income insecurity.

- "American Syndrome" and Political Roots of American Obesity (*Truthout* 2013 May[248]): "When we [look at the trends and causes of obesity], we will discover that ==the obesity epidemic in America is essentially a mental health problem==, whose underlying causes are economic and political. ... As more and more Americans have seen their standard of living sink and their stress factors increase, they have taken to the all-purpose, all-American sedative—food—in a big way."
- Obesity, diets, and social inequalities (*Nutr Rev* 2009 May[249]): "Obesity and type-2 diabetes follow a socioeconomic gradient. Highest rates are observed among groups with the lowest levels of education and income and in the most deprived areas. ... This article discusses obesity as an economic phenomenon. ==Obesity is the toxic consequence of economic insecurity and a failing economic environment==."
- Poverty is obesogenic (*Nutr Hosp* 2013 Sep[250]): "Many studies have shown an overall socio-economic gradient in obesity in modern industrialized societies. Rates tend to decrease progressively with increasing socio-economic status."
- Economic security and "scientifically educated individualism" are protective against obesity (*BMJ Open* 2014 May[251]): "This might suggest that economically secure, scientifically educated individualism may therefore be protective against obesity."

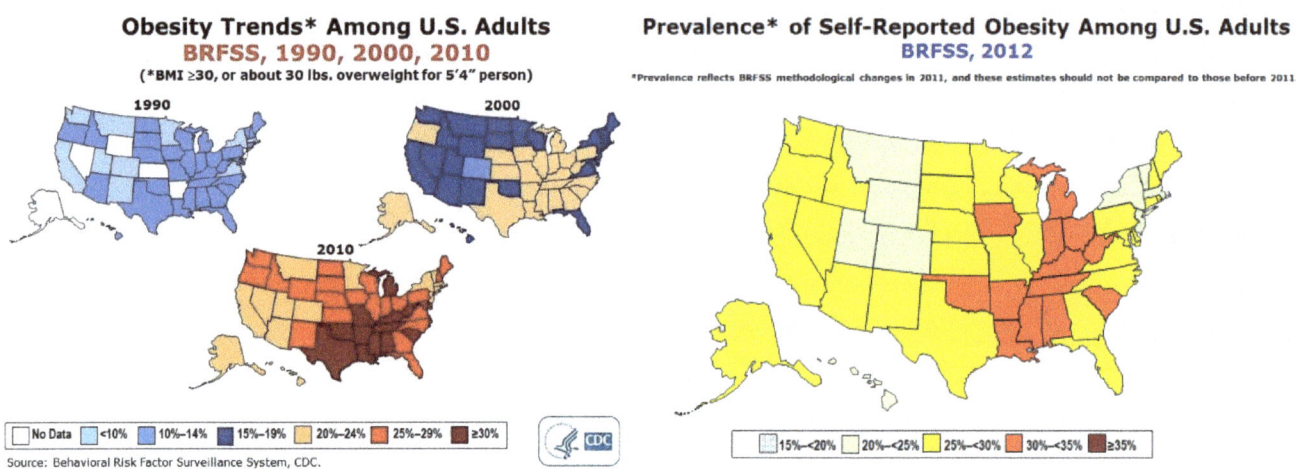

Obesity trends in the United States: The rapid obesification of the American population cannot be attributed to genetic causes; however it follows racial, economic, and political trends. Images from cdc.gov/obesity/data/adult.html 2014 Jul.

---

[248] Kihn ED. The Political Roots of American Obesity. *Truthout* 2013 May truth-out.org/opinion/item/16149-the-political-roots-of-american-obesity
[249] Drewnowski A. Obesity, diets, and social inequalities. *Nutr Rev*. 2009 May;67 Suppl 1:S36-9
[250] Pérez Rodrigo C. Current mapping of obesity. *Nutr Hosp*. 2013 Sep;28 Suppl 5:21-31
[251] Ulijaszek SJ. Do adult obesity rates in England vary by insecurity as well as by inequality? *BMJ Open*. 2014 May 13;4(5):e004430

Mini-Monograph: The Major Fatty Acids and End-products of Clinical Significance

The fatty acids of major importance and the ones discussed here are all polyunsaturated fatty acids, meaning that they have *several* carbon-to-carbon double bonds (i.e., C=C), which are vulnerable to oxidation, rancidification, and/or hydrogenation. Therefore, these fatty acids must be protected from oxygen, heat, light, and prolonged storage. Once structurally altered by oxygen, heat, or light, these fatty acids lose some or all of their biologic value, and they take on disease-promoting properties by interfering with fatty acid metabolism, altering cell membrane dynamics, and/or by having direct/indirect inflammatory and carcinogenic actions.

Fatty acids serve three primary biologic functions: 1) as cell membrane components that modulate membrane pliability and receptor sensitivity, 2) as precursors to potent biologic regulators such as prostaglandins and leukotrienes, and 3) as modulators of gene expression. Each fatty acid must be either provided by diet or manufactured from enzymatic conversion of its predecessor in order to carry out its physiologic role. Deficiency of any fatty acid results in impairment of physiologic function. These impairments begin subtly and often go unrecognized by clinicians who may then erroneously employ pharmacologic and surgical interventions to alleviate *diseases* that originate from *deficiencies* of fatty acids and other nutrients.

Polyunsaturated fatty acids (PUFA) are categorized based on the location of the first carbon-to-carbon double bond from the methyl group, which is located at the opposite end from the carboxyl carbon.[252] The major categories from a biological and nutritional standpoint are the omega-3 fatty acids (having the first carbon-to-carbon double bond starting at the third carbon from the methyl group) and the omega-6 fatty acids (having the first carbon-to-carbon double bond starting at the sixth carbon from the methyl group). The most commonly known member of the omega-9 group is oleic acid from olive oil; but it is of lesser biologic importance than the omega-3 and omega-6 fatty acids, which are the key determinants of the biologically powerful thromboxanes, leukotrienes, prostaglandins, and isoprostanes. The term "omega" is commonly represented as either "Ω" or "w" or "ω" or "n". For the sake of consistency and readability, I will use either the word "omega" or the symbol "n" in this text.

The general term "eicosanoids" is used to describe the various metabolic end products of 20-carbon fatty acid metabolism, including thromboxanes (TX), leukotrienes (LT), and prostaglandins (PG). Produced in minute quantities of approximately 1 milligram per day[253], prostaglandins are produced by nearly all mammalian cells; their production is not confined to leukocytes even though they are often associated with immune activation. Since they are produced and act locally at the site of metabolic activation, they are autocrine and paracrine rather than endocrine.[254] These chemicals have short half-lives, with thromboxanes existing only for a few seconds after production[255] while leukotrienes persist for as long as four hours.[256] While specific enzymes transform one fatty acid into another (within the same family, n-3 or n-6, respectively), the production of eicosanoids is *initiated by enzymes* but often *completed by non-specific, random interactions* dependent on free radicals and/or random conformational changes in enzymes and substrates.[257]

The two main families of bioactive fatty acids are the omega-3 and omega-6 families. These families have generally *opposing* effects to each other and therefore the quantitative balance of these fatty acids serves to dictate the body's ability to establish and retain homeostasis with regard to the modulation of cellular function in general and the production of thromboxanes, leukotrienes, and prostaglandins in particular.[258] With an excess of n-6 fatty acids and a deficiency of n-3 fatty acids, the human body fails to function optimally and the clinical result is an increase in the prevalence and severity of clinical diseases associated with imbalanced gene expression, cell membrane function, and eicosanoid production—namely cancer, heart disease, diabetes, arthritis, allergy, autoimmune diseases, depression, bipolar disorder, schizophrenia, and the long list of "diseases of Western civilization."[259]

---

[252] Erasmus U. *Fats that heal, fats that kill*. British Columbia Canada: Alive Books, 1993 Page 15-16
[253] Delvin TM. *Textbook of Biochemistry with Clinical Correlations*. New York: Wiley-Liss, 1997. Pages 431-441
[254] McGlivery RW. *Biochemistry: A Functional Approach. Third Edition*. Philadelphia: WB Saunders, 1983. Pages 747-750
[255] McGlivery RW. *Biochemistry: A Functional Approach. Third Edition*. Philadelphia: WB Saunders, 1983. Pages 747-750
[256] Delvin TM. *Textbook of Biochemistry with Clinical Correlations*. New York: Wiley-Liss, 1997. Pages 431-441
[257] Thuresson ED, Lakkides KM, Smith WL. Different catalytically competent arrangements of arachidonic acid within the cyclooxygenase active site of prostaglandin endoperoxide H synthase-1 lead to the formation of different oxygenated products. *J Biol Chem*. 2000 Mar 24;275(12):8501-7 jbc.org/cgi/reprint/275/12/8501
[258] Tapiero et al. Polyunsaturated fatty acids (PUFA) and eicosanoids in human health and pathologies. *Biomed Pharmacother*. 2002;56(5):215-22
[259] Price WA. *Nutrition and Physical Degeneration*. Santa Monica: Price-Pottinger Nutrition Foundation, 1945

Omega-3 fatty acids:
- **General properties**
    o The first double bond is at third carbon from the methyl group
    o **Primarily from flax seed and cold-water aquatic animals ("antifreeze" for deep water fish, seal, whale) and game animals, also from some leafy green vegetables in small amounts.**
    o Maintain cell membrane fluidity and tissue flexibility and elasticity due to markedly curved structure (maintains space between molecules) compared to saturated fatty acids (straight molecules are closely packed with less room for motion)
    o N-3 fatty acids consistently lower serum triglycerides levels in contrast to n-6 fatty acids, which generally cause serum triglycerides to increase.[260]
    o **Causes of n-3 deficiency include:**
        1. Low-fat diets (in general)
        2. Decreased intake of omega-3 (specifically)
        3. Increased intake of omega-6 (such as "to lower cholesterol")
        4. Intake of unnatural *trans*-fatty acids versus natural *cis*-fatty acids. *Trans*-fatty acids are found in hydrogenated oils (hydrogenation makes oil thicker, prevents oxidation, and "improves" taste), fried foods. *Trans*-PUFA increase LDL and reduce HDL.[261]
        5. Alteration of feed for farm animals (substitution of grasses, plants, insects with grains, which are high in n-6 FA), this is why wild game animals have more n-3
        6. High-fat diets if fats are imbalanced with excess of n-6 and trans-FA's
        7. Maldigestion and/or malabsorption
        8. Primary or secondary defects in enzyme function for the conversion of dietary precursors to the end-stage biologically-active fatty acids
    o **Clinical manifestations of deficiency of omega-3 fats are far more subtle than those associated with omega-6 deficiency: (in animal studies) reduced learning, impaired vision, polydypsia.** Given the importance of n-3 fatty acids in health and disease and the relative deficiency state which is the norm in America, we could also argue that deficiency of n-3 fatty acids predispose to the chronic degenerative diseases of cancer, diabetes, cardiovascular disease and to the more subtle functional problems of dermatitis and the epidemic of neurocognitive and neuropsychiatric disorders.
    o **Tissue levels are measurably changed within one week of supplementation and are restored to constant levels in 12 weeks of supplementation (per animal studies).** Not all manifestations of deficiency are corrected with supplementation, indicating that fatty acid deficiencies may leave permanent residual effects, particularly if deficiency occurs early in life during the time of rapid growth and development, especially of the brain.
- **Alpha-linolenic acid, linolenic acid, ALA, α-LNA, ALNA, 18:3n3**
    o **Essential fatty acid:** ALA is the parent fatty acid of the omega-3 class; it is the "first in line."
    o Sources include **flax seed oil (57% ALA)** and canola (rape seed) oil (9% ALA), soy oil, breast milk, English/black walnuts, soybeans, pine nuts, green vegetables, and beans.
    o ALA may theoretically be converted to EPA and DHA but this should not be expected to occur sufficiently in all patients at all times due to interindividual variations in enzyme activity and inadequate nutritional/cofactor status. To attain a measurable increase in EPA from ALA supplementation, approximately eleven-times (11x) the amount of ALA must be consumed to achieve a proportional response to that which can be achieved with direct supplementation of

---

[260] Simopoulos AP. Essential fatty acids in health and chronic disease. *Am J Clin Nutr*. 1999 Sep;70(3 Suppl):560S-569S
[261] Tapiero H, et al. Polyunsaturated fatty acids (PUFA) and eicosanoids in human health and pathologies. *Biomed Pharmacother*. 2002;56(5):215-22

EPA.[262] No increase in DHA has been observed in humans after supplementation of ALA; in fact, supplementation with flax seed oil has actually been shown to reduce DHA levels in humans.[263,264]
- Lipid-lowering effects are not seen with ALA supplementation and are only attained with the use of EPA and DHA; however ALA can reduce blood pressure.[265]
- ALA has potent anti-inflammatory benefits independent of its conversion to EPA or DHA.[266] The mechanism of action appears to be downregulation of NFkB rather than the direct modulation of eicosanoid biosynthesis. One study using flax oil as a source of ALA to treat rheumatoid arthritis found no clinical or biochemical benefit (i.e., no change in Hgb, CRP, ESR).[267]

- **Stearidonic acid, 18:4n3, octadecatetraenoic acid**
  - Small amount found in black currant oil
  - Human studies have found that stearidonic acid increases EPA 2x more efficiently than does ALA but does not increase DHA.[268]
  - Inhibits 5-lipoxygenase.[269]

- **N-3 Eicosatetraenoic acid, 20:4n3**
  - 20:4n-3 is eicosatetraenoic acid.[270,271]
  - The term "eicosatetraenoic acid" applies to both 20:4n6 (arachidonic acid) of the omega-6 fatty acid family[272] and 20:4n3 of the omega-3 fatty acid family.[273,274] Therefore, to avoid the confusion that would result from the use of the term "eicosatetraenoic acid" by itself, "n-6 eicosatetraenoic acid" should be used when referring to 20:4n6 (arachidonic acid) and "n-3 eicosatetraenoic acid" should be used when referring to 20:4n3.

- **Eicosapentaenoic acid, EPA, 20:5n3**
  - Effectively absent in vegan diets; the major dietary source is fish oil.
  - EPA can decrease production of DGLA.[275]
  - EPA doses of at least 4 grams per day are needed to increase bleeding time.[276]
  - EPA–derived eicosanoids have anti-inflammatory properties, including a reduction in the production of pro-inflammatory eicosanoids such as LT-B4, PAFs, and cytokines such as TNF-alpha and IL-1, and a large reduction in PG-E2 and TX-B2.[277]
  - Animal studies suggest that vitamin B-6 deficiency can reduce the function of delta-6-desaturase by 64% and lead to a reduction in EPA and DHA.[278]

---

[262] "Indu and Ghafoorunissa showed that while keeping the amount of dietary LA constant, 3.7 g ALA appears to have biological effects similar to those of 0.3 g long-chain n-3 PUFA with conversion of 11 g ALA to 1 g long-chain n-3 PUFA." Simopoulos AP. Essential fatty acids in health and chronic disease. *Am J Clin Nutr*. 1999 Sep;70(3 Suppl):560S-569S

[263] Saldeen T. *Health Effects of Fish Oil with a Focus on Natural, Stable, Fish Oil*. Buxton Road, New Mills, High Peak: Nutri Ltd. [Date unknown] page 33

[264] "Linear relationships were found between dietary alpha-LA and EPA in plasma fractions and in cellular phospholipids. … There was an inverse relationship between dietary alpha-LA and docosahexaenoic acid concentrations in the phospholipids of plasma, neutrophils, mononuclear cells, and platelets." Mantzioris E, et al. Differences exist in the relationships between dietary linoleic and alpha-linolenic acids and their respective long-chain metabolites. *Am J Clin Nutr*. 1995 Feb;61(2):320-4

[265] Simopoulos AP. Essential fatty acids in health and chronic disease. *Am J Clin Nutr*. 1999 Sep;70(3 Suppl):560S-569S

[266] "CONCLUSIONS: Dietary supplementation with ALA for 3 months decreases significantly CRP, SAA and IL-6 levels in dyslipidaemic patients. This anti-inflammatory effect may provide a possible additional mechanism for the beneficial effect of plant n-3 polyunsaturated fatty acids in primary and secondary prevention of coronary artery disease." Rallidis LS, Paschos G, Liakos GK, Velissaridou AH, Anastasiadis G, Zampelas A. Dietary alpha-linolenic acid decreases C-reactive protein, serum amyloid A and interleukin-6 in dyslipidaemic patients. *Atherosclerosis*. 2003 Apr;167(2):237-42

[267] "Thus, 3-month's supplementation with alpha-LNA did not prove to be beneficial in rheumatoid arthritis." Nordstrom DC, et al. Alpha-linolenic acid in the treatment of rheumatoid arthritis: a double-blind, placebo-controlled and randomized study: flaxseed vs. safflower seed. *Rheumatol Int*. 1995;14(6):231-4

[268] "RESULTS: Dietary SDA increased EPA and docosapentaenoic acid concentrations but not DHA concentrations in erythrocyte and in plasma phospholipids. The relative effectiveness of the tested dietary fatty acids in increasing tissue EPA was 1:0.3:0.07 for EPA:SDA:ALA." James MJ, Ursin VM, Cleland LG. Metabolism of stearidonic acid in human subjects: comparison with the metabolism of other n-3 fatty acids. *Am J Clin Nutr*. 2003 May;77(5):1140-5

[269] Guichardant M, Traitler H, Spielmann D, Sprecher H, Finot PA. Stearidonic acid, an inhibitor of the 5-lipoxygenase pathway. *Lipids*. 1993 Apr;28(4):321-4

[270] Tapiero H, et al. Polyunsaturated fatty acids (PUFA) and eicosanoids in human health and pathologies. *Biomed Pharmacother*. 2002;56(5):215-22

[271] Erasmus U. *Fats that heal, fats that kill*. British Columbia Canada: Alive Books, 1993 Page 276

[272] "5,8,11,14-eicosatetraenoic (20:4(n-6))" Mimouni V, Christiansen EN, Blond JP, Ulmann L, Poisson JP, Bezard J. Elongation and desaturation of arachidonic and eicosapentaenoic acids in rat liver. Effect of clofibrate feeding. *Biochim Biophys Acta*. 1991 Nov 27;1086(3):349-53

[273] Tapiero H, et al. Polyunsaturated fatty acids (PUFA) and eicosanoids in human health and pathologies. *Biomed Pharmacother*. 2002 Jul;56(5):215-22

[274] Erasmus U. *Fats that heal, fats that kill*. British Columbia Canada: Alive Books, 1993 Page 276

[275] Horrobin DF. Interactions between n-3 and n-6 essential fatty acids (EFAs) in the regulation of cardiovascular disorders and inflammation. *Prostaglandins Leukot Essent Fatty Acids*. 1991 Oct;44(2):127-31

[276] "A dose of 1.8 g EPA/d did not result in any prolongation in bleeding time, but 4 g/d increased bleeding time and decreased platelet count with no adverse effects. In human studies, there has never been a case of clinical bleeding…" Simopoulos AP. Essential fatty acids in health and chronic disease. *Am J Clin Nutr*. 1999 Sep;70(3 Suppl):560S-569S

[277] Tapiero H, et al. Polyunsaturated fatty acids (PUFA) and eicosanoids in human health and pathologies. *Biomed Pharmacother*. 2002 Jul;56(5):215-22

[278] Tsuge H, Hotta N, Hayakawa T. Effects of vitamin B-6 on (n-3) polyunsaturated fatty acid metabolism. *J Nutr*. 2000 Feb;130(2S Suppl):333S-334S

- o Children with allergies show altered fatty acid metabolism[279] that is not caused by impaired delta-6-desaturase activity and which results reduced EPA levels.[280]
- o N-6 fatty acids facilitate elongation of EPA to n-3 DPA.[281] Thus, anti-inflammatory EPA is depleted by consumption of proinflammatory n-6 fatty acids.
- o Evidence suggests that EPA must be incorporated into cell membrane phospholipids for its beneficial effects on eicosanoid metabolism to be realized. Administration of n-6 fatty acids removes EPA from cell membranes and relocates EPA from phospholipids into triacylglycerols. Therefore the benefits of EPA are mitigated by n-6 fatty acids, and thus "…dietary therapies designed to increase the EPA content of tissue phospholipids may need to focus on limiting n-6 fatty acid intake in addition to increasing EPA intake." [282]

- **DPA: n-3 docosapentaenoic acid, 22:5n3**
    - o Production is increased slightly with consumption of the n-3 precursor ALA.[283]
    - o Production can be increased with consumption of n-6 fatty acids.[284] The clinical implications of this finding are significant, because it implies that concomitant administration of n-6 fatty acids such as ALA and arachidonate with EPA would preferentially shuttle EPA to DPA, and therefore the formation of the beneficial EPA-derived eicosanoids would be reduced.
    - o The term "docosapentaenoic acid" can apply to both 22:5n3 of the omega-3 fatty acid family[285,286] and 22:5n6 of the omega-6 fatty acid family.[287,288,289] Because to use the term "docosapentaenoic acid" may be ambiguous, the terms "n-3 docosapentaenoic acid" should be used when discussing 22:5n3 and "n-6 docosapentaenoic acid" should be used when discussing 22:5n6.

- **DHA: docosahexaenoic acid, 22:6n-3**
    - o Found only in plants of the sea, phytoplankton/microalgae, and consumers of microalgae (such as fish)
    - o Essential for neural function, effectively absent in vegan diets, present in breast milk (low in vegetarians); major n-3 in tissues; component of phosphatidylethanolamine and phosphatidylserine; deficiency is associated with inadequate intake of DHA and/or deficient conversion from ALA or EPA.
    - o Animal studies have shown that induction of DHA deficiency causes memory deficits and a reduction in hippocampal cell size.[290]
    - o DHA is an important component of cell membranes and generally appears to improve cell membrane function via improving receptor function and signal transduction.
    - o DHA levels are reduced by ethanol consumption.[291]
    - o Animal studies suggest that vitamin B-6 deficiency can reduce the function of delta-6-desaturase by 64% and lead to a reduction in EPA and DHA.[292]

---

[279] Yu G, Bjorksten B. Serum levels of phospholipid fatty acids in mothers and their babies in relation to allergic disease. *Eur J Pediatr*. 1998 Apr;157(4):298-303
[280] Yu G, Bjorksten B. Polyunsaturated fatty acids in school children in relation to allergy and serum IgE levels. *Pediatr Allergy Immunol*. 1998 Aug;9(3):133-8
[281] "The major findings of this study were: 1) n-6 fatty acids markedly stimulated the elongation of EPA to 22:5..." Rubin D, Laposata M. Cellular interactions between n-6 and n-3 fatty acids: a mass analysis of fatty acid elongation/desaturation, distribution among complex lipids, and conversion to eicosanoids. *J Lipid Res*. 1992 Oct;33(10):1431-40
[282] Rubin D, Laposata M. Cellular interactions between n-6 and n-3 fatty acids: a mass analysis of fatty acid elongation/desaturation, distribution among complex lipids, and conversion to eicosanoids. *J Lipid Res*. 1992 Oct;33(10):1431-40
[283] Tarpila, et al, Adlercreutz H. The effect of flaxseed supplementation in processed foods on serum fatty acids and enterolactone. *Eur J Clin Nutr*. 2002 Feb;56(2):157-65
[284] Rubin D, Laposata M. Cellular interactions between n-6 and n-3 fatty acids: a mass analysis of fatty acid elongation/desaturation, distribution among complex lipids, and conversion to eicosanoids. *J Lipid Res*. 1992 Oct;33(10):1431-40
[285] "docosapentaenoic acid (22:5n-3)" Williard DE, Harmon SD, Kaduce TL, Preuss M, Moore SA, Robbins ME, Spector AA. Docosahexaenoic acid synthesis from n-3 polyunsaturated fatty acids in differentiated rat brain astrocytes. *J Lipid Res*. 2001 Sep;42(9):1368-76
[286] "…docosapentaenoic acid (22:5n-3)…" Takahashi R, Nassar BA, Huang YS, Begin ME, Horrobin DF. Effect of different ratios of dietary N-6 and N-3 fatty acids on fatty acid composition, prostaglandin formation and platelet aggregation in the rat. *Thromb Res*. 1987 Jul 15;47(2):135-46
[287] Retterstol K, Haugen TB, Christophersen BO. The pathway from arachidonic to docosapentaenoic acid (20:4n-6 to 22:5n-6) and from eicosapentaenoic to docosahexaenoic (20:5n-3 to 22:6n-3) studied in testicular cells from immature rats. *Biochim Biophys Acta*. 2000 Jan 3;1483(1):119-31
[288] "docosapentaenoic acid (DPAn-6)" Ahmad A, et al. A decrease in cell size accompanies a loss of docosahexaenoate in the rat hippocampus. *Nutr Neurosci* 2002;5:103-13
[289] "The desaturation of adrenic acid to n-6 docosapentaenoic acid was decreased in the normo- and hyperglycemic diabetic rats." Mimouni V, Narce M, Huang YS, Horrobin DF, Poisson JP. Adrenic acid delta 4 desaturation and fatty acid composition in liver microsomes of spontaneously diabetic Wistar BB rats. *Prostaglandins Leukot Essent Fatty Acids*. 1994 Jan;50(1):43-7
[290] Ahmad A, et al. A decrease in cell size accompanies a loss of docosahexaenoate in the rat hippocampus. *Nutr Neurosci*. 2002 Apr;5(2):103-13
[291] Pawlosky RJ, Bacher J, Salem N Jr. Ethanol consumption alters electroretinograms and depletes neural tissues of docosahexaenoic acid in rhesus monkeys: nutritional consequences of a low n-3 fatty acid diet. *Alcohol Clin Exp Res*. 2001 Dec;25(12):1758-65
[292] Tsuge H, Hotta N, Hayakawa T. Effects of vitamin B-6 on (n-3) polyunsaturated fatty acid metabolism. *J Nutr*. 2000 Feb;130(2S Suppl):333S-334S

- o Supplementation with EPA+DHA is generally safe and reduces all-cause mortality.[293]
- o In late 2003, bioactive metabolites of DHA were discovered. Previous to the publication of this research, production of bioactive metabolites of DHA via lipoxygenase and cyclooxygenase was unsuspected and/or unproved, and the anti-inflammatory biochemical and clinical effects of DHA were mostly thought to be due to alterations in membrane/receptor function and retroconversion to EPA. We now know that DHA is converted by several mechanisms (lipoxygenase, cyclooxygenase, random reactions, and cell-to-cell interactions) into docosatrienes and resolvins, which are described below.[294]

Bioactive and Clinically Significant End-products of Omega-3 Fatty Acids

End-products from n-3 fatty acids generally have what are considered "health-promoting effects" which are generally weaker than and opposite to the end-products of the major n-6 fatty acid, arachidonate. Additionally, since n-3 fatty acids compete with the same metabolizing enzymes as do the n-6 family of fatty acids, a major portion of the "clinical effectiveness" of n-3 fatty acids comes not from the production of n-3 end-products but rather from the *impairment of the n-6 cascade*.

- **Prostaglandin E-3 (PG-E3)**
  - o PG-E3 and EPA both reduce formation of arachidonate-derived eicosanoids[295]
- **Prostaglandin G-3 (PG-G3)**
  - o Formed from EPA by cyclooxygenase (COX)
- **Prostaglandin H-3 (PG-H3)**
  - o Formed from PG-G3 by peroxidase
- **Prostaglandin I-3 (PG-I3)**
  - o Decreases platelet aggregation[296]
  - o Promotes vasodilation[297]
  - o Possibly antiarrhythmic
  - o Probably contributes to the hypotensive effect of fish oil[298]
- **Thromboxane A-3 (TX-A3)**
  - o Biologically inert
- **Leukotriene B-5 (LT-B5)**
  - o Significantly weaker than LT-B4; "functionally attenuated"[299]
  - o May possess mild anti-inflammatory activity either directly or by reducing production of the more powerful arachidonate-derived LT-B4.[300]
- **Plasminogen activator inhibitor-1 (PAI-1)**
  - o Increased with fish oil supplementation to maintain hemostasis
- **Docosatrienes**
  - o Formed by (12-, 15-, 17-) lipoxygenase and cyclooxygenase-2 from DHA
  - o Potent inhibitors of TNFa
  - o Downregulate gene expression for proinflammatory IL-1
  - o Reduce neutrophil entry to sites of inflammation

---

[293] "The recent GISSI (Gruppo Italiano per lo Studio della Sopravvivenza nell'Infarto miocardico)-Prevention study of 11,324 patients showed a 45% decrease in risk of sudden cardiac death and a 20% reduction in all-cause mortality in the group taking 850 mg/d of omega-3 fatty acids." O'Keefe JH Jr, Harris WS. From Inuit to implementation: omega-3 fatty acids come of age. *Mayo Clin Proc*. 2000 Jun;75(6):607-14

[294] "These results indicate that DHA is the precursor to potent protective mediators generated via enzymatic oxygenations to novel docosatrienes and 17S series resolvins that each regulate events of interest in inflammation and resolution." Hong S, Gronert K, Devchand PR, Moussignac RL, Serhan CN. Novel docosatrienes and 17S-resolvins generated from docosahexaenoic acid in murine brain, human blood, and glial cells. Autacoids in anti-inflammation. *J Biol Chem*. 2003 Apr 25;278(17):14677-87

[295] Erasmus U. *Fats that heal, fats that kill*. British Columbia Canada: Alive Books, 1993 Page 278

[296] Horrobin DF. Ascorbic acid and prostaglandin synthesis. *Subcell Biochem*. 1996;25:109-15

[297] Horrobin DF. Ascorbic acid and prostaglandin synthesis. *Subcell Biochem*. 1996;25:109-15

[298] Du Plooy WJ, Venter CP, Muntingh GM, et al. The cumulative dose response effect of eicosapentaenoic and docosahexaenoic acid on blood pressure, plasma lipid profile and diet pattern in mild to moderate essential hypertensive black patients. *Prostaglandins Leukot Essent Fatty Acids* 1992 Aug;46(4):315-21

[299] Rubin D, Laposata M. Cellular interactions between n-6 and n-3 fatty acids: a mass analysis of fatty acid elongation/desaturation, distribution among complex lipids, and conversion to eicosanoids. *J Lipid Res*. 1992 Oct;33(10):1431-40

[300] Rubin D, Laposata M. Cellular interactions between n-6 and n-3 fatty acids. *J Lipid Res*. 1992 Oct;33(10):1431-40

- **Resolvins**
  - Derived from EPA and DHA via the COX-2 enzyme with production notably increased in the presence of low-dose aspirin
  - Downregulate cytokine expression, reduce neutrophil entry to sites of inflammation, and reduce inflammation-related pain
- **Neuroprotectin**
  - Neuroprotectin D1 (NPD1) is derived from DHA and exerts potent anti-inflammatory and anti-apoptotic/neuroprotective bioactivity
  - Other forms include Neuroprotectins A and B
- **Maresins**
  - Discovered in 2009 and generated by the 14-lipoxygenase pathway[301]
  - The term *maresins* is coined from **Ma**crophage-derived **res**olution of **in**flammation
  - Potent anti-inflammatory and proresolving properties similar to Resolvin E1
  - Maresin 1, MaR1, proved to be a potent mediator, stopping PMN infiltration and stimulating macrophage phagocytosis of apoptotic cells—*efferocytosis*.[302]
- **GPR-120—a fatty acid receptor mediating some of the anti-inflammatory and insulin-sensitizing benefits of n3 fatty acids**
  - As indicated by the title of the original research supervised by Olefsky[303] in 2010, G protein-coupled receptor 120 (GPR120) is an omega-3 fatty acid receptor mediating potent anti-inflammatory and insulin-sensitizing effects.

Beyond "anti-inflammation" to and understanding of the *active resolution of inflammation*

What began to be appreciated by the discovery of the docosatrienes, resolvins, and maresins is that resolution of inflammation is and can be an active process, not merely the fading of a proinflammatory response. The identification of these mediators as stimulators of active pro-resolution agents gives a new perspective on the resolution of inflammation and injury—that it can be actively stimulated rather than merely passively awaited.

---

[301] Serhan CN et al. Maresins: novel macrophage mediators with potent antiinflammatory and proresolving actions. *J Exp Med*. 2009 Jan 16;206(1):15-23

[302] "In cell biology, efferocytosis (from efferre, Latin for 'to take to the grave', 'to bury') is the process by which dying/dead cells (e.g. apoptotic or necrotic) are removed by phagocytic cells. It can be regarded as the 'burying of dead cells'. en.wikipedia.org/wiki/Efferocytosis 2014 May

[303] Oh DY, Talukdar S, Bae EJ, Imamura T, Morinaga H, Fan W, Li P, Lu WJ, Watkins SM, Olefsky JM. GPR120 is an omega-3 fatty acid receptor mediating potent anti-inflammatory and insulin-sensitizing effects. *Cell*. 2010 Sep 3;142(5):687-98

Chapter 4: Major Modifiable Factors in Systemic Inflammation

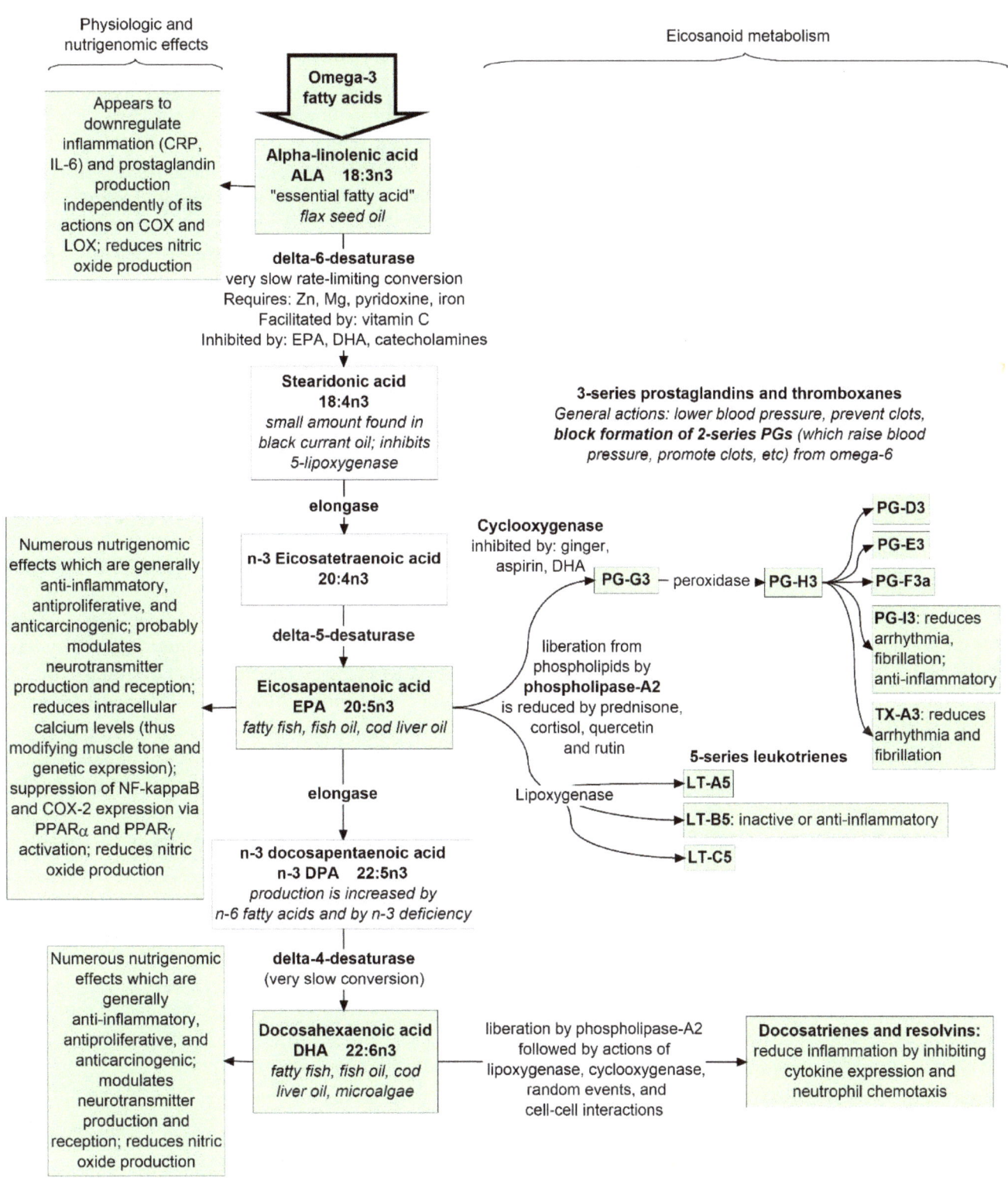

Metabolism of Omega-3 Fatty Acids and Related Eicosanoids: Health-promoting (i.e., either beneficial or neutral/blocking) fatty acids and metabolites are emphasized in the above diagram by the color green; obviously, n3 fatty acids are predominantly positive in their metabolic effects and associated health outcomes.

OMEGA-6—first double bond at 6th carbon from the methyl group
- **Linoleic acid, LA, 18:2n6, linoleate**
  - Essential fatty acid from nut, seed, and vegetable oils, especially safflower oil, sunflower oil, corn oil, walnut oil, sesame seed oil, LA is the parent fatty acid of the omega-6 class,
  - EPA and DHA decrease conversion of linoleate to arachidonate; high doses of LA inhibit conversion of alpha-LNA to EPA and DHA due to competition for delta-6 desaturase
  - Hydrogenated "trans" forms are common in processed and fried foods,
  - LA favors oxidative modification of LDL cholesterol, increases platelet response to aggregation, and suppresses the immune system.[304] Adipose LA levels are positively correlated with CVD.
  - Promotes metastasis and inflammation.
  - LA is the predominant PUFA in US diets. Daily intake of linoleic acid is approximately 10 grams, only a small amount of which is converted to arachidonate.[305]
  - LA effectively lowers cholesterol, but otherwise this fatty acid is consistently associated with exacerbation of cancer and inflammation and thus should be avoided.
  - LA undergoes oxidative metabolism by 15-lipoxygenase-1 to form 13-S-HODE[306], and this is discussed in greater detail later in this section
- **gamma (γ)-linolenic acid, GLA, 18:3n6, gamma-linolenate**
  - Formation is increased from linoleic acid by vitamin C[307]
  - Found in evening primrose oil, borage seed oil, hemp seed oil, and black currant seed oil
  - GLA restores action of delta-6-desaturase (D6D) in aging animals, suggesting that GLA intake should increase in older rats and humans
  - Useful in eczema for improvement in skin health and in diabetes especially for improvement in nerve function
  - GLA may facilitate the conversion of ALA to EPA and perhaps to DHA.
  - In patients who respond to GLA supplementation, we can reasonably hypothesize that they have impaired D-6-Desaturase activity since most patients have adequate dietary intake of LA. Therefore, by extension, we can suppose that their conversion of ALA to EPA is likewise impaired and that they may benefit from EPA supplementation.
  - Formation of GLA from LA is inhibited by EPA and other n-3 EFAs[308]
  - Overall, the weight of the research suggests that supplementation with GLA *does* lead to modest increases in arachidonate, despite the slow conversion of DGLA to arachidonate by delta-5 desaturase. Coadministration of EPA with GLA prevents any rise in arachidonate, as discussed later in this section.
- **Dihomo-gamma-linolenic acid, 20:3n6, DGLA, eicosatrienoic acid, eicosatrienoate**
  - DGLA eicosanoids have benefits for the cardiovascular system and have anti-inflammatory effects
  - Generally speaking, metabolites of DGLA are fewer in number and weaker in physiologic effect than the metabolites of arachidonic acid.
  - Vitamin C "has a significant effect in stimulating the conversion of DGLA into its metabolites..." at doses which are "...clinically relevant."[309]
  - DGLA levels are 34% lower than normal in patients with magnesium deficiency.[310]
  - Production is decreased with supplementation of ALA[311] and EPA and other n-3 EFAs except when GLA is provided directly[312]

---

[304] Simopoulos AP. Essential fatty acids in health and chronic disease. *Am J Clin Nutr*. 1999 Sep;70(3 Suppl):560S-569S
[305] Delvin TM. *Textbook of Biochemistry with Clinical Correlations*. New York: Wiley-Liss, 1997. Pages 431-441
[306] Shureiqi I, Lippman SM. Lipoxygenase modulation to reverse carcinogenesis. *Cancer Res*. 2001 Sep 1;61(17):6307-12
[307] Horrobin DF. Ascorbic acid and prostaglandin synthesis. *Subcell Biochem* 1996;25:109-15
[308] Horrobin DF. Interactions between n-3 and n-6 essential fatty acids (EFAs) in the regulation of cardiovascular disorders and inflammation. *Prostaglandins Leukot Essent Fatty Acids* 1991 Oct;44(2):127-31
[309] Horrobin DF. Ascorbic acid and prostaglandin synthesis. *Subcell Biochem*. 1996;25:109-15
[310] "...dihomogamma linoleic acid (20:3 n-6) was 34% lower..." Galland L. Impaired essential fatty acid metabolism in latent tetany. *Magnesium* 1985;4(5-6):333-8
[311] Simopoulos AP. Essential fatty acids in health and chronic disease. *Am J Clin Nutr*. 1999 Sep;70(3 Suppl):560S-569S
[312] Horrobin DF. Interactions between n-3 and n-6 essential fatty acids (EFAs) in the regulation of cardiovascular disorders and inflammation. *Prostaglandins Leukot Essent Fatty Acids*. 1991 Oct;44(2):127-31

- o Low levels of DGLA are associated with increased risk for stroke and myocardial infarction.[313] We could speculate that low levels of DGLA may be associated with pyridoxine or magnesium deficiency, of which are associated with cardiovascular disease.
- o DGLA metabolites reduce the formation of the arachidonate-derived 2-series prostaglandins, 4-series leukotrienes and platelet-activating factor.[314]
- **Arachidonic acid, 20:4n6, n-6 eicosatetraenoic acid, AA, ARA**
  - o Arachidonic acid is the predominant fatty acid in most tissues (diet-dependent!) acted upon by cyclooxygenase (to form prostaglandins and thromboxanes) and lipoxygenase (to form leukotrienes); it is the major n-6 in cell membranes and body tissues
  - o Liberated from phospholipids by phospholipase enzymes, most notably phospholipase A2.
  - o Most end-products of arachidonate metabolism are pro-inflammatory and are "in general harmful"[315] although arachidonate itself is a necessary component of phospholipids and sphingolipids in cell membranes.
  - o Arachidonate and its metabolites are referred to as eicosanoids.[316] Arachidonic acid is the predominant fatty acid in membrane phospholipids and is the preferred substrate for eicosanoid production relative to EPA.[317] Given that arachidonate's eicosanoids are biologically more powerful than those of EPA, we can accurately generalize that arachidonate and its respective prostaglandins and leukotrienes dominate the fatty acid and eicosanoid playground in both *quantitative* and *qualitative* respects. Therefore, successful intervention against arachidonate metabolism must consider 1) the quantity of arachidonate, 2) the balance of n-3 to n-6, and also 3) specific measures to hinder the production of the harmful arachidonate metabolites.
  - o Arachidonic acid is the direct precursor to the isoprostanes 8-iso prostaglandin-E2 (8-iso-PG-E2) and 8-iso prostaglandin-F2-alpha (8-iso-PG-F2-alpha), mediators that possess **inflammatory and hyperalgesic** properties and which are produced by the radical-mediated non-enzymatic peroxidation of arachidonate.[318] Inhibition of cyclooxygenase and/or lipoxygenase does not decrease the inflammatory and pain-producing effects of isoprostanes. Production of 8-iso-PG-F2-alpha is increased by and is a marker of oxidative stress. Obviously, inhibition of isoprostane formation is part of the biochemical and therefore clinical justification for antioxidant therapy in the treatment of painful orthopedic and rheumatic disorders. Supplemental ascorbic acid, tocopherols, and EPA have been shown to lower isoprostane levels in humans.
  - o Formation of arachidonate from DGLA is inhibited by EPA.[319]
  - o Formation of arachidonic metabolites is not increased by vitamin C.[320]
  - o The term "eicosatetraenoic acid" can apply to both 20:4n6 (arachidonic acid) of the omega-6 fatty acid family[321] and to 20:4n3 of the omega-3 fatty acid family.[322,323] Therefore, to avoid the confusion that would result from the use of the term "eicosatetraenoic acid" by itself, "n-6 eicosatetraenoic acid" should be used when referring to 20:4n6 (arachidonic acid) and "n-3 eicosatetraenoic acid" should be used when referring to 20:4n3.
  - o Liberation of arachidonic acid from membrane phospholipids phosphatidylcholine and phosphatidylinositol is increased by contact with IgE.[324] This finding presumably helps explain why inflammatory conditions are generally exacerbated by allergen exposure and why allergy

---

[313] Horrobin DF. Interactions between n-3 and n-6 essential fatty acids (EFAs) in the regulation of cardiovascular disorders and inflammation. *Prostaglandins Leukot Essent Fatty Acids* 1991 Oct;44(2):127-31
[314] Fan YY, Chapkin RS. Importance of dietary gamma-linolenic acid in human health and nutrition. *J Nutr*. 1998 Sep;128(9):1411-4
[315] Horrobin DF. Ascorbic acid and prostaglandin synthesis. *Subcell Biochem*. 1996;25:109-15
[316] Delvin TM. *Textbook of Biochemistry with Clinical Correlations*. New York: Wiley-Liss, 1997. Pages 431-441
[317] Rubin D, Laposata M. Cellular interactions between n-6 and n-3 fatty acids. *J Lipid Res*. 1992 Oct;33(10):1431-40
[318] Evans AR, et al. Isoprostanes, novel eicosanoids that produce nociception and sensitize rat sensory neurons. *J Pharmacol Exp Ther*. 2000 Jun;293(3):912-20
[319] Horrobin DF. Interactions between n-3 and n-6 essential fatty acids (EFAs) in the regulation of cardiovascular disorders and inflammation. *Prostaglandins Leukot Essent Fatty Acids* 1991 Oct;44(2):127-31
[320] Horrobin DF. Ascorbic acid and prostaglandin synthesis. *Subcell Biochem*. 1996;25:109-15
[321] "5,8,11,14-eicosatetraenoic (20:4(n-6))" Mimouni V, Christiansen EN, Blond JP, Ulmann L, Poisson JP, Bezard J. Elongation and desaturation of arachidonic and eicosapentaenoic acids in rat liver. Effect of clofibrate feeding. *Biochim Biophys Acta*. 1991 Nov 27;1086(3):349-53
[322] Tapiero H, et al. Polyunsaturated fatty acids (PUFA) and eicosanoids in human health and pathologies. *Biomed Pharmacother*. 2002 Jul;56(5):215-22
[323] Erasmus U. *Fats that heal, fats that kill*. British Columbia Canada: Alive Books, 1993 Page 276
[324] McGlivery RW. *Biochemistry: A Functional Approach. Third Edition*. Philadelphia: WB Saunders, 1983. Pages 747-750

elimination and anti-allergy immunomodulatory treatments result in a reduction in pain and inflammation.
- o Elevated ARA may lead to altered binding of hormones, growth factors, neurotransmitters, and common food antigen peptides.
- o Dietary ARA works synergistically with proinflammatory genotypes such as the variant 5-lipoxygenase alleles which are common in the general population: Africans (24%), Asians and Pacific Islanders (19.4%), other racial/ethnic groups (18.2%), Hispanics (3.6%), whites (3.1%), and the atherogenic effect of dietary arachidonic acid in these patients can be mitigated by dietary EPA.[325]
- **Adrenic acid, 22:4n6, docosatetraenoic acid**
  - o Little is known about this fatty acid.
  - o Concentrated in and may have a regulatory role in the adrenal glands.[326]
- **N-6 docosapentaenoic acid, 22:5n6**
  - o 22:5n6 is increased by n-3 fatty acid deficiency, especially in the brain cortex.[327]
  - o The term "docosapentaenoic acid" can apply to both 22:5n3 of the omega-3 fatty acid family[328,329] and to 22:5n6 of the omega-6 fatty acid family.[330,331,332] Therefore, because to use the term "docosapentaenoic acid" may be ambiguous, the terms "n-3 docosapentaenoic acid" should be used when discussing 22:5n3 and "n-6 docosapentaenoic acid" should be used when discussing 22:5n6.

DGLA metabolites formed by cyclooxygenase

- **Prostaglandin E-1 (PG-E1)**
  - o The main metabolite from DGLA.[333]
  - o Production is increased by vitamin C.[334]
  - o Decreases platelet aggregation.[335]
  - o Causes vasodilation.[336]
  - o Lowers blood pressure.[337]
  - o Inhibits cholesterol biosynthesis and lowers cholesterol levels in animals.[338]
  - o "A potent anti-inflammatory agent."[339]
  - o Probably the most potent PG with respect to bronchodilation.[340]
  - o Production is decreased by n-3 fatty acids.[341]
  - o May have a mood elevating effect insofar as levels are elevated in patients with mania, reduced in patients with depression, and are elevated by ethanol intake.[342]

---

[325] Dwyer JH, et al. Arachidonate 5-lipoxygenase promoter genotype, dietary arachidonic acid, and atherosclerosis. *N Engl J Med*. 2004 Jan 1;350(1):29-37
[326] Horrobin DF. Ascorbic acid and prostaglandin synthesis. *Subcell Biochem*. 1996;25:109-15
[327] Retterstol K, et al. The metabolism of 22:5(-6) and of docosahexaenoic acid [22:6(-3)] compared in rat hepatocytes. *Biochim Biophys Acta*. 1996 Oct 18;1303(3):180-6
[328] "docosapentaenoic acid (22:5n-3)" Williard DE, et al. Docosahexaenoic acid synthesis from n-3 polyunsaturated fatty acids in differentiated rat brain astrocytes. *J Lipid Res*. 2001 Sep;42(9):1368-76
[329] "...docosapentaenoic acid (22:5n-3)..." Takahashi R, et al. Effect of different ratios of dietary N-6 and N-3 fatty acids on fatty acid composition, prostaglandin formation and platelet aggregation in the rat. *Thromb Res*. 1987 Jul 15;47(2):135-46
[330] Retterstol K, Haugen TB, Christophersen BO. The pathway from arachidonic to docosapentaenoic acid (20:4n-6 to 22:5n-6) and from eicosapentaenoic to docosahexaenoic acid (20:5n-3 to 22:6n-3) studied in testicular cells from immature rats. *Biochim Biophys Acta*. 2000 Jan 3;1483(1):119-31
[331] "docosapentaenoic acid (DPAn-6)" Ahmad A, Murthy M, Greiner RS, Moriguchi T, Salem N Jr. A decrease in cell size accompanies a loss of docosahexaenoate in the rat hippocampus. *Nutr Neurosci*. 2002 Apr;5(2):103-13
[332] "The desaturation of adrenic acid to n-6 docosapentaenoic acid was decreased in the normo- and hyperglycemic diabetic rats." Mimouni V, et al. Adrenic acid delta 4 desaturation and fatty acid composition in liver microsomes of spontaneously diabetic Wistar BB rats. *Prostaglandins Leukot Essent Fatty Acids*. 1994 Jan;50(1):43-7
[333] Horrobin DF. Ascorbic acid and prostaglandin synthesis. *Subcell Biochem* 1996;25:109-15
[334] Horrobin DF. Ascorbic acid and prostaglandin synthesis. *Subcell Biochem*. 1996;25:109-15
[335] Horrobin DF. Interactions between n-3 and n-6 essential fatty acids (EFAs) in the regulation of cardiovascular disorders and inflammation. *Prostaglandins Leukot Essent Fatty Acids* 1991 Oct;44(2):127-31
[336] Tapiero H, et al. Polyunsaturated fatty acids (PUFA) and eicosanoids in human health and pathologies. *Biomed Pharmacother*. 2002 Jul;56(5):215-22
[337] Horrobin DF. Interactions between n-3 and n-6 essential fatty acids (EFAs) in the regulation of cardiovascular disorders and inflammation. *Prostaglandins Leukot Essent Fatty Acids* 1991 Oct;44(2):127-31
[338] Horrobin DF. Interactions between n-3 and n-6 essential fatty acids (EFAs) in the regulation of cardiovascular disorders and inflammation. *Prostaglandins Leukot Essent Fatty Acids* 1991 Oct;44(2):127-31
[339] Horrobin DF. Ascorbic acid and prostaglandin synthesis. *Subcell Biochem*. 1996;25:109-15
[340] Horrobin DF. Ascorbic acid and prostaglandin synthesis. *Subcell Biochem*. 1996;25:109-15
[341] Rubin D, Laposata M. Cellular interactions between n-6 and n-3 fatty acids: a mass analysis of fatty acid elongation/desaturation, distribution among complex lipids, and conversion to eicosanoids. *J Lipid Res*. 1992 Oct;33(10):1431-40
[342] Horrobin DF, Manku MS. Possible role of prostaglandin E1 in the affective disorders and in alcoholism. *Br Med J*. 1980 Jun 7;280(6228):1363-6

- Certain biological properties of PG-E1 are 20 times stronger than those of PG-E2.[343]
- PG-E1 inhibits vascular smooth muscle cell proliferation in vitro.[344]

DGLA metabolites formed by 15-lipoxygenase
- **15-hydroxy-eicosatrienoic acid, 15-OH-DGLA, 15-OH-20:3n-6, 15-HETrE**
  - Potent anti-inflammatory action and inhibition of arachidonic acid cascade via inhibition of 5-lipoxygenase and 12-lipoxygenase.[345,346]

Arachidonic acid metabolites formed by cyclooxygenase
- **Thromboxane A-2 (TX-A2)**
  - Causes platelet aggregation[347] and vasoconstriction.[348]
  - Promotes cardiac arrhythmias and hypertension.
  - Considered much more powerful than the thromboxanes derived from EPA and DGLA.
  - Precursor to TX-B2.
- **Thromboxane B2**
  - Inactive[349]
- **Prostaglandin I2, PG-I2, prostacyclin**
  - Commonly considered one of the only desirable/beneficial end-products of arachidonic acid metabolism[350] despite the little known fact that increases nociception and thus promotes hyperalgesia.[351]
  - Production is increased by vitamin C.[352]
  - Decreases platelet aggregation.
  - Causes vasodilation[353] and lowers blood pressure.[354,355]
  - Formed from PG-H2 via prostacyclin synthase.[356]
- **Prostaglandin D2, PG-D2**
  - Causes bronchoconstriction, smooth muscle contraction, and hypotension and is the major arachidonate-cyclooxygenase product produced in mast cells.[357]
  - Accentuates production of histamine and can trigger release of histamine from mast cells in the absence of IgE binding.
- **Prostaglandin E2, PG-E2**
  - Produced from arachidonic acid by cyclooxygenase. PG-E2 increases expression of cyclooxygenase and IL-6; thus inflammation manifested by an increase in PG-E2 leads to additive expression of cyclooxygenase, which further increases inflammation.[358]
  - Suppresses lymphocyte proliferation and natural killer cell activity[359]; appears to cause stimulation of "suppressor cells"
  - Released by tumor cells and suppressor cells; promotes chemotaxis; increases platelet aggregation

---

[343] Fan YY, Chapkin RS. Importance of dietary gamma-linolenic acid in human health and nutrition. *J Nutr.* 1998 Sep;128(9):1411-4
[344] Fan YY, Chapkin RS. Importance of dietary gamma-linolenic acid in human health and nutrition. *J Nutr.* 1998 Sep;128(9):1411-4
[345] Horrobin DF. Interactions between n-3 and n-6 essential fatty acids (EFAs) in the regulation of cardiovascular disorders and inflammation. *Prostaglandins Leukot Essent Fatty Acids* 1991 Oct;44(2):127-31
[346] Fan YY, Chapkin RS. Importance of dietary gamma-linolenic acid in human health and nutrition. *J Nutr.* 1998 Sep;128(9):1411-4
[347] Delvin TM. *Textbook of Biochemistry with Clinical Correlations.* New York: Wiley-Liss, 1997. Pages 431-441
[348] Horrobin DF. Ascorbic acid and prostaglandin synthesis. *Subcell Biochem* 1996;25:109-15
[349] Delvin TM. *Textbook of Biochemistry with Clinical Correlations.* New York: Wiley-Liss, 1997. Pages 431-441
[350] Horrobin DF. Ascorbic acid and prostaglandin synthesis. *Subcell Biochem.* 1996;25:109-15
[351] Evans AR, et al. Isoprostanes, novel eicosanoids that produce nociception and sensitize rat sensory neurons. *J Pharmacol Exp Ther.* 2000 Jun;293(3):912-20
[352] Horrobin DF. Ascorbic acid and prostaglandin synthesis. *Subcell Biochem.* 1996;25:109-15
[353] Horrobin DF. Ascorbic acid and prostaglandin synthesis. *Subcell Biochem.* 1996;25:109-15
[354] Delvin TM. *Textbook of Biochemistry with Clinical Correlations.* New York: Wiley-Liss, 1997. Pages 431-441
[355] Tapiero H, et al. Polyunsaturated fatty acids (PUFA) and eicosanoids in human health and pathologies. *Biomed Pharmacother.* 2002 Jul;56(5):215-22
[356] "Prostacyclin synthase catalyzes an intramolecular redox reaction in which prostaglandin endoperoxide, PGH2, is converted to prostacyclin." oxfordbiomed.com/pg61prossyn.html on September 6, 2006
[357] Peters SP, et al. The role of prostaglandin D2 in IgE-mediated reactions in man. *Trans Assoc Am Physicians.* 1982;95:221-8
[358] Bagga D, Wang L, Farias-Eisner R, Glaspy JA, Reddy ST. Differential effects of prostaglandin derived from omega-6 and omega-3 polyunsaturated fatty acids on COX-2 expression and IL-6 secretion. *Proc Natl Acad Sci U S A.* 2003 Feb 18;100(4):1751-6 pnas.org/cgi/reprint/100/4/1751.pdf
[359] Calder PC. Long-chain n-3 fatty acids and inflammation: potential application in surgical and trauma patients. *Braz J Med Biol Res.* 2003 Apr;36(4):433-46

- o Causes relaxation of bronchus and uterus smooth muscle in nonpregnant animals and uterine contractions in pregnant animals[360]
- o PG-E2 causes pain and also but increases the intensity and duration of pain sensations that are mediated by other triggers such as histamine and bradykinin[361]
- o Increases IgE production[362]
- o Increases vascular permeability and vasodilation thus enhancing edema[363]
- o Promotes action of epidermal growth factor[364]
- o Production is decreased by n-3 fatty acids[365]
- **Prostaglandin F2-alpha, PG-F2a, PG-F2α**
  - o Promotes bronchoconstriction and uterine contractions
  - o Increased levels associated with dysmenorrhea
  - o Increased production with vitamin C deficiency, formation is reduced by vitamin C, and low levels of vitamin C are seen in women with dysmenorrhea.[366]
  - o Promotes formation of MMP-2 and other collagenases that promote joint destruction in various types of arthritis and are required by metastasizing cancer cells to penetrate basement membranes
- **Prostaglandin G2 (PG-G2)**
  - o Induces rapid and irreversible platelet aggregation[367]
- **Prostaglandin H2 (PG-H2)**
  - o Induces rapid and irreversible platelet aggregation[368]

Linoleic acid metabolites formed by lipoxygenases
- **13-S-HODE, 13-S-hydroxyoctadecadienoic acid**
  - o 13-S-HODE is formed from linolenic acid by 15-LOX-1 and is generally considered to have anticancer actions[369]; 13-S-HODE inhibits ornithine decarboxylase[370]
  - o "12/15-LOX may cause mitochondrial dysfunction through its metabolites such as 13-S-hydroxyoctadecadienoic acid (13-S-HODE) and 12-Shydroxyeicosatetraenoic acid (12-S-HETE) which can cause mitochondrial degradation."[371]

Arachidonic acid metabolites formed by lipoxygenases
- **5-hydroperoxyeicosatetraenoic acid, 5-HPETE**
  - o HPETEs are converted to their respective HETEs either spontaneously or by peroxidases.[372]
  - o 5-hydroxyeicosatetraenoic acid is known to reduce the depolarization threshold of primary afferent neurons and may thus lead to pain
  - o Reinforces activation of 5-lipoxygenase
  - o May be directly cytotoxic
  - o Necessary for the formation of MMP-2 and other collagenases that promote joint destruction in various types of arthritis and are required by metastasizing cancer cells to penetrate basement membranes; formation is inhibited by the lipoxygenase inhibitors esculetin and caffeic acid[373]
  - o 5-HPETE is the major lipoxygenase product in inflamed tissues and promotes chemotaxis and neutrophil degranulation of lysosomal hydrolytic enzymes[374]

---

[360] McGlivery RW. *Biochemistry: A Functional Approach. Third Edition*. Philadelphia: WB Saunders, 1983. Pages 747-750
[361] Calder PC. Long-chain n-3 fatty acids and inflammation: potential application in surgical and trauma patients. *Braz J Med Biol Res*. 2003 Apr;36(4):433-46
[362] Calder PC. Long-chain n-3 fatty acids and inflammation: potential application in surgical and trauma patients. *Braz J Med Biol Res*. 2003 Apr;36(4):433-46
[363] Calder PC. Long-chain n-3 fatty acids and inflammation: potential application in surgical and trauma patients. *Braz J Med Biol Res*. 2003 Apr;36(4):433-46
[364] Tapiero H, et al. Polyunsaturated fatty acids (PUFA) and eicosanoids in human health and pathologies. *Biomed Pharmacother*. 2002;56(5):215-22
[365] Rubin D, Laposata M. Cellular interactions between n-6 and n-3 fatty acids: a mass analysis of fatty acid elongation/desaturation, distribution among complex lipids, and conversion to eicosanoids. *J Lipid Res*. 1992 Oct;33(10):1431-40
[366] Horrobin DF. Ascorbic acid and prostaglandin synthesis. *Subcell Biochem* 1996;25:109-15
[367] McGlivery RW. *Biochemistry: A Functional Approach. Third Edition*. Philadelphia: WB Saunders, 1983. Pages 747-750
[368] McGlivery RW. *Biochemistry: A Functional Approach. Third Edition*. Philadelphia: WB Saunders, 1983. Pages 747-750
[369] Shureiqi I, Lippman SM. Lipoxygenase modulation to reverse carcinogenesis. *Cancer Res*. 2001 Sep 1;61(17):6307-12
[370] Shureiqi I, Lippman SM. Lipoxygenase modulation to reverse carcinogenesis. *Cancer Res*. 2001 Sep 1;61(17):6307-12
[371] Mabalirajan U, Ghosh B. Mitochondrial dysfunction in metabolic syndrome and asthma. *J Allergy* (Cairo). 2013;2013:340476
[372] Delvin TM. *Textbook of Biochemistry with Clinical Correlations*. New York: Wiley-Liss, 1997. Pages 431-441
[373] Reich R, et al. Identification of arachidonic acid pathways required for the invasive and metastatic activity of malignant tumor cells. *Prostaglandins* 1996 Jan;51:1-17
[374] Delvin TM. *Textbook of Biochemistry with Clinical Correlations*. New York: Wiley-Liss, 1997. Pages 431-441

- 5-HPETE is considered to have pro-cancer actions and facilitates production of proteolytic enzymes that promote joint destruction and tumor invasiveness[375]
- **5-HETE, 5-S-HETE**
    - 5-HETE is considered to have pro-cancer actions by blocking apoptosis and promoting tumor growth[376]
- **8-S-HETE**
    - 8-S-HETE is genotoxic and promotes cancer development[377]
- **12-HPETE, 12-hydroperoxyeicosatetraenoic acid, 12-hydroperoxyeicosatetraenoate,**
    - 12-HPETE is the major lipoxygenase product in platelets and the pancreas[378]
- **12-R-HETE**
    - 12-R-HETE is produced by 12-R-LOX and promotes proliferation of colon cancer cells[379]
- **12-S-HETE**
    - 12-S-HETE promotes tumor growth by several mechanisms, including 1) "up-regulating adhesion molecules and increasing the adhesion of tumor cells to the microvessel endothelium," 2) "…promoting tumor spread,"" and 3) inhibiting apoptosis[380]
    - Expression of 12-S-LOX and presumably therefore production of 12-S-HETE is directly correlated with aggressiveness, stage, and grade in human prostate cancer[381]
    - "12/15-LOX may cause mitochondrial dysfunction through its metabolites such as 13-S-hydroxyoctadecadienoic acid (13-S-HODE) and 12-Shydroxyeicosatetraenoic acid (12-S-HETE) which can cause mitochondrial degradation."[382]
- **15-hydroperoxyeicosatetraenoic acid, 15-HPETE, 15-hydroperoxyeicosatetraenoate**
    - 15-HPETE is the major lipoxygenase product in eosinophils, T-lymphocytes, and the trachea[383]
- **15-S-HETE**
    - 15-S-HETE is formed from arachidonic acid by the action of 15-LOX-2 and appears to have anticancer action, yet the data on this are conflicting[384]
- **Leukotriene B4: LT-B4**
    - Promotes immunosuppression via inhibition of CD4 cells and promotion of proliferation of CD8 cells.[385]
    - Promotes edema: increases vascular permeability, enhances local blood flow, is a potent chemotactic agent for leukocytes,
    - Exacerbates tissue damage: induces release of lysosomal enzymes, increases production of reactive oxygen species, TNF-a, IL-1, and IL-6[386]
    - Associated with accelerated atherosclerosis in patients with proinflammatory variants of 5-lipoxygenase[387]
    - Production is increased by dietary arachidonic acid and production is reduced by EPA.[388]
    - LT-B4 inhibits apoptosis in cancer cells and is generally considered procarcinogenic.[389]
- **LT-C4 and LT-D4 and LT-E4:**
    - Promote muscle contraction, bronchoconstriction, intestinal muscle contraction,
    - Promote increased capillary permeability which results in edema
    - More powerful than histamine in promotion of "allergic" symptoms[390]
    - Patients with severe asthma have elevated levels of LT-E4 that are not reduced with steroid treatment.[391]

---

[375] "Specific metabolites of each pathway, i.e. PGF2 alpha and 5-HPETE, are able to transcend the block and restore collagenase production, invasiveness in vitro and metastatic activity in vivo." Reich et al. Identification of arachidonic acid pathways required for the invasive and metastatic activity of malignant tumor cells. *Prostaglandins* 1996 Jan;5:1-17
[376] Shureiqi I, Lippman SM. Lipoxygenase modulation to reverse carcinogenesis. *Cancer Res*. 2001 Sep 1;61(17):6307-12
[377] Shureiqi I, Lippman SM. Lipoxygenase modulation to reverse carcinogenesis. *Cancer Res*. 2001 Sep 1;61(17):6307-12
[378] Delvin TM. *Textbook of Biochemistry with Clinical Correlations*. New York: Wiley-Liss, 1997. Pages 431-441
[379] Shureiqi I, Lippman SM. Lipoxygenase modulation to reverse carcinogenesis. *Cancer Res*. 2001 Sep 1;61(17):6307-12
[380] Shureiqi I, Lippman SM. Lipoxygenase modulation to reverse carcinogenesis. *Cancer Res*. 2001 Sep 1;61(17):6307-12
[381] Shureiqi I, Lippman SM. Lipoxygenase modulation to reverse carcinogenesis. *Cancer Res*. 2001 Sep 1;61(17):6307-12
[382] Mabalirajan U, Ghosh B. Mitochondrial dysfunction in metabolic syndrome and asthma. *J Allergy* (Cairo). 2013;2013:340476
[383] Delvin TM. *Textbook of Biochemistry with Clinical Correlations*. New York: Wiley-Liss, 1997. Pages 431-441
[384] Shureiqi I, Lippman SM. Lipoxygenase modulation to reverse carcinogenesis. *Cancer Res*. 2001 Sep 1;61(17):6307-12
[385] Delvin TM. *Textbook of Biochemistry with Clinical Correlations*. New York: Wiley-Liss, 1997. Pages 431-441
[386] Calder PC. Long-chain n-3 fatty acids and inflammation: potential application in surgical and trauma patients. *Braz J Med Biol Res*. 2003 Apr;36(4):433-46
[387] Dwyer JH, et al. Arachidonate 5-lipoxygenase promoter genotype, dietary arachidonic acid, and atherosclerosis. *N Engl J Med*. 2004 Jan 1;350(1):29-37
[388] Dwyer JH, et al. Arachidonate 5-lipoxygenase promoter genotype, dietary arachidonic acid, and atherosclerosis. *N Engl J Med*. 2004 Jan 1;350(1):29-37
[389] Shureiqi I, Lippman SM. Lipoxygenase modulation to reverse carcinogenesis. *Cancer Res*. 2001 Sep 1;61(17):6307-12
[390] Delvin TM. *Textbook of Biochemistry with Clinical Correlations*. New York: Wiley-Liss, 1997. Pages 431-441
[391] Vachier I, et al. High levels of urinary leukotriene E4 excretion in steroid treated patients with severe asthma. *Respir Med*. 2003 Nov;97(11):1225-9

Metabolism of Omega-6 Fatty Acids and Related Eicosanoids: Health-promoting n6 fatty acids and derivatives are indicated by the green-colored background, while inflammatory and disease-promoting n6 fatty acids and derivatives are indicated by the red-colored background.

Important Enzymes in Fatty Acid Metabolism

Fatty acids are converted to other fatty acids in the same family by the desaturase and elongase enzymes. The major "direction" of these reactions is depicted in the diagrams; however these reactions, like nearly all enzymatic reactions, are reversible to a limited extent. Fatty acids are converted to biologically active end-products by enzymes such as the cyclooxygenases, lipoxygenases, cytochrome P-450 enzymes and by nonenzymatic conversion. Four important concepts need to be understood in relation to the enzymes that interconvert fatty acids:

1) **These enzymes do not work with equal efficiency**, and thus their end-products may not be produced in sufficient amounts to be biologically or clinically significant. Therefore, *on paper*, the cascade of fatty acid metabolism appears to flow easily from one fatty acid to its downstream progeny; in reality however, this process is often slow and therefore not immediately reliable when one is looking for rapid and reliable clinical results. The desaturase enzymes are slow and rate limiting, whereas the elongase enzymes function efficiently and rapidly. For example, Horrobin noted, "Because the 6-desaturation step is so rate-limiting, it is impossible to produce any significant elevation of DGLA levels in humans by increasing linoleic acid intake."[392]

2) **These enzymes are subject to significant interpatient variability** due to inherited and acquired factors that can reduce enzyme activity. For example, many patients (especially those with eczema and diabetes) have extreme reductions in the activity of delta-6-desaturase, the rate-limiting enzyme in the fatty acid cascades from ALA and LA. When delta-6-desaturase is slow to perform its conversions, synthesis of all downstream fatty acids is greatly reduced.

3) *These enzymes, like all enzymes, require cofactors.* If the patient is deficient in cofactors, the efficiency of enzymatic conversions is greatly impaired. Since micronutrient deficiencies are common even in developed countries, and since people can have clinically significant micronutrient deficiencies (i.e., "marginal malnutrition"[393]) yet still be "apparently healthy", a wise clinical strategy is to ensure that the patient's micronutrient status is adequate by encouraging the patient to consume a nutritious organic[394] whole foods diet along with a high-potency broad-spectrum multivitamin and multimineral supplement. Patients with magnesium deficiency show impaired fatty acid metabolism because desaturase enzymes are unable to function properly without sufficient magnesium.[395] Animal studies suggest that vitamin B-6 deficiency can reduce the function of delta-6-desaturase by 64% and lead to a reduction in EPA and DHA.[396]

4) **Substrates compete for enzymatic conversion.** In several instances, the same enzyme must act upon two different fatty acids in two different omega families. For example, delta-6-desaturase converts the omega-3 linolenic acid to stearidonic acid, yet this same enzyme also converts the omega-6 linoleic acid to gamma-linolenic acid. If the diet contains an absolute or relative excess of linoleic acid, then on a molecular and functional level, this excess linoleic acid will disproportionately utilize delta-6-desaturase and conversion of available linoleic acid to gamma-linolenic acid will be reduced. As reviewed by Dupont[397], "A competitive interaction between fatty acids exists so that those of the [alpha-linolenic acid, omega-3] family suppress the metabolism of those of the [linoleic acid, omega-6] family, and the [linoleic acid, omega-6] family suppress metabolism of the [linolenic acid, omega-3] family although less strongly. Both the [linoleic acid, omega-6] and [alpha-linolenic acid, omega-3] fatty acids suppress metabolism of the [oleic acid, omega-9] fatty acids." Stated more plainly by Pizzorno[398], "…a relative excess of one fatty acid will tend to hog an enzyme system, resulting in decreased conversion of the other fatty acids." In reviewing clinical evidence that EPA supplementation leads to significant reductions (50%) in DGLA levels, Horrobin[399] noted, "However, the n-3 EFAs are much more effective in inhibiting n-6 EFA metabolism than vice versa." A practical example: in a patient who is deficient in both omega-3 and omega-6 fatty acids, supplementation exclusively with flax oil will exacerbate the deficiency of gamma-linolenic acid.

---

[392] Horrobin DF. Interactions between n-3 and n-6 essential fatty acids (EFAs) in the regulation of cardiovascular disorders and inflammation. *Prostaglandins Leukot Essent Fatty Acids*. 1991 Oct;44(2):127-31
[393] Allen LH. The nutrition CRSP: what is marginal malnutrition, and does it affect human function? *Nutr Rev*. 1993 Sep;51(9):255-67
[394] Bob Smith. *Journal of Applied Nutrition* 1993; 45: 35-39
[395] Galland L. Impaired essential fatty acid metabolism in latent tetany. *Magnesium*. 1985;4(5-6):333-8
[396] Tsuge H, Hotta N, Hayakawa T. Effects of vitamin B-6 on (n-3) polyunsaturated fatty acid metabolism. *J Nutr*. 2000 Feb;130(2S Suppl):333S-334S
[397] Dupont J. Lipids. In: Brown ML (ed). *Present Knowledge in Nutrition. Sixth Edition*. Washington DC: International Life Sciences Institute;1990 page 62
[398] Pizzorno JE. *Total Wellness*. Rocklin: Prima; 1996 page 170
[399] Horrobin DF. Interactions between n-3 and n-6 essential fatty acids (EFAs) in the regulation of cardiovascular disorders and inflammation. *Prostaglandins Leukot Essent Fatty Acids*. 1991 Oct;44(2):127-31

- **Delta-6-desaturase (D6D):**
    - In omega-3 fatty acid metabolism, D6D converts linolenic acid to stearidonic acid. In omega-6 fatty acid metabolism, D6D converts linoleic acid to gamma-linolenic acid. D6D is the rate-limiting enzyme in fatty acid metabolism, meaning that it is the slowest functioning enzyme in the cascade of fatty acid conversions. Recall that in biochemistry the first enzyme in a series of biochemical reactions tends to be the rate-limiting enzyme for the sake of avoiding unnecessary downstream conversions. D6D is inhibited by trans fatty acids.[400] Action of this enzyme is increased during essential fatty acid deficiency.[401] Patients with eczema and diabetes have been noted to have defects in the function of D6D.[402]
    - Efficient function of D6D requires iron, magnesium, zinc, pyridoxine, niacin, and riboflavin. Administration of supraphysiologic doses of enzyme cofactors can improve function of defective or mutated enzymes.[403]
    - The catecholamines epinephrine and norepinephrine inhibit D5D and D6D.[404]
- **Delta-5-desaturase (D5D):**
    - In omega-6 fatty acid metabolism, D5D converts DGLA to arachidonic acid. However, this enzyme is slow, so that virtually all arachidonic acid found in body tissues originated from the consumption of land animal fats/meats[405] such as beef, liver, pork, lamb, and poultry. Additionally, some people (such as those with X-linked retinitis pigmentosa[406]) have reduced action of D5D and therefore have low levels of DHA. D5D is inhibited by EPA.[407] Released in increased amounts during stress and anxiety, the catecholamines epinephrine and norepinephrine inhibit D5D and D6D.[408]
- **Delta-4-desaturase**
    - Action of this enzyme is increased during essential fatty acid deficiency.[409]
- **Elongase**: These enzymes efficiently add carbon groups to the fatty acid chain.
- **Prostaglandin synthase complex (PGS)**: This is the major enzyme system that is responsible for prostaglandin biosynthesis. PGS includes phospholipase A2 and cyclooxygenase.[410]
- **Phospholipase-A2**
    - Crucial to the arachidonic acid cascade since cyclooxygenase can act only on free arachidonate (i.e., after arachidonate has been liberated from membrane phospholipids); this is the rate-limiting step in the formation of arachidonate-derived prostaglandins.[411]
    - Contact of IgE with mast cells stimulates the release of arachidonate, which must occur via phospholipase A2[412]
    - Inhibited by adrenal steroids (cortisol) and prednisone
- **Cyclooxygenase (COX) (also called "prostaglandin synthase" or "PGS" or "prostaglandin endoperoxide synthase")**
    - COX-1 is "constitutive" and is found in all cells, while COX-2 is inducible by stimulation from monocytes/macrophages following stimulation by PAF, IL-1, or bacterial lipopolysaccharide; its induction is inhibited by glucocorticoids.[413]
    - COX is irreversibly inhibited following acetylation by aspirin.

---

[400] Simopoulos AP. Essential fatty acids in health and chronic disease. *Am J Clin Nutr.* 1999 Sep;70(3 Suppl):560S-569S
[401] "The delta 4 desaturase activity is increased in essential fatty acid deficiency similar to delta 6 desaturase." Christophersen BO, Hagve TA, Christensen E, Johansen Y, Tverdal S. Eicosapentaenoic- and arachidonic acid metabolism in isolated liver cells. *Scand J Clin Lab Invest Suppl.* 1986;184:55-60
[402] "This concept is illustrated by atopic eczema and diabetes, which may represent inherited and acquired examples of inadequate delta-6-desaturation." Horrobin DF. Fatty acid metabolism in health and disease: the role of delta-6-desaturase. *Am J Clin Nutr.* 1993 May;57(5 Suppl):732S-736S
[403] Ames BN, et al. High-dose vitamin therapy stimulates variant enzymes with decreased coenzyme binding affinity (increased K(m)). *Am J Clin Nutr* 2002 Apr;75:616-58
[404] Mamalakis G, et al. Anxiety and adipose essential fatty acid precursors for prostaglandin E1 and E2. *J Am Coll Nutr.* 1998 Jun;17(3):239-43
[405] Pizzorno JE. *Total Wellness*. Rocklin: Prima; 1996 page 169
[406] Hoffman DR, et al. Impaired synthesis of DHA in patients with X-linked retinitis pigmentosa. *J Lipid Res* 2001 Sep;42(9):1395-401
[407] Barham JB, Edens MB, Fonteh AN, Johnson MM, Easter L, Chilton FH. Addition of eicosapentaenoic acid to gamma-linolenic acid-supplemented diets prevents serum arachidonic acid accumulation in humans. *J Nutr.* 2000 Aug;130(8):1925-31
[408] Mamalakis G, et al. Anxiety and adipose essential fatty acid precursors for prostaglandin E1 and E2. *J Am Coll Nutr.* 1998 Jun;17(3):239-43
[409] "The delta 4 desaturase activity is increased in essential fatty acid deficiency similar to delta 6 desaturase." Christophersen BO, et al. Eicosapentaenoic- and arachidonic acid metabolism in isolated liver cells. *Scand J Clin Lab Invest Suppl.* 1986;184:55-60
[410] Delvin TM. *Textbook of Biochemistry with Clinical Correlations*. New York: Wiley-Liss, 1997. Pages 431-441
[411] Delvin TM. *Textbook of Biochemistry with Clinical Correlations*. New York: Wiley-Liss, 1997. Pages 431-441
[412] McGlivery RW. *Biochemistry: A Functional Approach. Third Edition*. Philadelphia: WB Saunders, 1983. Pages 747-750
[413] Delvin TM. *Textbook of Biochemistry with Clinical Correlations*. New York: Wiley-Liss, 1997. Pages 431-441

- o The expression of COX is inhibited by glucocorticoids,[414] which also inhibit phospholipase A2.
- o **COX forms TXs and PGs, while LIPOX form LTs.**
- o The COX metabolite PG-F2alpha is necessary for the formation of matrix metalloproteinase-2 and other collagenases which are utilized for the destruction of connective tissue[415]
- o **COX is apparently activated by either n-6 fatty acids or the oxidized metabolites of n-6 fatty acids.[416] Therefore, consumption of n-6 fatty acids alone—*without trauma or inflammatory stimuli*—is sufficient for the increased production of the harmful arachidonate-derived prostaglandins and leukotrienes**. Thus, by definition, a diet high in n-6 fatty acids may subtly yet significantly promote pain, inflammation, joint destruction, and cancer.
- o A well-established consequence of inhibiting COX is that of increasing LIPOX metabolites. Inhibiting COX will decrease COX metabolites, yet will cause an increase in LIPOX metabolites because of increased substrate levels; i.e., the liberated arachidonate that is not metabolized by COX is now available to be metabolized by LIPOX. Thus, inhibiting COX produces a "metabolic shunt" effect that increases production of inflammatory mediators such as HETE and the leukotrienes. Additionally, inhibition of COX inhibits formation of the beneficial anti-inflammatory DGLA metabolites.
- o Arachidonate metabolites from COX function for the most part to increase inflammation and pain.[417]
- o Increased expression of COX-2 increases production of PG-E2 and has been associated with increased production of anti-apoptotic proteins and a reduction in pro-apoptotic proteins in cultured rat intestinal cells.[418]
- o The activity of lipoxygenase and cyclooxygenase produces reactive oxygen species (ROS) intermediates.
- o The paradox of how a single enzyme such as cyclooxygenase can produce such a wide array of metabolites from a single substrate such as arachidonic acid is solved by recognizing that arachidonate is three-dimensionally rearranged once within the cyclooxygenase enzyme and that these random arrangements favor the production of different metabolites by the preferential molecular modification of the original arachidonate.[419] Additionally, cyclooxygenase may become slightly rearranged as well, thus further promoting the heterogeneity of progeny.
- **Lipoxygenases**: a family of enzymes that form leukotrienes
    - o Corneal lipoxygenase is inhibited by vitamin C[420]
    - o The activity of lipoxygenase and cyclooxygenase produce ROS intermediates
    - o **5-lipoxygenase, 5-LOX**
        - This is a pro-inflammatory enzyme that has different basal levels of activity in different people and in different disease conditions. Proinflammatory variances of this enzyme are seen in Africans (24%), Asians and Pacific Islanders (19.4%), other racial/ethnic groups (18.2%), Hispanics (3.6%) and whites (3.1%) and are associated with accelerated atherosclerosis and elevations in CRP especially when the diet is high in arachidonic acid and low in EPA[421]

---

[414] Tapiero H, et al. Polyunsaturated fatty acids (PUFA) and eicosanoids in human health and pathologies. *Biomed Pharmacother*. 2002;56(5):215-22
[415] "Specific metabolites of each pathway, i.e. PGF2 alpha and 5-HPETE, are able to transcend the block and restore collagenase production, invasiveness in vitro and metastatic activity in vivo." Reich R, Martin GR. Identification of arachidonic acid pathways required for the invasive and metastatic activity of malignant tumor cells. *Prostaglandins* 1996 Jan;51(1):1-17
[416] "...due to activation of cyclooxygenase either by oxygenated metabolites of n-6 fatty acids or by the n-6 fatty acids themselves." Rubin D, Laposata M. Cellular interactions between n-6 and n-3 fatty acids: a mass analysis of fatty acid elongation/desaturation, distribution among complex lipids, and conversion to eicosanoids. *J Lipid Res*. 1992 Oct;33(10):1431-40
[417] Tapiero H, et al. Polyunsaturated fatty acids (PUFA) and eicosanoids in human health and pathologies. *Biomed Pharmacother*. 2002;56(5):215-22
[418] Tapiero H, et al. Polyunsaturated fatty acids (PUFA) and eicosanoids in human health and pathologies. *Biomed Pharmacother*. 2002;56(5):215-22
[419] Thuresson ED, Lakkides KM, Smith WL. Different catalytically competent arrangements of arachidonic acid within the cyclooxygenase active site of prostaglandin endoperoxide H synthase-1 lead to the formation of different oxygenated products. *J Biol Chem*. 2000 Mar 24;275(12):8501-7 jbc.org/cgi/reprint/275/12/8501
[420] Horrobin DF. Ascorbic acid and prostaglandin synthesis. *Subcell Biochem* 1996;25:109-15
[421] Dwyer JH, et al. Arachidonate 5-lipoxygenase promoter genotype, dietary arachidonic acid, and atherosclerosis. *N Engl J Med*. 2004 Jan 1;350(1):29-37

- 5-LOX has been described as "procarcinogenic" due to its role in producing LT-B4 which has mitogenic and anti-apoptotic actions[422]
- The 5-LOX metabolite 5-HPETE is necessary for the formation of matrix metalloproteinase-2 and other collagenases which are utilized for the destruction of connective tissue[423]

o **8-lipoxygenase, 8-LOX**
- 8-LOX is upregulated in animal models of cancer and has been described as "procarcinogenic" due to its role in producing 8-HETE, which has genotoxic effects and which is found in humans[424]

o **12-R-lipoxygenase, 12-R-LOX**
- 12-R-LOX has been described as "procarcinogenic" due to its role in producing 12-R-HETE[425]

o **12-S-lipoxygenase, 12-S-LOX**
- 12-S-LOX has been described as "procarcinogenic" due to its role in producing 12-S-HETE[426]
- Expression of 12-S-LOX is directly correlated with aggressiveness, stage, and grade in human prostate cancer[427]

o **15-lipoxygenase-1, 15-LOX-1**
- 15-LOX-1 metabolizes n-6 linoleic acid into 13-S-HODE, which appears to have *anti*cancer actions[428]

o **15-lipoxygenase-2, 15-LOX-2**
- 15-LOX-2 metabolizes n-6 arachidonic acid into 15-S-HETE, which appears to have *anti*cancer actions[429]

o **12/15-lipoxygenase, 12/15-LOX**
- Earlier works cited previously described 12 LOX and 15 LOX separately; more recent reviews have described "12/15-LOX" as a single enzyme; in this moment, whether this term is being used to describe the 12 and 15 forms *separately yet in conjunction* or as a different enzyme from the other 12 and 15 forms is not clear, and the differentiation may not be of practical clinical importance at this time. However, what is relevant is the connection between Western high-fat diets, LOX activity, and mitochondrial dysfunction as contributors to insulin resistance; an impressive review article published in 2013 by Mabalirajan and Ghosh[430] noted that high-fat Western diets (in animal models) lead to activation of 12/15-LOX and resulted in oxidative modification of fatty acids and sequential mitochondrial impairment, ER stress, UPR, and insulin resistance. Beyond the intellectual gratification of enhanced understanding, this data suggests that LOX inhibition—such as for example via ginger or bioavailable curcumin—might be an additional therapeutic strategy against organelle (e.g., mito and ER) dysfunction and subsequent pathoclinical complications.

---

[422] "These targets include procarcinogenic lipoxygenases (LOXs), including 5-, 8-, and 12-LOX, and anticarcinogenic LOXs, including 15-LOX-1 and possibly 15-LOX-2." Shureiqi I, Lippman SM. Lipoxygenase modulation to reverse carcinogenesis. *Cancer Res*. 2001 Sep 1;61(17):6307-12
[423] "Specific metabolites of each pathway, i.e. PGF2 alpha and 5-HPETE, are able to transcend the block and restore collagenase production, invasiveness in vitro and metastatic activity in vivo." Reich R, Martin GR. Identification of arachidonic acid pathways required for the invasive and metastatic activity of malignant tumor cells. *Prostaglandins* 1996 Jan;51(1):1-17
[424] Shureiqi I, Lippman SM. Lipoxygenase modulation to reverse carcinogenesis. *Cancer Res*. 2001 Sep 1;61(17):6307-12
[425] Shureiqi I, Lippman SM. Lipoxygenase modulation to reverse carcinogenesis. *Cancer Res*. 2001 Sep 1;61(17):6307-12
[426] Shureiqi I, Lippman SM. Lipoxygenase modulation to reverse carcinogenesis. *Cancer Res*. 2001 Sep 1;61(17):6307-12
[427] Reich R, et al. Identification of arachidonic acid pathways required for the invasive and metastatic activity of malignant tumor cells. *Prostaglandins* 1996 Jan;51(1):1-17
[428] Shureiqi I, Lippman SM. Lipoxygenase modulation to reverse carcinogenesis. *Cancer Res*. 2001 Sep 1;61(17):6307-12
[429] Shureiqi I, Lippman SM. Lipoxygenase modulation to reverse carcinogenesis. *Cancer Res*. 2001 Sep 1;61(17):6307-12
[430] Mabalirajan U, Ghosh B. Mitochondrial dysfunction in metabolic syndrome and asthma. *J Allergy* (Cairo). 2013;2013:340476

Additional Details: NFkB and Its Phytonutritional Modulation

Nuclear transcription factor kappaB (NFkB, NFkB) is one of several transcription factors which act as "facilitators" for the elaboration and amplification of specific gene products. In the case of NFkB, most of the genes that appear to be influenced are those that increase the production of pro-inflammatory mediators such as IL-2 (which increases production of collagen-digesting proteases), IL-6 (which then increases production of C-reactive protein), cyclooxygenase-2 (which then increases production of prostaglandins), lipoxygenase (which produces leukotrienes), and inducible nitric oxide synthase (for the production of nitric oxide), etc. Inhibition of NFkB is increasingly considered a major therapeutic goal in the treatment and prevention of a wide range of illnesses, including cancer, arthritis, autoimmune diseases, neurologic illnesses such as Alzheimer's and Parkinson's disease, and other "inflammatory" diseases.[431][432] While we as holistic clinicians work to address the underlying cause of the problem in a given patient, I believe that some degree of "suppression" of NFkB is therapeutically appropriate for at least two reasons: 1) it helps to limit tissue damage and to improve patient outcomes, and 2) suppression of NFkB helps to *break the vicious cycle* of positive feedback wherein *inflammation promotes more inflammation* by the NFkB stimulating effect of several of the products of NFkB activation: NFkB increases the production of IL-1, PG-E2, oxidative stress, TNF-a, and CRP—all of which work additively and synergistically to increase activation of NFkB. Therefore, regardless of the underlying cause, which may have already been addressed and eradicated, it is conceivable that some patients will suffer from inflammatory disorders simply because of the positive feedback that mediators have on the activation of NFkB, which then promotes more inflammation.

Schema of the NFkB pathway—from environmental triggers to clinical presentations: Notice the self-perpetuating cycle wherein inflammatory mediators activate NFkB for the formation of additional inflammatory mediators. From Vasquez 2005.[433]

Pharmaceutical companies are scrambling to develop clinically useful synthetic inhibitors of NFkB. These companies will eventually be successful in this endeavor, and we can also confidently predict that the pharmaceutical version of NFkB suppression will arrive with a plethora of adverse effects, most likely *because of the potency and specificity* of the drug. NFkB plays an important role in a wide range of normal, healthy physiologic processes, including the immune response to infectious diseases. We should therefore seek to *modulate* its function

---

[431] D'Acquisto F, May MJ, Ghosh S. Inhibition of Nuclear Factor Kappa B (NF-kB): An Emerging Theme in Anti-Inflammatory Therapies. *Mol Interv*. 2002 Feb;2:22-35
[432] Tak PP, Firestein GS. NFkB: a key role in inflammatory diseases. *J Clin Invest*. 2001 Jan;107(1):7-11 jci.org/cgi/content/full/107/1/7
[433] Vasquez A. Nutritional and Botanical Inhibition of NFkB, the Major Intracellular Amplifier of the Inflammatory Cascade. *Nutritional Perspectives* 2005;Jul:5-12

rather than sophomorically *suppress* its function. Fortunately, we can do this with several natural interventions, not the least of which are vitamin D[434,435], curcumin[436] (requires piperine for absorption[437]), lipoic acid[438], green tea[439], rosemary[440], grape seed extract[441], propolis[442], zinc[443], high-dose selenium[444], indole-3-carbinol[445,446], N-acetyl-L-cysteine[447], and resveratrol.[448,449] Other nutrients such as isohumulones from *Humulus lupulus*[450] and fatty acids inhibit NFkB *indirectly* via activation of peroxisome proliferator-activated receptors alpha (PPAR-α) and gamma (PPAR-γ). GLA activates PPAR-gamma and thereby inhibits NFkB[451], while (oxidized) EPA activates PPAR-alpha and thus inhibits NFkB[452]; these latter findings reflect a quantum leap in our understanding of the mechanisms of diet-induced anti-inflammation (i.e., anti-inflammatory nutrigenomics, or anti-inflammatory immunonutrigenomics) since they show that food constituents modify human physiology and phenotype at the genetic/pre-transcriptional level and not only at the metabolic/post-transcriptional level as was previously thought.

Almost certainly, many of the anti-inflammatory benefits of plant-based diets are partially resultant from the downregulation of NFkB by dietary phytonutrients, of which more than several thousand exist in complex and additive/synergistic combinations.[453] Notice that the above-mentioned suppressors of NFkB are mostly phenolic compounds that are naturally occurring in fruits, vegetables, herbs, and spices. A diet based upon fruits and vegetables would be naturally high in these compounds and would be likely to provide an anti-inflammatory influence on genetic expression. Indeed, this dietary and phytonutritional environment would be consistent with that in which human physiology evolved, to which it adapted, and upon which it thereby became dependent.[454,455] Relatedly, our epidemic of vitamin D deficiency[456] resultant from our artificial, indoor, clothed lifestyles

---

[434] "1Alpha,25-dihydroxyvitamin D3 (1,25-(OH)2-D3), active metabolite of vitamin D, can inhibit NFkB activity in human MRC-5 fibroblasts, targeting DNA binding of NFkB but not translocation of its subunits p50 and p65." Harant et al. 1Alpha,25-dihydroxyvitamin D3 decreases DNA binding of nuclear factor-kappaB. *FEBS Lett*. 1998;436:329-34

[435] "Thus, 1,25(OH)2D3 may negatively regulate IL-12 production by downregulation of NF-kB activation and binding to the p40-kB sequence." D'Ambrosio D, et al. Inhibition of IL-12 production by 1,25-dihydroxyvitamin D3. *J Clin Invest*. 1998 Jan 1;101(1):252-62

[436] "Curcumin, EGCG and resveratrol have been shown to suppress activation of NF-kappa B." Surh et al. Molecular mechanisms underlying chemopreventive activities of anti-inflammatory phytochemicals: down-regulation of COX-2 and iNOS through suppression of NF-kappa B activation. *Mutat Res*. 2001 Sep 1;480-481:243-68

[437] Shoba G, et al. Influence of piperine on the pharmacokinetics of curcumin in animals and human volunteers. *Planta Med*. 1998 May;64(4):353-6

[438] "ALA reduced the TNF-alpha-stimulated ICAM-1 expression in a dose-dependent manner, to levels observed in unstimulated cells. Alpha-lipoic acid also reduced NFkB activity in these cells in a dose-dependent manner." Lee HA, Hughes DA. Alpha-lipoic acid modulates NFkB activity in human monocytic cells by direct interaction with DNA. *Exp Gerontol*. 2002 Jan-Mar;37(2-3):401-10

[439] "In conclusion, EGCG is an effective inhibitor of IKK activity. This may explain, at least in part, some of the reported anti-inflammatory and anticancer effects of green tea." Yang F, Oz HS, Barve S, de Villiers WJ, McClain CJ, Varilek GW. The green tea polyphenol (-)-epigallocatechin-3-gallate blocks nuclear factor-kappa B activation by inhibiting I kappa B kinase activity in the intestinal epithelial cell line IEC-6. *Mol Pharmacol*. 2001 Sep;60(3):528-33

[440] "These results suggest that carnosol suppresses the NO production and iNOS gene expression by inhibiting NFkB activation, and provide possible mechanisms for its anti-inflammatory and chemopreventive action." Lo AH, Liang YC, Lin-Shiau SY, Ho CT, Lin JK. Carnosol, an antioxidant in rosemary, suppresses inducible nitric oxide synthase through down-regulating nuclear factor-kappaB in mouse macrophages. *Carcinogenesis*. 2002 Jun;23(6):983-91

[441] "Constitutive and TNFalpha-induced NFkB DNA binding activity was inhibited by GSE at doses > or =50 microg/ml and treatments for > or =12 h." Dhanalakshmi et al. Inhibition of NFkB pathway in grape seed extract-induced apoptotic death of human prostate carcinoma DU145 cells. *Int J Oncol*. 2003;23:721-7

[442] "Caffeic acid phenethyl ester (CAPE) is an anti-inflammatory component of propolis (honeybee resin). CAPE is reportedly a specific inhibitor of nuclear factor-kappaB (NFkB)." Fitzpatrick LR, Wang J, Le T. Caffeic acid phenethyl ester, an inhibitor of nuclear factor-kappaB, attenuates bacterial peptidoglycan polysaccharide-induced colitis in rats. *J Pharmacol Exp Ther*. 2001 Dec;299(3):915-20

[443] "Our results suggest that zinc supplementation may lead to downregulation of the inflammatory cytokines through upregulation of the negative feedback loop A20 to inhibit induced NFkB activation." Prasad AS, et al. Antioxidant effect of zinc in humans. *Free Radic Biol Med*. 2004 Oct 15;37(8):1182-90

[444] Note that the patients in this study received a very high dose of selenium: 960 micrograms per day. This is at the top—and some would say over the top—of the safe and reasonable dose for long-term supplementation. This study lasted for three months. "In patients receiving selenium supplementation, selenium NFkB activity was significantly reduced, reaching the same level as the nondiabetic control group. CONCLUSION: In type 2 diabetic patients, activation of NFkB measured in peripheral blood monocytes can be reduced by selenium supplementation, confirming its importance in the prevention of cardiovascular diseases." Faure P, et al. Selenium supplementation decreases nuclear factor-kappa B activity in peripheral blood mononuclear cells from type 2 diabetic patients. *Eur J Clin Invest*. 2004 Jul;34:475-81

[445] Takada Y, Andreeff M, Aggarwal BB. Indole-3-carbinol suppresses NF-{kappa}B and I{kappa}B{alpha} kinase activation causing inhibition of expression of NF-{kappa}B-regulated antiapoptotic and metastatic gene products and enhancement of apoptosis in myeloid and leukemia cells. *Blood*. 2005 Apr 5; [Epub ahead of print]

[446] "Overall, our results indicated that indole-3-carbinol inhibits NFkB and NFkB-regulated gene expression and that this mechanism may provide the molecular basis for its ability to suppress tumorigenesis." Takada Y, et al. Indole-3-carbinol suppresses NFkB and IkappaBalpha kinase activation, causing inhibition of expression of NFkB-regulated antiapoptotic and metastatic gene products and enhancement of apoptosis in myeloid and leukemia cells. *Blood*. 2005 Jul 15;106:641-9

[447] "CONCLUSIONS: Administration of N-acetylcysteine results in decreased nuclear factor-kappa B activation in patients with sepsis, associated with decreases in interleukin-8 but not interleukin-6 or soluble intercellular adhesion molecule-1. These pilot data suggest that antioxidant therapy with N-acetylcysteine may be useful in blunting the inflammatory response to sepsis." Paterson RL, Galley HF, Webster NR. The effect of N-acetylcysteine on nuclear factor-kappa B activation, interleukin-6, interleukin-8, and intercellular adhesion molecule-1 expression in patients with sepsis. *Crit Care Med*. 2003 Nov;31(11):2574-8

[448] "Resveratrol's anticarcinogenic, anti-inflammatory, and growth-modulatory effects may thus be partially ascribed to the inhibition of activation of NFkB and AP-1 and the associated kinases." Manna SK, Mukhopadhyay A, Aggarwal BB. Resveratrol suppresses TNF-induced activation of nuclear transcription factors NF-kappa B, activator protein-1, and apoptosis: potential role of reactive oxygen intermediates and lipid peroxidation. *J Immunol*. 2000 Jun 15;164(12):6509-19

[449] "Both resveratrol and quercetin inhibited NFkB-, AP-1- and CREB-dependent transcription to a greater extent than the glucocorticosteroid, dexamethasone." Donnelly LE, et al. Anti-inflammatory Effects of Resveratrol in Lung Epithelial Cells. *Am J Physiol Lung Cell Mol Physiol*. 2004 Oct;287(4):L774-83

[450] Yajima H, et al. Isohumulones, bitter acids derived from hops, activate both peroxisome proliferator-activated receptor alpha and gamma and reduce insulin resistance. *J Biol Chem*. 2004 Aug 6;279(32):33456-62. Epub 2004 Jun 3. jbc.org/cgi/content/full/279/32/33456

[451] "Thus, PPAR gamma serves as the receptor for GLA in the regulation of gene expression in breast cancer cells. " Jiang WG, et al. Peroxisome proliferator activated receptor-gamma (PPAR-gamma) mediates the action of gamma linolenic acid in breast cancer cells. *Prostaglandins Leukot Essent Fatty Acids*. 2000 Feb;62(2):119-27

[452] "...EPA requires PPARalpha for its inhibitory effects on NFkB." Mishra A, Chaudhary A, Sethi S. Oxidized omega-3 fatty acids inhibit NFkB activation via a PPARalpha-dependent pathway. *Arterioscler Thromb Vasc Biol*. 2004 Sep;24(9):1621-7. Epub 2004 Jul 1. atvb.ahajournals.org/cgi/content/full/24/9/1621

[453] "We propose that the additive and synergistic effects of phytochemicals in fruit and vegetables are responsible for their potent antioxidant and anticancer activities, and that the benefit of a diet rich in fruit and vegetables is attributed to the complex mixture of phytochemicals present in whole foods." Liu RH. Health benefits of fruit and vegetables are from additive and synergistic combinations of phytochemicals. *Am J Clin Nutr*. 2003 Sep;78(3 Suppl):517S-520S

[454] Heaney RP. Long-latency deficiency disease: insights from calcium and vitamin D. *Am J Clin Nutr*. 2003 Nov;78(5):912-9

[455] O'Keefe JH Jr, Cordain L. Cardiovascular disease resulting from a diet and lifestyle at odds with our Paleolithic genome. *Mayo Clin Proc*. 2004 Jan;79(1):101-8

[456] Thomas MK, et al. Hypovitaminosis D in medical inpatients. *N Engl J Med*. 1998 Mar 19;338(12):777-83

unquestionably contributes to our modern pro-inflammatory tendency, and vitamin D supplementation has already proven to be immunomodulating and anti-inflammatory in human clinical trials.[457,458,459]

Basic Physiology of NFkB: A Simplified Conceptual Model: "Indeed, the previous view that nutrients only interact with human physiology at the metabolic/post-transcriptional level must be updated in light of current research showing that nutrients can, in fact, modify human physiology and phenotype at the genetic/pre-transcriptional level." Quote and updated image from Vasquez A. Nutritional and Botanical Inhibition of NFkB, the Major Intracellular Amplifier of the Inflammatory Cascade. A Practical Clinical Strategy Exemplifying Anti-Inflammatory Nutrigenomics. *Nutritional Perspectives* 2005;July: 5-12

---

[457] Van den Berghe G, et al. Bone turnover in prolonged critical illness: effect of vitamin D. *J Clin Endocrinol Metab*. 2003 Oct;88(10):4623-32
[458] Hypponen E, et al. Intake of vitamin D and risk of type 1 diabetes: a birth-cohort study. *Lancet*. 2001 Nov 3;358(9292):1500-3
[459] Mahon BD, et al. Cytokine profile in patients with multiple sclerosis following vitamin D supplementation. *J Neuroimmunol*. 2003;134(1-2):128-32

Mini-Monograph: Food Allergy and Adverse Food Reactions: A few considerations and perspectives

"**Adverse food reactions**" is a broad and general category that includes food allergy, food sensitivity, and food intolerance. The term "food" here means anything that is ingested other than drugs and medications and includes food, drink, food additives, preservatives, and food dyes. Many studies in the medical literature underestimate the high prevalence and clinical importance of food allergies because of inconsistent terminology, imperfect laboratory assessments[460], and the assumption that an "apparently healthy" person would only be allergic/sensitive to one or two foods—this is an erroneous assumption considering that many patients with food allergy/sensitivity/intolerance must avoid several (common range 3-10) commonly eaten foods to obtain clinical response and maximal improvement.[461,462] Clinical practice differs from basic research in that we as clinicians must often do what is effective while having neither the need nor the luxury for determining the molecular and physiologic basis for the effectiveness of each treatment in each patient. Clinical research has scientifically proven that adverse food reactions, regardless of the underlying mechanism(s) or classification of allergy, intolerance, or sensitivity, can exacerbate a wide range of human illnesses, including thyroid disease[463], mental depression[464,465], asthma, rhinitis,[466] recurrent otitis media[467], migraine[468,469,470], attention deficit and hyperactivity disorders[471], epilepsy[472,473,474], gastrointestinal inflammation[475], hypertension[476], joint pain[477,478,479,480,481,482,483], and other health problems.

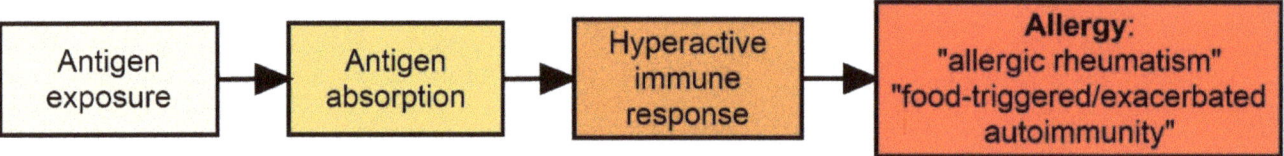

The common view of allergic phenomena: This model is incomplete and therefore inaccurate because it fails to include the prerequisite immune dysfunction and complex physiologic interconnections

"**Food allergy**" generally refers to adverse food reactions that are specifically immunoglobulin-mediated. Classically, food allergy is seen with immediate-onset allergy mediated via IgE antibodies which initiate mast cell degranulation and histamine release. The classic symptoms of immediate-onset allergies are skin rash, abdominal pain, angioedema, and bronchoconstriction. However, many doctors recognize the possibility of IgG-mediated allergies and suggest that these might be responsible for the delayed-onset or "hidden" food allergies which are clinically significant but more subtle and difficult to diagnose than the classic IgE-mediated allergies. The binding of antigens with immunoglobulins forms immune complexes that can deposit in parenchymal and synovial tissues where a localized immune response causes inflammation and organ dysfunction. "**Food sensitivity**" refers to immune-mediated adverse food reactions that are not antibody-mediated but are mediated by some other aspect of the immune/inflammatory system. An example of this is the increased production of specific prostaglandins in

---

[460] Bindslev-Jensen C, Skov PS, Madsen F, Poulsen LK. Food allergy and food intolerance--what is the difference? *Ann Allergy*. 1994 Apr;72(4):317-20
[461] Grant EC. Food allergies and migraine. *Lancet*. 1979 May 5;1(8123):966-9
[462] Speer F. Multiple food allergy. *Ann Allergy*. 1975 Feb;34(2):71-6
[463] Sategna-Guidetti C, et al. Prevalence of thyroid disorders in untreated adult celiac disease patients and effect of gluten withdrawal. *Am J Gastroenterol*. 2001;96:751-7
[464] Mills N. Depression and food intolerance: a single case study. *Hum Nutr Appl Nutr*. 1986 Apr;40(2):141-5
[465] Parker G, Watkins T. Treatment-resistant depression: when antidepressant drug intolerance may indicate food intolerance. *Aust N Z J Psychiatry*. 2002 Apr;36(2):263-5
[466] Speer F. The allergic child. *Am Fam Physician*. 1975 Feb;11(2):88-94
[467] Juntti H, Tikkanen S, Kokkonen J, et al. Cow's milk allergy is associated with recurrent otitis media during childhood. *Acta Otolaryngol*. 1999;119(8):867-73
[468] Monro J, Carini C, Brostoff J. Migraine is a food-allergic disease. *Lancet*. 1984 Sep 29;2(8405):719-21
[469] Egger J, Carter CM, Wilson J,et al. Is migraine food allergy? A double-blind controlled trial of oligoantigenic diet treatment. *Lancet*. 1983 Oct 15;2(8355):865-9
[470] Monro J, Brostoff J, Carini C, Zilkha K. Food allergy in migraine. Study of dietary exclusion and RAST. *Lancet*. 1980 Jul 5;2(8184):1-4
[471] Boris M, Mandel FS. Foods and additives are common causes of the attention deficit hyperactive disorder in children. *Ann Allergy*. 1994 May;72(5):462-8
[472] Egger J, Carter CM, Soothill JF, Wilson J. Oligoantigenic diet treatment of children with epilepsy and migraine. *J Pediatr*. 1989;114(1):51-8
[473] Pelliccia A, et al. Partial cryptogenetic epilepsy and food allergy/intolerance. Reflections on three clinical cases. *Minerva Pediatr*. 1999 May;51(5):153-7
[474] Frediani T, Lucarelli S, Pelliccia A, et al. Allergy and childhood epilepsy: a close relationship? *Acta Neurol Scand*. 2001 Dec;104(6):349-52
[475] Marr HY, Chen WC, Lin LH. Food protein-induced enterocolitis syndrome: report of one case. *Acta Paediatr Taiwan*. 2001;42(1):49-52
[476] Grant EC. Food allergies and migraine. *Lancet*. 1979 May 5;1(8123):966-9
[477] Golding DN. Is there an allergic synovitis? *J R Soc Med*. 1990 May;83(5):312-4
[478] Panush RS. Food induced ("allergic") arthritis: clinical and serologic studies. *J Rheumatol*. 1990 Mar;17(3):291-4
[479] Pacor ML, Lunardi C, Di Lorenzo G, Biasi D, Corrocher R. Food allergy and seronegative arthritis: report of two cases. *Clin Rheumatol*. 2001;20(4):279-81
[480] Schrander JJ, Marcelis C, de Vries MP, van Santen-Hoeufft HM. Does food intolerance play a role in juvenile chronic arthritis? *Br J Rheumatol*. 1997;36(8):905-8
[481] van de Laar MA, van der Korst JK. Food intolerance in rheumatoid arthritis. I. A double blind, controlled trial. *Ann Rheum Dis*. 1992 Mar;51(3):298-302
[482] Haugen MA, et al. A pilot study of the effect of an elemental diet in the management of rheumatoid arthritis. *Clin Exp Rheumatol*. 1994 May-Jun;12(3):275-9
[483] van de Laar MA, et al. Food intolerance in rheumatoid arthritis. II. Clinical and histological aspects. *Ann Rheum Dis*. 1992 Mar;51(3):303-6

food-induced irritable bowel syndrome.[484] **"Food intolerance"** refers to adverse food reactions which are associated with poor nutritional status and/or impaired hepatic detoxification and which are *not* immune-mediated. Classic and well-known examples of this category of adverse food reaction include MSG sensitivity (associated with deficiency of vitamin B-6 and subsequent defects in hepatic transamination), tyramine intolerance that can result in hypertension and headaches, and histamine intolerance that can result in bronchoconstriction.[485] From a practical clinical standpoint, the following facts are self-evident for any doctor working in the field of nutrition:

1. Some people have adverse food reactions from the foods that they eat.
2. Food-induced reactions may be either immediate-onset (i.e., within minutes) or delayed-onset (within days) of eating the triggering food.
3. The same patient might have immediate-onset reactions to food X with symptoms A and B and simultaneously have a delayed-onset reaction to food Y with symptom C.
4. Food X might cause symptoms D and E in one patient and symptoms F and G in another patient.
5. By avoiding allergens and/or improving immune function, many "diseases" go away without direct treatment and the patient experiences an improved state of health.
6. Failure to identify and avoid problematic foods combined with failure to correct the underlying immune dysfunction often makes the "disease" recalcitrant to remediation even with "generally effective" treatment. This has been demonstrated in migraine, hypertension[486], and drug-resistant mental depression.[487]

Approaching a more complete understanding of "allergy" in general and the "allergic" contribution to systemic inflammation and autoimmunity in particular: Simple and obvious though it may appear, the addition and acknowledgement of immune dysfunction to the schema of clinical allergy/inflammation contains a gateway for accessing more effective understandings and treatments for this common group of problems.

Food allergy both *results from* and *contributes to* immune dysfunction and a systemic proinflammatory state. Food allergy contributes to "autoimmunity" and musculoskeletal inflammation via several mechanisms, including but not limited to the following:

1. <u>Stimulation of cytokine release</u>: As will be discussed later, the term "superantigen" classically refers to microbial—viral, bacterial, or fungal—antigens which have the ability to induce production of excessive levels of cytokines and other inflammatory effectors[488], and superantigens appear to be involved in the

---

[484] "Food intolerance associated with prostaglandin production is an important factor in the pathogenesis of IBS." Jones VA, McLaughlan P, Shorthouse M, Workman E, Hunter JO. Food intolerance: a major factor in the pathogenesis of irritable bowel syndrome. *Lancet.* 1982 Nov 20;2(8308):1115-7
[485] Wantke F, Hemmer W, Haglmuller T, Gotz M, Jarisch R. Histamine in wine. Bronchoconstriction after a double-blind placebo-controlled red wine provocation test. *Int Arch Allergy Immunol.* 1996 Aug;110(4):397-400
[486] "When an average of ten common foods were avoided there was a dramatic fall in the number of headaches per month, 85% of patients becoming headache-free. The 25% of patients with hypertension became normotensive." Grant EC. Food allergies and migraine. *Lancet.* 1979 May 5;1(8123):966-9
[487] "The prevalence of food intolerance as a contributing factor to depressive disorders requires clarification. Clinicians should be aware of the possible syndrome and that it may be worsened by psychotropic medication." Parker G, Watkins T. Treatment-resistant depression: when antidepressant drug intolerance may indicate food intolerance. *Aust N Z J Psychiatry.* 2002 Apr;36(2):263-5
[488] "The basis of autoimmune disorders due to superantigen is due to greater stimulation of T-lymphocytes and elaborate cytokine production." Hemalatha V, Srikanth P, Mallika M. Superantigens - Concepts, clinical disease and therapy. *Indian J Med Microbiol* 2004;22:204-211

pathogenesis of inflammatory musculoskeletal disorders such as rheumatoid arthritis.[489,490] **In this section I propose that since food allergens appear capable of inducing cytokine production, they should in certain circumstances be considered "dietary superantigens"** since they invoke cytokine release similarly as do microbial superantigens. An important distinction here, however, is that microbial superantigens generally stimulate cytokine release as an inherent property in *all* patients, whereas **the production of cytokines by dietary (super)antigens is dependent on previous sensitization**; thus cytokine production by allergens is patient-dependent and not an inherent property of the allergen itself. **Mononuclear cells from egg-allergic patients produce much more proinflammatory cytokine (interferon) than do those from nonallergic patients.**[491] Similarly, **in children with autism, who commonly demonstrate immune dysfunction and neuroautoimmunity**[492]**, exposure to food allergens greatly increases cytokine release compared to controls**.[493] Food allergy, NFkB activation, cytokine release, and increased intestinal permeability form a self-perpetuating vicious cycle because consumption of dietary allergens causes damage to the intestinal mucosa and stimulates NFkB activation and cytokine release which then increases intestinal permeability, thus allowing for increased absorption of dietary and microbial immunogens for the perpetuation and exacerbation of allergy and immune dysfunction.[494] Proinflammatory cytokines would be expected to contribute to autoimmune disease induction via mechanisms such as bystander activation and increased autoantigen processing regardless of their original stimuli.

2. Immune complex formation and deposition: **Dietary antigen-antibody immune complexes are formed following the consumption of allergenic foods by patients with allergy to those foods**[495,496] and these anti-food and anti-IgE immune complexes contribute to allergic symptomatology by a mechanism that has been described as "chronic serum sickness."[497] These immune complexes are then deposited in the joints to localize the resultant proinflammatory response. In the study by Carini et al[498], the authors found that **patients with food-induced joint pain and inflammation had anti-IgE IgG antibodies which formed large immune complexes that were detectable in synovial fluid and which probably contributed to the arthritis**. Anti-IgE IgG antibodies are commonly elevated in patients with allergic/inflammatory diseases such as eczema[499], asthma[500], and Crohn's disease[501] and thus tissue damage in these conditions appears mediated at least in part by anti-immunoglobulin immune complexes (i.e., anti-IgE IgG complexed with IgE) rather than the classic antigen-antibody immune complexes. In this way, food allergies cause joint pain and inflammation by the deposition of immune complexes into the synovium and joint cartilage.[502] Conversely, the consumption of a relatively hypoallergenic diet reduces intake of food antigens and helps reduce IgE levels. This explains, in part, the success of hypoallergenic diets in the treatment of immune-

---

[489] "They also suggest that the etiology of RA may involve initial activation of V beta 14+ T cells by a V beta 14-specific superantigen with subsequent recruitment of a few activated autoreactive v beta 14+ T cell clones to the joints while the majority of other V beta 14+ T cells disappear." Paliard X, West SG, Lafferty JA, Clements JR, Kappler JW, Marrack P, Kotzin BL. Evidence for the effects of a superantigen in rheumatoid arthritis. *Science*. 1991 Jul 19;253(5017):325-9

[490] "Given that binding sites for superantigens have been mapped to the CDR4s of TCR beta chains, the synovial localization of T cells bearing V beta s with significant CDR4 homology indicates that V beta-specific T-cell activation by superantigen may play a role in RA." Howell MD, et al. Limited T-cell receptor beta-chain heterogeneity among interleukin 2 receptor-positive synovial T cells suggests a role for superantigen in rheumatoid arthritis. *Proc Natl Acad Sci*. 1991 Dec 1;88:10921-5

[491] "The levels of IFN-gamma production of only IL-2-stimulated or both ovalbumin-stimulated and IL-2-stimulated peripheral blood mononuclear cells from egg-sensitive patients with atopic dermatitis was significantly higher than that of healthy children and that of egg-sensitive patients with immediate allergic symptoms." Shinbara M, et al. Interferon-gamma and interleukin-4 production of ovalbumin-stimulated lymphocytes in egg-sensitive children. *Ann Allergy Asthma Immunol*. 1996;77(1):60-6

[492] "Autistic children, but not normal children, had antibodies to caudate nucleus (49% positive sera), cerebral cortex (18% positive sera) and cerebellum (9% positive sera)." Singh VK, Rivas WH. Prevalence of serum antibodies to caudate nucleus in autistic children. *Neurosci Lett*. 2004 Jan 23;355(1-2):53-6

[493] Jyonouchi H, Sun S, Itokazu N. Innate immunity associated with inflammatory responses and cytokine production against common dietary proteins in patients with autism spectrum disorder. *Neuropsychobiology*. 2002;46(2):76-84

[494] Ma TY, Iwamoto GK, Hoa NT, Akotia V, Pedram A, Boivin MA, Said HM. TNF-alpha-induced increase in intestinal epithelial tight junction permeability requires NF-kappa B activation. Am *J Physiol Gastrointest Liver Physiol*. 2004 Mar;286(3):G367-76 ajpgi.physiology.org/cgi/content/full/286/3/G367

[495] "Antigen entry and the formation of immune complexes occur in atopic subjects after food ingestion. ...Food allergic subjects showed, after food challenge, the presence of IgE and IgG immune complexes, which correlates with the subsequent occurrence of symptoms." Carini C, Brostoff J. Evidence for circulating IgE complexes in food allergy. *Ric Clin Lab*. 1987 Oct-Dec;17(4):309-22

[496] "Following challenge, immune complexes containing IgE, IgG, and antigen are detectable in the circulation. Their appearance correlates with the production of symptoms." Carini C, Brostoff J, Wraith DG. IgE complexes in food allergy. *Ann Allergy*. 1987 Aug;59(2):110-7

[497] Marinkovich V. "Immunology and Food Allergy" in "Applying Functional Medicine in Clinical Practice." Institute for Functional Medicine. Seattle, Washington: March 2005

[498] "In three food-allergic patients IgG anti-IgE was detectable in a complexed form in the serum samples examined before and after food challenge. The finding of IgG anti-IgE autoantibody in a group of patients with allergic arthralgia is quite exciting." Carini et al. Immune complexes in food-induced arthralgia. *Ann Allergy*. 1987 Dec;59(6):422-8

[499] "An IgG type of antibody directed against IgE has been studied in serum from healthy and allergic individuals. ... Significantly raised levels of anti-IgE autoantibody were found in patients suffering from atopic disorders in comparison to the controls." Carini et al. IgG autoantibody to IgE in atopic patients. *Ann Allergy*. 1988 Jan;60(1):48-52

[500] "Significantly enhanced levels of IgE/anti-IgE IC were detected in children with asthma." Ritter C, Battig M, Kraemer R, Stadler BM. IgE hidden in immune complexes with anti-IgE autoantibodies in children with asthma. *J Allergy Clin Immunol*. 1991 Nov;88(5):793-801

[501] "In CD sera no food-specific IgE could be detected, but levels of immune complexes of IgE and IgG anti-IgE autoantibodies were statistically significantly increased compared to healthy controls." Huber A, Genser D, Spitzauer S, Scheiner O, Jensen-Jarolim E. IgE/anti-IgE immune complexes in sera from patients with Crohn's disease do not contain food-specific IgE. *Int Arch Allergy Immunol*. 1998 Jan;115(1):67-72

[502] Inman RD. Antigens, the gastrointestinal tract, and arthritis. *Rheum Dis Clin North Am*. 1991 May;17(2):309-21

complex-mediated diseases such as mixed cryoglobulinemia[503,504], hypersensitivity vasculitis[505], and leukocystoclastic vasculitis with arthritis.[506] In patients with rheumatoid arthritis, the symptomatic and clinical improvement induced by hypoallergenic diets correlates with reductions in antibodies to food antigens.[507]

3. <u>Damage to the intestinal mucosa with resultant increased absorption of dietary and microbial antigens</u>: Consumption of food allergens increases intestinal permeability[508] and thus amplifies the absorption of intestinal contents—dietary and microbial antigens. Patients with food allergy have "leaky gut" that is exacerbated by consumption of allergenic foods; thus lactulose-mannitol assays can be used to assist the diagnosis of food allergy.[509,510] By increasing intestinal permeability, consumption of dietary antigens serves to exacerbate the adverse effects of gastrointestinal dysbiosis by increasing antigen and (anti)metabolite absorption. Since both dietary allergens and bacterial endotoxin stimulate production of cytokines[511], **concomitant exposure to both allergens and intra-intestinal endotoxin leads to an additive increase in proinflammatory cytokine production.**[512] Thus, **consumption of allergenic foods in the presence of gastrointestinal dysbiosis would be expected to lead to more severe and more diverse adverse physiologic and clinical consequences than would be experienced following exposure to either allergens or dysbiosis alone.**

4. <u>Dietary haptenization</u>: **Dietary antigens can complex with human tissues to form *neoantigens* that are immunostimulatory**. The best example of this appears to be the induction of autoimmunity by wheat-derived gliadin which haptenizes with intestinal tissue transglutaminase and other extracellular matrix proteins and results in the allergic-autoimmune disease celiac disease.[513,514] **The finding that gliadin proteins haptenize with collagen and can induce the formation of anti-collagen antibodies in humans**[515] **makes clear the pathomechanism by which "wheat allergy" can directly precipitate systemic musculoskeletal autoimmunity**. Once initiated and perpetuated by dietary gliadin from wheat, additional autoimmunity ensues (perhaps mediated directly by epitope spreading and/or indirectly by deposition of immune complexes) which is directed against various tissues, most notably the thyroid gland[516], brain[517],

and musculoskeletal system.[518] Given the association between lupus and celiac disease[519,520,521], we may speculate that allergy becomes systemic autoimmunity in certain circumstances and in susceptible patients.

- Review and proposal: Hapten exposure might predispose to atopic disease—the hapten-atopy hypothesis (*Trends Immunol* 2009 Feb[522] and SkinAndAllergyNews.com 2010 Oct[523]): Dr McFadden and his colleagues propose that **orally-consumed chemicals—commonly consumed as processed foods—bind to and alter endogenous proteins to result in hapten-protein neoantigens that stimulate immunologic disease, particularly allergic conditions** such as atopic dermatitis (eczema), asthma and seasonal respiratory allergies. Per an interview with Jancin, McFadden explained that "Haptens are low-molecular-weight organic chemicals that aren't allergenic on their own but can bind to a peptide or protein, thereby altering its configuration and rendering it foreign and allergenic. Examples of haptens include antibiotics and some other drugs, as well as chemicals present in toiletries, processed foods, powdered milk, preservatives used in vaccines, and metal jewelry. … **Various brands of powdered milk contain a mean of 12 haptens each.** … Also, epidemiologic studies show that certain maternal occupations predispose to the birth of atopic children. Among these occupations are hairdresser, beautician, cleaner, electroplater, bar staff, dental assistant, confectionary maker, and book binder. What these diverse occupations have in common is increased environmental exposure to haptens."

5. Dietary molecular mimicry: Just as microbes produce structures similar to human molecules which then incite a cross-reacting immune response—**molecular mimicry** (discussed elsewhere in this chapter in the section on dysbiosis)—certain dietary antigens appear capable of inducing cross reactions. For example, Vojdani et al[524] recently demonstrated **cross-reactivity between anti-gliadin antibodies and anti-cerebellar antibodies in an experimental model that may partly explain the anti-brain autoimmunity seen in autism.** Further expanding this concept of dietary molecular mimicry is the finding that "the virulence factor of C albicans-hyphal wall protein 1 (HWP1)-contains amino acid sequences that are identical or highly homologous to known coeliac disease-related alpha-gliadin and gamma-gliadin T-cell epitopes."[525] This raises three interrelated possibilities: 1) that gastrointestinal overgrowth of *Candida albicans* and the resultant elaboration of HWP1 and immunostimulation may result in sensitivity to gluten, particularly as HWP1 and gliadin are both substrates for transglutaminase, 2) that consumption of wheat gluten may trigger sensitivity to *Candida albicans*, and 3) that wheat gluten and *Candida albicans* must both be present for the development of celiac disease and the ensuant autoimmunity. Additional details on the ability of *C. albicans* to contribute to autoimmunity are discussed in the section on dysbiosis.

6. Enhanced processing of autoantigens: Food-allergic patients may produce autoimmunity-stimulating autoantigens following exposure to foods to which they are sensitized. This has been demonstrated in autistic children, **exposure of lymphocytes from autistic patients to dietary antigens (gliadin and casein peptides) stimulates production of autoantigens that presumably incite and perpetuate autoimmunity**.[526] Thus, at least in autistic patients, we have evidence that food allergy can segue into autoimmunity. This phenomenon is probably not restricted only to autistic patients, as suggested by the association between celiac disease and the systemic autoimmune disease lupus.[527,528,529]

---

[518] "JIA children have an increased prevalence of autoimmune thyroiditis, subclinical hypothyroidism and coeliac disease." Stagi S, Giani T, Simonini G, Falcini F. Thyroid function, autoimmune thyroiditis and coeliac disease in juvenile idiopathic arthritis. *Rheumatology* (Oxford). 2005 Apr;44(4):517-2
[519] Zitouni M, Daoud W, Kallel M, Makni S. Systemic lupus erythematosus with celiac disease: a report of five cases. *Joint Bone Spine*. 2004 Jul;71(4):344-6
[520] Komatireddy GR, Marshall JB, Aqel R, Spollen LE, Sharp GC. Association of systemic lupus erythematosus and gluten enteropathy. *South Med J*. 1995 Jun;88:673-6
[521] Rustgi AK, Peppercorn MA. Gluten-sensitive enteropathy and systemic lupus erythematosus. *Arch Intern Med*. 1988 Jul;148(7):1583-4
[522] McFadden JP, et al. Does hapten exposure predispose to atopic disease? The hapten-atopy hypothesis. *Trends Immunol*. 2009 Feb;30(2):67-74
[523] Article by Bruce Jancin of the Skin & Allergy News Digital Network; interview with Dr. John P. McFadden. Expert Analysis from the Annual Congress of the European Academy of Dermatology and Venereology: Exploring the Hapten Hypothesis of Atopic Disease. skinandallergynews.com/news/medical-dermatology/single-article/eadv-exploring-the-hapten-hypothesis-of-atopic-disease/e7df2851ed.html Posted 10/26/10 and accessed May 31, 2011.
[524] "This cross-reaction was further confirmed by DOT-immunoblot and inhibition studies. We conclude that a subgroup of patients with autism produce antibodies against Purkinje cells and gliadin peptides, which may be responsible for some of the neurological symptoms in autism." Vojdani A, O'Bryan T, Green JA, Mccandless J, Woeller KN, Vojdani E, Nourian AA, Cooper EL. Immune response to dietary proteins, gliadin and cerebellar peptides in children with autism. *Nutr Neurosci*. 2004 Jun;7:151-61
[525] "Subsequently, C albicans might function as an adjuvant that stimulates antibody formation against HWP1 and gluten, and formation of autoreactive antibodies against tissue transglutaminase and endomysium." Nieuwenhuizen WF, et al. Is Candida albicans a trigger in the onset of coeliac disease? *Lancet*. 2003;361(9375):2152-4
[526] Vojdani A, Pangborn JB, Vojdani E, Cooper EL. Infections, toxic chemicals and dietary peptides binding to lymphocyte receptors and tissue enzymes are major instigators of autoimmunity in autism. *Int J Immunopathol Pharmacol*. 2003 Sep-Dec;16(3):189-99
[527] Zitouni M, Daoud W, Kallel M, Makni S. Systemic lupus erythematosus with celiac disease: a report of five cases. *Joint Bone Spine*. 2004 Jul;71(4):344-6
[528] Komatireddy GR, Marshall JB, Aqel R, Spollen LE, Sharp GC. Association of systemic lupus erythematosus and gluten enteropathy. *South Med J*. 1995 Jun;88:673-6
[529] Rustgi AK, Peppercorn MA. Gluten-sensitive enteropathy and systemic lupus erythematosus. *Arch Intern Med*. 1988 Jul;148(7):1583-4

7. <u>Diet-derived xenobiotic immunotoxicity</u>: Foods commonly contain trace amounts of xenobiotics such as pesticides, fungicides, fumigants, fertilizers, preservatives, military propellants such as perchlorate[530], and toxic metals such as mercury. Some of these xenobiotics have been insufficiently studied in humans, while others such as mercury are well-known immunotoxins capable of inducing immune dysfunction which may contribute to autoimmunity. **Mercury poisoning/accumulation can occur in humans as a result of consumption of contaminated foods—especially seafood such as shark, swordfish, king mackerel, tilefish, and albacore ("white") tuna**[531], and the immunologic effects of organic and/or inorganic mercury include immunosuppression, immunostimulation, formation of antinucleolar antibodies targeting fibrillarin, and formation and deposition of immune-complexes, resulting in a syndrome called "mercury-induced autoimmunity" which can be induced by exposure of susceptible animals to mercury.[532] Mercury/"silver" amalgam dental fillings rank highly among the most significant source of mercury exposure in humans, and **implantation of mercury-silver dental amalgams in susceptible animals causes chronic stimulation of the immune system with induction of systemic autoimmunity**.[533] Besides being **a neurotoxin with no safe exposure limit**[534], **mercury is known to modify/antigenize endogenous proteins to promote autoimmunity**[535], and **mercury may also promote autoimmunity by contributing to a pro-inflammatory environment that awakens quiescent autoreactive immunocytes via bystander activation**[536] (detailed later). For example, administration of mercury to "susceptible" mice induces autoimmunity via modification of the nucleolar protein *fibrillarin*[537]; noteworthy in this regard is the fact that antifibrillarin antibodies are characteristic of the autoimmune disease **scleroderma**.[538] Mercury toxicity is commonly encountered in clinical practice (diagnosis and treatment are discussed later), and a recent study published in *JAMA* showed that 8% of American women of childbearing age have sufficient levels of mercury in their bodies to produce neurologic damage in their children.[539] **The mercury-based preservative thimerosol is a type-IV (delayed hypersensitivity) sensitizing agent**[540], and **recent research implicates mercury as an important contributor to the clinical manifestations of autism**[541,542] **and eczema.**[543] Preliminary clinical evidence shows that removal of mercury amalgams, particularly along with

---

[530] "The Bush administration has imposed a gag order on the U.S. Environmental Protection Agency from publicly discussing perchlorate pollution, even as two new studies reveal high levels of the rocket-fuel component may be contaminating the nation's lettuce supply." Peter Waldman. Rocket Fuel Residues Found in Lettuce: Bush administration issues gag order on EPA discussions of possible rocket fuel tainted lettuce. *Wall Street Journal*. See organicconsumers.org/toxic/lettuce042903.cfm, rhinoed.com/epa's_gag_order.htm, peer.org/press/508.html yubanet.com/artman/publish/article_13637.shtml

[531] Note cfsan.fda.gov/~dms/admehg3.html for the white-washed version; see ewg.org/issues/mercury/20040319/index.php for a more accurate and complete perspective.

[532] Havarinasab S, Hultman P. Organic mercury compounds and autoimmunity. *Autoimmun Rev*. 2005;4(5):270-5 generationrescue.org/pdf/havarinasab.pdf

[533] "We hypothesize that under appropriate conditions of genetic susceptibility and adequate body burden, heavy metal exposure from dental amalgam may contribute to immunological aberrations, which could lead to overt autoimmunity." Hultman P, Johansson U, Turley SJ, Lindh U, Enestrom S, Pollard KM. Adverse immunological effects and autoimmunity induced by dental amalgam and alloy in mice. *FASEB J*. 1994 Nov;8(14):1183-90 fasebj.org/cgi/reprint/8/14/1183

[534] University of Calgary Faculty of Medicine. How Mercury Causes Brain Neuron Degeneration commons.ucalgary.ca/mercury/

[535] Havarinasab S, Hultman P. Organic mercury compounds and autoimmunity. *Autoimmun Rev*. 2005 Jun;4(5):270-5

[536] "It is therefore theoretically possible that compounds present in vaccines such as thiomersal or aluminium hydroxyde can trigger autoimmune reactions through bystander effects." Fournie GJ, et al. Induction of autoimmunity through bystander effects: immunological disorders induced by heavy metals. *J Autoimmun*. 2001 May;16(3):319-26

[537] Nielsen JB, Hultman P. Mercury-induced autoimmunity in mice. *Environ Health Perspect*. 2002 Oct;110 Suppl 5:877-81

[538] "Since anti-fibrillarin antibodies are specific markers of scleroderma, the present animal model may be valuable for studies of the immunological aberrations which are likely to induce this autoimmune response." Hultman P, Enestrom S, Pollard KM, Tan EM. Anti-fibrillarin autoantibodies in mercury-treated mice. *Clin Exp Immunol*. 1989 Dec;78:470-7

[539] "However, approximately 8% of women had concentrations higher than the US Environmental Protection Agency's recommended reference dose (5.8 microg/L), below which exposures are considered to be without adverse effects. Women who are pregnant or who intend to become pregnant should follow federal and state advisories on consumption of fish." Schober SE, et al. Blood mercury levels in US children and women of childbearing age, 1999-2000. *JAMA*. 2003 Apr 2;289(13):1667-74

[540] "Thimerosal is an important preservative in vaccines and ophthalmologic preparations. The substance is known to be a type IV sensitizing agent. High sensitization rates were observed in contact-allergic patients and in health care workers who had been exposed to thimerosal-preserved vaccines." Westphal GA, et al. Homozygous gene deletions of the glutathione S-transferases M1 and T1 are associated with thimerosal sensitization. *Int Arch Occup Environ Health*. 2000 Aug;73(6):384-8

[541] Vojdani A, Pangborn JB, Vojdani E, Cooper EL. Infections, toxic chemicals and dietary peptides binding to lymphocyte receptors and tissue enzymes are major instigators of autoimmunity in autism. *Int J Immunopathol Pharmacol*. 2003 Sep-Dec;16(3):189-99

[542] Geier DA, Geier MR. A comparative evaluation of the effects of MMR immunization and mercury doses from thimerosal-containing childhood vaccines on the population prevalence of autism. *Med Sci Monit*. 2004 Mar;10(3):PI33-9. Epub 2004 Mar 1. medscimonit.com/pub/vol_10/no_3/3986.pdf

[543] Weidinger S, Kramer U, Dunemann L, Mohrenschlager M, Ring J, Behrendt H. Body burden of mercury is associated with acute atopic eczema and total IgE in children from southern Germany. *J Allergy Clin Immunol*. 2004 Aug;114(2):457-9

implementation of antioxidant therapy and/or mercury chelation, benefits the biochemical status and/or clinical course of autoimmune disease.[544,545]

8. <u>Diet-derived dysbiosis</u>: Induction and exacerbation of dysbiosis following chronic consumption of allergenic foods has been reported to occur in humans. Raw vegetables and salad greens are thoroughly contaminated with bacteria and occasionally other microbes. Food can be contaminated with pathogenic microbes via improper preparation, storage, or handling by chefs with contagious diseases and poor hygiene. An inflammatory "reactive" arthritis can result from consumption of food that is contaminated by microorganisms, most commonly *Salmonella*[546,547,548] and *Campylobacter* species.[549] Long-term autoimmune/inflammatory complications of gastrointestinal infections/colonization sourced from food include Reiter's syndrome, Guillain-Barre syndrome (peripheral nerve autoimmunity), uveitis, sacroiliitis, and ankylosing spondylitis.

9. <u>Diet-derived immunodysregulation</u>: Certain foods contain constituents that cause immune dysfunction and the induction or exacerbation of autoimmunity. L-Canavanine sulfate is a non-protein amino acid found in alfalfa sprouts which triggers a condition similar to systemic lupus erythematosus in monkeys[550,551] and which may exacerbate SLE in humans.

10. <u>Dietary xenobiotics</u>: Artificial sweeteners, thickeners, flavor enhancers, emulsifiers, and plasticizers can be found in foods, particularly those which are manufactured and processed. Some of these chemicals have the potential to alter immune mechanisms in favor of autoimmunity. These dietary xenobiotics may be particularly relevant for initiating and promoting Crohn's disease.[552]

11. <u>Immunogenicity induced by cooking—the Maillard reaction (non-enzymatic glycosylation)</u>: Heated exposure of lysine, arginine, and tryptophan to reducing sugars such as fructose and lactose results in the non-enzymatic binding (glycosylation) of the sugar with the amino acid. If the amino acid is a component of a protein, then the structure and antigenicity of the protein is altered as it is now a glycoprotein, which may either serve as a neoantigen or may increase the allergenicity of a protein that was previously hypoallergenic, as seen with the roasting of peanuts.[553,554] Glycoproteins formed from the baking and browning of foods are also called *glycotoxins* and are capable of exacerbating inflammation in patients with diabetes.[555] Similar to the formation of **glycotoxins** is the formation of **acrylamide**, a possible carcinogen, in fried and baked foods.

---

[544] Prochazkova J, Sterzl I, Kucerova H, Bartova J, Stejskal VD. The beneficial effect of amalgam replacement on health in patients with autoimmunity. *Neuro Endocrinol Lett.* 2004 Jun;25(3):211-8. See also: "The MELISA Test is reproducible, sensitive, specific, and reliable for detecting metal sensitivity in metal-sensitive patients." Valentine-Thon E, Schiwara HW. Validity of MELISA for metal sensitivity testing. *Neuro Endocrinol Lett.* 2003 Feb-Apr;24(1-2):57-64. See also: "The hypothesis that metal exposure from dental amalgam can cause ill health in a susceptible part of the exposed population was supported." Lindh U, et al. Removal of dental amalgam and other metal alloys supported by antioxidant therapy alleviates symptoms and improves quality of life in patients with amalgam-associated ill health. *Neuro Endocrinol Lett.* 2002 Oct-Dec;23(5-6):459-82 nel.edu/23_56/NEL235602A12_Lindh.htm and nel.edu/pdf_w/23_56/NEL235602A12_Lindh_wr.pdf

[545] "This study documents objective biochemical changes following the removal of these fillings along with other dental materials, utilizing a new health care model of multidisciplinary planning and treatment." Huggins HA, Levy TE. Cerebrospinal fluid protein changes in multiple sclerosis after dental amalgam removal. *Altern Med Rev.* 1998 Aug;3(4):295-300 thorne.com/altmedrev/.fulltext/3/4/295.pdf

[546] "We describe the case of a patient who became ill with Salmonella Blockley food poisoning while working in Cyprus in August 1994. As his diarrhoea resolved he began to suffer from lower limb joint pains which were diagnosed as acute salmonella reactive arthritis." Wilson IG, Whitehead E. Long-term post-Salmonella reactive arthritis due to Salmonella Blockley. *Jpn J Infect Dis.* 2004 Oct;57(5):210-1

[547] "Reactive joint symptoms after food-borne Salmonella infection may be more frequent than previously thought. The duration of diarrhea is strongly correlated with the occurrence of joint symptoms." Locht H, et al. High frequency of reactive joint symptoms after an outbreak of Salmonella enteritidis. *J Rheumatol.* 2002 Apr;29(4):767-71

[548] Leirisalo-Repo M, et al. Long-term prognosis of reactive salmonella arthritis. *Ann Rheum Dis.* 1997 Sep;56(9):516-20

[549] "Campylobacter jejuni is the most commonly reported bacterial cause of foodborne infection in the United States. Adding to the human and economic costs are chronic sequelae associated with C. jejuni infection--Guillian-Barre syndrome and reactive arthritis." Altekruse SF, Stern NJ, Fields PI, Swerdlow DL. Campylobacter jejuni--an emerging foodborne pathogen. *Emerg Infect Dis.* 1999 Jan-Feb;5(1):28-35

[550] "L-Canavanine sulfate, a constituent of alfalfa sprouts, was incorporated into the diet and reactivated the syndrome in monkeys in which an SLE-like syndrome had previously been induced by the ingestion of alfalfa seeds or sprouts." Malinow MR, Bardana EJ Jr, Pirofsky B, Craig S, McLaughlin P. Systemic lupus erythematosus-like syndrome in monkeys fed alfalfa sprouts: role of a nonprotein amino acid. *Science.* 1982 Apr 23;216(4544):415-7

[551] "Occurrence of autoimmune hemolytic anemia and exacerbation of SLE have been linked to ingestion of alfalfa tablets containing L-canavanine." Alcocer-Varela J, et al. Effects of L-canavanine on T cells may explain the induction of systemic lupus erythematosus by alfalfa. *Arthritis Rheum.* 1985 Jan;28(1):52-7

[552] "Various food additives, especially emulsifiants, thickeners, surface-finishing agents and contaminants like plasticizers share structural domains with mycobacterial lipids. It is therefore hypothesized, that these compounds are able to stimulate by molecular mimicry the CD1 system in the gastrointestinal mucosa and to trigger the pro-inflammatory cytokine cascade." Traunmuller F. Etiology of Crohn's disease: Do certain food additives cause intestinal inflammation by molecular mimicry of mycobacterial lipids? *Med Hypotheses.* 2005;65(5):859-64

[553] "Roasted peanuts exhibited a higher level of IgE binding, which was correlated with a higher level of AGE adducts. We concluded that there is an association between AGE adducts and increased IgE binding (i.e., allergenicity) of roasted peanuts." Chung SY, Champagne ET. Association of end-product adducts with increased IgE binding of roasted peanuts. *J Agric Food Chem.* 2001 Aug;49(8):3911-6

[554] "The data presented here indicate that thermal processing may play an important role in enhancing the allergenic properties of peanuts and that the protein modifications made by the Maillard reaction contribute to this effect." Maleki SJ, Chung SY, Champagne ET, Raufman JP. The effects of roasting on the allergenic properties of peanut proteins. *J Allergy Clin Immunol.* 2000 Oct;106(4):763-8

[555] "A study now reveals that the consumption of foods rich in browned and oxidized products (so-called glycotoxins) induces a chronic inflammatory state in diabetic individuals." Monnier VM, Obrenovich ME. Wake up and smell the maillard reaction. *Sci Aging Knowledge Environ.* 2002 Dec 18;2002(50):pe21

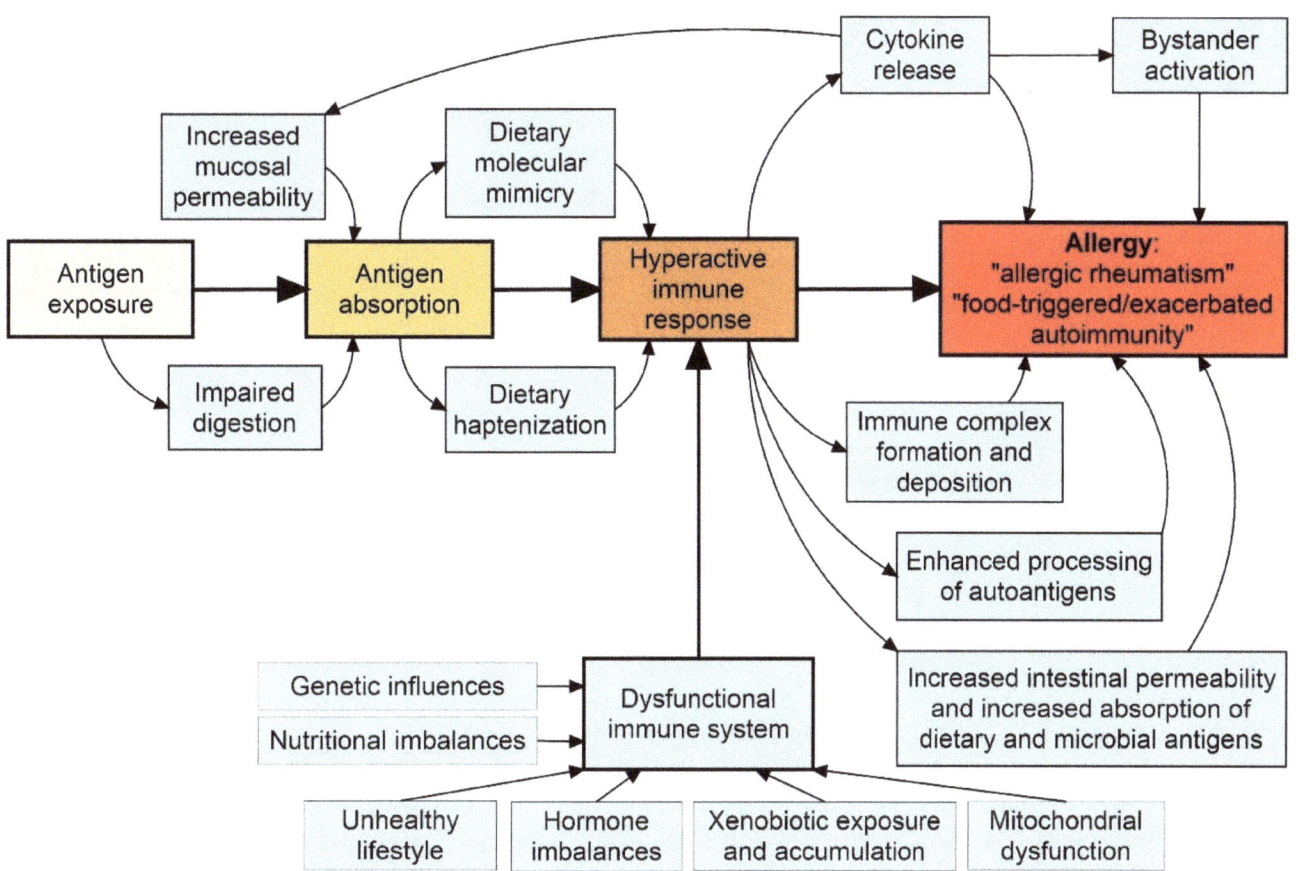

Approaching a More Comprehensive Understanding of "Food Allergy" and Its Contribution to Immune Dysfunction and Musculoskeletal Inflammation: Useful as an example of a more profound understanding of "allergy", this diagram is self-explanatory.

Common allergy treatments advocated by the pharmaceutical industry create an overly simplistic and inaccurate view of the allergic process which obfuscates the identification and correction of the underlying processes, only two of which are antigen exposure and histamine release. Nutritionally-oriented doctors, too, often emphasize the identification and elimination of allergen exposure as the sole means of addressing allergic diathesis with the presumption that allergen avoidance cures the allergy. These simplistic models and the incomplete treatments based upon them fail to address the underlying cause of the allergic phenomenon: immune dysfunction. Allergic manifestations always require at least two factors: 1) exposure of the antigen to the immune system (antigen absorption) and 2) a dysfunctional immune system that "overreacts" to the otherwise benign antigen. Allergy treatment that fails to address the underlying immune dysfunction is incomplete. Allergy treatment that addresses the underlying immune dysfunction has the opportunity to correct the *total problem*, rather than merely reducing the manifestations of the problem. Therefore, treatment of the allergic diathesis must always address issues of antigen exposure, antigen absorption, *and the dysfunctional immune system* that results in the hyperactive immune response that we call "allergy." Elimination of either antigen exposure or antigen absorption eliminates allergic manifestations, but does not necessarily correct the underlying immune defect(s). Complete correction of the underlying immune defect obviates the need for the identification and avoidance of the allergen. In clinical practice, a combination of both approaches—allergen avoidance and immune modulation—is the most effective approach, affording relatively high effectiveness in symptom reduction even with only modest compliance.

Orthomolecular Immunomodulation: The Author's Approach to Alleviating Allergy
My clinical approach to improving immune function in patients with allergy begins with supplementation of vitamin E, CoQ-10, vitamin B-12, vitamin C, bioflavonoids, honey, and fish oil. Thereafter, I look at hormones,

particularly DHEA, estrogen (quantitative and qualitative), testosterone, and cortisol. I also look at diet and bowel health with respect to putrefaction and intestinal permeability. Although rarely powerful when used in isolation, these treatments when used in combinations tailored to the individual patient often result in an impressive reduction in allergic manifestations even when allergen avoidance is either not pursued or not feasible. The process of alleviating allergic disorders is, however, arduous and time-consuming unless the doctor uses a group of protocols such as those described herein which address the most common contributing factors to allergic problems. Here I extend my previous three-step process[556] into a four-tiered approach, with the fourth step including selected pharmaceutical drugs.

Step 1: From initial patient assessment to the first phase of treatment
In a patient with presumed "allergy" who is in otherwise good health, following a basic health assessment and exclusion of significant disease, I begin by correcting problems that are common to patients with allergy. Minor improvements in allergy symptoms as a result of a low-cost low-risk interventions can be multiplied with a specified group of interventions; we aim for a modest improvement with several treatments rather than a "silver bullet" miracle cure with a single intervention. For example, 10% improvement in symptoms may be insignificant in itself; however a 10% improvement from six interventions results in a 60% improvement and enhances patient confidence long enough for other interventions and assessments to be implemented, if necessary. The goal with the first step of treatment is to correct the most common and most likely problems, namely fatty acid imbalances, micronutrient deficiencies, phytonutrient insufficiencies, and dysbiosis.

- Avoidance of suspected food allergens: The most common allergens are wheat, cow's milk, and eggs; however any patient can be allergic to any food. It is not uncommon for patients to have to avoid up to 10 foods before attaining maximal improvement, and up to 85% of migraine patients can be cured of their headaches by the use of allergy avoidance alone.[557] Food allergy avoidance for 1 month helps achieve symptomatic relief and allows the gut to heal and the immune system to recalibrate. The diet should emphasize consumption of lean meats, fruits, vegetables, nuts, seeds, and berries to ensure a systemic anti-inflammatory effect and increased consumption of anti-inflammatory phytonutrients, especially flavonoids. High-glycemic foods are avoided as are "food additives" such as tartrazine, which is known to exacerbate allergic asthma. Some foods like tuna, certain cheeses and wines are high in histamine; frequent consumption of these foods by an allergic individual is analogous to adding fuel to a fire that the patient is simultaneously trying to extinguish. Recall that in breast-feeding infants, the mother will have to consume a hypoallergenic diet to prevent passage of allergens[558] and allergen-antibody immune complexes[559] in breast milk.
- Rotation diet: While select foods should be completely avoided, the remaining foods that are consumed should be rotated in and out of the diet with a periodicity of 3-5 days. Patients should avoid "dietary monotony"[560] by consuming a variety of foods. By rotating different foods in and out of the diet, patients are more likely to consume a nutritious diet and are less likely to develop or perpetuate food allergies.
- Probiotics: Supplementation with probiotics (beneficial strains of bacteria and yeast) appears to improve intestinal barrier function, promote microecological balance in the gastrointestinal tract, modulate immune function—specifically by inducing the Treg phenotype, and thus reduce manifestations of allergic disease.[561,562,563]

---

[556] Vasquez A. Improving neuromusculoskeletal health by optimizing immune function and reducing allergic reactions. *Nutritional Perspectives* 2005; October: 27-35, 40
[557] Grant EC. Food allergies and migraine. *Lancet.* 1979 May 5;1(8123):966-9
[558] "In all, clinical disappearance of symptoms was observed after removal of milk from the mother's diet and/or elimination from the child's diet of any cow's-milk-based hypoallergenic formula." Barau E, Dupont C. Allergy to cow's milk proteins in mother's milk or in hydrolyzed cow's milk infant formulas as assessed by intestinal permeability measurements. *Allergy.* 1994 Apr;49(4):295-8
[559] The finding of egg-allergen immune complex in breast milk implies 1) egg protein escapes complete digestion/degradation in the gastrointestinal tract, 2) egg protein is absorbed intact through the mucosa, 3) egg protein escapes filtration by the liver, 4) egg protein stimulates formation IgA immune complexes, and 5) egg-IgA immune complexes are secreted in milk which would then expose the infant to both allergen and immune complex, possibly resulting in clinical disease. Hirose J, et al. Occurrence of the major food allergen, ovomucoid, in human breast milk as an immune complex. *Biosci Biotechnol Biochem.* 2001 Jun;65(6):1438-40
[560] Pelchat ML, Schaefer S. Dietary monotony and food cravings in young and elderly adults. *Physiol Behav.* 2000 Jan;68(3):353-9
[561] Majamaa H, Isolauri E. Probiotics: a novel approach in the management of food allergy. *J Allergy Clin Immunol* 1997 Feb;99(2):179-85
[562] von der Weid T, Ibnou-Zekri N, Pfeifer A. Novel probiotics for the management of allergic inflammation. *Dig Liver Dis.* 2002 Sep;34 Suppl 2:S25-8
[563] "The administration of probiotics, strains of bacteria from the healthy human gut microbiota, have been shown to stimulate antiinflammatory, tolerogenic immune responses, the lack of which has been implied in the development of atopic disorders. Thus probiotics may prove beneficial in the prevention and alleviation of allergic disease." Rautava S, Isolauri E. The development of gut immune responses and gut microbiota: effects of probiotics in prevention and treatment of allergic disease. *Curr Issues Intest Microbiol.* 2002 Mar;3(1):15-22

- Vitamin C: A recent clinical trial showed that 2 grams per day of ascorbic acid reduced blood histamine levels by 38%.[564] Cathcart hypothesized that high doses of vitamin C (i.e., bowel tolerance) may impair the adsorption of IgE with allergens and thus retard the allergic cascade from being initiated.[565] Either of these two mechanisms, perhaps in addition to other mechanisms, may explain the anti-allergy effects of ascorbic acid.[566]
- CoQ-10: CoQ-10 levels are low in approximately 40% of patients with allergies, according to a small study conducted by Folkers and Pfeiffer.[567] Asthmatics also have lower levels of CoQ-10 compared to healthy people.[568] In my experience, clinical improvement is commonly seen in allergic patients after supplementation with CoQ-10. I generally prescribe 100-300mg/day of CoQ-10 for adults.

> **CoQ-10 for allergy treatment**
> The mechanisms involved with this benefit are likely mediated primarily via improved mitochondrial function which ultimately manifests as reduced inflammation, oxidant stress, and enhanced Treg formation, as well as direct inhibition of NFkB by CoQ-10.

- Vitamin E: Vitamin E has been shown to reduce IgE levels in humans and to reduce the manifestations of allergy-related disease.[569] I commonly prescribe 800-2,000 IU per day of mixed tocopherols with approximately 40% gamma tocopherol for patients with allergy.
- Bioflavonoids: Bioflavonoids stabilize mast cell membranes and thus reduce the liberation of histamine. Additionally, quercetin and catechin inhibit the action of histidine decarboxylase, which converts histidine into histamine. Many fruits, vegetables, and herbal teas are excellent sources of flavonoids, which can also be consumed in the form of tablets and capsules.
- Vitamin B-12: Vitamin B-12 has been shown to reduce physiologic manifestations of allergy in ovalbumin-sensitized mice.[570] Since vitamin B-12 is safe, non-toxic, and bioavailable when administered orally in large doses to humans, I commonly prescribe 2,500-5,000 mcg per day for allergic patients for a one-month trial. Although the benefit of vitamin B-12 in patients with sulfite-sensitive asthma is biochemically mediated rather than immunologically mediated[571], this research adds tangential support to the use of high-dose vitamin B-12 in selected patients with allergy (particularly asthma), at least for a short-term clinical trial. Hydroxocobalamin and methylcobalamin are preferred over cyanocobalamin due to the content of cyanide in the latter.[572]

Step 2: Additional interventions for moderate or unresponsive allergies: For patients who do not respond sufficiently to the first phase of treatment, the following interventions can be considered.
- Pancreatic and proteolytic enzymes: Pancreatic enzymes have been shown to alleviate symptoms of food allergy in a controlled clinical trial.[573] Administration of enzyme preparations can alleviate intestinal and extra-intestinal manifestations of food allergy.[574] Proteolytic enzymes are safe and effective for the relief of musculoskeletal pain, as reviewed later in this text and elsewhere.[575] When taken with food, pancreatic/proteolytic enzymes facilitate hydrolysis of proteins, fats, and carbohydrates and are then absorbed into the systemic circulation for an anti-inflammatory effect. Although individual enzymes may be used in isolation, enzyme therapy is generally delivered in the form of polyenzyme preparations containing pancreatin, bromelain, papain, amylase, lipase, trypsin and alpha-chymotrypsin.

---

[564] "Chemotaxis was inversely correlated to blood histamine (r = -0.32, p = 0.045), and, compared to baseline and withdrawal values, histamine levels were depressed 38% following VC supplementation. ... These data indicate that VC may indirectly enhance chemotaxis by detoxifying histamine in vivo." Johnston CS, Martin LJ, Cai X. Antihistamine effect of supplemental ascorbic acid and neutrophil chemotaxis. *J Am Coll Nutr*. 1992 Apr;11(2):172-6
[565] "Allergic and sensitivity reactions are frequently ameliorated and sometimes completely blocked by massive doses of ascorbate. I now hypothesize that one mechanism in blocking of allergic symptoms is the reducing of the disulfide bonds between the chains in antibody molecules making their bonding antigen impossible." Cathcart RF 3rd. The vitamin C treatment of allergy and the normally unprimed state of antibodies. *Med Hypotheses*. 1986 Nov;21(3):307-21
[566] Bucca C, Rolla G, Oliva A, Farina JC. Effect of vitamin C on histamine bronchial responsiveness of patients with allergic rhinitis. *Ann Allergy*. 1990 Oct;65(4):311-4
[567] Ye CQ, et al. A modified determination of coenzyme Q10 in human blood and CoQ10 blood levels in diverse patients with allergies. *Biofactors*. 1988 Dec;1(4):303-6
[568] Gazdik F, et al. Decreased levels of coenzyme Q(10) in patients with bronchial asthma. *Allergy*. 2002 Sep;57(9):811-4
[569] Tsoureli-Nikita E, et al. Evaluation of dietary intake of vitamin E in the treatment of atopic dermatitis. *Int J Dermatol*. 2002 Mar;41(3):146-50
[570] "We infer that Cbl administration significantly reduced the IL-2 concentration, and secondarily the IL-4, IgE and histamine concentrations." Funada U, Wada M, Kawata T, Tanaka N, Tadokoro T, Maekawa A. Effect of cobalamin on the allergic response in mice. *Biosci Biotechnol Biochem* 2000 Oct;64(10):2053-8
[571] Anibarro B, et al. Asthma with sulfite intolerance in children: a blocking study with cyanocobalamin. *J Allergy Clin Immunol*. 1992 Jul;90(1):103-9
[572] Freeman AG. Cyanocobalamin--a case for withdrawal: discussion paper. *J R Soc Med*. 1992 Nov;85(11):686-7
[573] Raithel M, Weidenhiller M, Schwab D, Winterkamp S, Hahn EG. Pancreatic enzymes: a new group of antiallergic drugs? *Inflamm Res*. 2002 Apr;51 Suppl 1:S13-4
[574] Gaby AR. Pancreatic enzymes block food allergy reactions. *Townsend Letter for Doctors and Patients* townsendletter.com/Nov_2002/gabyliteraturereview1102.htm
[575] Vasquez A. Improving overall health while safely and effectively treating musculoskeletal pain. *Nutritional Perspectives* 2005; 28: 34-38, 40-42

- NFkB inhibitors: The clinical significance of NFkB and its phytonutritional modulation is detailed later in this book and elsewhere.[576] Nutrients that can be used to downregulate inflammatory responses are vitamin D, curcumin (requires piperine for absorption), lipoic acid, green tea, rosemary, grape seed extract, propolis, resveratrol, selenium, zinc, and N-acetyl-cysteine.
- Eradication of harmful intestinal yeast, bacteria, and other "parasites": I have seen several patients become cured of their "allergies" once we eradicated the dysbiotic bacteria, yeast, amoebas, or other microorganisms from their gastrointestinal tract. Intestinal colonization with harmful bacteria/yeast/protozoa/amebas can cause mucosal injury and result in macromolecular absorption and thus promotes immune sensitization to dietary antigens; in these situations, correction of dysbiosis via eradication of harmful microorganisms can lead to an impressive reduction in food-associated allergic phenomena. Although many indirect mechanisms will be discussed later, the most direct means by which dysbiosis may contribute to "allergy" is via endogenous formation of histamine via bacterial histidine decarboxylase. Galland and Lee[577] reported that eradication of *Giardia lamblia* in patients with chronic digestive complaints lessened the severity of food intolerance/allergy in 54% of patients. The supremely important topic of gastrointestinal dysbiosis is detailed later in this chapter.

Step 3: Treatment for severe allergies: For some patients with severe allergies, we start with selected treatments from Step 2 or Step 3 on the first visit *in addition to* the treatments included in Step 1. Implementation is customized based on history, examination, laboratory findings, and the doctor's experience and good judgment.
- Calcium and magnesium butyrate: Butyrate is a short-chain fatty acid which can be obtained from 1) a limited number of foods, namely butter, 2) intestinal fermentation of carbohydrates by probiotic bacteria, and 3) use of nutritional supplements. It is increasingly well-established that probiotic bacteria have immune-normalizing and "anti-allergy" effects, and this benefit is probably mediated at least in part by probiotic production of butyrate. The mechanisms of the anti-allergy effect of butyrate are manifold, and as a fatty acid butyrate activates peroxisome-proliferator activated receptor-alpha (PPAR-alpha) and thereby results in an immunomodulatory action and a suppressive effect on NFkB.[578,579] Butyrate is also a primary fuel for enterocytes and may improve enterocyte metabolism for the normalization of intestinal permeability. In the treatment of patients with inflammatory bowel disease, 4 grams per day of orally administered butyrate salts safely improves the action of mesalamine[580] as does topical application of butyrate in distal ulcerative colitis.[581] As a normal dietary component and product of the gastrointestinal tract, supplemental calcium and magnesium salts of butyrate are safe and effective for human consumption at doses of 1,000 – 4,500 mg butyrate per day for the alleviation of allergic diseases.[582,583]
- Purified chondroitin sulfate and glucosamine sulfate: Doctors and patients everywhere should already know that chondroitin sulfate and glucosamine sulfate are safe and effective for the treatment of osteoarthritis. Furthermore, purified chondroitin sulfate is cardioprotective and that it helps to reduce the vessel occlusion characteristic of atherosclerosis.[584] Additionally, new experimental evidence shows that chondroitin sulfate and glucosamine sulfate can inhibit allergic reactions.[585] With this in mind, it is reasonable to speculate that many arthritic patients who respond to glucosamine and chondroitin may actually be responding to the anti-allergy benefits of chondroitin and glucosamine *rather than* or *in addition to* the "cartilage building" properties of these supplements. Furthermore, there is evidence that purified chondroitin sulfate can act as a "decoy" and reduce adhesion of harmful bacteria; the role of harmful gastrointestinal bacteria in the genesis and perpetuation of joint pain and inflammation will be discussed in the next article in this series. For now, it will suffice to say that occult gastrointestinal infections (i.e.,

---

[576] Vasquez A. Nutritional and botanical inhibition of NFkB, the major intracellular amplifier of the inflammatory cascade. *Nutritional Perspectives*, July 2005:5-12.
[577] Galland L, Lee M. Abstract #170 High frequency of giardiasis in patients with chronic digestive complaints. *Am J Gastroenterol* 1989;84:1181
[578] Zapolska-Downar D, Siennicka A, Kaczmarczyk M, Kolodziej B, Naruszewicz M. Butyrate inhibits cytokine-induced VCAM-1 and ICAM-1 expression in cultured endothelial cells: the role of NFkB and PPARalpha. *J Nutr Biochem*. 2004 Apr;15(4):220-8
[579] Luhrs H, et al. Butyrate inhibits NFkB activation in lamina propria macrophages of patients with ulcerative colitis. *Scand J Gastroenterol*. 2002 Apr;37(4):458-66
[580] Vernia P, et al. Combined oral sodium butyrate and mesalazine treatment compared to oral mesalazine alone in ulcerative colitis. *Dig Dis Sci*. 2000 May;45:976-81
[581] Vernia P, et al. Topical butyrate improves efficacy of 5-ASA in refractory distal ulcerative colitis: results of a multicentre trial. *Eur J Clin Invest*. 2003 Mar;33(3):244-8
[582] Neesby TE. Method for desensitizing the gastrointestinal tract from food allergies. United States Patent 4,721,716. January 26, 1988
[583] Neesby TE. Method for desensitizing the gastrointestinal tract from food allergies. United States Patent 4,735,967. April 5, 1988
[584] Morrison LM, Enrick N. Coronary heart disease: reduction of death rate by chondroitin sulfate A. *Angiology*. 1973 May;24(5):269-87
[585] Theoharides TC, Bielory L. Mast cells and mast cell mediators as targets of dietary supplements. *Ann Allergy Asthma Immunol*. 2004 Aug;93(2 Suppl 1):S24-34

gastrointestinal dysbiosis) are a major contributor to the systemic pain and inflammation seen in conditions such as rheumatoid arthritis and ankylosing spondylitis.
- Hormones: DHEA, progesterone, testosterone, and cortisol tend to be lower in allergic/autoimmune individuals than in healthy controls. I use either serum testing and/or 24-hour urine samples before prescribing hormones, though I will empirically use progesterone in a woman or a 3-month trial of DHEA in a man with allergies if I find sufficient indications and no contraindications. Treatment is customized per patient. I discuss the hormonal contributions to autoimmunity later in this chapter under the heading of "orthoendocrinology." As I have noted previously[586], much of what applies to "allergy" also applies to "autoimmunity" and *vice versa*; they are both manifestations of immune dysfunction.

> **Nutritional immunomodulation for the treatment of "allergies"**
>
> Very importantly, the new treatment approach of "nutritional immunomodulation" as described in this textbook is a very important advance in the treatment of allergic conditions; this approach stimulates phenotypic switching in favor of regulatory T-cells (Treg) and thereby supports natural, endogenous anti-inflammatory anti-allergy anti-autoimmune benefits. This current section outlines my anti-allergy approach as originally printed in 2005-2006 and while still useful, it should be used in conjunction with the more advanced information now presented in this book generally (with an emphasis on antidysbiotic and orthoendocrinology interventions) and with the most recent version of the nutritional immunomodulation protocol.
>
> Vasquez A. Improving neuromusculoskeletal health by optimizing immune function and reducing allergic reactions: a review of 16 treatments and a 3-step clinical approach. *Nutritional Perspectives* 2005; Oct

Step 4: Drug treatments: We must acknowledge a place for drug therapy in patients with recalcitrant or severe allergies.
- Prednisone: For patients with allergies that are inconsolable, prednisone becomes a reasonable consideration. The lowest effective dose should be used for the shortest possible period of time. Discontinuation of treatment that has lasted longer than 4 days must be gradual in order to avoid adrenal insufficiency. Topical rather than systemic therapy should be used when appropriate.
- Sodium cromoglycate: Cromoglycate is a mast cell stabilizer which can be applied nasally for allergic rhinitis (Nasalcrom) or taken orally (Gastrocrom) by patients with food allergy to inhibit the local response to type-1 allergies.[587] The drug is poorly absorbed; therefore its anti-allergy effect is mediated at the gastrointestinal mucosa even though the benefits are systemic. Although not officially "approved" in the US for the treatment of food allergy, numerous studies support its use for this purpose.[588] Cromoglycate has been shown to reduce allergy-induced migraine[589] and eczema[590] and prevent the formation of immune complexes following the consumption of allergenic foods. In addition to preventing the allergic phenomena related directly to the consumption of allergenic foods, an additional mechanism of action of sodium cromoglycate is probably that it reduces the allergy-induced increase in intestinal permeability[591] and thereby prohibits absorption of bacterial and other microbial antigens and metabolites; stated differently, some of the manifestations attributed to "food allergy" are probably not mediated by the response to food allergens directly but result from the adverse immunologic and metabolic responses toward gut-derived microbial antigens and metabolites which are absorbed in increased amounts following the consumption of allergenic foods which increase intestinal permeability and absorption of "foreign" and "toxic" intraluminal contents which would have otherwise been excluded. Common doses for children are 100 mg 30 minutes before food (up to 400 mg per day) and 100-200 mg qid for adults 30 minutes before meals. Capsules or ampules should be mixed in plain water before consumption.

---

[586] Vasquez A. "Inflammation and Autoimmunity: A Functional Medicine Approach." David S. Jones, MD (Editor-in-Chief). *Textbook of Functional Medicine*. Gig Harbor, WA; Institute for Functional Medicine: 2006, pages 409-417. These ideas have been further developed in my own books and presentations.
[587] drugs.com/MMX/Cromolyn_Sodium.html Accessed November 24, 2005
[588] "Both the clinician's and patient's preferences and the clinician's evaluation of the specific response to challenge showed a significant benefit from SCG." Dannaeus A, Foucard T, Johansson SG. The effect of orally administered sodium cromoglycate on symptoms of food allergy. *Clin Allergy*. 1977 Mar;7(2):109-15
[589] "Immune complexes were not produced in those patients who were protected by sodium cromoglycate. These observations confirm that a food-allergic reaction is the cause of migraine in this group of patients." Monro J, Carini C, Brostoff J. Migraine is a food-allergic disease. *Lancet*. 1984 Sep 29;2(8405):719-21
[590] "The same atopic patients pretreated with oral sodium cromoglycate had less antigen entry, diminished immune-complex formation, and no atopic symptoms." Paganelli R, Levinsky RJ, Brostoff J, Wraith DG. Immune complexes containing food proteins in normal and atopic subjects after oral challenge and effect of sodium cromoglycate on antigen absorption. *Lancet*. 1979 Jun 16;1(8129):1270-2
[591] "It is suggested that a local IgE-mediated mechanism acts as a "trigger" for the entry of antigen and the formation of immune complexes by altering the permeability of the gut mucosa. The resulting delayed onset symptoms could be viewed as a form of serum sickness with few or many target organs affected." Carini C, Brostoff J, Wraith DG. IgE complexes in food allergy. *Ann Allergy*. 1987 Aug;59(2):110-7

- Leukotriene antagonists: Montelukast (Singulair®, Merck) is an orally active leukotriene receptor antagonist that blocks leukotriene D4 from the cysteinyl leukotriene CysLT-1 receptor and thereby reduces vasodilation, eosinophilic inflammation, and vascular hyperpermeability. Montelukast is used in the medical treatment of asthma, rhinitis, and eczema.

Objective means for the identification of allergens: skin-prick testing, serum IgE and IgG assays, double-blind placebo-controlled food challenges, and the elimination and challenge technique
- Skin prick testing: IgE-dependent immediate-onset allergies as assessed with a skin-prick test are indicative of immediate-onset allergy to the particular allergen, and provide the identity of the allergen, quantification of the severity of the allergic response, *and evidence of underlying immune dysfunction*. Skin-prick testing does not assess for delayed-onset allergies, thus leaving at least one class of adverse food reactions literally unassessed.
- Allergen-specific serum levels of IgE and IgG: Elevated serum levels of IgE and IgG, which are identified as specific for certain foods, also provide the identity of the allergen *and evidence of underlying immune dysfunction*. These "objective" tools are part of the clinician's repertoire for identifying food allergens, while keeping in mind that both skin-prick testing and serum testing are prone to both false positives and false negatives. Serum IgE testing does not assess IgG-mediated allergies, nor does it assess for sensitivity (immune but not immunoglobulin-mediated responses) or intolerance, which tends to be biochemical rather than immunologic. IgG assays and the subclasses of IgG-4 assays have not gained acceptance for their sensitivity or specificity, even though clinicians order them and patients pay for them.
- Double-blind placebo-controlled food challenge: Another commonly mentioned objective means for identifying food allergens is the "double-blind placebo-controlled food challenge" (DBPCFC) wherein food is administered a double-blind fashion with placebo control generally via either capsules or nasogastric tube. Unfortunately, DBPCFC is commonly considered the gold standard for the identification of particular allergens and the establishment of an allergic diathesis. This is unfortunate because the hospital admission and associated costs are expensive, cumbersome and therefore inaccessible for most patients. Some patients will have a false-negative response when challenged with isolated foods because of the lack of "accessory antigens", "accomplice antigens", or "bystander antigens."[592] Some patients will have adverse food reactions only when foods are eaten either with *high frequency* or in *specific combinations* or when *gastrointestinal problems* (e.g., dysbiosis or increased intestinal permeability) are present at the same time as the food challenge. For example, while the patient may tolerate eggs alone and wheat alone without the manifestation of allergic symptoms, the additive insult of the combination of both eggs and wheat may cause sufficient intestinal damage and/or immune activation that clinical manifestations become apparent. With single food challenges given with **DBPCFC**, "real life" situations are not reproduced, and false negative results may erroneously suggest that either the patient has no allergies or that a particular food is not offensive.
- Elimination and challenge: The "**elimination and challenge**" technique (more accurately described as "avoidance and challenge") requires that the patient first clear the diet of all possible offending foods, either by **fasting** or by **consuming a simple diet of unlikely-to-be-allergenic foods**, such as the classic triad of rice, lamb, and pears or a relatively hypoallergenic hydrolyzed formula such as Vivonex. After 7-14 days of elimination (i.e., avoidance) *and the clearing of symptoms thought to be allergy-mediated*, an offending food is reintroduced by intense consumption (i.e., eaten with every meal) for a period of up to two days. Every two to four days, a new food is added back into the diet, and a correlation is searched for between consumption of a given food and the exacerbation of symptoms. If the symptoms do not abate or disappear with the fasting/elimination phase, then confirming the nature of the disorder as allergic is more difficult and determining the identity of the allergen is additionally unlikely. However, in some cases, clinical signs and symptoms that are indeed allergy-mediated will fail to regress significantly during the brief washout period. This is because the underlying tissue damage is too great to be healed in such a short time. A good example is the thyroid disease induced by gluten-containing grains in people with the severe gluten allergy called

---

[592] "The mechanisms of enhanced permeability to specific and bystander antigens have been delineated as well as the molecular events involved in the sequential phases of allergic reactions." Heyman M. Gut barrier dysfunction in food allergy. *Eur J Gastroenterol Hepatol*. 2005 Dec;17(12):1279-1285

celiac disease; simply avoiding gluten for 1-2 weeks does not restore endocrine function because the body needs more time to reacquire homeostasis and to heal injured tissues. A common scenario is one in which symptoms remit during fasting/elimination and then return *gradually* rather than *immediately* when the offending food is eaten. In these situations, the most likely explanations are either 1) a threshold of time was necessary for physiologic abnormalities (e.g., immune complex deposition, increased intestinal permeability, dysbiosis, accumulative immune stimulation) to culminate in the reproduction of symptoms, or 2) synergistic factors may have to be combined in order to produce the symptoms of allergy, such as the induction of IgE-mediated increased intestinal permeability by food R which then leads to the increased absorption of food S, to which the peripheral immune system then responds with an IgG-mediated reaction with resultant clinical manifestations. In the latter case, food R or food S *when eaten alone or on a rotation basis* may be insufficient to produce allergic manifestations, but the combination of R+S, which would not be identified with skin-prick testing, serum tests, or one-at-a-time DBPCFC, may produce allergic manifestations. Since, in real life, foods are eaten in combination when they cause allergic disease (e.g. a headache or joint pain after eating a hamburger with wheat/gluten, cheese/milk, mayonnaise/egg, and pickle/tartrazine/yeast), a reasonable conclusion is that foods will have to be avoided in specific combinations to attain maximal improvement in allergic symptoms since complex foods probably work synergistically to produce allergic manifestations in affected people. Creating chronological distance between the consumption of allergenic foods explains the success of the **rotation diets** in alleviating allergic manifestations, but it does little to address the underlying immune dysfunction other than to reduce the total allergenic load to which the immune system is exposed. **Intestinal dysbiosis** can also increase intestinal permeability and result in increased absorption of food antigens and depletion of detoxification co-factors, which can mimic or perpetuate immune-mediated food allergies; correction of the dysbiosis can (*begin to* or *immediately*) normalize immune function and eliminate symptoms *attributed to* or *triggered by* the consumption of specific foods.

Objective Assessments for Adverse Food Reactions—A Quick Clinical Guide

	Advantages	Disadvantages
Skin-prick testing	<ul><li>Proves presence of allergic diathesis.</li><li>Identifies allergen that is being responded to by IgE-mediated reaction.</li><li>Can be used for both food and inhalant allergies.</li></ul>	<ul><li>Numerically impossible to test for all probable allergens due to method of testing, which can be quite painful</li><li>Allergen preparations may not contain full spectrum of immunogenic epitopes that are present in "real food" thus patient may not respond to offensive food, resulting in clinically relevant false negative results.</li><li>Subcutaneous injection is not the natural or physiologic route of allergen exposure.</li><li>Does not assess for IgG or other delayed-onset allergies, thus resulting in clinically relevant false negative results.</li><li>Does not assess for reactions that are mediated by immune complexes, thus resulting in clinically relevant false negative results.</li><li>Procedure is moderately expensive.</li><li>Does not assess for intolerances or biochemical perturbations, thus resulting in clinically relevant false negative results.</li></ul>
Serum IgE assay	<ul><li>Identifies allergen that is being responded to by IgE-mediated reaction.</li><li>Can be used for both food and inhalant allergies.</li><li>Procedure is relatively painless and provides "objective evidence" of food allergies.</li></ul>	<ul><li>Numerically impossible to test for all probable allergens due to method of testing.</li><li>Allergen preparations may not contain full spectrum of immunogenic epitopes that are present in "real food" thus patient may not respond to offensive food, resulting in clinically relevant false negative results.</li><li>Does not assess for IgG or other delayed-onset allergies, thus resulting in clinically relevant false negative results.</li><li>Does not assess for reactions that are mediated by IgG, IgM, or IgA immune complexes, thus resulting in clinically relevant false-negative results.</li><li>Does not assess for intolerances or biochemical perturbations, thus resulting in clinically relevant false negative results.</li></ul>
Serum IgG4 assay	<ul><li>Identifies allergen that is being responded to by IgG-mediated reaction.</li><li>Mostly used in an attempt to identify delayed-onset food allergies.</li><li>Procedure is relatively painless.</li><li>Procedure provides "objective evidence" of food allergies.</li></ul>	<ul><li>Numerically impossible to test for all probable allergens due to method of testing.</li><li>Allergen preparations may not contain full spectrum of immunogenic epitopes that are present in "real food" thus patient may not respond to offensive food, resulting in clinically relevant false negative results.</li><li>Does not assess for IgE or other immediate-onset allergies, thus resulting in clinically relevant false negative results.</li><li>Does not assess for reactions that are mediated by immune complexes, thus resulting in clinically relevant false negative results.</li><li>Procedure is moderately expensive.</li><li>Does not assess for intolerances or biochemical perturbations, thus resulting in clinically relevant false negative results.</li><li>The clinical relevance of IgG4 antibodies to food is controversial.[593]</li></ul>

---

[593] "...it seems unlikely that increased IgG4 antibody levels against egg white is a cause of egg hypersensitivity, and one should pay much attention to IgG1 antibodies ...it is possible that increased IgG4 may reduce the effect of complement-fixing antibodies like IgG1 and/or interfere the action of IgE antibodies." Nakagawa T. Egg white-specific IgE and IgG subclass antibodies and their associations with clinical egg hypersensitivity. *N Engl Reg Allergy Proc.* 1988 Jan-Feb;9(1):67-73

Objective Assessments for Adverse Food Reactions—A Quick Clinical Guide *continued*

	Advantages	Disadvantages
Double-blind placebo-controlled food challenges	<ul><li>Allows for control of interfering factors.</li><li>Removes psychological cues and triggers that can be mistakenly interpreted as adverse food reactions.</li><li>Procedure provides "objective evidence" of food allergies.</li></ul>	<ul><li>Setting and experiment are artificial and not representative of the real environment in which the patient lives and is exposed to allergen(s).</li><li>Testing of single antigens alone is not reflective of real life wherein antigens are consumed in combination.</li><li>Numerically impossible to test for all probable allergens due to method of testing.</li><li>Allergen preparations may not contain full spectrum of immunogenic epitopes that are present in "real food" thus patient may not respond to offensive food, resulting in clinically relevant false negative results.</li><li>Procedure is time-consuming and cumbersome and requires the preparation of both food challenge and placebo, which are administered either by capsules or by nasogastric tube.</li><li>Due to small quantity of allergen and limited time of observation, does not assess for reactions that are quantity-dependent, delayed-onset, or mediated by immune complexes, thus resulting in clinically relevant false negative results.</li><li>Procedure is moderately expensive.</li><li>Does not assess for intolerances or biochemical perturbations, thus resulting in clinically relevant false negative results.</li></ul>
Elimination and challenge	<ul><li>Represents "real life" situations with psychological influences, daily stress, and combinations of foods.</li><li>No financial cost.</li><li>Easy to implement for motivated patients.</li><li>Trains patients to be active in their healthcare and to learn how to diagnose and treat themselves—the true goals of wellness promotion.</li><li>Allows patients and clinicians to assess for dysbiotic food reactions secondary to nonspecific SIBO (e.g., bloating and flatulence), H2S toxicity secondary to sulfur-reducing bacteria (e.g., myalgia, dyscognition, hypothermia), or D-lactate toxicity (e.g., headache and dyscognition).</li></ul>	<ul><li>Compliance is a challenge for unmotivated or undisciplined patients.</li><li>Identification of offending allergen may take time and repeated cycles of elimination and challenge before the allergen is conclusively identified.</li></ul>

❶ Food ❷ Infections ❸ Nutri-immunomod ❹ Dysmetab ❺ Stress/Sleep/Socio/Surg/Sup ❻ Endo ❼ Xeno

❷ Infections & Dysbiosis:
Subclinical Infections & Persistent Microbial Colonization

> **Major Concepts in this Section**
> This section reviews in detail the mechanisms by which dysbiosis—also described as multifocal polydysbiosis, subclinical infections, microbial colonizations—contributes to immune dysfunction that results in systemic inflammation generally and rheumatic diseases specifically. Understanding this section and taking appropriate clinical action is of the highest importance in the successful treatment of inflammatory/rheumatic disorders. Readers of this section must attain 1) an appreciation of the mechanisms by which microbes and their molecular effects contribute to pro-inflammatory immune dysfunction, and 2) an appreciation that exclusive therapeutic focus on the eradication of microbe is fraught with inefficacy if it fails to address the intrinsic patient-specific imbalances that allowed that individual patient to be susceptible to microbe-induced inflammation and immune imbalance. "Dysbiosis" is not simply about the effects of microbes in inflammatory disease, the detection and eradication of those microbes. Although this section focuses on microbes and their effects, detection, and treatment, the complete treatment of dysbiosis needs to contain three major components: ❶ microbe-specific treatment, ❷ restoration of immune function and other means by which to make the human host less hospitable to re-colonization, ❸ promotion of immune and inflammatory tolerance.

Multifocal Dysbiosis: A Major Promoter of Chronic Inflammation and "Autoimmunity"
Microbes contribute to noninfectious human diseases—including chronic inflammation and autoimmunity—by mechanisms which are *numerous, complex, direct* and *indirect*. For the purposes of this discussion, I will use a broad definition of dysbiosis that implies "a relationship of non-acute host-microorganism interaction that adversely affects the human host"; the subtype of dysbiosis can be distinguished based on location: gastrointestinal, orodental, sinorespiratory, genitourinary, dermal, or environmental. Patients may have more than one dysbiotic loci at a time with microbes from more than one kingdom. One of the best clinical examples of autoimmunity/inflammation perpetuated by multifocal dysbiosis is Behcet's syndrome, characterized by subclinical pulmonary infection (sinorespiratory dysbiosis) with *Chlamydia pneumonia*[594], cutaneous colonization (dermal dysbiosis) with *Staphylococcus aureus*[595], and orodental dysbiosis with *Streptococcus sanguis*.[596] Combine with multifocal dysbiosis a few pro-rheumatic genetic traits (especially HLA-B27) and subclinical proinflammatory nutritional imbalances[597], and it becomes easy to see why rheumatic diseases are generally still considered "idiopathic" when reviewed from a reductionistic medical paradigm that fails to appreciate the interconnected and "holistic" web of influences that synergize to produce systemic inflammation. For the majority of patients in outpatient clinical practice, the location of their dysbiosis is the gut, which is easily assessed with specialized stool testing and parasitology examinations, and which is easily treated with oral botanical antimicrobials and dietary modification. In my own clinical practice, I consider stool testing extremely valuable and estimate that 80% of parasitology examinations return with at least one clinically-relevant abnormality. ==I will demonstrate in this section that testing for and treating dysbiosis is absolutely essential in patients with chronic fatigue, fibromyalgia, autoimmunity, and any type of so-called "chronic inflammatory disease"==—the latter is more wisely termed ==*sustained inflammatory response*==.

Readers should appreciate that the "total dysbiotic load" (TDL) or "total microbial load" (TML) from all sources—skin, gastrointestinal tract, genitourinary tract, sinorespiratory tract, orodental cavity, environment, and

---

[594] "These finding provide serological evidence of chronic C. pneumoniae infection in association with Behcet's disease." Ayaslioglu E, Duzgun N, Erkek E, Inal A. Evidence of chronic Chlamydia pneumoniae infection in patients with Behcet's disease. *Scand J Infect Dis*. 2004;36(6-7):428-30
[595] "Staphylococcus aureus (41/70, 58.6%, p = 0.008) and Prevotella spp (17/70, 24.3%, p = 0.002) were significantly more common in pustules from BS patients..." Hatemi G, et al. The pustular skin lesions in Behcet's syndrome are not sterile. *Ann Rheum Dis*. 2004 Nov;63(11):1450-2
[596] "These data indicate that the BD patients are infected with IgA protease-producing S. sanguis strains, which cause an increase of IgA titer against these organisms and IgA protease antigen." Yokota K, Oguma K. IgA protease produced by Streptococcus sanguis and antibody production against IgA protease in patients with Behcet's disease. *Microbiol Immunol*. 1997;41(12):925-31
[597] Seaman DR. The diet-induced proinflammatory state: a cause of chronic pain and other degenerative diseases? *J Manipulative Physiol Ther*. 2002 Mar-Apr;25:168-79

any subclinical parenchymal/tissue foci—contributes to the total inflammatory load (TIL) and total xenobiotic load (TXL) which the immune system must process and which the hepatobiliary system must detoxify, respectively.

At least 70% of patients with chronic arthritis are carriers of "silent infections", according to a 1992 article published in the peer-reviewed medical journal *Annals of the Rheumatic Diseases*.[598] A 2001 article in this same journal which focused exclusively on five bacteria showed that **56% of patients with idiopathic inflammatory arthritis had gastrointestinal or genitourinary dysbiosis**.[599] Indeed, published research strongly and consistently indicates that bacteria, yeast/fungi, amebas, protozoa, and other "parasites" (rarely including helminths/worms) are underappreciated causes of neuromusculoskeletal inflammation. This section will explain the mechanisms by which **silent infections**, **noninfectious microbial colonization**, and **dysbiosis** can cause and perpetuate numerous health problems, and I will also discuss basic assessment and treatment measures that can be used clinically to help patients with microbe-induced musculoskeletal inflammation.

A problem that plagues many healthcare providers of all professions is that most doctors are still under the spell of the "Pasteurian paradigm of infectious disease", namely that pathogenic microorganisms cause *disease* by causing "*infection*." Relatedly, Koch's Postulates first published in 1884 held that "the organism must be found in all animals suffering from the disease, but not in healthy animals" and "the cultured organism should cause disease when introduced into a healthy animal."[600] Such contributions by Pasteur, Koch, and other researchers were essential in providing a preliminary understanding of the role of microorganisms in the genesis of human disease; however, we must appreciate that these simplistic, linear, and rather primitive models do not suffice for explaining all microbe-induced disorders. The major problems with the paradigms proposed by Pasteur and Koch are that both of these models fail to appreciate 1) adverse microbe-host interactions which may not *result in* nor *result from* a true "infection" (thus refuting the Pasteurian paradigm), and 2) the importance of the patient's biochemical individuality and genetic uniqueness which influence the clinical manifestations of dysbiosis-induced disease such that a) not all patients exposed to a pathogenic microbe will express the stereotypic disease, and b) some patients exposed to microorganisms that are generally considered benign commensals will produce a dramatic inflammatory response which results in clinical disease (thus refuting Koch's postulates). Supported amply by the research reviewed herein, **healthcare providers have an obligation to move beyond these simplistic "pathogenic" "infection-based" models of microorganism-induced disease to apprehend the more common "functional" disorders that can result from exposure to microbes.** Readers will note that these new concepts and ideas are amply supported by the references to the biomedical research that are included in the footnotes.[601,602]

> **Dysbiosis definitions and descriptions**
>
> **Dysbiosis**: A relationship of non-acute non-infectious host-microorganism interaction that adversely affects the human host.
>
> **Dysbiosis subtypes** (based on location):
> 1. Orodental
> 2. Sinorespiratory
> 3. Gastrointestinal
> 4. Parenchymal, tissue
> 5. Genitourinary
> 6. Cutaneous
> 7. Environmental
>
> **Multifocal dysbiosis**: A clinical condition characterized by a patient's having more than one foci/location of dysbiosis; generally the adverse physiologic and clinical consequences are additive and synergistic.
>
> **Polydysbiosis**: Concurrent dysbiosis with microbes of different species.

One of the common rhetorical positions espoused by undertrained skeptics is, "If infections caused autoimmunity, then antibiotics would cure autoimmune disease." This rhetoric is biophysiologically illogical for several reasons:

1. First, autoimmunity may be incited by microbes and then persist in the absence of those same microbes; when a hammer breaks a window, removing the hammer does not repair the window. Autoimmunity—whether induced by xenobiotics or microorganisms—may have a tendency to persist due to the immune sensitization toward autoantigens that have been haptenized, exposed, or otherwise immunogenized, and

---

[598] "At the time of initial evaluation, 57 (69%) of the patients with oligoarthritis and 4/20 (20%) of the control subjects were carriers of clinically silent infections." Weyand CM, Goronzy JJ. Clinically silent infections in patients with oligoarthritis: results of a prospective study. *Ann Rheum Dis*. 1992 Feb;51(2):253-8
[599] Fendler C, et al. Frequency of triggering bacteria in patients with reactive arthritis and undifferentiated oligoarthritis and the relative importance of the tests used for diagnosis. *Ann Rheum Dis*. 2001 Apr;60(4):337-43 ard.bmjjournals.com/cgi/content/full/60/4/337
[600] Koch's Postulates. encyclopedia.thefreedictionary.com/Koch%27s+postulates Accessed October 4, 2005
[601] Noah PW. The role of microorganisms in psoriasis. *Semin Dermatol*. 1990 Dec;9(4):269-76
[602] Samarkos M, Vaiopoulos G. The role of infections in the pathogenesis of autoimmune diseases. *Curr Drug Targets Inflamm Allergy*. 2005 Feb;4(1):99-10

due to the secondary endocrinologic changes and xenobiotic accumulation that have been induced by the disease process and which perpetuate the dysregulated proinflammatory state. The autoimmune "reactive arthritis" that follows microbial infection responds only partially to early antibiotic treatment[603], thus indicating that microbe-induced musculoskeletal inflammation—once induced—may persist despite [supposedly] effective antimicrobial treatment. **Pro-inflammatory antigens can persist in synovial immunocytes for years following a bacterial infection that results in chronic inflammatory arthritis.**[604] Conversely, the observation that antimicrobial intervention, particularly with more powerful treatments, can significantly reduce (not eliminate) the development of "autoimmune" phenomena in patients following bacterial infection[605] appears to indicate that 1) microorganisms, particularly bacteria, contribute directly to the genesis of specific inflammatory/autoimmune disorders, and that 2) antimicrobial treatment of autoimmune disorders is warranted.

> **Mechanisms of autoimmunity-induction by microorganisms**
>
> "Infectious agents can cause **autoimmune disease by different mechanisms**, which fall into two categories: *antigen specific* in which pathogen products or elements have a central role e.g. **superantigens** or epitope **(molecular) mimicry**, and *antigen non-specific* in which the pathogen provides the appropriate inflammatory setting for **bystander activation**."
>
> Samarkos, Vaiopoulos. The role of infections in the pathogenesis of autoimmune diseases. *Curr Drug Targets Inflamm Allergy*. 2005 Feb

2. Second, all clinicians are aware that no antimicrobial treatment eradicates *all* microbes from *all* surfaces; for example, an orally administered broad-spectrum antibiotic is not appropriate for eradicating a fungal infection located in the sinuses. **Microbial drug resistance is an increasingly large problem in outpatient and hospital-based medicine**[606] where antimicrobial drug therapies are the mainstay treatment of bacterial infections and no consideration is given to effective botanical antimicrobials (reviewed later) and to strengthening host defenses (described throughout this text and particularly in sections on diet and immunonutrition).

3. Third, the administration of antimicrobial therapeutics of a limited scope for a limited time may allow the dysbiosis to return when the antimicrobials are discontinued. The autoimmune condition problem may continue or recur despite even "appropriate" antimicrobial treatment if the duration of antimicrobial treatment is too brief.

4. Fourth, even when the microbe is eradicated, its antigens may persist. **Microbial antigens can persist within the human body for years following clearance of the primary infection.**[607,608,609]

5. ==Fifth, the microbe-autoimmunity model of autoimmune disease induction does not state that microbes are the *sole cause* of autoimmunity. What I have documented here with an abundance of research is that **microbes are a major contributor to autoimmunity** and that **dysbiosis works in concert with hormonal abnormalities, xenobiotic immunotoxicity, food intolerances, and a proinflammatory lifestyle which synergize to create proinflammatory immune dysfunction that happens to destroy body tissues in a phenomenon that gets labeled "autoimmunity."**==

Despite the ability of autoimmunity/inflammation to persist despite the eradication of causative microorganisms, clinicians (and patients) will be pleased to learn that effective oligomicrobial eradication can result in dramatic clinical improvements in patients with autoimmunity. This observation is not merely anecdote from practicing clinicians; **published research and relatively large clinical trials are increasingly documenting that comprehensive antimicrobial treatments do indeed *promote regression* and *initiate cure*** in a growing list of previously "untreatable" autoimmune diseases.

---

[603] Laasila K, Laasonen L, Leirisalo-Repo M. Antibiotic treatment and long term prognosis of reactive arthritis. *Ann Rheum Dis*. 2003 Jul;62(7):655-8
[604] "Extensive bacterial cultures of the synovial fluid were negative…We conclude that in patients with reactive arthritis after yersinia infection, microbial antigens can be found in synovial-fluid cells from affected joints." Granfors et al. Yersinia antigens in synovial-fluid cells from patients with reactive arthritis. *N Engl J Med* 1989;320:216-2
[605] Yli-Kerttula et al. Effect of a three month course of ciprofloxacin on the late prognosis of reactive arthritis. *Ann Rheum Dis*. 2003 Sep;62:880-4 ard.bmjjournals.com/cgi/content/full/62/9/880
[606] Sharma R, Sharma CL, Kapoor B. Antibacterial resistance: Current problems and possible solutions. *Indian J Med Sci* 2005 Dec 27;59:120-129
[607] Inman RD. Antigens, the gastrointestinal tract, and arthritis. *Rheum Dis Clin North Am*. 1991 May;17(2):309-21
[608] "These samples were studied by immunochemical techniques for the presence of Yersinia antigens at the beginning of infection and up to 4 years thereafter… This study has, for the first time, directly demonstrated that bacterial antigens persist for a long time in patients who develop ReA after Y. enterocolitica O:3 infection." Granfors K, Merilahti-Palo R, Luukkainen R, Mottonen T, Lahesmaa R, Probst P, Marker-Hermann E, Toivanen P. Persistence of Yersinia antigens in peripheral blood cells from patients with Yersinia enterocolitica O:3 infection with or without reactive arthritis. *Arthritis Rheum*. 1998 May;41(5):855-62
[609] "Extensive bacterial cultures of the synovial fluid were negative…We conclude that in patients with reactive arthritis after yersinia infection, microbial antigens can be found in synovial-fluid cells from affected joints." Granfors et al. Yersinia antigens in synovial-fluid cells from patients with reactive arthritis. *N Engl J Med* 1989;320:216-2

Dysbiotic inflammation—beyond the microbe: Often what we find when working with autoimmune/inflammatory patients is that they are having a pathogenic inflammatory response to a nonpathogenic microbe. Remember, we are not looking for classic "infection" here; we are looking to determine which underlying disruptions may be exacerbating inflammation and the patient's symptomatology. We have to look beyond the disease-associated characteristics of the microbe to see the patient's individualized response to the microbe. Dysbiosis in one patient may present with dermatitis, while [what appears to be] the same microbial imbalance in another patient can present as peripheral neuropathy or inflammatory arthritis.

Mechanisms of Autoimmune Disease Induction by Microorganisms

I have identified at least seventeen mechanisms by which microorganisms can cause immune dysfunction that promotes musculoskeletal inflammation. Each of the following exemplifies a mechanism by which microbes can cause "disease" without causing an "infection." Mechanisms by which microorganisms can contribute to musculoskeletal inflammation without causing "infection" include but are not limited to the following:

1. Molecular mimicry: Several microbes have peptides and other structures that resemble or "mimic" the peptides and cell structures found in human tissues. Thus, when the immune system fights against the microbe, the antibodies and T-cells can "cross-react" with the tissues of the human host. In this way, the immune system begins attacking the human body, which is otherwise an innocent bystander—the victim of "friendly fire."[610] As reviewed by Ringrose[611], evidence clearly indicates that specific microbial proteins have amino acid homology with human proteins and/or that homologous bacterial peptides appear to

---

[610] Wucherpfennig KW. Mechanisms for the induction of autoimmunity by infectious agents. *J Clin Invest*. 2001 Oct;108(8):1097-104 jci.org/cgi/reprint/108/8/1097
[611] Ringrose JH. HLA-B27 associated spondyloarthropathy, an autoimmune disease based on crossreactivity between bacteria and HLA-B27? *Ann Rheum Dis*. 1999 Oct;58(10):598-610 ard.bmjjournals.com/cgi/content/full/58/10/598

stimulate (auto)immunity toward similar neighboring human peptides. Therefore the two underlying bases for autoimmune induction by molecular mimicry—namely 1) homology between human and microbial amino acid sequences, and 2) stimulation of immunity against human peptides—do indeed occur *in vivo*. **Molecular mimicry is strongly implicated in the pathogenesis of reactive arthritis and ankylosing spondylitis.**[612,613]

- Psoriasis and molecular mimicry—Ex vivo experimental study using human T-cells (*Clin Exp Immunol* 1999 Sep[614]): The authors of this paper introduce their topic by noting that psoriasis is an inflammatory disease mediated largely by T-cells in the skin and that psoriasis has a strong association with infections by group-A beta-hemolytic streptococci bacteria, also known as *Streptococcus pyogenes*. The authors cite their previous work which showed that patients with active psoriasis have Th1-like cells that respond to a 20 amino acid (AA) sequence shared between a protein made by streptococcal bacteria (M protein) that has the same AA sequence as the human protein found in the skin named keratin, specifically keratin 17. ("Keratin" is a group of fibrous structural proteins forming the key structural material of the outer layer of human skin; keratin is also the key structural component of hair and nails. Keratin 17 is not expressed in normal skin except for hair follicles, sweat/sebaceous glands, and basal cells in the scalp; however, keratin 17 is expressed in suprabasal keratinocytes in lesional psoriatic skin, thus making its presence in skin a unique feature of psoriasis lesions. Increased production of keratin 17 can be induced by the pro-inflammatory cytokines gamma-interferon, which plays a key role as a mediator of psoriatic inflammation, and IL-6, which is abundant in psoriatic lesions. Langerhans cells are the dendritic cells of the epidermis; as such, they function as antigen-presenting cells (APC). Given that keratin within skin cells exists as an intracellular structural (cytoskeletal) protein, its ability to be exposed to the immune system is required for it to function as an autoantigen, a target of self-induced immunologic attack. The authors of this paper note that "cytoplasmic processes of Langerhans cells can extend into the cytoplasm of adjacent keratinocytes with frequent absence of intervening plasma membranes at the apices of these processes"; thus these epidermal APCs can uptake and present antigen via MHC class 1 and class 2 molecules to CD8 and CD4 T-cells, respectively.) These same Th1-like cells are deleted following treatment with ultraviolet B (UVB) radiation that induces clinical remission; the fact that the disappearance of these cells correlates with clinical improvement following treatment implies that these cells may have a direct causative role in the skin inflammation of psoriasis. In the ex vivo experiment, the authors took T-cells from the blood of 17 psoriatic patients and 17 healthy controls and then challenged these T-cells with keratin peptides and M-peptides to monitor for increased production of gamma-interferon [IFNg]), which implies specificity for the corresponding amino acid sequences. Results of the investigation showed that the most frequent and strongest responses were observed to a peptide from keratin 17 that shares a specific AA sequence with M-protein. Specifically, the overlapping AA sequence is A-L-E-E-A-N. In fact, T-cell responses to the ALEEAN sequence were stronger than to the corresponding M-peptide containing the ALEEAN sequence; this implies that sensitized T-cells preferentially attack keratin rather than the bacterial peptide. The ALEEAN sequence present in keratin 17 is also found in keratin subtype 14, which is overexpressed in psoriatic skin; thus, for T-cells already primed to respond to ALEEAN following exposure to *Streptococcus pyogenes*, the dual exposure to ALEEAN in keratins 14 and 17—both of which are uniquely present in psoriatic skin—may promote localized attack by T-cells against keratinocytes, i.e., immune cross-reactivity via molecular mimicry. UVB treatment abolished

Molecular mimicry in psoriatic skin and bacterial proteins
These amino acid sequences are found both in human keratin and M-protein from the bacteria *Streptococcus pyogenes*. 1. ALEEAN, 2. LRR-LD, 3. AKLEA, 4. AKLEAE. Gudmundsdottir et al. Is an epitope on keratin 17 a major target for autoreactive T lymphocytes in psoriasis? *Clin Exp Immunol*. 1999 Sep

---

[612] "HLA-B27 and proteins from enteric bacteria are structurally related, in a manner that may affect T cell response to enteric pathogens." Inman RD, Scofield RH. Etiopathogenesis of ankylosing spondylitis and reactive arthritis. *Curr Opin Rheumatol*. 1994 Jul;6(4):360-70

[613] "With respect to bacterial infection, recent findings in bacterial antigenicity, host response through interactions of antigen-presenting cells, T cells, and cytokines are providing new understanding of host-pathogen interactions and the pathogenesis of arthritis." Kim TH, Uhm WS, Inman RD. Pathogenesis of ankylosing spondylitis and reactive arthritis. *Curr Opin Rheumatol*. 2005 Jul;17(4):400-5

[614] Gudmundsdottir AS, et al. Is an epitope on keratin 17 a major target for autoreactive T lymphocytes in psoriasis? *Clin Exp Immunol*. 1999 Sep;117(3):580-6

T-cell responses to keratin and M protein, while responses to other bacterial antigens (streptokinase [SK] and streptodornase [SD]) were not affected. The authors conclude, "These findings are consistent with the notion that AA sequences which keratin has in common with M-protein may be a major target for autoreactive T cells in psoriasis." Per Table 2 of their article, 13 of 17 psoriatic patients demonstrated a T-cell response to peptide 146-K17 (from human keratins subtypes 14 and 17) contrasted to only 4 of 17 healthy controls; interestingly, three patients and eight controls showed no responses to either keratin or M protein. This lack of perfect concordance indicates that molecular mimicry and the resulting immune cross-reaction does not account for the entirety of the pathogenesis of psoriasis, or that ❶ the research methods employed in the study were imperfect resulting in a few false negatives and/or false positives, or ❷ seasonal variation in streptococcal infections caused varying intensities of immune responsiveness, ❸ seasonal vitamin D fluctuations caused varying intensities of immune responsiveness, ❹ that a variable unaccounted for (e.g., sun exposure, medication use, etc) influenced these results, or that ❺ other nonstreptococcal infections/microbes—as very well documented by Noah and colleagues[615]—and dysbiotic microbial relationships may have been causative in some cases of psoriasis. Readers and clinicians should note that the ALEEAN sequence is not the only sequence shared between human keratin and staphylococcal M-protein; other homologous sequences include LRR-LD, AKLEA, and AKLEAE.

Peptide identification and source	Peptide amino acid (AA) sequence
Peptide 146-M from *Streptococcus pyogenes*	**AKKQVEKALEEANSKLAALE**
Peptide 146-M49 from *Streptococcus pyogenes*	AKKKVEADLAEANSKLQALE
Peptide 146-K17* from human keratin subtypes 14 and 17	**SYLDKVRALEEANADLEVK**
Peptide 146-K9 from human keratin	SYLDKVQALEEANNDLENKI

Data from Figure 1 and Table 1 of Gudmundsdottir et al. *Clin Exp Immunol*. 1999 Sep;117(3):580-6
* Based on the frequency of IFN-g-producing T-cells of patients and controls after stimulation with M- and keratin peptides sharing the ALEEAN sequence, peptide 146-K17 is the only peptide which elicited significantly stronger responses in psoriatic patients than in healthy controls

- <u>Psoriasis and molecular mimicry—Psoriasis is an autoimmune disease caused in whole or in part by molecular mimicry. (*Trends Immunol* 2009 Oct[616])</u>: The authors of this paper note that T cells in psoriatic lesions are oligoclonal and that these T-cells recognize amino acid sequences (determinants) common to streptococcal M-protein and human skin keratin; they propose that CD8(+) T cells in psoriatic epidermis respond mainly to such determinants. Further, they note that streptococcal peptidoglycan may act as an adjuvant for this immune response and that, likewise, a streptococcal superantigen may promote an inflammatory/cytokine milieu that advances skin-homing of tonsillar T cells. They conclude their abstract/summary by stating that if the above bases are correct, then "tonsillectomy should be associated with fewer T cells that recognize keratin and streptococcal determinants." These conclusions are conceptually consistent with previously published literature, in particular the work of Noah and colleagues[617], which has also emphasized the microbial link to psoriasis and has noted the documented benefit of tonsillectomy. I included citation to this article for the additional reason that it is one of the first articles to boldly state *in its title* that molecular mimicry is a defining pathoetiologic aspect of psoriasis, thus emphasizing the role of this mechanism in the condition previously acquiesced by the medical profession to the realms of esotericity and idiopathicity in order to justify perpetual pharmaceuticalization of these patients.[618]

---

[615] Rosenberg EW, Noah PW, Skinner RB Jr. Microorganisms and psoriasis. *J Natl Med Assoc*. 1994 Apr;86(4):305-10
[616] Valdimarsson et al. Psoriasis--as an autoimmune disease caused by molecular mimicry. *Trends Immunol*. 2009 Oct;30(10):494-501
[617] Rosenberg EW, Noah PW, Skinner RB Jr. Microorganisms and psoriasis. *J Natl Med Assoc*. 1994 Apr;86(4):305-10
[618] Vasquez A. Twilight of the Idiopathic Era and the Dawn of New Possibilities in Health and Healthcare. *Naturopathy Digest* 2006 Mar

2. Superantigens: Many viral, bacterial, and fungal microbes produce superantigens—molecules which are capable of causing widespread, nonspecific, and unregulated proinflammatory immune activation. One of the hallmarks of superantigens is their ability to induce polyclonal T- and B-lymphocyte activation and the production of excessive levels of cytokines and other inflammatory effectors.[619] Solanki et al[620] described superantigens as "microbial or viral toxins" which behave as "immunostimulatory molecules" and "extremely potent polyclonal T-cell mitogens" which "bind major histocompatibility complex (MHC) class-II molecules without any prior processing and stimulate large number of T cells (up to 20% of all T cells)" due to "their **unique ability to cross-link MHC class II [found on antigen-presenting cells] and the T-cell receptor (TCR),** forming a trimolecular complex."; these authors concisely note that superantigens "activate antigen-presenting dendritic cells by producing increased expression of HLA-DR antigen and co-stimulatory molecules (CD54, CD83 and CD86) and the production of tumor necrosis factor TNF-alpha [as well as TNF-beta, IL-2, and gamma-interferon]." Obviously, when the body is in such a state of unregulated inflammation *combined with simultaneous bacterial antigen presentation*, inevitably some of this inflammation will affect the structures of the musculoskeletal system especially because articular tissues are predisposed to immune attack due to their proclivity to retain antigens and immune complexes[621,622]; the resulting inflammatory response is further exaggerated/exacerbated by superantigen-driven immunostimulation. Several research groups have found evidence of superantigen involvement in the pathogenesis of rheumatoid arthritis.[623,624] Superantigens can be categorized as ❶ **endogenous superantigens**—these are encoded by viruses such as Epstein-Barr virus, ❷ **exogenous superantigens**—these are elaborated by bacteria and include staphylococcal enterotoxins and streptococcal pyrogenic exotoxins, and ❸ **B-cell superantigens**—these predominantly stimulate B-cells to produce antibodies/immunoglobulins; an example of a B-cell superantigen is staphylococcal proteins A and Fv. Very noteworthy is the fact that superantigens, which are directly immunologically active at very low concentrations, are resistant to degradation by protein-digesting enzymes (proteases) and that they are absorbed intact directly through the skin and mucosal surfaces; therefore, a direct positive relationship is likely to exist between microbial production and physiologic effects of superantigens.

> **Important concepts about superantigens**
> Bacteria and other microorganisms (microbes) can each produce several—not just one—superantigens. The implications are that 1) one single microbe can promote inflammation and immune dysfunction via elaboration of several different superantigens, and that 2) researchers have to test for several superantigens per microbe per patient per disease in order to fully appreciate the role of a microbe's superantigen repertoire in association with a particular disease. Further adding to the complexity of these associations is the fact that other molecules—beside and beyond the classic/known/prototypic superantigens—can also contribute to pro-inflammatory immune dysfunction; bacterial DNA is known to be immunostimulatory.

- Skin disorders and superantigens—Superantigens in dermatologic diseases. (*Dermatology Online Journal* 2008 Feb[625]): In this excellent review of molecular biology and clinical disorders, the authors note that microbial superantigens are associated with many important clinical disease that affect the skin, including staphylococcal toxic shock syndrome, staphylococcal scalded skin syndrome, guttate psoriasis, psoriasis vulgaris (chronic plaque psoriasis), Kawasaki syndrome, atopic dermatitis, cutaneous T-cell lymphoma, and acute juvenile pityriasis rubra pilaris. The authors state, "Evidence shows that T-cells in psoriasis are triggered by conventional antigens and superantigens. It is suggested that although **the process is initiated by bacterial superantigens, molecular mimicry**

---

[619] "The basis of autoimmune disorders due to superantigen is due to greater stimulation of T-lymphocytes and elaborate cytokine production." Hemalatha V, Srikanth P, Mallika M. Superantigens - Concepts, clinical disease and therapy. *Indian J Med Microbiol* 2004;22:204-211
[620] Solanki LS, Srivastava N, Singh S. Superantigens: a brief review with special emphasis on dermatologic diseases. *Dermatology Online Journal* 2008 Feb 28;14(2):3
[621] Inman RD. Antigens, the gastrointestinal tract, and arthritis. *Rheum Dis Clin North Am*. 1991 May;17(2):309-21
[622] "Other factors, like the specific properties of synovial vessels and the adhesion molecules responsible for synovium-specific homing, will contribute to the guiding of the monocytes from the mucosal areas into the joints." Wuorela M, Tohka S, Granfors K, Jalkanen S. Monocytes that have ingested Yersinia enterocolitica serotype O:3 acquire enhanced capacity to bind to nonstimulated vascular endothelial cells via P-selectin. *Infect Immun*. 1999 Feb;67(2):726-32 iai.asm.org/cgi/content/full/67/2/726
[623] "They also suggest that the etiology of RA may involve initial activation of V beta 14+ T cells by a V beta 14-specific superantigen with subsequent recruitment of a few activated autoreactive v beta 14+ T cell clones to the joints while the majority of other V beta 14+ T cells disappear." Paliard X, West SG, Lafferty JA, Clements JR, Kappler JW, Marrack P, Kotzin BL. Evidence for the effects of a superantigen in rheumatoid arthritis. *Science*. 1991 Jul 19;253(5017):325-9
[624] "Given that binding sites for superantigens have been mapped to the CDR4s of TCR beta chains, the synovial localization of T cells bearing V beta s with significant CDR4 homology indicates that V beta-specific T-cell activation by superantigen may play a role in RA." Howell MD, Diveley JP, Lundeen KA, Esty A, Winters ST, Carlo DJ, Brostoff SW. Limited T-cell receptor beta-chain heterogeneity among interleukin 2 receptor-positive synovial T cells suggests a role for superantigen in rheumatoid arthritis. *Proc Natl Acad Sci U S A*. 1991 Dec 1;88(23):10921-5
[625] Solanki LS, Srivastava N, Singh S. Superantigens: a brief review with special emphasis on dermatologic diseases. *Dermatology Online Journal* 2008 Feb 28;14(2):3

between the bacterial antigens and keratin 17 leads to activation of autoreactive T-cells and persistence of disease." The authors note that all streptococci secrete SPEC, a superantigen known to stimulate marked expansion of T-cells which display a particular marker "Vβ2"; these Vβ2 T-cells are found in increased quantities in acute skin lesions of patients with guttate psoriasis.

- Psoriasis and superantigens—High prevalence of Staphylococcus aureus cultivation and superantigen production in patients with psoriasis. (*Eur J Dermatol* 2009 May[626]): This excellent research—conducted in by assessing the skin and nasal cavities (nostrils, nares) of 50 psoriatics and 50 healthy controls—demonstrates the following associations between psoriasis and active colonization with the bacteria *Staphylococcus aureus*:

  ❶ Psoriatic skin lesions have more *Staphylococcus aureus* than does nearby unaffected skin: In patients with psoriasis, skin lesions are more likely to culture *Staphylococcus aureus* (64%) than is the unaffected non-lesional skin (14%).

  ❷ Psoriatic patients are more likely to harbor *Staphylococcus aureus* in their nares/nostrils than are healthy people: "*Staphylococcus aureus* was cultivated from the nares in 25 (50%) of 50 patients with psoriasis and in 17 (34%) of 50 healthy controls."

  ❸ The *Staphylococcus aureus* found at the site of psoriatic lesions is more likely to be a strain of bacteria that produces distinct toxins: "In psoriasis patients, 31 (96.8%) out of the 32 strains isolated from the lesional skin and 3 (42.3%) out of the 7 strains isolated from the non-lesional skin were toxigenic (p = 0.01)." This means that psoriasis is quantitatively (more bacteria) and qualitatively (more toxin-producing bacteria) linked with *Staphylococcus aureus*. A very important contribution of this study is the finding that *Staphylococcus aureus* produces numerous—not only one—superantigens capable of inducing a significant part of the pathophysiology of psoriasis; these superantigens can be described as "non-classical superantigens" such as methicillin resistance gene (*mecA*), *etb*, *eta* and *see* as well as "classical superantigens such as *sea*, *seb*, *sec*, *sed* and *tst*.

  ❹ The *Staphylococcus aureus* found in the nares/nostrils of psoriatic patients is more likely to be a strain of bacteria that produces distinct toxins: "Isolated strains from the nares were toxigenic in 96% (24/25) for patients with psoriasis and in 41.2% (7/17) for healthy controls, respectively (p = 0.006)." A strong correlation of approximately 70% was found between the *Staphylococcus aureus* in the nares and on the skin of patients with psoriasis; this means that cross-contamination from skin to nares and from nares to skin is very likely.

  ❺ Psoriatic patients with lesions that culture positive for *Staphylococcus aureus* have worse disease activity than psoriatic patients with negative cultures: "Patients with cultivation-positive in lesional skin had a significantly higher PASI score than patients who were cultivation-negative in lesional skin (8.28 +/- 3.97 vs. 5.89 +/- 2.98, p = 0.031)." More *Staphylococcus aureus* in psoriasis lesions could be cause (i.e., the *Staphylococcus aureus* are directly contributing to the psoriatic lesions) or effect (i.e., the psoriatic lesions are more likely to become colonized with *Staphylococcus aureus*). However, given the established molecular role of superantigens in two primary hallmarks of psoriasis—inflammation and cytokine-induced cellular hyperproliferation—the most logical interpretation is that the association between *Staphylococcus aureus* and psoriasis is causal rather than casual.

  The authors conclude by stating, "Our results confirm that *S. aureus* colonization and its toxigenic-strains are associated with psoriasis. According to our findings, non-classical superantigens such as methicillin resistance gene (*mecA*), *see* and *etb* may also be associated with psoriasis."

3. Enhanced production/processing of autoantigens: When the immune system perceives the presence of microbial molecules, mechanisms are enhanced which facilitate the processing and presentation of preexistent antigens to the immune system, which then targets these antigens for destruction. Of course, this is beneficial when fighting a true infection; but recent evidence shows that chronic silent infections can

---

[626] Balci et al. High prevalence of Staphylococcus aureus cultivation and superantigen production in patients with psoriasis. *Eur J Dermatol*. 2009 May-Jun;19(3):238-42

facilitate the processing and presentation of the body's own antigens (autoantigens) which are then attacked. Clinically, we see the immune system attacking the body, and we call this an "autoimmune disease" even though the original cause of the problem may have been an occult infection or exposure to specific microbial molecules. Ringrose et al[627] showed that infecting HLA-B27-positive human cells with *Salmonella typhimurium* and *Shigella flexneri* caused these cells to express autoantigens, namely human histone H3, human ribosomal protein S17 (two separate amino acid sequences) and the heavy chain of HLA-B27. A similar phenomenon has been demonstrated in autistic children wherein patients exposed to bacterial antigens (streptokinase), toxic chemicals (Thimerosal, ethyl-mercury), and dietary antigens (gliadin and casein peptides) produce autoantigens that appear capable of inciting and perpetuating autoimmunity.[628] **Therefore, we have experimental evidence with human cells *in vitro* which demonstrates that *enhanced processing of autoantigens* occurs following exposure to bacterial antigens, dietary allergens, and xenobiotics.**

- Psoriasis and microbially-evoked autoantigens—Ex vivo experimental study using human T-cells (see especially *Clin Exp Immunol* 1999 Sep[629]): Amino acid sequences in skin keratin subtypes 14 and 17 have homology with peptides from the bacterium *Streptococcus pyogenes*, thereby providing clear evidence of molecular mimicry between an infectious agent and chronic human disease, as reviewed in a previous section. Evidence has shown that psoriatic patients have T-cells which specifically target keratin 17 thereby indicating that keratin 17 serves as an autoantigen in psoriasis; Johnston et al[630] wrote, "…psoriatic individuals have CD8(+) T cells that recognize keratin self-antigens." As noted earlier in this chapter, increased production of keratin 17 can be induced by the pro-inflammatory cytokines gamma-interferon, which plays a key role as a mediator of psoriatic inflammation, and IL-6, which is abundant in psoriatic lesions. Factors that can increase IFN-g and/or IL-6 production are numerous and include such phenomena as infection, injury, obesity, and consumption of a pro-inflammatory diet; increased production of IFN-g and IL-6 is characteristic of nearly any immune response and is certainly not specific to psoriasis or any other rheumatic condition. As noted previously, the ALEEAN sequence present in keratin 17 is also found in keratin subtype 14, which is overexpressed in psoriatic skin; thus, for T-cells already primed to respond to ALEEAN following exposure to *Streptococcus pyogenes*, the dual exposure to ALEEAN in keratins 14 and 17—both of which are uniquely present in psoriatic skin—may promote localized attack by T-cells against keratinocytes, i.e., immune cross-reactivity via molecular mimicry. The data support the following:

  ❶ Exposure to microbes induces IFNg and/or IL-6: IFN-g and IL-6 production is increased during overt or occult infection/colonization/dysbiosis, such as with *Streptococcus pyogenes* and other pathogenic microorganisms.

  ❷ Increased production of IFN-g and IL-6 increases production of keratin-17: Increased production of IFN-g and IL-6 increases production of keratin-17.

  ❸ Keratin-17 is an autoantigen in psoriatic skin: Keratin-17 is a clinically-important autoantigen in psoriasis based on its location, molecular homology with proteins made by *Streptococcus pyogenes* which is a known trigger in psoriasis, and the identification of T-cells which are specifically responsive to keratin-17.

  ❹ Therefore, microbial exposure → IFN-g and IL-6 → increased keratin-17 = increased autoantigen production induced by pro-inflammatory cytokines induced by microbial exposure.

  ❺ Furthermore, increased production of autoantigen keratin-17 by IFN-g and IL-6 is probably not microbe-dependent. Of note, obesity in general and visceral adipose tissue in particular are causally associated with increased production of these inflammatory cytokines. If non-microbial induction of IFN-g and IL-6 can stimulate increased production of autoantigen

---

[627] Ringrose et al. Influence of infection of cells with bacteria with reactive arthritis on peptide repertoire presented by HLA-B27. *J Med Microbiol* 2001 Apr:385-9
[628] Vojdani et al. Infections, toxic chemicals and dietary peptides binding to lymphocyte receptors and tissue enzymes are major instigators of autoimmunity in autism. *Int J Immunopathol Pharmacol*. 2003 Sep-Dec;16(3):189-99
[629] Gudmundsdottir AS, et al. Is an epitope on keratin 17 a major target for autoreactive T lymphocytes in psoriasis? *Clin Exp Immunol*. 1999 Sep;117(3):580-6
[630] Johnston A, et al. Peripheral blood T cell responses to keratin peptides that share sequences with streptococcal M proteins are largely restricted to skin-homing CD8(+) T cells. *Clin Exp Immunol*. 2004 Oct;138(1):83-93 ncbi.nlm.nih.gov/pmc/articles/PMC1809187/pdf/cei0138-0083.pdf

keratin-17, then we would expect conditions such as obesity/hyperadiposity to be associated with more severe psoriasis; indeed this appears to be the case, as recently shown in studies showing that obese young women are at increased risk for severe psoriasis[631] and that weight loss treatments can improve psoriasis.[632]

4. <u>Bystander activation</u>: Evidence suggests that we all have immunocytes capable of attacking our body tissues, and thus we all have the potential to develop autoimmune disease. Normally, these autoreactive cells are kept anergic, dormant, quiescent, and otherwise inactive through various mechanisms that regulate the immune system; in this way, such autoreactive cells can be considered "bystanders" because they are not really doing anything and are basically "standing by." Bystander activation occurs when these cells are awakened by the cascade of inflammatory processes that occur as a result of superantigen exposure, molecular mimicry, immune complex deposition, or xenobiotic immunotoxicity. Bystander activation appears to contribute to the development of certain **autoimmune conditions, such as drug-induced lupus**[633], and it may be a contributing pathogenic mechanism in **heavy/toxic metal-induced autoimmunity**.[634]

    - <u>Psoriasis and bystander activation—Keratinocytes are immunologically active cells that present bacterial-derived superantigens to T lymphocytes. (*J Dermatol Sci* 1993 Oct[635])</u>: Most doctors and researchers have believed that epidermal keratinocytes were relatively passive components of the outer layers of the skin where these cells form a mechanical barrier against injury and infection; likewise, their role in skin diseases was considered passive, with keratinocytes acting as passive targets and "**innocent bystanders**." However, newer research mandates that we reclassify keratinocytes from passive barrier cells to "fully fledged members of the immune system (i.e. immunocytes)" based on the findings that keratinocytes produce important cytokines, adhesion molecules, and mononuclear cell chemotactic factors. Activated keratinocytes "can initiate and perpetuate the inflammatory and immunological reactions in the skin which contribute to the pathobiology of psoriasis." Specifically, cytokine-activated keratinocytes can present bacterial superantigens to T-cells, resulting in activation and proliferation of these effectors of psoriasis.

    - <u>Thyroid autoimmunity induced by hepatitis C virus via bystander activation—Binding of hepatitis C virus E2 protein to thyroid cells may cause thyroid autoimmunity via bystander activation (*J Autoimmun* 2008 Dec[636])</u>: Hepatitis C virus (HCV) infection is well-known to be causally associated with thyroid autoimmunity (e.g., Hashimoto's thyroiditis) but the molecular mechanism by which this association manifests has not been previously elucidated. In this study, researchers Akeno, Blackard, and Tomer showed that thyroid cells express a surface receptor called CD81, which is a binding site for the HCV protein E2. When HCV E2 binds to CD81, the proinflammatory cytokine IL-8 is produced. These authors concluded, "In summary, we have shown that CD81 is expressed in thyroid cells and can bind HCV envelope protein E2 leading to IL-8 production. These data suggest that local effects of HCV proteins can induce thyroiditis by bystander activation mechanisms." Although their conclusion might be premature insofar as their data showed deductive probability rather than objective certainty, it may be considered pragmatically sufficient.

5. <u>Haptenization and the formation of neoantigens/neoautoantigens</u>: ==A nonantigenic microbial molecule may bind to a nonantigenic human molecule and result in the formation of a new hybridized or "haptenized" molecule—neoantigen—which stimulates immunologic attack.== Haptenization may be the underlying

---

[631] "Multivariate analysis demonstrated an association between excess increase in body mass index and psoriasis in females only." Bryld LE, et al. High body mass index in adolescent girls precedes psoriasis hospitalization. *Acta Derm Venereol*. 2010 Sep;90(5):488-93

[632] "There are two recent reports of chronic severe psoriasis improving with weight loss after Roux-en-Y gastric bypass surgery. We have observed two patients with body mass indices greater than 50 kg/m(2) who had marked improvement in their psoriasis after gastric bypass surgery." Hossler EW, Maroon MS, Mowad CM. Gastric bypass surgery improves psoriasis. *J Am Acad Dermatol*. 2010 Jul 21

[633] "Several mechanisms for induction of autoimmunity will be discussed, including bystander activation of autoreactive lymphocytes due to drug-specific immunity or to non-specific activation of lymphocytes, direct cytotoxicity with release of autoantigens and disruption of central T-cell tolerance." Rubin RL. Drug-induced lupus. *Toxicology*. 2005 Apr 15;209(2):135-47

[634] "It is therefore theoretically possible that compounds present in vaccines such as thiomersal or aluminium hydroxyde can trigger autoimmune reactions through bystander effects." Fournie GJ, et al. Induction of autoimmunity through bystander effects. *J Autoimmun*. 2001 May;16(3):319-26

[635] Nickoloff BJ, et al. Activated keratinocytes present bacterial-derived superantigens to T lymphocytes: relevance to psoriasis. *J Dermatol Sci*. 1993 Oct;6(2):127-33

[636] Akeno N, Blackard JT, Tomer Y. HCV E2 protein binds directly to thyroid cells and induces IL-8 production: a new mechanism for HCV induced thyroid autoimmunity. *J Autoimmun*. 2008 Dec;31(4):339-44 ncbi.nlm.nih.gov/pmc/articles/PMC2641008/pdf/nihms84111.pdf

mechanism by which viruses induce autoimmunity[637] and appears to be a primary mechanism by which *Staphylococcus aureus* contributes to autoimmune vasculitis in Wegener's granulomatosis, namely by producing an antigenic acid phosphatase enzyme which binds with human endothelial cells by a charge interaction—the resultant hybrid/hapten/neoantigen formed by the antigen-endothelium complex becomes the target of immune attack, thus creating the phenomenon of "autoimmunity" and the clinical consequences of vasculitis.[638] Similarly, Hwp1 (Hyphal wall protein-1) of *Candida albicans* is a substrate for the tissue transglutaminase enzyme and cross-links with proteins in the mammalian mucosa[639]; the resultant neoantigen that results from this microbe-human haptenization would be a prime candidate to incite autoimmunity, as has been demonstrated by the transglutaminase-mediated haptenization of gliadin with human collagen *in vivo*.[640,641] In fact, since both Hwp1 and gliadin are substrates for tissue transglutaminase, *Candida albicans* may be synergistic with gluten/gliadin in the production of the systemic inflammatory/autoimmune/allergic condition known as celiac disease[642]; this may exemplify the interrelated nature of dysbiosis, food allergy, and autoimmunity. Lastly, since many toxic metals, xenobiotics, and drugs appear to trigger autoimmunity via haptenization[643,644,645], the adverse effects of these toxicants will be enhanced by microbe-induced alterations in xenobiotic detoxification and/or the proinflammatory effects of peptidoglycans, exotoxins, endotoxins, lipoteichoic acid, and other antigens and superantigens. In a recent animal study, exposure to bacterial endotoxin exacerbated metal-induced autoimmunity.[646] Endotoxin from gram-negative bacteria impairs detoxification by inhibiting the first cytochrome-p450-mediated step of detoxification[647]; this inhibition of detoxification increases the risk for drug toxicity and chemical accumulation. Bacteria can also adversely affect detoxification by elaborating beta-glucuronidase in the lumen of the intestine which cleaves bile-secreted toxins from their water-soluble conjugation moieties, resulting in increased "enterohepatic recycling"[648] or "enterohepatic recirculation"[649] as discussed below; increased re-exposure to previously detoxified endogenous and exogenous toxins can result in an upregulation of Phase 1 (cytochrome-p450-mediated biotransformation) leading to the formation of reactive intermediates and a condition commonly described by clinicians as "imbalanced detoxification" or "pathological detoxification."

- Wegener's granulomatosis and bacterial enzyme haptenization—Staphylococcal enzyme acid phosphatase binds to (i.e., haptenizes) endothelial cells via charge interaction in Wegener's vasculitis (*Clin Exp Immunol* 2000 Mar[650]): Wegener's granulomatosis is an autoimmune vasculitic condition with a high mortality; the majority of untreated patients die an average of 5 months following

---

[637] Van Ghelue M, et al. Autoimmunity to nucleosomes related to viral infection: a focus on hapten-carrier complex formation. *J Autoimmun*. 2003;20(2):171-82
[638] Brons RH, Bakker HI, Van Wijk RT, et al. Staphylococcal acid phosphatase binds to endothelial cells via charge interaction; a pathogenic role in Wegener's granulomatosis? *Clin Exp Immunol*. 2000 Mar;119(3):566-73 blackwell-synergy.com/doi/abs/10.1046/j.1365-2249.2000.01172.x
[639] "By serving as a microbial substrate for epithelial cell transglutaminase, Hwp1 (Hyphal wall protein 1) of Candida albicans participates in cross-links with proteins on the mammalian mucosa." Staab JF, et al. Expression of transglutaminase substrate activity on Candida albicans germ tubes through a coiled, disulfide-bonded N-terminal domain of Hwp1 requires C-terminal glycosylphosphatidylinositol modification. *J Biol Chem*. 2004 Sep 24;279(39):40737-47 jbc.org/cgi/content/full/279/39/40737
[640] "Our findings firstly demonstrated that gliadin was directly bound to tTG in duodenal mucosa of coeliacs and controls, and the ability of circulating tTG-autoantibodies to recognize and immunoprecipitate the tTG-gliadin complexes." Ciccocioppo R, Di Sabatino A, Ara C, Biagi F, Perilli M, Amicosante G, Cifone MG, Corazza GR. Gliadin and tissue transglutaminase complexes in normal and coeliac duodenal mucosa. *Clin Exp Immunol*. 2003 Dec;134(3):516-24
[641] "Thus, modification of gluten peptides by tTG, especially deamidation of certain glutamine residues, can enhance their binding to HLA-DQ2 or -DQ8 and potentiate T cell stimulation. Furthermore, tTG-catalyzed cross-linking and consequent haptenization of gluten with extracellular matrix proteins allows for storage and extended availability of gluten in the mucosa." Dieterich W, Esslinger B, Schuppan D. Pathomechanisms in celiac disease. *Int Arch Allergy Immunol*. 2003 Oct;132(2):98-108
[642] "Subsequently, C albicans might function as an adjuvant that stimulates antibody formation against HWP1 and gluten, and formation of autoreactive antibodies against tissue transglutaminase and endomysium." Nieuwenhuizen WF, et al. Is Candida albicans a trigger in the onset of coeliac disease? *Lancet*. 2003;361(9375):2152-4
[643] Rao T, Richardson B. Environmentally induced autoimmune diseases: potential mechanisms. *Environ Health Perspect*. 1999 Oct;107 Suppl 5:737-42
[644] "Here, Peter Griem and colleagues focus on several aspects of neoantigen formation by xenobiotics: metabolism of xenobiotics into reactive, haptenic metabolites; polymorphisms of metabolizing enzymes; induction of costimulatory signals; and sensitization of T cells." Griem P, Wulferink M, Sachs B, Gonzalez JB, Gleichmann E. Allergic and autoimmune reactions to xenobiotics: how do they arise? *Immunol Today*. 1998 Mar;19(3):133-4
[645] "It appears that the patients' antibodies recognize epitopes consisting of the TFA group plus associated structural features of the protein carriers (100 kDa, 76 kDa, 59 kDa, 57 kDa and 54 kDa), not the TFA hapten alone." Kenna JG, et al. Metabolic basis for a drug hypersensitivity: antibodies in sera from patients with halothane hepatitis recognize liver neoantigens that contain the trifluoroacetyl group derived from halothane. *J Pharmacol Exp Ther*. 1988 Jun;245(3):1103-9 As an extension of this work, also see: "These investigations have further revealed that the antibodies are directed against distinct polypeptide fractions (100 kDa, 76 kDa, 59 kDa, 57 kDa, 54 kDa) that have been covalently modified by the reactive trifluoroacetyl halide metabolite of halothane." Satoh H, et al. Human anti-endoplasmic reticulum antibodies in sera of patients with halothane-induced hepatitis are directed against a trifluoroacetylated carboxylesterase. *Proc Natl Acad Sci* 1989 Jan;86(1):322-6 pnas.org/cgi/reprint/86/1/322
[646] Abedi-Valugerdi M, Nilsson C, Zargari A, Gharibdoost F, DePierre JW, Hassan M. Bacterial lipopolysaccharide both renders resistant mice susceptible to mercury-induced autoimmunity and exacerbates such autoimmunity in susceptible mice. *Clin Exp Immunol*. 2005 Aug;141(2):238-47
[647] Shedlofsky SI, et al, Blouin RA. Endotoxin administration to humans inhibits hepatic cytochrome P450-mediated drug metabolism. *J Clin Invest*. 1994 Dec;94:2209-14
[648] "Enterohepatic recycling occurs by biliary excretion and intestinal reabsorption of a solute, sometimes with hepatic conjugation and intestinal deconjugation. ... Of particular importance is the potential amplifying effect of enterohepatic variability in defining differences in the bioavailability, apparent volume of distribution and clearance of a given compound." Roberts et al. Enterohepatic circulation: physiological, pharmacokinetic and clinical implications. *Clin Pharmacokinet* 2002;41:751-90
[649] Liska DJ. The detoxification enzyme systems. *Altern Med Rev*. 1998 Jun;3(3):187-98
[650] Brons RH, Bakker HI, Van Wijk RT, et al. Staphylococcal acid phosphatase binds to endothelial cells via charge interaction; a pathogenic role in Wegener's granulomatosis? *Clin Exp Immunol*. 2000 Mar;119(3):566-73

diagnosis, and 2-year survival without treatment is 10%. Histologically, the condition demonstrates focal accumulations of inflammation and immune cell activity (i.e., granulomas); however, the main clinical concern is the vasculitis in general and in particular the vasculitis affecting the kidneys and which commonly leads to kidney failure, a leading cause of death in affected patients. This excellent study by Brons and coworkers shows that the bacteria *Staphylococcus aureus* produces an enzyme—acid phosphatase—which binds to endothelial cells, the cells that form the inner linings of arteries and all blood vessels. This positively-charged enzyme has also been shown to bind to the renal basement membrane, a target of immune attack in inflammatory/autoimmune renal diseases described as crescentic glomerulonephritis, a type of immune-mediated renal disease seen in several autoimmune conditions such as Goodpasture syndrome, IgA nephropathy, and systemic lupus erythematosus. Because the staphylococcal acid phosphatase is a foreign non-self protein, the human immune system forms antibodies against it; these antibodies are measurable in the blood of patients with Wegener's vasculitis. Thus, when the staphylococcal acid phosphatase binds to endothelial cells, the antibodies directed against the acid phosphatase induce a vigorous immune response and inflammatory reaction on the surface of the vessel wall—this is the hallmark of vasculitis. The authors conclude that "Since antibodies directed against staphylococcal acid phosphatase are present in patients with WG and these antibodies recognize endothelial cell-bound staphylococcal acid phosphatase, we suggest that the results published in this study support the hypothesis that staphylococcal acid phosphatase may play a role in the initiation of vasculitis and glomerulonephritis in patients with WG by acting as a planted antigen." For this discussion, "planted antigen" and "hapten" are synonymous and interchangeable.

6. <u>Peptidoglycans, teichoic acid, and exotoxins from gram-positive bacteria</u>: Peptidoglycan (PG), a major cell-wall component of Gram-positive bacteria. Peptidoglycans from gram-positive bacteria such as group-A streptococci can cause malaise, fever, dermatosis, tenosynovitis, cryoglobulinemia (an immune complex disease), and arthritis.[651] Experimental arthritis can be induced in animals by exposing them to group-B streptococci isolated from the nasopharynx of human patients with rheumatoid arthritis.[652] *Staphylococcus aureus* is a gram-positive bacterium, certain strains of which produce the toxic shock syndrome toxin-1 (TSST-1) that causes scalded skin syndrome, toxic shock syndrome, and food poisoning; other strains of *Staphylococcus aureus* that do not produce TSST-1 are also capable of causing toxic shock syndrome from colonization of bone, vagina, wounds, or rectum.[653] Experimental evidence has shown that peptidoglycan-polysaccharide complexes from "good" and "normal" bacteria such as Bifidobacteria and *Lactobacillus casei* can also induce an inflammatory arthritis; this speaks against the "more is better" approach to probiotic supplementation and also demonstrates how **bacterial overgrowth of the small bowel (detailed later) can induce joint pain and inflammation even in the absence of so-called "pathogens."**[654,655]
    - <u>Psoriasis and peptidoglycans</u>—Peptidoglycan appears to be a major causative factor for psoriasis (*Trends Immunol* 2006 Dec[656]): Peptidoglycan is a major cell-wall component of Gram-positive bacteria and has been detected within antigen-presenting cells of patients with psoriasis. Furthermore, the skin of patients with psoriasis shows Th1 cells that are specifically responsive to streptococcal and/or staphylococcal peptidoglycans; this indicates that peptidoglycan is probably an important T-cell stimulator which contributes to psoriasis. Additionally, patients with psoriasis appear to be genetically predisposed to disorders associated with peptidoglycans because their immune cells are altered in such a way as to allow for enhanced T-cell response to the bacterial antigens such as peptidoglycans. The authors conclude, "These observations suggest that peptidoglycan is a major

---

[651] "A characteristic intermittent neutrophilic dermatosis, associated with polyarthritis, tenosynovitis, malaise, fever, and cryoglobulinemia, occurs in 20% of patients who undergo ileojejunal bypass surgery for the treatment of morbid obesity... Peptidoglycans from numerous intestinal bacteria...are suggested as causative of the toxic and immunologic features of this syndrome." Ely PH. The bowel bypass syndrome: a response to bacterial peptidoglycans. *J Am Acad Dermatol*. 1980 Jun;2(6):473-87
[652] "The origin of rheumatoid arthritis (RA) is in our opinion a bacterial infection." Svartz N. The origin of rheumatoid arthritis. *Rheumatology*. 1975;6:322-8
[653] Shandera WX, Moran A. "Infectious diseases: viral and rickettsial." In Tierney LM, McPhee SJ Papadakis MA (eds). *Current Medical Diagnosis and Treatment. 44th Edition*. New York: Lange; 2005, page 1356-8
[654] Simelyte E, et al. Bacterial cell wall-induced arthritis: chemical composition and tissue distribution of four Lactobacillus strains. *Infect Immun*. 2000 Jun;68(6):3535-40
[655] Toivanen P. Normal intestinal microbiota in the aetiopathogenesis of rheumatoid arthritis. *Ann Rheum Dis*. 2003;62:807-11 ard.bmjjournals.com/cgi/reprint/62/9/807
[656] Baker BS, Powles A, Fry L. Peptidoglycan: a major aetiological factor for psoriasis? *Trends Immunol*. 2006 Dec;27(12):545-51

etiological factor for psoriasis and emphasize the importance of peptidoglycan in bacterial-infection-induced inflammatory disease."

- <u>Psoriasis and peptidoglycans—Patients with cutaneous and arthritic psoriasis have elevated IgA antibodies against streptococcal peptidoglycan-polysaccharide. (*Clin Exp Rheumatol* 1997 Jul-Aug[657])</u>: Patients with psoriasis and psoriatic arthritis have elevated IgA levels specific to streptococcal peptidoglycan-polysaccharide (PG-PS); antibody levels do no vary with disease severity. Very remarkably, the authors concluded by stating, "**The results suggest chronic mucosal stimulation of lymphocytes by long-lived streptococcal antigens in patients with psoriasis...**" Readers should appreciate that the evidence linking psoriasis with mucosal infections with the streptococcal bacteria is consistent and very strong. The mucosal surfaces of the nose, sinuses, and throat are the most common locations for chronic streptococcal bacteria colonization/dysbiosis.

- <u>Psoriasis and peptidoglycans and teichoic acid—Contribution of *Staphylococcus aureus* cell wall products teichoic acid and peptidoglycan to immunoglobulin (IgE, IgA, IgG) synthesis and CD23 expression in patients with atopic dermatitis (*Immunology* 1992 Jan[658])</u>: Patients with the inflammatory pruritic skin condition atopic dermatitis (eczema) have increased skin and nasal colonization with the bacteria *Staphylococcus aureus* and that the immune response induced by living or dead *Staphylococcus aureus* differs in eczema patients from that seen in normal healthy patients; in patients with eczema, exposure to fragments of *Staphylococcus aureus* actually causes immunosuppression (reductions in IgA and IgG) rather than the expected immune upregulation that should occur following exposure to a pathogenic microbe. Furthermore, in patients with eczema, exposure to *Staphylococcus aureus* cell wall fragments causes increased production of IgE and histamine, two pathophysiologic factors inextricably associated with the skin inflammation and discomfort/itchiness of eczema. The finding that bacterial cell wall fragments can lead to reduced production of IgA and IgG implies that mucous membrane and/or skin colonization with *Staphylococcus aureus* (and perhaps *Bordetella pertussis*, *Haemophilus influenzae* and Gram-negative bacteria which produce lipopolysaccharide [LPS]) can promote local and systemic immune suppression which favors (poly)microbial colonization and persistence while also contributing to skin inflammation and irritation via enhanced production of IgE and histamine. Readers should appreciate that psoriatic patients also have increased nasal and skin colonization with *Staphylococcus aureus* and that psoriasis—like eczema—is a chronic inflammatory skin disorder; thus, *Staphylococcus aureus* probably acts via similar molecular mechanisms to produce these two disorders, which differ from each other yet at the same time can be seen as variants on the theme of microorganism-triggered "patterns of inflammation."

- <u>Rheumatoid arthritis and peptidoglycans: Normal intestinal bacteria appear to contribute to rheumatoid arthritis and other inflammatory [joint] diseases (*Ann Rheum Dis* 2003 Sep[659])</u>: In this article Professor Toivanen reviews 61 published articles to advance the model of inflammatory disease induction by bacteria, particularly what might generally be considered normal intestinal bacteria. Professor Toivanen notes several interesting items of fact: ❶ bacteria that are genetically identical per PCR testing can have subtle differences in their peptidoglycan structure, and these minute differences in peptidoglycan structure [perhaps due to epigenetic factors] can effect profound differences in pathophysiologic responses, i.e., either promoting or suppressing inflammatory responses by the immune system, ❷ bacterial peptidoglycan can stimulate the production of the autoantibody **rheumatoid factor**, which for many decades was considered the primary serologic diagnostic marker for rheumatoid arthritis (80% positivity), and which is present in other autoimmune disorders such as Sjogren's syndrome (70% positivity), and which contributes directly to joint and tissue injury and inflammation via direct deposition, particularly in the form of immune complexes, and ❸ peptidoglycans induce inflammatory responses following binding with Toll-like receptor 2 (TLR-2). Three successive sentences are particularly worthy of quotation:

---

[657] Rantakokko K, et al. Antibodies to streptococcal cell wall in psoriatic arthritis and cutaneous psoriasis. *Clin Exp Rheumatol*. 1997 Jul-Aug;15(4):399-404
[658] Neuber K, König K. Effects of Staphylococcus aureus cell wall products (teichoic acid, peptidoglycan) and enterotoxin B on immunoglobulin (IgE, IgA, IgG) synthesis and CD23 expression in patients with atopic dermatitis. *Immunology*. 1992 January; 75(1): 23–28 ncbi.nlm.nih.gov/pmc/articles/PMC1384797/
[659] Toivanen P. Normal intestinal microbiota in the aetiopathogenesis of rheumatoid arthritis. *Ann Rheum Dis*. 2003 Sep;62(9):807-11

"The ability of bacterial cell walls to induce chronic, erosive arthritis was first described in the rat by using *Streptococcus pyogenes*. Self-perpetuating arthritis, closely resembling human rheumatoid arthritis by histological criteria, develops in susceptible rat strains after a single intraperitoneal injection of the bacterial cell wall. In addition to *Streptococcus pyogenes*, several bacterial species representing Lactobacillus, Bifidobacterium, Eubacterium, Collinsella, and Clostridium have been observed to have a similar ability."

The important observation that, in experimental models with genetically susceptible animals, chronic inflammatory arthritis can be induced by a one-time exposure to commonly encountered bacteria provides clear objective proof that bacteria and—importantly—their nonviable cell wall fragments can induce chronic inflammatory disease. Readers should note the evidence showing that *Streptococcus pyogenes* can contribute to inflammatory *arthritis* in certain models, while contributing to inflammatory *dermatitis* in others.

- Skin disorders and peptidoglycans—Beta-blocking drugs and bacterial peptidoglycan promote Th1-mediated inflammatory responses in skin (*Brain Behav Immun* 2008 Jan[660]): The authors of this paper note that many inflammatory diseases such as psoriasis, atopic dermatitis, lichen planus, and vitiligo have also been associated with emotional stress and local alterations of the sympathetic (adrenergic) nervous system. Using a unique experimental model, the authors show that peptidoglycan from Gram-positive bacteria—but not lipopolysaccharide from Gram-negative bacteria—promoted a local Th1-type proinflammatory response. Based on the responses elicited by adrenergic receptor (AR)-blocking drugs, the authors conclude that the Th1 polarization is mediated by inhibition of both beta1- and beta2-AR. The local pro-inflammatory response includes enhanced local expression of IFN-gamma, IL-12 and IL-23 as well as of IFN-beta and CXCR3 ligands. The local inflammatory response resulted in an increase of antigen-positive plasmacytoid dendritic cells (pDCs) in the draining lymph node. In sum, these results suggest that "altered sympathetic nervous activity together with selected pattern recognition receptors activation might serve as initiation and/or persistence factors for numerous Th1-sustained inflammatory skin diseases." Psoriasis is a known Th1-sustained inflammatory skin disease; more recent research has demonstrated a strong Th-17 component as well.

7. Endotoxins (lipopolysaccharide) from gram-negative bacteria: Many different species of gram-negative bacteria produce endotoxin, also known as bacterial lipopolysaccharide (LPS). Even in the absence of viable bacteria, the exposure of humans to endotoxin, say for example by intravenous administration for the purpose of experimentation, produces a wide range of adverse physiologic consequences, including 1) triggering an acute proinflammatory response resembling febrile illness or sepsis, 2) increasing intestinal permeability, causing "leaky gut"[661], 3) inhibiting hepatic detoxification[662], 4) disrupting the blood-brain barrier and promoting neurodegeneration via neuroinflammation.[663,664,665] The pathophysiologic effects of endotoxin/LPS are often *similar to* and *synergistic with* those of superantigens to effect altered tissue function and widespread inflammation. **LPS and antigens from gram-negative bacteria (in the absence of viable bacteria) exacerbate arthritis in experimental models[666] and trigger inflammatory arthropathy (reactive arthritis) in humans.[667]**

- Psoriasis and lipopolysaccharide from Gram-negative bacteria—Proposed explanation for the exacerbation of psoriasis in AIDS with a discussion of substance P and gram-negative bacteria

---

[660] Manni M, Maestroni GJ. Sympathetic nervous modulation of the skin innate and adaptive immune response to peptidoglycan but not lipopolysaccharide: involvement of beta-adrenoceptors and relevance in inflammatory diseases. *Brain Behav Immun*. 2008 Jan;22(1):80-8

[661] "After endotoxin administration systemic absorption and excretion of lactulose increased almost two-fold... These data suggest that a brief exposure to circulating endotoxin increases the permeability of the normal gut." O'Dwyer et al. A single dose of endotoxin increases intestinal permeability in healthy humans. *Arch Surg*. 1988 Dec;123:1459-64

[662] Shedlofsky SI, et al, Blouin RA. Endotoxin depresses hepatic cytochrome P450-mediated drug metabolism in women. *Br J Clin Pharmacol*. 1997 Jun;43(6):627-32

[663] "Following administration of lipopolysaccharide (LPS) to immunized mice, antibodies gain access to the brain. They bind preferentially to hippocampal neurons and cause neuronal death with resulting cognitive dysfunction and altered hippocampal metabolism..." Kowal C, et al. Cognition and immunity; antibody impairs memory. *Immunity*. 2004 Aug;21(2):179-88 immunity.com/content/article/abstract?uid=PIIS1074761304001980

[664] Fassbender K, et al . The LPS receptor (CD14) links innate immunity with Alzheimer's disease. *FASEB J*. 2004 Jan;18(1):203-5. fasebj.org/cgi/reprint/03-0364fjev1

[665] Laflamme N, Rivest S. Toll-like receptor 4: the missing link of the cerebral innate immune response triggered by circulating gram-negative bacterial cell wall components. *FASEB J*. 2001 Jan;15(1):155-163 fasebj.org/cgi/reprint/15/1/155.pdf

[666] "The results showed that administration of LPS was followed by reactivation of AIA in a dose-related fashion." Yoshino S, Yamaki K, Taneda S, Yanagisawa R, Takano H. Reactivation of antigen-induced arthritis in mice by oral administration of lipopolysaccharide. *Scand J Immunol*. 2005 Aug;62(2):117-22

[667] "Extensive bacterial cultures of synovial fluid were negative...We conclude that in patients with reactive arthritis after yersinia infection, microbial antigens can be found in synovial-fluid cells from affected joints."Granfors et al.Yersinia antigens in synovial-fluid cells from patients with reactive arthritis. *N Engl J Med* 1989;320:216-2

(*Autoimmunity* 2004 Feb[668]): The author of this paper proposes that the well-known induction or exacerbation of psoriasis by HIV infection may be due to a variety of factors, including ❶ increased colonization of skin by *Staphylococcus aureus*, ❷ increased release of substance P by immunocytes rather than neurons, and ❸ increased infections/colonization with Gram-negative bacteria which elaborate endotoxin/lipopolysaccharide, which is potently pro-inflammatory. Also proposed is the model of a vicious cycle wherein psoriatic lesions produce substance P, which then promotes HIV replication and exacerbation of HIV-related disease, which then leads to exacerbations of psoriasis, which leads to more substance P elaboration and HIV replication. Other researchers have noted that psoriatic lesions show increased nerve growth and increased elaboration from nerves of substance P, which is a pro-inflammatory neuropeptide.[669]

- Psoriasis and endotoxin/LPS from Gram-negative bacteria—Improvement of psoriasis with cholestyramine (*Arch Dermatol* 1982 Mar[670]): In this letter to the editor, the authors report the rapid improvement of psoriasis after the oral administration of cholestyramine resin in five patients with psoriasis. The rationale for this intervention is to reduce the patient's total inflammatory load by reducing the amount of bacterial endotoxin/LPS absorbed from the gastrointestinal tract. Five patients were treated with oral cholestyramine 4 grams 4 times daily and topical chlorhexidine soap.

- Psoriasis—Endotoxin/lipopolysaccharide (LPS) from intestinal Gram-negative bacteria and the effect of binding with orally administered bile acids (*Pathophysiology* 2003 Dec[671]): This is an impressively large and impressively innovative study. The authors tested the hypothesis that an insufficiency in bile acid production by the liver results in increased bacterial endotoxin absorption from the intestines and that this endotoxin contributes to the immune dysfunction and systemic inflammation of psoriasis. The authors note that, under normal conditions, bile acids secreted from the hepatobiliary system act as detergents by degrading intestinal endotoxins and thereby protecting the host from their pathophysiologic sequelae. Bile acids thereby participate in "physico-chemical defense" by splitting endotoxin/lipopolysaccharide into nontoxic fragments and thus preventing the consequent release of inflammatory cytokines. In this clinical trial, total of 800 psoriasis patients participated in the study and 551 were treated with oral bile acid (dehydrocholic acid) supplementation for 1-8 weeks. Treatment efficacy was evaluated clinically and by use of the standard Psoriasis Area Severity Index (PASI) score. The authors note remarkable improvement; "During this treatment, 434 patients (78.8%) became asymptomatic. Of 249 psoriatics receiving the conventional therapy, only 62 (24.9%) showed clinical recovery during the same period of time (P<0.05)." Patients with more acute and short-term psoriasis showed very high rates of improvement; 95% of these patients had resolution of their psoriasis. After two years of treatment, 319 of 551 (57.9%) psoriasis patients treated with bile acids were asymptomatic, compared to only 15 of 249 (6.0%) patients receiving the standard drug treatment. As for the subset of patients with acute psoriasis, at the end of two years, 147 of 184 (79.9%) of psoriatic patients treated with bile acids were asymptomatic; only 10 of 139 (7.2%) acute psoriasis patients receiving standard drug treatment were cured. The authors summarize, "To conclude, the results obtained suggest that psoriasis can be treated with success by oral bile acid supplementation presumably affecting the microflora and endotoxins released and their uptake in the gut." These findings are consistent with the facts that ❶ psoriasis manifests most obviously as dermal hyperproliferation induced by cytokines and that ❷ endotoxin/LPS is one of the most powerful inducers of cytokine release.

- Psoriasis: 6 of 11 (54%) patients were shown to have endotoxinemia—measurable blood levels of bacterial lipopolysaccharide/endotoxin from Gram-negative bacteria (*Archives of Dermatology* 1982 Mar[672]): The authors introduce their letter by stating, "Our interest in the possibility of endotoxemia

---

[668] Namazi MR. Paradoxical exacerbation of psoriasis in AIDS: proposed explanations including the potential roles of substance P and gram-negative bacteria. *Autoimmunity*. 2004 Feb;37(1):67-71
[669] "Indeed, we have noted marked proliferation of nerve fibers in transplanted psoriatic plaques compared with the few nerves in transplanted normal human skin. By double label immunofluorescence staining, we have further demonstrated that in these terminal cutaneous nerves there is a marked upregulation of neuropeptides, such as substance P and calcitonin gene-related protein." Raychaudhuri SP, Raychaudhuri SK. Role of NGF and neurogenic inflammation in the pathogenesis of psoriasis. *Prog Brain Res*. 2004;146:433-7
[670] Skinner RB, Rosenberg EW, Belew PW, Marley WM. Improvement of psoriasis with cholestyramine. [letter] *Arch Dermatol*. 1982 Mar;118(3):144
[671] Gyurcsovics K, Bertók L. Pathophysiology of psoriasis: coping endotoxins with bile acid therapy. *Pathophysiology*. 2003 Dec;10(1):57-61
[672] Belew PW, Rosenberg EW, Skinner RB Jr, Marley WM. Endotoxemia in psoriasis. *Arch Dermatol*. [Letter] 1982 Mar;118(3):142-3

in psoriasis followed recent demonstrations of alterations in levels of alternative complement pathway components and of circulating IgA immune complexes in psoriasis. Endotoxin and immune IgA complexes each activate the alternative complement pathway." These authors report finding **circulating blood levels of endotoxin/lipopolysaccharide in 6 of 11 (54%) of their tested psoriatic patients**. Research laboratory methods are described.

- Psoriasis—Use of cholestyramine to bind intestinal endotoxin, and nutrient treatment of severe psoriasis in alcoholics (*J Drugs Dermatol* 2010 Apr[673]): Alcoholism increases the risk of initiation/exacerbation of psoriasis by as much as 800%, with the effect being strongest in men. Of course, alcoholism causes other health problems, too; notable for this discussion are ❶ increased intestinal permeability leading to bacterial endotoxin absorption, and ❷ vitamin and mineral deficiencies commonly causing elevated homocysteine levels and hypomagnesemia, respectively. The two patients in this 2-case report and brief review were treated with magnesium 600 mg, folic acid 5 mg, pyridoxine 100 mg, and cobalamin 1 mg in addition to routine topical and oral medications for psoriasis, acute infections (one patient was treated with Bactrim for MRSA); one patient was treated with cholestyramine 4 grams 4 times per day for 5 days repeated for 3 courses. In the discussion section of the article, the authors review that alcoholism causes increased intestinal permeability and resultant increased absorption of endotoxin with immunogenic/inflammatory consequences. Additionally, cholestyramine while being appropriate for alcoholics to bind endotoxin might exacerbate magnesium deficiency via reduced intestinal absorption (i.e., binding) and by increased urinary excretion, the latter according to an animal study. As has been noted elsewhere, the authors of this report note that both psoriatics and alcoholics tend to have higher levels of homocysteine; less widely appreciated is the fact that homocysteine primes neutrophils for inflammatory responses, tissue homing, and induction of increased oxidative stress and tissue damage, some of which is relevant and somewhat specific for the pathogenesis of psoriasis. A separate publication cited by these authors noted that homocysteine levels correlated positively and folate levels correlated negatively with the severity and extent of psoriasis. Homocysteine causes intracellular depletion of magnesium; this problem is ameliorated by supplementation with magnesium, folate, pyridoxine, and cobalamin. Not mentioned in this report is the possibility that hypomagnesemia contributes to psoriasis via enhancement of neurogenic inflammation, and that folate and other coenzymes are necessary for the epigenetic modifications (most obviously, DNA methylation) that might favorably influence the psoriatic and proinflammatory phenotype.

8. Immunostimulation by bacterial DNA: **Bacterial DNA stimulates a proinflammatory response that is comparable to that induced by endotoxin/LPS.** Exposure to single-stranded *bacterial* DNA induces formation of antibodies against single-stranded *mammalian* DNA. These findings may be particularly relevant to patients with systemic lupus erythematosus—a disorder for which the pathogenic hallmark is the formation of anti-DNA antibodies—since these patients have an impaired ability to clear bacterial DNA from the serum and therefore experienced prolonged pro-inflammatory stimulation when exposed to bacterial DNA.[674] Chronic exposure to immunostimulating antigens is a recognized means for the induction of autoimmunity in animal models.

- Psoriasis and immunostimulation via bacterial DNA—Enhanced activation of blood mononuclear cells in patients with psoriasis vulgaris mediated by streptococcal antigen with bacterial DNA (*J Invest Dermatol* 2009 Nov[675]): The authors note that streptococcal infection has an intimate relationship with psoriasis even though the specific role of streptococcal DNA has not been previously clarified. Therefore, these researchers investigated the effect of streptococcal DNA on lymphocyte proliferation and activation as well as cytokine secretion in psoriasis. As has been previously reported by other

---

[673] Aronson PJ, Malick F. Towards rational treatment of severe psoriasis in alcoholics: report of two cases. *J Drugs Dermatol*. 2010 Apr;9(4):405-8
[674] "The immunostimulatory activities of bacterial DNA are varied and encompass the mitogenicity of B cells and the induction of cytokines including IFN-α/β, IFN-γ, tumor necrosis factor alpha, interleukin 6 (IL-6), and IL-12 (17, 21, 23). Together, these activities resemble those of endotoxin..." Pisetsky DS. Antibody responses to DNA in normal immunity and aberrant immunity. *Clin Diagn Lab Immunol*. 1998 Jan;5(1):1-6 cvi.asm.org/cgi/reprint/5/1/1
[675] Cai YH, Lu ZY, Shi RF, Xue F, Chen XY, Pan M, Yuan WR, Xu H, Li WP, Zheng J. Enhanced proliferation and activation of peripheral blood mononuclear cells in patients with psoriasis vulgaris mediated by streptococcal antigen with bacterial DNA. *J Invest Dermatol*. 2009 Nov;129:2653-60

researchers, the authors of this paper also found that peripheral blood mononuclear cells (PBMCs) from psoriatic patients had higher proliferative responses upon stimulation by streptococcal antigens (SA) when compared with those from healthy individuals. Pretreatment of the streptococcal antigens with an enzyme that degrades DNA (DNase-1) reduced the amount of immune stimulation elicited following exposure of immune cells to streptococcal antigens, thus implicating streptococcal DNA as having an important role in the induction of the pro-inflammatory response elicited by streptococcal antigens in psoriatic immune cells. The authors conclude, "This study demonstrates the integral function of SA, particularly streptococcal DNA, in the pathogenesis of psoriasis."

9. <u>Activation of Toll-like receptors (TLR) and NFkB (NFkB)</u>: Microbial products such as peptidoglycans and endotoxins (as well as others) promote inflammation and arthritogenesis by activating receptors and nuclear transcription factors with the resultant non-specific upregulation of proinflammatory genetic expression. Nuclear transcription factor kappaB (NFkB) is considered one of the most important nuclear transcription factors for stimulating genetic expression of proinflammatory genes, and NFkB is activated by microbes and their structures including viruses and endotoxins.[676] Similar to NFkB are the Toll-like receptors (TLRs), which promote an inflammatory response by NFKB-dependent and NFKB-independent pathways following exposure to microbial structures including but not limited to peptidoglycans and lipopolysaccharides.[677] About a dozen different TLRs have been identified, and these play an important role in the joint destruction seen in the classic example of dysbiotic arthropathy—rheumatoid arthritis.[678] From a nutritional perspective, we see that **Toll-like receptor activity is stimulated by saturated fatty acids and inhibited by polyunsaturated fatty acids, especially the omega-3 fatty acid docosahexaenoic acid.**[679] Likewise, NFkB activity can be modulated by numerous nutrients as I have reviewed later in this text and elsewhere.[680] Of course, nutritional, botanical, or pharmacologic modulation of inflammation should not supersede investigation and correction of the underlying cause(s) of inflammation.

  - <u>Psoriasis and bacterial activation of TLRs and NFkB—Toll-like receptors in skin</u> (*Adv Dermatol* 2008[681]): The author cites research showing that keratinocytes in **psoriatic lesions have increased levels of TLRs 1, 2, 4, 5 and 9 compared with normal skin**; this suggests the probability of enhanced responsiveness to microbial immunogens. Whether this upregulated expression of TLRs is a nonspecific response to inflammation or a specific response to the presence of microorganisms is not clear; however what is very obvious is that the presence of microbe-sensing TLRs with the presence of additional bacteria on the skin of psoriatic patients certainly provides a well-set stage for dermatologic inflammation. "Thus," the author notes, "TLR activation may also play a role in the pathophysiology of psoriasis by exacerbating the disease process." Also noted is the very important observation that **the antimicrobial peptide cathelicidin (LL-37), which is found at high levels in psoriatic skin, can convert non-stimulatory self-DNA into a potent activator of TLR-9** on dendritic cells (plasmacytoid DCs) resulting in production of IFN-alpha, leading to the conclusion that "This may be one important mechanism of how **TLRs can promote autoimmunity in psoriasis**." Per review by Lamphier et al[682], TLR-9 is expressed intracellularly and is activated in response to DNA, in particular DNA containing unmethylated CpG motifs that are more prevalent in microbial than mammalian DNA; however, under certain conditions, TLR-9 can recognize self-DNA and this may promote immune responses against DNA such as noted in the autoimmune disease systemic lupus erythematosus (SLE) particularly as TLR-9 binds rather indiscriminately to a broad range of DNAs. Notice the implications and four-step stream of probable events: ❶ microbe-induced skin inflammation and tissue injury → ❷ upregulation of TLRs (esp. TLR-9) and antimicrobial peptides (esp. cathelicidin) → ❸ cathelicidin-induced conversion of nonoffensive self-DNA into an autoinflammatory immunogen, which then potently activates the already upregulated TLR-9 = ❹

---

[676] Tak PP, Firestein GS. NFkB: a key role in inflammatory diseases. *J Clin Invest*. 2001;107(1):7-11 jci.org/cgi/content/full/107/1/7
[677] Armant MA, Fenton MJ. Toll-like receptors: a family of pattern-recognition receptors in mammals. *Genome Biol*. 2002 Jul 29;3(8):REVIEWS3011
[678] Ospelt C, et al. Toll-like receptors in rheumatoid arthritis joint destruction mediated by two distinct pathways. *Ann Rheum Dis*. 2004 Nov;63 Suppl 2:ii90-ii91
[679] Lee JY, Sohn KH, Rhee SH, Hwang D. Saturated fatty acids, but not unsaturated fatty acids, induce the _expression of cyclooxygenase-2 mediated through Toll-like receptor 4. J Biol Chem. 2001 May 18;276(20):16683-9. Epub 2001 Mar 2 jbc.org/cgi/content/full/276/20/16683
[680] Vasquez A. Reducing pain and inflammation naturally - part 4: nutritional and botanical inhibition of NFkB, the major intracellular amplifier of the inflammatory cascade. A practical clinical strategy exemplifying anti-inflammatory nutrigenomics. *Nutritional Perspectives*, July 2005:5-12.
[681] Miller LS. Toll-like receptors in skin. *Adv Dermatol*. 2008;24:71-87
[682] Lamphier MS, Sirois CM, Verma A, Golenbock DT, Latz E. TLR9 and the recognition of self and non-self nucleic acids. *Ann N Y Acad Sci*. 2006 Oct;1082:31-43

thereby, microbial inflammation results in autoimmunity/autoinflammation (to self-DNA). **A well-known function of TLRs is, via their transmembrane domain and a cytoplasmic tail domain that is homologous to the interleukin-1 receptor, the initiation of various intracellular signaling cascades, including activation of nuclear factor-kB (NFkB), which is a key transcription factor that promotes transcription of genes coding for pro-inflammatory molecules** such as cytokines, chemokines, co-stimulatory molecules (needed for immune responsiveness), and adhesion molecules (needed for the homing of immunocytes to inflamed/damaged tissue).

10. <u>Immune complex formation and deposition</u>: Chronic infection generally results in the increased production of immune complexes, which are polymeric antigen-antibody combinations. Antigen-antibody combinations are formed almost anytime the humoral immune system is fighting against a virus, bacteria, yeast, or food allergen. Although essential for the destruction and clearance of pathogenic antigens, immune complexes pose a problem for the body due to 1) the difficulty in clearing them from the systemic circulation, and 2) their proclivity for deposition in the skin and joints.[683] Indeed, **immune complexes are significant contributors to most "autoimmune" diseases; immune complex deposition is responsible for triggering joint inflammation in rheumatoid arthritis**[684] **and for the facial rash and many of the other clinical manifestations which characterize systemic lupus erythematosus (SLE, lupus).** Immune complex deposition directly contributes to the renal disease and vasculitis common in patients with autoimmune disease. Patients with autoimmune disease commonly have circulating IgM and IgA antibodies against bacteria from the gastrointestinal and genitourinary tracts[685] clearly indicating an active immune response against these bacteria and suggesting breaches in mucosal integrity. Since IgA-containing immune complexes are cleared from the serum by hepatocytes and are secreted intact into the bile[686,687,688], hepatobiliary phytostimulation may thereby produce an anti-rheumatic benefit; however, this hypothesis requires serologic and outcomes-based validation in a clinical trial.[689]

- Psoriasis and immune complexes—Circulating IgA immune complexes in patients with psoriasis (*J Invest Dermatol* 1983 Jun[690]): Using a sensitive and specific Raji cell radioimmunoassay, authors of this study analyzed the sera of 35 patients with psoriatic arthritis for IgA-containing circulating immune complexes (IgA-CIC). Additionally, measurements for circulating immune complexes (CIC) containing IgG or IgM were performed using the 125I-Clq binding assay and the Raji IgG radio-immunoassay. Results showed that, **"Twenty-eight of thirty five (80%) patients with PsA were found to have IgA-containing circulating immune complexes.** In contrast, only 13 of 35 (37%) had IgG-containing circulating immune complexes detected using the Raji IgG assay and 10 of 33 (33%) had IgG- or IgM-containing immune complexes detected using the 125I-Clq binding assay." Frequency, level, or subclass of immune complexes did not correlate with different types or severities of cutaneous psoriasis. However, **the level of IgA-CIC did significantly correlate with the severity of psoriatic arthritis**—higher levels of IgA-CIC corresponded with more severe psoriatic arthritis. The authors concluded, "The finding of IgA-containing circulating immune complexes in 80% of patients with psoriatic arthritis as well as the significantly higher levels of these complexes in the patients with more severe arthritis suggests that IgA-containing circulating immune complexes may play a role in the pathogenesis of psoriatic arthritis." Generally speaking, because IgA is the subclass of antibody/immunoglobulin that is used to defend mucosal surfaces such as the mouth, throat,

---

[683] Inman RD. Antigens, the gastrointestinal tract, and arthritis. *Rheum Dis Clin North Am*. 1991 May;17(2):309-21
[684] Abramson SB. Mediators of inflammation, tissue destruction, and repair: cellular constituents." In Klippel JH. *Primer on the rheumatic diseases. 11th edition*. Atlanta: Arthritis Foundation; 1997, page 39
[685] "IgM and IgA anti-Proteus antibodies were significantly higher in patients with RF-positive RA compared with all other patient groups." Newkirk MM, et al. Elevated levels of IgM and IgA antibodies to Proteus mirabilis and IgM antibodies to Escherichia coli are associated with early rheumatoid factor (RF)-positive rheumatoid arthritis. *Rheumatology* 2005;44:1433-41
[686] "Clearance of IgA immune complexes was delayed after bile duct ligation." Harmatz PR, Kleinman RE, Bunnell BW, McClenathan DT, Walker WA, Bloch KJ. The effect of bile duct obstruction on the clearance of circulating IgA immune complexes. *Hepatology*. 1984 Jan-Feb;4(1):96-100
[687] Lemaitre-Coelho I, et al. High levels of secretory IgA and free secretory component in the serum of rats with bile duct obstruction. *J Exp Med*. 1978 Mar 1;147(3):934-9
[688] "CONCLUSIONS: Biliary obstruction secondary to both calculus or malignancy of the hepatobiliary system causes suppression of bile IgA secretion and elevated serum level of secretory IgA. Bile secretory IgA secretion recovers with endoscopic drainage of the obstructed system." Sung JJ, Leung JC, Tsui CP, Chung SS, Lai KN. Biliary IgA secretion in obstructive jaundice: the effects of endoscopic drainage. *Gastrointest Endosc* 1995 Nov;42:439-44
[689] Vasquez A. Do the Benefits of Botanical and Physiotherapeutic Hepatobiliary Stimulation Result From Enhanced Excretion of IgA Immune Complexes? *Naturopathy Digest* 2006; January: naturopathydigest.com/archives/2006/jan/vasquez_immune.php
[690] Hall RP, Peck GL, Lawley TJ. Circulating IgA immune complexes in patients with psoriasis. *J Invest Dermatol*. 1983 Jun;80(6):465-8

respiratory tract, and the gastrointestinal and genitourinary tracts, elevations of IgA and IgA-CIC naturally encourage physicians to strongly consider microbial colonization of one or more mucosal surfaces. Additionally, since IgA-CIC are cleared by the liver for excretion into the bile and therefore into the intestines, additional attention (phytotherapeutic and physiologic) to ensuring optimal hepatobiliary and intestinal functions is likely to be of clinical benefit.[691]

- Psoriasis and immune complexes—IgA-containing immune complexes in patients with psoriatic arthritis (*Clin Exp Rheumatol* 1984 Jul-Sep-5[692]): In this study, blood samples from 21 patients with psoriasis were examined for the presence of IgA-CIC using the Raji IgA radioimmunoassay. Further, the Raji IgG radioimmunoassay and 125I-Clq binding assay were used to detect IgG-CIC and IgM-CIC. Results from the patients with psoriatic arthritis were contrasted against results from 25 patients with various nonpsoriatic hyperkeratotic skin disorders. Patients were given systemic therapy with etretinate (20 patients) or 13-cis-retinoic acid (1 patient)[Note 693]; blood from of 15 patients treated with etretinate were studied before, during, and after therapy. Whereas fourteen of 21 (67%) patients with psoriasis had evidence of IgA-CIC during the course of their disease, only 1 of 25 patients (4%) with other hyperkeratotic skin disorders showed this finding. Among the psoriatic patients, only 2 of 19 (11%) had evidence of IgG-CIC using the Raji IgG assay, and only 1 of 19 (5%) had evidence of IgG-CIC or IgM-CIC using the 125I-Clq binding assay. As was found in their previous study[694], these authors again showed a positive correlation between the extent of *psoriatic* disease and the level of IgA-CIC. Among 15 patients followed during therapy, results showed that levels of IgA-CIC did not change in response to positive response to treatment. Thus, given the correlation of IgA-CIC with the severity of psoriatic arthritis, the lack of correlation of IgA-CIC with improvement, and the lack of correlation of IgG-CIC and IgM-CIC with psoriasis, the authors concluded that, "...IgA-containing CIC are not directly related to the cutaneous manifestations of psoriasis, but may be important in the modification of immune or inflammatory responses in these patients." Another more likely explanation in the opinion of the current author (Dr Vasquez) is that IgA-CIC contribute to and represent the underlying pathophysiology of psoriasis (i.e., mucosal colonization with antigenic microbes and/or exposure to dietary antigens) which exists in proportion to the severity of the illness (i.e., serving as a reflection of both antigenic stimulation and abnormally increased mucosal permeability) and which persists despite clearance of skin lesions (i.e., the most superficial manifestation of the illness).

11. <u>Antimetabolites</u>: Yeast and bacteria can produce certain molecules which *jam up, monkey wrench*, or otherwise interfere with normal human cellular metabolism. The best example is **D-lactic acid**, which impairs human metabolic pathways that are designed to work with the "human" form of this metabolite—the levo isomer—L-lactic acid. Commonly resulting in headache, fatigue, depression, and sometimes death, D-lactic acidosis is extensively well documented in the medical research literature and commonly occurs in association with bacterial overgrowth of the intestine, particularly following intestinal bypass surgery.[695] Other antimetabolites produced from (intestinal) microbes which are associated with human disease and dysfunction include **ammonia, tryptamine, tyramine, octopamine, mercaptes, aldehydes, alcohol (ethanol), tartaric acid, indolepropionic acid, indoleacetic acid, skatole, indole, putrescine, and cadaverine**. Many of these metabolites are seen in higher amounts in patients with migraine, depression, weakness, confusion, schizophrenia, agitation, hepatic encephalopathy, chronic arthritis and rheumatoid arthritis. **Gut-derived neurotoxins** from bacteria and yeast may contribute to autistic symptomatology[696,697], and case reports have consistently demonstrated that excess absorption of bacterial

---

[691] Vasquez A. Do the Benefits of Botanical and Physiotherapeutic Hepatobiliary Stimulation Result From Enhanced Excretion of IgA Immune Complexes? naturopathydigest.com/archives/2006/jan/vasquez_immune.php
[692] Hall RP, Gerber LH, Lawley TJ. IgA-containing immune complexes in patients with psoriatic arthritis. *Clin Exp Rheumatol*. 1984 Jul-Sep;2(3):221-5
[693] Of note, etretinate is an aromatic retinoid which was approved for severe psoriasis in 1986 and removed from the Canadian market in 1996 and the United States market in 1998 due to the high risk of birth defects; it has been somewhat replaced by acitretin, a safer metabolite of etretinate. 13-cis-retinoic acid is more commonly known as isotretinoin and is available by prescription; like other synthetic variants of vitamin A, it is highly teratogenic (ie, isotretinoin causes severe birth defects.).
[694] Hall RP, Gerber LH, Lawley TJ. IgA-containing immune complexes in patients with psoriatic arthritis. *Clin Exp Rheumatol*. 1984 Jul-Sep;2(3):221-5
[695] "D-Lactic acidosis is a potentially fatal clinical condition seen in patients with a short small intestine and an intact colon. Excessive production of D-lactate by abnormal bowel flora overwhelms normal metabolism of D-lactate and leads to an accumulation of this enantiomer in the blood." Vella A, Farrugia G. D-lactic acidosis: pathologic consequence of saprophytism. *Mayo Clin Proc*. 1998 May;73(5):451-6
[696] Sandler RH, Finegold SM, Bolte ER, et al. Short-term benefit from oral vancomycin treatment of regressive-onset autism. *J Child Neurol*. 2000 Jul;15(7):429-35
[697] Shaw et al. Increased urinary excretion of analogs of Krebs cycle metabolites and arabinose in two brothers with autistic features. *Clin Chem* 1995;41(8Pt1):1094-104

metabolites can alter behavior in humans and result in acute neurocognitive decline and behavioral abnormalities in children.[698] **Hydrogen sulfide**, produced by intestinal bacteria such as *Citrobacter freundii*[699], is a mitochondrial poison[700] and is strongly associated with disease activity in ulcerative colitis.[701] Degradation of tryptophan by bacterial tryptophanase predisposes to a "functional tryptophan deficiency" and may result in insufficiency of serotonin which would contribute to hyperalgesia, depression, impaired adrenal responsiveness[702] ("hypoadrenalism"), and insomnia; **indole** and **skatole**, which are gut-derived bacterial degradation products of tryptophan, produce an inflammatory arthritis identical to rheumatoid arthritis in animal models.[703,704]

- Increased D-lactic acid intestinal bacteria in chronic fatigue syndrome (*In Vivo* 2009 Jul[705]): These researchers begin by noting that the symptoms of cognitive dysfunction and neurological impairment which are commonly seen in patients with chronic fatigue syndrome (CFS) are also classic presenting complaints in patients with D-lactic acidosis, which is always caused by bacterial overgrowth of the small bowel and/or (more rarely) by the patient's inability to metabolize/detoxify products of bacterial metabolism produced in the small and/or large bowel. The authors report finding a **significant increase of Gram-positive facultative anaerobic fecal microorganisms** in 108 CFS patients as compared to 177 control subjects. Specifically, they found that, "The viable count of D-lactic acid producing *Enterococcus* and *Streptococcus* spp. in the fecal samples from the CFS group (3.5 x 10(7) cfu/L and 9.8 x 10(7) cfu/L respectively) were significantly higher than those for the control group (5.0 x 10(6) cfu/L and 8.9 x 10(4) cfu/L respectively). **Readers should note that this is approximately a 10-fold increase in *Enterococcus* and a 1,000-fold increase in *Streptococcus* in the CFS group compared with the control group. These Gram-positive bacteria produced not only more lactic acid in general but specifically they produced more of the dextro isomer D-lactic acid** than the Gram negative *Escherichia coli*. The authors correctly conclude that these findings "might explain not only neurocognitive dysfunction in CFS patients but also mitochondrial dysfunction, these findings may have important clinical implications." A note of personal experience: the current author (Dr Vasquez) had one event of severe headache and dyscognition following consumption of a prebiotic (FOS) supplement during my 6-year bout with a CFS-related condition; from this experience, I furthered my understanding of dysbiosis and would continue to do so for the following 10 years. Of further note, based on my personal experience and review of the biomedical literature, I proposed in my CME monograph *Musculoskeletal Pain: Expanded Clinical Strategies* (2008, Institute for Functional Medicine) that D-lactic acidosis was one of the pathophysiologic mechanisms by which microbial overgrowth of the intestines causes fibromyalgia; I was therefore gratified to see this article—published in 2009, nearly 2 years after I had proposed this mechanism—verifying my hypothesis.

- Short bowel syndrome and D-lactic acidosis: Case report (*Arch Dis Child* 1980 Oct[706]): The three-sentence abstract of this case report reads, "Metabolic acidosis in a 3-year-old child with short bowel syndrome led to the discovery of massive D-lactic aciduria. After normalization of the intestinal bacterial flora, D-lactate disappeared together with the acidosis. Dysbacteriosis with excessive production of D-lactate by intestinal bacteria (unidentified) and subsequent absorption explains this

---

[698] "The neurological features consisted of a depressed conscious state, confusion, aggressive behaviour, slurred speech and ataxia. The organic acid profile of urine demonstrated increased amounts of lactic, 3-hydroxypropionic, 3-hydroxyisobutyric, 2-hydroxyisocaproic, phenyllactic, 4-hydroxyphenylacetic and 4-hydroxyphenyllactic acids. Of the lactic acid 99% was D-lactic acid." Haan et al. Severe illness caused by products of bacterial metabolism in child with short gut. *Eur J Pediatr*. 1985;144:63-5
[699] Lennette (editor in chief). *Manual of Clinical Microbiology. 4th Edition*. Am Soc Microbiology: 1985, p 269. Also indstate.edu/thcme/micro/GI/general/sld038.htm 2005 Oct
[700] "Treatment of H2S poisoning may benefit from interventions aimed at minimizing ROS-induced damage and reducing mitochondrial damage." Eghbal MA, Pennefather PS, O'Brien PJ. H2S cytotoxicity mechanism involves reactive oxygen species formation and mitochondrial depolarisation. *Toxicology*. 2004 Oct 15;203(1-3):69-76
[701] "CONCLUSIONS: Metabolic effects of sodium hydrogen sulfide on butyrate oxidation along the length of the colon closely mirror metabolic abnormalities observed in active ulcerative colitis, and increased production of sulfide in ulcerative colitis suggests that the action of mercaptides may be involved in the genesis of ulcerative colitis." Roediger WE, et al. Reducing sulfur compounds of the colon impair colonocyte nutrition: implications for ulcerative colitis. *Gastroenterology* 1993 Mar;104:802-9
[702] "This hypothesis is supported by the findings in chronic MS patients of a significantly diminished adrenal cortisol reactivity to insulin-induced hypoglycemia which is considered a stress response mediated through the 5-HT system. Consequently, since patients with MS exhibit an abnormal response to stress it follows that increased tryptophan availability through dietary supplementation would diminish their vulnerability to psychological stress." Sandyk R. Tryptophan availability and the susceptibility to stress in multiple sclerosis: a hypothesis. *Int J Neurosci*. 1996 Jul;86(1-2):47-53
[703] Nakoneczna I, Forbes JC, Rogers KS. The arthritogenic effect of indole, skatole and other tryptophan metabolites in rabbits. *Am J Pathol*. 1969 Dec;57(3):523-38
[704] Rogers KS, Forbes JC, Nakoneczna I. Arthritogenic properties of lipophilic, aryl molecules. *Proc Soc Exp Biol Med*. 1969 Jun;131(2):670-2
[705] Sheedy JR, et al. Increased d-lactic acid intestinal bacteria in patients with chronic fatigue syndrome. *In Vivo*. 2009 Jul-Aug;23(4):621-8
[706] Schoorel EP, Giesberts MA, Blom W, van Gelderen HH. D-Lactic acidosis in a boy with short bowel syndrome. *Arch Dis Child*. 1980 Oct;55(10):810-2

unusual cause of metabolic acidosis." Note the use of the term "dysbacteriosis" which is more commonly abbreviated to "dysbiosis", with the latter term being more accurate in terms of its nonspecificity since the disease-producing microbes may be from several different kingdoms. The young boy in this case report underwent bowel resection secondary to multiple congenital malformations and complications from infection, i.e., mesenteric thrombosis tertiary to dehydration secondary to infectious diarrhea. After several episodes of neurocognitive dysfunction including weakness and dyspnea, the child was eventually diagnosed with multiple nutritional deficiencies, malabsorption, and lactic acidosis secondary to intestinal overgrowth of Gram-positive D-lactate-producing bacteria and an insufficiency of Gram-negative bacteria. The child was treated only with probiotic supplementation—no antibiotics were given—and D-lactate levels fell quickly within 4 days and were virtually undetectable by day 11. Thus, probiotic therapy alone may be sufficient treatment for some cases of D-lactic acidosis, particularly when an "insufficiency dysbiosis" of beneficial bacteria and a relative or absolute "overgrowth dysbiosis" of harmful bacteria coexist.

12. <u>Autointoxication, auto-brewery syndrome, hepatic encephalopathy</u>: The term "autointoxication" fell out of favor among American allopaths in the 1940s despite the recognition and objective documentation that systemically absorbed microbial metabolites/toxins from the colon could adversely affect systemic health, particularly neurocognitive function.[707] "Hepatic encephalopathy"—classically characterized by elevated serum ammonia which is a direct and surrogate marker for putrefactive dysbiosis overwhelming hepatic detoxification capacity and impaired neurotransmission, respectively—seems to be one of the currently acceptable terms for this phenomenon, and probably the condition exists among some outpatients to a milder degree than that which is classically seen in patients with fulminant liver failure—I first published that sentence in early 2006[708], and in 2014 I worked with a patient who proved this to be true:

Clinical Case **Elevated plasma ammonia in a 45yo male with gastrointestinal dysbiosis**: These laboratory results from April 2014 show elevated plasma/serum ammonia in a 45yo previously athletic male suffering with a 2-year history of debilitating fatigue and neuromuscular disorder; the patient has no history of liver disease, and all other laboratory testing is remarkably normal. Iron overload was excluded (ferritin level ranging from 49-81 ng/ml on several occasions); copper overload was excluded (normal ceruoplasmin and serum copper). Other testing showed a remarkably elevated urine DHPPA (3,4 dihydroxyphenylpropionic acid), which is produced by various bacteria from dietary chlorogenic acid, sourced from a wide variety of fruits, vegetables, tea and coffee; elevated DHPPA is an objective marker consistent with SIBO—small intestine bacterial overgrowth. Tartaric acid is found in small/modest amounts in fruits such as grapes, bananas, and tamarinds but elevated levels in urine generally correlate with fungal/yeast overgrowth of the intestines. Of additional note, this patient was unlikely to be biotin deficient per daily supplementation of approximately 2 mg/d; nevertheless, we increased biotin intake to 5 mg/d while treating with laxative doses of ascorbic acid each morning followed later in the day by berberine 1500 mg/d, time-released emulsified oregano oil 600 mg/d, and low-fermentation diet. These treatments and especially the addition of azithromycin 250 mg/d per high antibody titers against *Chlamydophila pneumoniae* (discussed in Chapters 1 [laboratory assessments] and 4 [dysbiosis] lead to important clinical improvements.

Results dated 2014 Apr

Test Name: AMMONIA (P)

Analyte Name	Units	Ref Range	04/11/14
AMMONIA (P)	UMOL/L	< OR = 47	58 (H)

Results dated 2013 Aug

Dihydroxyphenylpropionic Acid (DHPPA)	19.1	<= 5.3
Tartaric Acid	32	<= 15

---
[707] Person JR, Bernhard JD. Autointoxication revisited. *J Am Acad Dermatol*. 1986;15(3):559-63
[708] Vasquez A. Nutritional and Botanical Treatments against "Silent Infections" and Gastrointestinal Dysbiosis. *Nutritional Perspectives* 2006; January

Recognition that excess or abnormal microbes in the gut could cause neuropsychiatric symptoms contributed to the rationale for the use of colonic irrigation in clinical practice which was fully endorsed by the American Medical Association in a position paper published in 1932.[709] Concurrently, an article published in the *New England Journal of Medicine*[710] in this same year documented the clinical benefits of colonic irrigation in patients with mental disease; the treatment was deemed effective against most cases of dementia, depression, neurosis and many cases of irritability, headaches, and hypertension. Enemas and colonics, which promote hepatobiliary detoxification[711,712] and cleanse the bowel of harmful microbes, were valued by clinicians as a cure or adjunctive treatment for numerous systemic diseases.[713] Although the term "autointoxication" is eschewed as "unscientific", all medical professionals recognize that gastrointestinal dysbiosis—particularly generalized overgrowth of yeast and bacteria—can cause clinical conditions characterized by inflammatory vasculitis, dermatitis, arthritis as well as neurological symptoms ranging from confusion and disorientation to somnolence and death. Of a less dramatic but much more frequent note, bacterial overgrowth of the small bowel is also a cause of gastroesophageal reflux disease (GERD) because products of bacterial fermentation relax the lower esophageal sphincter[714] and retard intestinal transit[715]; ameliorating the intestinal bacterial overgrowth by simply "starving" the bacteria of carbohydrate by implementation of a **low-carbohydrate diet** alleviates GERD symptoms and substantiates the cause-and-effect relationship.[716,717]

One of the liver's chief functions is that of "detoxifying" environmentally ingested and endogenously produced metabolites and toxins, including those of microbial origin produced de novo within the gastrointestinal tract. The metabolic activity of the microbial population within the intestinal lumen is quantitatively enormous, physiologically important, and clinically significant; an estimated ten trillion microorganisms reside within the intestinal lumen of each human. Being very small of course creates very large surface-to-volume ratios for microorganisms; if we take as given that an average bacterium of spherical shape has surface area of approximately 12 micrometers squared, then multiplying this surface area by 10 trillion in order to give some appreciation of the mass of lipopolysaccharide and peptidoglycan mass yields a surface area of 120 trillion micrometers squared or 120 billion meters squared, equal to approximately 29,652,645 acres or 12,000,000 hectares. Given that the total surface of the bacterial community is constantly being shed and replaced by individual microbes throughout each unit of time and also per death of each microbe, then the "functional surface area" of the microbial population is massive beyond comprehension, leaving unquantifiable debris to be either physically excluded or immunologically processed. In addition to this "physical debris", microbes secrete even more metabolic molecules, some of which are intentionally and directly toxic and all of which have to be processed/detoxified/eliminated if and when they are absorbed systemically. As stated previously in this chapter, readers should appreciate that the "total dysbiotic load" (TDL) from all sources—skin, gastrointestinal tract, genitourinary tract, sinorespiratory tract, orodental cavity, environment, and any subclinical parenchymal foci—contributes to the total inflammatory load (TIL) and total xenobiotic load (TXL) which the immune system must process and which the hepatobiliary system must detoxify.

In a review article[718] published in 2010 which applies specifically to the gastrointestinal subtype of dysbiosis, the authors start their paper by stating, "Detoxification of gut-derived toxins and microbial

---

[709] Bastedo WA. Colon irrigations: their administration therapeutic applications and dangers. *Journal of the American Medical Association* 1932;98:734-6
[710] Marshall HK, Thomson CR. Colon irrigation in the treatment of mental disease. N Engl J Med 1932; 207 (Sept 8): 454-7
[711] Garbat, AL, Jacobi, HG: Secretion of Bile in Response to Rectal Installations. *Arch Intern Med* 1929; 44: 455-462
[712] "Caffeine enemas cause dilation of bile ducts, which facilitates excretion of toxic cancer breakdown products by the liver and dialysis of toxic products from blood across the colonic wall. The therapy must be used as an integrated whole." Gerson M. The cure of advanced cancer by diet therapy. *Physiol Chem Phys*. 1978;10(5):449-64
[713] Snyder RG. The value of colonic irrigations in countering auto-intoxication of intestinal origin. *Medical Clinics of North America* 1939; May:781-788
[714] "In summary, we have shown that colonic fermentation, through the production of SCFAs, exerts a controlled feedback on LES motor function." Piche T, et al. Modulation by colonic fermentation of LES function in humans. *Am J Physiol Gastrointest Liver Physiol*. 2000 Apr;278(4):G578-84
[715] "Altered gastrointestinal motility and sensation, changed activity of the central nervous system, and increased sympathetic drive and immune activation may be understood as consequences of the host response to SIBO." Lin HC. Small intestinal bacterial overgrowth: a framework for irritable bowel syndrome. *JAMA*. 2004 Aug 18;292(7):852-8
[716] "These data suggest that a very low-carbohydrate diet in obese individuals with GERD significantly reduces distal esophageal acid exposure and improves symptoms." Austin GL, et al. A very low-carbohydrate diet improves gastroesophageal reflux and its symptoms. *Dig Dis Sci*. 2006 Aug;51(8):1307-12
[717] "The 5 individuals described in these case reports experienced resolution of GERD symptoms after self-initiation of a low-carbohydrate diet." Yancy WS Jr, et al. Improvement of gastroesophageal reflux disease after initiation of a low-carbohydrate diet: five brief case reports. *Altern Ther Health Med*. 2001 Nov-Dec;7(6):120, 116-9
[718] Szabo G, Bala S, Petrasek J, Gattu A. Gut-liver axis and sensing microbes. *Dig Dis*. 2010;28(6):737-44

products from gut-derived microbes is a major role of the liver. While the full repertoire of gut-derived microbial products that reach the liver in health and disease is yet to be explored, the levels of bacterial lipopolysaccharide (LPS), a component of Gram-negative bacteria, is increased in the portal and/or systemic circulation in several types of chronic liver diseases." The total metabolic and toxic load from the microbes in the gut can be of such a volume that the body's ability to detoxify/metabolize these toxins is overwhelmed.

- Autointoxication, auto-brewery syndrome: A child with ethanol intoxication secondary to bacterial/fungal overgrowth of the intestines (*J Pediatr Gastroenterol Nutr* 2001 Aug[719]): In this case report and review of the literature, the authors begin their article by noting that, "The term **auto-brewery syndrome** has been used to describe patients who become repeatedly inebriated after ingestion of food of high carbohydrate nature in the presence of abnormal yeast proliferation, particularly of *Candida* species." The case report centers on a 13-year-old girl who had bowel resection for important reasons when a neonate and who later had "recurrent episodes of bizarre behavior, somnolence, disorientation, and a fruity odor of her breath and was suspected to be abusing alcohol." **The young girl was diagnosed with alcohol intoxication when ethanol blood levels were repeatedly elevated in the range of 250 mg/dL to 350 mg/dL**; she persistently denied any intake of alcoholic beverages. Readers should note that in most states in the United States, a blood alcohol concentration (BAC) of or greater than 100 mg/dL is the legal definition of intoxication and drunkenness.[720] The young girl's father—a physician—began testing the girl's breath alcohol level at home and noticed a strong correlation between her elevated ethanol levels and the intake of carbohydrate-rich meals or fructose-containing drinks, such as fruit juices. The girl was treated empirically for bacterial overgrowth of the intestines with courses of the anti-bacterial drugs Bactrim, Flagyl, and Augmentin and attained zero benefit. The girl was then submitted for underwent upper gastrointestinal endoscopy study to obtain aspirates for microbial analysis; the aspirate grew abundant *Candida glabrata* and *Sacchromyces cerevisiae*. **Sensitivity-directed treatment with fluconazole resolved all symptoms and prevented recurrence of the elevated ethanol levels**. The combination of bacterial with fungal overgrowth was likely synergistic; bacterial LPS blocked Cyp450 detoxification and thereby heightened sensitivity to the fungally-produced ethanol.

13. Dysbiotic arthropathy, dysbiotic dermatitis, dysbiotic vasculitis (etc): Current terms for this condition include "bowel-associated dermatosis-arthritis syndrome"[721], "intestinal arthritis-dermatitis syndrome"[722], and "bypass disease"[723]—all of which are largely mediated by the gut-derived absorption of microbial antigens, mucosal and systemic antibody formation, and antigen-antibody binding in the circulation and tissues followed by systemic deposition of circulating immune complexes in skin, joints, kidneys, and vascular endothelium.

Intestinal arthritis-dermatitis syndrome: rheumatic-inflammatory complications of gastrointestinal dysbiosis-induced systemic inflammation and immune complex deposition

1. **Arthritis***‡ —Most commonly of the peripheral joints but may also include the spine and sacroiliac joints; may be destructive or nondestructive, with or without RF and serologic evidence of immune complex mediation such as hypocomplimentemia
2. **Dermatitis***‡ —"The most common non-articular inflammatory findings in patients with intestinal bypass arthritis involve the skin, reported in as many as 77% of patients." Rashes may be urticarial, maculopapular, papulovesicular or vesiculopustular affecting any part of the face, trunk or extremities
3. Myalgia
4. Myositis, polymyositis‡
5. Pleuritis‡
6. Pericarditis‡
7. Raynaud's phenomenon
8. Vasculitis, leukocytoclastic angiitis*‡
9. Oral ulceration‡
10. Tenosynovitis
11. Paresthesias, peripheral neuropathy*
12. Carpal tunnel syndrome

* Note that these are common clinical manifestations of underlying immune complex pathophysiology.
‡ Note that many of these clinical manifestations of bypass-induced intestinal dysbiosis are clinical manifestations of—and indeed components of the diagnostic criteria for—prototypic autoimmune diseases such as systemic lupus erythematosus.

Ross et al. Jejunoileal bypass arthritis. *Baillieres Clin Rheumatol*. 1989 Aug

---

[719] Dahshan et al. Auto-brewery syndrome in a child with short gut syndrome: case report and review of the literature. *J Pediatr Gastroenterol Nutr*. 2001 Aug;33:214-5
[720] Cohen JS. (Plantz SH, Talavera F, Anker A, editors). Alcohol Intoxication. emedicinehealth.com/alcohol_intoxication/page2_em.htm June 9, 2011
[721] Jorizzo JL, et al. Bowel-bypass syndrome without bowel bypass. Bowel-associated dermatosis-arthritis syndrome. *Arch Intern Med*. 1983 Mar;143(3):457-61
[722] Stein HB, Schlappner OL, Boyko W, Gourlay RH, Reeve CE. The intestinal bypass: arthritis-dermatitis syndrome. *Arthritis Rheum*. 1981 May;24(5):684-90
[723] Utsinger PD. Systemic immune complex disease following intestinal bypass surgery: bypass disease. *J Am Acad Dermatol*. 1980 Jun;2(6):488-95

- <u>Authoritative review: Jejunoileal bypass arthritis (*Baillieres Clin Rheumatol* 1989 Aug[724])</u>: In this 17-page review chapter, authors Ross, Scott, and Pincus discuss the allopathic medicosurgical use of jejunoileal bypass, a surgical procedure wherein the jejunum is connected to the terminal ileum, thereby bypassing the absorptive surface of the jejunum, causing a surgically-induced malabsorption and diarrhea-induced nausea and anorexia which results in weight loss for the "treatment" of obesity. The procedure was used on more than 100,000 patients between the years 1954-1983 when it was discarded due to the high rates of clinically important post-operative complications, noted in up to 58% of patients. Interestingly, studying the rheumatologic complications of jejunoileal bypass contributed to scientific knowledge about the relationship of microbial dysbiosis and inflammatory diseases, particularly skin inflammation and joint inflammation; the authors write, "However, important advances in the understanding of inflammatory joint disease emerged from studies of the prominent rheumatologic complication of intestinal bypass known as the **arthritis-dermatitis syndrome**. Furthermore, the symptoms of "**bypass arthritis**" have been recognized in individuals who have not undergone intestinal bypass, but who had perturbations of intestinal anatomy secondary to postoperative, inflammatory or diverticular conditions." The pathophysiology of bypass arthritis-dermatitis syndrome is straightforward and linear and easy to understand: ❶ altered intestinal structure and function leads to bacterial overgrowth and compromise of the intestinal mucosa, ❷ bacterial overgrowth and compromise of the intestinal mucosa leads to increased absorption of bacteria and bacterial antigens, perhaps as well as food antigens, ❸ increased absorption of bacteria and bacterial antigens leads to antibody formation, ❹ combination of bacterial antigens with antibodies leads to immune complex formation, ❺ immune complexes have a biologic proclivity for deposition in the joints, vessels, kidneys, skin, alveoli, and serosal surfaces, ❻ deposition of immune complexes in any tissue results in a localized immune response with resultant inflammation regardless of the primary origin of the antigens from the overgrowth/overcolonization of bacteria. Per the authors, "The pathogenesis of intestinal bypass arthritis involves bacterial overgrowth and mucosal alterations in the defunctionalized segment of small intestine, i.e., the 'blind loop'. ... "The blunted villi allow increased absorption of bacteria and bacterial products, leading to dissemination of high molecular weight immune complexes containing bacterial products." These "immune complexes of enteric antigens" are then deposited in the joints, skin, vessels, kidneys, and pulmonary alveoli to produce arthritis, dermatitis, vasculitis, nephritis, and pneumonitis, respectively.

  > **The molecular evidence**
  > Immune complexes in intestinal bypass arthritis contain IgG, IgM, and IgA antibodies directed against bacterial antigens from *E. coli*, *Bacteroides*, *Lactobacilli*, and Group D (gamma) streptococcus.
  >
  > Ross e al. *Baillieres Clin Rheumatol*. 1989 Aug

  New-onset inflammatory joint symptoms are noted in 6-52% of patients following jejunoileal bypass. Most commonly the inflammatory arthritis is seen in females, and the presentation "mimics early rheumatoid arthritis" with involvement of the hands, wrists, and knees and less commonly the spine and sacroiliac joints. Morning stiffness—a finding classic for inflammatory joint disease—is common. The arthritis is generally nondestructive; however, some post-bypass patients will develop periarticular erosions and sclerosis—findings common to rheumatoid arthritis. Tests for antinuclear antibodies (ANA), rheumatoid factor (RF), and serum complement are generally normal, but some patients will develop cryoglobulinemia due to immune complex formation and others positive for HLA-B27 will develop spondylitis. "Therefore", the authors note in 1989, "the diagnosis of intestinal bypass arthritis remains primarily clinical." Very interestingly, one patient developed "classic rheumatoid arthritis with erosions and rheumatoid factors following jejunoileal bypass. ... ...the patient experienced complete remission of musculoskeletal disease soon after revision [surgical reversal] of the bypass..." The vast majority (up to 77%) of patients with bypass-induced dysbiotic arthritis develop skin inflammation alongside; "The most common non-articular inflammatory

---

[724] Ross CB, Scott HW, Pincus T. Jejunoileal bypass arthritis. *Baillieres Clin Rheumatol*. 1989 Aug;3(2):339-55

findings in patients with intestinal bypass arthritis involve the skin, reported in as many as 77% of patients. ... Typical rashes may be urticarial, maculopapular, papulovesicular or vesiculopustular... Any part of the face, trunk or extremities may be involved."

Beside and beyond the merely symptomatic treatments such as NSAIDs—which notoriously increase intestinal permeability and may therefore contribute to the pathophysiology of intestinal dysbiosis—ultimate treatments for bypass dermatitis-arthritis syndrome are either antimicrobial therapy to eradicate the intestinal bacterial overgrowth or surgical restoration of the original intestinal anatomy. Impressively, surgical restoration of normal anatomy can completely resolve the condition within 48 hours, thereby proving the cause-and-effect relationship. **Broad-spectrum antimicrobial drugs are use empirically: tetracycline, metronidazole, trimethoprim/sulphamethoxazole, and clindamycin.** Oral corticosteroids may be used to help control the inflammation; adverse effects including exacerbation of diabetes and hypertension, as well as promotion of additional bacterial overgrowth due to intestinal immunosuppression are well-known. Importantly, "bowel bypass disease without bowel bypass" can occur secondary to any condition that promotes bacterial overgrowth of the intestines and the resultant immune complex formation; the term used to describe this phenomenon is "bowel-associated dermatitis and arthritis."

> **Dysbiosis-induced immune complex formation and deposition accounts for the primary underlying pathophysiology of bypass arthritis and arthritis-dermatitis syndrome**
>
> "The pathogenesis of intestinal bypass arthritis involves bacterial overgrowth and mucosal alterations in the defunctionalized segment of small intestine, i.e., the 'blind loop'. ... "The blunted villi allow increased absorption of bacteria and bacterial products, leading to dissemination of high molecular weight immune complexes containing bacterial products." These "immune complexes of enteric antigens" are then deposited in the joints, skin, vessels, kidneys, and pulmonary alveoli to produce arthritis, dermatitis, vasculitis, nephritis, and pneumonitis, respectively.
>
> Ross et al. *Baillieres Clin Rheumatol.* 1989 Aug

- Pro-inflammatory effect of *Lactobacillus rhamnosus Lcr35* (*PLoS One* 2011 Apr[725]): This experimental study shows that some intestinal bacteria—in this case, a specific strain of *Lactobacillus* identified as *Lactobacillus rhamnosus Lcr35*—can incite a proinflammatory effect. The possibility exists that the physiologic consequences of an individual bacteria might be different *in vivo* when intermixed with the effects of other microbes; however, the most reasonable interpretation of this data is that *Lactobacillus rhamnosus* promotes inflammation and should therefore be avoided in patients already experiencing excessive inflammation. The authors introduce their paper appropriately by stating, "Some [probiotic] strains modulate the cytokine production of dendritic cells (DCs) in vitro and induce a regulatory response, while others induce conversely a pro-inflammatory response." Results of this experiment showed that, by use of DNA microarray and qRT-PCR analysis, the probiotic induced a large-scale change in gene expression (nearly 1,700 modulated genes, with 3-fold changes), but only with high doses (multiplicity of infection [MOI] of 100x [range 0.01 to 100]). Flow cytometry analysis showed an upregulated expression of CD86, CD83, HLA-DR and TLR4 and reduced expression of DC-SIGN, MR and CD14. Cytokine measurements showed strong dose-dependent increases in pro-Th1/Th17 cytokine levels (TNFα, IL-1β, IL-12p70, IL-12p40 and IL-23) contrasted with only a slight increase in anti-inflammatory IL-10. The authors concluded therefore that, "The probiotic *L. rhamnosus Lcr35* [leads to], at high doses, to the semi-maturation of the [dendritic] cells and to a strong pro-inflammatory effect." This article is noteworthy for showing the molecular evidence of dose-dependent inflammation induction by a bacterium generally considered to be among a group of beneficial bacteria; many people consider "*Lactobacillus*" as a group to be exclusively beneficial while this evidence demonstrates pro-inflammatory effects. Bacterial overgrowth of the small bowel (aka, small intestine bacterial overgrowth [SIBO]) commonly includes a mix of Gram-negatives with Gram-positives, anaerobes with aerobes, and so-called "beneficial" bacteria along with pathogens and potential pathogens.

---

[725] Evrard B, et al. Dose-Dependent Immunomodulation of Human Dendritic Cells by the Probiotic Lactobacillus rhamnosus Lcr35. *PLoS One*. 2011 Apr 18;6(4):e18735

Chapter 4: Major Modifiable Factors in Systemic Inflammation

Interconnected pathways Involved in dysbiosis-induced musculoskeletal inflammation/autoimmunity:
"What I talk about is only what I have lived through. If you have not lived through something, it is not true." Kabir (1440-1518), Indian poet

15. <u>Damage to the intestinal mucosa</u>: One of the indirect ways by which gastrointestinal microbes can cause non-infectious disease is by damaging the intestinal mucosa, a situation which results in "leaky gut." The increased absorption of molecular debris from the gut—"antigen overload" from otherwise benign yeast, bacteria, and foods—results in systemic inflammation[726] and immune activation[727], which contribute to enhanced autoantigen processing and bystander activation as discussed above. Exacerbations and relapse of the autoimmune diseases ulcerative colitis and Crohn's disease are preceded by increases in intestinal permeability; this is direct evidence of "leaky gut" preceding clinical disease.[728] Evidence of "leaky gut" is seen in several systemic inflammatory disorders, including asthma[729], eczema[730], psoriasis[731], Behcet's disease[732], seronegative spondyloarthritis[733] and ankylosing spondylitis[734] and nearly all of the so-called "idiopathic" juvenile arthropathies such as enteropathic spondyloarthropathy and oligoarticular juvenile idiopathic arthritis.[735] A "leaky gut" type of intestinal disease (protein-losing enteropathy) occurs in some patients with lupus.[736]

- <u>Intestinal permeability in patients with psoriasis (*J Dermatol Sci* 1991 Jul[737])</u>: In this study of 15 psoriatic patients and 15 healthy volunteers, intestinal permeability was evaluated using the 51Cr-labeled EDTA absorption test. 24-h urine excretion of 51Cr-EDTA from psoriatic patients was 2.46% which was significantly higher than the results from controls at 1.95% and therefore indicated increased intestinal permeability among patients with psoriasis. Clinical implications of these results include 1) that psoriasis not merely a skin condition and that it affects other vital structures, in this instance, the gastrointestinal tract, and 2) that enhanced intestinal absorption of food antigens and microbial metabolites and immunogenic debris is ensured among psoriatic patients and would be expected to contribute to systemic inflammation and immunologic sensitization. This study was published in 1991 and used urinary measurement of orally administered 51Cr-EDTA to determine intestinal permeability; in modern outpatient practice, we use the lactulose-mannitol assay as a more sensitive and reliable indicator of mucosal permeability status.

- <u>Skin diseases and intestinal permeability—Small intestinal permeability in dermatological disease</u> (*Quarterly Journal of Medicine* 1985 Sep[738]): The authors of this study assessed small intestinal permeability using the cellobiose/mannitol differential sugar absorption test (using urinary excretion of absorbed cellobiose and mannitol to determine intestinal permeability). Test subjects included 62 patients with atopic eczema, 29 with psoriasis, and 18 with dermatitis herpetiformis. Results of testing were *generally* unremarkable among *most* psoriatics and eczema patients when compared to the control population. However, some patients showed distinct abnormalities. Among the 62 patients with eczema, 7 (11%) had abnormal cellobiose/mannitol absorption as measured by urinary excretion; 6 of these patients underwent jejunal biopsy, and one patient was found to have celiac disease. Among the 29 patients with psoriasis, 7 (24%) had abnormal cellobiose/mannitol recovery. Among the 18 patients with dermatitis herpetiformis, 11 (61%) had abnormal cellobiose/mannitol recovery; this is not surprising give the intimate causative association between celiac disease and dermatitis herpetiformis. Thus, reasonable interpretations of this data are that ❶ a clinically significant number

---

[726] Campbell DI, Elia M, Lunn PG. Growth faltering in rural Gambian infants is associated with impaired small intestinal barrier function, leading to endotoxemia and systemic inflammation. *J Nutr*. 2003 May;133(5):1332-8

[727] "Altered gastrointestinal motility and sensation, changed activity of the central nervous system, and increased sympathetic drive and immune activation may be understood as consequences of the host response to SIBO." Lin HC. Small intestinal bacterial overgrowth: a framework for understanding irritable bowel syndrome. *JAMA*. 2004 Aug 18;292(7):852-8 This is one of few articles that I would describe as "brilliant" from the pages of *JAMA*—definitely worth reading by everyone who had or has a gastrointestinal tract or who treats patients who do.

[728] Wyatt J, Vogelsang H, Hubl W, Waldhoer T, Lochs H. Intestinal permeability and the prediction of relapse in Crohn's disease. *Lancet*. 1993 Jun 5;341(8858):1437-9

[729] Hijazi Z, et al. Intestinal permeability is increased in bronchial asthma. *Arch Dis Child*. 2004 Mar;89(3):227-9

[730] Ukabam SO, Mann RJ, Cooper BT. Small intestinal permeability to sugars in patients with atopic eczema. *Br J Dermatol*. 1984 Jun;110(6):649-52

[731] "The 24-h urine excretion of 51Cr-EDTA from psoriatic patients was 2.46 +/- 0.81%. These results differed significantly from controls (1.95 +/- 0.36%; P less than 0.05)." Humbert P, Bidet A, Treffel P, Drobacheff C, Agache P. Intestinal permeability in patients with psoriasis. *J Dermatol Sci*. 1991 Jul;2(4):324-6

[732] Fresko I, et al. Intestinal permeability in Behcet's syndrome. *Ann Rheum Dis*. 2001 Jan;60(1):65-6

[733] Di Leo V, D'Inca R, Bettini MB, Podswiadek M, Punzi L, Mastropaolo G, Sturniolo GC. Effect of Helicobacter pylori and eradication therapy on gastrointestinal permeability. Implications for patients with seronegative spondyloarthritis. *J Rheumatol*. 2005 Feb;32(2):295-300

[734] "Patients with AS have altered small intestinal, but not gastric, permeability. NSAID use cannot explain all the abnormality. Bowel permeability abnormalities, possibly genetically determined, may antedate development of bowel or joint symptoms." Vaile JH, Meddings JB, Yacyshyn BR, Russell AS, Maksymowych WP. Bowel permeability and CD45RO expression on circulating CD20+ B cells in patients with ankylosing spondylitis and their relatives. *J Rheumatol*. 1999 Jan;26(1):128-35

[735] Picco P, et al. Increased gut permeability in juvenile chronic arthritides. A multivariate analysis of diagnostic parameters. *Clin Exp Rheumatol*. 2000 Nov-Dec;18:773-8

[736] "Fourteen cases of primary lupus-associated protein-losing enteropathy have now been reported in the English-language literature." Perednia DA, Curosh NA. Lupus-associated protein-losing enteropathy. *Arch Intern Med*. 1990 Sep;150(9):1806-10

[737] Humbert P, Bidet A, Treffel P, Drobacheff C, Agache P. Intestinal permeability in patients with psoriasis. *J Dermatol Sci*. 1991 Jul;2(4):324-6

[738] Hamilton I, Fairris GM, Rothwell J, Cunliffe WJ, Dixon MF, Axon AT. Small intestinal permeability in dermatological disease. *Q J Med*. 1985 Sep;56(221):559-67

of patients with eczema, psoriasis, and dermatitis herpetiformis have abnormal intestinal permeability, ❷ that these "skin conditions" and apparent "dermatological diseases" are systemic disorders which commonly occur with gastrointestinal components, and ❸ given the important role of intestinal mucosa integrity as a barometer of health and as a determinant of systemic inflammation and immune responses, attention to gastrointestinal (dys)function in these patients is worthy of additional investigation by researchers and attention by clinicians. This study was published in 1985 and used urinary measurement of orally administered cellobiose and mannitol to determine intestinal permeability; in modern outpatient practice, we use the lactulose and mannitol assay as a more sensitive and reliable indicator of mucosal permeability status.

16. Insufficiency dysbiosis—an absolute or relative lack of beneficial bacteria: Clinicians performing stool tests on a regular basis—current author included—commonly find that patients simultaneously have—in addition to other problems—"too many bad bacteria and not enough good bacteria", as is commonly explained to patients. An insufficiency of beneficial bacteria leads to increased bacterial translocation, reduced colonization resistance, and failure to induce regulatory T-cells; all of these contribute to systemic inflammation. Beneficial bacteria in general exert many positive benefits for the host which might be summarized as follows: ❶ maintaining the health and permeability integrity of the mucosa, ❷ providing fuel—butyrate—for enterocytes and specifically colonocytes, ❸ maintaining a slightly acidic pH due to elaboration of metabolic acids, ❹ blocking colonization by harmful yeasts and bacteria via several mechanisms such as by *directly* producing antimicrobial factors and *indirectly* inducing enhanced secretion of secretory IgA from mucosal plasma cells, ❺ metabolism/processing of phytonutrients for absorption and enhanced physiologic function, ❻ co-feeding other probiotic bacteria, for example, Bifidobacteria convert carbohydrate substrate to lactate and acetate which are then further metabolized by *Lactobacillus* into butyrate; in this way, probiotic bacteria "support each other" and are dependent/interdependent, ❼ maintaining a favorable biochemical and immunologic milieu for other beneficial bacteria, ❽ promoting elaboration of anti-inflammatory cytokines and suppression of pro-inflammatory cytokines, specifically inducing tolerogenic DCs producing lowered amounts of pro-inflammatory IFN-gamma and elevated amounts of anti-inflammatory IL-10, ❾ helping to ameliorate allergy in general and food allergy in particular by the above mechanisms, and ❿ promoting maturation of undifferentiated/naïve T-cells into regulatory T-cells (Treg) for the suppression/modulation of pro-inflammatory Th17-cells which are some of the primary pathologic effectors of autoimmune-mediated tissue damage, particularly in multiple sclerosis. Induction of Foxp3+ Treg from mature Th2-type memory T-cells by use of combination treatment including retinoic acid (an active form of vitamin A) has been performed experimentally[739], probably occurs in vivo in humans, and is reviewed elsewhere in this book. Several of these aforementioned mechanisms are well-known and/or self-evident; however, induction of Treg by probiotics is a relatively new concept and is of supreme clinical importance and will be given additional detail here:

- Probiotic induction of Treg and DCreg: Generation of regulatory dendritic cells and CD4+Foxp3+ T cells by probiotics administration suppresses immune disorders (*Proc Natl Acad Sci USA* 2010 Feb[740]): In this study, the authors used a probiotic mixture which was found to achieve several very important

> **Probiotic mutualism via cross-feeding ultimately affects human gene expression, enterocyte health, and intestinal permeability**
>
> Oral supplementation with synbiotics provides inulin and fructooligosaccharides to *Bifidobacterium* and *Lactobacillus* which partially metabolize carbohydrate substrates to acetate and lactate which then serve as substrate for butyrogenic microbes such as *Roseburia intestinalis* and *Anaerostipes caccae* for the production of butyrate, which provides anti-inflammatory nutrigenomic benefits via suppression of NFkB, serves as a major fuel source for enterocytes especially colonocytes, and improves epithelial barrier integrity by modulating the expression of certain tight junction proteins such as cingulin, intercellular ZO (zonula occludens) proteins, and occludin. In this way, one can see how food intake influences/supports microbial mutualism for production of a metabolite that affects the tissue physiology and cellular molecular biology of the human host.
>
> Bosscher et al. Food-based strategies to modulate the composition of the intestinal microbiota and their associated health effects. *J Physiol Pharmacol.* 2009 Dec

---

[739] Kim BS, et al. Conversion of Th2 memory cells into Foxp3+ regulatory T cells suppressing Th2-mediated allergic asthma. *Proc Natl Acad Sci* 2010 May 11;107:8742-7
[740] Kwon HK, Lee CG, So JS, Chae CS, Hwang JS, Sahoo A, Nam JH, Rhee JH, Hwang KC, Im SH. Generation of regulatory dendritic cells and CD4+Foxp3+ T cells by probiotics administration suppresses immune disorders. *Proc Natl Acad Sci USA*. 2010 Feb 2;107(5):2159-64

goals: ❶ up-regulate CD4(+)Foxp3(+) regulatory T cells (Tregs) from the CD4(+)CD25(-) population, ❷ induced both T-cell and B-cell hyporesponsiveness, ❸ down-regulated T helper (Th) 1, Th2, and Th17 cytokines without apoptosis induction—the significance here is that the goal is to regulate and modulate the immune system, not induce death in key elements, and ❹ increased the suppressor activity of naturally occurring CD4(+)CD25(+) Tregs. The authors note that conversion of T-cells into Foxp3(+) Tregs is directly mediated by regulatory dendritic cells (DCreg) that express high levels of IL-10, TGF-beta, COX-2, and indoleamine 2,3-dioxygenase (IDO)—an enzyme involved in tryptophan degradation and the expression of which is very important for the formation of DCregs and therefore Tregs—and they also note that therapeutic benefits in animal models of experimental inflammatory bowel disease, atopic dermatitis, and rheumatoid arthritis is associated with and likely directly due to the enrichment of CD4(+)Foxp3(+) Tregs in the inflamed regions, following their maturation/promotion in the environment of the GALT—gut-associated lymphoid tissue.

- Probiotic induction of anti-inflammatory IL-10: Oral probiotic administration induces interleukin-10 production and prevents spontaneous autoimmune diabetes in the NOD mouse (*Diabetologia* 2005 Aug[741]): Researchers used the probiotic supplement VSL#3 on diabetes-prone mice (the non-obese diabetic [NOD] mouse develops a spontaneous form of autoimmune diabetes similar to the human disease). Results showed that probiotic administration prevented diabetes development in NOD mice and that the mice treated with the probiotic "showed reduced insulitis and a decreased rate of beta cell destruction. Prevention was associated with an increased production of IL-10 from Peyer's patches and the spleen and with increased IL-10 expression in the pancreas, where IL-10-positive islet-infiltrating mononuclear cells were detected." This is a very interesting experiment showing that marrow-derived immunocytes are re-programmed in gut-associated lymphoid tissue (GALT) and subsequently redistribute to the periphery to effect cellular immunomodulation and thereby prevent autoimmune-mediated tissue injury.

- Probiotic induction via IL-10 of Treg: Alleviation of experimental autoimmune encephalomyelitis by probiotics (*PLoS One* 2010 Feb[742]): Experimental autoimmune encephalomyelitis (EAE) is the experimental animal model of the human disease multiple sclerosis (MS), a chronic inflammatory autoimmune disease of the central nervous system (CNS). The authors note that, "One potential therapeutic strategy for MS is to induce regulatory cells that mediate immunological tolerance." Probiotics, including lactobacilli, have been shown to have immunomodulatory activity. Accordingly, they tested various *Lactobacillus* strains for suppression of EAE; tested strains included *L. paracasei DSM 13434, L. plantarum DSM 15312* and *DSM 15313*, each of which reduced inflammation in CNS and autoreactive T cell responses. The research showed that "***L. paracasei* and *L. plantarum DSM 15312* induced CD4(+)CD25(+)Foxp3(+) regulatory T cells (Tregs)** in mesenteric lymph nodes (MLNs) and enhanced production of serum TGF-beta1, while ***L. plantarum DSM 15313* increased serum IL-27 levels.**" Work by other researchers has shown that IL-27 suppresses Th17 activity while apparently promoting Th1 activity. Very interestingly and of high clinical importance is the finding that "each monostrain probiotic failed to be therapeutic in diseased mice, while a mixture of the three lactobacilli strains suppressed the progression and reversed the clinical and histological signs of EAE." As would be expected in a classic scenario, *Lactobacillus*-induced suppressive activity "correlated with attenuation of pro-inflammatory Th1 and Th17 cytokines followed by IL-10 induction in MLNs, spleen and blood." In a separate experiment, the researchers showed **that IL-10-producing CD4(+)CD25(+) Tregs played the main role in the anti-inflammatory effects induced by probiotic administration.**

---

[741] Calcinaro F, et al. Oral probiotic administration induces interleukin-10 production and prevents spontaneous autoimmune diabetes in the non-obese diabetic mouse. *Diabetologia*. 2005 Aug;48(8):1565-75
[742] Lavasani S, et al. A novel probiotic mixture exerts a therapeutic effect on experimental autoimmune encephalomyelitis mediated by IL-10 producing regulatory T cells. *PLoS One*. 2010 Feb 2;5(2):e9009

17. <u>Inhibition of detoxification</u>: **All clinicians must appreciate that bioaccumulation of toxic chemicals can trigger autoimmunity.**[743,744,745] Examples of this include the increased autoimmunity seen in humans exposed to pesticides[746,747], the scleroderma-like disease that results from exposure to vinyl chloride[748], the association of mercury and pesticide exposure with lupus[749], and the well-recognized connection between drug and chemical exposure and various autoimmune syndromes such as drug-induced lupus.[750] Indeed, more than 40 pharmaceutical drugs are known to cause drug-induced lupus, and bystander activation appears to be one of the primary mechanisms involved.[751] Thus having established the general premise that chemical exposure can cause autoimmune disease, it seems logical and probable that anything which would inhibit the body's ability to detoxify these chemicals would likewise increase the risk for autoimmunity. Stated differently, factors that inhibit detoxification and which therefore increase the body-burden of immunotoxic xenobiotics would serve to indirectly contribute to immunodysfunction and the resultant autoimmunity. Indeed, **patients with lupus and systemic sclerosis show defects in detoxification**[752]**, and different detoxification defects have been documented in patients with ankylosing spondylitis.**[753] Surmounting detoxification defects and xenobiotic exposure by the use of comprehensive detoxification programs (discussed later) is clinically beneficial.[754,755,756,757] Dysbiotic bacterial overgrowth of the gastrointestinal tract directly impairs detoxification via the following four mechanisms:

❶ <u>Cytochrome P450/phase-1 inhibition</u>: Bacterial lipopolysaccharide (endotoxin) has been shown to significantly impair Phase 1 of chemical detoxification.[758] Obviously when major cytochrome p450 pathways are inhibited by endotoxin, then detoxification/biotransformation of xenobiotics and drugs is greatly impaired.[759] The logical extrapolation is that these chemicals would accumulate in the body and promote immunologic and/or neurogenic sensitization.[760]

❷ <u>Deconjugation and enterohepatic recirculation</u>: Several species of bacteria produce deconjugating enzymes (such as beta-glucuronidase) that cleave previously "detoxified" toxins

---

[743] "Autoimmunity due to chemical exposure was evidenced by elevation of TA1 phenotype frequencies and presence of rheumatoid factor, immune complexes, ANA, and anti myelin basic protein antibodies. We conclude that chemical exposure may induce immune abnormalities including immune suppression and autoimmunity." Vojdani A, Ghoneum M, Brautbar N. Immune alteration associated with exposure to toxic chemicals. *Toxicol Ind Health* 1992;8:239-253

[744] Crinnion WJ. Results of a decade of naturopathic treatment for environmental illnesses. *J Naturopathic Med* 1994;17:21-27

[745] Crinnion WJ. Environmental medicine, part one: the human burden of environmental toxins and their common health effects. *Altern Med Rev*. 2000 Feb;5(1):52-63 thorne.com/altmedrev/.fulltext/5/1/52.pdf See also: Crinnion WJ. Environmental medicine, part 2 - health effects of and protection from ubiquitous airborne solvent exposure. *Altern Med Rev*. 2000 Apr;5(2):133-43 thorne.com/altmedrev/.fulltext/5/2/133.pdf

[746] "IgG levels decreased with increasing p,p'-DDE levels, with a statistically significant decrease of approximately 50% in the highest two categories of exposure. Sixteen (12%) were positive for antinuclear antibodies... These analyses provide evidence that p,p'-DDE modulates immune responses in humans." Cooper GS, et al. Associations between plasma DDE levels and immunologic measures in African-American farmers in North Carolina. *Environ Health Perspect*. 2004 Jul;112(10):1080-4

[747] "Twelve individuals who were exposed to chlorpyrifos were studied 1-4.5 y following exposure to determine changes in the peripheral immune system. The subjects were found to have a high rate of atopy and antibiotic sensitivities, elevated CD26 cells (p < .01), and a higher rate of autoimmunity, compared with two control groups." Thrasher JO, Madison R, Broughton A. Immunologic abnormalities in humans exposed to chlorpyrifos: preliminary observations. *Arch Environ Health* 1993;48:89-93

[748] "Vinyl chloride (VC) monomer can induce a scleroderma-like syndrome in a proportion of workers exposed to it during production of polyvinyl chloride." Black CM, Welsh KI, Walker AE, et al. Genetic susceptibility to scleroderma-like syndrome induced by vinyl chloride. *Lancet*. 1983 Jan 1;1(8314-5):53-5

[749] "...reported occupational exposure to mercury (OR 3.6), mixing pesticides for agricultural work (OR 7.4), and among dental workers (OR 7.1). ...these associations were fairly strong and statistically significant..." Cooper et al. Occupational risk factors for development of systemic lupus erythematosus. *J Rheumatol*. 2004 Oct;31:1928-33

[750] Hess EV. Environmental chemicals and autoimmune disease: cause and effect. *Toxicology*. 2002 Dec 27;181-182:65-70

[751] "Drug-induced lupus has been reported as a side-effect of long-term therapy with over 40 medications... Several mechanisms for induction of autoimmunity will be discussed, including bystander activation of autoreactive lymphocytes due to drug-specific immunity or to non-specific activation of lymphocytes, direct cytotoxicity with release of autoantigens ..." Rubin RL. Drug-induced lupus. *Toxicology*. 2005;209(2):135-47

[752] "The observed increased frequencies of the CYP1A1 mutant Val-allele and the slow actylator phenotype in idiopathic autoimmune disease support our concept that in slow acetylators non-acetylated xenobiotics may accumulate and are subsequently metabolized by other enzymes into reactive intermediates. Thus, enhanced formation of reactive metabolites could alter self-proteins..." von Schmiedeberg S, et al. Polymorphisms of the xenobiotic-metabolizing enzymes CYP1A1 and NAT-2 in systemic sclerosis and lupus erythematosus. *Adv Exp Med Biol*. 1999;455:147-52

[753] "Homozygosity for poor metabolizer alleles was found to be associated with AS... Significant within-family association of CYP2D6*4 alleles and AS was demonstrated. Weak linkage was also demonstrated between CYP2D6 and AS. We postulate that altered metabolism of a natural toxin or antigen by the CYP2D6 gene may increase susceptibility to AS." Brown MA, et al. Polymorphisms of the CYP2D6 gene increase susceptibility to ankylosing spondylitis. *Hum Mol Genet*. 2000 Jul 1;9(11):1563-6

[754] Crinnion WJ. Results of a decade of naturopathic treatment for environmental illnesses. *J Naturopathic Med* 1994;17:21-27

[755] Crinnion WJ. Environmental medicine, part one: the human burden of environmental toxins and their common health effects. *Altern Med Rev*. 2000 Feb;5(1):52-63 thorne.com/altmedrev/.fulltext/5/1/52.pdf See also: Crinnion WJ. Environmental medicine, part 2 - health effects of and protection from ubiquitous airborne solvent exposure. *Altern Med Rev*. 2000 Apr;5(2):133-43 thorne.com/altmedrev/.fulltext/5/2/133.pdf

[756] Krop J. Chemical sensitivity after intoxication at work with solvents: response to sauna therapy. *J Altern Complement Med*. 1998 Spring;4(1):77-86

[757] "Retesting following the detoxification program showed significantly improved scores on: three memory tests, block design, trails B, and embedded figures. Thus, there was significant reversibility of impairment after the detoxification interval." Kilburn KH, Warsaw RH, Shields MG. Neurobehavioral dysfunction in firemen exposed to polycholorinated biphenyls (PCBs): possible improvement after detoxification. *Arch Environ Health*. 1989 Nov-Dec;44(6):345-50

[758] Shedlofsky et al. Endotoxin administration to humans inhibits hepatic cytochrome P450-mediated drug metabolism. *J Clin Invest*. 1994 Dec;94(6):2209-14

[759] "CONCLUSIONS: These data show that endotoxin-induced inflammation decreases hepatic cytochrome P450-mediated metabolism of selected probe drugs in women as it does in men." Shedlofsky et al. Endotoxin depresses hepatic cytochrome P450-mediated drug metabolism in women. *Br J Clin Pharmacol*. 1997 Jun;43(6):627-32

[760] "The sick building syndrome and multiple chemical sensitivity syndrome have been defined as clinical entities in which exposure to chemical inhalants gives rise to disease. Current data on the existence of chemical irritant receptors in the airway and skin are discussed; neurogenic inflammation arising from stimulation of chemical irritant receptors is a possible model to explain many of the aspects of chemical sensitivities." Meggs WJ. Neurogenic inflammation and sensitivity to environmental chemicals. *Environ Health Perspect*. 1993 Aug;101(3):234-8

from their water-soluble moieties thus allowing the toxin to be reabsorbed in a mechanism termed "enterohepatic recycling"[761] or "enterohepatic recirculation."[762]

❸ Increased intestinal permeability: Damage to the intestinal mucosa increases absorption of intraluminal contents and thus increase the toxic load placed on the detoxification mechanisms, which are mostly located in the liver; eventually these pathways become depleted, rendering the host susceptible to the consequences of nutritional depletion and impaired detoxification.[763]

❹ Constipation: Bacterial overgrowth can lead to excess production of methane which causes constipation[764] and thus increases the "toxic load" in the colon which then increases the load on the liver via the portal circulation. Likewise, hydrogen sulfide also promotes constipation; however, often, constipation leads to laxation/diarrhea once a sufficient amount of microbial toxins/debris/metabolites have accumulated.

> **Immune alteration associated with exposure to toxic chemicals**
>
> "Autoimmunity due to chemical exposure was evidenced by elevation of TA1 phenotype frequencies and presence of rheumatoid factor, immune complexes, ANA, and antimyelin basic protein antibodies. **We conclude that chemical exposure may induce immune abnormalities including immune suppression and autoimmunity.**"
>
> Vojdani et al. Immune alteration associated with exposure to toxic chemicals. *Toxicol Ind Health*. 1992 Sep-Oct

Taken together, these enterometabolic mechanisms are consistent with the observance of increased risk for xenobiotic-associated diseases such as breast cancer[765,766] and Parkinson's disease[767,768] in patients with chronic constipation. With regard to Phase-1 acetylation, Evans[769] noted in a review published in 1984 that slow acetylation has been strongly noted in patients with Gilbert's disease and also bladder cancer, whereas the rapid acetylator phenotype is associated with diabetes mellitus. We would expect that patients with endotoxin-producing bacterial overgrowth of the small intestine would be more susceptible to the chemical accumulation that leads to multiple chemical sensitivity syndrome (MCS) and the xenobiotic-induced immune dysfunction that may result. In my own clinical practice, I have seen many patients with multiple chemical sensitivity respond very favorably to the eradication of their intestinal bacterial overgrowth, and I consider this treatment essential for all patients with autoimmune disease.

- Psoriasis—Genetic variants in drug metabolizing enzymes as risk factors for psoriasis (*Journal of Investigative Dermatology* 2003 May[770]): Foreign chemicals (xenobiotics) and drugs such as antimalarials and beta-blockers can trigger the onset or exacerbation of psoriasis; other exposures such as lithium, ACE inhibitors, nonsteroidal anti-inflammatory drugs, terbinafine, cigarette smoking, and heavy consumption of alcohol are also associated with the onset and exacerbation of psoriasis. Abnormalities in detoxification processes, such as different metabolic efficiencies caused by variant alleles of xenobiotic metabolizing enzymes, often leads to the accumulation of xenobiotics and/or their reactive metabolites. Accumulation of xenobiotics and/or their metabolites in tissues can result in the formation of neoantigens (i.e., haptens) and/or the exposure of cryptic peptides (e.g., autoantigens); these neoantigens and exposed autoantigens can then initiate and stimulate an aggressive T-cell response, resulting in tissue inflammation and injury. In this study, the authors analyzed xenobiotic-metabolizing enzymes in 327 Caucasian psoriasis patients and 235 control persons. Gene variants were tested for four phase I (oxidation) enzymes and three phase II (conjugation) enzymes. CYP1A1 alleles *2A and *2C were found more often in healthy controls,

---

[761] "Enterohepatic recycling occurs by biliary excretion and intestinal reabsorption of a solute, sometimes with hepatic conjugation and intestinal deconjugation. ... Of particular importance is the potential amplifying effect of enterohepatic variability in defining differences in the bioavailability, apparent volume of distribution and clearance of a given compound." Roberts et al. Enterohepatic circulation: physiological, pharmacokinetic and clinical implications. *Clin Pharmacokinet*. 2002;41:751-90
[762] Liska DJ. The detoxification enzyme systems. *Altern Med Rev*. 1998 Jun;3(3):187-98
[763] Lunn PG, Northrop-Clewes CA, Downes RM. Intestinal permeability, mucosal injury, and growth faltering in Gambian infants. *Lancet*. 1991 Oct 12;338(8772):907-1
[764] Lin HC. Small intestinal bacterial overgrowth: a framework for understanding irritable bowel syndrome. *JAMA*. 2004 Aug 18;292(7):852-8
[765] "These observations are consistent with an hypothesized association between constipation and increased risk of breast cancer." Micozzi MS, Carter CL, Albanes D, Taylor PR, Licitra LM. Bowel function and breast cancer in US women. *Am J Public Health*. 1989 Jan;79(1):73-5
[766] Petrakis NL, King EB. Cytological abnormalities in nipple aspirates of breast fluid from women with severe constipation. *Lancet*. 1981 Nov 28;2(8257):1203-4
[767] "...lower frequency bowel movements predict the future risk of PD. ...They also hypothesize that some yet undefined toxins break through the mucosal barrier of the intestine and are incorporated into the axon terminal of the vagus nerve and transported in a retrograde manner to the vagus nucleus." Ueki A, Otsuka M. Life style risks of Parkinson's disease: association between decreased water intake and constipation. *J Neurol*. 2004 Oct;251 Suppl 7:vII18-23
[768] "CONCLUSIONS: Findings indicate that infrequent bowel movements are associated with an elevated risk of future PD." Abbott RD, et al. Frequency of bowel movements and the future risk of Parkinson's disease. *Neurology*. 2001 Aug 14;57(3):456-62
[769] Evans DA. Survey of the human acetylator polymorphism in spontaneous disorders. *J Med Genet*. 1984 Aug;21(4):243-53
[770] Richter-Hintz D, et al. Allelic variants of drug metabolizing enzymes as risk factors in psoriasis. *J Investigative Dermatology*. 2003 May;120(5):765-70

suggesting a protective role for these gene variants. The authors note that no significant difference between patients and controls could be found for the phase I alleles 1B1*1, 1B1*3, 2E1*1A, and 2E1*5B nor for the phase II enzymes GSTT1 or NQOR when considered in isolation. However, an increased risk for psoriasis was associated with genetic variations in GSTM1 and with heterozygosity for CYP2C19 alleles *1A and *2A. The combination of CYP1A1*1A (reduced enzyme activity) with CYP2C19*1A increased the odds ratio (OR) in favor of psoriasis by 3.3 (OR=3.3) while the combination of CYP1A1*1A with GSTM1 increased the OR to 4.84. CYP1A1*2C encodes for an enzyme of greater detoxification activity and reduces the risk for developing psoriasis (OR=0.44). The authors conclude, "This is the first large-scale study on these enzymes and the results obtained support the concept that **different activities of metabolizing enzymes can contribute to disease etiology and progression**." This article supports the concept that genetic/inheritable abnormalities in detoxification abilities can increase the risk for developing psoriasis; if the increased risk is indeed due to the defective detoxification and not due to the gene products themselves per se, then any condition—importantly for this discussion the influence of bacteria—that alters detoxification could also increase the risk for psoriasis. The best singular example of this reality is the inhibition of CYP enzymes by bacterial endotoxin/lipopolysaccharide.

- Psoriasis—Evidence of impaired Phase-1 acetylation in psoriatics and psoriatics with psoriatic siblings (*Dermatologica* 1989[771]): Researchers conducting this study assessed acetylation ability using sulfamethazine as a probe in 64 psoriatic patients and in. Among the 157 normal control subjects, 90 (57.3%) were slow acetylators. Among the 64 psoriatic patients, 40 (62.5%) were slow acetylators. Among the 27 psoriatic patients who had a sibling with psoriasis, 22 (81%) were slow acetylators (p less than 0.05). The authors concluded, "**Slow acetylator phenotype may be a genetic risk factor for the development of psoriasis**." Interestingly, the slow acetylator phenotype noted above to be associated with psoriasis is also, per a 1984 review by Evans[772], associated with diabetes mellitus; clinical-epidemiologic research has consistently linked psoriasis and diabetes mellitus.

Impaired detoxification and illness

Clinically, three patterns of impaired detoxification are important and are particularly worthy of our attention:
1. <u>Slow CYP activation</u>: If "Phase-1" is slow, then toxins cannot be cleared from the system, and they accumulate. This leads to adverse effects from the toxins or the medications to which the patient is exposed. Patients with slow CYP activation are prone to adverse medication responses and environmental sensitivity because they are unable to normally clear drugs and chemicals from their system.
2. <u>Fast CYP activation</u>: If "Phase-1" is too fast, then toxins are converted into "reactive intermediates" which can bind to DNA or other cellular structures, resulting in genetic mutations or neoantigenization/haptenization. Patients with too-fast CYP activation may have more beneficial or adverse effects from medication if taking a medication that requires activation by the liver for function, or they may have less beneficial or adverse effects from medication if taking a medication that is inactivated by CYP oxidation.
3. <u>Slow Phase-2 conjugation</u>: Conjugation is the second phase of detoxification following Phase-1 oxidation. If Phase-2 is too slow in relation to Phase-1, we call this "imbalanced detoxification" or "pathological detoxification" because the reactive intermediates produced from Phase-1 oxidation cannot be cleared from the body yet are capable of binding to DNA and other vitally crucial cellular structures. Patients with slow Phase-2 conjugation are prone to adverse medication responses and environmental sensitivity because they are unable to normally clear drugs and chemicals from their system.

Variations in the rate and therefore quality and quantity of detoxification are induced by genetic variations and factors in the environment such as chemical exposures, gastrointestinal dysbiosis, nutrient status, and the consumption of specific foods. Each component of detoxification has several different subcomponents and therefore complex combinations of "too fast" and "too slow" can and do occur. However, **the final consequence of most types of altered detoxification is toxin accumulation**.

---

18. <u>Impairment of mucosal and systemic defenses</u>: Microbial colonization of mucosal surfaces can result in impaired local immunity by causing loss of protective secretory IgA or by causing direct tissue damage that results in increased absorption of microbial, dietary, or environmental antigens. Several

---

[771] Jiménez-Nieto LC, Ladero JM, Fernández-Gundín MJ, Robledo A. Acetylator phenotype in psoriasis. *Dermatologica*. 1989;178(3):136-7
[772] Evans DA. Survey of the human acetylator polymorphism in spontaneous disorders. *J Med Genet*. 1984 Aug;21(4):243-53

microorganisms such as *Entamoeba histolytica*[773], *Streptococcus sanguis*[774], and *Candida albicans*[775] externalize a protein-digesting enzyme (proteinase) that "digests" defensive immunoglobulins, including secretory IgA and humoral immunoglobulins. The proteinases produced by *Candida* are capable of lysing not only sIgA but also keratin and collagen[776], obviously providing for a breach of protection from other infections and antigens. In this way, mucosal microbial colonization with yeast/bacteria that secrete proteases/proteinases can "open the door" to previously excluded microbes or antigens to promote the resultant "infection" or "allergy", respectively. Furthermore, because IgA is destroyed by the protease, the infection is allowed to fester, resulting in on-going immune stimulation and its consequences such as bystander activation. This may explain why women with chronic vaginal candidiasis, which always implies chronic yeast overgrowth of the intestine[777], have nearly double the incidence of allergic rhinitis compared to patients without chronic yeast overgrowth.[778] Further supporting the link between yeast and allergy is another recent study showing that allergy/atopy is more common in patients with chronic yeast infections.[779] *Candida* produces an immunotoxin called "gliotoxin", which suppresses human immune function.[780] The combination of mucosal damage, destruction of sIgA, immunosuppression, and microbial overgrowth synergize to sensitize the systemic immune system toward allergic and proinflammatory disease.[781] Lastly, bacterial proteases work synergistically with biofilm formation to nullify immunologic attack (via immunosuppression and cytokine inactivation) and are important for the establishment of chronic mucosal colonization.[782] Impairment of mucosal defenses and—o a lesser extent systemic defenses has been sufficiently reviewed in this paragraph such that additional disease-specific discussions are unnecessary.

19. <u>Impairment of mucosal digestion by microbial proteases and inflammation</u>: Similar to the degradation of human IgA by microbial proteases/proteinases is the degradation of mucosal digestive enzymes such as the disaccharidases (sucrase, maltase, lactase, and isomaltase) and dipeptidases. First, impaired digestion of carbohydrates skews the intestinal milieu toward one favorable to bacterial/yeast overgrowth by increasing the levels of carbohydrate substrate upon which microbes feed. Impaired peptide breakdown promotes immune sensitization, protein malnutrition, and putrefaction. Second, inflammation resultant from intestinal dysbiosis further impairs carbohydrate digestion via downregulation of sucrase-isomaltase gene expression by inflammatory cytokines.[783] Third, destruction of microvilli exacerbates loss of mucosal enzymes and leads to additional malabsorption, maldigestion, and increased macromolecular absorption, such as seen in patients with intestinal giardiasis.[784] Impairment/reduction of disaccharidases and dipeptidases is also seen in patients with inflammatory bowel disease.[785]

20. <u>Inflammation-induced endocrine dysfunction</u>: Although research in this area is less conclusive, the pattern of emerging research indicates that the multifaceted phenomenon of inflammation, particularly the elaboration of cytokines, alters endocrine function, and these inflammation-induced endocrine alterations further promote additional musculoskeletal inflammation. Endocrine changes induced by chronic

---

[773] Kelsall BL, Ravdin JI. Degradation of human IgA by Entamoeba histolytica. *J Infect Dis*. 1993 Nov;168(5):1319-22

[774] "These data indicate that the BD patients are infected with IgA protease-producing S. sanguis strains, which cause an increase of IgA titer against these organisms and IgA protease antigen." Yokota K, Oguma K. IgA protease produced by Streptococcus sanguis and antibody production against IgA protease in patients with Behcet's disease. *Microbiol Immunol*. 1997;41(12):925-31

[775] Kaminishi H, Miyaguchi H, Tamaki T, et al. Degradation of humoral host defense by Candida albicans proteinase. *Infect Immun*. 1995 Mar;63(3):984-8

[776] "The enzymes produced by these yeasts are all carboxyl proteinases capable of degrading secretory IgA, the major immunoglobulin of mucous membranes. Some have keratino- or collagenolytic activity." Douglas LJ. Candida proteinases and candidosis. *Crit Rev Biotechnol*. 1988;8(2):121-9

[777] "The results showed that if C albicans was cultured from the vagina, it was always found in the stool... The gut-reservoir concept may well apply to other forms of candidiasis." Miles MR, Olsen L, Rogers A. Recurrent vaginal candidiasis. Importance of an intestinal reservoir. *JAMA*. 1977 Oct 24;238(17):1836-7

[778] Moraes PS. Recurrent vaginal candidiasis and allergic rhinitis: a common association. *Ann Allergy Asthma Immunol*. 1998 Aug;81(2):165-9

[779] Neves NA, Carvalho LP, De Oliveira MA, et al. Association between atopy and recurrent vaginal candidiasis. *Clin Exp Immunol*. 2005 Oct;142(1):167-71

[780] "This study suggests a previously unrecognized potential virulence factor of C. albicans that could contribute to persistence of yeast colonization or recurrence of symptomatic infection through diminished host resistance." Shah et al. Effect of gliotoxin on human polymorphonuclear neutrophils. *Infect Dis Obstet Gynecol* 1998;6:168-75

[781] "Studies performed in humans show that selective IgA deficiency, preterm delivery, intestinal helminth infection and type of feeding during the neonatal period may influence antigen uptake by the intestinal epithelium. These conditions...may cause increased absorption of intraluminal antigens and result in the triggering of allergic type responses." Reinhardt MC. Macromolecular absorption of food antigens in health and disease. *Ann Allergy*. 1984 Dec;53(6 Pt 2):597-601

[782] "The two proteases, alkaline protease and elastase, inhibit the function of the cells of the immune system (phagocytes, NK cells, T cells), inactivate several cytokines (IL-1, IL-2, IFN-r, TNF), cleave immunoglobulins and inactivate complement. Inhibition of the local immune response by bacterial proteases provides an environment for the colonization and establishment of chronic infection." Kharazmi A. Mechanisms involved in the evasion of the host defence by Pseudomonas aeruginosa. *Immunol Lett*. 1991 Oct;30(2):201-5

[783] Ziambaras T, Rubin DC, Perlmutter DH. Regulation of sucrase-isomaltase gene expression in human intestinal epithelial cells by inflammatory cytokines. *J Biol Chem*. 1996 Jan 12;271(2):1237-42 jbc.org/cgi/content/full/271/2/1237

[784] Buret AG. Immunopathology of giardiasis. *Mem Inst Oswaldo Cruz*. 2005 Mar;100 Suppl 1:185-90 scielo.br/pdf/mioc/v100s1/v100ns1a31.pdf

[785] "A significant reduction of the specific activity of disaccharidases (lactase, sucrase and trehalase) in jejunal mucosal homogenate occurred in patients with inflammatory bowel disease. ... Several dipeptidases such as glycyl-leucine, leucyl-glycine, glycyl-glycine and valyl-proline hydrolase activities were lower in patients with inflammatory bowel disease than in controls." Arvanitakis C. Abnormalities of jejunal mucosal enzymes in ulcerative colitis and Crohn's disease. *Digestion*. 1979;19(4):259-66

inflammation include increased production of proinflammatory **prolactin**, reduced production of anti-inflammatory and immunoregulatory **cortisol** and **androgens**. The effects of altered endocrine function is discussed in the following section detailing orthoendocrinology. The link between dysbiosis and inflammation-induced changes in endocrine status has only recently begun to be documented, and some of these conclusions are logical though somewhat speculative. However, the nature of holistic healthcare requires us to consider *all* potentially significant contributions and interconnections, and thus microbe-endocrine links are briefly outlined here based on *highly suggestive*—yet not *wholly conclusive*—data. What is very clear is that autoimmune patients have alterations in hypothalamic-pituitary-adrenal/gonadal function. What is not yet clear is whether or not these are primary initiators of disease or secondary results of the disease process. Here I propose that both of these statements are true, namely that 1) endocrine dysfunction predisposes to the immune dysfunction that results in autoimmunity, and that 2) systemic inflammation further exacerbates endocrine dysfunction. Further, I speculate and add that 3) in some patients, chronic dysbiosis and subclinical inflammation and bacterial endotoxinemia/exotoxinemia can initiate the endocrine dysfunction and pro-inflammatory state that can eventually cross a diagnostic threshold to become overt clinical autoimmunity. Research support is provided here:

- Altered hypothalamic responsiveness and circadian rhythm: The region of the basal hypothalamus is not protected by the blood-brain barrier and is sensitive and vulnerable to substances in the blood.[786] Because of this, hypothalamic and thus pituitary responses can be tuned to and/or altered by circulating prostaglandins, cytokines, and bacterial endotoxins and exotoxins. Patients with rheumatoid arthritis show hypothalamic/endocrine disturbances including blunted responsiveness to ACTH, abnormal circadian rhythm of prolactin and cortisol, and abnormalities in growth hormone secretion.[787] Furthermore, arginine vasopressin (AVP) is secreted from the hypothalamus in response to stress, is inherently pro-inflammatory, and is capable of augmenting prolactin secretion to further increase inflammation.[788]

- Irritable bowel syndrome as a clinical model of intestinal bacterial overgrowth dysbiosis: Dysregulation of the hypothalamic-pituitary-adrenal (HPA) axis in irritable bowel syndrome (*Journal of Neurogastroenterology and Motility* 2009 Feb[789]): In order to utilize irritable bowel syndrome (IBS) as a model of dysbiosis (subtype: microbial overgrowth within the intestines) and to thereby describe the hypothalamic and neuro-endocrine alterations as exemplifications of dysbiosis-induced alterations in neuro-endocrine function, a brief review to (re)acquaint readers with the fundamental cause of IBS will be provided (part 1) which will be followed by a brief overview of the neuro-endocrine abnormalities caused by dysbiosis in this condition (part 2). ❶ IBS was erroneously assumed to be enigmatic and esoteric by clinicians well-versed in the idiopathic ideology of allopathic/pharmacocentric medicine; meanwhile, the fact seemed quite obvious to the rest of us that so-called IBS was simply a manifestation of small intestine bacterial overgrowth (SIBO). Thankfully, the correct viewpoint—after years of clinical validation in integrative practices—has finally received widespread publication, although not necessarily widespread acceptance by scientific nihilists and therapeutic obstructionists. The masterful review by Lin[790] "Small intestinal bacterial overgrowth: a framework for understanding irritable bowel syndrome" published in *JAMA-Journal of the American Medical Association* in 2004 should have laid to rest the search for the major direct cause of IBS, particularly since follow-up studies using orally-administered nonabsorbable antibiotics[791,792,793,794] have shown consistent benefit despite the limited

---

[786] Waxman SG. *Clinical Neuroanatomy 25th Edition*. McGraw Hill Medical, New York, 2003, p 160
[787] Anisman H, et al. Neuroimmune mechanisms in health and disease: 2. Disease. *CMAJ*. 1996 Oct 15;155(8):1075-82
[788] Chikanza et al. Hypothalamic-pituitary-mediated immunomodulation: arginine vasopressin is a neuroendocrine immune mediator. *Br J Rheumatol*. 1998 Feb;37:131-6
[789] Chang L, et al. Dysregulation of the hypothalamic-pituitary-adrenal (HPA) axis in irritable bowel syndrome. *Neurogastroenterol Motil*. 2009 Feb;21(2):149-59
[790] Lin HC. Small intestinal bacterial overgrowth: a framework for understanding irritable bowel syndrome. *JAMA*. 2004 Aug 18;292(7):852-8
[791] Esposito I, de Leone A, Di Gregorio G, Giaquinto S, de Magistris L, Ferrieri A, Riegler G. Breath test for differential diagnosis between small intestinal bacterial overgrowth and irritable bowel disease: an observation on non-absorbable antibiotics. *World J Gastroenterol*. 2007 Dec 7;13(45):6016-21
[792] Peralta S, Cottone C, Doveri T, Almasio PL, Craxi A. Small intestine bacterial overgrowth and irritable bowel syndrome-related symptoms: experience with Rifaximin. *World J Gastroenterol*. 2009 Jun 7;15(21):2628-31
[793] Majewski M, McCallum RW. Results of small intestinal bacterial overgrowth testing in irritable bowel syndrome patients: clinical profiles and effects of antibiotic trial. *Adv Med Sci*. 2007;52:139-42
[794] Cuoco L, Salvagnini M. Small intestine bacterial overgrowth in irritable bowel syndrome: a retrospective study with rifaximin. *Minerva Gastroenterol Dietol*. 2006 Mar;52(1):89-95

scope of the pharmacologic intervention, failure to perform microbial identification and sensitivity testing, and the general failure to use probiotic therapy and dietary improvements which are required to (re)establish eubiosis. Thus, having established IBS to be a manifestation of intestinal dysbiosis generally and SIBO—or more accurately SIMO for "small intestinal microbial overgrowth" since the microbes may be yeast/fungi, amoebas or protozoas rather than exclusively bacteria—specifically, let us now look at the hypothalamic abnormalities seen in patients with "SIMO-induced IBS" (redundancy noted). ❷ Chang et al[795] in 2009 found evidence HPA axis dysregulation in women with IBS without psychiatric comorbidity as evidenced by SIMO-IBS patients' significantly lower basal secretion of adrenocorticotrophic hormone (ACTH) with slightly elevated and asynchronic secretion of cortisol contrasted with the findings in the control group. FitzGerald et al[796] showed that "women with IBS display blunted ACTH and cortisol responses to the LP (lumbar puncture used as a psychological stressor) along with a profile of affective responsiveness suggestive of chronic psychosocial stress, although no CRF (corticotrophin-releasing hormone in cerebrospinal fluid) differences between groups are observed." Whether these hypothalamic-pituitary dysfunctions are a contributing cause to or a result of SIMO-IBS could only be established by clinical trials with a 5-part protocol (i.e., 1. assessment of normal subjects, 2. intentional induction of SIMO-IBS, 3. reassessment, 4. successful treatment, 5. reassessment) which would be logistically cumbersome and ethically untenable.

- Increased production of prolactin: Prolactin is a highly proinflammatory hormone produced by the anterior pituitary gland as well as by peripheral lymphocytes. As a model of infection-induced inflammation, **sepsis is generally associated with increased prolactin production in humans**.[797] Prolactin levels increase due to chronic psychoemotional stress. **The classic exemplification of dysbiosis-induced musculoskeletal inflammation—reactive arthritis—is frequently associated with hyperprolactinemia.**[798]
    - Infection-induced arthritis: Elevated prolactin in reactive arthritis (*J Rheumatol* 1994 Jul[799]): Without any question whatsoever, reactive arthritis—formerly called Reiter's syndrome—is one of the prototypes of inflammatory arthritis and "autoimmunity" triggered by microorganisms, whether as an acute infection such as a urinary tract infection or gastroenteritis or as a chronic subclinical infection. This classic association—that between the microbe and the induction of arthritis and systemic inflammation—is discussed in all textbooks of pathology and all thorough textbooks of microbiology; it is therefore a matter of "medical fact." Therefore, the identification of hormonal abnormalities in patients with this prototypic microbe-induced autoimmune/inflammatory syndrome would be supportive of either/both of the following: ❶ microbial infection or colonization can result in hormone imbalances, such as elevated prolactin, and/or ❷ hormone imbalances such as elevated prolactin function synergistically with microbial colonization to result in systemic inflammation and dysbiotic rheumatism. In this study, the authors measured serum prolactin (PRL) in patients with reactive arthritis and groups of other patients. Results showed that elevated PRL levels > 20 ng/ml were found in 9 of 25 (36%) patients with reactive arthritis but almost none of the other patients. Furthermore, a direct positive correlation between serum prolactin levels and the clinical intensity of conjunctivitis, urethritis, dysentery, and uveitis was noted.
- Reduced production of cortisol: Cortisol is an immunoregulatory hormone which tends to suppress excess immune activity, and relative reductions in cortisol production are commonly seen in patients with autoimmunity and allergic disorders.[800,801] **Cortisol production is reduced by chronic**

---

[795] Chang L, et al. Dysregulation of the hypothalamic-pituitary-adrenal (HPA) axis in irritable bowel syndrome. *Neurogastroenterol Motil.* 2009 Feb;21(2):149-59
[796] FitzGerald LZ, Kehoe P, Sinha K. Hypothalamic--pituitary-- adrenal axis dysregulation in women with irritable bowel syndrome in response to acute physical stress. *West J Nurs Res.* 2009 Nov;31(7):818-36
[797] "Prolactin levels are regularly elevated in sepsis…" Dennhardt et al. Patterns of endocrine secretion during sepsis. *Prog Clin Biol Res* 1989;308:751-6
[798] "Hyperprolactinemia (PRL > 20 ng/ml) was found in 9 of 25 (36%) patients with RS." Jara et al. Hyperprolactinemia in Reiter's syndrome. *J Rheumatol* 1994;21:1292-7
[799] Jara et al. Hyperprolactinemia in Reiter's syndrome. *J Rheumatol.* 1994 Jul;21(7):1292-7
[800] "Yet evidence that patients with rheumatoid arthritis improved with small, physiologic dosages of cortisol or cortisone acetate was reported over 25 years ago, and that patients with chronic allergic disorders or unexplained chronic fatigue also improved with administration of such small dosages was reported over 15 years ago..." Jefferies WM. Mild adrenocortical deficiency, chronic allergies, autoimmune disorders and the chronic fatigue syndrome: a continuation of the cortisone story. *Med Hypotheses.* 1994 Mar;42(3):183-9 thebuteykocentre.com/Irish_%20Buteykocenter_files/further_studies/med_hyp2.pdf and members.westnet.com.au/pkolb/med_hyp2.pdf
[801] "The etiology of rheumatoid arthritis …explained by a combination of three factors: (i) a relatively mild deficiency of cortisol, …, (ii) a deficiency of DHEA, …and (iii) infection by organisms such as mycoplasma,..." Jefferies WM. The etiology of rheumatoid arthritis. *Med Hypotheses.* 1998 Aug;51(2):111-4

psychoemotional stress[802], and the stress of chronic inflammation due to dysbiosis and the resultant disease, pain, disability, and disfigurement may impair normal endocrine function.

- Allergies, autoimmunity, and fatigue-related syndromes—Mild adrenocortical deficiency and the work of Jefferies (*Med Hypotheses* 1994 Mar[803]): In his textbook *Safe Uses of Cortisol* and peer-reviewed articles, Jefferies has been the strongest proponent of the idea that patients with chronic allergies, autoimmune disorders, and chronic fatigue syndrome have mild adrenocortical deficiency resulting in low physiologic reserve and immune abnormalities that would be better treated with physiologic doses of bioidentical cortisol rather than high doses of synthetic cortisol mimetics. Dr Jefferies approach—using physiologic amounts of cortisol at doses less than 20 mg per day—does not cause adrenal suppression or adverse effects which are commonly seen when synthetic cortisol mimetics such as prednisone are used. Allergies and autoimmune disorders are commonly treated with synthetic cortisol mimetics as part of standard medical practice; this can be viewed as appreciation for the role of cortisol in immunomodulation. Relatedly, a clinical trial by Cleare et al[804] among patients with chronic fatigue syndrome (CFS) showed that low-dose cortisol in amounts of 5-10 mg per day provided significant benefit.

- Reduced production and bioavailability of androgens—testosterone and/or dehydroepiandrosterone (DHEA): High-intensity stress associated with military training leads to 60-80% reductions in androgens[805]; the chronic stress and pain associated with musculoskeletal inflammation may contribute to a similar profile on a subacute and chronic basis. Hyperprolactinemia further complicates this problem by simulating hepatic production of sex hormone binding globulin (SHBG) which adsorbs androgens and reduces their bioavailability. Indeed, the clinical manifestations of hypogonadism—including probably inflammatory/rheumatic complications—can be seen despite adequate production of androgens when elevated prolactin stimulates increased SHBG production and results in reduced bioavailability of androgens.[806]

  - Inflammatory bowel disease and dysbiosis—Patients with chronic inflammatory bowel disease have low levels of DHEA (*Clin Exp Rheumatol* 1998 Sep-Oct[807]): Readers should note that both of the major forms of inflammatory bowel disease (IBD)—Crohn disease (CD) and ulcerative colitis (UC)—are very closely associated with gastrointestinal dysbiosis; in fact, a very strong case can be made that IBD is one of the prototypic manifestations of gastrointestinal dysbiosis.[808] In this study, DHEA-sulfate (DHEA-s) levels were measured in blood from 112 patients with IBD (66 with CD and 46 with UC), and the levels were compared with those in 80 healthy controls. DHEA-s concentrations were measured in tissue samples from 40 patients (28 patients with IBD and 12 with other bowel disorders) who had undergone intestinal surgery. Results of these analyses showed that average blood DHEA-s were markedly lower in the two IBD groups (1350 nmol/l in UC and 1850 nmol/l in CD vs. 3300 nmol/l in controls); readers should note that the DHEA-s levels in the IBD patients were roughly half—50%—of normal. Andus et al[809] showed that DHEA 200mg/d provided important benefits for patients with treatment-resistant IBD.

---

[802] "Prolonged psychological stress is associated with a transient suppression of the HPA axis, manifested by low morning cortisol and reduced cortisol response to ACTH. The reduction of cortisol response is sufficient to cause false diagnosis of HPA insufficiency." Zarkovic M, Stefanova E, Ciric J, Penezic Z, Kostic V, Sumarac-Dumanovic M, Macut D, Ivovic MS, Gligorovic PV. Prolonged psychological stress suppresses cortisol secretion. *Clin Endocrinol* (Oxf). 2003 Dec;59(6):811-6

[803] Jefferies WM. Mild adrenocortical deficiency, chronic allergies, autoimmune disorders and the chronic fatigue syndrome. *Med Hypotheses*. 1994 Mar;42(3):183-9

[804] Cleare AJ, et al. Low-dose hydrocortisone in chronic fatigue syndrome: a randomised crossover trial. *Lancet*. 1999 Feb 6;353(9151):455-8

[805] "Plasma levels of testosterone, free testosterone, dehydroepiandrosterone, 17 alpha-hydroxyprogesterone, and androstenedione decreased by 60-80% during the course." Opstad PK. Androgenic hormones during prolonged physical stress, sleep, and energy deficiency. *J Clin Endocrinol Metab*. 1992 May;74(5):1176-83

[806] "The pitfalls of measuring only total serum testosterone are illustrated by a 52 year old man whose hyperprolactinaemia was associated with normal total serum testosterone but a raised sex-hormone-binding globulin, giving a low free testosterone. Prolactin suppression with bromocriptine normalized sex-hormone-binding globulin and free testosterone..." Hardy KJ, Seckl JR. Endocrine assessment of impotence--pitfalls of measuring serum testosterone without sex-hormone-binding globulin. *Postgrad Med J*. 1994 Nov;70(829):836-7

[807] de la Torre B, Hedman M, Befrits R. Blood and tissue dehydroepiandrosterone sulphate levels and their relationship to chronic inflammatory bowel disease. *Clin Exp Rheumatol*. 1998 Sep-Oct;16(5):579-82

[808] Tamboli CP, Neut C, Desreumaux P, Colombel JF. Dysbiosis in inflammatory bowel disease. *Gut*. 2004 Jan;53(1):1-4

[809] Andus T, et al. Patients with refractory Crohn's disease or ulcerative colitis respond to dehydroepiandrosterone. *Aliment Pharmacol Ther*. 2003 Feb;17(3):409-14

- HIV/AIDS—Testosterone deficiency is common in men and women infected with HIV (*Clin Infect Dis* 2001 Sep[810]): The authors note, "Androgen deficiency is a common endocrine abnormality among men and women with human immunodeficiency virus (HIV) infection. … The most useful laboratory indicator is the serum bioavailable (free) **testosterone** concentration." Clinical benefits of the correction of hypoandrogenism—specifically serum free testosterone and/or serum total testosterone—include improvements in lean body mass, energy, quality of life, and mood-depression scores.

In conclusion, **this survey of the literature has supported the concept that dysbiosis can contribute to systemic pain, inflammation, and immune activation by numerous mechanisms, and that many of these "silent infections" are self-perpetuating by inducing alterations in local milieu and systemic immunity**. Clinical experience has demonstrated again and again that eradicating dysbiosis helps normalize immune function, alleviate autoimmunity and allergy, reduce inflammation, improve detoxification, and to help "cure" people of their previously "incurable" multiple chemical sensitivity, environmental illness, and autoimmunity.

---

[810] Mylonakis et al. Diagnosis and treatment of androgen deficiency in human immunodeficiency virus-infected men and women. *Clin Infect Dis*. 2001 Sep 15;33:857-64

The Seven Main Loci of Dysbiosis

For a microorganism to induce a systemic proinflammatory immunodysregulatory response in a human, the microbe or its metabolic products must be exposed to a susceptible host. Non-infectious microbial overgrowth can occur inside the body (gastrointestinal, sinus, respiratory tract and lungs, genitourinary, or orodental), on the surface of the body (dermal), or outside of the body (environmental). The adverse physiologic and clinical effects can be similar regardless of the location of the microorganism. The term "dysbiosis" is classically applied to harmful, non-infectious relationships between the human host and yeast, bacteria, protozoans, amoebas, or other "parasites" located specifically in the gastrointestinal tract, and "dysbiosis" is now an accepted term in the medical literature.[811] However, we must also appreciate that harmful, noninfectious microbe-host interactions can also occur when microbes are localized in the sinuses, oral cavity, genitourinary tract, skin, and in the external environment. I prefer to use a broad definition of dysbiosis that implies "a relationship of non-infectious host-microorganism interaction that adversely affects the human host" and then to specify the subtype based on the location: gastrointestinal, oral, sinus, genitourinary, dermatologic, or environmental. Gastrointestinal dysbiosis is clearly the prototype for understanding other types of dysbiosis; this is because it seems to be the most common form of dysbiosis, perhaps due to the large numbers and types of microbes in the gut and the extensive surface area of the gastrointestinal tract. Clinicians must appreciate the anatomical interconnections that can segue one type of loci of dysbiosis into another. Orodental dysbiosis may result in gastrointestinal dysbiosis if the microbes can survive in the gastrointestinal tract. Sinus dysbiosis could likewise drain into the lungs and gastrointestinal tract. In women, close relationships between gastrointestinal dysbiosis and vaginal dysbiosis are well documented.[812] Bacterial and fungal superantigens from the surrounding environment can contribute to a proinflammatory response in the lungs and on the skin and which becomes systemic, leading to autoimmunity.[813,814]

Correlation of Dysbiosis with Autoimmune and Rheumatic Diseases

Disease & dysbiosis	Gastro-intestinal	Orodental	Sino-respiratory	Genito-urinary	Tissue	Cutaneous	Environ-mental
SLE	+		+				
RA	✓	✓	✓	✓	+ osteomyel		
ReA	✓		✓	✓	✓ pneumonia		
Psor	✓	✓	✓	✓		✓	✓
PM-DM	+	+	+				
Spond-AS	✓			✓			
Sclerod	+						
Weg	+	✓	✓				
Vasc	✓				✓ viral hep		
Sarc			✓				
Behc		✓	✓			✓	
Neuro	✓			✓			✓

✓ = Positive research and clinical evidence in humans; + = Weak research in humans, substantive research in animal models, biologic plausibility; N = Negative findings; No correlation; SLE = lupus; RA = rheumatoid arthritis; ReA = reactive arthritis; Psor = Psoriasis or psoriatic arthritis; PM-DM = polymyositis/dermatomyositis; PMR = polymyalgia rheumatica; Sjo = Sjogren's syndrome; Spond-AS = spondyloarthropathy and ankylosing spondylitis; Sclerod = scleroderma; Weg = Wegener's granulomatosis; Vasc = vasculitis; Sarc = sarcoidosis; Behc = Behcet's syndrome; Neuro = neurologic autoimmunity, which is not detailed in this text.

---

[811] Tamboli CP, Neut C, Desreumaux P, Colombel JF. Dysbiosis in inflammatory bowel disease. *Gut*. 2004 Jan;53(1):1-4
[812] "The results showed that if C albicans was cultured from the vagina, it was always found in the stool... The gut-reservoir concept may well apply to other forms of candidiasis." Miles MR, Olsen L, Rogers A. Recurrent vaginal candidiasis. Importance of an intestinal reservoir. *JAMA*. 1977 Oct 24;238(17):1836-7
[813] Campbell AW, Thrasher JD, Madison RA, Vojdani A, Gray MR, Johnson A. Neural autoantibodies and neurophysiologic abnormalities in patients exposed to molds in water-damaged buildings. *Arch Environ Health*. 2003 Aug;58(8):464-74
[814] Gray et al. Mixed mold mycotoxicosis: immunological changes in humans following exposure in water-damaged buildings. *Arch Environ Health* 2003 Jul;58:410-20

Gastrointestinal Dysbiosis: Overview of the Prototype of All Forms of Dysbiosis

We all have bacteria and occasionally small quantities of yeast in our intestines, and this is normal and generally healthy. However, problems arise when these yeast/bacteria become imbalanced or when *harmful* yeast, bacteria, parasites take up residence within the gut. Particularly in the European research literature, this condition has been more widely researched and described as "dysbacteriosis" or "dysbacterosis."[815] These latter terms are somewhat unfortunate because they imply that the problem has a *bacterial* origin, which is partially (and therefore significantly) misleading since dysbiosis commonly involves bacteria *and yeast* (including but not limited to *Candida albicans*) and commonly other harmful non-bacterial microbes such as *Giardia lamblia, Blastocystis hominis, Endolimax nana, Entamoeba histolytica* and a cast of other malcontents that adversely affect the overall health of their human host.[816] "Candidiasis" and yeast-related problems have been described in the research literature and general press.[817] Dysbiosis is probably a major aspect of the phenomenon that was previously referred to in the medical literature as "autointoxication" and which was effectively treated with dietary modifications, nutritional supplementation, and colonic irrigation.[818] **Given that endotoxin/lipopolysaccharide is one of the major activators of nuclear factor kappa-B (NFkB)[819], and that NFkB activation is a major rate-limiting step in the production of proinflammatory cytokines and in the induction of proinflammatory enzymes such as cyclooxygenase, lipoxygenase, and inducible nitric oxide synthase,[820] then the link between dysbiosis and systemic inflammation becomes clear: gastrointestinal bacterial overgrowth leads to excess production and absorption of endotoxin, which then initiates immune dysfunction and a systemic proinflammatory response.** Intestinal overgrowth of gram-negative bacteria is, in this author's opinion, highly problematic since endotoxin/lipopolysaccharide, of which there are varying degrees of toxicity, can cause intestinal inflammation, leaky gut, inhibition of hepatic detoxification, hyperalgesia[821], brain dysfunction[822] and immune dysfunction by acting as superantigens.[823] **Indeed, many of the systemic manifestations associated with dysbiosis are clearly not mediated by the infecting organism but are mediated by the host response to microbial toxins and to the systemic dysfunction induced by increased intestinal permeability and subsequent alterations in hepatic and immune function. Thus, the sequelae of dysbiosis are mediated by alterations in human physiology rather than being directly caused by the microbe.** Current research has linked several microbes with human autoimmune/inflammatory diseases, for example *Entamoeba histolytica* has been linked with Henoch Schonlein purpura[824], *Klebsiella pneumoniae* with ankylosing spondylitis[825], *Proteus mirabilis* with rheumatoid arthritis[826,827] and ankylosing spondylitis[828], *Pseudomonas aeruginosa* with multiple sclerosis[829], and *Helicobacter pylori* with reactive arthritis.[830]

---

[815] Lizko NN. Problems of microbial ecology in man space mission. *Acta Astronaut.* 1991;23:163-9
[816] Galland L. Intestinal protozoan infection is a common unsuspected cause of chronic illness. *J Advancement Med.* 1989;2: 539-552
[817] Crook W. The Yeast Connection. Professional Books. Jackson. Tennessee. 1983
[818] "The writer has observed numerous cases suffering from such conditions as chronic arthritis, hypertension, coronary disease, chronic abdominal distention, constipation, and colitis, in which the element of constipation, auto-intoxication and possible colon infection seemed to play a prominent part, which responded very satisfactorily to colonic irrigations after failure to improve following the usual forms of medical treatment." Snyder RG. The value of colonic irrigations in countering auto-intoxication of intestinal origin. *Medl Clin North America* 1939; May: 781-788
[819] D'Acquisto F, May MJ, Ghosh S. Inhibition of Nuclear Factor Kappa B (NF-B). *Mol Interv.* 2002 Feb;2(1):22-35 molinterv.aspetjournals.org/cgi/content/full/2/1/22
[820] Tak PP, Firestein GS. NFkB: a key role in inflammatory diseases. *J Clin Invest.* 2001 Jan;107(1):7-1 jci.org/cgi/content/full/107/1/7
[821] "We have recently shown that 'illness'-inducing agents, such as intraperitoneally administered lipopolysaccharide (LPS; bacterial endotoxin), can produce prolonged hyperalgesia." Watkins et al. Illness-induced hyperalgesia is mediated by spinal neuropeptides and excitatory amino acids. *Brain Res.* 1994 Nov 21;664(1-2):17-24
[822] "The immunogen E. coli lipopolysaccharide (LPS, endotoxin) has been widely used to stimulate immune/inflammatory responses both systemically and in the CNS... LPS appears to release glutamate, which then acts at non-NMDA receptors to remove the voltage-sensitive Mg2+ block of NMDA receptors, thus permitting NMDA receptors to be activated..." Wang et al. The bacterial endotoxin lipopolysaccharide causes rapid inappropriate excitation in rat cortex. *J Neurochem.* 1999 Feb;72:652-60
[823] "Superantigens are potent activators of CD4+ T cells, causing rapid and massive proliferation of cells and cytokine production... Superantigens have also been implicated in acute diseases such as food poisoning and TSS, and in chronic diseases such as psoriasis and rheumatoid arthritis." Torres BA, Kominsky S, Perrin GQ, Hobeika AC, Johnson HM. Superantigens: the good, the bad, and the ugly. *Exp Biol Med* (Maywood). 2001 Mar;226(3):164-76
[824] Demircin G, Oner A, Erdogan O, Bulbul M, Memis L. Henoch Schonlein purpura and amebiasis. *Acta Paediatr Jpn.* 1998 Oct; 40(5): 489-91
[825] Ahmadi K, et al. Antibodies to Klebsiella pneumoniae lipopolysaccharide in patients with ankylosing spondylitis. *Br J Rheumatol.* 1998 Dec;37(12):1330-3
[826] Ebringer A, Rashid T, Wilson C. Rheumatoid arthritis: proposal for the use of anti-microbial therapy in early cases. *Scand J Rheumatol* 2003;32(1):2-11
[827] Rashid T, et al. Proteus IgG antibodies and C-reactive protein in English, Norwegian and Spanish patients with rheumatoid arthritis. *Clin Rheumatol* 1999;18(3):190-5
[828] Wilson C, et al. Cytotoxicity responses to Peptide antigens in rheumatoid arthritis and ankylosing spondylitis. *J Rheumatol* 2003 May;30(5):972-8
[829] Hughes LE, et al. Antibody responses to Acinetobacter spp. and Pseudomonas aeruginosa in multiple sclerosis: prospects for diagnosis using the myelin-acinetobacter-neurofilament antibody index. *Clin Diagn Lab Immunol.* 2001 Nov;8(6):1181-8
[830] "... HP may be included in the list of possible arthritis triggering microbes."Melby et al.Helicobacter pylori--a trigger of reactive arthritis?*Infection*.1999;27:252-5

Gastrointestinal Dysbiosis: Subtypes and Categorization
Building upon a previous four-subtype categorization proposed by Galland[831], here I describe six different types of gastrointestinal dysbiosis:
1. Insufficiency dysbiosis: This results when there is an insufficient quantity of the "good bacteria." Absence of "good bacteria" such as *Bifidobacteria* and *Lactobacillus* leaves the gastrointestinal tract vulnerable to colonization with pathogens and is associated with increased risk for bacterial overgrowth and other intestinal diseases. Furthermore, **beneficial bacteria in the intestines helps to normalize systemic immune response and promote proper digestion, elimination and nutrient absorption**. Numerous scientific studies have documented the powerful benefits of supplementing with good bacteria (probiotics), supporting their growth with fermentable carbohydrates such as inulin and fructooligosaccharides (prebiotics), and by co-administering probiotics with prebiotics (synbiotics).
2. Bacterial overgrowth: This is a quantitative excess of yeast and bacteria in the gut. Bacterial overgrowth of the small bowel is a well-established medical problem that is particularly common in patients who are diabetic, elderly, immunosuppressed (such as with corticosteroids/prednisone[832,833]), naturally hypochlorhydric or iatrogenically hypochlorhydric due to "antacid" drugs.[834] This commonly results in gas, bloating, malabsorption, constipation and/or diarrhea, "irritable bowel syndrome", as well as myalgias and systemic immune activation.[835] **Animal studies have proven that peripheral arthritis can activated/reactivated by inducing bacterial overgrowth of the small bowel; endotoxins and other microbial products stimulate a systemic proinflammatory state which re-activates inflammation of joints and periarticular structures**.[836] Bacterial overgrowth of the small intestine is seen in 84% of patients with irritable bowel syndrome[837] and in **100% of patients with fibromyalgia**.[838] Researchers recently demonstrated that endotoxins can lead to impairment of muscle function and a lowered lactate threshold[839], thereby explaining the link between intestinal dysbiosis and chronic musculoskeletal pain that is not responsive to drugs or manual therapies. Drs. Over and Bucknall[840] describe a patient with **systemic sclerosis** who achieved **long-term remission** of her disease following **antibiotic treatment for intestinal bacterial overgrowth**. Bacterial overgrowth generally leads to pathologically synergistic clinical effects mediated by fermentation, putrefaction, constipation, increased enterohepatic recycling, bile acid deconjugation, malabsorption (particularly fat-soluble nutrients and vitamin B-12), nutritional deficiencies, sugar cravings, increased intestinal permeability, immune complex formation, and induction of a systemic proinflammatory response with immune complexes that is particularly prone to manifest as vasculitis and arthritis.[841,842,843]
3. Immunosuppressive dysbiosis: Some microbes, particularly yeast, produce toxins that suppress immune function. The immunosuppressive mycotoxin produced by *Candia albicans* is called gliotoxin[844], and it is

---

[831] Attributed to Galland L. "Fire in the belly: update on gut fermentation." Presented to Great Lakes Association of Clinical Medicine, circa 1996. Also, personal email from Leo Galland dated October 28, 2005: "I have used the concept of 4 types of dysbiosis (putrefaction, fermentation, depletion and immune activation forms) in several presentations and in one written document."
[832] "A 63-year-old man with systemic lupus erythematosus and selective IgA deficiency developed intractable diarrhoea the day after treatment with prednisone, 50 mg daily, was started. The diarrhoea was considered to be caused by bacterial overgrowth and was later successfully treated with doxycycline." Denison H, Wallerstedt S. Bacterial overgrowth after high-dose corticosteroid treatment. *Scand J Gastroenterol*. 1989 Jun;24(5):561-4
[833] "These bacteria also translocated to the mesenteric lymph nodes in mice injected with cyclophosphamide or prednisone." Berg RD, Wommack E, Deitch EA. Immunosuppression and intestinal bacterial overgrowth synergistically promote bacterial translocation. *Arch Surg*. 1988 Nov;123(11):1359-64
[834] Saltzman JR, Russell RM. Nutritional consequences of intestinal bacterial overgrowth. *Compr Ther*. 1994;20(9):523-30
[835] Lin HC. Small intestinal bacterial overgrowth: a framework for understanding irritable bowel syndrome. *JAMA*. 2004 Aug 18;292(7):852-8
[836] Lichtman SN, Wang J, Sartor RB, Zhang C, Bender D, Dalldorf FG, Schwab JH. Reactivation of arthritis induced by small bowel bacterial overgrowth in rats: role of cytokines, bacteria, and bacterial polymers. *Infect Immun*. 1995 Jun;63(6):2295-301
[837] Lin HC. Small intestinal bacterial overgrowth: a framework for understanding irritable bowel syndrome. *JAMA*. 2004 Aug 18;292(7):852-8
[838] Pimentel et al. A link between irritable bowel syndrome and fibromyalgia may be related to findings on lactulose breath testing. *Ann Rheum Dis*. 2004 Apr;63(4):450-2
[839] Bundgaard H, Kjeldsen K, Suarez Krabbe K, et al. Endotoxemia stimulates skeletal muscle Na+-K+-ATPase and raises blood lactate under aerobic conditions in humans. *Am J Physiol Heart Circ Physiol*. 2003 Mar;284(3):H1028-34. ajpheart.physiology.org/cgi/reprint/284/3/H1028
[840] Over et al. Regression of skin changes in patient with systemic sclerosis following treatment for bacterial overgrowth with ciprofloxacin. *Br J Rheumatol* 1998;37:696
[841] Lin HC. Small intestinal bacterial overgrowth: a framework for understanding irritable bowel syndrome. *JAMA*. 2004 Aug 18;292(7):852-8
[842] Zaidel O, Lin HC. Uninvited guests: the impact of small intestinal bacterial overgrowth on nutrition. *Practical Gastroenterology* 2003; 27(7):27-34
[843] "The initial skin changes were frankly vasculitic with 'target' lesions, whilst older lesions showed a psoriasiform scale and a tendency to central clearing. The illness was associated with raised levels of IgM and IgG containing circulating immune complexes and deposition of IgM and IgG in the dermis." Fairris GM, Ashworth J, Cotterill JA. A dermatosis associated with bacterial overgrowth in jejunal diverticula. *Br J Dermatol*. 1985 Jun;112(6):709-13
[844] "Candida albicans is known to produce gliotoxin, which has several prominent biological effects, including immunosuppression." Shah DT, Jackman S, Engle J, Larsen B. Effect of gliotoxin on human polymorphonuclear neutrophils. *Infect Dis Obstet Gynecol*. 1998;6(4):168-75

produced at the site of yeast overgrowth, thus suppressing local—and possibly, systemic—immune function.[845] Since secretory IgA is the first line of defense against allergens and infections in the gastrointestinal tract, its destruction by microbes such as *Candida albicans* and *Entamoeba histolytica* retards this immune barrier, and this can be considered a form of local immunosuppression.

4. <u>Hypersensitivity/allergic dysbiosis</u>: **Some people have an exaggerated immune response to otherwise "normal" yeast and bacteria. In this situation, we have to eradicate their "normal" yeast or bacteria in order to alleviate their hypersensitivity reaction.** The best example of this is the **severe intestinal inflammation that some patients develop in response to intestinal colonization with *Candida albicans***, which is generally considered "nonpathogenic" in small amounts. In susceptible patients, *Candida* can induce a severe local inflammatory reaction, such as colitis, that only remits with antifungal treatment.[846] **Gastrointestinal overgrowth of *Candida albicans* and *C. glabrata* caused near-fatal hypersensitivity alveolitis that remitted with eradication of gastrointestinal candidiasis**.[847] Some women become "allergic" to their own vaginal *Candida albicans*[848]; undoubtedly there are also men who are likewise allergic to their own intestinal yeast. In patients with lupus, gastrointestinal bacteria are abnormal (decreased colonization resistance[849]), and it is possible that gastrointestinal bacteria in these patients may translocate into the systemic circulation to induce formation of antibodies that cross-react with double-stranded DNA to produce the clinical manifestations of the disease.[850,851] With regard to dermal dysbiosis, **most (57%) of patients with atopic dermatitis show evidence of IgE-mediated histamine release (i.e., "allergy") to exotoxins secreted from *Staphylococcus aureus***, which commonly colonizes eczematous skin[852]; in other words: most eczema patients are allergic to their own dermal bacteria and can thus be said to have *hypersensitivity dermal dysbiosis*.

5. <u>Inflammatory dysbiosis and reactive arthritis</u>: People with specific genotypes and HLA markers are susceptible to a proinflammatory "autoimmune" syndrome that occurs following exposure to specific microbial molecules that are structurally similar to human body tissues—a phenomenon previously described as molecular mimicry. The best-known example of systemic musculoskeletal inflammation caused by microbial exposure is "reactive arthritis" such as Reiter's syndrome, which is classically seen in patients with the genotype HLA-B27 following urogenital exposure to *Chlamydia trachomatis*.

6. <u>Amoebas, cysts, protozoas, and other parasites</u>: In this case when we use the term "parasites'" we are not talking about worms/helminths, *per se*, although these are occasionally found with parasitology examinations. Certain microorganisms are not consistent with optimal health and should be eliminated even though the microbe is not classically identified as a "pathogen." Interestingly, 97% of patients severely infected with the gastrointestinal "parasite" *Entamoeba histolytica* develop self-destructive ANCA[853], suggesting the possibility that this microbe can induce or sustain autoimmunity.

Gastrointestinal Dysbiosis: Assessments

- <u>History</u>: Clinicians should suspect gastrointestinal dysbiosis in their patients with gas, bloating, alternating constipation/diarrhea, irritable bowel syndrome, fibromyalgia, chronic fatigue syndrome, multiple chemical sensitivity, severe allergies, and autoimmunity, especially Crohn's disease, ulcerative colitis, rheumatoid arthritis, and ankylosing spondylitis. Frequent gas and bloating indicates excess gastrointestinal fermentation by yeast and/or overgrowth of aerobic bacteria. Abdominal pain, chronic constipation, and/or diarrhea are clear

---

[845] "Based on the recent finding that C. albicans is able to produce an immunosuppressive mycotoxin, gliotoxin, we analyzed vaginal samples of 3 women severely symptomatic for vaginal candidiasis and found that they contained significant levels of gliotoxin." Shah DT, Glover DD, Larsen B. In situ mycotoxin production by Candida albicans in women with vaginitis. *Gynecol Obstet Invest*. 1995;39(1):67-9

[846] Doby T. Monilial esophagitis and colitis. *J Maine Med Assoc*. 1971 May;62(5):109-14

[847] "We conclude that the disease was induced by C.a.-antigen reaching the lungs from the intestinal tract via the bloodstream." Schreiber J, Struben C, Rosahl W, Amthor M. Hypersensitivity alveolitis induced by endogenous candida species. *Eur J Med Res*. 2000 Mar 27;5(3):126

[848] Ramirez De Knott HM, et al. Cutaneous hypersensitivity to Candida albicans in idiopathic vulvodynia. *Contact Dermatitis*. 2005 Oct;53(4):214-8

[849] "Colonization Resistance (CR)...tended to be lower in active SLE patients than in healthy individuals. This could indicate that in SLE more and different bacteria translocate across the gut wall due to a lower CR. Some of these may serve as polyclonal B cell activators or as antigens cross-reacting with DNA." Apperloo-Renkema HZ, Bootsma H, Mulder BI, Kallenberg CG, van der Waaij D. Host-microflora interaction in systemic lupus erythematosus (SLE): colonization resistance of the indigenous bacteria of the intestinal tract. *Epidemiol Infect*. 1994;112(2):367-73

[850] "The lower IgG antibacterial antibody titres in active SLE might possibly result from sequestration of these IgG antibodies in immune complexes, indicating a possible role for antibacterial antibodies in exacerbations of SLE." Apperloo-Renkema HZ, Bootsma H, Mulder BI, Kallenberg CG, van der Waaij D. Host-microflora interaction in systemic lupus erythematosus (SLE): circulating antibodies to the indigenous bacteria of the intestinal tract. *Epidemiol Infect*. 1995 Feb;114(1):133-41

[851] Pisetsky DS. Antibody responses to DNA in normal immunity and aberrant immunity. *Clin Diagn Lab Immunol* 1998;5:1-6

[852] "These data indicate that a subset of patients with AD mount an IgE response to SEs that can be grown from their skin." Leung DY, et al. Presence of IgE antibodies to staphylococcal exotoxins on the skin of patients with atopic dermatitis. Evidence for a new group of allergens. *J Clin Invest*. 1993 Sep;92(3):1374-80

[853] George J, Levy Y, Kallenberg CG, Shoenfeld Y. Infections and Wegener's granulomatosis--a cause and effect relationship? *QJM*. 1997 May;90(5):367-73

indications for stool testing; however, clinicians must remember that **many very heavily colonized patients will have no gastrointestinal symptoms**. Thus, **assessment and treatment for gastrointestinal dysbiosis is *not un*necessary simply because the patient lacks gastrointestinal symptoms**.
- **Breath testing**: Bacterial overgrowth of the small bowel can be objectively documented with measurement of a **post-carbohydrate hydrogen/methane breath test**, but I consider a history of postprandial gas and bloating to be sufficiently diagnostic.
- **Lactulose-mannitol assay for "leaky gut"**: The intestinal wall should function as a tightly regulated barrier that accomplishes two tasks: 1) **efficient absorption** of nutrients, and 2) **selective exclusion** of antigens, foreign debris, microbes and microbial antigens, and indigestible food residues. Compromise of the intestinal barrier results in impairments in nutrient absorption and/or toxin exclusion. Impaired nutrient absorption predisposes to and commonly results in micro- or macro-nutrient deficiencies. Impaired exclusion results in increased absorption of microbes, antigens, waste products, and debris into the systemic circulation. This phenomenon of altered intestinal permeability is referred to in the lay public and increasingly in the medical literature as "leaky gut" or "leaky gut syndrome."[854,855] In many patients this injury is occult, and **they have no gastrointestinal symptoms at all**; other patients may have a spectrum of signs and symptoms including diarrhea, constipation, abdominal pain, fatigue, general malaise, dyscognition, and an increase in the number and severity of food allergies, food sensitivities, and food intolerances. The **lactulose and mannitol assay** evaluates paracellular (pathologic) and transcellular (physiologic) absorption, respectively; and an increased lactulose:mannitol ratio is a non-specific finding that indicates gastrointestinal damage, generally due to 1) enterotoxin consumption such as with alcohol or NSAIDs, 2) malnutrition, 3) food allergy including celiac disease, 4) inflammatory bowel disease, and/or 5) dysbiosis—excess/harmful yeast, bacteria, or parasites. **Recall that "leaky gut" is only a symptom or manifestation of another, larger problem**.

Clinical Case Highly abnormal lactulose-mannitol ratio in a patient with idiopathic peripheral neuropathy prior to comprehensive stool analysis and parasitology showing intestinal dysbiosis: This 40-yo man presented with a multiyear history of periodic febrile exacerbations of peripheral neuropathy that would cause severe paresthesias and motor deficits. Food allergy and intestinal dysbiosis are the most obvious probable etiologies; dysbiosis was confirmed with laboratory testing showing *Pseudomonas*.

---

[854] Hollander D. Intestinal permeability, leaky gut, and intestinal disorders. *Curr Gastroenterol Rep.* 1999 Oct;1(5):410-6
[855] Keshavarzian A, Holmes EW, Patel M, Iber F, Fields JZ, Pethkar S. Leaky gut in alcoholic cirrhosis. *Am J Gastroenterol.* 1999 Jan;94(1):200-7

Gastrointestinal Dysbiosis, "Leaky Gut" and Impaired Detoxification: A Sample Model of Interconnected Scenarios and Some Clinical Remediation: Therapeutic considerations are italicized and highlighted in green while "entry points" are colored in yellow, and clinical manifestations are mostly colored in red. This diagram—made by Dr Vasquez at age 28y after several years of chronic fatigue and dysbiosis—was published for the first time in *Integrative Orthopedics* 2004 and is presented here virtually without change, excepting colorization. "And when a person goes through fire for his teaching [education], what does that prove? It is more meaningful—truly—when out of one's own burning cometh one's own teaching!" Nietzsche FW. *Thus Spoke Zarathustra*. Part 26

- **Comprehensive stool analysis and comprehensive parasitology**: The single best test for the assessment of gastrointestinal dysbiosis is a comprehensive stool analysis and comprehensive parasitology examination performed by a specialty laboratory that provides bacterial culture, yeast culture, microscopic exam, and measurement of sIgA to assess mucosal immune response, along with markers of inflammation such as lactoferrin, calprotectin, and/or lysozyme. Comprehensive parasitology examinations (x3) to assess for bacteria, yeast, and parasites should be followed by culture and sensitivity to fine-tune the identification of the microbes and to guide treatment. These tests should be performed by a specialty laboratory rather than a regular medical or hospital laboratory. Additional markers can help put microbiological findings into the proper context; for example, in a patient with no "pathogens" other than normal *Candida albicans*, the finding of an exaggerated inflammatory response suggests a hypersensitivity/allergic dysbiosis that should be eradicated. **Stool testing must be performed by a specialty laboratory** because the quality of testing provided by most standard "medical labs" and hospitals is completely inadequate. Initial samples should be collected on three separate occasions by the patient and each sample should be analyzed separately by the laboratory. Important qualitative and quantitative markers include the following:
    - Beneficial bacteria (" probiotics"): Microbiological testing should quantify and identify various beneficial bacteria, which should be present at "+4" levels on a 0-4 scale.
    - Harmful and potentially harmful bacteria, protozoans, amebas, etc.: Questionable or harmful microbes should be eradicated even if they are not identified as true pathogens in the paleo-classic Pasteurian/Kochian sense.[856]
    - Yeast and mycology: At least two tests must be performed for a complete assessment: 1) yeast culture, and 2) microscopic examination for yeast elements. (See Chapter 1 for additional discussion.)
    - Microbial sensitivity testing: An important component to parasitology testing is the determination of which anti-microbial agents (natural and synthetic) the microbe is sensitive to. This helps to guide and enhance the effectiveness of anti-microbial therapy.
    - Secretory IgA: SIgA levels are elevated in patients who are having an immune response to either food or microbial antigens.[857] Thus, in a patient with minimal dysbiosis, say for example with *Candida albicans*, an elevated sIgA can indicate that the patient is having a hypersensitivity reaction to an otherwise benign microbe—in this case, eradication of the microbe is warranted and may result in a positive clinical response. Low sIgA suggests either primary or secondary immune defect such as selective sIgA deficiency[858] or malnutrition, stress, prednisone/corticosteroids, or possibly mycotoxicosis (immunosuppression due to fungal immunotoxins).
    - Short-chain fatty acids: These are produced by intestinal bacteria. Quantitative excess indicates bacterial overgrowth of the intestines, while insufficiency indicates a lack of probiotics or an insufficiency of dietary substrate, i.e., soluble fiber. Abnormal patterns of individual short-chain fatty acids indicate qualitative/quantitative abnormalities in gastrointestinal microflora, particularly anaerobic bacteria that cannot be identified with routine bacterial cultures.
    - Beta-glucuronidase: This is an enzyme produced by several different intestinal bacteria. High levels of beta-glucuronidase in the intestinal lumen serve to nullify the benefits of detoxification (specifically glucuronidation) by cleaving the toxicant from its glucuronide conjugate. This can result in re-absorption of the toxicant through the intestinal mucosa which then re-exposes the patient to the toxin that was previously detoxified ("enterohepatic recirculation" or "enterohepatic recycling"[859]). This is an exemplary aspect of "auto-intoxication" that results in chronic fatigue and upregulation of Phase 1 detoxification systems (chapter 4 of *Integrative Rheumatology*).
    - Lactoferrin: The iron-binding glycoprotein lactoferrin is an inflammatory marker that helps distinguish functional disorders (i.e., IBS) from more serious diseases (i.e., IBD).

---

[856] Vasquez A. Nutritional and Botanical Treatments Against "Silent Infections" and Gastrointestinal Dysbiosis. *Nutr Perspect* 2006; Jan
[857] Quig DW, Higley M. Noninvasive assessment of intestinal inflammation: IBD vs. IBS. *Townsend Letter for Doctors and Patients* 2006;Jan:74-5
[858] "Selective IgA deficiency is the most common form of immunodeficiency. Certain select populations, including allergic individuals, patients with autoimmune and gastrointestinal tract disease and patients with recurrent upper respiratory tract illnesses, have an increased incidence of this disorder." Burks AW Jr, Steele RW. Selective IgA deficiency. *Ann Allergy*. 1986;57:3-13
[859] Parker et al.Enterohepatic recycling of phenolphthalein, morphine, lysergic acid diethylamide (LSD) and diphenylacetic acid in the rat. *Xenobiotica*. 1980;10:689-70

- o <u>Lysozyme</u>: Elevated in proportion to intestinal inflammation in dysbiosis and IBD.
- o <u>Other markers</u>: Other markers of digestion, inflammation, and absorption are reported with the more comprehensive panels performed on stool samples. These tests are not always necessary, but such additional information is always helpful when working with complex patients. These markers are relatively self-explanatory and/or are described on the results of the test by the laboratory.

Orodental Dysbiosis

- **Introduction**: The human oral cavity is heavily populated by microbes, and these microbes and their products such as endotoxin can enter the bloodstream to induce a proinflammatory response via "metastatic infection" and "**metastatic inflammation**", respectively.[860] The systemic inflammatory response triggered by mild oral/dental "infections" is now believed to exacerbate conditions associated with inflammation, such as cardiovascular disease and diabetes mellitus.[861] **Patients with rheumatoid arthritis have heightened antibody levels against common oral bacteria. IgG levels against** *Porphyromonas gingivalis, Prevotella melaninogenica, Bacteroides forsythus,* **and** *Prevotella intermedia* **were found to be significantly higher in RA patients when compared with those of controls**.[862] In the first human clinical trial to test the hypothesis that treatment of orodental dysbiosis would provide subjective and objective clinical benefits for patients with RA, Al-Katma et al[863] showed that **periodontal treatment consisting of scaling/root planing and oral hygiene instruction reduced symptom scores and ESR levels in patients with RA**.

- **Assessments**: Obviously, any major microbial infestations of the mouth, such as gingivitis or thrush, need to be treated regardless of the presence or absence of systemic inflammatory disease. **Culture of mouth, throat, dentures for yeast and bacteria can be performed** (see Noah[864]). Palpation/provocation of the gums and teeth should not cause pain; the presence of pain suggests underlying inflammation, which in turn indicates underlying infection. If flossing causes bleeding and pain, this is indicative of unhealthy gums due to an overgrowth of bacteria below the gum line. Mild gum regression and the development of deep dental pockets is an indication for intervention with fastidious oral hygiene and professional dental care. Patients with systemic disease including chronic unwellness may have asymptomatic infections of the mandible that can only be detected with non-standard imaging techniques such as computer-enhanced mandibular ultrasound.[865]

- **Specific treatment considerations**: A professional cleaning by a dentist or oral hygienist is a reasonable start. Thereafter, twice-daily brushing, flossing, and the use of an antiseptic mouthwash and a plaque-removing solution should be employed. To improve understand and compliance, clinicians should instruct patients that the purpose of flossing is not to remove food but to disrupt microbial biofilms. Toothbrushes should be periodically disinfected and replaced. Electric toothbrushes are more efficient than manual toothbrushes, and three-dimensional and ultrasound toothbrushes can cleanse below the gum line. Avoiding sucrose and refined carbohydrates is essential. Sugar-free chewing gums help to reduce bacterial loads at least in part by stimulating saliva production, and chewing gums with xylitol significantly reduce bacterial colonization of the oral cavity.[866,867] Immunonutrition as described later should be used to improve overall systemic defenses; particular consideration should be given to glutamine, bovine colostrum and IgG, and thymus extract—the latter per an animal study of experimental dental disease showing administration of thymus extract normalized immune function and reduced orodental dysbiosis.[868]

---

[860] Li X, Kolltveit KM, Tronstad L, Olsen I. Systemic diseases caused by oral infection. *Clin Microbiol Rev*. 2000 Oct;13(4):547-58 cmr.asm.org/cgi/content/full/13/4/547
[861] Amar S, Han X. The impact of periodontal infection on systemic diseases. *Med Sci Monit*. 2003 Dec;9(12):RA291-9 medscimonit.com/pub/vol_9/no_12/3776.pdf
[862] Ogrendik M, Kokino S, Ozdemir F, et al. Serum antibodies to oral anaerobic bacteria in patients with rheumatoid arthritis. *MedGenMed*. 2005 Jun 16;7(2):2
[863] "There was a statistically significant difference in DAS28 (4.3 +/- 1.6 vs. 5.1 +/- 1.2) and erythrocyte sedimentation rate (31.4 +/- 24.3 vs. 42.7 +/- 22) between the treatment and the control groups." Al-Katma et al. Control of periodontal infection reduces the severity of active rheumatoid arthritis. *J Clin Rheumatol*. 2007 Jun;13:134-7
[864] Noah PW. The role of microorganisms in psoriasis. *Semin Dermatol*. 1990 Dec;9(4):269-76
[865] "Through-transmission alveolar ultrasonography (TAU) is a novel imaging modality in dental medicine. A brief introduction to through-transmission ultrasonography (TTU) is followed by a description of the first commercially available TAU device, the Cavitat CAV 4000 (Cavitat Medical Technologies, Inc., Alba, TX)." Imbeau J. Introduction to through-transmission alveolar ultrasonography (TAU) in dental medicine. *Cranio*. 2005 Apr;23(2):100-12. Cavitat Medical Technologies appears to have been involved in some litigation and regulatory issues and may have closed per internet information and fda.gov/ohrms/dockets/dailys/01/aug01/080801/cp0001.pdf surveyed 2014 Jan.
[866] "Chewing 100% xylitol gum caused significant reductions on salivary MS scores (p < 0.025) which was little different from the 55% xylitol group. The results suggest that the use of xylitol chewing gum can reduce the levels of MS in plaque and saliva." Thaweboon S, Thaweboon B, Soo-Ampon S. The effect of xylitol chewing gum on mutans streptococci in saliva and dental plaque. *Southeast Asian J Trop Med Public Health*. 2004 Dec;35(4):1024-7
[867] "Especially xylitol-containing chewing gum may significantly reduce the growth of mutans streptococci and dental plaque which may be associated with dental caries." Makinen KK, Isotupa KP, Makinen PL, Soderling E, Song KB, Nam SH, Jeong SH. Six-month polyol chewing-gum programme in kindergarten-age children: a feasibility study focusing on mutans streptococci and dental plaque. *Int Dent J*. 2005 Apr;55(2):81-8
[868] Manti et al. Effects of immunomodulating agent on peripheral blood lymphocytes and subgingival microflora in ligature-induced periodontitis. *Infect Immun* 1984;45:172-9

Sinorespiratory Dysbiosis

- **Introduction**: Sinorespiratory dysbiosis refers to adverse health consequences resultant from noninfectious colonization of the respiratory tract. Patients with acute and chronic rhinosinusitis commonly display a rich mixture of bacteria and fungi in their sinuses. Regarding bacteria, both anaerobic and aerobic bacteria are seen, as are gram-positives such as *Staphylococcus aureus*, *Streptococcus* sp, Peptococcus/Peptostreptococcus, and gram-negative (endotoxin-producing) species including *Klebsiella pneumoniae*, *Proteus mirabilis*, *Bacteroides*, *Haemophilus parainfluenzae*, and *Haemophilus influenzae*.[869,870] Regarding fungi, **almost all patients with chronic sinus congestion have occult fungal sinus infections**, as shown in a landmark article wherein the authors concluded, "Fungal cultures of nasal secretions were positive in 202 (96%) of 210 consecutive chronic rhinosinusitis patients."[871] **Reactive arthritis** and **cutaneous vasculitis** have been reported in an HLA-B27-negative patient with *Chlamydia pneumoniae* pneumonia.[872] Perhaps the best current exemplification of the link between sinus infections and chronic inflammatory disease is seen in patients with **Wegener's granulomatosis**, who have a high incidence of sinus colonization with *Staphylococcus aureus*. In these patients, *Staphylococcus aureus* produces a superantigen as well as an antigenic acid phosphatase which induces autoimmune vasculitis, nephritis, the production of antineutrophil anticytoplasmic antibody (ANCA), and the formation of immune complexes. **Antimicrobial treatment to eradicate *Staphylococcus aureus* results in clinical remission of the "autoimmune" disease**[873], **thus proving the microbe-autoimmune link.** Increased nasal colonization with *Staphylococcus aureus* has also been documented in other inflammatory/autoimmune diseases, including **systemic lupus erythematosus**[874] and **psoriasis.**[875]

- **Assessments**: Several studies documenting fungal and bacterial colonization of the sinuses have used diagnostic/surgical techniques that are not routinely available to clinicians working in outpatient settings. **Nasal swab and culture, throat culture for bacteria and yeasts should be performed** (see Noah[876]). Accessing the sinuses is generally not feasible on a clinical/nonsurgical basis. Response to antimicrobial treatment implies cure of the occult infection. In severe cases, MRI or CT can be used to assess for occult infectious sinusitis.

DrV's favorite way of explaining dysbiosis: "Often what we find when working with autoimmune/inflammatory patients is that they are having a pathogenic inflammatory response to *nonpathogenic* microbes."

Research that exemplifies this concept:

- "Saint Louis University researchers have analyzed the microbiomes of people with chronic rhinosinusitis and healthy volunteers and found evidence that some chronic sinus issues may be the result of inflammation triggered by an immune response to otherwise harmless microorganisms in the sinus membranes.
- "Further study findings suggested that bacteria and fungi are not causing an infection in the sinuses, but rather, that the immune system was responding to commensals, microorganisms that, themselves, do not harm the human body.
- "When the immune system reacts in a hyper-responsive way, unnecessarily fighting off a harmless microorganism, it can initiate an immune response like inflammation. The body can then get locked into a cycle where inflammation generates more inflammation, causing a chronic condition.
- "Patients with CRS are hyper-responsive to normal microbiota," said Aurora. "Our take-home message is that the problem doesn't lie in the microbiota. The inflammatory response and the resulting damage from the prolonged inflammation are caused by the body's own immune response to harmless microbiota."

Harmless Members of Microbiome Spark Immune Reaction. sciencedaily.com/releases/2013/12/131219134455.htm Dec. 19, 2013. Original source: With Sinus Study, SLU Investigators Add Immune System Dimension to Discussion of Microbiota and Disease. slu.edu/x89847.xml

---

[869] "Aspirates of 72 chronically inflamed maxillary sinuses were processed for aerobic and anaerobic bacteria. Bacterial growth was present in 66 of the 72 specimens (92%).... The predominant anaerobic organisms were anaerobic cocci and Bacteroides sp, and the predominant aerobes or facultatives were Streptococcus sp and Staphylococcus aureus." Brook I. Bacteriology of chronic maxillary sinusitis in adults. *Ann Otol Rhinol Laryngol.* 1989 Jun;98(6):426-8
[870] "The most frequently isolated bacteria were Streptococcus viridans, Klebsiella pneumoniae, Proteus mirabilis, and Hemophilus parainfluenzae." Jiang RS, Hsu CY, Leu JF. Bacteriology of ethmoid sinus in chronic sinusitis. *Am J Rhinol.* 1997 Mar-Apr;11(2):133-7
[871] Ponikau JU, et al. The diagnosis and incidence of allergic fungal sinusitis. *Mayo Clin Proc.* 1999 Sep;74(9):877-84
[872] "Here we present the case history of a patient with C. pneumoniae community acquired pneumonia (CAP) who subsequently developed a ReA and a cutaneous vasculitis." Cascina et al. Cutaneous vasculitis and reactive arthritis following respiratory infection due to Chlamydia pneumoniae. *Clin Exp Rheumatol.* 2002;20(6):845-7
[873] Popa et al. Staphylococcus aureus and Wegener's granulomatosis. *Arthritis Res.* 2002;4(2):77-9 arthritis-research.com/content/4/2/077
[874] Medline abstract from Polish research: "In 9 from 14 patients with (64.3%) a.b. very massive growth of Staphylococcus aureus in culture from vestibulae of the nose swab was, in other cultures very massive growth of physiological flora was seen. ...clinical significance of asymptomatic bacteriuria and pathogenic bacteria colonisation of nostrils as a precedence to symptomatic infections needs further investigations." Koseda-Dragan M, Hebanowski M, Galinski J, Krzywinska E, Bakowska A. [Asymptomatic bacteriuria in women diagnosed with systemic lupus erythematosus (SLE)] *Pol Arch Med Wewn.* 1998 Oct;100(4):321-30.
[875] "The nasal carriage rate of Staphylococcus aureus in psoriatics was higher ...." Singh G, Rao DJ. Bacteriology of psoriatic plaques. *Dermatologica.* 1978;157(1):21-7
[876] Noah PW. The role of microorganisms in psoriasis. *Semin Dermatol.* 1990 Dec;9(4):269-76. Utterly brilliant work.

- **Specific treatment considerations**: Systemic antibiotics are commonly used by allopaths when treating sinus infections. Nasal lavage with saline is highly efficacious for relieving sinus congestion.[877] The basic solution is approximately one cup of warm water with one-half teaspoon of salt (sodium chloride) and one-half teaspoon baking soda (sodium bicarbonate). Distilled, bottled, or otherwise filtered and purified water may be preferred to avoid the microbial contaminants that are found in municipal tap water. To this can be added antimicrobial botanicals such as berberine, hyperforin (highly effective against *Staphylococcus aureus*[878]), artemisinin, and others (discussed later) as well as diluted iodine[879] and powdered Nystatin (sugar-free only.) Irrigation with a bulb syringe (such as used to clear an infant's nostrils) or Neti lota pot (aka: Neti pot, or Jala neti pot) can be performed by the patient while leaning over the sink. In the author's experience, 10-15 drops of povidone iodine 10% solution can be added to one cup of nasal lavage; higher amounts of iodine cause a burning sensation. Irrigating while kneeling with the head on the floor is the most effective technique for irrigating the maxillary sinuses and frontal recess; however most techniques are inefficient for accessing the sphenoid and frontal sinuses.[880] Nasal sprays and nebulizers with saline and/or antimicrobial herbs and medications can also be utilized.[881] However, clinicians and patients must remember that the creation of microbial imbalance is possible in the sinuses just as it is in the gastrointestinal tract; thus, the use of an antibacterial agent may result in fungal overgrowth or proliferation of resistant microbes. Patients with sinus dysbiosis can integrate antimicrobial sinus lavage into their daily hygiene routine, e.g., as at the same time they brush their teeth in the morning and evening. Perhaps we will find that many cases of recalcitrant gastrointestinal dysbiosis have recurred because of the gastrointestinal "seeding" of microbes from the sinorespiratory tract.

Tissue Dysbiosis, Parenchymal Dysbiosis

- **Introduction**: Infections and microbial colonization of internal organs is generally incompatible with life and unlikely to be a silent/asymptomatic locus of inflammatory stimuli due to the appropriate febrile response that typically characterizes such infections. However, exceptions to these rules do exist, and infections of parenchymal tissue—especially of liver or bone—have been reported as initiators/mimickers of systemic rheumatic/inflammatory disease. **Viral hepatitis may present with polyarthropathy while the hepatitis is asymptomatic and serum levels of liver enzymes are within normal limits**; in these cases, the underlying dysbiosis/infection is identified with the use of specific serologic testing.[882] **Polyarteritis nodosa** is an autoimmune/inflammatory vasculitic syndrome strongly associated with hepatitis B infection, and 90% of patients with the immune complex vasculitis cryoglobulinemia have hepatitis C.[883] Robertson and Hickling[884] describe the case of a young girl who was **tentatively diagnosed with juvenile rheumatoid arthritis before being more accurately diagnosed with "recurrent multifocal osteomyelitis."** Dysbiosis (characterized by the acute nature of the microbial colonization) can segue into a true "infection." An advantage to the term *dysbiosis* in this situation is that it

> "Blood Microbiota Dysbiosis" is Associated with the Onset of Cardiovascular Events in a Large Population
> "The main finding of the study is that a dysbiosis in blood microbiota, defined by a decrease in blood bacterial DNA content and an increase in the proportion of Proteobacteria phylum within blood microbiota, predicts long-term cardiovascular prognosis."
> Amar J, et al. *PLoS ONE* 2013:8(1); e54461

---

[877] "Endonasal irrigations with salt solutions are effective in the treatment of chronic sinusitis..." Bachmann G, Hommel G, Michel O. Effect of irrigation of the nose with isotonic salt solution on adult patients with chronic paranasal sinus disease. *Eur Arch Otorhinolaryngol*. 2000 Dec;257(10):537-41
[878] Schempp CM, Pelz K, Wittmer A, Schopf E, Simon JC. Antibacterial activity of hyperforin from St John's wort, against multiresistant Staphylococcus aureus and gram-positive bacteria. *Lancet*. 1999 Jun 19;353(9170):2129
[879] "Gargling with povidone-iodine before oral intubation reduces the transport of bacteria into the trachea." Ogata J, Minami K, Miyamoto H, Horishita T, Ogawa M, Sata T, Taniguchi H. Gargling with povidone-iodine reduces the transport of bacteria during oral intubation. *Can J Anaesth*. 2004 Nov;51(9):932-6 cja-jca.org/cgi/content/full/51/9/932 See also: "...a technique with facial, nasal vestibule and nasal cavity disinfection with a povidone-iodine solution followed by a cleansing of the nasal cavity (N = 87 patients and 166 samples)." Rombaux P, Collet S, Hamoir M, Eloy P, Bertrand B, Jamart F, Gigi J. The role of nasal cavity disinfection in the bacteriology of chronic sinusitis. *Rhinology*. 2005 Jun;43(2):125-9
[880] "...nasal douching while kneeling with the head on the floor...Nasal douches are more effective in distributing irrigation solution to the maxillary sinus and frontal recess.This should be the method of choice for irrigating these areas."Wormald et al.Comparative study of three methods of nasal irrigation.*Laryngoscope* 2004;114:2224-7
[881] "Therapy with a 4-week course of large-particle nebulized aerosol therapy improves symptomatology and objective parameters of rhinosinusitis in patients refractory to surgical and medical therapies. Addition of tobramycin appears of minimal benefit." Desrosiers MY, Salas-Prato M. Treatment of chronic rhinosinusitis refractory to other treatments with topical antibiotic therapy delivered by means of a large-particle nebulizer: results of a controlled trial. *Otolaryngol Head Neck Surg*. 2001 Sep;125(3):265-9
[882] "HCV arthritis should be considered in the differential diagnosis of seronegative arthritis of undetermined etiology even in the setting of normal liver chemistries." Akhtar AJ, Funnye AS. Hepatitis C virus associated arthritis in absence of clinical, biochemical and histological evidence of liver disease--responding to interferon therapy. *Med Sci Monit*. 2005 Jul;11(7):CS37-9 medscimonit.com/pub/vol_11/no_7/6300.pdf
[883] Tierney ML. McPhee SJ, Papadakis MA (eds). *Current Medical Diagnosis and Treatment 2006. 45th edition*. New York; Lange Medical Books: 2006, pages 844-850
[884] Robertson LP, Hickling P. Chronic recurrent multifocal osteomyelitis is a differential diagnosis of juvenile idiopathic arthritis. *Ann Rheum Dis*. 2001 Sep;60(9):828-31

encourages clinicians to search for inflammation-generating microbial foci that may exist despite the absence of organ failure or classic/standard characteristics associated with parenchymal infection.
- **Assessments**: Given the increasing prevalence of viral hepatitis and its protean manifestations, specific serologic testing for viral hepatitis is warranted in patients with constitutional symptoms and inflammatory/idiopathic arthralgia. Likewise, occult osteomyelitis—particularly of the mandible—is increasingly appreciated, particularly as newer imaging techniques are facilitating detection. Bone scans can detect clinically occult bone infections.
- **Specific treatment considerations**: Microbial identification, sensitivity, patient profile and status.
    - Involvement of tissue bacteria in the onset of diabetes in humans (*Diabetologia* 2011 Dec[885]): "RESULTS: We analysed 3,280 participants without diabetes or obesity at baseline. **The 16S rDNA concentration was higher in those destined to have diabetes**. No difference was observed regarding obesity. However, the 16S rDNA concentration was higher in those who had abdominal adiposity at the end of follow-up. The adjusted OR for incident diabetes and for abdominal adiposity were 1.35 and 1.18, respectively. Moreover, pyrosequencing analyses showed that participants destined to have diabetes and the controls shared a core blood microbiota, mostly composed of the Proteobacteria phylum (85-90%). "CONCLUSIONS/INTERPRETATION: 16S rDNA was shown to be an independent marker of the risk of diabetes. These findings are **evidence for the concept that tissue bacteria are involved in the onset of diabetes in humans**."
    - Example of tissue dysbiosis: Chronic bacterial infections/dysbiosis in the intervertebral discs of patients with chronic low back pain and disc herniation: Research published in 2013 showed that 46% of patients with chronic low back pain and lumbar disc herniations harbored chronic microbial infections within their intervertebral discs; these infections/colonizations were most commonly and significantly due to anaerobic bacteria (predominantly *Propionibacterium acnes*) while fewer patients carried aerobic bacteria in their disc material and these aerobic infections/colonizations appeared to be of lesser significance with regard to induction of pain and bone edema.[886] Antibiotic treatment (amoxicillin with clavulanic acid for 100 days) of patients with chronic low back pain was shown to provide important dose-dependent clinical benefit at the end of 100 days of treatment with benefits durable and progressive for one year[887]; impressive clinical response—approximately 50% reductions in pain and disability—following antimicrobial therapy was seen in 80% of patients in this research touted as "worthy of a Nobel Prize."[888]

Genitourinary dysbiosis
- **Introduction**: All doctors know that genitourinary infection with *Chlamydia trachomatis* can produce inflammatory arthropathy—"**reactive arthritis**"—and result in the condition previously known as Reiter's syndrome.[889] Often fatal, **toxic shock syndrome results from the absorption of toxins and superantigens from *Staphylococcus aureus* directly through the genitourinary mucosa**. In a study of 234 patients with inflammatory arthritis, 44% of patients had a silent genitourinary infection, mostly due to *Chlamydia, Mycoplasma,* or *Ureaplasma*.[890] Men with chronic prostatitis have elevated endotoxin levels in their expressed prostatic secretions[891], and plasma endotoxin levels are elevated in all types of chronic urinary tract infections[892],

---

[885] Amar et al. Involvement of tissue bacteria in the onset of diabetes in humans: evidence for a concept. *Diabetologia*. 2011 Dec;54(12):3055-61
[886] "In total, microbiological cultures were positive in 28 (46 %) patients. Anaerobic cultures were positive in 26 (43 %) patients, and of these 4 (7 %) had dual microbial infections, containing both one aerobic and one anaerobic culture." Albert HB, Lambert P, Rollason J, et al. Does nuclear tissue infected with bacteria following disc herniations lead to Modic changes in the adjacent vertebrae? *Eur Spine J*. 2013 Apr;22(4):690-6
[887] Albert HB, Sorensen JS, Christensen BS, Manniche C. Antibiotic treatment in patients with chronic low back pain and vertebral bone edema (Modic type 1 changes): a double-blind randomized clinical controlled trial of efficacy. *Eur Spine J*. 2013 Apr;22(4):697-707
[888] Sample I. Antibiotics could cure 40% of chronic back pain patients. theguardian.com/society/2013/may/07/antibiotics-cure-back-pain-patients
[889] Kobayashi S, Kida I. Reactive arthritis: recent advances and clinical manifestations. *Intern Med*. 2005;44:408-12 jstage.jst.go.jp/article/internalmedicine/44/5/408/_pdf
[890] "Urogenital swab cultures showed a microbial infection in 44% of the patients with oligoarthritis (15% Chlamydia, 14% Mycoplasma, 28% Ureaplasma), whereas in the control group only 26% had a positive result (4% Chlamydia, 7% Mycoplasma, 21% Ureaplasma)." Erlacher L, et al. Reactive arthritis: urogenital swab culture is the only useful diagnostic method for the detection of the arthritogenic infection in extra-articularly asymptomatic patients with undifferentiated oligoarthritis. *Br J Rheumatol*. 1995 Sep;34(9):838-42 rheumatology.oxfordjournals.org/cgi/content/abstract/34/9/838
[891] Dai YP, Sun XZ, Zheng KL. Endotoxins in the prostatic secretions of chronic prostatitis patients. *Asian J Androl*. 2005 Mar;7:45-7 blackwell-synergy.com/toc/ajan/7/1
[892] "RESULTS: The mean plasma endotoxin concentrations in patients with sterile pyuria, chronic complicated cystitis, acute uncomplicated pyelonephritis or acute exacerbation of chronic complicated pyelonephritis, chronic complicated pyelonephritis, and acute bacterial prostatitis or epididymitis were significantly higher than those in healthy individuals and in patients with acute uncomplicated cystitis." Et al. Plasma endotoxin concentrations in patients with urinary tract infections. *Int J Urol*. 1995 Sep;2(4):238-42

thus clearly demonstrating the *systemic* inflammatory nature of these *localized* infections. **Microbial contamination of the genitourinary tract can cause a systemic pro-inflammatory arthritogenic response.**[893]

> **Reactive arthritis: urogenital swab culture to detect arthritogenic infection(s)**
>
> "Urogenital swab culture is a sensitive diagnostic method to identify the triggering infection in reactive arthritis. ... Urogenital swab cultures showed a microbial infection in 44% of the patients with oligoarthritis (15% Chlamydia, 14% Mycoplasma, 28% Ureaplasma), whereas in the control group only 26% had a positive result (4% Chlamydia, 7% Mycoplasma, 21% Ureaplasma)."
>
> Erlacher et al. *Br J Rheumatol*. 1995 Sep

- **Assessments**: Basic assessment begins with a serum chemistry/metabolic panel to assess basic renal function, CBC to screen for any signs of classic infection, and urinalysis to assess for WBC, mucus, leukocyte esterase, bacteria and other basic markers. Serum tests for STDs can be performed. Urethral/vaginal swab for culture and DNA polymerase chain reaction is generally sufficient for the detection of the majority of urogenital infections. **Culture and sensitivity testing should be performed for all organisms from clean-catch urine specimens; assessment of sexual partners is advised** (see excellent review by Noah[894]). Women should undergo complete pelvic examinations, and men should undergo assessment of expressed prostatic secretions. Similar to the protocol evaluation of men with elevated PSA, a clinical trial of antibiotics/antimicrobials may reduce systemic inflammation and thereby implicate a dysbiotic stimulus to the inflammation.

- **Specific treatment considerations**: Asymptomatic genitourinary colonization with immunodysregulatory and arthritogenic dysbiotic microbes is impressively common; sufficiently common to warrant routine/empiric treatment. In women, particular attention must be given to correcting gastrointestinal dysbiosis due to the close anatomical proximity and therefore microbiologic communication between the anus (and therefore gastrointestinal tract) and vagina.[895] Sexual partners should be tested; barrier methods (e.g., condoms) and postponement of oral-genital contact should be discussed to reduce transmission/cross-contamination during treatment. Orally administered products including Uva Ursi[896], buchu[897] and cranberry[898], ciprofloxacin, metronidazole, are commonly used for genitourinary infections/colonizations.
    - Reactive arthritis induced by bacterial vaginosis (*Int J Prev Med* 2013 Jul[899]): Paraphrased from the abstract with additional information from the complete text and additional sources: The authors report a 42-year-old woman with **reactive arthritis induced by bacterial vaginosis who presented with oligoarthritis, arthralgia, and enthesitis**—the classic musculoskeletal manifestations of reactive arthritis and findings consistent (as perceived by some clinicians) with seronegative rheumatoid arthritis. She had zero history of diarrhea or dysuria or vaginal secretion, or sexually transmitted infections (STIs). Laboratory tests were normal except for a high erythrocyte sedimentation rate (ESR). Her pelvic examination revealed homogeneous white grey and malodorous vaginal discharge on the vaginal wall and Pap smear and Gram-stained smear of vaginal swab was consistent with bacterial vaginosis. "On physical examination, she had difficulty walking due to heel pain, a fever (38.8 degrees Celsius = 101.84 degrees Fahrenheit), swelling of her right ankle and right metatarsophalangeal joints." She responded to **metronidazole therapy [dose and duration not specified in article; however, treatment for bacterial vaginosis per *Epocrates*[900] "metronidazole 500 mg PO q12h x7 days; Info: may also consider 250 mg PO q8h x7 days in pregnant pts"]** and her six-month follow up hasn't shown recurrence of arthritis. As reactive arthritis (ReA) is a paradigm of a rheumatic disease in which the initiating infectious cause is known, so early use of antimicrobial drugs may prevent the development of musculoskeletal symptoms which are triggered by infections.

---

[893] Erlacher et al. Reactive arthritis: urogenital swab culture is the only useful diagnostic method for the detection of the arthritogenic infection in extra-articularly asymptomatic patients with undifferentiated oligoarthritis. *Br J Rheumatol*. 1995 Sep;34(9):838-42
[894] Noah PW. The role of microorganisms in psoriasis. *Semin Dermatol*. 1990 Dec;9(4):269-76
[895] "The results showed that if C albicans was cultured from the vagina, it was always found in the stool... The gut-reservoir concept may well apply to other forms of candidiasis." Miles MR, Olsen L, Rogers A. Recurrent vaginal candidiasis. Importance of an intestinal reservoir. *JAMA*. 1977 Oct 24;238(17):1836-7
[896] Yarnell E. Botanical medicines for the urinary tract. *World J Urol*. 2002 Nov;20(5):285-93
[897] "Buchu preparations are now used as a diuretic and for a wide range of conditions including stomach aches, rheumatism, bladder and kidney infections and coughs and colds." Simpson D. Buchu--South Africa's amazing herbal remedy. *Scott Med J* 1998 Dec;43(6):189-91
[898] Lynch DM Cranberry for prevention of urinary tract infections. *Am Fam Physician*. 2004 Dec 1;70(11):2175-7 aafp.org/afp/20041201/2175.pdf
[899] Aminzadeh Z, Fadaeian A. Reactive arthritis induced by bacterial vaginosis: prevention with an effective treatment. *Int J Prev Med*. 2013 Jul;4(7):841-4
[900] https://online.epocrates.com/noFrame/showPage.do?method=drugs&MonographId=256&ActiveSectionId=10 2014 Jan

Cutaneous Dysbiosis, Dermal Dysbiosis

- **Introduction**: Microorganisms from dermal infections such as acne can incite systemic inflammation either by dermal absorption of bacterial[901] and fungal[902] (super)antigens and by serving as loci for metastatic infections which produce septic arthritis.[903] **Patients with the autoimmune vasculitic syndrome known as Behcet's disease are more likely to develop arthritis if their skin lesions are infected, thus implicating absorption of an inflammatory immunogen**.[904] Most (57%) of patients with atopic dermatitis show evidence of IgE-mediated histamine release (i.e., "allergy") to exotoxins secreted from *Staphylococcus aureus*, which commonly colonizes eczematous skin[905]; in other words: most eczema patients are allergic to their own dermal bacteria and can thus be said to have *hypersensitivity dermal dysbiosis*.

- **Assessments**: Routine physical examination of the skin and scalp is generally sufficient to screen for obvious infections and any lesions that may be presumed to be colonized. Dermal scrapings and swabs are taken for bacterial, viral, and fungal cultures and microscopic examination. Skin/nail culture, Giemsa staining, culture of lesioned skin on blood agar, MacConkey agar, Sabouraud plates can be performed; see the review by Noah[906] for additional details. For many patients, especially those with atopic dermatitis, treatment can be empiric, per the protocol that follows, and clinically effective antimicrobial and immunorestorative treatment confirms the diagnosis of dysbiosis retrospectively; in other words, a successful clinical intervention—*therapeutic trial*—can provide diagnostic data—*diagnostic trial*.

- **Specific treatment considerations**: Topical and/or systemic antimicrobial treatment along with immunonutrition (detailed later) may be necessary for complete treatment of patients with inflammation perpetuated by dermal dysbiosis. Topical *Mahonia/Berberis aquifolium* is effective for dermal psoriasis[907] via its combined anti-inflammatory and antimicrobial benefits. Other botanical antimicrobials available in topical creams, gels, and soaps include grape seed extract, artemesinin from *Artemisia annua*, and tea tree oil. A complete outline of therapeutic interventions is as follows:

    1. Orally administered antimicrobial drugs to reduce total microbial load (TML), especially targeting *Staphylococcus aureus*: For example, cephalexin 50 mg/kg per day (maximum of 2 g/day), divided into 3 daily doses, for 2 weeks.[908]

    2. Intranasal antimicrobial treatment: Topical 5% povidone iodine is the fastest, most broadly antimicrobial, and least expensive; mupirocin ointment has been used in several studies.[909] Patients and their household members are instructed to apply intranasal treatment twice daily for five consecutive days of each month.

    3. Diluted bleach bath to reduce the total microbial load (TML) on the skin: Detailed in the accompanying textbox and in the following summaries:
        - Efficacy and safety of sodium hypochlorite (bleach) baths in patients with moderate to severe atopic dermatitis in Malaysia (*J Dermatol* 2013 Sep[910]): *Staphylococcus aureus* on skin and in nares contributes to disease pathogenesis in atopic dermatitis (AD). Patients between 2 and 30 years old with moderate to severe AD were enrolled in a prospective, randomized, placebo-controlled study. Patients soaked in diluted bleach (treatment) or distilled water baths (placebo) for 10 min, twice a week for 2 months. Patients in the treatment group showed significant reductions in Eczema Area and Severity Index (EASI) scores. **A 41.9% reduction in S. aureus density from baseline was seen**

---

[901] Delyle LG, Vittecoq O, Bourdel A, Duparc F, Michot C, Le Loet X. Chronic destructive oligoarthritis associated with Propionibacterium acnes in a female patient with acne vulgaris: septic-reactive arthritis? *Arthritis Rheum*. 2000 Dec;43(12):2843-7
[902] Hemalatha V, Srikanth P, Mallika M. Superantigens - Concepts, clinical disease and therapy. *Indian J Med Microbiol* 2004;22:204-211
[903] Schaeverbeke T, Lequen L, de Barbeyrac B, Labbe L, Bebear CM, Morrier Y, Bannwarth B, Bebear C, Dehais J. Propionibacterium acnes isolated from synovial tissue and fluid in a patient with oligoarthritis associated with acne and pustulosis. *Arthritis Rheum*. 1998 Oct;41(10):1889-93
[904] Diri E, Mat C, Hamuryudan V, Yurdakul S, Hizli N, Yazici H. Papulopustular skin lesions are seen more frequently in patients with Behcet's syndrome who have arthritis: a controlled and masked study. *Ann Rheum Dis*. 2001 Nov;60(11):1074-6
[905] "These data indicate that a subset of patients with AD mount an IgE response to SEs that can be grown from their skin." Leung DY, et al. Presence of IgE antibodies to staphylococcal exotoxins on the skin of patients with atopic dermatitis. *J Clin Invest*. 1993 Sep;92(3):1374-80
[906] Noah PW. The role of microorganisms in psoriasis. *Semin Dermatol*. 1990 Dec;9(4):269-76
[907] "Taken together, these clinical studies conducted by several investigators in several countries indicate that Mahonia aquifolium is a safe and effective treatment of patients with mild to moderate psoriasis." Gulliver WP, Donsky HJ. A report on three recent clinical trials using Mahonia aquifolium 10% topical cream and a review of the worldwide clinical experience with Mahonia aquifolium for the treatment of plaque psoriasis. *Am J Ther*. 2005 Sep-Oct;12(5):398-406
[908] Huang JT et al. Treatment of Staphylococcus aureus colonization in atopic dermatitis decreases disease severity. *Pediatrics*. 2009 May;123(5):e808-14
[909] Huang JT et al. Treatment of Staphylococcus aureus colonization in atopic dermatitis decreases disease severity. *Pediatrics*. 2009 May;123(5):e808-14
[910] Wong SM, et al R. Efficacy and safety of sodium hypochlorite (bleach) baths in patients with moderate to severe atopic dermatitis in Malaysia. *J Dermatol*. 2013 Sep 20

at 1 month further reducing to 53.3% at 2 months. Equal numbers of patients in both groups experienced mild side-effects. This study demonstrates that **diluted bleach baths clinically improved AD in as little as 1 month**. No patient withdrew from the treatment arm because of intolerance to the baths.
    - Treatment of Staphylococcus aureus colonization in atopic dermatitis decreases disease severity (*Pediatrics* 2009 May[911]): "METHODS: A randomized, investigator-blinded, placebo-controlled study was conducted with 31 patients, 6 months to 17 years of age, with moderate to severe atopic dermatitis and clinical signs of secondary bacterial infections. All patients received **orally administered cephalexin for 14 days** and were assigned randomly to receive **intranasal mupirocin ointment** treatment and **sodium hypochlorite (bleach) baths** (treatment arm) or intranasal petrolatum ointment treatment and plain water baths (placebo arm) for 3 months. The primary outcome measure was the Eczema Area and Severity Index score. RESULTS: The prevalence of community-acquired methicillin-resistant S aureus in our study (7.4% of our S aureus-positive skin cultures and 4% of our S aureus-positive nasal cultures) was much lower than that in the general population with cultures at Children's Memorial Hospital (75%-85%). **Patients in the group that received both the dilute bleach baths and intranasal mupirocin treatment showed significantly greater mean reductions from baseline in Eczema Area and Severity Index scores**, compared with the placebo group, at the 1-month and 3-month visits. The mean Eczema Area and Severity Index scores for the head and neck did not decrease for patients in the treatment group, whereas scores for other body sites (submerged in the dilute bleach baths) decreased at 1 and 3 months, in comparison with placebo-treated patients.
4. <u>Nutritional immunorestoration</u>: Patient-appropriate doses of vitamin A (not beta-carotene), zinc, vitamin D3, glutamine, arginine, etc.
5. <u>Environmental decontamination</u>: For example, bed sheets, towels, clothing, and furniture should all be cleaned thoroughly, preferably with an antimicrobial agent (as appropriate) such as bleach, alcohol, or povidone iodine. Clothes, bedding, and the environments in the car, home, and work should be disinfected and/or routinely washed; see section on *environmental dysbiosis*.

"Bleach bath" treatment for dermal dysbiosis

- Fill the bathtub with lukewarm water: approximately 40 gallons of water,
- Stir in one-quarter to one-half cup of common bleach (sodium hypochlorite 5-6% solution) solution to the bath water; the goal is to make a modified Dakin's solution with a final concentration of about 0.005%,
- Have patients soak in the chlorinated water for 5 to 10 minutes,
- Rinse thoroughly and pat (not rub) dry; use skin creams and emollients/moisturizers (if any) as usual,
- Perform bleach baths 2–3 times a week or as prescribed by the physician.
- Do not apply nondiluted bleach to skin; diluted bleach solution is generally well tolerated (same hypochlorite concentration as swimming pool water) but may likewise cause dryness and irritation, especially at skin lesions; avoid use or use extra caution in patients with contact allergy to chlorine.

Krakowski AC, et al. Management of atopic dermatitis in the pediatric population. *Pediatrics*. 2008 Oct

---

Environmental dysbiosis

- **Introduction**: Patients may develop inflammation/autoimmunity from exposures to microbial toxins from their home, work, or recreational environments. Many microorganisms, particularly yeasts/molds, defend themselves via elaboration of toxins to fend off other microbes that might otherwise invade their territory. Environmental and occupational researchers appreciate that **yeast/mold commonly elaborate immunomodulating bioaerosols, while gram-negative bacteria exude endotoxin, which is a common contaminant of "house dust."**[912] We may reasonably speculate that a susceptible person might have a systemic inflammatory response from the inhalation of bioaerosols and/or endotoxin in the air of their home and/or work environments. **Airborne immunogens include fungi, bacteria, actinomycetes, endotoxin, ß(1,3)-**

---

[911] Huang JT, et al. Treatment of Staphylococcus aureus colonization in atopic dermatitis decreases disease severity. *Pediatrics*. 2009 May;123(5):e808-14
[912] Douwes J, et al. Bioaerosol health effects and exposure assessment: progress and prospects. *Ann Occup Hyg*. 2003 Apr;47(3):187-200

glucans, peptidoglycans, microbial volatile organic compounds (MVOC), and mycotoxins.[913] "Toxic mold syndrome" and more recently "mixed mold mycotoxicosis"[914] describes patients with systemic health problems resultant from exposure to fungal bioaerosols, classically associated with mold-contaminated buildings following water damage. Such individuals develop systemic autoimmunity that resembles **multiple sclerosis** and **chronic inflammatory polyneuropathy** mediated in part by antibodies against endogenous neuronal structures.[915] Additional evidence proves that **mold exposure can lead to proinflammatory immune activation and resultant multisystem (especially neurologic) autoimmunity**.[916] This is yet another example of how microorganisms can cause human disease without causing "infection." Obviously, patients with inflammatory lung disorders such as asthma, idiopathic pulmonary fibrosis, and especially **acute pulmonary hemorrhage in infants**[917] are candidates for environmental evaluation and intervention. Patients with **Crohn's disease** are well-known to have exquisite sensitivity to the yeast *Saccharomyces cerevisiae*, and a few doctors have reported improvement in Crohn's patients following environmental disinfection. Of related interest is the finding that intraperitoneal exposure of autoimmune-prone mice to fungal components stimulates **autoimmune arthritis resembling rheumatoid arthritis**.[918]

- **Assessments**: Location-specific exacerbation of symptoms is an important historical indicator. Home, work, and recreational environments can be surveyed for microbial contamination, particularly mold. Pier-and-beam homes should be inspected for mold and water in the crawlspace; likewise, attics should be inspected for occult leaks and mold. Mold plates, Petri dishes, and filter cartridges can be used to identify airborne microbes. *Fusarium*, *Trichoderma*, and *Stachybotrys* produce mycotoxins.[919] Thorough cleaning/sanitization of wigs, shoes, furniture, whirlpool/pool water should be implemented; again, see the review by Noah.[920]
- **Specific treatment considerations**: Walls, windows, utility closets, bathrooms, and under-sink cabinets should be assessed for mold and thoroughly cleaned. High-efficiency air filters can be used in the HVAC system; stand-alone air purifiers and dehumidifiers can be used. Bedding, sheets, blankets, pillows, carpets, furniture and drapes should be inspected for contamination and thoroughly cleaned. Eucalyptus oil can be added to washing detergent to kill dust mites[921], as described in the following section. Buildings may have to be professionally and thoroughly remediated; on occasion, people will need to change to different work areas (i.e., new office space, work from home, change jobs) or—if the home is affected—relocate to a new living space.
    - Building-associated neurological damage modeled in human cells (*Mycopathologia* 2010 Dec[922]): "Damage to human neurological system cells resulting from exposure to mycotoxins confirms a previously controversial public health threat for occupants of water-damaged buildings. ... Damage to the neurological system can result from exposure to trichothecene mycotoxins in the indoor environment. This study demonstrates that neurological system cell damage can occur from satratoxin H exposure to neurological cells at exposure levels that can be found in water-damaged buildings contaminated with fungal growth. The constant activation of inflammatory and apoptotic pathways at low levels of exposure in human brain capillary endothelial cells, astrocytes, and neural progenitor cells may amplify devastation to neurological tissues and lead to neurological system cell damage from indirect events triggered by the presence of trichothecenes."

---

[913] Douwes J, et al. Bioaerosol health effects and exposure assessment: progress and prospects. *Ann Occup Hyg*. 2003 Apr;47(3):187-200
[914] Gray MR, et al. Mixed mold mycotoxicosis: immunological changes in humans following exposure in water-damaged buildings. *Arch Environ Health*. 2003;58:410-20
[915] "The authors concluded that exposure to molds in water-damaged buildings increased the risk for development of neural autoantibodies, peripheral neuropathy, and neurophysiologic abnormalities in exposed individuals." Campbell AW, Thrasher JD, Madison RA, Vojdani A, Gray MR, Johnson A. Neural autoantibodies and neurophysiologic abnormalities in patients exposed to molds in water-damaged buildings. *Arch Environ Health*. 2003 Aug;58(8):464-74
[916] "Abnormally high levels of ANA, ASM, and CNS myelin (immunoglobulins [Ig]G, IgM, IgA) and PNS myelin (IgG, IgM, IgA)... showing an increased risk for autoimmunity. ...exposure to mixed molds and their associated mycotoxins in water-damaged buildings leads to multiple health problems involving the CNS and the immune system... Mold exposure also initiates inflammatory processes." Gray MR, Thrasher JD, Crago R, Madison RA, Arnold L, Campbell AW, Vojdani A. Mixed mold mycotoxicosis: immunological changes in humans following exposure in water-damaged buildings. *Arch Environ Health*. 2003 Jul;58(7):410-20
[917] "Mean colony counts for all fungi averaged 29227 colony-forming units (CFU)/m3 in homes of patients and 707 CFU/m3 in homes of controls... Conclusion Infants with pulmonary hemorrhage and hemosiderosis were more likely than controls to live in homes with toxigenic S atra and other fungi in the indoor air." Etzel RA, et al. Acute pulmonary hemorrhage in infants associated with exposure to Stachybotrys atra and other fungi. *Arch Pediatr Adolesc Med*. 1998 Aug;152(8):757-62
[918] Yoshitomi H, Sakaguchi N, Kobayashi K, et al. A role for fungal {beta}-glucans and their receptor Dectin-1 in the induction of autoimmune arthritis in genetically susceptible mice. *J Exp Med*. 2005 Mar 21;201(6):949-60 jem.org/cgi/content/full/201/6/949
[919] Am Acad Pediatrics.Toxic effects of indoor molds. Committee on Environ Health. *Pediatrics* 1998;101(4p1):712-4
[920] Noah PW. The role of microorganisms in psoriasis. *Semin Dermatol*. 1990 Dec;9(4):269-76
[921] Tovey et al. Simple washing procedure with eucalyptus oil for controlling house dust mites and allergens in clothing bedding. *J Allergy Clin Immunol* 1997;100:464-6
[922] Karunasena E, Larrañaga MD, Simoni JS, Douglas DR, Straus DC. Building-associated neurological damage modeled in human cells: a mechanism of neurotoxic effects by exposure to mycotoxins in the indoor environment. *Mycopathologia*. 2010 Dec;170(6):377-90

- Changes in pro-inflammatory cytokines in association with exposure to moisture-damaged building microbes (*Eur Respir J* 2001 Dec[923]): "In the present study, the authors compared the respiratory symptoms, the production of inflammatory mediators interleukin (IL)-1, IL-4, IL-6, tumor necrosis factor-alpha (TNF-alpha) and cell count in nasal lavage fluid and induced sputum samples of subjects working in moisture-damaged and control school buildings. … The authors found a significant elevation of IL-1, TNF-alpha and IL-6 in nasal lavage fluid and IL-6 in induced sputum during the spring term in the subjects from the moisture-damaged school building compared to the subjects from the control building. The exposed workers reported sore throat, phlegm, eye irritation, rhinitis, nasal obstruction and cough in parallel with these findings. The present data suggests an association between microbial exposure, and symptoms as well as changes in pro-inflammatory mediators detected from both the upper and lower airways."

- Co-cultivated damp building related microbes *Streptomyces californicus* and *Stachybotrys chartarum* induce immunotoxic and genotoxic responses via oxidative stress (*Inhal Toxicol* 2009 Aug[924]): "Oxidative stress has been proposed to be one mechanism behind the adverse health outcomes associated with living in a damp indoor environment. In the present study, the capability of damp building-related microbes *Streptomyces californicus* and *Stachybotrys chartarum* to induce oxidative stress was evaluated in vitro. In addition, the role of oxidative stress in provoking the detected cytotoxic, genotoxic, and inflammatory responses was studied by inhibiting the production of reactive oxygen species (ROS) using N-acetyl-l-cysteine (NAC). RAW264.7 macrophages were exposed in a dose- and time-dependent manner to the spores of co-cultivated *S. californicus* and *S. chartarum*, to their separately cultivated spore-mixture, or to the spores of these microbes alone. … **All the studied microbial exposures triggered oxidative stress and subsequent cellular damage in RAW264.7 macrophages**. The ROS scavenger, NAC, prevented growth arrest, apoptosis, DNA damage, and cytokine production induced by the co-culture since it reduced the intracellular level of ROS within macrophages. In contrast, the DNA damage and cell cycle arrest induced by the spores of *S. californicus* alone could not be prevented by NAC. Bioaerosol-induced oxidative stress in macrophages may be an important mechanism behind the frequent respiratory symptoms and diseases suffered by residents of moisture damaged buildings. Furthermore, microbial interactions during co-cultivation stimulate the production of highly toxic compound(s) which may significantly increase oxidative damage."

- Chlamydophila pneumoniae antibodies in office workers with and without inflammatory rheumatic diseases in a moisture-damaged building (*Eur J Clin Microbiol Infect Dis* 2005 Mar[925]): "In the study reported here, we evaluated the serum samples obtained from 18 of the office workers, both at work and following a vacation period of 2–4 weeks' duration. **Among the 18 employees, seven had rheumatic diseases and two had upper and lower respiratory symptoms**, while nine employees had no diseases or prolonged respiratory symptoms. All of the subjects were female and their mean age at the time of the study was about 50 years. … The elevated antibody levels in the employees we tested might have been caused by prolonged exposure to *C. pneumoniae* or some immunologically active part(s) of the microbe. **The clustering of inflammatory rheumatic diseases among individuals in moisture damaged buildings is rare and its causes are not known. We suggest that *C. pneumoniae* or some other microbe(s) capable of producing similar antibody reactions and living possibly within amoebae potentially cause these clusters**."

- Inflammatory mediators in nasal lavage, induced sputum and serum of employees with rheumatic and respiratory disorders (*Eur Respir J* 2001 Sep[926]): "Exposure to microbes present in mold-damaged buildings has been linked to increased frequency of various inflammatory diseases. The current study examined differences in inflammatory mediators in nasal lavage (NAL), induced sputum (IS) and serum of occupants with rheumatic or respiratory disorders and their controls, all working in the same

---

[923] Purokivi et al. Changes in pro-inflammatory cytokines in association with exposure to moisture-damaged building microbes. *Eur Respir J*. 2001 Dec;18(6):951-8
[924] Markkanen Penttinen P, Pelkonen J, Tapanainen M, Mäki-Paakkanen J, Jalava PI, Hirvonen MR. Co-cultivated damp building related microbes Streptomyces californicus and Stachybotrys chartarum induce immunotoxic and genotoxic responses via oxidative stress. *Inhal Toxicol*. 2009 Aug;21(10):857-67
[925] Seuri M, Paldanius M, Leinonen M, Roponen M, Hirvonen MR, Saikku P. Chlamydophila pneumoniae antibodies in office workers with and without inflammatory rheumatic diseases in a moisture-damaged building. *Eur J Clin Microbiol Infect Dis*. 2005 Mar;24(3):236-7
[926] Roponen et al. Inflammatory mediators in nasal lavage, induced sputum and serum of employees with rheumatic and respiratory disorders. *Eur Respir J* 2001;18:542-8

moisture-damaged building. ... Concentrations of NO, interleukin (IL)-1, IL-4, IL-6 and tumor necrosis factor-alpha in NAL, IS and serum (excluding NO and IL-1) of the subjects were measured during an occupational exposure period and the vacation period without such exposure. **The concentrations of IL-4 in NAL fluid were significantly higher among all occupants during the working period (geometric mean 8.5 microg** x mL(-1), range 0-206.5 microg x mL(-1)), as **compared to that during vacation (0.4 microng** x mL(-1) range 0-3.7 pg x mL(-1)) (p = 0.008). Absence from the work environment also significantly diminished reporting of symptoms. IL-4 levels in the serum of case subjects were significantly higher than in controls. Moreover, employees with respiratory symptoms had markedly higher exhaled NO values than their controls (p = 0.028). In summary, these data suggest that mediators in nasal lavage samples reflect the occupational exposure to molds, whereas possible indicators of existing disorders are detectable in serum."

- Joint symptoms and diseases associated with moisture damage in a health center (*Clin Rheumatol* 2003 Dec[927]): "Rheumatic diseases do not usually cluster in time and space. It has been proposed that **environmental exposures may initiate autoimmune responses.** We describe a cluster of rheumatic diseases among a group of health center employees who began to complain of symptoms typically related to moldy houses, including mucocutaneous symptoms, nausea and fatigue, within a year of moving into a new building. Dampness was found in the insulation space of the concrete floor below ground level. **Microbes indicating mold damage and actinobacteria were found in the flooring material and in the outer wall insulation.** ... All 34 subjects working at the health center had at least some rheumatic complaints. Two fell ill with a typical rheumatoid factor (RF)-positive **rheumatoid arthritis** (RA), and 10 had **arthritis that did not conform to any definite arthritic syndrome** (three met the classification criteria for RA). Prior to moving into the problem building one subject had suffered **reactive arthritis**, which had then recurred. Another employee had undiagnosed **ankylosing spondylitis** and later developed **psoriatic arthritis**, and another developed **undifferentiated vasculitis**. A total of 16 subjects developed **joint pains**, 11 of these after beginning work at the health center. Three subjects developed **Raynaud's symptom**. Fourteen cases had elevated levels of **circulating immune complexes** in 1998, 17 in 1999, but there were only three cases in 2001, when the health center had been closed for 18 months. **The high incidence of joint problems among these employees suggests a common triggering factor for most of the cases. As some of the symptoms had tended to subside while the health center was closed, the underlying causes are probably related to the building itself** and possibly to the **abnormal microbial growth in its structures.**"

---

[927] Luosujärvi RA, et al. Joint symptoms and diseases associated with moisture damage in a health center. *Clin Rheumatol*. 2003 Dec;22(6):381-5

Cleaning the home/work/recreational environment of microbial contaminants

Household "dust" is actually a complex mixture of microscopic particles such as fabric fragments (from bedding, carpet, clothing, etc.), pollen (from outdoor plants), dirt (which has settled from the air), dead skin cells (from humans and pets), bacteria and mold, and the feces of dust mites and other insects. Since dust, especially the feces from dust mites, is very allergenic, particularly for patients with eczema. Reducing the amount of "dust" in a home environment involves 3 general steps:

1. **Dust, mold, and chemical removal**
    - Cleaning: Periodically, use a damp cloth on furniture to remove dust that accumulates.
    - Vacuuming: Vacuum the floors/carpet and ensure that the vacuum is equipped with an *allergy filter* or HEPA filter to ensure that the dust is not simply transposed from the floor back into the air and onto furniture, bedding, and clothes. In severe cases, patients with inflammatory disorders, allergies/eczema, and environmental sensitivity may choose to have carpets removed and replaced either with a low-offgassing/outgassing flooring such as bamboo hardwoods or ceramic tile.
    - Exclude pollen/mold: Close doors and windows on days the pollen/mold count is high.
    - Pet control: If you have pets, it is often helpful to 1) wash them regularly, 2) keep them off the bedding, and/or 3) allow them to stay outdoors as much as is possible and practical.
    - Using air filters for the central cooling/heating unit: Consider the "Filterete Allergen Reducing Filter" from 3M (comes with a purple label); more expensive and effective options are available for complicated cases.
    - Vinyl/hypoallergenic mattress cover: Buy and use a simple hypoallergenic or vinyl mattress cover to eliminate exposure to years of accumulated dust inside the mattress which is slept on for 8 hours each night. The goal is create an airtight seal around the mattress to contain the dust and antigens. Vinyl mattress covers are inexpensive and widely available.
2. **Reducing the amount of moisture in the air**. Ideally, the steam from bathing and cooking areas should be vented outdoors so that moisture does not accumulate inside the living area. Moisture is necessary for dust mites and mold to live and to create allergens; if the air is very moist then the inflammation-producing activities of the dust mites and mold are stimulated. Conversely, by reducing the humidity in the air, we are able to impair the microbes and thus reduce the amount of antigens. Reducing the amount of moisture in the air by use of an electric dehumidifier may be necessary to help reduce the amount of both dust allergen and mold in a home.
3. **Wash clothes/linens with eucalyptus oil to eliminate dust mites**: The combination of 1) hot water, 2) detergent, and 3) eucalyptus oil is an effective and natural way to get rid of dust mites and dust allergens. As validated by research published in *Journal of Allergy and Clinical Immunology*[928], this is an effective technique for killing and eliminating dust mites from clothing and bed sheets. "Bi-O-Klean Hand Dishwashing Liquid" available at Whole Foods Market or "Kit liquid dishwashing detergent concentrate" meet the criteria for the selection of a detergent for this purpose. Eucalyptus oil must never be applied to the skin or taken internally.

Metric measurements from the original study	"American" unit translation	One-half recipe
1. **Eucalyptus oil**: 100 mL	6 tablespoons or 3.4 oz.	3 tablespoons or 1½ oz.
2. **Detergent**: 25 mL liquid concentrated dishwashing detergent	1 ½ tablespoons or 0.8 oz.	¾ tablespoons or 0.4 oz.
3. **Warm water** (30°C): 50 Liters	86°F water: 13 gallons	86°F water: 6 gallons
4. **Soak clothing/bedding in hot detergent-eucalyptus solution for 15-30 minutes, then wash in machine as usual.**		

---

[928] 1) When mixed, the oil-detergent mixture should dissolve to form a clear homogenous solution, and 2) five mL (1 teaspoon) of the mixture stirred with 200 mL (6 oz.) of water should form a "milky, opaque solution that is stable (does not "break oil") for at least 10 minutes." Tovey ER, McDonald LG. A simple washing procedure with eucalyptus oil for controlling house dust mites and their allergens in clothing and bedding. *J Allergy Clin Immunol*. 1997 Oct;100(4):464-6

Problematic Bacteria, Yeast, and Parasites: A Listing of Commonly Encountered Dysbiotic Microorganisms

All of the following yeast, bacteria, and "parasites" have been observed in various patients in my private practice of chiropractic and naturopathic medicine. Even though several of these microbes are considered nonpathogenic by outdated medical paradigms[929,930,931] that are still hypnotized by Pasteur and Koch (i.e., the "external invader paradigm"), their presence is generally inconsistent with optimal health and their eradication is rewarding for both doctor and patient. In other words, **even if a microbe is not a true pathogen and is thus not a therapeutic target from a *disease-oriented paradigm*, we as clinicians are still justified in eradicating it from our chronically ill patient from a *wellness-oriented paradigm* because we know that 1) eradicating potentially harmful bacteria will do no harm to the patient, and 2) in many cases—indeed *the majority* of cases—patients experience a significant and sustained clinical improvement regardless of their presenting complaint, thus implying a causal relationship between the microbe and the non-infectious illness.**

The following microbes are commonly detected with stool testing performed by a specialty laboratory. **One of the benefits of specialized stool testing is that it allows the presence of microbes to be determined within a context that evaluates the patient's individualized response.** For example, the finding of a mild degree of *Candida albicans* ("+1" on a 0-4 scale) might be considered insignificant; however if no other pathogens are identified, and the secretory IgA, lactoferrin, and lysozyme levels are elevated, then the clinician is justified in determining that the patient is having a hypersensitivity reaction to an otherwise "benign" yeast. **Remember, we are not looking for classic "infection" here; we are looking to determine which underlying disruptions may be exacerbating inflammation and the patient's symptomatology.** We have to look beyond the *disease-associated characteristics of the microbe* to see *the patient's individualized response to the microbe*. **Often what we find when working with autoimmune/inflammatory patients is that they are having a *pathogenic inflammatory response* to a *nonpathogenic* microbe.** When reading the following table, rather than focusing on the details, readers should read the information with due diligence with the final goal being not the memorization of microbe-disease associations but rather the concept that microbial colonization is a sufficient trigger for induction of inflammation and the clinical appearance of many "autoimmune disorders." The distinguishing characteristic that differentiates "an idiopathic autoimmune disease" from "microbe-triggered reactive arthritis" is not the biochemistry of the inflammatory cascade nor the pathohistologic findings; but rather, the defining characteristic of reactive arthritis is the presence of an identified microbial exposure. Therefore, the practical distinction is made by the clinician—not the disease entity itself. If the physician searches for and empirically treats the microbial triggers for most "idiopathic inflammatory disorders" and "autoimmune diseases", then that clinician will—in the words of Henry David Thoreau in *Walden*—"meet with a success unexpected in common hours."

Commonly Encountered Dysbiotic Microorganisms—*alphabetized listing*

Dysbiotic microbe	Pathophysiology and clinical manifestations
Aeromonas hydrophila	• *Aeromonas hydrophila* can cause colitis and should therefore be eradicated immediately upon detection.[932]
Blastocystis hominis	• Commonly asymptomatic; can cause abdominal pain, nausea, vomiting, diarrhea, weight loss[933,934], fever, chills, malaise, anorexia, flatus, eosinophilia[935] • Fecal leukocytes are occasionally seen[936]; can cause colitis[937]

---

[929] "...standard of care in developed countries is to maintain schizophrenia patients on neuroleptics, this practice is not supported by the 50-year research record for the drugs. ...this paradigm of care worsens long-term outcomes, ... 40% of all schizophrenia patients would fare better if they were not so medicated." Whitaker R. The case against antipsychotic drugs: a 50-year record of doing more harm than good. *Med Hypotheses*. 2004;62:5-1 psychrights.org/Research/Digest/Chronicity/50yearecord.pdf
[930] Hyman M. Paradigm shift: the end of "normal science" in medicine understanding function in nutrition, health, and disease. *Altern Ther Health Med*. 2004;10:10-5,90-4
[931] Heaney RP. Vitamin D, nutritional deficiency, and the medical paradigm. *J Clin Endocrinol Metab* 2003;88:5107-8 jcem.endojournals.org/cgi/content/full/88/11/5107
[932] Farraye FA, Peppercorn MA, Ciano PS, Kavesh WN. Charles A. Segmental colitis associated with Aeromonas hydrophila. *Am J Gastroenterol*. 1989 Apr;84(4):436-8
[933] O'Gorman MA, et al. Prevalence and characteristics of Blastocystis hominis infection in children. *Clin Pediatr* (Phila) 1993 Feb;32(2):91-6
[934] Telalbasic S, Pikula ZP, Kapidzic M. Blastocystis hominis may be a potential cause of intestinal disease. *Scand J Infect Dis* 1991;23(3):389-90
[935] Sheehan DJ, Raucher BG, McKitrick JC. Association of Blastocystis hominis with signs and symptoms of human disease. *J Clin Microbiol*. 1986;24(4):548-50
[936] Diaczok BJ, Rival J. Diarrhea due to Blastocystis hominis: an old organism revisited. *South Med J* 1987 Jul;80(7):931-2
[937] Russo AR, Stone SL, Taplin ME, Snapper HJ, Doern GV. Presumptive evidence for Blastocystis hominis as a cause of colitis. *Arch Intern Med*. 1988 May;148(5):1064

Commonly Encountered Dysbiotic Microorganisms — *alphabetized listing, continued*

Microbe	Pathophysiology and clinical manifestations
Candida albicans and other yeasts	• Although normal in small amounts ("+1"), excess *Candida* in the intestines is never a sign of optimal health. Patients may have mild general symptoms such as fatigue and dyscognition ("brain fog"); gas and intestinal bloating following consumption of carbohydrates are common. • *Candida* produces an immunosuppressive myotoxin called gliotoxin as well as an IgA-destroying protease and can cause watery diarrhea, particularly in elderly, ill, and immunosuppressed patients.[938] • *Candida* is always present in the gastrointestinal tract of women with recurrent yeast vaginitis.[939] • Some people have an inflammatory hypersensitivity to *Candida*, as it can cause **local allergic dermatitis/mucositis**[940], **colitis**[941], and **pulmonary inflammation (hypersensitivity alveolitis** from gastrointestinal colonization).[942] • Other yeasts such as *Candida parapsilosis* and *Geotrichum capitatum* are occasionally seen and should be eradicated.
Citrobacter rodentium *Citrobacter freundii*	• *Citrobacter freundii* is a gram-negative anaerobe; it produces pro-inflammatory endotoxin. • *Citrobacter* species may cause **gastroenteritis** in humans[943] • Most strains of *Citrobacter freundii* produce hydrogen sulfide[944] which interferes with mitochondrial function and energy production and may be a major causative molecule in **ulcerative colitis**.[945] • Animal studies have shown that this bacterium can induce an intense inflammatory response in the gastrointestinal tract that resembles **inflammatory bowel disease**.[946] • Gastrointestinal dysbiosis with *Citrobacter freundii* may be causative in so-called "rheumatoid arthritis" in some patients.[author's experience]
Dientamoeba fragilis	• *Dientamoeba fragilis* is a flagellate protozoan that can cause **diarrhea, abdominal pain, nausea, vomiting, fatigue, malaise, eosinophilia, urticaria, pruritus and/or weight loss**. It is commonly associated with pinworm infection and may produce a clinical picture that mimics **food allergy, colitis, or eosinophilic enteritis**.[947]

---

[938] Gupta TP, Ehrinpreis MN. Candida-associated diarrhea in hospitalized patients. *Gastroenterology* 1990 Mar;98(3):780-5
[939] Miles MR, Olsen L, Rogers A. Recurrent vaginal candidiasis. Importance of an intestinal reservoir. *JAMA*. 1977 Oct 24;238(17):1836-7
[940] Ramirez De Knott HM, McCormick TS, et al. Cutaneous hypersensitivity to Candida albicans in idiopathic vulvodynia. *Contact Dermatitis*. 2005 Oct;53(4):214-8
[941] Doby T. Monilial esophagitis and colitis. *J Maine Med Assoc*. 1971 May;62(5):109-14
[942] "We conclude that the disease was induced by C.a.-antigen reaching the lungs from the intestinal tract via the bloodstream." Schreiber J, Struben C, Rosahl W, Amthor M. Hypersensitivity alveolitis induced by endogenous candida species. *Eur J Med Res*. 2000 Mar 27;5(3):126 Stunningly brilliant article.
[943] "Members of this genus can cause neonatal meningitis and, perhaps, gastroenteritis in both children and adults." Lipsky BA, Hook EW 3rd, Smith AA, Plorde JJ. Citrobacter infections in humans: experience at the Seattle Veterans Administration Medical Center and a review of the literature. *Rev Infect Dis*. 1980 Sep-Oct;2:746-60
[944] Lennette EH (editor in chief). *Manual of Clinical Microbiology. Fourth Edition*. Washington DC; American Society for Microbiology: 1985, page 269. See also web.indstate.edu/thcme/micro/GI/general/sld038.htm Accessed 10/27/2005
[945] "CONCLUSIONS: Metabolic effects of sodium hydrogen sulfide on butyrate oxidation along the length of the colon closely mirror metabolic abnormalities observed in active ulcerative colitis, and the increased production of sulfide in ulcerative colitis suggests that the action of mercaptides may be involved in the genesis of ulcerative colitis." Roediger et al. Reducing sulfur compounds of the colon impair colonocyte nutrition: implications for ulcerative colitis. *Gastroenterology*. 1993 Mar;104(3):802-9
[946] Higgins LM, Frankel G, Douce G, Dougan G, MacDonald TT. Citrobacter rodentium infection in mice elicits a mucosal Th1 cytokine response and lesions similar to those in murine inflammatory bowel disease. *Infect Immun*. 1999 Jun;67(6):3031-9 iai.asm.org/cgi/reprint/67/6/3031.pdf
[947] Cuffari C, Oligny L, Seidman EG. Dientamoeba fragilis masquerading as allergic colitis. *J Pediatr Gastroenterol Nutr*. 1998 Jan;26(1):16-20

Commonly Encountered Dysbiotic Microorganisms—*alphabetized listing*, continued

Microbe	Pathophysiology and clinical manifestations
Endolimax nana	• *Endolimax nana*, a protozoa, has a world-wide distribution and is commonly considered an harmless commensal of the intestine.[948] • Intestinal infection with *Endolimax nana* can cause a **peripheral arthropathy** that is clinically similar to **rheumatoid arthritis** and which remits with effective parasite eradication.[949] • In my own clinical practice, I have seen several cases of intestinal colonization with *Endolimax nana* in patients who presented with **chronic fatigue, myalgia, eczema,** and especially refractory **chronic vaginitis.**
Entamoeba histolytica	• Induces tissue damage, **amebic colitis,** and **liver abscess.**[950] • Associated with **Henoch Schonlein purpura** in a single case report[951] • **Amebic colitis** may be misdiagnosed as **ulcerative colitis.**[952] • May contribute to **irritable bowel syndrome, rheumatoid arthritis, fibromyalgia, food allergy,** or **multiple chemical sensitivity** and can **exacerbate HIV infection.**[953] • Hepatic infection is associated with induction of antineutrophil cytoplasmic antibodies (ANCA) such as seen with the vasculitic disease Wegener's granulomatosis.[954]
Gamma *strep* *Enterococcus*	• "Gamma strep", *Enterococcus faecalis*, and *Streptococcus faecalis* are somewhat interchangeable terms.[955,956,957] These terms refer to gram-positive *Enterococcus* species such as *Enterococcus faecalis*, which cause **urinary tract infections, bacteremia, intra-abdominal infections, and endocarditis.** • Enterococci produce **lipoteichoic acid** which is proinflammatory in a manner similar to endotoxin from gram-negative bacteria, and these gram-positive bacteria also appear to produce a superantigen.[958] • "Gamma strep" is commonly identified in stool tests of patients with **chronic unwellness and fatigue.**
Giardia lamblia "Beaver fever"	• Causatively associated with **abdominal pain, diarrhea, constipation, bloating, chronic fatigue, and food allergy/intolerance.**[959] • May contribute to **irritable bowel syndrome, rheumatoid arthritis, food allergy,** or **multiple chemical sensitivity.**[960] • Extraintestinal symptoms of gastrointestinal *Giardia* infection can include **fever, maculopapular rashes, geographic tongue, pulmonary infiltrates, lymphadenopathy, polyarthritis, aphthous ulcers, and urticaria.**[961]

---

[948] Information available at www2.provlab.ab.ca/bugs/webbug/parasite/artifact/enana.htm as of December 26, 2003
[949] "Endolimax nana grew on stool culture. Both the patient's diarrhea and arthritis responded effectively to therapy with metronidazole. The diagnosis of parasitic rheumatism was made in retrospect." Burnstein SL, Liakos S. Parasitic rheumatism presenting as rheumatoid arthritis. *J Rheumatol.* 1983 Jun;10(3):514-5
[950] Huston CD. Parasite and host contributions to the pathogenesis of amebic colitis. *Trends Parasitol.* 2004 Jan; 20(1): 23-6
[951] Demircin G, Oner A, Erdogan O, Bulbul M, Memis L. Henoch Schonlein purpura and amebiasis. *Acta Paediatr Jpn.* 1998 Oct; 40(5): 489-91
[952] Galland L. Intestinal protozoan infection is a common unsuspected cause of chronic illness. *J Advancement Med.* 1989;2: 539-552
[953] Galland L. Intestinal protozoan infection is a common unsuspected cause of chronic illness. *J Advancement Med.* 1989;2: 539-552
[954] George J, et al. Infections and Wegener's granulomatosis--a cause and effect relationship? *QJM.* 1997 May;90(5):367-73 qjmed.oxfordjournals.org/cgi/reprint/90/5/367
[955] "Figure 38: "Gamma *Streptococcus*" : *Enterococcus faecalis*" and "The genus *Enterococcus* was once a part of the *Streptococcus* genus, was considered a "gamma *Streptococcus* species." microbelibrary.org/asmonly/details_print.asp?id=1986&lang
[956] "Enterococcus faecalis. Synonyms: group D strep, Streptococcus faecalis. Classification: facultative anaerobic, gram+ bacteria, cocci." medinfo.ufl.edu/year2/mmid/bms5300/bugs/strfaeca.html
[957] "Microscopically, Gram-positive cocci occurring in chains or pairs with individual cells being somewhat elongated can be presumed to be streptococci or enterococci." members.tripod.com/piece_de_resistance/SAARS/bugs/menteroc.htm
[958] Lynn E. Hancock and Michael S. Gilmore. Department of Microbiology and Immunology, University of Oklahoma Health Sciences Center. Pathogenicity of Enterococci published in "Gram-Positive Pathogens" edited by Fischetti V et al. w3.ouhsc.edu/enterococcus/lynn_revirew.asp
[959] Galland L, Lee M. #170 High frequency of giardiasis in patients with chronic digestive complaints. *Am J Gastroenterol* 1989;84:1181
[960] Galland L. Intestinal protozoan infection is a common unsuspected cause of chronic illness. *J Advancement Med.* 1989;2: 539-552
[961] Corsi A, et al. Ocular changes associated with Giardia lamblia infection in children. *Br J Ophthalmol.* 1998 Jan;82:59-62 bjo.bmjjournals.com/cgi/content/full/82/1/59

Commonly Encountered Dysbiotic Microorganisms—*alphabetized listing, continued*

Microbe	Pathophysiology and clinical manifestations
Giardia lamblia [continued from previous page]	• **Ocular complications** from gastrointestinal infection include iridocyclitis, choroiditis, retinal hemorrhages, anterior and posterior uveitis, retinal vasculitis, and "salt and pepper" retinal degeneration. These complications are most likely due to deposition of **immune complexes** in the retinal epithelium.[962] • Reported to have caused numerous cases of **reactive arthritis (peripheral arthritis and/or sacroiliitis)** in patients who are either positive or negative for HLA-B27[963]; "beaver fever" is a cause of reactive arthritis.[964] • Antigen detection appears superior to microscopic examination for detection.[965]
Hafnia alvei	• *Hafnia alvei* is a gram-negative bacterium capable of causing **reactive arthritis** from gastrointestinal infection; the reactive arthritis associated with *Hafnia alvei* occurs without association with HLA-B27.[966]
Helicobacter pylori	• *H. pylori* is a gram-negative endotoxin-producing rod that causes stomach ulcers and appears to cause **reactive arthritis** in some patients.[967] • *H. pylori* colonization is increased in patients with **scleroderma**.[968] • *H. pylori* is commonly found in the middle ear of patients with acute otitis media.[969] • Strongly and causatively associated with Raynaud's syndrome/phenomenon.
Klebsiella pneumoniae	• Many cases of gastrointestinal colonization with this microorganism produce no acute gastrointestinal symptoms such as nausea, vomiting, constipation, or diarrhea. Patients may have mild general symptoms such as fatigue and dyscognition ("brain fog"). • Can cause **diarrhea**[970] and **acute gastroenteritis**.[971] • Associated with **reactive arthritis** such as **ankylosing spondylitis**.[972] • Gram-negative bacteria, produces endotoxin/lipopolysaccharide that is capable of impairing cytochrome p-450 and **reducing hepatic clearance and urinary/biliary excretion of drugs**.[973]

---

[962] "The retinal changes associated with giardiasis are more than likely caused by immune mechanisms. Wania reported that circulating immune complexes were found in all of the patients with ocular complications he examined." Corsi A, Nucci C, Knafelz D, Bulgarini D, Di Iorio L, Polito A, De Risi F, Ardenti Morini F, Paone FM. Ocular changes associated with Giardia lamblia infection in children. *Br J Ophthalmol*. 1998 Jan;82(1):59-62 bjo.bmjjournals.com/cgi/content/full/82/1/59
[963] Layton et al. Sacroiliitis in an HLA B27-negative patient following giardiasis. *Br J Rheumatol*. 1998;37:581-3 rheumatology.oxfordjournals.org/cgi/reprint/37/5/581
[964] "Giardia lamblia infection is rarely associated with adult reactive arthritis. We report first North American case and review pediatric and adult literature. Antimicrobial treatment is essential to eradicate the parasite and control the arthritis." Tupchong et al. Beaver fever--a rare cause of reactive arthritis. *J Rheumatol* 1999;26:2701-2
[965] "For all patients, microscopy was uniformly negative, but 6 of 13 patients were antigen positive... Giardiasis, an increasing problem in family practice, should be considered early in patients with GI disturbances. New, sensitive immunodiagnostic tests that usually require a single specimen are more useful than microscopy." Chappell CL, Matson CC. Giardia antigen detection in patients with chronic gastrointestinal disturbances. *J Fam Pract*. 1992 Jul;35(1):49-53
[966] Toivanen P, Toivanen A. Two forms of reactive arthritis? *Ann Rheum Dis*. 1999 Dec;58(12):737-41 ard.bmjjournals.com/cgi/content/full/58/12/737 See also: Newmark JJ, Hobbs WN, Wilson BE. Reactive arthritis associated with Hafnia alvei enteritis. *Arthritis Rheum*. 1994 Jun;37(6):960
[967] "Our findings suggest that HP may be included in the list of possible arthritis triggering microbes." Melby KK, Kvien TK, Glennas A. Helicobacter pylori--a trigger of reactive arthritis? *Infection*. 1999;27(4-5):252-5
[968] "Patients with SSc have H. pylori infection at a higher prevalence than the general population." Yazawa N, Fujimoto M, Kikuchi K, et al. High seroprevalence of Helicobacter pylori infection in patients with systemic sclerosis: association with esophageal involvement. *J Rheumatol*. 1998 Apr;25(4):650-3
[969] "Twelve of 15 smears for MEE were positive for HP by immunohistochemistry and 14 by Giemsa that were Gram-negative." Morinaka S, Tominaga M, Nakamura H. Detection of Helicobacter pylori in the middle ear fluid of patients with otitis media with effusion. *Otolaryngol Head Neck Surg*. 2005 Nov;133(5):791-4
[970] Niyogi SK, Pal A, Mitra U, Dutta P. Enteroaggretative Klebsiella pneumoniae in association with childhood diarrhoea. *Indian J Med Res* 2000 Oct;112:133-4
[971] Ananthan et al. Enterotoxigenicity of Klebsiella pneumoniae associated with childhood gastroenteritis in Madras, India. *Jpn J Infect Dis* 1999 Feb;52(1):16-7
[972] Ahmadi et al. Antibodies to Klebsiella pneumoniae lipopolysaccharide in patients with ankylosing spondylitis. *Br J Rheumatol*. 1998 Dec;37(12):1330-3
[973] Hasegawa T, Takagi K, Kitaichi K. Effects of bacterial endotoxin on drug pharmacokinetics. *Nagoya J Med Sci* 1999 May;62(1-2):11-28

Commonly encountered dysbiotic microorganisms—*alphabetized listing*, continued

Microbe	Pathophysiology and clinical manifestations
Proteus mirabilis	• Gram-negative bacteria, produces endotoxin/lipopolysaccharide.[974] • Gastrointestinal and urinary tract colonization is associated with **rheumatoid arthritis**[975,976] and **ankylosing spondylitis**.[977] • In one of my patients, GI dysbiosis with *Proteus* incited **"idiopathic inflammatory polyneuropathy"** that disappeared within one month of parasite eradication and which coincided with normalization of hsCRP.
Pseudomonas aeruginosa	• *Pseudomonas aeruginosa* is a gram-negative bacterium, produces endotoxin[978] and can cause antibiotic-associated diarrhea.[979,980] • Many cases of gastrointestinal colonization with this microorganism produce no acute gastrointestinal symptoms such as nausea, vomiting, constipation, or diarrhea. Patients may have mild general symptoms such as fatigue and dyscognition ("brain fog"). • Patients with **multiple sclerosis** show evidence of a heightened immune response against *Pseudomonas aeruginosa*, consistent with cross-reactivity.[981]

Comprehensive Stool Analysis / Parasitology x3

MICROBIOLOGY

Bacteriology Culture

Beneficial flora		Imbalances		Dysbiotic flora	
Bifidobacter	4+	Haemolytic E. coli	4+	Pseudomonas sp.	4+
E. coli	4+	Gamma strep	2+		
Lactobacillus	2+				

Mycology (Yeast) Culture

Normal flora		Dysbiotic flora
Candida glabrata	1+	
Rhodotorula sp.	1+	

Stool culture results showing overgrowth of *Pseudomonas* in a patient with sensorimotor peripheral neuropathy—immunorestoration, immunomodulation, and antimicrobial therapy resulted in sustained remission of fatigue, periodic fever, and neuropathy: *Psuedomonas aeruginosa* shows cross-reactivity with human neuronal tissues.[982,983] Note also the abnormal yeast, consistent with GI immunosuppression.

---

[974] Kondakova et al. Structural and serological studies of the O-antigen of Proteus mirabilis O-9. *Carbohydr Res* 2003 May 23;338(11):1191-6
[975] Ebringer A, Rashid T, Wilson C. Rheumatoid arthritis: proposal for the use of anti-microbial therapy in early cases. *Scand J Rheumatol* 2003;32(1):2-11
[976] Rashid T, et al. Proteus IgG antibodies and C-reactive protein in English, Norwegian and Spanish patients with rheumatoid arthritis. *Clin Rheumatol* 1999;18(3):190-5
[977] Wilson C, Rashid T, Tiwana H, et al. Cytotoxicity responses to Peptide antigens in rheumatoid arthritis and ankylosing spondylitis. *J Rheumatol* 2003 May;30(5):972-8
[978] Bergan T. Pathogenetic factors of Pseudomonas aeruginosa. *Scand J Infect Dis Suppl.* 1981;29:7-12
[979] Kim et al. Pseudomonas aeruginosa as a potential cause of antibiotic-associated diarrhea. *J Korean Med Sci.* 2001 Dec;16(6):742-4
[980] Porco et al. Pseudomonas aeruginosa as a cause of infectious diarrhea successfully treated with oral ciprofloxacin. *Ann Pharmacother.* 1995 Nov;29(11):1122-3
[981] Hughes LE, Bonell S, Natt RS, et al. Antibody responses to Acinetobacter spp. and Pseudomonas aeruginosa in multiple sclerosis: prospects for diagnosis using the myelin-acinetobacter-neurofilament antibody index. *Clin Diagn Lab Immunol.* 2001 Nov;8(6):1181-8
[982] Hughes LE, Bonell S, Natt RS, et al. Antibody responses to Acinetobacter spp. and Pseudomonas aeruginosa in multiple sclerosis: prospects for diagnosis using the myelin-acinetobacter-neurofilament antibody index. *Clin Diagn Lab Immunol.* 2001 Nov;8(6):1181-8 cvi.asm.org/content/8/6/1181.full.pdf
[983] Hughes LE, Smith PA, Bonell S, Natt RS, Wilson C, Rashid T, Amor S, Thompson EJ, Croker J, Ebringer A. Cross-reactivity between related sequences found in Acinetobacter sp., Pseudomonas aeruginosa, myelin basic protein and myelin oligodendrocyte glycoprotein in multiple sclerosis. *J Neuroimmunol.* 2003 Nov;144:105-15

Commonly encountered dysbiotic microorganisms—*alphabetized listing*, *continued*

Dysbiotic microbe	Pathophysiology and clinical manifestations
Segmented filamentous bacteria (SFB)	• **Segmented filamentous bacteria (SFB)** are *unculturable* **Gram-positive** spore-forming rods most closely related to the genus Clostridium; within a short period of time, SFB rapidly took the spotlight of microbial fame when several articles were published showing the ability of SFB to **induce highly pathogenic Th-17 cells**[984,985], known for their involvement in diabetes mellitus and especially their prime role in **autoimmune diseases such as rheumatoid arthritis, multiple sclerosis, and psoriasis.** SFB have been noted in humans by Caselli et al[986] who documented SFB-like organisms in histological slides of ileo-cecal valves in patients with ulcerative colitis; in their small study of 18 patients, they noted " SFB-like organisms are more often seen and in much greater density in patients with UC than in control cases without bowel inflammation, while they are never found in CD patients. ... As both **antibiotics and probiotics have previously proved to be active against SFB in mice**, we suggest that therapeutic manipulation of SFB might be tried in UC patients." • Orally administered vancomycin is one of the only and quite likely the best of anti-SFB antimicrobial agents suitable for human clinical outpatient use; in my recent clinical experience with this agent, I have found that low-modest doses —even as low as 125 mg/d for months at a time— promote notable benefit (e.g., major clinical improvement and reduction in serum CCP) with no detectable adverse effect. Empiric use (i.e., without laboratory identification of SFB in particular or a targeted bacterium in general) of oral vancomycin has shown noteworthy benefit in autism[987] and primary sclerosing cholangitis (PSC)[988]—in PSC, highly noteworthy and consistent with my own clinical experience is the fact that lower-dose oral vancomycin appears to be safer and more clinically effective than a higher dose. Oral vancomycin generally has zero-low intestinal absorption and systemic bioavailability.[989] However, several case reports of adverse effects (including allergy/hypersensitivity, anaphylaxis, red man syndrome) following oral vancomycin make clear the fact that some patients absorb an amount worthy of clinical consideration; absorption is increased in patients with bowel inflammation, and clearance is reduced (thus serum levels and risk for adverse effects are higher) in patients with renal insufficiency.[990] Quite obviously, any plan to change gastrointestinal microbial flora must also ❶ aim for the eradication of multiple disease-inducing agents (i.e., rarely only one microbial offender is responsible; often multiple antimicrobial agents will have to be used), ❷ unfailingly include and emphasize a plant-based gluten-free diet (which generally does not have to be and in many cases should not be vegan or completely vegetarian), ❸ generally include probiotic therapy via direct supplementation, and ❹ generally be implemented for many months (some clinical cases will respond brilliantly to only a few days or weeks of treatment, while all cases will require long-term preservation of eubiosis for maintenance of optimal immunoinflammatory outcomes). Since berberine is also effective against Gram-positive microbes, one might consider using berberine additionally or alternatively against SFB despite the lack of supporting evidence from a microbiologic standpoint; the clinical efficacy and safety of berberine (500 mg BID-TID for 3 months) is well documented in recent clinical trials in patients with dyslipidemia and diabetes mellitus type-2.

---

[984] Ivanov II, Littman DR. Segmented filamentous bacteria take the stage. *Mucosal Immunol.* 2010 May;3(3):209-12
[985] Ivanov II, Atarashi K, Manel N et al. Induction of intestinal Th17 cells by segmented filamentous bacteria. *Cell.* 2009 Oct 30;139(3):485-98
[986] Caselli et al. Segmented filamentous bacteria-like organisms in histological slides of ileo-cecal valves in patients with UC. *Am J Gastroenterol.* 2013 May;108(5):860-1
[987] "The vancomycin dose was 500 mg/day..." Sandler et al. Short-term benefit from oral vancomycin treatment of regressive-onset autism. *J Child Neurol* 2000 Jul:429-35
[988] Oral vancomycin 125mg or 250 mg QID. Tabibian et al. Vancomycin metronidazole patients primary sclerosing cholangitis. *Aliment Pharmacol Ther* 2013 Mar;604-1
[989] "Orally administered vancomycin at 125 mg 4 times daily was not absorbed from the gastrointestinal tract." Rao et al. Systemic absorption of oral vancomycin in patients with Clostridium difficile infection. *Scand J Infect Dis.* 2011 May;43(5):386-8
[990] Osawa R, Kaka AS. Maculopapular rash induced by oral vancomycin. *Clin Infect Dis.* 2008 Sep 15;47(6):860-1

Commonly encountered dysbiotic microorganisms—*alphabetized listing*, continued

Dysbiotic microbe	Pathophysiology and clinical manifestations
Staphylococcus aureus *Staphylococcus epidermidis*	• **Any and all *Staphylococcus aureus* should be eradicated immediately due to the well-known inflammatory consequences of the toxins and superantigens this bacterium produces.** *Staphylococcus aureus* is a gram-positive bacterium, certain strains of which produce the toxic shock syndrome toxin-1 (TSST-1) that produces scalded skin syndrome, toxic shock syndrome, and food poisoning; other strains of *Staphylococcus aureus* that do not produce TSST-1 are also capable of causing toxic shock syndrome from colonization of bone, vagina, wounds, or rectum.[991] • Gastrointestinal colonization with *Staphylococcus aureus* is a known cause of **acute colitis**[992], and nasal carriage of this bacterium is documented in patients with several autoimmune disorders, including **Wegener's granulomatosis**[993], **systemic lupus erythematosus**[994] and **psoriasis**.[995, 996] • *Staphylococcus aureus* can trigger **reactive arthritis**.[997] • *Staphylococcus epidermidis* can trigger **reactive arthritis and sacroiliitis**.[998] • Patients with **Behcet's syndrome** commonly have skin lesions that are colonized by *Staphylococcus aureus*.[999] • Most (57%) of patients with **atopic dermatitis** show evidence of IgE-mediated histamine release (i.e., "allergy") to exotoxins secreted from *Staphylococcus aureus*, which commonly colonizes eczematous skin[1000]; in other words: most eczema patients are allergic to their own dermal bacteria and can thus be said to have *hypersensitivity dermal dysbiosis*.

---

[991] Shandera WX, Moran A. "Infectious diseases: viral and rickettsial." In Tierney LM, McPhee SJ Papadakis MA (eds). Current Medical Diagnosis and Treatment. 44th edition. New York: Lange; 2005, page 1356-8

[992] Watanabe H, Masaki H, Asoh N, Watanabe K, Oishi K, Kobayashi S, Sato A, Nagatake T. Enterocolitis caused by methicillin-resistant Staphylococcus aureus: molecular characterization of respiratory and digestive tract isolates. *Microbiol Immunol.* 2001;45(9):629-34 jstage.jst.go.jp/article/mandi/45/9/629/_pdf

[993] Popa ER, et al. Staphylococcus aureus and Wegener's granulomatosis. *Arthritis Res.* 2002;4(2):77-9 arthritis-research.com/content/4/2/077

[994] Medline abstract from Polish research: "In 9 from 14 patients with (64.3%) a.b. very massive growth of Staphylococcus aureus in culture from vestibulae of the nose swab was, in other cultures very massive growth of physiological flora was seen. ...clinical significance of asymptomatic bacteriuria and pathogenic bacteria colonisation of nostrils as a precedence to symptomatic infections needs further investigations." Koseda-Dragan M, Hebanowski M, Galinski J, Krzywinska E, Bakowska A. [Asymptomatic bacteriuria in women diagnosed with systemic lupus erythematosus (SLE)] Pol Arch Med Wewn. 1998 Oct;100(4):321-30.

[995] "Nasal carriage rate of Staphylococcus aureus in psoriatics was higher than control groups."Singh et al. Bacteriology of psoriatic plaques. *Dermatologica* 1978;157:21-7

[996] "In this study, S aureus was present in more than 50% of patients with AD and PS. We found that the severity of AD and PS significantly correlated to enterotoxin production of the isolated S aureus strains." Tomi NS, Kranke B, Aberer E. Staphylococcal toxins in patients with psoriasis, atopic dermatitis, and erythroderma, and in healthy control subjects. *J Am Acad Dermatol.* 2005 Jul;53(1):67-72

[997] "CONCLUSION--Reactive arthritis may rarely follow Staph aureus infection. HLA-B27 negativity may be associated with a self limited arthritis in these cases." Siam AR, Hammoudeh M. Staphylococcus aureus triggered reactive arthritis. *Ann Rheum Dis.* 1995 Feb;54(2):131-3

[998] "We report an unusual case of a patient with SE bacteriaemia, who developed elbow arthritis, asymmetrical sacroiliitis, keratoderma and restrictive cardiomyopathy." Giordano N, et al. Reactive arthritis by staphylococcus epidermidis: report of an unusual case. *Clin Rheumatol.* 1996;15(1):59-61

[999] "At least one type of microorganism was grown from each pustule. Staphylococcus aureus (41/70, 58.6%, p = 0.008) and Prevotella spp (17/70, 24.3%, p = 0.002) were significantly more common in pustules from BS patients, and coagulase negative staphylococci (17/37, 45.9%, p = 0.007) in pustules from acne patients. CONCLUSIONS: The pustular lesions of BS are not usually sterile." Hatemi G, et al. The pustular skin lesions in Behcet's syndrome are not sterile. *Ann Rheum Dis.* 2004 Nov;63(11):1450-2

[1000] "These data indicate that a subset of patients with AD mount an IgE response to SEs that can be grown from their skin." Leung DY, et al. Presence of IgE antibodies to staphylococcal exotoxins on the skin of patients with atopic dermatitis. Evidence for a new group of allergens. *J Clin Invest.* 1993 Sep;92(3):1374-80

Commonly encountered dysbiotic microorganisms—*alphabetized listing*, continued

Microbe	Pathophysiology and clinical manifestations
Streptococcus pyogenes Group A *streptococci*	• Intestinal overgrowth of this bacterium, which produces peptidoglycans, can cause **dermatosis, inflammatory polyarthritis, tenosynovitis, malaise, fever, and cryoglobulinemia**.[1001] • Non-infectious manifestations precipitated by infection with *S. pyogenes* include **autoimmune neuropsychiatric disorders** (including obsessive-compulsive disorder and Sydenham's chorea), **dystonia, glomerulonephritis, and reactive arthritis**.[1002] • Group A streptococci can cause **reactive arthritis** in humans.[1003] • *Streptococcus pyogenes* is a very likely trigger of **psoriasis**[1004]; chronic penicillin treatment leads to clinical improvement of recalcitrant psoriasis.[1005] • Certain strains of *S. pyogenes* produce an exotoxin that can cause toxic shock syndrome.[1006]

Clinical Benefits of Identifying and Eradicating Dysbiosis

In the previous section, I described the biochemical/physiologic mechanisms by which microorganisms can contribute to disease *without causing a classic "infection"* and promote systemic inflammation and human disease. Thus having developed the precept that **microorganisms can cause inflammatory disease by noninfectious means**, I will (re)state here that the cure of human disease by eradication of harmful microbes is not a requirement to prove the validity of this thesis. Inflammation and autoimmunity are self-perpetuating phenomena that can persist despite the effective eradication of the principle cause, and research has demonstrated that microbial antigens can remain present in synovial fluid for several years after the eradication of the primary infection.[1007] With that said, we are fortunate to observe that **many patients with autoimmunity are indeed benefited and occasionally "cured" by removal of instigating microbes**. I have seen this on numerous occasions in my clinical practice, and this phenomenon has also been documented in the research literature. Examples published in the research include the amelioration of one patient's scleroderma with the eradication of intestinal bacterial overgrowth[1008], the amelioration of Wegener's granulomatosis with antimicrobial therapy against *Staphylococcus aureus*[1009,1010], and the alleviation of inflammatory arthritis following the use of antibiotics against genitourinary *Chlamydia trachomatis* and gastrointestinal *Salmonella enteritidis, Yersinia enterocolitica, Shigella flexneri* or *Campylobacter jejuni*.[1011] Treatments for addressing dysbiosis and its numerous sequelae are described in the pages/sections that follow.

> **Landmark work by Dr Patricia Noah**
> "We have repeatedly observed psoriatic flares associated with microbial infection, sequestered antigen, and colonization. **Removal of these microbial foci results in clearing of the disease.**"
>
> Patricia Noah PhD from University of Tennessee College of Medicine. *Semin Dermatol.* 1990

Natural Treatments for the Eradication of Dysbiosis and Related Immune-Complex Diseases

Although antimicrobial drugs may be used, these are not universally curative and are not necessarily "more powerful" or "more effective" than natural treatments. Treatments for gastrointestinal dysbiosis may be somewhat

---

[1001] Ely PH. The bowel bypass syndrome: a response to bacterial peptidoglycans. *J Am Acad Dermatol.* 1980 Jun;2(6):473-87
[1002] Hahn RG, Knox LM, Forman TA. Evaluation of poststreptococcal illness. *Am Fam Physician.* 2005 May 15;71(10):1949-54 aafp.org/afp/20050515/1949.pdf
[1003] "We present a patient whose clinical features are more consistent with post-streptococcal reactive arthritis than acute rheumatic fever." Howell EE, Bathon J. A case of post-streptococcal reactive arthritis. *Md Med J.* 1999 Nov-Dec;48(6):292-4
[1004] "These findings justify the hypothesis that S pyogenes infections are more important in the pathogenesis of chronic plaque psoriasis than has previously been recognized, and indicate the need for further controlled therapeutic trials of antibacterial measures in this common skin disease." El-Rachkidy RG, et al. Increased Blood Levels of IgG Reactive with Secreted Streptococcus pyogenes Proteins in Chronic Plaque Psoriasis. *J Invest Dermatol.* 2007 Mar 8
[1005] "Total duration of the study was two years. Initially benzathine penicillin 1.2 million units, was given I.M. AST fortnightly. After 24 weeks benzathine penicillin was reduced to 1.2 million units once a month... Significant improvement in the PASI score was noted from 12 weeks onwards. All patients showed excellent improvement at 2 years." Saxena VN, Dogra J. Long-term use of penicillin for the treatment of chronic plaque psoriasis. *Eur J Dermatol.* 2005 Sep-Oct;15(5):359-62
[1006] Chikkamuniyappa S. Streptococcal toxic shock syndrome and sepsis manifesting in a patient with chronic rheumatoid arthritis. *Dermatol Online J.* 2004 Jul 15;10(1):7
[1007] "Extensive bacterial cultures of synovial fluid were negative... We conclude that in patients with reactive arthritis after yersinia infection, microbial antigens can be found in synovial-fluid cells from affected joints."Granfors et al.Yersinia antigens in synovial-fluid cells from patients with reactive arthritis. *N Engl J Med* 1989;320:216-2
[1008] Over et al. Regression of skin changes in patient with systemic sclerosis following treatment for bacterial overgrowth with ciprofloxacin. *Br J Rheumatol* 1998;37:696
[1009] Popa et al. Staphylococcus aureus and Wegener's granulomatosis. *Arthritis Res.* 2002;4(2):77-9 arthritis-research.com/content/4/2/077
[1010] George J, Levy Y, Kallenberg CG, Shoenfeld Y. Infections and Wegener's granulomatosis--a cause and effect relationship? *QJM.* 1997 May;90(5):367-73
[1011] Kobayashi et al. Reactive arthritis: recent advances and clinical manifestations. *Intern Med.* 2005 May;44:408-12 jstage.jst.go.jp/article/internalmedicine/44/5/408/_pdf

summarized as follows: *"Starve, Poison, Crowd, Purge, and Support Immunity."* The following concepts and therapeutics are particularly—though not exclusively—relevant for the treatment of *gastrointestinal* dysbiosis.

1. **Diet modifications (*"starve the microbes"*)**: The diet plan should ensure **avoidance of sugar**, grains, soluble fiber, gums, prebiotics, and dairy products since these contain **fermentable carbohydrates that promote overgrowth of bacteria and other microorganisms in the gut**. Short-term **fasting** starves intestinal microbes, temporarily eliminates dietary antigens, alleviates "autointoxication", and stimulates the humoral immune system in the gut to more effectively destroy local microbes.[1012,1013] Thus, implementation of the "**specific carbohydrate diet**" popularized by Gottschall[1014] along with periodic fasting, which has obvious anti-inflammatory benefits[1015], can be used therapeutically in patients with conditions associated with dysbiosis-induced inflammation. Plant-based low-carbohydrate diets can lead to favorable changes in the quality and quantity of intestinal microflora. Hypoallergenic diets are proven beneficial for the treatment of the **immune complex disease** called mixed cryoglobulinemia.[1016,1017]

2. **Antimicrobial treatments (*"poison the microbes, not the patient"*)**: Anti-microbial herbs can be used which directly kill or strongly inhibit the intestinal microbes. The most commonly used and well-documented botanicals in this regard are listed in the section below. Antimicrobial treatment is frequently continued for 1-3 months, and co-administration of drugs can be utilized when appropriate. Sometimes antimicrobial drugs are necessary, especially for acute and severe infections; often nutritional and botanical interventions are safer and more effective. Although these herbs are generally taken orally, some of them can also be applied topically (in a cream or lotion), and nasally (in a saline water lavage, as detailed previously). Botanical medicines are generally used in combination, and lower doses of each can be used when used in combination compared to the doses that are necessary when the herbs are used in isolation.

   - **Oregano oil in an emulsified and time-released tablet**: Botanical oils that are not emulsified do not attain maximal dispersion in the gastrointestinal tract; products that are not time-released may be absorbed before reaching the colon in sufficient concentrations. Emulsified oil of oregano in a time-released tablet is proven effective in the eradication of harmful gastrointestinal microbes, including *Blastocystis hominis, Entamoeba hartmanni,* and *Endolimax nana*.[1018] An in vitro study[1019] and clinical experience support the use of emulsified oregano against *Candida albicans*. The common dose is 600 mg per day in divided doses for at least 6 weeks.[1020]

   - **Berberine**: Berberine is an alkaloid extracted from plant such as *Berberis vulgaris,* and *Hydrastis canadensis,* and it shows effectiveness against *Giardia, Candida,* and *Streptococcus* in addition to its direct anti-inflammatory and antidiarrheal actions. Oral dose of 400 mg/d had been common for adults[1021] until newer research showed that berberine 1,000-1,500 mg/d for 3 months was safe and impressively effective for the treatment of dyslipidemia, dysglycemia, metabolic syndrome, diabetes type-2; berberine is more effective dose-for-dose than is metformin.[1022] Topical *Mahonia/Berberis aquifolium* is effective for dermal psoriasis[1023] via its combined anti-inflammatory and antimicrobial benefits.

   - *Artemisia annua*: Artemisinin has been safely used for centuries in Asia for the treatment of malaria[1024,1025], and it also has **effectiveness against anaerobic bacteria** due to the pro-oxidative sesquiterpene

---

[1012] Trollmo C, Verdrengh M, Tarkowski A. Fasting enhances mucosal antigen specific B cell responses in rheumatoid arthritis. *Ann Rheum Dis*. 1997 Feb;56(2):130-4
[1013] Ramakrishnan T, Stokes P. Beneficial effects of fasting and low carbohydrate diet in D-lactic acidosis associated with short-bowel syndrome. *JPEN J Parenter Enteral Nutr*. 1985 May-Jun;9(3):361-3
[1014] Gottschall E. *Breaking the Vicious Cycle: Intestinal Health Through Diet*. Kirkton Press; Rev edition (August 1, 1994)
[1015] "The pooling of these studies showed a statistically and clinically significant beneficial long-term effect." Muller H, de Toledo FW, Resch KL. Fasting followed by vegetarian diet in patients with rheumatoid arthritis: a systematic review. *Scand J Rheumatol*. 2001;30(1):1-10
[1016] "CONCLUSION: These data show that an LAC diet decreases the amount of circulating immune complexes in MC and can modify certain signs and symptoms of the disease." Ferri C, Pietrogrande M, Cecchetti R, et al. Low-antigen-content diet in the treatment of patients with mixed cryoglobulinemia. *Am J Med*. 1989 Nov;87:519-24
[1017] Pietrogrande M, Cefalo A, Nicora F, Marchesini G. Dietetic treatment of essential mixed cryoglobulinemia. *Ric Clin Lab*. 1986 Apr-Jun;16(2):413-6
[1018] Force M, Sparks WS, Ronzio RA. Inhibition of enteric parasites by emulsified oil of oregano in vivo. *Phytother Res*. 2000 May;14(3):213-4
[1019] Stiles JC, Sparks W, Ronzio RA. The inhibition of Candida albicans by oregano. *J Applied Nutr* 1995;47:96–102
[1020] Force M, Sparks WS, Ronzio RA. Inhibition of enteric parasites by emulsified oil of oregano in vivo. *Phytother Res*. 2000 May;14(3):213-4
[1021] Berberine. *Altern Med Rev*. 2000 Apr;5(2):175-7 thorne.com/altmedrev/.fulltext/5/2/175.pdf
[1022] Yin et al. Efficacy of berberine in patients with type 2 diabetes mellitus. *Metabolism*. 2008 May;57(5):712-7. See also Kong et al. Berberine is a novel cholesterol-lowering drug working through a unique mechanism distinct from statins. *Nat Med*. 2004 Dec;10(12):1344-51
[1023] "Taken together, these clinical studies conducted by several investigators in several countries indicate that Mahonia aquifolium is a safe and effective treatment of patients with mild to moderate psoriasis." Gulliver WP, Donsky HJ. A report on three recent clinical trials using Mahonia aquifolium 10% topical cream and a review of the worldwide clinical experience with Mahonia aquifolium for the treatment of plaque psoriasis. *Am J Ther*. 2005 Sep-Oct;12(5):398-406
[1024] Dien TK, et al. Effect of food intake on pharmacokinetics of oral artemisinin in healthy Vietnamese subjects. *Antimicrob Agents Chemother*. 1997 May;41(5):1069-72
[1025] Giao PT, et al. Artemisinin for treatment of uncomplicated falciparum malaria: is there a place for monotherapy? *Am J Trop Med Hyg*. 2001 Dec;65(6):690-5

endoperoxide. In a recent study treating patients with malaria, "the adult artemisinin dose was 500 mg; children aged < 15 years received 10 mg/kg per dose" and thus the dose for an 80-lb child would be 363 mg per day by these criteria.[1026] I commonly use **artemisinin at 100 mg twice per day (with other antimicrobial botanicals such as berberine) in divided doses for adults with dysbiosis**. One of the additional benefits of artemisinin is its systemic bioavailability.

- St. John's Wort (*Hypericum perforatum*): Best known for its antidepressant action, **hyperforin from *Hypericum perforatum* also shows impressive antibacterial action, particularly against gram-positive bacteria such as *Staphylococcus aureus*, *Streptococcus pyogenes* and *Streptococcus agalactiae*.** According to in vitro studies, the lowest effective hyperforin concentration is 0.1 mcg/mL against *Corynebacterium diphtheriae* with increasing effectiveness against multiresistant *Staphylococcus aureus* at higher concentrations of 100 mcg/mL.[1027] Since oral dosing with hyperforin can result in serum levels of 500 nanogram /mL (equivalent to 0.5 microgram/mL) then it is possible that high-dose hyperforin will have systemic antibacterial action. Regardless of its possible systemic antibacterial effectiveness, **hyperforin should clearly have antibacterial action when applied "topically" such as when it is taken orally against gastric and upper intestinal colonization.** Extracts from St. John's Wort hold particular promise against multidrug-resistant *Staphylococcus aureus*[1028] and perhaps *Helicobacter pylori*.[1029]

- Myrrh (*Commiphora molmol*): Myrrh is remarkably effective against parasitic infections.[1030] A recent clinical trial against **schistosomiasis**[1031] showed "The parasitological cure rate after three months was 97.4% and 96.2% for *S. haematobium* and *S. mansoni* cases with the marvelous clinical cure without any side-effects."[1032]

- Bismuth: Bismuth is commonly used in the empiric treatment of diarrhea (e.g., "Pepto-Bismol") and is commonly combined with other antimicrobial agents to reduce drug resistance and increase antibiotic effectiveness.[1033]

- Peppermint (*Mentha piperita*): Peppermint shows antimicrobial and antispasmodic actions and has demonstrated clinical effectiveness in patients with bacterial overgrowth of the small bowel.

- Uva Ursi: Uva ursi can be used against gastrointestinal pathogens on a limited basis per culture and sensitivity findings; its primary historical and modern use is as a urinary antiseptic which is effective only when the urine pH is alkaline.[1034] Components of uva ursi potentiate antibiotics.[1035] **This herb has some ocular and neurologic toxicity and should be used with professional supervision for low-dose and/or short-term administration only.**[1036]

- Garlic: Garlic shows *in vitro* antimicrobial action against numerous microorganisms, including *H. pylori*, *Pseudomonas aeruginosa*, and *Candida albicans*, and this effect is mediated *directly* via microbicidal actions as well as *indirectly* via dissolution of microbial biofilms[1037] and inhibition of quorum sensing.[1038] However, since the antimicrobial components of garlic are likely absorbed in the upper gastrointestinal tract, I propose that it is unlikely that garlic can exert a clinically significant anti-dysbiotic effect in the lower small intestine and colon. In fact, two studies in humans have shown that—despite its *in vitro* effectiveness

---

[1026] Giao PT, Binh TQ, Kager PA, Long HP, Van Thang N, Van Nam N, de Vries PJ. Artemisinin for treatment of uncomplicated falciparum malaria: is there a place for monotherapy? *Am J Trop Med Hyg*. 2001 Dec;65(6):690-5 ajtmh.org/cgi/reprint/65/6/690
[1027] Schempp et al. Antibacterial activity of hyperforin from St John's wort, against multiresistant Staphylococcus aureus and gram-positive bacteria. *Lancet*. 1999;353:2129
[1028] Gibbons S, Ohlendorf B, Johnsen I. The genus Hypericum--a valuable resource of anti-Staphylococcal leads. *Fitoterapia*. 2002 Jul;73(4):300-4
[1029] "A butanol fraction of St. John's Wort revealed anti-Helicobacter pylori activity with MIC values ranging between 15.6 and 31.2 microg/ml." Reichling J, Weseler A, Saller R. A current review of the antimicrobial activity of Hypericum perforatum L. *Pharmacopsychiatry*. 2001 Jul;34 Suppl 1:S116-8
[1030] El Baz, et al. Clinical and parasitological studies on efficacy of Mirazid in treatment of schistosomiasis haematobium in Tatoon. *J Egypt Soc Parasitol* 2003;33:761-76
[1031] Schistosomiasis. dpd.cdc.gov/dpdx/HTML/Schistosomiasis.htm
[1032] Abo-Madyan AA, Morsy TA, Motawea SM. Efficacy of Myrrh in the treatment of schistosomiasis (haematobium and mansoni) in Ezbet El-Bakly, Tamyia Center, El-Fayoum Governorate, Egypt. *J Egypt Soc Parasitol*. 2004 Aug;34(2):423-46
[1033] Veldhuyzen van Zanten SJ, Sherman PM, Hunt RH. Helicobacter pylori: new developments and treatments. *CMAJ*. 1997;156(11):1565-74
[1034] Yarnell E. Botanical medicines for the urinary tract. *World J Urol*. 2002 Nov;20(5):285-93
[1035] Shimizu M, Shiota S, Mizushima T, Ito H, Hatano T, Yoshida T, Tsuchiya T. Marked potentiation of activity of beta-lactams against methicillin-resistant Staphylococcus aureus by corilagin. *Antimicrob Agents Chemother*. 2001 Nov;45(11):3198-201 aac.asm.org/cgi/reprint/45/11/3198
[1036] "A 56-year-old woman who ingested uva ursi for 3 years noted a decrease in visual acuity within the past year. Ocular examination including fluorescein angiography revealed a typical bull's-eye maculopathy bilaterally." Wang L, Del Priore LV. Bull's-eye maculopathy secondary to herbal toxicity from uva ursi. *Am J Ophthalmol*. 2004 Jun;137:1135-7
[1037] "Sub-MICs of allicin also diminished the biofilm formations by S. epidermidis." Perez-Giraldo C, et al. In vitro activity of allicin against Staphylococcus epidermidis and influence of subinhibitory concentrations on biofilm formation. *J Appl Microbiol*. 2003;95(4):709-11
[1038] "The results indicate that a QS-inhibitory extract of garlic renders P. aeruginosa sensitive to tobramycin, respiratory burst and phagocytosis by PMNs, as well as leading to an improved outcome of pulmonary infections." Bjarnsholt T, et al. Garlic blocks quorum sensing and promotes rapid clearing of pulmonary Pseudomonas aeruginosa infections. *Microbiology*. 2005 Dec;151(Pt 12):3873-80. The in vivo portion of this study was performed in lab animals, not humans.

against *H. pylori*—garlic is ineffective in the treatment of gastric *H. pylori* colonization.[1039,1040] While these studies argue against the use of garlic as antimicrobial monotherapy, the possibility remains that garlic may enhance the clinical effectiveness of other antimicrobial therapeutics via its aforementioned ability to weaken microbial biofilms and to impair quorum sensing, which otherwise serve to protect yeast/bacteria from immune attack and from antibacterial/antifungal therapeutics.

- **Cranberry**: Particularly effective for the prevention and adjunctive treatment of urinary tract infections, mostly by inhibiting adherence of *E. coli* to epithelial cells.[1041]
- **Thyme (*Thymus vulgaris*)**: Thyme extracts have direct antimicrobial actions and also potentiate the effectiveness of tetracycline against drug-resistant *Staphylococcus aureus*.[1042] Thyme also appears effective against *Aeromonas hydrophila*.[1043]
- **Clove (*Syzygium* species)**: Clove's eugenol has been shown in animal studies to have a potent antifungal effect.[1044]
- **Anise**: Although it has weak antibacterial action when used alone, anise does show in vitro activity against molds.[1045]
- **Buchu/betulina**: Buchu has a long history of use against urinary tract infections and systemic infections.[1046]
- **Caprylic acid and undecylenic acid**: Caprylic acid is a medium chain fatty acid that is commonly used in patients with dysbiosis, particularly that which has a fungal/yeast component. Beside empiric use, caprylic acid may be indicated by culture-sensitivity results provided with comprehensive parasitology. When bacterial/fungal sensitivity tests indicate caprylic acid, many clinicians prefer to use undecylenic acid which is reportedly up to six times more powerful than caprylic acid.[1047] Commercial preparations delivering 50 mg undecylenic acid per gelcap can be taken orally in doses of 3-5 gelcaps three times per day. Anti-candidal action has been reported[1048], and my impression is that undecylenic acid is among the more valuable therapeutics in the treatment of gastrointestinal dysbiosis.
- **Dill (*Anethum graveolens*)**: Dill shows activity against several types of mold and yeast.[1049]
- **Brucea javanica**: Extract from *Brucea javanica* fruit shows *in vitro* activity against *Babesia gibsoni*, *Plasmodium falciparum*[1050], *Entamoeba histolytica*[1051] and *Blastocystis hominis*.[1052,1053]
- **Acacia catechu**: *Acacia catechu* shows moderate *in vitro* activity against *Salmonella typhi*.[1054]

3. *Oral administration of proteolytic enzymes*: The use of polyenzyme therapy in patients with dysbiotic inflammation is justified for at least four reasons. First, orally administered proteolytic enzymes are efficiently absorbed by the gastrointestinal tract into the systemic circulation[1055] to then provide a **clinically significant**

[1039] "This study did not support a role for either garlic or jalapenos in the treatment of H. pylori infection. Caution must be used when attempting to extrapolate data from in vitro studies to the in vivo condition." Graham et al. Garlic or jalapeno peppers for treatment of Helicobacter pylori infection. *Am J Gastroenterol*. 1999 May;94(5):1200-2
[1040] "Five patients completed the study. There was no evidence of either eradication or suppression of H. pylori or symptom improvement whilst taking garlic oil." McNulty CA, et al. A pilot study to determine the effectiveness of garlic oil capsules in the treatment of dyspeptic patients with Helicobacter pylori. *Helicobacter*. 2001;6(3):249-53
[1041] Lynch DM. Cranberry for prevention of urinary tract infections. *Am Fam Physician*. 2004 Dec 1;70(11):2175-7 aafp.org/afp/20041201/2175.pdf
[1042] Fujita M, Shiota S, Kuroda T, Hatano T, Yoshida T, Mizushima T, Tsuchiya T. Remarkable synergies between baicalein and tetracycline, and baicalein and beta-lactams against methicillin-resistant Staphylococcus aureus. *Microbiol Immunol*. 2005;49(4):391-6
[1043] "...thyme essential oil showed the greatest inhibition against A. hydrophila." Fabio A, Corona A, Forte E, Quaglio P. Inhibitory activity of spices and essential oils on psychrotrophic bacteria. *New Microbiol*. 2003 Jan;26(1):115-20
[1044] Chami N, et al. Antifungal treatment with carvacrol and eugenol of oral candidiasis in immunosuppressed rats. *Braz J Infect Dis*. 2004 Jun;8(3):217-26
[1045] "Anise oil was not particularly inhibitory to bacteria (inhibition zone, approximately 25 mm); however, anise oil was highly inhibitory to molds." Elgayyar M, et al. Antimicrobial activity of essential oils from plants against selected pathogenic and saprophytic microorganisms. *J Food Prot*. 2001 Jul;64(7):1019-24
[1046] "Buchu preparations are now used as a diuretic and for a wide range of conditions including stomach aches, rheumatism, bladder and kidney infections and coughs and colds." Simpson D. Buchu--South Africa's amazing herbal remedy. *Scott Med J* 1998 Dec;43(6):189-91
[1047] Undecylenic acid. Monograph. *Altern Med Rev*. 2002 Feb;7(1):68-70 thorne.com/altmedrev/.fulltext/7/1/68.pdf
[1048] McLain N, et al. Undecylenic acid inhibits morphogenesis of Candida albicans. *Antimicrob Agents Chemother*. 2000 Oct;44(10):2873-5
[1049] "Antimicrobial testings showed high activity of the essential A. graveolens oil against the mold Aspergillus niger and the yeasts Saccharomyces cerevisiae and Candida albicans." Jirovetz L, Buchbauer G, Stoyanova AS, Georgiev EV, Damianova ST. Composition, quality control, and antimicrobial activity of the essential oil of long-time stored dill (Anethum graveolens L.) seeds from Bulgaria. *J Agric Food Chem*. 2003 Jun 18;51(13):3854-7
[1050] Murnigsih T, Subeki, Matsuura H, et al. Evaluation of the inhibitory activities of the extracts of Indonesian traditional medicinal plants against Plasmodium falciparum and Babesia gibsoni. *J Vet Med Sci*. 2005 Aug;67(8):829-31 jstage.jst.go.jp/article/jvms/67/8/829/_pdf
[1051] Wright CW, O'Neill MJ, Phillipson JD, Warhurst DC. Use of microdilution to assess in vitro antiamoebic activities of Brucea javanica fruits, Simarouba amara stem, and a number of quassinoids. *Antimicrob Agents Chemother*. 1988 Nov;32(11):1725-9
[1052] "Dichloromethane and methanol extracts from the Brucea javanica seed and a methanol extract from Quercus infectoria nut gall showed the highest activity." Sawangjaroen N, Sawangjaroen K. The effects of extracts from anti-diarrheic Thai medicinal plants on the in vitro growth of the intestinal protozoa parasite: Blastocystis hominis. *J Ethnopharmacol*. 2005 Apr 8;98(1-2):67-72
[1053] "The crude extracts of Coptis chinensis (CC) and Brucea javanica (BJ) were found to be most active against B. hominis." Yang LQ, et al. In vitro response of Blastocystis hominis against traditional Chinese medicine. *J Ethnopharmacol*. 1996 Dec;55(1):35-42
[1054] "Moderate antimicrobial activity was shown by Picorhiza kurroa, Acacia catechu, ..." Rani P, Khullar N. Antimicrobial evaluation of some medicinal plants for their anti-enteric potential against multi-drug resistant Salmonella typhi. *Phytother Res*. 2004 Aug;18(8):670-3
[1055] Liebow C, Rothman SS. Enteropancreatic Circulation of Digestive Enzymes. *Science* 1975; 189(4201): 472-474

anti-inflammatory benefit as I reviewed recently.[1056] Second and more specifically, oral administration of proteolytic enzymes is generally believed to effect a **reduction in immune complexes and their clinical consequences**[1057], and immune complexes are probably a major mechanism of dysbiosis-induced disease and are pathogenic in rheumatoid arthritis[1058] and many other autoimmune diseases such as systemic lupus erythematosus, dermatomyositis, Sjogren's syndrome, and polyarteritis nodosa.[1059] Third, proteolytic enzymes have been shown to **stimulate immune function**[1060] and may thereby promote clearance of occult infections. Fourth, **proteolytic enzymes inhibit formation of microbial biofilms** and increase immune penetration and the effectiveness of antimicrobial therapeutics.[1061] Although individual enzymes may be used in isolation, enzyme therapy is generally delivered in the form of polyenzyme preparations containing pancreatin, bromelain, papain, amylase, lipase, trypsin and alpha-chymotrypsin.[1062]

4. **Probiotic supplementation ("*crowd out the bad with the good*")**: Given that "healthy" intestinal bacteria can alleviate disease and promote normal immune function[1063], then it is conversely true that a condition of harmful or suboptimal intestinal bacteria could promote disease and lead to immune dysfunction. For patients with gastrointestinal and genitourinary dysbiosis, supplementation with *Bifidobacteria*, *Lactobacillus*, and perhaps *Saccharomyces* and other beneficial strains is mandatory. The wide-ranging and well-documented benefits seen with probiotic supplementation provide direct support for the importance of microbial balance in health and disease. Supplementation with probiotics (live bacteria) is the best option, however prebiotics (such as fructooligosaccharides), and synbiotics (probiotics + prebiotics) may also be used. Synbiotic supplementation has been shown to reduce endotoxinemia and clinical symptoms in 50% of patients with minimal hepatic encephalopathy[1064], and probiotic supplementation safely ameliorated the adverse effects of bacterial overgrowth in a clinical study of patients with renal failure.[1065]

5. **Immunonutrition**: Obviously, the diet should be nutritious and free of sugars and other "junk foods" that promote inflammation and suppress immune function.[1066] Especially in patients with gastrointestinal dysbiosis, vitamin and mineral supplementation should be used to counteract the effects of malabsorption, maldigestion, and hypermetabolism that accompany immune activation. Additionally, oral glutamine in doses of six grams three times daily can help normalize intestinal permeability, enhance immune function, and improve clinical outcomes in severely ill patients.[1067] Zinc and vitamin A supplementation are each well known to support immune function against infection. Selenium has anti-inflammatory and antiviral actions.[1068] Vitamin D supplementation reduces inflammation, protects against autoimmunity, and promotes immunity against viral and bacterial infections.[1069] Supplementation with IgG from bovine colostrum can also provide benefit against chronic and acute infections.[1070,1071] Extracts from bovine thymus are safe for clinical use in humans and have shown anti-infective and anti-inflammatory benefits in elderly patients[1072] as well as antirheumatic/anti-inflammatory benefits in patients with autoimmune diseases[1073,1074,1075]; in an animal study of experimental

---

[1056] Vasquez A. Improving overall health while safely and effectively treating musculoskeletal pain. *Nutritional Perspectives* 2005; 28: 34-38, 40-42
[1057] Galebskaya LV, Ryumina EV, Niemerovsky VS, Matyukov AA. Human complement system state after wobenzyme intake. *VESTNIK MOSKOVSKOGO UNIVERSITETA. KHIMIYA*. 2000. Vol. 41, No. 6. Supplement. Pages 148-149
[1058] Edwards JC, Cambridge G. Rheumatoid arthritis: the predictable effect of small immune complexes in which antibody is also antigen. *Br J Rheumatol*. 1998 Feb;37(2):126-30 rheumatology.oxfordjournals.org/cgi/reprint/37/2/126
[1059] Jancar S, Sanchez Crespo M. Immune complex-mediated tissue injury: a multistep paradigm. *Trends Immunol*. 2005 Jan;26(1):48-55
[1060] Zavadova E, Desser L, Mohr T. Stimulation of reactive oxygen species production and cytotoxicity in human neutrophils in vitro and after oral administration of a polyenzyme preparation. *Cancer Biother*. 1995 Summer;10(2):147-52
[1061] "The enzymes were shown to inhibit the biofilm formation. When applied to the formed associations, the enzymes potentiated the effect of antibiotics on the bacteria located in them." Tets VV, et al. [Impact of exogenic proteolytic enzymes on bacteria][Quote from abstract; article in Russian] *Antibiot Khimioter*. 2004;49(12):9-13
[1062] Vasquez A. Improving overall health while safely and effectively treating musculoskeletal pain. *Nutritional Perspectives* 2005; 28: 34-38, 40-42
[1063] Isolauri E, Sutas Y, Kankaanpaa P, Arvilommi H, Salminen S. Probiotics: effects on immunity. *Am J Clin Nutr*. 2001 Feb;73(2 Suppl):444S-450S
[1064] Liu Q, et al. Synbiotic modulation of gut flora: effect on minimal hepatic encephalopathy in patients with cirrhosis. *Hepatology*. 2004 May;39(5):1441-9
[1065] Simenhoff ML, Dunn SR, Zollner GP, Fitzpatrick ME, Emery SM, Sandine WE, Ayres JW. Biomodulation of the toxic and nutritional effects of small bowel bacterial overgrowth in end-stage kidney disease using freeze-dried Lactobacillus acidophilus. *Miner Electrolyte Metab*. 1996;22(1-3):92-6
[1066] Seaman DR. The diet-induced proinflammatory state: a cause of chronic pain and other degenerative diseases? *J Manipulative Physiol Ther*. 2002 Mar-Apr;25:168-79.
[1067] Miller AL. Therapeutic considerations of L-glutamine: a review of the literature. *Altern Med Rev*. 1999 Aug;4(4):239-48
[1068] Beck MA. Nutritionally induced oxidative stress: effect on viral disease. *Am J Clin Nutr*. 2000 Jun;71(6 Suppl):1676S-81S
[1069] Vasquez A, Manso G, Cannell J. The clinical importance of vitamin D (cholecalciferol). *Altern Ther Health Med*. 2004 Sep-Oct;10(5):28-36
[1070] Mero A, Kahkonen J, Nykanen T, Parviainen T, Jokinen I, Takala T, Nikula T, Rasi S, Leppaluoto J. IGF-I, IgA, and IgG responses to bovine colostrum supplementation during training. *J Appl Physiol*. 2002 Aug;93(2):732-9 jap.physiology.org/cgi/content/full/93/2/732
[1071] "The preparation has high antibacterial antibody titres, and a high capacity for the neutralization of bacterial toxins. It is well tolerated and highly effective in the treatment of severe diarrhoea, e.g. in AIDS patients." Stephan et al. Antibodies from colostrum in oral immunotherapy. *J Clin Chem Clin Biochem*. 1990 Jan;28(1):19-23
[1072] Pandolfi et al. T-dependent immunity in aged humans. Clinical and immunological evaluation after three months of thymic extract. *Thymus* 1983;5:235-40
[1073] Lavastida MT, Goldstein AL, Daniels JC. Thymosin administration in autoimmune disorders. *Thymus*. 1981 Feb;2(4-5):287-95
[1074] Thrower PA, Doyle DV, Scott J, Huskisson EC. Thymopoietin in rheumatoid arthritis. *Rheumatol Rehabil*. 1982 May;21(2):72-7
[1075] Malaise et al. Treatment of active rheumatoid arthritis with intravenous injections of thymopentin. *Lancet* 1985;1:832-6

dental disease, administration of thymus extract was shown to normalize immune function and reduce orodental dysbiosis.[1076]

6. **Hepatobiliary stimulation for IgA-complex removal**: The binding of immunoglobulin A (IgA) with antigen creates IgA immune complexes that contribute to tissue destruction by complement activation (alternate pathway) and other pathomechanisms in IgA nephropathy[1077], Henoch-Schonlein purpura[1078], rheumatoid vasculitis[1079], lupus[1080], and Sjogren's syndrome.[1081] Autoreactive IgA antibodies are a characteristic of lupus and Sjogren's syndrome[1082] and correlate strongly with disease activity in rheumatoid arthritis.[1083] **Immune complexes containing secretory IgA that has been reabsorbed from mucosal surfaces mediate many of the clinical phenomenon of dysbiosis-related musculoskeletal disease[1084], and these same IgA-containing immune complexes are eliminated from the systemic circulation via the liver and biliary system[1085,1086], thus providing the rationale for the use of botanicals and physiotherapeutics that promote liver function and bile flow in the treatment of IgA-mediated inflammatory disorders.** Numerous experimental studies in animals have shown that circulating IgA immune complexes are taken up by hepatocytes and then secreted into the bile for elimination.[1087,1088] The fact that bile duct obstruction retards systemic clearance of IgA immune complexes and that **normalization/optimization of bile flow reduces serum IgA levels by enhancing biliary excretion in animals[1089,1090] and humans[1091]** proves the importance of ensuring optimal hepatobiliary function and supports the use of botanical and physiological therapeutics that facilitate bile flow. A 1929 clinical study with human patients published in *Archives of Internal Medicine* provided irrefutable radiographic documentation that **therapeutic enemas safely and effectively stimulate bile flow for 45-60 minutes following administration[1092]**, and this finding, along with the obvious quantitative reduction in intestinal microbes induced by such "cleansing", helps explain the reported benefits of colonics/enemas in patients with systemic illness[1093,1094,1095,1096] and other immune-complex associated diseases such as cancer.[1097] Validation of this concept is demonstrated by the significant efficacy of immunoadsorption[1098] and plasmapheresis[1099,1100]

[1076] Manti F, Kornman K, Goldschneider I. Effects of an immunomodulating agent on peripheral blood lymphocytes and subgingival microflora in ligature-induced periodontitis. *Infect Immun*. 1984 Jul;45(1):172-9 pubmedcentral.gov/articlerender.fcgi?tool=pubmed&pubmedid=6234232

[1077] "...it is likely that the usual instance of IgA-associated glomerulonephritis is due to deposition of circulating immune complexes containing IgA." McPhaul JJ Jr. IgA-associated glomerulonephritis. *Annu Rev Med*. 1977;28:37-42

[1078] "... it is generally considered to be an immune complex-mediated disease characterized by the presence of polymeric IgA1 (pIgA1)-containing immune complexes predominantly in dermal, gastrointestinal, and glomerular capillaries. ...also been observed in the kidneys of patients with liver cirrhosis, dermatitis herpetiformis, celiac disease, and chronic inflammatory disease of the lung. " Rai A, Nast C, Adler S. Henoch-Schonlein purpura nephritis. *J Am Soc Nephrol*. 1999 Dec;10(12):2637-44

[1079] Voskuyl AE, Hazes JM, Zwinderman AH, Paleolog EM, van der Meer FJ, Daha MR, Breedveld FC. Diagnostic strategy for the assessment of rheumatoid vasculitis. *Ann Rheum Dis*. 2003 May;62(5):407-13 ard.bmjjournals.com/cgi/reprint/62/5/407

[1080] Sikander FF, Salgaonkar DS, Joshi VR. Cryoglobulin studies in systemic lupus erythematosus. *J Postgrad Med* 1989;35:139-43

[1081] Pourmand N, Wahren-Herlenius M, Gunnarsson I, et al. Ro/SSA and La/SSB specific IgA autoantibodies in serum of patients with Sjogren's syndrome and systemic lupus erythematosus. *Ann Rheum Dis*. 1999 Oct;58(10):623-9 ard.bmjjournals.com/cgi/content/full/58/10/623

[1082] Pourmand et al. Ro/SSA and La/SSB specific IgA autoantibodies in serum of patients with Sjogren's syndrome and systemic lupus erythematosus. *Ann Rheum Dis*. 1999 Oct;58(10):623-9

[1083] Jonsson T, Valdimarsson H. What about IgA rheumatoid factor in rheumatoid arthritis? *Ann Rheum Dis*. 1998 Jan;57(1):63-4

[1084] Inman RD. Antigens, the gastrointestinal tract, and arthritis. *Rheum Dis Clin North Am*. 1991 May;17(2):309-21

[1085] Russell MW, Brown TA, Claflin JL, Schroer K, Mestecky J. Immunoglobulin A-mediated hepatobiliary transport constitutes a natural pathway for disposing of bacterial antigens. *Infect Immun*. 1983 Dec;42(3):1041-8 pubmedcentral.gov/articlerender.fcgi?tool=pubmed&pubmedid=6642659

[1086] "The liver therefore appears to be singularly capable of transporting both free and complexed IgA into its secretion, the bile." Russell MW, Brown TA, Mestecky J. Preferential transport of IgA and IgA-immune complexes to bile compared with other external secretions. *Mol Immunol*. 1982 May;19(5):677-82

[1087] "These results indicate that mouse hepatocytes are involved in the uptake and hepatobiliary transport of pIgA and pIgA-IC of low mol. wt." Phillips JO, Komiyama K, Epps JM, Russell MW, Mestecky J. Role of hepatocytes in the uptake of IgA and IgA-containing immune complexes in mice. *Mol Immunol*. 1988 Sep;25(9):873-9

[1088] "Thus hepatobiliary transport appears to be the major pathway for the clearance of both IgA IC and free IgA from the circulation." Brown TA, Russell MW, Kulhavy R, Mestecky J. IgA-mediated elimination of antigens by the hepatobiliary route. *Fed Proc*. 1983 Dec;42(15):3218-21

[1089] "Clearance of IgA immune complexes was delayed after bile duct ligation." Harmatz PR, Kleinman RE, Bunnell BW, McClenathan DT, Walker WA, Bloch KJ. The effect of bile duct obstruction on the clearance of circulating IgA immune complexes. *Hepatology*. 1984 Jan-Feb;4(1):96-101

[1090] Lemaitre-Coelho I, et al. High levels of secretory IgA and free secretory component in the serum of rats with bile duct obstruction. *J Exp Med*. 1978 Mar 1;147:934-9

[1091] "CONCLUSIONS: Biliary obstruction secondary to both calculus or malignancy of the hepatobiliary system causes suppression of bile IgA secretion and elevated serum level of secretory IgA. Bile secretory IgA secretion recovers with endoscopic drainage of the obstructed system." Sung JJ, Leung JC, Tsui CP, Chung SS, Lai KN. Biliary IgA secretion in obstructive jaundice: the effects of endoscopic drainage. *Gastrointest Endosc*. 1995 Nov;42(5):439-44

[1092] Garbat AL, Jacobi HG. Secretion of Bile in Response to Rectal Installations. *Arch Intern Med* 1929; 44: 455-462

[1093] Crinnion WJ. Results of a decade of naturopathic treatment for environmental illnesses. *J Naturopathic Med* 1994;17:21-27

[1094] Snyder RG. The value of colonic irrigations in countering auto-intoxication of intestinal origin. *Medical Clinics of North America* 1939; May: 781-788

[1095] Marshall HK, Thomson CR. Colon irrigation in the treatment of mental disease. *N Engl J Med* 1932; 207 (Sept 8): 454-7

[1096] Bastedo WA. Colon irrigations: their administration, therapeutic applications, and dangers. *Journal of the American Medical Association* 1932; 98(9): 734-6

[1097] Gonzalez NJ, Isaacs LL. Evaluation of pancreatic proteolytic enzyme treatment of adenocarcinoma of the pancreas, with nutrition and detoxification support. *Nutr Cancer*. 1999;33(2):117-24

[1098] Braun N, Erley C, Klein R, Kotter I, Saal J, Risler T. Immunoadsorption onto protein A induces remission in severe systemic lupus erythematosus. *Nephrol Dial Transplant*. 2000 Sep;15(9):1367-72 ndt.oxfordjournals.org/cgi/reprint/15/9/1367

[1099] Santos-Ocampo AS, Mandell BF, Fessler BJ. Alveolar hemorrhage in systemic lupus erythematosus: presentation and management. *Chest*. 2000 Oct;118(4):1083-90 chestjournal.org/cgi/content/full/118/4/1083

[1100] Choi BG, Yoo WH. Successful treatment of pure red cell aplasia with plasmapheresis in a patient with systemic lupus erythematosus. *Yonsei Med J*. 2002 Apr;43(2):274-8 eymj.org/2002/pdf/04274.pdf (techniques for removing immune complexes) in patients with lupus. Furthermore, this directly supports the naturopathic concept of "treating the liver" in patients with systemic disease by the use of dietary and botanical therapeutics that stimulate bile flow, such as beets, ginger[1101], curcumin/turmeric[1102], *Picrorhiza*[1103], milk thistle[1104], *Andrographis paniculata*[1105], and *Boerhaavia diffusa*.[1106] Investigation of an antirheumatic benefit from phytophysiotherapeutic hepatobiliary stimulation is worthy of clinical trials with pre- and post-intervention measurement of serum immune complexes and other clinical indexes.[1107]

7. **Ensure generous bowel movements and consider therapeutic purgatives** (*purge: to free from impurities*): Dysbiotic patients should consume a low-fermentation fiber-rich diet that allows for 1-2 very generous bowel movements per day. Constipation must absolutely be eliminated—pun intended; for patients being treated for dysbiosis of any type, constipation is absolutely unacceptable, since the gastrointestinal tract provides the largest burden of pro-inflammatory (e.g., endotoxin, bacterial DNA) and anti-metabolic (e.g., D-lactate, H2S) microbial debris and metabolites. Patients with severe or recalcitrant dysbiosis can start the day with a laxative dose of ascorbic acid (e.g., 20-60 grams with 4 cups of water) and should expect liquid diarrhea within 30-60 minutes. The goal here is purgative physical removal of enteric microbes; in high concentrations, ascorbic acid has a direct antibacterial effect. Magnesium in elemental doses of 500-1,500 mg also helps soften stool and promote laxation. One-two cups of coffee promotes the laxative effect and provides some sense of pleasure to an otherwise not-so-pleasant experience; however, dysbiosis-affected patients often feel impressively better following therapeutic laxation. Rapid-acting antimicrobials, such as iodine/iodide, can be coadministered. Electrolyte replacement, for example with salted vegetable juice, is advisable for patients using therapeutic laxation on a regular basis.

2013 INTERNATIONAL CONFERENCE ON HUMAN NUTRITION AND FUNCTIONAL MEDICINE
PORTLAND OREGON CONVENTION CENTER • SEPTEMBER 25-29, 2013

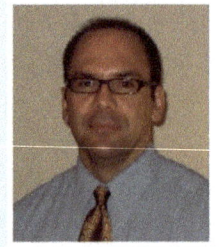

Antirheumatic Use of Antimicrobial Drugs with Neuroendocrine Interventions in the Treatment of Autoimmunity
Alex Vasquez D.C., N.D., D.O., F.A.C.N.

2013 presentation and slides:
- Presentation slides: CreateSpace.com/4478800
- Video access: vimeo.com/ichnfm/drv2013dysbiosisdrugs
- Password: DrV2013DysbiosisDrugs.

The clinical implementation of an anti-dysbiosis program must be tailored to the patient's overall condition and his/her willingness to implement the above-mentioned treatment options. Some patients are only willing to take a few treatments, while empowered autonomous nonmasochistic patients are more willing to do **whatever is necessary** in order to regain their health, even if it means taking numerous supplements, improving diet, starting/ending the day with enemas, and making appropriate changes in lifestyle and relationships to improve immune function. To the extent that we *first, do no harm*, all of the above-mentioned therapeutic interventions are reasonable "alternatives" to life-long medicalization, surgery, and immune-system destroying high-dose chemotherapy, which is astoundingly expensive, highly hazardous, and incompletely effective. **Patients**

[1101] "Further analyses for the active constituents of the acetone extracts through column chromatography indicated that [6]-gingerol and [10]-gingerol, which are the pungent principles, are mainly responsible for the cholagogic effect of ginger." Yamahara J, Miki K, Chisaka T, Sawada T, Fujimura H, Tomimatsu T, Nakano K, Nohara T. Cholagogic effect of ginger and its active constituents. *J Ethnopharmacol*. 1985;13(2):217-25

[1102] "On the basis of the present findings, it appears that curcumin induces contraction of the human gall-bladder." Rasyid A, Lelo A. The effect of curcumin and placebo on human gall-bladder function: an ultrasound study. *Aliment Pharmacol Ther*. 1999 Feb;13(2):245-9

[1103] "Significant anticholestatic activity was also observed against carbon tetrachloride induced cholestasis in conscious rat, anaesthetized guinea pig and cat. Picroliv was more active than the known hepatoprotective drug silymarin." Saraswat B, Visen PK, Patnaik GK, Dhawan BN. Anticholestatic effect of picroliv, active hepatoprotective principle of Picrorhiza kurrooa, against carbon tetrachloride induced cholestasis. *Indian J Exp Biol*. 1993 Apr;31(4):316-8

[1104] "We conclude that SIL counteracts TLC-induced cholestasis by preventing the impairment in both the BS-dependent and -independent fractions of the bile flow." Crocenzi FA, Sanchez Pozzi EJ, Pellegrino JM, Rodriguez Garay EA, Mottino AD, Roma MG. Preventive effect of silymarin against taurolithocholate-induced cholestasis in the rat. *Biochem Pharmacol*. 2003 Jul 15;66(2):355-64

[1105] "Andrographolide from the herb Andrographis paniculata (whole plant) per se produces a significant dose (1.5-12 mg/kg) dependent choleretic effect (4.8-73%) as evidenced by increase in bile flow, bile salt, and bile acids in conscious rats and anaesthetized guinea pigs." Shukla B, Visen PK, Patnaik GK, Dhawan BN. Choleretic effect of andrographolide in rats and guinea pigs. *Planta Med*. 1992 Apr;58(2):146-9

[1106] "The extract also produced an increase in normal bile flow in rats suggesting a strong choleretic activity." Chandan BK, Sharma AK, Anand KK. Boerhaavia diffusa: a study of its hepatoprotective activity. *J Ethnopharmacol*. 1991 Mar;31(3):299-307

[1107] Vasquez A. Do the Benefits of Botanical and Physiotherapeutic Hepatobiliary Stimulation Result From Enhanced Excretion of IgA Immune Complexes? *Naturopathy Digest* 2006; January: naturopathydigest.com/archives/2006/jan/vasquez_immune.php with autoimmune diseases have numerous, largely untapped options for the treatment of their autoimmune diseases; therefore, (pseudo)justifying lethal and expensive and devastating medical interventions on the basis of a "lack of other treatment alternatives"[1108] when reasonable, safe, and effective options have not been implemented is scientifically inaccurate, ethically untenable, and medicolegally questionable.

Santiago De Compostela: "Many chains have been laid upon man so that he should no longer behave like an animal, and he has in truth become gentler, more spiritual, more joyful, more reflective than any other animal is. Now, however, he suffers: from having worn his chains for so long, from being deprived for so long of clean air and free movement. These chains are those heavy and pregnant errors contained in the conceptions of morality, religion and metaphysics. Only when this sickness from one's chains has also been overcome will the first great goal have truly been attained: the separation of man from the animals. We stand now in the midst of our work of removing these chains, and we need to proceed with the greatest caution." Nietzsche FW. *Human, All Too Human*, Section: The Wanderer and His Shadow

---

[1108] Binks M, Passweg JR, Furst D, et al. Phase I/II trial of autologous stem cell transplantation in systemic sclerosis: procedure related mortality and impact on skin disease. *Ann Rheum Dis*. 2001 Jun;60(6):577-84 ard.bmjjournals.com/cgi/content/full/60/6/577

❶ Food ❷ Infections ❸ Nutri-immunomod ❹ Dysmetab ❺ Stress/Sleep/Socio/Surg/Sup ❻ Endo ❼ Xeno

❸ Nutritional Immunomodulation:
Nutritional Interventions to Induce Regulatory T-cells (Treg)

> **Major Concepts in this Section**
>
> "Inflammatory balance" is largely a biochemical endpoint whereas "immune balance" refers more directly to immunophenotypic predominance. In this section, I will outline a nutrition-based clinical protocol for the induction of active cell-mediated anti-inflammation via selective induction of regulatory T-cells ("Treg"). The goal with this component of the functional Inflammology protocol is to utilize the body's own immunomodulating ability by providing the appropriate nutritional climate for epigenetic upregulation of expression of the transcription factor FoxP3, which is the main identifier of the Treg phenotype. Components of this protocol are proven to provide clinical benefit; this nutritional immunomodulation protocol performs best when utilized within an intact functional inflammology protocol, as described throughout this chapter.

Anti-inflammatory/anti-allergy/antirheumatic nutritional immunomodulation: Although the term "nutritional immunomodulation" can be used to include nearly any dietary pattern or nutrient intake that has a meaningful effect on immune function (in which case, the term would encompass the totality of all food and nutrient intake), in this section I will use the term to specifically denote epigenetic induction of regulatory T-cells (Treg) from their precursors—the undifferentiated (indicated by the number zero, or "0") naïve T-helper cells—known as Th0 cells. This is a new, exciting, and remarkably well-documented therapeutic tool that we now have in our food-based armamentarium in the battles against common immune diseases such as metabolic inflammation (e.g., diabetes mellitus and the metabolic syndrome), allergy (e.g., asthma) and autoimmunity (e.g., psoriasis, rheumatoid arthritis, SLE, and multiple sclerosis). For this discussion of nutritional immunomodulation, readers need a practical understanding of the following cell types, their nutritional influences and physiologic/pathologic effects:

> **Treg/Th17 imbalance = autoimmunity**
> "Imbalance between effector and regulatory T-cells (Treg) underlies the loss of immune-tolerance to self-antigens in autoimmune disease."
> Holder et al. *J Autoimmun*. 2014 Feb

- CD3(+)CD4(-)CD8(-) double negative T cells: These cells arrived from the bone marrow to the thymus, but have not yet been fully "programed" for their ultimate functions; however, these cells are not benign and appear to contribute to autoimmune-type inflammation via necrotic-inflammatory cell death via a mechanism that is activated by mitochondrial dysfunction: activation of mTOR.
- Th0—naive T-cells: These cells have been "partially programmed" to become effector cells, particularly Th1, Th2, Th17, or T-regulatory cells.
- Th1 cells: Contribute to cell-mediated "chronic inflammation."
- Th2 cells: Contribute to antibody-mediated inflammation, allergies, and formation of autoreactive antibodies such as ANA.
- Th17 cells: Contribute very significantly to autoimmune-type inflammation as seen in SLE and multiple sclerosis.
- T-regulatory cells (Treg): Treg are immunomodulatory and generally anti-inflammatory; they dampen the activity of Th1, Th2, Th17 cells, and thereby promote *active* anti-inflammation and immune tolerance to self and environment. Treg surface markers are CD4 and CD25; the transcription factor is FOXp3. Two main subtypes of Treg exist: "natural Tregs" (nTregs) are thymically derived; "induced Tregs" (iTregs) are converted in the periphery in the gastrointestinal associated lymphoid tissue (GALT) from CD4+ CD25- Foxp3- effector T-cells (Teffs). Clinicians need to pay attention to the fact that dietary interventions (or dietary negligence) can affect GALT function and directly and potently promote Treg induction (or Th17 induction); furthermore, iTregs maintain their induced Treg phenotype and function only if the conditions for such are favorable—namely: proper nutritional environment in the absence of microbial pathogens.

Again, the fact that the distinction between Treg (immune tolerance) and Th17 (inflammation, autoimmunity) occurs in the GALT makes the importance of diet and gastrointestinal eubiosis/dysbiosis so obvious that refutation of the importance of these environmental determinants for shaping immunologic health is on the verge of being obscene. Further, the facts that nTreg cells produce TGF-beta and iTreg cells produce IL-10 gives prominence to iTreg for active immunosuppression and thus gives prominence to the following nutritional immunomodulation protocol as a key component of any modern treatment plan for inflammatory, allergic, or autoimmune disease.

- γδ T cells, gamma delta T cells: Gamma-delta T-cells are notorious for their promotion of autoimmunity and allergic inflammation, at least in part via their production of IL-17; one animal study has shown that the population of gamma-delta T-cells is doubled by consumption of genetically modified food (corn).

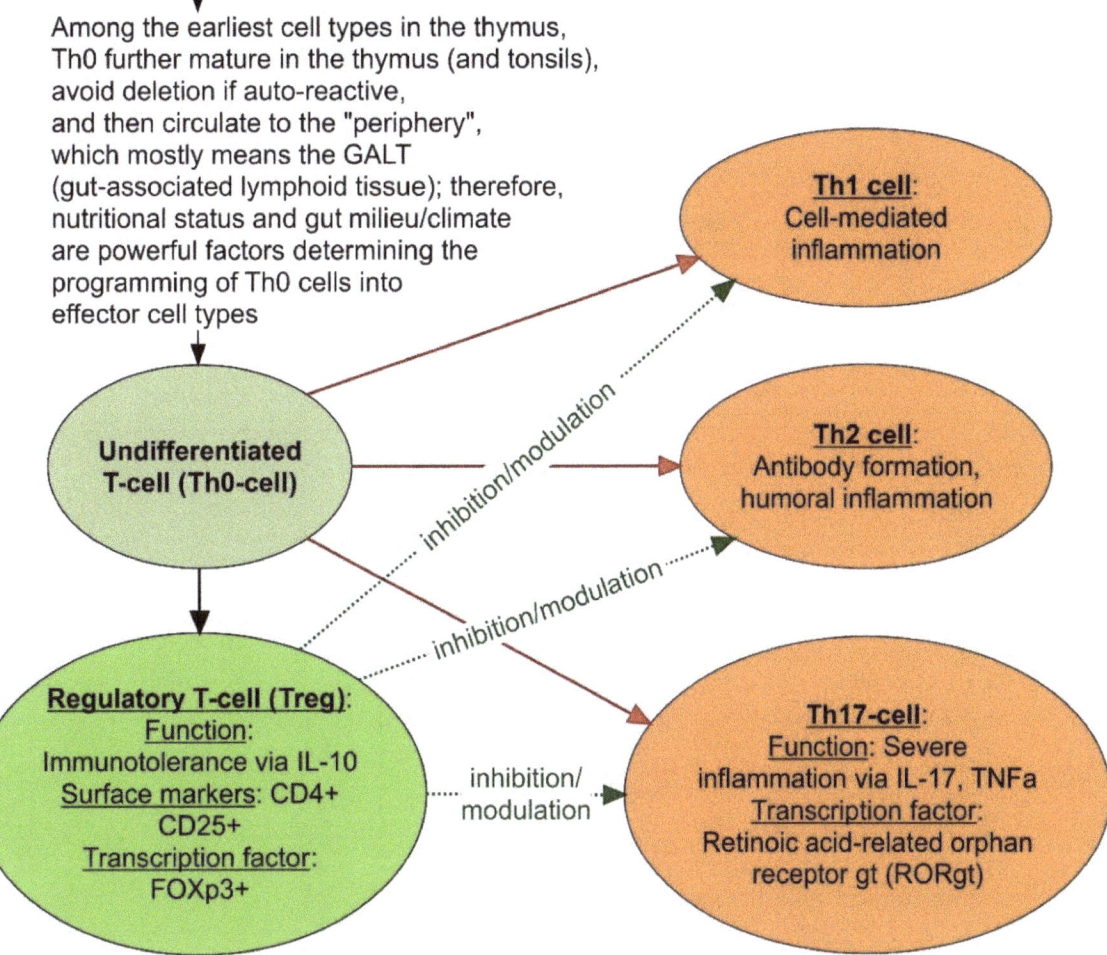

Immunophenotype determination per inflammatory/microbial/nutritional climate: The cytokine climate, nutritional status, and microbial balance determine which immunocyte phenotype will be selected. If the climate is "hostile" then pro-inflammatory immunocytes will be selected; if nutritional needs are met and the internal milieu is relatively un-inflamed and un-infected, then tolerogenic T-regulatory cells will predominate. Thus, when dealing with disorders of sustained inflammation/allergy/autoimmunity, the task of the physician is to create or re-create the conditions for immunotolerance to predominate. Regulatory T-cells (Treg) provide anti-inflammatory immunomodulation and are characterized by the surface markers CD4 CD25 and transcription factor FOXp3 while Th-17 cells promote severe inflammation, autoimmunity, and are marked by the transcription factor RORγt—retinoic acid-related orphan receptor γt, also known as RORC in humans.

DrV's "recipe" for optimized induction of the Treg phenotype is as follows: I first published this protocol in 2012 in *Functional Immunology and Nutritional Immunomodulation*[1109], and I am happy to see that clinical trials have now validated the last outstanding component of the protocol; thus now all components of the protocol are supported by clinical trials in humans. Of additional note regarding the induction of Treg versus Th-17 cells, I have chosen to not discuss transforming growth factor-β (TGF-β, TGF-beta) since this cytokine is clearly nondeterministic with regard to Treg/Th-17 induction; TGF-beta can stimulate both/either Treg/Th-17 induction depending on other cytokines and determinants, and thus these deciding factors should be the recipients of our attention.

- Mitochondrial optimization, mTOR inhibition: Recently, mitochondrial dysfunction in general and mTOR activation in particular has been shown to inhibit induction of Treg cells; inhibition of mTOR with NAC 4,800mg/d in divided doses was shown to inhibit mTOR and promote induction of the FoxP3 phenotype Treg cells and result in clinical alleviation of disease in patients with SLE. My basic, foundational, and initial protocol for optimizing mitochondrial function includes: carbohydrate avoidance and/or MTC/caprylate supplementation to enhance endogenous production of BHB, moderate physical exercise/activity 1 h/d, CoQ10 100 mg/d, NAC 1,500 mg TID, lipoic acid 200-400 mg TID, acetyl-carnitine 1 g BID-QID, and biotin 1-10 mg/d.
    - N-acetylcysteine reduces disease activity by blocking mammalian target of rapamycin in T cells from systemic lupus erythematosus patients (*Arthritis Rheum* 2012 Sep[1110]): "NAC up to 2.4 gm/day was tolerated by all patients, while 33% of those receiving 4.8 gm/day had reversible nausea. ... Considered together, 2.4 gm and 4.8 gm NAC reduced the SLEDAI score after 1 month, 2 months, 3 months (P = 0.0030), and 4 months; the BILAG score after 1 month and 3 months; and the FAS score after 2 months and 3 months. NAC increased Δψm [mitochondrial inner membrane potential] in all T cells, profoundly reduced mTOR activity, enhanced apoptosis, reversed expansion of CD4-CD8- T cells, stimulated FoxP3 expression in CD4+CD25+ T cells, and reduced anti-DNA production. CONCLUSION: This pilot study suggests that NAC safely improves lupus disease activity by blocking mTOR in T lymphocytes."
- Biotin: Normal dietary intake of biotin is less than 97.5 microg (0.4 micromol); genotropic biotinopathy is treated with pharmacological/supranutritional doses of biotin 5–20 mg/d in children and adults while some patients may require higher doses of 40–200 mg/d.[1111] Biotin is necessary for histone biotinylation; the effect is dose-dependent, regional, and repressive[1112], notably of TNF-alpha gene transcription—correspondingly, biotin deficiency promotes inflammation while biotin supplementation reduces inflammation.[1113]
    - Biotin deficiency up-regulates and biotin supplementation reduces TNF-alpha production in murine macrophages (*J Leukoc Biol* 2008 Apr): Significant decreases in serum biotin levels have been reported in patients with chronic inflammatory diseases. Cell proliferation and biotinylation of intracellular proteins were decreased significantly in biotin-deficient cells compared with biotin-sufficient cells, and this corresponded with significantly higher production and mRNA expression of TNF-alpha. TNF-alpha induction by biotin deficiency was down-regulated by biotin supplementation in vitro and in vivo. These results show that biotin deficiency up-regulates TNF-alpha production and that biotin supplementation down-regulates TNF-alpha production, suggesting that biotin status may influence inflammatory diseases.
    - Biotin supplementation at a pharmacologic dose decreases proliferation rates of human peripheral blood mononuclear cells (PBMC) and decreases cytokine release (*J Nutr* 2001 May[1114]): Oral administration of biotin 756.1 microg/d (3.1 micromol/d) for 14 d "caused a significant decrease of PBMC proliferation. At 2 d after mitogen stimulation, [3H]thymidine uptake by postsupplementation PBMC was 66 % of the uptake by presupplementation PBMC. Similarly, concentrations of interleukin-1β (2 d after mitogen) and interleukin-2 (1 d after mitogen) in media

---

[1109] Vasquez A. *Functional Immunology and Nutritional Immunomodulation*. Published June 5, 2012, ISBN-10: 1477603859, ISBN-13: 978-1477603857
[1110] Lai ZW et al. N-acetylcysteine reduces disease activity by blocking mammalian target of rapamycin in T cells from systemic lupus erythematosus patients: a randomized, double-blind, placebo-controlled trial. *Arthritis Rheum*. 2012 Sep;64(9):2937-46
[1111] Baumgartner MR. Vitamin-responsive disorders: cobalamin, folate, biotin, vitamins B1 and E. *Handb Clin Neurol*. 2013;113:1799-810
[1112] Hassan YI, Zempleni J. A novel, enigmatic histone modification: biotinylation of histones by holocarboxylase synthetase. *Nutr Rev*. 2008 Dec;66(12):721-5
[1113] Kuroishi T, Endo Y, Muramoto K, Sugawara S. Biotin deficiency up-regulates TNF-alpha production in murine macrophages. *J Leukoc Biol*. 2008 Apr;83(4):912-20
[1114] Per the authors 2.46 micromol = 600 microg, and thus 3.1 micromol = 756.1 microg. Zempleni J, Helm RM, Mock DM. In vivo biotin supplementation at a pharmacologic dose decreases proliferation rates of human peripheral blood mononuclear cells and cytokine release. *J Nutr*. 2001 May;131(5):1479-84

from postsupplementation PBMC were 65% and 44%, respectively, of those for presupplementation PBMC. ... Overall, this study provides evidence that administration of pharmacologic doses of biotin [756.1 microg/d] for 14 d decreases PBMC proliferation and synthesis of interleukin-1β and interleukin-2." These impressive results show that low-dose orally administered biotin reduces monocyte proliferation by -34%, IL-1 by -35%, and IL-2 by -56%.

- Vitamin E: The *gamma* form of tocopherol inhibits cyclooxygenase and has anti-inflammatory activity.[1115] Alpha-tocopherol has been shown to decrease CRP levels in patients with CVD and in those with risk factors for CVD; alpha-tocopherol inhibits protein kinase C, 5-lipoxygenase, tyrosine-kinase, and cyclooxygenase-2.[1116] Clinical trials and case reports have demonstrated benefit of vitamin E supplementation in patients with rheumatoid arthritis[1117,1118], spondylosis[1119] and osteoarthritis[1120], and autoimmune diseases including scleroderma, discoid lupus erythematosus, porphyria cutanea tarda, vasculitis, and polymyositis.[1121,1122,1123] In 2013, we as clinicians gained valuable insight into the mechanism of action of vitamin E thanks to the work of Salinthone et al[1124] who showed that, rather than functioning simply/solely as an antioxidant, vitamin E significantly raises cyclic adenosine monophosphate (cAMP) levels and thereby has an anti-inflammatory effect; they showed that "vitamin E resulted in a greater than 2-fold increase in cAMP level (29.19 pmol/mg protein) compared to baseline. Lipoic acid was used as a positive control, which generated 45.49 pmol/mg protein of cAMP." Elevation of cAMP—such as by alpha-tocopherol and lipoic acid—results in a dose-dependent inhibition of inflammatory IL-2 and IL-17 cytokine generation and by this mechanism—additive/synergistic with the antioxidant and mitochondrial-supportive effects—reduces inflammation. Most cAMP-elevating agents demonstrate anti-inflammatory actions by increasing production of anti-inflammatory IL-10 and reducing production of pro-inflammatory TNF-alpha.[1125]

Vitamin E nutritional immunomodulation
Vitamin E increases:
• IL-10
• Antioxidant defenses
• Mitochondrial performance
Vitamin E decreases:
• Protein kinase C
• 5-lipoxygenase
• Tyrosine-kinase
• Cyclooxygenase-2
• IL-2
• IL-17
• TNF-alpha
• IgE
• CRP
• Serum AGE

    - Vitamin E for atopic dermatitis and effect on immunoglobulin E (*Int J Dermatol*. 2002 Mar[1126]): This notable placebo (PL)-controlled study used "natural origin" vitamin E (VE) 400 IU (268 mg) in 96 subjects with atopic dermatitis and for 8 months and found that "23 of the 50 subjects treated with VE showed great improvement, compared to only one in the PL group; and almost complete remission of atopic dermatitis in seven of the 50 subjects in the VE group, but none in the PL group. ... Subjects with great improvement and near remission of atopic dermatitis in the VE group demonstrated a decrease of 62% in serum IgE levels based on initial conditions, while, in subjects taking PL, the difference was approximately 34.4%. ... A remarkable improvement in facial

---

[1115] Jiang Q, Christen S, Shigenaga MK, Ames BN. gamma-tocopherol, the major form of vitamin E in the US diet, deserves more attention. *Am J Clin Nutr* 2001;74(6):714-22
[1116] Singh et al. Vitamin E, oxidative stress, and inflammation. *Annu Rev Nutr*. 2005;25:151-74
[1117] Helmy M, Shohayeb M, Helmy MH, el-Bassiouni EA. Antioxidants as adjuvant therapy in rheumatoid disease. A preliminary study. *Arzneimittelforschung*. 2001;51(4):293-8
[1118] Edmonds SE, et al. Putative analgesic activity of repeated oral doses of vitamin E in the treatment of rheumatoid arthritis. *Ann Rheum Dis*. 1997 Nov;56(11):649-55
[1119] "Vitamin E administration at a dose of 100 mg daily for three weeks resulted in a significant increase in serum vitamin E level accompanied by complete relief of pain... The results therefore strongly indicate that vitamin E is effective in curing spondylosis and most probably due to its antioxidant activity." Mahmud Z, Ali SM. Role of vitamin A and E in spondylosis. *Bangladesh Med Res Counc Bull*. 1992 Apr;18(1):47-59. See also "The results of this double-blind controlled clinical trial showed that vitamin E was superior to placebo with respect to the relief of pain (pain at rest, pain during movement, pressure-induced pain) and the necessity of additional analgesic treatment. Improvement of mobility was better in the group treated with vitamin E." Blankenhorn G. [Clinical effectiveness of Spondyvit (vitamin E) in activated arthroses. A multicenter placebo-controlled double-blind study] [Article in German—information from abstract] *Z Orthop Ihre Grenzgeb* 1986;124:340-3. See also This is a very interesting study because the clinical response to vitamin E was proportional to the increase in plasma levels of vitamin E, thus confirming the dose-response relationship that implies causality as well as indicating that the failure of such treatment in some patients may be due to malabsorption or unquenchable systemic oxidative stress rather than the inefficacy of vitamin E supplementation, per se. "There were no significant differences in the efficacy of the two drugs, although one patient of the V-group refused further treatment after 8 days because of inefficacy. V reduced or abolished the pain at rest in 77% (D in 85%), the pain on pressure in 67% (D in 50%), and the pain on movement in 62% (D in 63%). Both treatments appeared to be equally effective in reducing the circumference of the knee joints (p = 0.001) and the walking time (p less than 0.001) and in increasing the joint mobility (p less than 0.002)." Scherak O, et al. [High dosage vitamin E therapy in patients with activated arthrosis] [Article in German—information from abstract] *Z Rheumatol*. 1990 Nov-Dec;49(6):369-73
[1120] Machtey I, Ouaknine L. Tocopherol in Osteoarthritis: a controlled pilot study. *J Am Geriatr Soc*. 1978 Jul;26(7):328-30
[1121] Killeen RN, Ayres S Jr, Mihan R. Polymyositis: response to vitamin E. *South Med J*. 1976 Oct;69(10):1372-4
[1122] Ayres S Jr, Mihan R. Lupus erythematosus and vitamin E: an effective and nontoxic therapy. *Cutis*. 1979 Jan;23(1):49-52, 54
[1123] Ayres S Jr, Mihan R. Is vitamin E involved in the autoimmune mechanism? *Cutis*. 1978 Mar;21(3):321-5
[1124] Salinthone et al. α-Tocopherol stimulates cyclic AMP production in human peripheral mononuclear cells and alters immune function. *Mol Immunol*. 2013 Mar;53(3):173-8
[1125] Eigler et al. Anti-inflammatory activities of cAMP-elevating agents: enhancement of IL-10 synthesis and suppression of TNF production. *J Leukoc Biol*. 1998 Jan;63(1):101-7
[1126] Tsoureli-Nikita et al. Evaluation of dietary intake of vitamin E in the treatment of atopic dermatitis: a study of the clinical course and evaluation of the immunoglobulin E serum levels. *Int J Dermatol*. 2002 Mar;41(3):146-50

erythema, lichenification, and the presence of apparently normal skin was reported. Eczematous lesions healed mostly as a result of decreased pruritus."
- o No effect of ineffective nondescript vitamin E supplementation on nasal symptoms and specific IgE levels in patients with perennial allergic rhinitis (*Ann Allergy Asthma Immunol.* 2006 Jan[1127]): This clinical trial by Velazquez et al showed no benefit of "vitamin E 400 IU/d" in symptoms nor IgE levels; importantly however, 1) the authors did not specify the type or source of "vitamin E" that was used and therefore we might assume that it was the inexpensive ineffective DL racemic mixture, 2) serum lipid peroxides did not change, thus strongly suggesting inefficacy and lack of potency of the vitamin E supplement used, and 3) the study was conducted in an industrial region of Mexico City, an area internationally notorious for severe airborne pollution. Further differentiating this study and greatly reducing the opportunity to observe efficacy was the assessment of specific (very limited) IgE rather than total IgE.

- Transgenic food avoidance: Per the animal study summarized below, the finding that GMO corn—but not natural corn—lead to increases in IL-6 (which promotes Th-17 cell development, as well as cardiometabolic disease) and gamma-delta T cells (which also produce tissue-damaging IL-17) is sufficient to mechanistically connect GMO foods with inflammatory and dysmetabolic disease in humans. Thus, the implications of this data are that, given that gamma-delta T-cells make IL-17, currently the most notorious cytokine in autoimmune inflammation, humans should avoid GMO foods.
  - o Intestinal and peripheral immune response to MON810 maize ingestion in weaning and old mice (*J Agric Food Chem* 2008 Dec[1128]): The authors' abstract understates the importance of their findings, noting immune system abnormalities and an increase in the pro-inflammatory cytokine IL-6 following consumption of GMO corn compared with natural corn. The increase in IL-6 is by itself significant, given the role of inflammation in essentially all human diseases and the ability of IL-6 to induce Th-17 phenotype characteristic of more severe allergic and autoimmune diseases. However, per my reading of the full text of the article, I find this article to sound the alarm on GMO foods per the authors' report, "One of the more recurrent alterations in lymphocyte phenotypes observed in this study was an increase in the TCRγδ+ (gamma-delta T-cells) population. A high percentage of these lymphocytes are localized in the gut and … γδT cells seem to be important regulatory elements of the immune system, being capable of modulating inflammatory response associated with infectious agents and autoantigens. Higher numbers of γδT cells have been observed in humans with asthma, in intraepithelial lymphocytes (IELs) of children with untreated food allergy, and in the duodenum of children with juvenile idiopathic arthritis or connective tissue disease with gastrointestinal symptoms." Further, gamma-delta T-cells are known to secrete IL-17, the cytokine responsible for the massive tissue damage seen in autoimmune diseases such as multiple sclerosis, rheumatoid arthritis, and psoriasis, and which is also elevated in autism.[1129]

- Sodium avoidance: Sodium—independent from the chloride anion—induces the Th17 phenotype via induction of serum glucocorticoid kinase 1 (SGK1) which stabilizes the IL-23 receptor necessary for maintaining the Th17 phenotype and inflammatory disease.
  - o Sodium drives autoimmune disease by induction of pathogenic TH17 cells (*Nature* 2013 Apr[1130]): Changes in environmental factors must ultimately be driving the marked increase in the incidence of autoimmune diseases in the past half-century. "The newly identified population of interleukin (IL)-17-producing CD4(+) helper T cells (TH17 cells) has a pivotal role in autoimmune diseases. … Here we show that increased salt (sodium chloride, NaCl) concentrations found locally under physiological conditions in vivo markedly boost the induction of murine and human TH17 cells. … The TH17 cells generated under high-salt conditions display a highly pathogenic and stable phenotype characterized by the upregulation of the pro-inflammatory cytokines GM-CSF, TNF-α

[1127] Montaño Velázquez BB, et al. Vitamin E effects on nasal symptoms and serum specific IgE levels in patients with perennial allergic rhinitis. *Ann Allergy Asthma Immunol*. 2006 Jan;96(1):45-50
[1128] Finamore et al. Intestinal and peripheral immune response to MON810 maize ingestion in weaning and old mice. *J Agric Food Chem*. 2008 Dec 10;56(23):11533-9
[1129] Al-Ayadhi LY, Mostafa GA. Elevated serum levels of interleukin-17A in children with autism. *J Neuroinflammation*. 2012 Jul 2;9:158
[1130] Kleinewietfeld et al. Sodium chloride drives autoimmune disease by the induction of pathogenic TH17 cells. *Nature*. 2013 Apr 25;496(7446):518-22

and IL-2. ... Thus, increased dietary salt intake might represent an environmental risk factor for the development of autoimmune diseases through the induction of pathogenic TH17 cells."
- Induction of pathogenic TH17 cells by sodium (*Nature* 2013 Apr[1131]): "TH17 cells (interleukin-17 (IL-17)-producing helper T cells) are highly proinflammatory cells that are critical for clearing extracellular pathogens and for inducing multiple autoimmune diseases. IL-23 has a critical role in stabilizing and reinforcing the TH17 phenotype by increasing expression of IL-23 receptor (IL-23R) and endowing TH17 cells with pathogenic effector functions." Here, the researchers discovered that serum glucocorticoid kinase 1 (SGK1), a serine/threonine kinase, is critical for regulating IL-23R expression and stabilizing the TH17 cell phenotype and that a modest increase in salt concentration induces SGK1 expression, promotes IL-23R expression and enhances TH17 cell differentiation in vitro and in vivo, accelerating the development of autoimmunity. "These data demonstrate that SGK1 has a critical role in the induction of pathogenic TH17 cells and provide a molecular insight into a mechanism by which an environmental factor such as a high salt diet triggers TH17 development and promotes tissue inflammation."

- **Probiotics**: Molecular signatures from probiotic bacteria synergize to promote epigenetic induction of Treg cells; probiotic metabolites—particularly butyrate—also promote the histone acetylation which is a common theme in FoxP3 induction.

> **Probiotic regulatory immunomodulation**
> Components:
> 1. *Lactobacillus acidophilus* (LA),
> 2. *Lactobacillus casei* (LC),
> 3. *Lactobacillus reuteri* (LR),
> 4. *Bifidobacterium bifidium* (BB),
> 5. *Streptococcus thermophilus* (ST).
>
> Effects:
> - Induction of T-cell and B-cell hyporesponsiveness,
> - Suppression of Th1, Th2, and Th17 cytokines,
> - Induction and maintenance of CD4(+)Foxp3(+) Tregs,
> - Alleviation of intestinal hyperpermeability, allergy, inflammation, autoimmunity.
>
> Noted: Kwon et al, *Proc Natl Acad Sci* 2010 Feb

- Probiotics induce Treg at the expense of Th-1/2/17 (*Clin Exp Allergy* 2014 Apr[1132]): "There is emerging evidence that resident symbionts induce tolerogenic gut-associated Treg cells and dendritic cells that ensure the preferential growth of symbionts; keeping pathogenic strains in check and constraining proinflammatory Th1, Th2 and Th17 clones."
- Regulatory dendritic cells and CD4+Foxp3+ T cells by probiotics administration suppresses immune disorders (*Proc Natl Acad Sci* 2010 Feb[1133]): "Administration of probiotics had therapeutical effects in experimental inflammatory bowel disease, atopic dermatitis, and rheumatoid arthritis. The therapeutic effect of the probiotics is associated with enrichment of CD4(+)Foxp3(+) Tregs in the inflamed regions. Collectively, the administration of probiotics that enhance the generation of rDCs and Tregs represents an applicable treatment of inflammatory immune disorders."

- **Lipoic acid**: LA is an antioxidant and direct inhibitor of NFkB; a clinical trial in humans with multiple sclerosis showed that lipoic acid 400mg PO TID reduced IL-17 levels by 35-50%—the clinical importance of this is massive, given that IL-17 is a major effector of tissue destruction in autoimmune diseases.
  - Lipoic acid attenuates inflammation via cAMP and protein kinase A signaling (*PLoS One* 2010 Sep[1134]): "Oral administration of 1200 mg LA to MS subjects resulted in increased cAMP levels in PBMCs four hours after ingestion. Average cAMP levels in 20 subjects were 43% higher than baseline. ... [In vitro] We show that LA reduces IL-6 production in a dose-dependent manner...Pretreatment with 50 and 100 μg/ml LA prior to LPS stimulation resulted in reduced IL-6 levels by 19 and 34%, respectively. ... Stimulation with anti-CD3/CD28 resulted in dramatic and statistically significant increases in IL-17 levels compared to untreated controls. Pretreatment with 50 and 100 μg/ml LA inhibited IL-17 production by 35 and 50%, respectively. Collectively, these data indicate that LA exerts anti-inflammatory functions in part by inhibiting IL-6 and IL-17

[1131] Wu et al. Induction of pathogenic TH17 cells by inducible salt-sensing kinase SGK1. *Nature.* 2013 Apr 25;496(7446):513-7
[1132] West CE et al. The gut microbiota and its role in the development of allergic disease: a wider perspective. *Clin Exp Allergy.* 2014 Apr 29
[1133] Kwon et al. Generation of regulatory dendritic cells and CD4+Foxp3+ T cells by probiotics administration suppresses immune disorders. *Proc Natl Acad Sci* 2010 Feb 2;107(5):2159-64
[1134] Salinthone S, et al. Lipoic acid attenuates inflammation via cAMP and protein kinase A signaling. *PLoS One.* 2010 Sep 28;5(9). pii: e13058

synthesis. ... Collectively, the data presented here indicate that LA inhibits T cell proliferation and activation....Collectively, the cytokine data suggest that LA is exerting its anti-inflammatory effects by lowering the concentrations of pro-inflammatory cytokines (IL-6 and IL-17) while possibly having a biphasic effect on IL-10."

- Vitamin A, retinoic acid, RA: Retinoic acid is required for Treg induction and for maintenance of Treg phenotype, especially in an inflammatory/IL-6 milieu. Vitamin A enhances histone acetylation at the promoter region of the Foxp3 gene, thereby enhancing FOXp3 transcription and the resultant Treg phenotype. Many patients have insufficient intake of preformed vitamin A and must therefore use oral vitamin A supplementation; relatedly, 27-45% of women (volunteers from UK) are "slow converters" of beta-carotene to vitamin A, and they must likewise supplement with vitamin A in order to meet physiologic needs.[1135] Hypothyroidism also impairs conversion of beta-carotene to vitamin A; zinc is also needed for this conversion. Women who are pregnant or might become pregnant are generally advised to keep vitamin A intake below 8,000-9,000 IU/day from all sources. When treating acute viral infections, I have traditionally used a time-limited loading dose of 100,000-300,000 IU/d for 7-10 days followed by a maintenance dose of 10,000-25,000 IU/d for children and adults; I think this is a reasonable approach for the rapid repletion of vitamin A stores for the treatment of acute illness. However, after seeing the success of two clinical trials demonstrating successful FOXp3 and Treg induction in humans with inflammatory diseases following vitamin A 25,000 IU/d, I am inclined to describe the loading dose as optional, particularly for patients wary of the vitamin A headache, which can occur with loading dose without real vitamin A overload or toxicity (i.e., some patients get a headache from high-dose vitamin A supplementation even after the first day, when they are clearly *not* vitamin A toxic). Vitamin A toxicity is monitored clinically with six main findings: "two pains"—bone pain and headache, "two skins"—dry skin and chapped lips, and "two labs"—elevated GGT and triglycerides. The *in vitro* data showing that vitamin A promotes the Treg phenotype is impressively strong; the clinical data that is accumulating is showing that vitamin A supplementation promotes improved Treg/Th-17 balance in humans.

> **Vitamin A: clinical pearls and observations**
> - Use vitamin A *with* or *following* vitamin D, or start with a low dose of vitamin A: Preformed vitamin A should not be used without concomitant or previous supplementation with physiologic doses of vitamin D3. What may possibly occur in patients with inflammatory/autoimmune diseases who are deficient in both vitamin A and vitamin D is that monotherapy with vitamin A partly restores immune function but does so in a way that is skewed toward Th17 responses due to the lack of vitamin D3; the resulting clinical exacerbation may be a form of (analogous to) what we might call *nutritionally-induced immune reconstitution inflammatory syndrome* (IRIS, or in this case nIRIS). Another clinical approach is to avoid the loading dose of vitamin A unless the patient is already replete with vitamin D. Noted is the fact that studies using vitamin A 25,000 IU/d in the treatment of inflammatory disease for Treg induction have *not* observed disease flares.
> - Acute loading dose is not necessary: The vitamin A loading dose commonly used for acute viral infections is not necessary when vitamin A is being used for FOXp3 and Treg induction.
> - Early headache with vitamin A loading dose does not indicate "vitamin A toxicity": Some patients are intolerant of high-dose vitamin A, especially if given in an emulsified form (thus with better absorption). Vitamin A loading dose is really only indicated when a rapid response is needed, as with acute viral infections, not with long-term immunomodulation.

  o Retinoic acid stabilizes antigen-specific regulatory T-cell function in autoimmune hepatitis type 2 (*J Autoimmun* 2014 Feb[1136]): This study is not a clinical trial; data are in vitro / ex vivo. The authors introduce their paper with a clear summary, "Imbalance between effector and regulatory T-cells (Treg) underlies the loss of immune-tolerance to self-antigens in autoimmune disease" and they go on to note that "In autoimmune hepatitis type 2 (AIH-2), effector CD4 T-cell immune responses to cytochrome P450IID6 (CYP2D6) are permitted by **numerically** and **functionally** impaired Treg. ... Treg exposure to inflammatory challenge results in decreased suppressive function and up-regulation of Th1/Th2/Th17 transcription factors both in health and AIH-2. ... inflammation-

---

[1135] "The extent to which β-carotene is converted to vitamin A is highly variable between well-nourished healthy individuals. This variable response to β-carotene has led to the characterization of the poor [slow] converter phenotype in 27–45% of volunteers in double-tracer studies." Leung WC et al. Two common single nucleotide polymorphisms in the gene encoding beta-carotene 15,15'-monooxygenase alter beta-carotene metabolism in female volunteers. *FASEB J*. 2009 Apr;23(4):1041-53

[1136] Holder BS et al. Retinoic acid stabilizes antigen-specific regulatory T-cell function in autoimmune hepatitis type 2. *J Autoimmun*. 2014 Feb 21. pii: S0896-8411(14)00040-7 induced decrease in Treg function is also abrogated by retinoic acid (RA) / rapamycin (RP) in health and RA in patients."

- o All-trans retinoic acid sustains the stability and function of natural regulatory T cells in an inflammatory milieu (*J Immunol* 2010 Sep[1137]): "Recent studies have demonstrated that plasticity of naturally occurring CD4(+)Foxp3(+) regulatory T cells (nTregs) may account for their inability to control chronic inflammation in established autoimmune diseases. All-trans retinoic acid (atRA), the active derivative of vitamin A, has been demonstrated to promote Foxp3(+) Treg differentiation and suppress Th17 development. In this study, we report a vital role of atRA in sustaining the stability and functionality of nTregs in the presence of IL-6. We found that nTregs treated with atRA were resistant to Th17 and other Th cell conversion and maintained Foxp3 expression and suppressive activity in the presence of IL-6 in vitro. atRA decreased IL-6R expression and signaling by nTregs. Of interest, adoptive transfer of nTregs even from arthritic mice treated with atRA suppressed progression of established collagen-induced arthritis. We suggest that nTregs treated with atRA may represent a novel treatment strategy to control established chronic immune-mediated inflammatory diseases."
- o Clinical use of vitamin A supplementation on retinoic acid-related orphan receptor γt (RORγt) and interleukin-17 (IL-17) gene expression in Avonex-treated multiple sclerosis patients (*J Mol Neurosci* 2013 Nov[1138]): Patients received retinyl palmitate 25,000 IU/d per day for 6 months; results showed that vitamin A downregulates IL-17 gene expression (reported as 1.7-fold reduction) and RORγt gene expression (reported as 50-fold reduction). The authors proudly state, "An attractive feature of our survey is that, for the first time in the world, an assessment of the effect of retinyl palmitate supplementation on IL-17 gene expression in multiple sclerotic patients has been performed. Results of our study show that supplementation with vitamin A decreases IL-17 and RORγt gene expression significantly, while there was no change at the end of the study in the placebo group."
- o Clinical use of vitamin A supplementation for Foxp3 induction in atherosclerotic patients (*J Nutrigenet Nutrigenomics* 2013 Jan[1139]): Patients with atherosclerosis and healthy controls received retinyl palmitate 25,000 IU/d for 4 months. The levels of Foxp3 expression increased significantly in both groups, more so in the patients with atherosclerosis (10-fold to 14-fold) than in healthy controls (5-fold to 7-fold) as expected. The authors concluded that "...vitamin A has the effect of increasing expression of regulatory T cells, it can be concluded that supplementation with vitamin A in atherosclerotic patients may be effective in slowing disease progression. No adverse effects were reported.
- **Inflammation reduction**: Reducing inflammation in general and IL-6, IL-17, and TNFa in particular is important for decreasing induction of inflammatory phenotypes—Th1, Th2, Th17—and optimizing induction of Treg. Of clinical importance are the following facts: summarized as *inflammation becomes a vicious cycle*, and therefore the clinician's task is to break these cycles as effectively and consistently as possible using wide range of modalities:
  - o IL-6 vicious cycle: IL-6 promotes Th-17 induction, and the Th-17 phenotype directly/indirectly promotes additional IL-6 production; in my earlier review of NFkB, I noted that IL-6 and TNF-alpha both stimulate NFkB activation, leading to a vicious cycle of inflammation,
  - o IL-17 is the main cytokine causing tissue damage: IL-17 is the effector of tissue damage, and tissue damage then causes additional immune response and subsequent cytokine release,
  - o IL-21 vicious cycle: IL-21 promotes Th-17 induction; the Th-17 phenotype produces IL-21[1140],
  - o TNF-alpha vicious cycle: TNFa promotes Th-17 induction; Th-17 phenotype produces TNFa.

Thus, means to reduce IL-6, IL-17, and TNFa help to break the vicious cycles of inflammation, such means include but are not limited to:

[1137] Zhou X et al. Cutting edge: all-trans retinoic acid sustains stability and function of natural regulatory T cells in inflammatory milieu. *J Immunol*. 2010 Sep;185:2675-9
[1138] Mohammadzadeh Honarvar N et al. The effect of vitamin A supplementation on retinoic acid-related orphan receptor γt (RORγt) and interleukin-17 (IL-17) gene expression in Avonex-treated multiple sclerotic patients. *J Mol Neurosci*. 2013 Nov;51(3):749-53
[1139] Mottaghi et al. Influence of vitamin A supplementation on Foxp3 and TGF-ß gene expression in atherosclerotic patients. *J Nutrigenet Nutrigenomics*. 2012;5(6):314-26
[1140] Korn et al. IL-17 and Th17 Cells. *Annu Rev Immunol*. 2009;27:485-517

- o IL-6 reduction: IL-6 can be reduced by multivitamin/mineral supplementation, CoQ10, vitamin D, low-carbohydrate diets, moderate exercise, weight loss, lipoic acid, antidysbiosis/antimicrobial treatments as needed; vitamin A helps maintain iTreg phenotype and activity in an inflammatory milieu,
- o IL-17 reduction: IL-17 can be reduced by lipoic acid (per in vitro and ex vivo research),
- o IL-21 reduction: Animal studies have shown that vitamin D deficiency increases responsiveness to IL-21 (pro-inflammatory effect), and that vitamin D supplementation reduces responsiveness to IL-21 (anti-inflammatory effect),
- o TNF-alpha reduction: TNFa can be reduced by fish oil and biotin (per in vitro and ex vivo research),
- Vitamin D3: Several clinical trials in humans have shown that vitamin D3 supplementation (detailed previously and throughout in this textbook) induces higher number and function of Treg cells within approximately 1 month in adult humans who are "apparently healthy" and those who have autoimmune diseases such as multiple sclerosis (MS) and systemic lupus erythematosus (SLE, lupus).
    - o Small study shows that vitamin D increases anti-inflammatory IL-10 and reduces frequency of pro-inflammatory Th-17 cells (*Mult Scler* 2012 Dec[1141]): Four healthy individuals (n=4) took 5000-10,000 IU/day of vitamin D over 15 weeks, after which serum 25(OH) vitamin D levels rose significantly from baseline, with a corresponding increase in IL-10 production by peripheral blood mononuclear cells and a reduced frequency of Th17 cells.
    - o Vitamin D supplementation increases regulatory T cells in apparently healthy subjects (*Isr Med Assoc J* 2010 Mar[1142]): In this study, most "healthy" subjects were vitamin D deficient at the start of this study, then received one dose of vitamin D 140,000 IU (nonphysiologic dosing) and were not corrected to optimal vitamin D status. Nonetheless, participants showed an increase in Tregs.
    - o T-cell modulating effects of high dose vitamin D3 supplementation in multiple sclerosis (*PLoS One* 2010 Dec[1143]): N=15 RRMS patients were supplemented with 20,000 IU/d vitamin D3 for 12 weeks. "All patients finished the protocol without side-effects, hypercalcemia, or hypercalciuria. The median vitamin D status increased from 50 nmol/L (31-175) at week 0 to 380 nmol/L (151-535) at week 12 (P<0.001). During the study, 1 patient experienced an exacerbation of MS and was censored from the T cell analysis. The proportions of (naïve and memory) CD4+ Tregs remained unaffected. Although Treg suppressive function improved in several subjects, this effect was not significant in the total cohort. An increased proportion of IL-10+ CD4+ T cells was found after supplementation."
    - o One of the most important studies ever ignored: Intake of vitamin D and risk of type 1 diabetes *Lancet* 2001 Nov[1144]): This is one of the most important studies ever published in medicine and nutrition, showing that among more than 10,000 infants, vitamin D supplementation 2,000 IU/d for the first year of life showed complete safety and a dose-dependent reduction in autoimmune type-1 diabetes mellitus up to -78% over 30 years of follow-up. If any drug showed this level of safety, affordability, and efficacy, its use would almost certainly be medically and legally mandatory; the continued ignoring of this data by the medical/pediatrician/ObGyn communities is one of many nutritional-medical travesties in medicine and healthcare.

> **Vitamin D prevention of autoimmune diabetes: lessons learned and ignored**
> - More than 10,000 human infants were to receive 2,000 IU/d of vitamin D for the first year of life,
> - No report of adverse effects.
> - Dose-dependent reduction in autoimmune diabetes up to -78% with 30 years of follow-up,
> - Published in *The Lancet*
> - Virtually completely ignored by the medical and healthcare community
>
> Hyppönen et al. *Lancet*. 2001 Nov

- o Vitamin D restores Treg:Th17 balance in patients with SLE (*Arthritis Res Ther* 2012 Oct[1145]): Cholecalciferol 100,000 IU per week for 4 weeks followed by 100,000 IU of cholecalciferol per

---

[1141] Allen AC et al. A pilot study of the immunological effects of high-dose vitamin D in healthy volunteers. *Mult Scler*. 2012 Dec;18(12):1797-800
[1142] Prietl et al. Vitamin D supplementation and regulatory T cells in apparently healthy subjects: vitamin D for autoimmune diseases? *Isr Med Assoc J*. 2010;12:136-9
[1143] Smolders J et al. Safety and T cell modulating effects of high dose vitamin D3 supplementation in multiple sclerosis. *PLoS One*. 2010 Dec 13;5(12):e15235
[1144] Hyppönen et al. Intake of vitamin D and risk of type 1 diabetes: a birth-cohort study. *Lancet*. 2001 Nov 3;358(9292):1500-3
[1145] Terrier B et al. Restoration of regulatory and effector T cell balance and B cell homeostasis in systemic lupus erythematosus patients through vitamin D supplementation. *Arthritis Res Ther*. 2012 Oct 17;14(5):R221

month for 6 months in 20 SLE patients with hypovitaminosis D resulted in increased serum 25(OH)D levels from 18 ng/mL to 51 ng/mL at 2 months and to 41 ng/mL. "Vitamin D was well tolerated and induced a preferential increase of naïve CD4+ T cells, an increase of regulatory T cells and a decrease of effector Th1 and Th17 cells. Vitamin D also induced a decrease of memory B cells and anti-DNA antibodies."

- Fatty acids—N3 fatty acids and GLA: N3 fatty acids and n6 GLA have shown the ability to reduce the biochemical and clinical manifestations of inflammatory and autoimmune diseases. At first (i.e., in the 1980s-1990s) we thought this was primarily mediated via enzyme and prostaglandin competition, and then later (> years 2000s) we added nutrigenomic and resolvin (et al) effects; by now (> year 2013) we are inclined to include Treg/Th17 modulation as a component of the effectiveness of CFAT—combination fatty acid therapy—via interaction with the human fatty acid receptors, which are all-to-commonly known by the popular and animal-specific (because this is where most basic science research is performed) name of PPAR—peroxisome proliferator-activated receptors. Students and clinicians can easily recall the relative specificity of fatty acids for PPARs by remembering that PPAR-*gamma* is activated by n6 *gamma*-linolenic acid, GLA, while EPA activates PPAR-alpha. Given then that PPAR-*gamma* is activated by *gamma*-linolenic acid, and given that PPAR-gamma activation promotes dendritic cells to produce retinoic acid (vitamin A) to induce Tregs[1146], then a logical deduction is that GLA (especially with additional vitamin A, or—at the very least—a diet high in plant material for provision of beta-carotene) should help induce Treg for the control of inflammation/autoimmunity. Increased dietary intake of n3 fatty acids has been shown to reduce the incidence of autoimmune diabetes in humans, suggesting n3FA-mediated immunomodulation, not merely anti-inflammation.
- Infection/dysbiosis clearance: Gastrointestinal dysbiosis prompts formation of pro-inflammatory effector cells: Th1, Th2, Th17. Therefore, eliminating/reducing problematic microbes and promoting systemic eubiosis is important for inducing immunophenotype balance. I am particularly interested in and impressed by the role of segmented filamentous bacteria (SFB) in this regard (detailed in the section on dysbiosis in this book).
- Green tea: Green tea component EGCG induces Treg cells. Patients are recommended to have two cups per day and/or use standardized oral supplementation (caffeinated or decaffeinated).
    - Treg induction by green tea polyphenol EGCG (*Immunol Lett* 2011 Sep[1147]): "Regulatory T cells (Treg) are critical in maintaining immune tolerance and suppressing autoimmunity. The transcription factor Foxp3 serves as a master switch that controls the development and function of Treg. Foxp3 expression is epigenetically regulated by DNA methylation, and DNA methyltransferase (DNMT) inhibitors can induce Foxp3 expression in naive CD4(+) T cells. We showed that EGCG, a major green tea polyphenol, could act as a dietary DNMT inhibitor, and induced Foxp3 and IL-10 expression in CD4(+) Jurkat T cells at physiologically relevant concentrations in vitro. We further showed that mice treated with EGCG in vivo had significantly increased Treg frequencies and numbers in spleen and lymph nodes and had inhibited T cell response. Induction of Foxp3 expression correlated with a concomitant reduction in DNMT expression and a decrease in global DNA methylation. Our data suggested that EGCG can induce Foxp3 expression and increase Treg frequency via a novel epigenetic mechanism. ...the ability of dietary agents to target similar mechanisms offers opportunities for potentially sustained and longer-term exposures with lower toxicity [compared with drugs]."
    - Green tea EGCG ameliorates obesity and autoinflammatory arthritis by altering T-cell balance (*Immunol Lett* 2014 Jan[1148]): Paraphrasing the authors: Epigallocatechin-3-gallate (EGCG) is the most biologically active catechin in green tea and has therapeutic effects in autoinflammatory diseases

---

[1146] "Overall, our present results suggest that PPARγ ligation may be an important factor in stimulating DCs to produce RA and that the associated ability to enhance generation of iTregs may be one mechanism by which PPARγ ligands can ameliorate autoimmune diseases." Housley et al. PPARgamma regulates retinoic acid-mediated DC induction of Tregs. *J Leukoc Biol*. 2009 Aug;86(2):293-301
[1147] Wong et al. Induction of regulatory T cells by green tea polyphenol EGCG. *Immunol Lett*. 2011 Sep 30;139(1-2):7-13
[1148] Byun et al. Epigallocatechin-3-gallate ameliorates both obesity and autoinflammatory arthritis aggravated by obesity by altering the balance among CD4+ T-cell subsets. *Immunol Lett*. 2014 Jan-Feb;157(1-2):51-9

and obesity. Obesity is an inflammatory condition because of the inflammatory cytokines and higher Th1 cell differentiation detected in both obese animals and humans. In this work using animal models of diet-induced obesity and obesity+RA, EGCG reduced the body weight and fat infiltration in liver tissue while improving serum lipid profiles in obese mice and induced a higher Treg/Th17 cell ratio in obese and obese+RA mice. "Thus, EGCG has an anti-inflammatory effect by suppressing STAT3 proteins and Th17-cell differentiation. EGCG thus shows promise for treating autoimmune conditions related to STAT3 or Th17 cells, such as metabolic syndrome, inflammatory arthritis, and some neoplastic diseases."

Nutritional immunomodulation of immunophenotype via induction of Treg phenotype: Specific nutrients and an anti-inflammatory milieu promote immune tolerance and avoidance of allergic, inflammatory, and autoimmune diseases by several mechanisms, including induction of Treg phenotype for suppression of Th-1/2/17 hyperactivity.

Case Report **Remarkable nutritional cure of ~18 years of untreatable psoriasis**: Paradoxically, many of us in the clinical nutrition field have been employing components of nutritional immunomodulation for many years without fully realizing the mechanisms behind the clinical benefits that we consistently observed. I recall the case of a young woman I treated in approximately 2003 for her then 18-year history of treatment-resistant full-body psoriasis; her recovery was so rapid and nearly complete that the case has always stood out in my memory. This case (included below) was published in print and on the internet in 2005 in the professional magazine *Nutritional Wellness*[1149] in a discussion of my 5-part nutrition protocol (detailed in the previous section of this chapter); an updated version of the case is provided here:

- Case: This is a 17-year-old woman with head-to-toe psoriasis since childhood. She wears long pants and long-sleeved shirts year-round to conceal her skin lesions, and the psoriasis is a major interference to her social life. Palliative medications have ceased to help. I recall the first time that I saw this patient, I either thought to myself or said aloud, "This psoriasis looks like a second-degree burn" because the inflammation was pervasive, extremely red/erythematous, and had caused thickening of the skin.
- Treatment: The Paleo-Mediterranean diet[1150] was implemented, with an emphasis on food allergy identification. We used a multivitamin-mineral supplement with 200 mcg selenium to compensate for the nutritional insufficiencies and selenium deficiency common in patients with psoriasis; likewise, 10 mg of folic acid was added to address the relative vitamin deficiencies and elevated homocysteine common in these patients.[1151] Fish oil and GLA from

---

[1149] Vasquez A. Implementing the Five-Part Nutritional Wellness Protocol for the Treatment of Various Health Problems. *Nutritional Wellness* 2005 Nov
[1150] Vasquez A. Revisiting the Five-Part Nutritional Wellness Protocol: The Supplemented Paleo-Mediterranean Diet. *Nutritional Perspectives* 2011 January
[1151] Vanizor Kural B, et al. Plasma homocysteine and its relationships with atherothrombotic markers in psoriatic patients. *Clin Chim Acta* 2003;332(1-2):23-3.

borage oil was used for the anti-inflammatory and skin-healing benefits.[1152] Vitamin E (1,200 IU of mixed tocopherols) and lipoic acid (1,000 mg per day) were added for their anti-inflammatory benefits and to combat the oxidative stress that is characteristic of psoriasis.[1153] Of course, probiotics were used to modify gut flora, which is commonly deranged in patients with psoriasis.[1154]

- Results: Within a few weeks, this patient's "lifelong psoriasis" was essentially gone. Food allergy identification and avoidance played a major role in the success of this case; in her case, the offending food was chicken broth. When I saw the patient again nine months later for her second visit, she had no visible evidence of psoriasis. Her "medically untreatable" condition was essentially cured by the use of my basic protocol, with the addition of a few extra nutrients. At the second visit—approximately 4-5 weeks after the first visit—I recall saying to the patient, "You no longer have skin lesions consistent with the diagnosis of psoriasis."
- New perspective and mechanisms of effectiveness: The success of this case was effected via nutritional immunomodulation. Without knowing I was doing so, I had implemented nearly a perfect recipe for induction of Treg cells for the endogenous suppression of pathogenic Th17-mediated inflammation.

Rx and rationale at the time	Actual nutritional immunomodulation
Cod liver oil for anti-inflammatory EPA and DHA	❶ vitamin A, ❷ vitamin D, ❸ EPA and DHA in the cod liver oil stimulated induction of Treg cells to provide endogenous cell-mediated anti-inflammation; retinoic acid and vitamin D both inhibit pathogenic Th17 cells and promote Treg, and the effect is likely additive/synergistic, particularly given vitamin D's ability to lower IL-6,
Paleo diet for general health promotion, increased intake of potassium relative to sodium	Elimination of wheat, common allergens, and increased consumption of vegetables promoted ❹ anti-inflammatory climate and modified gastrointestinal bacteria; ❺ sodium avoidance
Lipoic acid for antioxidant and anti-NFkB activity	❻ 35-50% reduction in IL-17; ❼ lipoic acid also helps to optimize mitochondrial function an effect which is expected to promote Treg,
Probiotics for global benefit	❽ Probiotics promote Treg
Vitamin E for antioxidant/anti-inflammatory benefit	New data published in 2014 shows that alpha-tocopherol increases cAMP and thereby reduces IL-6 and IL-17 in a manner similar to that of lipoic acid

Nutritional Immunomodulation: Induction of Treg at the expense/suppression of Th-1/2/17

1. Mitochondrial optimization
2. Biotin
3. E-vitamin
4. Sodium avoidance
5. Transgenic food avoidance
6. Probiotics
7. Lipoic acid
8. A-vitamin
9. Infection/dysbiosis clearance
10. D-vitamin
11. Fatty acids: EPA-DHA and GLA
12. IL-6 reduction: create overall antiinflammatory milieu for Treg induction
13. Green tea

DrV's nutritional immunomodulation protocol: The new (Jun 2014) acronym is "My BEST PLAID FIG."

[1152] Vasquez A. New insights into fatty acid supplementation and its effect on eicosanoid production and genetic expression. *Nutritional Perspect* 2005: Jan: 5-16
[1153] Kokcam I, Naziroglu M. Antioxidants and lipid peroxidation status in the blood of patients with psoriasis. *Clin Chim Acta* 1999;289(1-2):23-31
[1154] Waldman A, et al. Incidence of Candida in psoriasis: a study on the fungal flora of psoriatic patients. *Mycoses* 2001;44(3-4):77-81.

❶ Food ❷ Infections ❸ Nutri-immunomod ❹ Dysmetab ❺ Stress/Sleep/Socio/Surg/Sup ❻ Endo ❼ Xeno

❹ Dysmetabolism & Dysfunctional Organelles: Mitochondrial Dysfunction, Endoplasmic Reticulum Stress and the Unfolded Protein Response:

Common Causative, Contributing, and Consequential Components of Cardiometabolic Syndrome, Hypertension, Neurodegeneration, Inflammation, Allergy and Autoimmunity

Major Concepts in this Section
This section introduces the concept of *dysmetabolism* and then uses the best described components of *organelle dysfunction*—mitochondrial dysfunction and endoplasmic reticulum stress (and the consequent unfolded protein response)—to concretely demonstrate the mechanisms of and solutions to subcellular dysfunction. Numerous diagrams—including concept images, flowcharts, scanning electron micrographs—are provided to facilitate and expedite the reader's apprehension of these complex, important and ultimately simple clinical entities. Following the briefest introduction, mitochondrial dysfunction is described in sufficient clinical detail followed by a practical protocol for its remediation; that section is followed by a similar "problem and solution" review of endoplasmic reticulum stress and unfolded protein response.

Dysmetabolism & Organelle Dysfunction:
Endoplasmic reticulum stress, Mitochondrial dysfunction

The Six Fundamental
Vicious Cycles (∞) of Metabolic Inflammation:
1) MitoDys ∞ ERS-UPR
2) MitoDys ∞ Inflammation
3) ERS-UPR ∞ Inflammation
4) Inflammation ∞ Oxidative Stress
5) Oxidative stress ∞ MitoDys
6) Oxidative stress ∞ ERS-UPR

Oxidant stress:
Increased production of ROS / depletion of antioxidant protection

Inflammation:
Cytokine production with resultant cellular dysfunction and tissue destruction

Conceptual diagram demonstrating the major components and vicious cycles of dysmetabolism, organelle dysfunction, and the inflammatory and oxidative consequences: This diagram allows us to appreciate the following vicious cycles, discussed in the text and respective citations:
1. Endoplasmic reticulum stress causes mitochondrial dysfunction, and mitochondrial dysfunction (MitoDys) causes endoplasmic reticulum stress (ERS).
2. MitoDys causes inflammation, and inflammation causes MitoDys.
3. ERS causes inflammation, and inflammation causes ERS.
4. Inflammation causes oxidative stress, and oxidative stress causes inflammation.
5. Oxidative stress causes MitoDys, and MitoDys causes oxidative stress.
6. Oxidative stress causes ERS, and ERS causes oxidative stress.

Major Concepts in this Section on Mitochondrial Dysfunction

Mitochondria do much more than simply produce ATP; they also sense and respond to nutritional status (not simply metabolize available carbon substrates), sense and respond to microbes, are vulnerable to the presence of bacteria and viruses, create reactive oxygen (ROS) and nitrogen species (RNS), are involved in the secretion and reception of insulin, and can promote inflammation and immune imbalance via elaboration of cytokines and Th-17 cells, respectively. Mitochondria are also key players in the determination of the timing and type of cell death, whether by apoptosis or necrosis. When mitochondria are functioning "normally" and "optimally", the various roles of mitochondria can be said to be mostly efficient and beneficent; however, when mitochondria become injured, impaired, or otherwise "dysfunctional" then the ATP-producing and other roles played by mitochondria are adversely affected to the detriment of the human host. The physiologic roles and consequences of dysfunction are outlined in the table below:

Physiologic roles of mitochondria	Consequences of mitochondrial dysfunction
1) Efficiently produce ATP	Inefficient production of ATP with reduced total output.
2) Sense and respond to microbes	Exaggerated response to microbes with inefficient and excessive immune and inflammatory responses.
3) Theoretically, mitochondria perform normal duties especially ATP production without regard for infectious disease status	Mitochondria can be destroyed by infectious agents, such as herpes simplex virus; other microbes and their products (such as bacterial endotoxin) cause mitochondrial dysfunction.
4) Create ROS and RNS as a side-effect of metabolism	Produce excessive ROS and RNS which leads to damage at four levels: 1) mitochondrial—e.g., mitochondrial inner membrane (MIM) and mitochondrial DNA, 2) cellular—e.g., nuclear DNA, 3) tissue—e.g., substantia nigra in Parkinson's disease, 4) systemic—e.g., measureable alterations in oxidative markers, such as TBARS and GSH. Note that oxidative damage to the MIM causes increased oxidant production via dysfunction of the ETC, thereby creating a vicious cycle.
5) Secretion and reception of insulin	Mitochondrial dysfunction contributes to the "diabetic phenotype of hyperglycemia" via impaired pancreatic secretion of insulin and also by impaired peripheral reception of insulin.
6) Normally, mitochondria should not have an appreciable or adverse effect on immune and inflammatory balance	Mitochondrial dysfunction in general and mitochondrial hyperpolariziation in particular promote increased production of inflammatory cytokines, cyclooxygenase, and Th-17 cells while retarding induction of Treg cells.
7) Mitochondrial-triggered apoptosis needs to be appropriately timed per cell.	An excess of apoptosis leads to premature tissue failure, while a failure of cell-killing and relative immortalization of cells contributes to autoimmunity and also cancer. Inflammatory cell death—necrosis—promotes additional inflammation via DAMP-receptor activation; this is noted as a consequence of mitochondrial dysfunction in autoimmune diseases such as SLE.

The three most classic characteristics of mitochondrial dysfunction are ❶ impaired ATP production: reduced efficiency and reduced amount of ATP production, ❷ increased free radical production, and ❸ increased inflammatory tendency, via chemical and enzymatic mediators (such as cytokines and cyclooxygenase, respectively) and cellular effectors (especially Th-17 cells). Given the consequences (introduced above) and high prevalence of mitochondrial disorders in routine outpatient clinical practice, physicians need to appreciate the practical, efficient, and effective, clinical means by which mitochondrial function can be restored, protected, and optimized.

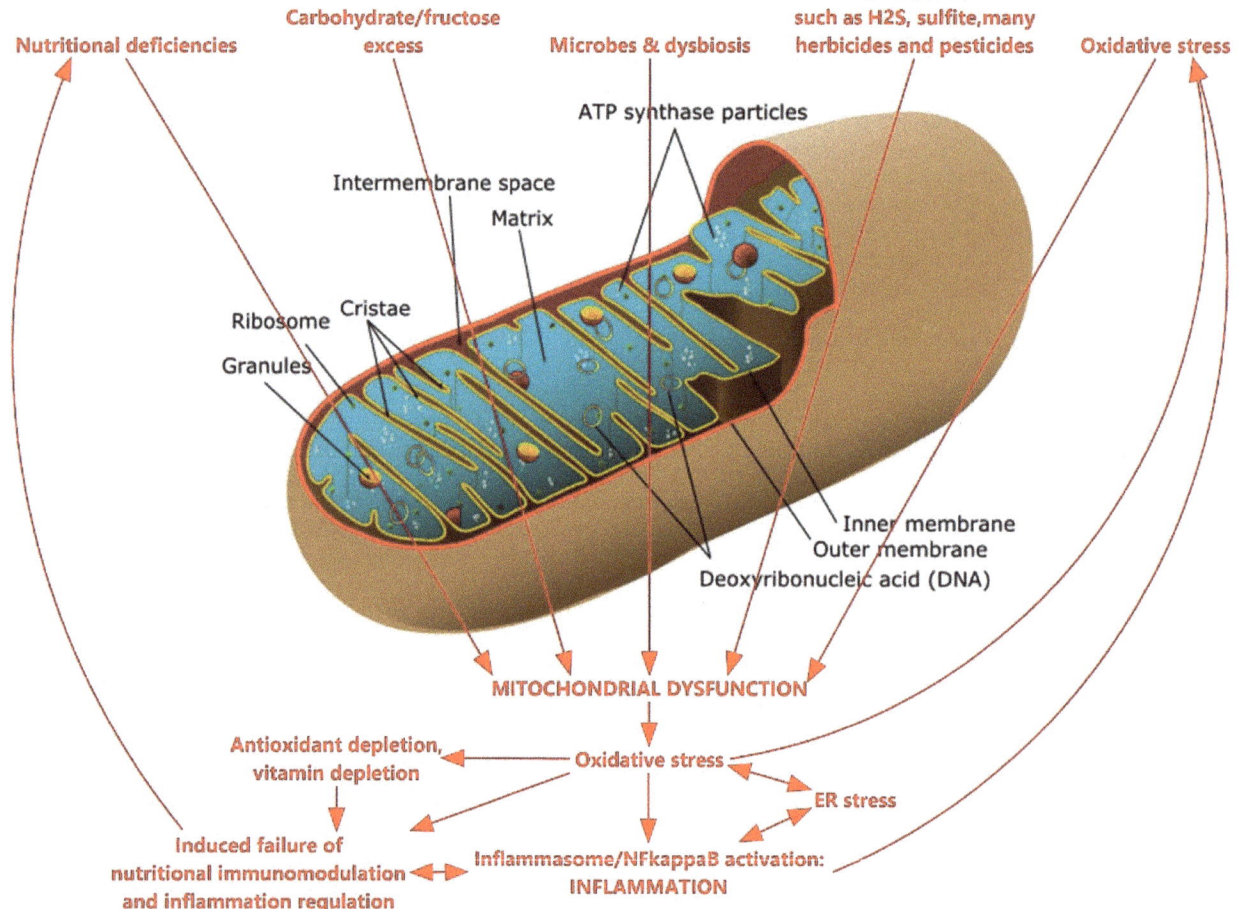

Schematic overview of mitochondrial dysfunction's major causes and consequences: Notice the presence of vicious cycles whereby cause becomes consequence, and then consequence becomes cause. Several dietary, nutritional, botanical, pharmaceutical/microbiologic, and sociopolitical interventions are obvious from the diagram.

Mitochondria—Re-Introduction and New Perspectives:
- Production of cellular energy in the form of ATP: Mitochondria are organelles ("small organs") within each cell that produce the majority of cellular energy for biochemical reactions and cellular processes. The primary fuel used by cells of the body is ATP—adenosine triphosphate. Everyone who has studied mitochondria—ranging from high-school and undergraduate students of Biology all the way to doctorate-level medical/healthcare professionals—is familiar with the fact that mitochondria make ATP; in fact, for most people, whether they are general public or doctors, this is all they know about mitochondria. New research, however, has shown us that mitochondria have many roles in addition to their ability to produce cellular energy. Most importantly, mitochondria are now known to play important roles in perpetuating chronic inflammation, responding to microbial infections, triggering of cell death, and controlling various metabolic processes.[1155,1156]
- Perpetuation of chronic inflammation: Most relevant to the focus of this work on clinical conditions related to inflammation is the fact that mitochondria have the ability to trigger inflammatory responses via activation of the nuclear transcription factor kappa-B (NFkB). Transcription factors are intracellular molecules that bind to the genetic material (DNA) in the nucleus of the cell to influence the activation or transcription of specific genes; in this case the transcription factor kappaB is most notorious for its activation of genes that promote inflammatory responses—necessary for short-term responses to injury or infection, but harmful when protracted and nonspecific. In this way, certain types of mitochondrial stimulation/activation/dysfunction can

---

[1155] Pieczenik SR, Neustadt J. Mitochondrial dysfunction and molecular pathways of disease. *Exp Mol Pathol*. 2007 Aug;83(1):84-92
[1156] Green DR, Galluzzi L, Kroemer G. Mitochondria and the autophagy-inflammation-cell death axis in organismal aging. *Science*. 2011 Aug 26;333(6046):1109-12

contribute to "chronic inflammation"; conversely, interventions that restore/improve proper mitochondrial function have generally been shown to provide anti-inflammatory benefits.

- <u>Responsiveness to microbial infections</u>: Very interestingly, mitochondria have the ability to sense and respond to microbial infections, particularly infections due to viruses and Gram-negative bacteria. This may be related to the evolutionary origin of mitochondria, which is generally perceived to be that of aerobic bacteria that formed a symbiotic intercellular relationship with eukaryotic cells; the primitive bacteria would have needed the ability to respond to stresses in its environment, particularly potential invasion by or competition from infectious agents.
- <u>Triggering of cell death via apoptosis and/or necrosis</u>: Mitochondria are known to play a dual role in relation to a particular form of cell death called "apoptosis" which can be thought of as a peaceful/programmed/noninflammatory death of a cell (in contrast to "necrosis" which is inflammatory cellular death, and "autoschizis" which is cellular self-destruction through progressive fragmentation such as seen in cancer cells, for example, following administration of vitamins C and K3[1157]). Mitochondria have a two-part function, either promoting or resisting cell death; stated more simply and clearly: mitochondria play a role in keeping healthy cells alive, while promoting the death/apoptosis of unhealthy/dysfunctional/malignant cells. Mitochondrial dysfunction, as should be expected, impairs normal function and thus leads to the opposite of what we normally expect from mitochondria. In mitochondrial dysfunction, instead of promoting the death of dysfunctional cells, these cells become immortal and resistant to death; examples of this are autoreactive cells and cancer cells, which should have been "killed off" by apoptosis before being allowed to accumulate to such an extent that they cause harm to the host, either by autoimmunity or malignancy, respectively. In mitochondrial dysfunction, instead of keeping healthy cells alive, mitochondria promote the death of otherwise healthy cells; e.g., the loss of neurons that help control movement or which contribute to learning and thinking, thus resulting in Parkinson's disease or Alzheimer's disease, respectively.
- <u>Contribution to control of various metabolic processes</u>: Mitochondria play an integral role in several physiologic processes, including blood pressure control and blood glucose control. The release of insulin from the beta-cells in the pancreas is triggered by a cascade of events beginning with elevated levels of blood glucose and resulting in the entry of calcium into these cells with subsequent release of insulin into the blood; thus, mitochondrial dysfunction results in impaired pancreatic responsiveness to elevated glucose levels, thereby contributing to the complex condition we know as type-2 diabetes mellitus. Mild impairment of muscle contractility in the heart, which can be due to mitochondrial dysfunction and nutrient deficiencies/imbalances, leads to reduced heart function, which causes reflex activation of the sympathetic nervous system—the "panic response" of the nervous system that causes the "fight or flight" phenomenon. Chronic low-level activation of the sympathetic nervous system promotes several adverse effects associated with stress/fight/flight/panic, including elevated blood pressure (hypertension), activation of the renin-aldosterone system (water retention), vasoconstriction (reduced peripheral circulation) and hypercoagulability (promotion of blood clots, thrombosis). Natural treatments that restore or support mitochondrial function generally lower blood pressure in hypertensives, reduce blood glucose levels in diabetics, and reduce markers of inflammation in healthy patients as well as patients with inflammatory diseases; these examples will be further detailed throughout the multivolume textbook of <u>Inflammation Mastery</u> starting in 2014.

An accurate contemporary understanding of mitochondria in clinical medicine requires ❶ an updated conceptual appreciation of the roles of mitochondria in normal physiology and the consequences of mitochondrial dysfunction and the implications for various diagnoses and disease states, ❷ a "detailed familiarity" with ATP-producing processes and pathways, of which five are most important: 1) glycolysis, 2) pyruvate dehydrogenase, 3) Krebs cycle, citric acid cycle, 4) electron transport chain, and 5) alternate fuel (e.g., fructose, ketones, fatty acids, amino acids, ethanol) inputs into glycolysis and the citric acid cycle, and ❸ knowledge about how to improve/restore/optimize mitochondrial function—a customizable clinical strategy.

[1157] Lasalvia-Prisco et al. Serum markers variation consistent with autoschizis induced by ascorbic acid-menadione in patients with prostate cancer. *Med Oncol.* 2003;20(1):45-52

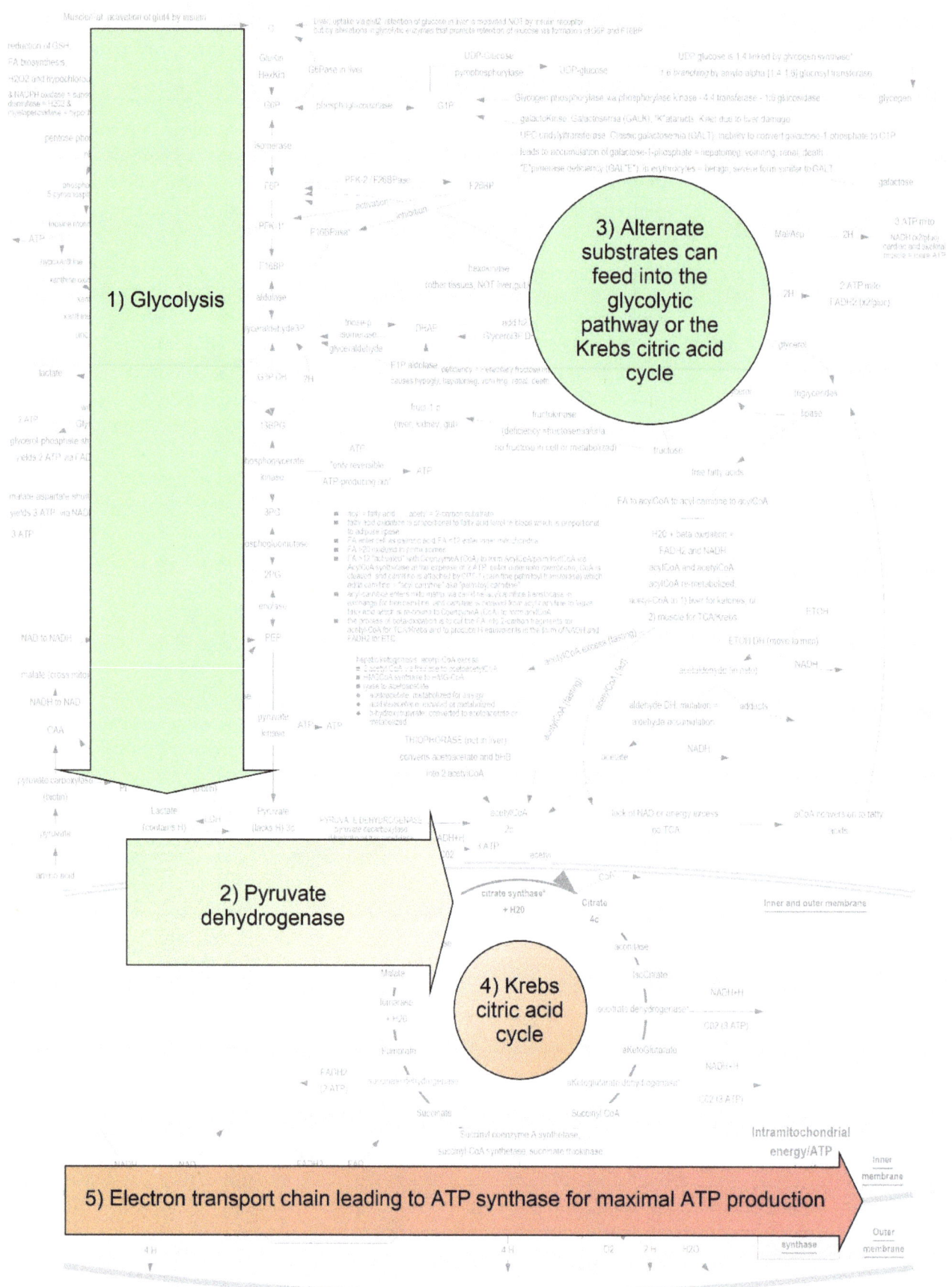

Conceptual overview of 1) glycolysis, 2) pyruvate dehydrogenase complex, 3) the accessory pathways that feed into the glycolysis or Krebs' cycle, 4) Krebs' citric acid cycle, and 5) electron transport chain: Clinical implications are discussed in the text.

Chapter 4: Major Modifiable Factors in Systemic Inflammation

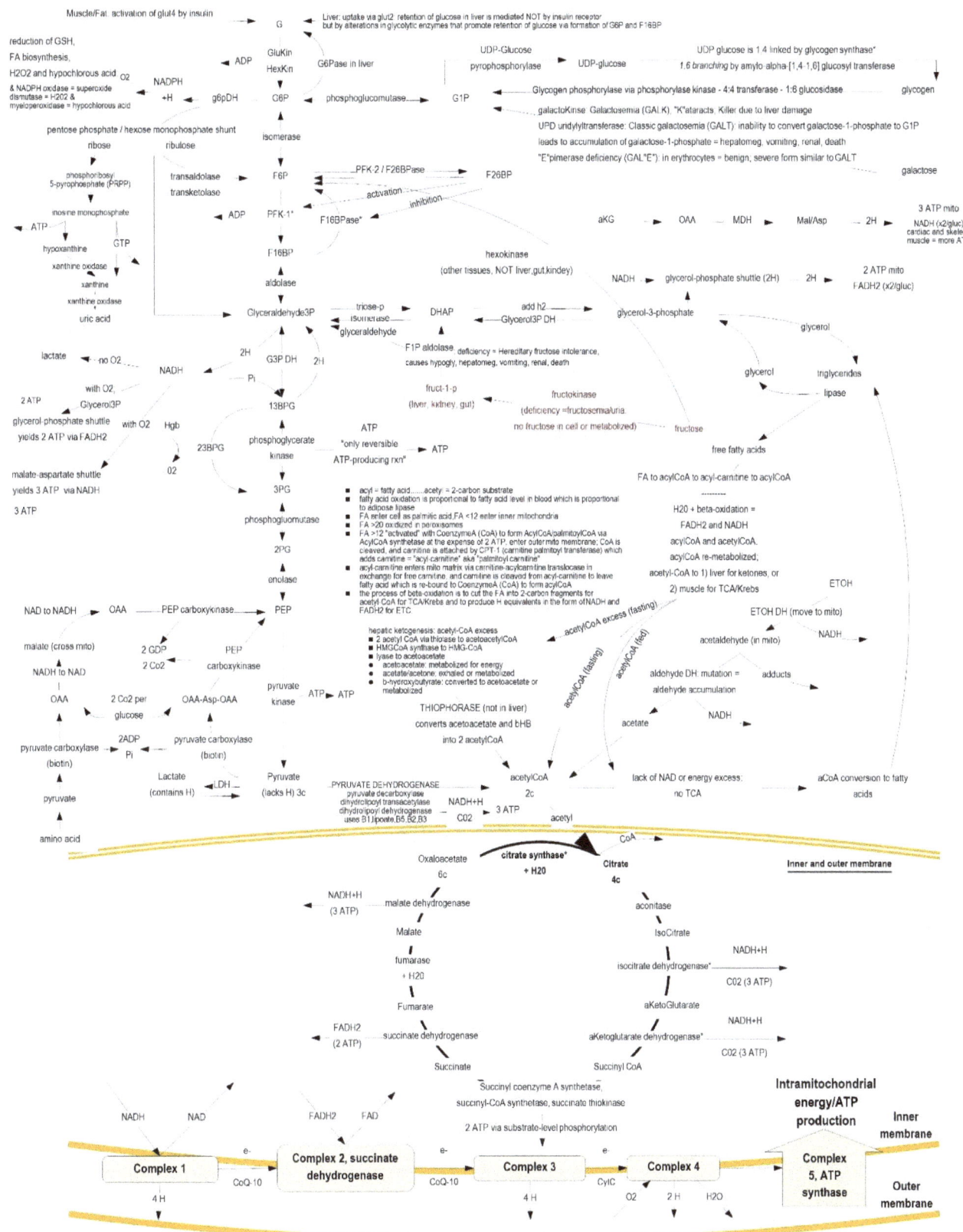

Detailed overview of glycolysis, pyruvate dehydrogenase complex, accessory input pathways, Krebs' cycle, and ETC: Note that the entry of fructose into the pathway via fructokinase to produce fructose-1-phosphate (colored in red) costs ATP, and thereby overconsumption of fructose—most obviously and specifically in the form of high-fructose corn syrup—causes ATP depletion with resultant metabolic and inflammatory consequences which promote insulin resistance and hypertension. These and other clinical implications are discussed in the text.

Krebs cycle, citric acid cycle: Excellent review diagram respectfully used from and credited to the open-access resource en.wikipedia.org/wiki/Citric_acid_cycle.[1158] Note per the diagram (colored in blue) the importance of vitamin B3—niacin/niacinamide. Not depicted here but of particular importance is the input of glutamate via conversion by glutamate dehydrogenase into alpha-ketoglutarate; of high clinical relevance is the inhibition of glutamate dehydrogenase by (dietary) sulfite, which results in a massive reduction in ATP production and helps explain the migraine-generating and inflammation-exacerbating effect of dietary sulfites in susceptible persons, particularly those with primary and secondary mitochondrial defects.

Krebs cycle enzymes, with a (partial) listing of cofactors and other comments and considerations:
- **Pyruvate dehydrogenase (complex)**: This is not a single enzyme but rather an "enzyme complex" with several subunits, each with its own nutritional cofactor. Vitamin B1 (thiamine pyrophosphate): pyruvate dehydrogenase subunit requires B1. Lipoic acid: dihydrolipoyl transacetylase subunit requires lipoic acid. Vitamin B2: dihydrolipoyl dehydrogenase subunit requires B2 and B3; also, B2 is needed for formation of NADH. Vitamin B3: dihydrolipoyl dehydrogenase subunit requires B2 and B3. Vitamin B5 (?): In medical school (class of 2010) we were taught by a respectable/multipublished mitochondrial researcher that pantothenic acid—vitamin B5—was also required for this step.
- **Citrate synthase**: Irreversible reaction. [no coenzyme noted]
- **Aconitase**: Isomeration reaction. [no coenzyme noted]

[1158] "Citric acid cycle with aconitate 2" by Narayanese, WikiUserPedia, YassineMrabet, TotoBaggins - biocyc.org/META/NEW-IMAGE?type=PATHWAY&object=TCA. Image adapted from :Image:Citric acid cycle noi.svg(uploaded to Commons by wadester16). Licensed under Creative Commons Attribution-Share Alike 3.0 via Wikimedia Commons - commons.wikimedia.org/wiki/File:Citric_acid_cycle_with_aconitate_2.svg#mediaviewer/File:Citric_acid_cycle_with_aconitate_2.svg.

- **Isocitrate dehydrogenase**: Vitamin B3: conversion of isocitrate to oxalosuccinate produces NADH. Magnesium or manganese[1159]
- **Alpha-ketoglutarate dehydrogenase (complex), oxoglutarate dehydrogenase (complex)**: Vitamin B3: produces NADH, Vitamin B1 (thiamine pyrophosphate): oxoglutarate dehydrogenase, Lipoic acid: dihydrolipoyl succinyltransferase, Vitamin B2: dihydrolipoyl dehydrogenase subunit requires; also, B2 is needed for formation of NADH. *Comment*: This is not a single enzyme but rather an "enzyme complex" with several subunits, each with its own nutritional cofactor; one of the main end-products is the formation of NADH from B3. Glutamate is converted to alpha-ketoglutarate by glutamate dehydrogenase, which is blocked by sulfite, which is itself derived from certain foods and medications and which can also be chelated by hydroxocobalamin; excess sulfite impairs formation of alpha-ketoglutarate and can reduce ATP production by more than 50%.[1160]
- **Succinyl-CoA synthetase**: [no coenzyme noted]
- **Succinate dehydrogenase, succinate-coenzyme Q reductase, Complex 2 of the ETC**: This is a complex enzyme with several subunits. Uses oxidized CoQ-10 in the form of ubiquinone to form the reduced form ubiquinol. This is the only enzyme complex that participates in both the citric acid cycle and the electron transport chain. CoQ-10: enzyme binds directly with CoQ-10, Vitamin B2: a flavoprotein is part of the enzyme's structure, Iron: an iron-sulfur protein is part of the enzyme's structure, Cardiolipin (containing the fatty acid DHA) and phosphatidylethanolamine (which can contain DHA, arachidonic acid, and/or oleic acid) are components of two hydrophobic membrane anchor subunits.
- **Fumarase**: Vitamin B3: produces NADH; however, the enzyme itself appears to function without cofactors or coenzymes.
- **Malate dehydrogenase**: Vitamin B3: produces NADH

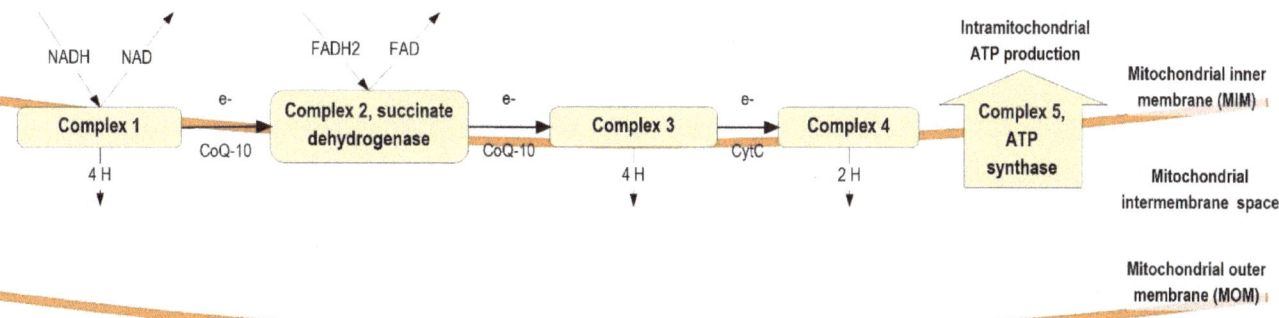

Electron transport chain (ETC) structure, with additional emphasis on the "nonstructure" of the innermembrane space created by the inner and outer mitochondrial membranes, permeability of both of which must be tightly regulated for optimal mitochondrial performance, including but not limited to ATP production: The semi-contained mitochondrial intermembrane space allows the accumulation of protons from the electron transport chain (ETC) to concentrate into a "pressurized" electromechanical gradient that powers ETC Complex #5, also called ATP synthase. ATP synthase is powered via the transmittal of protons from their high concentration gradient in the intermembrane space through the structure of the ATP synthase enzyme, which acts as a "pore" or "pressure valve" allowing protons to move to an area of lesser concentration inside the mitochondria. If the ATP synthase enzyme is bypassed due to a defective or "leaky" inner membrane that allows protons to leak back into the mitochondria, then the production of cellular energy will be reduced, leading to metabolic impairments such as increased free radical production (as the ETC works harder to compensate for reduced efficiency) and clinical manifestations such as fatigue, dyscognition, and muscle (e.g., heart) impairment including body aches and pains consistent with clinical presentations of fibromyalgia and chronic fatigue syndrome. Transmembrane potential of the mitochondrial inner membrane (MIM) is essential for the electromechanical gradient that drives ATP synthase; compromise of this membrane due to dietary faults (e.g., fatty acid deficiency, antioxidant deficiency) or biochemical faults (e.g., overproduction of free radicals which damage the MIM) will lead to hyperpermeability of the MIM ("leaky mitochondria") and reduced ATP synthesis. Clinical implications and interventions are discussed in the text; most of the clinical work with regard to nutritional optimization of the MIM has been led by Professor Garth Nicolson PhD.

[1159] en.wikipedia.org/wiki/Isocitrate_dehydrogenase#Detailed_mechanism Accessed April 2012
[1160] "Intracellular ATP measured 3 h later was significantly depleted by 100 μM sulfite, with about 50–60% decrease in both [neural and hepatic] cell lines." Zhang X, Vincent AS, Halliwell B, Wong KP. A mechanism of sulfite neurotoxicity: direct inhibition of glutamate dehydrogenase. *J Biol Chem*. 2004 Oct 8;279(41):43035-45

A Practical, Cost-Effective, Safe, Ethical Clinical Approach to Improving Mitochondrial Function—DrV's Strategy Suitable for Most Cases of Mitochondrial Dysfunction Seen in General Outpatient Practice

Mitochondrial disorders can be categorized based on the underlying etiology or combination of etiologies:

1) <u>Primary/genotropic mitochondrial disorders</u>: These can range from mild to severe, from occult to life-threatening, and although usually apparent in infancy-childhood, these primary/genotropic disorders can present later in adult life. Manifestations can be generalized affecting multiple organ systems or specific to one system—most commonly either the heart or central nervous system. Due to their rarity, severity, and need for specialist management, these primary/genotropic disorders are not the focus of the following section, although much of the information will be relevant, and conceptually and clinically applicable. For example, the rather common *and notably mild* primary/genotropic mitochondrial disorders associated with migraine headaches are a clear example of a heritable/primary/genotropic mitochondriopathy that responds very well to the interventions described below, especially nutrients that support the electron transport chain (ETC), namely coenzyme Q10 (CoQ-10), riboflavin, magnesium as discussed and cited below. In the main, primary/genotropic mitochondrial disorders are relatively rare.

2) <u>Secondary/acquired mitochondrial disorders</u>: Mitochondrial performance can be severely impaired by secondary/acquired conditions, such as exposure to certain pharmaceutical drugs, toxic industrial chemicals, toxic metals, and bacterial or viral infections; these types of mitochondrial disorders have been previously underappreciated but are progressively gaining a foothold in the consciousness of researchers and clinicians worldwide. These secondary/acquired mitochondrial disorders can affect anyone at any time. The clinical strategy for these conditions should be obvious, focusing on the support of optimal mitochondrial function (outlined below) while eliminating the problematic infection and/or toxic exposure (customized per patient's exposure). Importantly, secondary/acquired mitochondrial disorders are increasingly recognized as common (as more physicians become aware of the clinical frequency and implications of mitochondrial dysfunction) and are becoming more common (as our environment becomes more polluted with herbicides, pesticides, and other persistent organic pollutants as a result of governmental-political failure to regulate industry and protect humanity from unfettered corporate profiteering.

3) <u>Mixed-etiology (perhaps also called tertiary) mitochondrial disorders</u>: Of course, a patient could have both a primary/genotropic disorder along with a secondary/acquired mitochondrial disorder. The classic example of this combination is migranogenic mitochondrial impairment (primary disorder) exacerbated by one or more secondary disorders such as microbial colonization, a pro-inflammatory diet, or nutrient (e.g., magnesium) deficiency; this model helps explain—and place into perspective—the hereditary and environmental contributions to such mixed-etiology mitochondrial disorders.

When possible, the cause of the mitochondrial dysfunction should be treated directly; however, in practical reality of clinical practice, we often have to use an empirical and eclectic approach. Note that eclecticism and empiricism are not the same as random and illogical; even when using an empirical and eclectic approach, we clinicians can choose among the more efficacious and applicable interventions per research and nuances of patient history and assessment. For more complicated or severe cases, we can use laboratory assessments, depending on the problem suspected clinically; however, more skilled and experienced clinicians tend to find that laboratory tests for the assessment of mitochondrial function are not needed on a routine basis. On the contrary, the vast majority of mitochondrial dysfunction observed or suspected in routine outpatient clinical practice can be treated without mitochondria-specific, time-consuming, resource-depleting, and treatment-delaying laboratory assessments.

Understanding mitochondrial function for clinical intervention: As a group of intracellular organelles numbering from—for example, and not including the zero per erythrocyte—200 per cell in the biceps to 3,500 per cardiomyocyte, **mitochondria are a heterogeneous group**, populated by those with a theoretical optimal performance ("Olympians") down to those with cell-threatening and body-damaging effects ("misfits"). The mitochondrial population must therefore be occasionally culled for the health of the cell and of the larger organism.[1161] Generally, the interconnected eliminative and regenerative processes can be described with the following terminology; additional terms are also listed here for convenience.

1) <u>Fusion</u>: The binding of two mitochondria into one single mitochondria,
2) <u>Reallocation/partitioning</u>: The redistribution of "better" and "worse" mitochondrial components into regions that will eventually split to generate progeny.
3) <u>Fission</u>: The splitting of the large mitochondrion into two daughter mitochondria: 90% of the time, both offspring will be sufficiently healthy and will have benefitted from the reallocation of genetic and structural material, while approximately 10% of the time, one mitochondrion will have received the better components and thus has significantly improved function, and the other ("the runt") will have been allocated a disproportionate share of the damaged/expended/oxidized mitochondrial goods and will therefore have severely impaired function, which targets it for destruction via mitophagy.
4) <u>Mitophagy/autophagy</u>: Targeted destruction of dysfunctional mitochondria; this can occur following the fusion-fission cycle or likely—in the case of a severely dysfunctional *misfit* mitochondria—directly, i.e., without preceding fusion and fission. Although destruction/removal often has a negative connotation (perhaps mostly in Western cultures unconsciously dominated by the Greek-Roman "progressive and additional" Apollonian ideal without the balancing "regressive and subtractive" Dionysian construct), readers should appreciate that mitophagy is necessary for sustaining cellular and organismal health; defects in mitophagy are inconsistent with health and survival. As discussed below, **some significant benefits derived from carbohydrate restriction, fasting, and exercise are mediated by the promotion of mitophagy**, because mild cellular stresses prompt the fusion/fission/mitophagy process, which generally leads to enhanced health and performance of the remaining mitochondrial population, also referred to *en masse* as the "mitochondrial mass." Obviously, if mitophagy proceeds unchecked, then cells will lose the mitochondria's ability to form sufficient ATP and carry out other functions, and cell death will result. In sum: **Insufficient mitophagy promotes oxidative and inflammatory injury, while excess mitophagy leads to insufficient production of ATP and causes cell death and resultant tissue/organism failure**.
5) <u>Biogenesis</u>: Just as mitophagy can occur without a preceding fusion-fission cycle, so can fission; if a mitochondrion is a reasonably robust *Olympian* and if it is stimulated by intracellular signals indicating sufficient nutrients and need are present, it can split, accumulate nutrients, and grow, thus contributing directly to an enhanced mitochondrial population and expanded mitochondrial biomass.

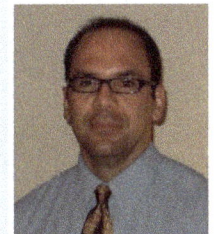

2013 INTERNATIONAL CONFERENCE ON HUMAN NUTRITION AND FUNCTIONAL MEDICINE
PORTLAND OREGON CONVENTION CENTER • SEPTEMBER 25-29, 2013

Mitochondrial Nutrition *and Beyond*:
Mitochondrial Optimization for Optimal Health
- Brief introduction and review
- Mitochondrial interventions

Alex Vasquez D.C., N.D., D.O., F.A.C.N.

2013 presentation and slides:
- Presentation slides: CreateSpace.com/4478800
- Video access: vimeo.com/ichnfm/2013mito-drv
- Password: DrV_mito_protocol2013
- Album access: vimeo.com/album/3033545
- Password: DrV_Mito_and_More

[1161] Twig G, et al. Mitochondrial fusion, fission and autophagy as a quality control axis: the bioenergetic view. *Biochimica et Biophysica Acta* 2008 May; 1777: 1092–1097

6) Δψm, MIM transmembrane potential (MIMtmp): MIM transmembrane potential (MIMtmp) is a quantification of proton concentration in the intermembrane space. For optimal mitochondrial performance, MIMtmp needs to be conceptually "in the middle"—neither too high nor too low.

- **Excess MIM transmembrane potential—mitochondrial hyperpolarization—essentially turns off ETC flow and "shuts down" or "hibernates" the mitochondria, which is now resistant to triggering of apoptosis, thus promoting cell immortalization seen in cancer, autoimmunity, and vascular smooth muscle hyperproliferation**: Excessive polarization of the transmembrane potential (MIM hyperpolarization, MIMhp) can be caused by LPS activation of TLR, and it can also be caused by immune activation itself, with the latter resulting in a vicious cycle because immune activation causes MIMhp which then triggers activation of mTOR, which promotes additional inflammation and autoimmunity as well as resistance to apoptosis, allowing autoreactive lymphocytes to evade deletion. While mitochondrial hyperpolarization impairs apoptosis, cell death via necrosis is enhanced, and this "inflammatory death" of immunocytes contributes to total inflammatory load since necrotic debris from cells and mitochondria activates damage associated molecular pattern (DAMP) receptors which promote inflammation.

> **MIM hyperpolarization is characteristic of cancer and autoimmunity, with the latter secondary to mTOR activation and its inhibition of FoxP3+ Treg generation**
> - "Maximal hyperpolarization stalls respiration and oxidative phosphorylation, essentially "*shutting off mitochondria*" and shifting energy production to the cytoplasm, with glycolysis becoming the primary source of ATP. A glycolytic phenotype is associated with resistance to apoptosis, in part because the "inactive" hyperpolarized mitochondria cannot induce apoptosis. The majority of human cancers are characterized by hyperpolarized mitochondria, and this metabolic remodeling might be the basis of the Warburg effect in cancer."*
> - "Mitochondrial hyperpolarization and the resultant ATP depletion sensitize T cells for necrosis, which may significantly contribute to inflammation in patients with SLE."**
>
> *Michelakis ED. Mitochondrial medicine: a new era in medicine. *Circulation*. 2008 May **Gergely et al. Mitochondrial hyperpolarization and ATP depletion in patients with SLE. *Arthritis Rheum*. 2002 Jan

- **Insufficient MIM transmembrane potential** "deflates" the proton gradient that is needed to drive ATP synthase; an excessive reduction triggers MTP-mediated apoptosis: A reduction in MIMtmp can be caused by 1) reduced Krebs' and/or ETC performance causing reduced proton generation, or by leakage of protons back through the MIM via 2) unregulated *basal* transmembrane permeability ("leaky mitochondria") due to oxidative damage to the MIM or dietary lack of appropriate fatty acids and phospholipids for MIM structure and maintenance, 3) heightened *augmented physiologic* channel-mediated transmembrane conductance via UPC (uncoupling proteins) or the dreaded MTP (mitochondrial transition pore) which is activated by reduced MIMtmp and leads to further rapid "deflating" of the mitochondria, spewing of apoptotic mediators to the cytoplasm and resultant cell death, 4) artificial *pharmacologic/xenobiotic* ionophore-mediated transmembrane conductance via substances such as salicylate and 2,4-dinitrophenol, and/or possibly 5) leakiness of the MOM, which is generally incompatible with mitochondrial and cell survival. **When MIMtmp is reduced by whatever means, then ATP synthase's rotary catalysis of ATP production will be reduced, thus severely compromising the generation of cellular energy.**

Conceptually and therefore practically, clinicians benefit from organizing information into categories that can then be subdivided into individual therapeutics; the three main categories of "interventional mitochondrial medicine" as I am defining it are ❶ therapeutic mitophagy—interventions which support therapeutic mitophagy such as carbohydrate/calorie restriction and physical exercise, ❷ mitochondrial support and stimulation—nutritional/phytonutritional support of biochemical processes (e.g., Krebs' cycle and ETC) and physiologic processes (e.g., biogenesis), and ❸ therapeutic disinhibition—removing the obstacles to mitochondrial performance such as xenobiotics and infections. Practically and respectively, these three steps are applied as 1) lifestyle, 2) supplementation, and 3) removal; skilled clinicians should be able to address each of these components simultaneously, prioritizing each particular treatment plan per the needs and responses of the patient. Students/clinicians implementing these protocols should already be familiar with dosing and administration and therefore such information is not included here; further, doses have to be modified per patient not simply based on age, weight, renal function, and (poly)pharmacy, but also per the level of need for and engagement with the overall treatment plan. With regard to the latter two considerations, the dose, duration, and variety of interventions is determined by severity of the illness(es) and the willingness vs resistance of the patient to do the whole program or simply a fewer parts of it. Indeed, doing every aspect of every component of the FINDSEX protocol would be prohibitively expensive and impractically time-consuming for most patients; here, physicians will have to guide patients to the most effective and necessary components of the protocol to customize the plan for the needs, abilities, and nuances of each patient.

❶ **Therapeutic mitophagy *via lifestyle*:** My concept of "therapeutic mitophagy" is this: the intentional induction/promotion of mitophagy—for either/both of the following: reduction in mitochondrial mass for a reduction in inflammatory signaling and oxidant production, and the "culling of the mitochondrial herd" to eliminate the lower-performing mitochondria. Carbohydrate restriction and moderate exercise are two safe and universally available and affordable means to therapeutically/intentionally induce mitophagy and achieve numerous anti-oxidant and anti-inflammatory benefits.

1. **Carbohydrate restriction/avoidance, fasting, ketogenic diet**:
   - Mitochondrial mechanism(s): High dietary loads of carbohydrates overwhelm the nonregulated enzymatic systems involved in substrate conversion, leading to what can be described as a short-term "mitochondrial burnout" due to excess subsequent free radical generation; evidence of this appears quite clear, with an irrefutable collection of data from human trials showing that 100g glucose leads to oxidative stress, antioxidant depletion, a measurable inflammatory response, and immune/phagocytic suppression. Conversely, carbohydrate restriction promotes mitochondrial function generally by allowing mitochondria to adapt to being fueled by a variety of sources (leading to structural reorganization of ETC supercomplex assembly[1162]), rather than the "easy currency" and "quick fix" of carbohydrate; specifically, carbohydrate restriction promotes ketogenesis and resultant endogenous production of beta-hydroxy-butyrate (bHB) which stimulates complexes 3 and 4 of the ETC. Whereas consumption/provision of "simple" carbohydrates appears to overwhelm mitochondria and lead to oxidative stress and inflammation; carbohydrate avoidance and promotion of a mildly ketotic state have the opposite effects—anti-inflammatory and antioxidant benefits. The mild stress of caloric/carbohydrate restriction prompts a wide range of physiologic adaptations, one of which is mitophagy, which has the overall effect of reducing oxidant stress and pro-inflammatory signaling.
   - Clinical benefits: Carbohydrate avoidance—and its physiologic converse of ketogenesis promotion—demonstrates an unsurpassed cure rate of hypertension and diabetes mellitus type-2. Carbohydrate avoidance promotes endogenous antioxidant defenses, systemic anti-inflammation, longevity in multiple species, and a rejuvenative phenotype via—among several other means—histone acetylation.
2. **Exercise**:
   - Mitochondrial mechanism(s): Improves oxygen delivery via vasodilation and increased cardiovascular output (heart rate × stroke volume). Promotes mito-availability of magnesium due to systemic alkalinization secondary to physiologic hyperventilation and resultant respiratory alkalosis; alkalinity promotes renal retention of magnesium and increases intracellular uptake of magnesium thereby increasing magnesium's availability to various enzymes, including the phosphorylating ATP synthase. The stress of exercise prompts a wide range of physiologic adaptations, one of which is mitophagy, which has the overall effect of reducing oxidant stress and pro-inflammatory signaling; exercise also promotes mitochondrial biogenesis and induction/upregulation of ATP-producing substrate-converting enzymes.
   - Clinical benefits: Weight loss, anti-inflammation via elaboration of myokines and via reduction in (visceral) adipose), enhanced insulin responsiveness via muscle uptake of glucose as well as increased elaboration of GLUT-4 receptors, reduced mental depression and psychological dependency, enhanced appearance and self-esteem, likely increased competence and intelligence via skill-building and exercise-induced neurogenesis assuming that one is in [has created for oneself] an environment conducive to intellectual optimization; obviously, this requires more than simply the provision of exercise for neurogenesis and synaptic plasticity; one must give these new neuroconnections something to ponder and perform.

[1162] Lapuente-Brun et al. Supercomplex assembly determines electron flux in the mitochondrial electron transport chain. *Science*. 2013 Jun 28;340(6140):1567-70

❷ **Mitochondrial support** *via supplementation*: Many interventions are available which serve to either support or stimulate mitochondrial function. Simply "stimulating" mitochondrial function would likely be a bad idea if a sizeable portion of the individual's mitochondrial population is dysfunctional; stimulating dysfunctional mitochondria would be expected to promote inflammation and oxidative stress. Clinicians should seek to—as we say in naturopathic medicine—*reestablish the foundation for* (mitochondrial) *health* before employing attempts at mitochondrial stimulation or interventions that promote biogenesis. Thus, in this second category, I will list—in somewhat of a prioritized sequence—those therapeutics which generally support and can later be used to optimize mitochondrial function generally and ATP production specifically. The prioritization of these is somewhat—but not entirely—conceptual; the actual "priority" is the one-many that will best benefit the individual patient.

3. <u>Five-Part Supplemented Paleo-Mediterranean Diet</u>[1163]: **Plant-based protein-adequate organic diet supplemented with vitamins, minerals, fatty acids, and probiotics.**
    - <u>Mitochondrial mechanism(s)</u>: Vitamins (coenzymes) and minerals (cofactors) must be present in sufficient amounts in order for biochemical reactions to proceed with health-optimizing efficiency; nutritional deficiencies impair biochemical efficiency and initiate the progressive reductions in cellular function that initiates/promotes/mimics and contributes to various disease states. Most people are nutrient deficient and should take a multivitamin and multimineral supplement[1164,1165], and people with metabolic impairments such as those due to single nucleotide polymorphisms (SNPs) will need to use "high-dose vitamin therapy" for the duration of their lives in order to stimulate their variant enzymes[1166] and—speaking casually—push sluggish enzymes to complete their reactions. More specifically, B1 (thiamine), B2 (riboflavin), B3 (niacin), B5 (pantothenate), and lipoic acid are required components for the pyruvate dehydrogenase complex[1167] which transfers/converts pyruvate made in the cytoplasm into acetyl-CoA in the mitochondria. B2 is required for the formation of flavin adenine dinucleotide (FAD), and B3 is required for the formation of niacinamide adenine dinucleotide (NAD)—both of these constituents are absolutely required for mitochondrial production of ATP. Further, B2 is a cofactor for glutamate dehydrogenase which converts glutamate to alpha-ketoglutarate for use in the Krebs' cycle. Magnesium is required for phosphorylation reactions, e.g., phosphorylation of ADP to ATP by Complex 5—ATP synthase. Antioxidants, such as tocopherols in general (especially gamma) and tocopherol succinate in particular, help to protect oxidation-vulnerable phospholipids and nuclear and mitochondrial DNA. For general biochemical and antioxidant "support" of mitochondrial function, and for the prevention and treatment of mitochondrial disorders—regardless of cause—routine use of a high-quality broad-spectrum multivitamin and multimineral supplement is reasonable.
    - <u>Clinical benefits</u>: B1 improves renal function in DM. B2 improves mood, especially in women, and doses of 400mg daily are remarkably effective for migraine prophylaxis with the most likely effect being mediated via improved function of ETC Complex #2. B3 is also effective against migraine, perhaps partly via vasodilation, but more likely via stimulation of ETC Complex #1. The vitamin CoQ-10 is necessary for ETC Complexes #1-3. These and other nutrient-specific locations are illustrated in the diagram below of the ETC.

4. <u>Coenzyme-Q10</u>: CoQ-10 would have received better public acceptance if Folkers had named it "vitamin Q" instead of "coenzyme Q", per his own admission.
    - <u>Mitochondrial mechanism(s)</u>: Transfers electrons between complexes 1, 2, and 3. Functions as lipid-soluble antioxidant. Direct anti-inflammatory effect via inhibition of NFkB.
    - <u>Clinical benefits</u>: The single most effective "vitamin" treatment for hypertension; alleviates hypertension and insulin resistance probably via improvement of mitochondrial function. Remarkably effective for migraine prophylaxis in adults and children; clinical benefits also shown for Parkinson's disease and Huntington's disease (delayed progression) and asthma (reduced medication dependency). The best nutritional treatment for renal insufficiency is CoQ-10 100-300mg/d and thiamine 100mg TID.

[1163] Vasquez A. Revisiting the Five-Part Nutritional Wellness Protocol: The Suppplemented Paleo-Mediterranean Diet. *Nutritional Perspectives* 2011 Jan: 19-25 ichnfm.org/faculty/vasquez/pdf/vasquez_2011_five-part_protocol_revisited.pdf
[1164] Fletcher RH, Fairfield KM. Vitamins for chronic disease prevention in adults: clinical applications. *JAMA*. 2002 Jun 19;287(23):3127-9
[1165] Heaney RP. Long-latency deficiency disease: insights from calcium and vitamin D. *Am J Clin Nutr*. 2003 Nov;78(5):912-9
[1166] Ames et al. High-dose vitamin therapy stimulates variant enzymes with decreased coenzyme binding affinity (increased K(m)). *Am J Clin Nutr*. 2002 Apr;75:616-58
[1167] My source of information on this list of coenzymes is my professor in medical school at UNTHSC, Ladislav Dory PhD. I realize some might debate this list of cofactors; but likewise my professor—based on his intimate work with mitochondria—would likely refute those debates. So, I think this list is reasonable for purposes presented here.

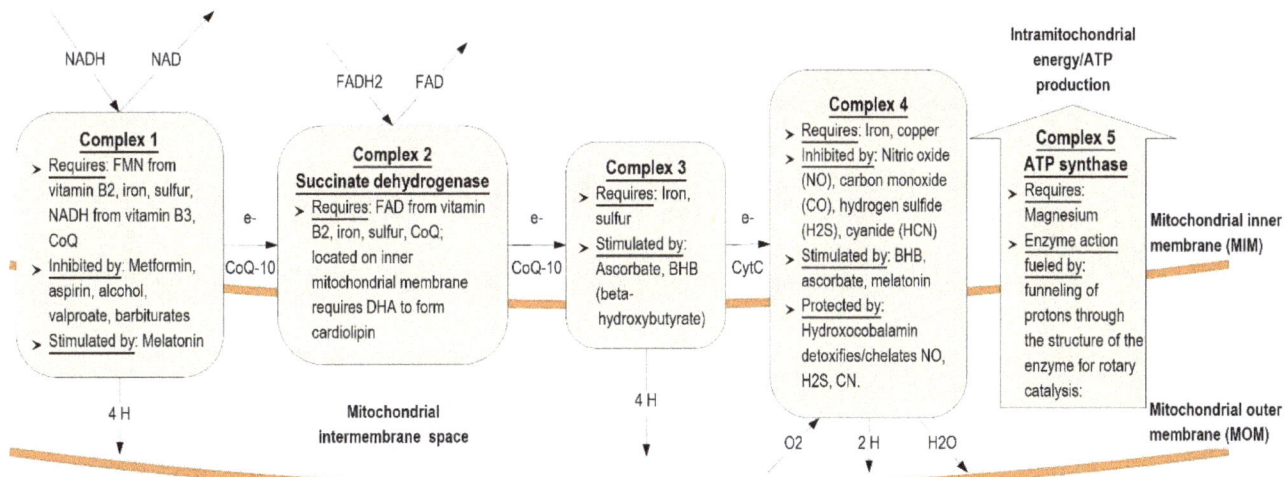

Electron transport chain (ETC) with some requirements, inhibitors, stimulators, and protectors: Clinical implications are obvious from the diagram and are additionally discussed in the text.

5. **"Vitamin E"**: What is meant here by "vitamin E" is mixed tocopherols with at least 40% gamma-tocopherol; additionally, alpha-tocopherol succinate has been described as being somewhat "mitochondria specific" and might be used alongside mixed tocopherols. A reasonable *supplemental* dose of tocopherols is 400 IU/d while a more assertive *interventional* dose is 1,200-1,600 IU/d.
   - Mitochondrial mechanism(s): Generalized anti-inflammatory and anti-oxidant effects; specifically helps to protect cell membranes in general and mitochondrial membranes in particular.
   - Clinical benefits: Anti-inflammatory and immune-modulating effects (e.g., reductions in IgE in patients with eczema, and reductions in ANA in patients with various autoimmune diseases). Alleviates pain in osteoarthritis; can help to restore/normalize mitochondrial function in patients with mitochondrial disease. Important experimental (not clinical) research published in 2013 by Salinthone et al[1168] showed for the first time that (alpha) tocopherol raises cAMP and has a potent anti-inflammatory effect, with a notable maximal reduction of PHA-stimulated IL-17 production by 73-79% in human peripheral blood mononuclear cells (PBMC); of additional note and importance, the authors report their findings using various other nutrients on cAMP production, "cAMP levels were 7.56, 10.57, 14.23 and 5.21 pmol/mg protein for GSE, EGCG, ascorbic acid, and resveratrol, respectively. Conversely, treatment with α-tocopherol resulted in a greater than 2-fold increase in cAMP level (29.19 pmol/mg protein) compared to baseline. Lipoic acid was used as a positive control, which generated 45.49 pmol/mg protein of cAMP."

6. **Lipoic acid**:
   - Mitochondrial mechanism(s): Coenzyme for various enzymatic reactions, including pyruvate dehydrogenase. Water-soluble and lipid-soluble antioxidant. Anti-inflammatory benefits via direct inhibition of NFkB as well as via reductions in IL-17.
   - Clinical benefits: Diabetic neuropathy, hypertension, diabetes mellitus type-2. Per the work of Bruce Ames and based largely on animal studies, we note that lipoic acid and acetyl-L-carnitine function additively/synergistically and should generally be used together. Lipoic acid has a short half-life and should therefore be administered in divided doses throughout the day, e.g., 300-400mg TID-QID.

7. **L-carnitine and Acetyl-L-carnitine (the "carnitines")**: 2-4 g/d
   - Mitochondrial mechanism(s): L-carnitine is required for mitochondrial beta-oxidation of long-chain fatty acids for ATP production; long-chain fatty acids must be in the form of esters of L-carnitine (acylcarnitines) in order

---

[1168] Salinthone et al. α-Tocopherol stimulates cyclic AMP production in human peripheral mononuclear cells and alters immune function. *Mol Immunol*. 2013 Mar:173-8 to enter the mitochondrial matrix where beta-oxidation occurs.[1169] Carnitines also lessen the cellular load of ceramide—inhibition of ceramide-generating sphingomyelinase has been documented, and promotion of ceramide degradation is hypothesized—thereby improving cellular metabolic function and reducing the secondary inflammation.

- Clinical pearl: One might reasonably wonder how/why supplementation with "carnitines" can be of benefit among patients who are well-nourished via dietary protein intake from animal sources; the answer is found in the fact that the metabolic impairment caused by the Westernized diet (notably high in both sugars and fats, especially saturated fats) leads to abnormalities in lipid deposition which demonstrate several abnormal characteristics and can thus be termed *metabolic dyslipidosis*, which I describe in the following way: *quantitative*—excess total fat, *qualitative*—notable accumulation of fatty acids that have physiologic consequences: notably palmitate and ceramide, *altered*—in obesity and insulin resistance, fats are altered biochemically for example by oxidation via oxidative stress or hydroperoxidation via lipoxygenase and are therefore chemically altered and abnormal, *locational*—inside parenchymal cells (not simply adipocytes) where they lead to metabolic impairments such as endoplasmic reticulum stress and mitochondrial dysfunction. Hence, in disorders associated with endoplasmic reticulum stress, mitochondrial dysfunction, insulin resistance, cardiomyopathy, and biological aging, supplemental carnitines can help rectify abnormal intracellular lipid accumulation/deposition via promotion of mitochondrial metabolism (beyond "fat burning" and more toward "trash burning") thereby alleviating part of the fuel overload problem that triggers metabolic impairment and its inflammatory consequences.

> **Multiple benefits of carnitines**
> "In humans and experimental models, carnitines have several activities that might influence aging. Fatty acid peroxidation proved depleted, and **carnitines restored the phospholipid composition of mitochondrial membranes and enhanced the cellular energetics in mitochondria**, increasing cytoplasmic acetyl-coenzyme A concentrations through the higher availability of **acetyl** groups. In addition, **carnitines stabilized cell membrane fluidity by regulating phospholipid levels** and **reduced ceramide production and insulin-like growth factor**, preventing cellular death and apoptosis."
> Cavallini et al, *Urology* 2004 Apr

- Clinical benefits of carnitine supplementation: Alzheimer's disease, hypertension, insulin resistance, Peyrone's disease, erectile dysfunction. Per Bruce Ames and based largely on animal studies, we note that lipoic acid and acetyl-L-carnitine function additively/synergistically and should be used together for optimal benefit.
    - In vitro study: L-carnitine prevents doxorubicin-induced apoptosis of cardiac myocytes via inhibition of ceramide generation (*FASEB J* 1999 Sep[1170]): This study showed that L-carnitine blocked ceramide production via sphingomyelinase following metabolic stress induced by doxorubicin/Adriamycin. The authors wrote, "Moreover, in vitro studies conducted on cell extracts or with purified acid sphingomyelinase demonstrated that L-carnitine exerted a dose-dependent, sphingomyelinase inhibitory effect (through V(max) reduction). Taken together, these findings show that by inhibiting a (perhaps novel) drug-activated acid sphingomyelinase and ceramide generation, L-carnitine can prevent doxorubicin-induced apoptosis of cardiac myocytes."
    - Clinical trial and proof of principle: Carnitines versus testosterone in the treatment of sexual dysfunction, depressed mood, and fatigue associated with male aging (*Urology* 2004 Apr[1171]): 120 male ~66yo patients were randomized into three groups: 1) testosterone (undecanoate, oral) 160 mg/day, 2) propionyl-L-carnitine 2 g/day plus acetyl-L-carnitine 2 g/day, 3) placebo for 6 months. "Testosterone and carnitines significantly improved the peak systolic velocity, end-diastolic velocity, resistive index, nocturnal penile tumescence, International Index of Erectile Function score, Depression Melancholia Scale score, and fatigue scale score. Carnitines proved significantly more active than testosterone in improving nocturnal penile tumescence and International Index of Erectile Function score. Testosterone significantly increased the prostate volume and free and total testosterone levels and significantly lowered serum luteinizing hormone; carnitines did not. CONCLUSIONS: Testosterone and, especially, carnitines proved to be active drugs for the therapy of symptoms associated with male aging." Very importantly, all of the men in this study—per inclusion criteria—demonstrated decreased libido and erectile quality, depressed mood and intellectual concentration ability, irritability, fatigue,

---

[1169] Linus Pauling Institute Micronutrient Information Center. L-Carnitine. lpi.oregonstate.edu/infocenter/othernuts/carnitine/
[1170] Andrieu-Abadie N, et al. L-carnitine prevents doxorubicin-induced apoptosis of cardiac myocytes: role of inhibition of ceramide. *FASEB J*. 1999 Sep;13(12):1501-10
[1171] Cavallini G, Caracciolo S, Vitali G, Modenini F, Biagiotti G. Carnitine versus androgen administration in the treatment of sexual dysfunction, depressed mood, and fatigue associated with male aging. *Urology*. 2004 Apr;63(4):641-6

and free testosterone lower than 6 pg/mL (normal range 8.7 to 54.7 pg/mL); despite the fact that they were all fatigued, depressed, and hypogonadal, carnitines 4g/d proved more effective than testosterone. Of additional note, this article repeatedly and uniquely emphasized that "carnitines" serve, via promotion of acetyl groups into Krebs cycle, to enhance ATP production and reduce ROS production, e.g., "*Carnitines boost the increase and transport of acetyl groups, thereby enhancing Krebs cycle and aerobic metabolism*" and "*Carnitines restore [normalize] the ROS physiologic concentration by acting on the Krebs cycle.*" This study showed that partial restoration of metabolic function using very simple nutritional intervention—two forms of L-carnitine 4g/d—is clinically effective and in fact more effective than testosterone for improving mood and sexual health in elderly hypogonadal men.

8. **Biotin: 2-10 mg/d (rarely up to 200 mg/d)**
   - Mitochondrial mechanism(s): The water-soluble nutrient biotin, generally classified as a B-complex vitamin, is required by all organisms but is synthesized only by "lower" organisms such as bacteria, yeast, molds, algae, and some plants; therefore, it is essential that humans have an adequate external source of the nutrient. Normal dietary intake of biotin is less than 97.5 microg (0.4 micromol); biotin absorption/bioavailability from oral administration is nearly 100% even with pharmacologic dosing[1172] thus indicating that parenteral administration is largely unnecessary except in the rarest of cases. Biotin performs its biochemical functions via attachment to proteins (biotinylation) such as enzymes and histones; attachment occurs via holocarboxylase synthetase and release via biotinidase. Biotin is an enzyme cofactor for the following five enzymes: (1 and 2) *Acetyl-CoA carboxylase I and II* for binding bicarbonate to acetyl-CoA to form malonyl-CoA. Malonyl-CoA is required for the synthesis of fatty acids. The former is crucial in cytosolic fatty acid synthesis, and the latter functions in regulating mitochondrial fatty acid oxidation. (3) *Pyruvate carboxylase* for gluconeogenesis, (4) *Methylcrotonyl-CoA carboxylase* for catabolism of leucine, (5) *Propionyl-CoA carboxylase* for the metabolism of certain amino acids, cholesterol, and odd-chain fatty acids.[1173] Genotropic defects in either the *attaching* holocarboxylase synthetase or the *releasing* biotinidase leads to –as would be expected– metabolic impairments (metabolic acidosis, neurologic and dermatologic disorders), the severity of which is dependent on the degree of enzyme impairment; biotinidase deficiency leads to biotin depletion due to failure of biotin recycling and failure to detach biotin from dietary proteins. Genotropic biotinopathy is treated with pharmacological/supranutritional doses of biotin 5–20 mg/d in children and adults; some patients may require higher doses of 40–200 mg/d.[1174] Secondary/acquired biotin deficiency is caused by insufficient/blocked dietary intake/absorption (e.g., due to raw egg white, malabsorption, long-term parenteral nutrition), increased need during pregnancy (note that biotin deficiency is teratogenic and occurs in humans[1175,1176]), excess loss with hemodialysis, or drug-induced depletion as with long-term anticonvulsant therapy—note that pharmacologic anticonvulsant therapy commonly causes deficiency of folate and cholecalciferol as well, with the latter two deficiencies contributing to increased seizure activity and therapeutic recalcitrance. Biotinylation of histones affects gene transcription in a manner similar (in concept) to the better known means of methylation and acetylation; in the case of histone biotinylation, the effect is dose-dependent, regional, and repressive[1177], notably of TNF-alpha gene transcription.[1178] Since biotin is a small molecule that can bind to many proteins without affecting biological activity, the finding of biotin-binding antibodies/immunoglobulins (BBI) is not surprising. A low percentage (3-6%) of the population has biotin-

> **Benefits of biotin**
> Biotin is a nontoxic water-soluble vitamin necessary for several metabolic pathways, mitochondrial fatty acid oxidation, and repression of TNF-alpha gene transcription.

[1172] "Biotin was administered orally (2.1, 8.2, or 81.9 micromol) or intravenously (18.4 micromol) to 6 healthy adults in a crossover design with > or =2 wk between each biotin administration. Before and after each administration, timed 24-h urine samples were collected. Urinary recoveries of biotin plus metabolites were similar (approximately 50%) after the 2 largest oral doses and the 1 intravenous dose, suggesting 100% bioavailability of the 2 largest oral doses… Our data provide evidence that oral biotin is completely absorbed even when pharmacologic doses are administered. Zempleni et al. Bioavailability of biotin given orally to humans in pharmacologic doses. *Am J Clin Nutr* 1999;69:504-8
[1173] lpi.oregonstate.edu/infocenter/vitamins/biotin/ Reviewed 2014 Jun
[1174] Baumgartner MR. Vitamin-responsive disorders: cobalamin, folate, biotin, vitamins B1 and E. *Handb Clin Neurol*. 2013;113:1799-810
[1175] "Biotin deficiency is teratogenic in several mammalian species. ... The conclusion that marginal biotin deficiency occurs frequently in the first trimester further raises concern about potential human teratogenicity." Mock et al. Marginal biotin deficiency during normal pregnancy. *Am J Clin Nutr*. 2002 Feb;75(2):295-9
[1176] "Taken together, such studies provide evidence that a substantial proportion of pregnant women are marginally biotin deficient. In mice, degrees of biotin deficiency that are metabolically similar to those seen in pregnant women are very teratogenic. Moreover, in mice, a marginal degree of biotin deficiency in the dam causes a much more severe degree of deficiency in the fetus. These observations further raise concerns that biotin deficiency does occur and does cause human birth defects." Mock DM. Marginal biotin deficiency is common in normal human pregnancy and is highly teratogenic in mice. *J Nutr*. 2009 Jan;139(1):154-7
[1177] Hassan YI, Zempleni J. A novel, enigmatic histone modification: biotinylation of histones by holocarboxylase synthetase. *Nutr Rev*. 2008 Dec;66(12):721-5
[1178] Kuroishi T, Endo Y, Muramoto K, Sugawara S. Biotin deficiency up-regulates TNF-alpha production in murine macrophages. *J Leukoc Biol*. 2008 Apr;83(4):912-20

binding IgM antibodies[1179] while the incidence of BBI is markedly higher in patients with metabolic/inflammatory/allergic/autoimmune diseases; given the role of biotin in mitochondrial function and suppression of TNF-alpha transcription, this finding warrants clinical consideration. Muratsugu et al[1180] quantified biotin-binding IgG, IgA, IgM among healthy and infirmed patients to find that while levels were generally low in the healthy population and within the IgM subclass, both biotin-binding IgA and *especially* biotin-binding IgG were impressively higher (frequency and quantity) among patients with bronchial asthma, atopic dermatitis, epilepsy, and juvenile rheumatoid arthritis (IgG range of positivity: 28-62%) compared with levels among the apparently healthy (7%); biotin-binding IgM was *lower* among infirmed than healthy. Likewise, Nagamine et al (1994)[1181] found a higher prevalence of BBI in patients with Grave's thyropathy (47% vs 10% in nonGrave's). The question then becomes whether this finding is an *insignificant epiphenomenon*, a *pathogenic cause or consequence*, or *if a subclass might even be protective*; the former hypothesis—that BBI are a clinically insignificant epiphenomenon—appears to be the victor. Muratsugu M et al (op cit) concluded, "The clinical significance of biotin-binding immunoglobulin is not clear at the present time…" Nagamine et al (op cit 1994) found "no significant relationship between BBI prevalence and thyroid hormone concentrations, anti-thyroglobulin antibody (TGAb) or anti-thyroid microsomal antibody (McAb) titers. In addition, biotin levels in peripheral blood and red blood cells and biotinidase activity did not differ in the BBI detected and non-detected groups"; this data strongly suggests that although BBI are found in patients with thyroid autoimmunity, these BBI are not of pathogenic and clinical significance. Nagamine et al (1996)[1182] studied the prevalence of biotin-binding immunoglobulin in patients with allergic and autoimmune diseases and found a higher prevalence of BBI among patients with Crohn's disease, ulcerative colitis, atopic dermatitis, lupus, progressive systemic sclerosis; however, the lack of clinical correlation and the lack of correlation with serum biotin levels and clinical biotin status again appear to indicate that that BBI are a clinically insignificant epiphenomenon and—therefore—that biotin supplementation is not contraindicated in patients with (or without) BBI. Supranutritional biotin supplementation might provide clinical benefits via maintenance of mitochondrial performance and—*of potentially massive importance*—nutraceutical suppression of TNF-alpha transcription; in support of this component of anti-inflammatory/antirheumatic nutritional immunomodulation is the finding that **orally-administered biotin supplementation can decrease proliferation rates of peripheral blood mononuclear cells and decreases cytokine release in humans**.

- Clinical benefits of biotin supplementation:
    - Biotin supplementation at a pharmacologic dose decreases proliferation rates of human peripheral blood mononuclear cells (PBMC) and decreases cytokine release (*J Nutr* 2001 May[1183]): Oral administration of biotin 756.1 microg/d (3.1 micromol/d) for 14 d "caused a significant decrease of PBMC proliferation. At 2 d after mitogen stimulation, [3H]thymidine uptake by postsupplementation PBMC was 66 % of the uptake by presupplementation PBMC. Similarly, concentrations of interleukin-1β (2 d after mitogen) and interleukin-2 (1 d after mitogen) in media from postsupplementation PBMC were 65% and 44%, respectively, of those for presupplementation PBMC. … Overall, this study provides evidence that administration of pharmacologic doses of biotin [756.1 microg/d] for 14 d decreases PBMC proliferation and synthesis of interleukin-1β and interleukin-2." These are very impressive results, showing that a modest dose of orally administered biotin reduces monocyte proliferation by -34%, IL-1 by -35%, and IL-2 by -56%.
    - Drug-induced biotin deficiency in children with valproic acid (VPA) monotherapy (*Epilepsia*. 2001 Oct[1184]): "Strong inverse correlations were observed between liver enzymes and VPA blood levels with the activity of the enzyme. Additionally, no inhibitory effect on biotinidase activity was found, when the enzyme was incubated in vitro with high (1.2 mM) concentrations of the drug. Skin lesions (seborrheic rash, alopecia) were improved in our patients after biotin (10 mg/day) supplementation. It

---

[1179] "These IgM antibodies were present in 3% adults regardless of age, but were rarely found in children." Chen T et al. Biotin IgM antibodies in human blood: a previously unknown factor eliciting false results in biotinylation-based immunoassays. *PLoS One*. 2012;7(8):e42376
[1180] Muratsugu M et al. Quantitation of biotin-binding immunoglobulins G, A, and M in Human Sera Using F(ab')2anti-human immunoglobulin-coated microplates. *Biol Pharm Bull*. 2008 Mar;31(3):507-10
[1181] Nagamine et al. Clinical evaluation of biotin-binding immunoglobulin in patients with Graves' disease. *Clin Chim Acta*. 1994 Apr;226(1):47-54
[1182] Nagamine T et al. Prevalence of biotin-binding immunoglobulin in patients with allergic and autoimmune diseases. *Clin Chim Acta*. 1996 Feb 28;245(2):209-17
[1183] Per the authors 2.46 micromol = 600 microg, and thus 3.1 micromol = 756.1 microg. Zempleni J, Helm RM, Mock DM. In vivo biotin supplementation at a pharmacologic dose decreases proliferation rates of human peripheral blood mononuclear cells and cytokine release. *J Nutr*. 2001 May;131(5):1479-84
[1184] Schulpis KH et al. Low serum biotinidase activity in children with valproic acid monotherapy. *Epilepsia*. 2001 Oct;42(10):1359-62

is suggested that VPA impairs the liver mitochondrial function, resulting in a low biotinidase activity and or biotin deficiency." What interested me most about this article was the mention of drug-induced biotin deficiency/dysfunction and the connection with mitochondrial dysfunction; the full text of the article did not provide (likely through no fault of the authors) additional explication but rather a correlative hypothesis that "A possible speculation, as regards the VPA mechanism over biotinidase activity, could be related with an expected impairment of a number of carboxylases involved in the biotin cycle of mitochondrial function. Finally, the absence on an in vitro effect of the drug on biotinidase reinforces the suggestion that an indirect mechanism takes place between VPA and the enzyme." Biotinidase activity was dose-dependently reduced by approximately 20-80% *in vivo* despite the fact that the enzyme was not inhibited by the drug *in vitro*; therefore, VPA "somehow" causes impaired enzyme transcription or production, which the authors related to impaired mitochondrial function.

- o Chromium and biotin improves coronary risk factors in hypercholesterolemic type 2 diabetes mellitus (*J Cardiometab Syndr*. 2007 Spring[1185]): "The authors report here a randomized, double-blind placebo-controlled trial (N=348; chromium picolinate and biotin combination [CPB]: 226, placebo: 122; T2DM participants with hemoglobin A1c [HbA1c] >or=7%) evaluating the effects of CPB on lipid and lipoprotein levels. Participants were randomly assigned (2:1 ratio) to receive either CPB (600 microg chromium as chromium picolinate and 2 mg biotin) … In the primary analysis, CPB lowered HbA1c (P<.05) and glucose (P<.02) significantly compared with the placebo group. No significant changes were observed in other lipid levels. In participants with HC and T2DM, significant changes in total cholesterol and low-density lipoprotein cholesterol (LDL-C) levels and atherogenic index were observed in the CPB group (P<.05). Significant decreases in LDL-C, total cholesterol, HbA1c, and very low-density cholesterol levels (P<.05) were observed in the CPB group taking statins. CPB treatment was well tolerated with no adverse effects, dissimilar from those associated with placebo. These data suggest that intervention with CPB improves cardiometabolic risk factors."
- o Chromium picolinate and biotin combination improves glucose metabolism in treated, uncontrolled overweight/obese patients with type-2 diabetes (*Diabetes Metab Res Rev* 2008 Jan-Feb): N = 447 subjects with poorly controlled type 2 diabetes (HbA(1c) > or = 7.0%) were enrolled and received either chromium picolinate (600 microg Cr(+3)) with biotin (2 mg), or matching placebo, for 90 days in combination with stable oral anti-diabetic agents (OADs). … Change in HbA(1c) was significantly different between treatment groups (p = 0.03). HbA(1c) in the chromium picolinate/biotin group decreased 0.54%. The decrease in HbA(1c) was most pronounced in chromium picolinate/biotin subjects whose baseline HbA(1c) > or = 10%, and highly significant when compared with placebo (-1.76% vs - 0.68%; p = 0.005). Fasting glucose levels were reduced in the entire chromium picolinate/biotin group versus placebo (-9.8 mg/dL vs 0.7 mg/dL; p = 0.02). Reductions in fasting glucose were also most marked in those subjects whose baseline HbA(1c) > or = 10.0%, and significant when compared to placebo (-35.8 mg/dL vs. 16.2 mg/dL; p = 0.01). Treatment was well tolerated with no adverse effects dissimilar from placebo.

9. **Magnesium (Mg):** 600 mg/d or bowel tolerance; urinary alkalinization is important for cellular uptake
   - Mitochondrial mechanism(s): Magnesium plays a pivotal role in formation of the transition state of ATP synthase enzyme (complex 5) where ATP is synthesized from ADP and inorganic phosphate.[1186]
   - Clinical benefits: Hypertension, seizures/epilepsy, migraine and all types of headaches, insulin resistance, heart failure, depression, anxiety, bruxism and muscle cramps. Mg alleviates neurogenic inflammation in animal models.

10. **Medium-chain triglycerides (MTC):** dose varies per source and concentration (e.g., crude food extract versus purified concentrate), but generally 1-2 TBS = 15-30 ml = 14-28 g lipid = 100-200 calories; true toxicity is very low; gastrointestinal intolerance / diarrhea occurs with very large doses; margin of safety is very high

---

[1185] Albarracin C et al. Combination of chromium and biotin improves coronary risk factors in hypercholesterolemic type 2 diabetes mellitus. *J Cardiometab Syndr*. 2007;2(2):91-7
[1186] Ko YH, Hong S, Pedersen PL. Chemical mechanism of ATP synthase. *J Biol Chem*. 1999 Oct 8;274(41):28853-6

- Mitochondrial mechanism(s): MTC and the ketone bodies (KB) into which they are converted are clearly the preferred fuel source for most mitochondria under normal conditions. MTC and KB actually improve mitochondrial function via upregulation/induction of key enzymes and ETC complexes 3 and 4; in contrast to CHO such as fructose which cause mitochondrial damage, MTC and KB improve and restore mitochondrial function while serving as a fuel source. Beta-hydroxybutyrate (bHB) bolsters antioxidant defenses and promotes histone acetylation for induction of a rejuvenative phenotype.
- Clinical benefits: Administration of MTC (e.g., coconut oil), caprylic acid and relative derivatives, and/or fasting—which promotes endogenous bHB production—leads to clinical improvements in and alleviation of Alzheimer's disease, asthma and various inflammatory disorders. Note that ketogenic therapy is the most safe and effective treatment for both chronic epilepsy and status epilepticus.

11. **Resveratrol: 250 mg/d or more**
    - Mitochondrial mechanism(s): Resveratrol promotes mitochondrial biogenesis, hence is reputation for being the botanical mimic of exercise. Additionally, resveratrol also has some anti-oxidant and anti-inflammatory actions; paradoxically, resveratrol may have an estrogenic effect at the level of the estrogen receptor while also suppressing activity of aromatase.
    - Clinical benefits: Improvement in endothelial function; cardioprotective benefits.

12. **DHA (docosahexaenoic acid) from fish oil or blue-green algae: 500-2,000 mg/d or more**
    - Mitochondrial mechanism(s): DHA becomes integrated into the phospholipid phosphatidylserine, which is the structural anchor for succinate dehydrogenase—a key enzyme in the Krebs' cycle and ETC (complex 2).
    - Clinical benefits: Anti-inflammatory, cardioprotective, neuroprotective, improves cardiovascular health, improves brain function in various neuropsychiatric disorders such as depression, anxiety, bipolar, schizophrenia.

13. **Optimization of iron status—avoiding iron deficiency (both systemic and cerebral) while also avoiding iron overload**: Iron deficiency impairs mitochondrial function because iron is needed for several biochemical reactions in the electron transport chain; conversely, iron overload also impairs mitochondrial function due to free radical damage. The amount of iron in the body can be accurately determined by the blood test "serum ferritin." Per my publications on this topic and review of the literature (more than 300 papers read), optimal iron status correlates with a serum ferritin of 40-70 ng/ml; the only exception to this rule appears to be a subset of patients with restless leg syndrome (RLS) who have a defect in the transport of iron into the brain, such that they need higher levels of iron correlating with a serum ferritin up to 120 ng/ml. Stated again and differently, some patients with RLS have a defect in the transport of iron into the brain, and this defect can be overcome by allowing the patient to have higher-than-normal levels of iron, up to 120 ng/ml. Iron overload is a common problem, too, either due to lifestyle factors such as overconsumption of alcohol and/or iron-rich foods such as beef and liver, or due to diseases such as type-2 diabetes, metabolic syndrome, or the genetic iron-accumulation disorder hemochromatosis, which is one of the most common genetic diseases seen in humans with a frequency of approximately 1 per 200-250 in the general population. Hereditary iron overload disorders are seen in people of all genetic backgrounds and ethnicities; they appear most common in persons of African descent (perhaps as high as 1 per 80 persons). Serum ferritin levels higher than 200 ng/ml in a woman or 300 ng/ml in a man strongly suggest the probability of excess iron and warrant evaluation and treatment, even in the absence of clinical pathology[1187]; overt pathologic damage caused by iron is generally seen with ferritin values greater than 1,000 mcg/L. [Note: when discussing ferritin, the measurement units mcg/L and ng/ml are equivalent.]

    > **Optimal iron status is necessary for optimal mitochondrial function**
    > - Measure serum ferritin: For most patients, optimal iron status correlates with a serum ferritin of 40-70 ng/ml.
    > - Avoid iron deficiency: Iron is a required component of cytochrome C in the electron transport chain (ETC) that produces ATP.
    > - Avoid iron overload: Excess iron causes free radical damage that impairs mitochondrial function.

    - Mitochondrial mechanism(s): Iron is necessary for ETC complexes 3 and 4; iron deficiency causes ETC dysfunction, which generally results in reduced ATP formation and increased oxidant formation. Iron overload promotes lipid oxidation and DNA damage, both of which can contribute to mitochondrial impairment. Iron

---

[1187] Barton JC, McDonnell SM, Adams PC, et al. Management of hemochromatosis. *Ann Intern Med.* 1998 Dec 1;129(11):932-9

obviously plays other roles, such as formation of hemoglobin, synthesis of dopamine, function of thyroid hormones, fatty acid metabolism, etc.
- Clinical benefits: Patients feel better when their iron status is optimized so that they are neither iron-deficient nor iron-overloaded. For most patients, optimal iron status correlates with a serum ferritin of 40-70 ng/ml.

14. **N-Acetyl-Cysteine (NAC)**:
    - Mitochondrial mechanism(s): NAC provides cysteine for GSH production. NAC also inhibits NFkB. NAC inhibits viral replication (e.g., HIV) more effectively than and independently from its conversion to GSH. Recently, NAC at relatively high doses of 4,800mg/d in divided doses was shown to modulate mitochondrial hyperpolarization (by dissociating the generally resultant mTOR activation) and lead to very important clinical and immunological improvements in patients with SLE; NAC was shown to be safe and well-tolerated by all SLE patients up to 2.4g/d with reversible nausea in 33% of patients receiving 4.8g/d. This study by Lai, Hanczko, Bonilla, et al[1188] is truly a landmark contribution and advance in the field of rheumatology and immunology because it proves 1) that mitochondrial dysfunction directly leads to an autoimmune phenotype, and 2) that inhibition of mTOR by NAC is safe and effective in patients with SLE; important insights from this remarkable work are as follows:

    > **Mechanistic and clinical proof that mitochondrial dysfunction directly contributes to autoimmunity**
    >
    > "Similar to the effect of rapamycin, suppression of mTOR by NAC was accompanied by increased FoxP3 expression in CD4+/CD25+ T cells. These results suggest that the effect of NAC on the immune system is 1) cell type-specific and 2) it occurs through disconnecting the activation of mTOR from the elevation of $\Delta\psi_m$ in lupus T cells, similar to the effect of rapamycin."
    >
    > Lai et al. *Arthritis Rheum* 2012 Sep

    - NAC 4,800mg/d in divided doses proved safe and clinically beneficial in patients with SLE, leading to reductions in disease activity and ANA levels.
    - Mitochondrial hyperpolarization (MHP) causes mTOR activation which in turn suppresses the expression of the FoxP3 transcription factor necessary for induction of T-regulatory cells. Note that the mTOR activation is the cause of the FoxP3 suppression; ironically, NAC actually increases MHP but dissociates it from mTOR by having a greater effect on and via mTOR suppression. The nutritional supplement NAC works in a similar manner as does the immunosuppressive drug rapamycin, with a mechanism of suppression of mTOR and the effect of enhancing endogenous anti-inflammatory immunomodulation via CD4+ CD25+ FoxP3+ T-regulatory cells. Stated again and differently, NAC paradoxically worsens mitochondrial hyperpolarization in patients with SLE but does so at the same time that it has a more significant impact on mTOR; NAC's rapamycin-like targeting of mTOR dissociates mitochondrial hyperpolarization from mTOR activation. The reduction in mTOR activity (which is of greater consequence than the increase in MIM polarization) allows enhanced expression of FoxP3 for increased elaboration of T-regulatory cells, thereby providing endogenous immunoregulation.
    - "MHP of lupus T cells, which most prominently affects DN [double-negative, autoimmunity-promoting] T cells, was associated with resistance to activation-induced apoptosis. In 27 SLE patients receiving daily NAC doses of 1.2 g, 2.4 g, and 4.8 g considered together, both **spontaneous and CD3/CD28-induced apoptosis of DN T cells were markedly increased** and the **expansion of these cells was effectively reversed**. The **elimination of DN T cells, which are known promote anti-DNA autoantibody production by B cells**, is likely to contribute to reduced anti-DNA titers and to the efficacy of NAC.
    - "The therapeutic importance of NAC for SLE is reflected by: 1) achieving clinical improvement in two validated disease activity scores within 3 months; 2) diminishing fatigue (21), which is considered the most disabling symptom in a majority of SLE patients (22); 3) absence of significant side-effects; and 4) affordability of this medication. A monthly supply of 600-mg NAC capsules (120–240 capsules) costs $15–$30 on the retail market. This sharply contrasts with average annual direct medical costs estimated

---

[1188] Lai ZW, Hanczko R, Bonilla E, et al. N-acetylcysteine reduces disease activity by blocking mammalian target of rapamycin in T cells from systemic lupus erythematosus patients: a randomized, double-blind, placebo-controlled trial. *Arthritis Rheum*. 2012 Sep;64(9):2937-46 to be ~$22,580 per patient in 2009.Thus, the cost of NAC at $180–$360/year would be negligible in comparison to the overall expenditures to society and the expected benefit in reducing the need for vastly more expensive medications burdened with potentially serious side-effects."

15. <u>**General antioxidant support**</u>: Naturally-derived antioxidants in general tend to have anti-inflammatory, disease-alleviating, and health-promoting benefits; much of the benefit from eating a complex plant-based diet is derived from the additive and synergistic biochemical and physiologic benefits provided by phytonutrients, of which 5,000-8,000 exist.[1189] Hence, as I have stated and published for many years, the best approach is a plant-based diet that provides adequate protein, reduces intake of starchy phytonutrient-deficient carbohydrates such as wheat/rye/barley/potatoes, and to which is added a broad-spectrum high-potency multivitamin and multimineral supplementation.[1190]

- <u>Mitochondrial mechanism(s)</u>: Speaking generally, broadly, and accurately, we can estimate that anti-inflammatory and antioxidant therapeutics/diets/interventions/supplements will tend to improve mitochondrial function; some might argue against this by stating that oxidative stress induces hormesis to which I'll reply that chronic/sustained/long-term minute-by-minute adaptation is not possible because adaptive mechanisms are not long to be depleted. I think a better approach is to provide sufficient and perhaps supraphysiologic antioxidant support via diet and supplements and to then punctuate that biochemical bliss reasonable bouts of hormetic shock such as fasting, exercise, and ethanol to which defensive/adaptive mechanisms can respond—this is the best of both words, to which a few exceptions are noted, such as blunting of physiologic responsiveness to exercise with antioxidant supplementation in patients with DM-2/MetSyn. Identical arguments are valid or invalid within different clinical contexts, and the argument in favor of high(er) dosing of antioxidants is—as logically anticipated—more easily made when treating *autoimmune/hyperinflammatory/hyperoxidative* patients with more severe oxidant and inflammatory stress.

- <u>Clinical benefits</u>: Paraphrasing Dr Bruce Ames: Mitochondrial oxidative decay is a major contributor to aging and is accelerated by many common micronutrient deficiencies; an optimum intake of micronutrients can "tune-up mitochondrial metabolism" and give a marked increase in health, particularly for the poor, elderly, and obese, at little cost.[1191]

<u>Mitochondrial dysfunction as cause and consequence of oxidative stress and inflammation</u>:
Clinical implications are obvious from the diagram and are additionally discussed in the text.

[1189] Liu RH. Health benefits of fruit and vegetables are from additive and synergistic combinations of phytochemicals. *Am J Clin Nutr*. 2003 Sep;78(3 Suppl):517S-520S
[1190] Vasquez A. Revisiting the Five-Part Nutritional Wellness Protocol. *Nutr Perspect* 2011 Jan: 19-25
[1191] Ames BN, Atamna H, Killilea DW. Mineral and vitamin deficiencies can accelerate the mitochondrial decay of aging. *Mol Aspects Med*. 2005 Aug-Oct;26(4-5):363-78

16. **General anti-inflammatory support**:
    - <u>Mitochondrial mechanism(s)</u>: Pro-inflammatory cytokines such as interferon (IFN)-gamma, interleukin (IL)-1b, and tumor necrosis factor (TNF)-alpha impair mitochondrial function via cytokine-stimulated iNOS-induced nitric oxide (NO) production[1192], and mitochondrial dysfunction increases elaboration of ROS which act as signaling molecules to increase the production of pro-inflammatory cytokines[1193]; additively, mitochondrial dysfunction also increases cellular sensitivity to pro-inflammatory cytokines.[1194] Obviously, the stage is thus set for a self-perpetuating cycle.
    - <u>Clinical benefits</u>: Vitamin D3 supplementation, low-carbohydrate diets, and multivitamin-multimineral supplementation are excellent examples of anti-inflammatory interventions that are safe and effective. Additional anti-inflammatory benefit can be obtained by eradicating dysbiotic infections, correcting hormone imbalances, reducing obesity, etc. *Refer to my NFkB mini-monograph earlier in Chapter 4*.

17. **High-salicylate diet and/or low-dose aspirin to provide salicylate for ionophore alleviation of mitochondrial hyperpolarization—hypothesis**:
    - <u>Mitochondrial mechanism(s)</u>: To the best of my knowledge, I am the first to propose that the well-documented benefits of plant-based diets against cancer and autoimmunity may stem in part from the ionophore action of salicylate against mitochondrial hyperpolarization which is common both in cancer and autoimmunity.
    - <u>Clinical benefits</u>: High-plant diets and low-dose aspirin have shown benefit against inflammatory and malignant diseases; what I propose here is that part of the mechanism may be that of alleviation of mitochondrial hyperpolarization by the ionophore action of salicylic acid, a well-absorbed phytochemical that is believed to be significantly responsible for the health-promoting and anticancer benefits of plant-based diets.

18. **Alkalinization, acid-base balance, pH**: Several general statements can be made on this topic that are true and which will serve as an introduction to the topic of acid-base balance in the body. Although I initially approached this topic of acid-base balance with some skepticism and disregard, I have come to have profound and deep respect for this simple concept and intervention that provides numerous very important clinical benefits. Overall, the human body produces and excess of acidic substances that require balancing via internal buffering systems and also via dietary consumption of alkalinizing base-forming substances. The *internal* buffering systems succeed at keeping the acid-base balance within a range compatible for survival; *internal* buffering systems include control of respiratory rate, and the adaptations of the kidneys. The *external* buffering system of dietary consumption of foods that have an alkalinizing effect help to fine-tune the pH of the body in very important ways. My description is: *internal* acid-base buffering via respiration and renal adaptation sustains *life*, while the *external* acid-base buffering of dietarily consumed alkalinizing substances sustains *health*. The Western diet promotes diet-induced metabolic acidosis, while a plant-based Paleolithic diet or vegetarian diet promotes alkalinization.
    - <u>Mitochondrial mechanism(s)</u>: Alkalinization promotes renal retention and cellular uptake of magnesium, which is an essential nutrient for efficient action of complex 5, ATP synthase. In neurons, magnesium along with zinc also provide partial blockade of NMDA receptor channeling of calcium; high-levels of intracellular calcium ("intracellular hypercalcinosis"[1195]) promote inflammation and cause mitochondrial stress.
    - <u>Clinical benefits</u>: In sum, the benefits of slight alkalinization to achieve a urine pH of 7.5-8.5 include:
        - Increased renal retention of potassium, calcium, and magnesium
        - Increased (11%) intracellular uptake and retention of magnesium
        - Increased excretion of toxins and xenobiotics[1196]
        - Reduction in serum cortisol
        - Improved markers of bone health: reduced bone breakdown
        - Increased serum endorphins, which elevate mood, alleviate pain, and reduce addictiveness.

[1192] "These data suggest that IL-1b–induced NO production in cardiac myocytes lowers energy production and myocardial contractility through a direct attack on the mitochondria, rather than through cGMP-mediated pathways." Tatsumi T, Matoba S, Kawahara A, et al. Cytokine-induced nitric oxide production inhibits mitochondrial energy production and impairs contractile function in rat cardiac myocytes. *J Am Coll Cardiol*. 2000 Apr;35(5):1338-46
[1193] Naik E, Dixit VM. Mitochondrial reactive oxygen species drive proinflammatory cytokine production. *J Exp Med*. 2011 Mar 14;208(3):417-20
[1194] "… mitochondrial dysfunction could amplify the responsiveness to cytokine-induced chondrocyte inflammation through ROS and NF-κB activation." Vaamonde-Garcia et al. Mitochondrial dysfunction increases inflammatory responsiveness to cytokines in human chondrocytes. *Arthritis Rheum* 2012 Sep:2927-36
[1195] Vasquez A. Intracellular Hypercalcinosis. *Naturopathy Digest* 2006 naturopathydigest.com/archives/2006/sep/vasquez.php
[1196] Proudfoot AT, Krenzelok EP, Vale JA. Position Paper on urine alkalinization. *J Toxicol Clin Toxicol*. 2004;42(1):1-26

19. **Melatonin support, including sleep, 5HTP, dietary tryptophan such as whey protein isolate**:
    - Mitochondrial mechanism(s): Melatonin stimulates complexes 1 and 4 of the ETC; melatonin is also a powerful antioxidant. Melatonin also has an immune-stimulating action that shows clinical effectiveness against infections but which warrants caution for patients with allergy/autoimmunity.
    - Clinical benefits: Physiologic dose is 200 mcg/night; clinical doses range from 200mcg-40mg taken at night before bedtime. Benefits are noted in cancer (enhanced survival), fibromyalgia migraine (reduced pain), hypertension (mild reductions in pressure), and of course jet-lag and insomnia (resynchronization and sleep). With regard to improving sleep, some patients respond better to lower doses <3mg/night while higher doses >6mg/night can have a paradoxical effect of impairing sleep; further, some patients may experience impairment of libido and/or exacerbation of fatigue/depression—in case of the latter, early morning exercise and exposure to bright full-spectrum light are beneficial.
20. **Phospholipid replacement therapy**:
    - Mitochondrial mechanism(s): Because the function of the ETC-ATPase is completely dependent on the integrity of the inner mitochondrial membrane, and because oxidative damage and/or biochemical defects in phospholipid composition (e.g., due to poor nutrition and insufficient intake of proper fatty acids) impair function of the ETC and reduce transmembrane potential, phospholipid replacement therapy has conceptual validity, and clinical trials have proven its merit. Professor Dr Garth Nicolson[1197] deserves most of the credit for bringing this concept and application to clinical practice, and his research articles and clinical presentation from the 2013 International Conference on Human Nutrition and Functional Medicine (along with presentations and articles from Drs Hirshey, Gonzalez, and Vasquez) are online: ICHNFM.org/events/MitochondrialMedicine/
    - Clinical benefits: Phospholipid replacement therapy—whether with soy lecithin or with proprietary phospholipid formulations—has proven in animal studies and human clinical trials to improve health in general and mitochondrial performance in particular.
        - Lipid Replacement Therapy for replacing damaged lipids in cellular membranes and organelles and restoring function (*Biochim Biophys Acta* 2014 Jun[1198]): "Various chronic clinical conditions are characterized by membrane damage, mainly oxidative but also enzymatic, resulting in loss of cellular function. This is readily apparent in mitochondrial inner membranes where oxidative damage to phospholipids like cardiolipin and other molecules results in loss of trans-membrane potential, electron transport function and generation of high-energy molecules. Recent clinical trials have shown the benefits of Lipid Replacement Therapy in restoring mitochondrial function and reducing fatigue in aged subjects and patients with a variety of clinical diagnoses that are characterized by loss of mitochondrial function and include fatigue as a major symptom."
21. **Oxygen, deep breathing, exercise, hyperbaric oxygen**:
    - Mitochondrial mechanism(s): Oxygen is the molecular "magnet" which pulls protons through the ETC for the formation of water. Without oxygen to receive mitochondrial protons, mammalian cellular respiration ceases. Mild/moderate exercise promotes physiologic hyperventilation and increased cardiac output, increasing blood/nutrient and oxygen delivery to issues while also promoting systemic alkalinization via respiratory alkalosis. Hyperbaric oxygen can be used to "force" oxygen into underperfused tissues and to maximize oxygen-to-cell delivery thereby promoting mitochondrial function; excess oxygen therapy can have a detrimental effect via increased free radical production and also via promotion of vascular hyperproliferation, as noted in the treatment of the retinopathy of prematurity.
    - Clinical benefits: People feel better when they exercise and breathe deeply; doing so regularly improves mitochondrial performance.
22. **Ginkgo, Ginkgo biloba**:
    - Mitochondrial mechanism(s): Antioxidant, vasodilator, specifically improves mitochondria function.
    - Clinical benefits: Alleviation of intermittent claudication, erectile dysfunction, fibromyalgia (combination nutritional intervention with CoQ10), improved cognition and alleviation of dementia and depression.

[1197] Nicolson GL. Mitochondrial dysfunction and chronic disease: treatment with natural supplements. *Altern Ther Health Med*. 2014 Winter;20 Suppl 1:18-25
[1198] Nicolson GL, Ash ME. Lipid Replacement Therapy: a natural medicine approach to replacing damaged lipids in cellular membranes and organelles and restoring function. *Biochim Biophys Acta*. 2014 Jun;1838(6):1657-79

❸ **Mitochondrial disinhibition *via elimination of infections and xenobiotics***: If a patient has mitochondrial dysfunction not caused mostly by genetic mutations (e.g., low likelihood of inherited or spontaneous mitochondrial disease) nor by the biochemical impairment caused by coenzyme and cofactor deficiencies (e.g., let's assume the patient is well-nourished and is taking a high-potency broad-spectrum multivitamin and multimineral supplement), then we must ask, "What *exogenous* factors can cause mitochondrial impairment?" Beyond diet-induced impairment of mitochondrial function via consumption of simple carbohydrates (and resultant oxidative stress, fuel overload, ceramide, etc) and nutritional deficiencies (nutritional mitochondriopathy), many patients also demonstrate mitochondrial impairment due to microbes (microbial mitochondriopathy) and xenobiotics (xenobiotic mitochondriopathy).[1199]

23. **Detoxification, avoidance of toxins (xenobiotics) that impair mitochondrial function**:
    - Mitochondrial mechanism(s): Many persistent organic pollutants (POPs) such as pesticides (e.g., dieldrin) and dioxin-related compounds cause mitochondrial impairment.
    - Clinical benefits: Xenobiotic mitochondriopathy is noted in Parkinson's disease, as well as insulin resistance and metabolic syndrome. Detoxification is promoted by oral chlorella supplementation, exercise, nutritional supplementation (e.g., NAC for GSH protection and conjugation) as discussed elsewhere in this textbook.
        o Eat organic foods to reduce pesticide/herbicide exposure (*Environ Res* 2014 Jul[1200]): "CONCLUSIONS: The consumption of an organic diet for one week significantly reduced organophosphate pesticide exposure in adults."
        o "Effects of the Roundup and glyphosate on mitochondrial oxidative phosphorylation" (*Chemosphere* 2005 Dec[1201]): In this study, the researcher used and named a specific brand of chemical formulation. "Roundup stimulates succinate-supported respiration twice, with simultaneous collapse of transmembrane electrical potential, while glyphosate used in the same concentrations does not induce any significant effect. Additionally, Roundup depresses state 3 respiration by about 40%, at 15 mM, whereas uncoupled respiration in the presence of FCCP is depressed by about 50%. Depression of uncoupled respiratory activity is mediated through partial inhibition of mitochondrial complexes II and III, but not of complex IV. The phosphorylative system was affected by both a direct and an indirect effect on the F0F1 ATPase activity. The addition of uncoupled concentrations of Roundup to Ca2+-loaded mitochondria treated with Ruthenium Red resulted in non-specific membrane permeabilization, as evidenced by mitochondrial swelling... Therefore, the uncoupling of oxidative phosphorylation is also related to the non-specific membrane permeabilization induced by Roundup. Glyphosate alone does not show any relevant effect on the mitochondrial bioenergetics, in opposition to Roundup formulation products. ... these results question the safety of Roundup on animal health."
        o Glyphosate is a mitochondrial toxin (*Environ Toxicol Pharmacol* 2012 Sep[1202]): This study was performed on the human epidermal cell line HaCaT to examine the cytotoxic effects of glyphosate; researchers "observed an increase in the number of early apoptotic cells at a low cytotoxicity level (15%), and then, a decrease, in favor of late apoptotic and necrotic cell rates for more severe cytotoxicity conditions. At the same time, we showed that the glyphosate-induced mitochondrial membrane potential disruption could be a cause of apoptosis in keratinocyte cultures."
        o Glyphosate herbicide is synergistic with common additives to effect mitochondrial toxicity (*Toxicol In Vitro*. 2013 Feb[1203]): Glyphosate shows less toxicity alone than when combined with a surfactant, at which point the combination of chemicals is cytotoxic. TN-20 is a common surfactant in glyphosate herbicides. This research shows that the combination of glyphosate with the TN-20 surfactant leads to increased caspase activity (a sign of cell death via apoptosis) and reduced mitochondrial membrane potential. "The results support the possibility that mixtures of glyphosate and TN-20 aggravate mitochondrial damage and induce apoptosis and necrosis. Throughout this process, TN-20 seems to

---

[1199] Vasquez A. Mitochondrial medicine arrives to prime time in clinical care. *Altern Ther Health Med*. 2014 Winter;20 Suppl 1:26-30 ichnfm.org/events/MitochondrialMedicine
[1200] Oates et al. Reduction in urinary organophosphate pesticide metabolites in adults after a week-long organic diet. *Environ Res*. 2014 Jul;132:105-11
[1201] Peixoto F. Comparative effects of the Roundup and glyphosate on mitochondrial oxidative phosphorylation. *Chemosphere*. 2005 Dec;61(8):1115-22
[1202] Heu et al. Glyphosate-induced epidermal cell death: involvement of mitochondrial and oxidative mechanisms. *Environ Toxicol Pharmacol*. 2012 Sep;34(2):144-53
[1203] Kim et al. Mixtures of glyphosate and surfactant TN20 accelerate cell death via mitochondrial damage-induced apoptosis and necrosis. *Toxicol In Vitro* 2013 Feb:191-7

disrupt the integrity of the cellular barrier to glyphosate uptake, promoting glyphosate-mediated toxicity."
- o **Major pesticides are more toxic to human cells than their declared active principles** (*Biomed Res Int* 2014 Feb[1204]): Pesticides are used throughout the world as mixtures called formulations. They contain adjuvants, which are often kept confidential and are called "inerts" by the manufacturing companies, plus a declared active principle, which is usually tested alone. In this study, adjuvants were more cytotoxic than the declared active components of the pesticides/herbicides through the disruption of membrane and mitochondrial respiration. "Despite its relatively benign reputation, Roundup was among the most toxic herbicides and insecticides tested." hindawi.com/journals/bmri/2014/179691/

24. **Eradication of gastrointestinal dysbiosis & small intestine bacterial overgrowth (SIBO)**:
    - Mitochondrial mechanism(s): Dysbiotic bacteria in the intestines impair systemic mitochondrial function via gut-to-systemic absorption of D-lactic acid, hydrogen sulfide, and endotoxin/LPS.
    - Clinical benefits: Chronic fatigue syndrome, fibromyalgia, migraine headaches; pathophysiology, assessments, and treatments for dysbiosis are detailed elsewhere in this textbook.

25. **Eradication/suppression of any persistent "internal" infections**: Essentially any chronic infection will be associated with immune activation and thus inflammation and elaboration of cytokines; both inflammation as a general process and the elaboration of specific cytokines are known to impair mitochondrial function. Furthermore, some microorganism capable of causing chronic infections such as *Chlamydophila pneumoniae* (CP) are called "obligate intracellular bacteria/parasites" because these microbes are incapable of producing their own energy in the form of ATP and thus they must siphon cellular fuel from the host they have infected. Chronic viral infections—particularly those persistent infections caused by members of the herpes family of viruses—should be tested for with blood tests from a standard medical lab; assertive non-drug treatment to suppress viral replication should be implemented for 2-6 months and then serologic (blood) tests can be repeated to determine success of viral suppression. Pathophysiology, assessments, and treatments for dysbiosis are detailed throughout this textbook; note the section on laboratory assessments in Chapter 1. The following table provides examples of pathogens, assessments, and interventions.
    - Mitochondrial mechanism(s): Many microbes—especially those that cause long-term occult/silent infections—impair mitochondrial function; I have referred to this as microbial mitochondriopathy[1205] and have provided additional details and mechanisms in other sections of this book.
    - Clinical benefits: Eradicating mitochondria-impairing microbes with nutritional immunorestoration and/or direct antimicrobial interventions allows restoration and normalization of mitochondrial performance.
        - o **Bacterial toxins impair mitochondrial function** (*IUBMB Life* 2012 May[1206]): "Bacterial toxins have been shown to be targeted to the matrix, inner membrane, and outer membrane. The major class of toxins and effectors targeted to mitochondria are predicted to form pores..."
        - o **Viral toxins impair mitochondrial function** (*Infect Disord Drug Targets* 2012 Feb[1207]): "Viral products alter oxidative balance, mitochondrial permeability transition pore, mitochondrial membrane potential, electron transport and energy production. Moreover, viruses may cause the Warburg Effect, in which metabolism is reprogrammed to aerobic glycolysis as the main source of energy. ... A large number of viral products localize in mitochondria and interact with cellular mitochondrial proteins."
        - o **Viruses induce mitochondrial dysfunction** to promote viral replication, thereby leading to additional mitochondrial dysfunction (*Int J Biochem Cell Biol* 2013 Jan[1208]): "Increase in MMP, disrupts Δψm [MIM transmembrane potential] and affects mitochondrial bioenergetics. Viruses have developed strategies to modulate MMP and to effectively control cell death. In this regard, anti- or pro-apoptotic viral proteins co-opt host mitochondria to modulate MMP, affecting mitochondrial bioenergetics in favor of replication."

[1204] Mesnage et al. Major pesticides are more toxic to human cells than their declared active principles. *Biomed Res Int*. 2014;2014:179691
[1205] Vasquez A. Mitochondrial medicine arrives to prime time in clinical care. *Altern Ther Health Med*. 2014 Winter;20 Suppl 1:26-30 ichnfm.org/events/MitochondrialMedicine
[1206] Jiang et al. Hijacking mitochondria: bacterial toxins that modulate mitochondrial function. *IUBMB Life*. 2012 May;64(5):397-401
[1207] Williamson et al. Viral product trafficking to mitochondria, mechanisms and roles in pathogenesis. *Infect Disord Drug Targets*. 2012 Feb;12(1):18-37
[1208] El-Bacha T, Da Poian AT. Virus-induced changes in mitochondrial bioenergetics as potential targets for therapy. *Int J Biochem Cell Biol*. 2013 Jan;45(1):41-6

Microbial Mitochondriopathy—Introduction to key examples of common clinical relevance

Microbes capable of contributing to fatigue, mitochondrial dysfunction, and energy impairment due to chronic occult/silent infections in humans	Sample interventions
• <u>HSV</u>—herpes simplex viruses types 1 and 2: Although infection with HSV is common, higher antibody titers correlate with higher levels of viral replication; thus [nutritional] treatments should be implemented to reduce viral replication in order to improve energy levels and avoid illness associated with HSV-1 (and to a lesser extent HSV-2) such as Alzheimer's disease, risk of which correlates with IgM antibodies to HSV.[1209] Generally, testing IgG antibodies is sufficient. **HSV infection kills mitochondria by destroying mitochondrial DNA.**[1210]	**DrV's antiviral protocol**[1211]: • <u>Vitamin A</u>: Acute infections are treated with 100,000 international units limited to 7-10 days only followed by daily maintenance dosage • <u>Vitamin D3</u>: 10,000 IU/d for 10 days followed by daily maintenance dosage • <u>Selenium</u>: 600 mcg/d • <u>Lipoic acid</u>: 200 to 400 mg three times per day • <u>NAC</u>: 1,500 mg 2 to 3 times per day between meals • <u>Melatonin</u>: 3-20 mg HS • <u>Licorice</u>: tea or capsules; monitor for hypertension and hypokalemia with extended use • <u>CoQ-10</u>: 100-300mg to protect mitochondria and avoid virus-induced fatigue
• <u>CMV</u>—cytomegalovirus: Another member of the herpes family of viruses, chronic low-grade CMV infection is very common in humans; IgG antibodies or more direct tests (no perfect test exists) should be performed, nutritional viral suppression implemented, and antibodies are then retested. **CMV infection causes mitochondrial dysfunction.**[1212]	
• <u>HHV-6</u>—Human herpes virus type-6: Associated with chronic fatigue syndrome, a condition known to be associated with mitochondrial dysfunction. **Proteins of HHV-6 infection alter mitochondrial membrane potential and cause mitochondrial dysfunction.** Generally, testing IgG antibodies is sufficient.	
• <u>EBV</u>—Epstein Barr virus: EBV is the cause of infectious mononucleosis, a common illness experienced by most people throughout the world. While most patients recover uneventfully from the infection, some patients appear to harbor a chronic ongoing infection with EBV as evidenced by a combination of several laboratory tests available for antibodies and antigens. **Patients who develop chronic fatigue following EBV infection show evidence of alterations in mitochondrial function.**[1213]	
• <u>CP</u>—*Chlamydophila pneumoniae*: "**Chlamydiae are obligate intracellular gram-negative bacteria and are dependent on the host cell for ATP.** Thus, chlamydial infection may alter the intracellular levels of ATP and affect all energy-dependent processes within the cell."[1214] IgG titers of 1/64 to 1/256 suggest of chronic infection and consideration for treatment.[1215]	• <u>NAC</u>: 1,000 mg 2 to 3 times per day between meals • <u>Long-term azithromycin</u>: 250-500mg every-other-day for 4-6 months then retest titer

---

[1209] Letenneur L, et al. Seropositivity to herpes simplex virus antibodies and risk of Alzheimer's disease: a population-based cohort study. *PLoS One*. 2008;3(11):e3637
[1210] "Mitochondria have crucial roles in the life and death of mammalian cells, and help to orchestrate host antiviral defences. Here, we show that the ubiquitous human pathogen herpes simplex virus (HSV) induces rapid and complete degradation of host mitochondrial DNA during productive infection of cultured mammalian cells." Saffran HA, Pare JM, Corcoran JA, Weller SK, Smiley JR. Herpes simplex virus eliminates host mitochondrial DNA. *EMBO Rep*. 2007 Feb;8(2):188-9
[1211] Citations for the antiviral protocol are detailed in Vasquez A. *Chiropractic and Naturopathic Mastery of Common Clinical Disorders* (2009) and will likely be updated and expanded in Volume 2 of the new *Inflammation Mastery* series; Volume 2 is anticipated in 2015.
[1212] McCormick et al. Disruption of mitochondrial networks by human cytomegalovirus UL37 gene product. *J Virol*. 2003 Jan;77(1):631-41
[1213] "A comparison of gene expression profiles early and late following EBV infection revealed that those who did not recover had differentially expressed genes implicating mitochondrial perturbations with fatty acid metabolism, mitochondrial function and apoptosis pathways." Vernon SD, Whistler T, Cameron B, et al. Preliminary evidence of mitochondrial dysfunction associated with post-infective fatigue after acute infection with Epstein Barr virus. *BMC Infect Dis*. 2006 Jan 31;6:15
[1214] Yaraei K, et al. Effect of Chlamydia pneumoniae on cellular ATP content in mouse macrophages: role of Toll-like receptor 2. *Infect Immun*. 2005 Jul;73(7):4323-6
[1215] Ben-Yaakov et al. Prevalence of antibodies to Chlamydia pneumoniae in an Israeli population without clinical evidence of respiratory infection. *J Clin Pathol* 2002 May:355-8

26. **Avoidance of dietary sulfite, eradication of H2S-producing dysbiosis, and/or chelation/detoxification of sulfite and H2S with hydroxocobalamin**: Sulfite is a substance found naturally and in significant amounts in some foods such as dried fruit and red wine; it is also added to some foods and drugs as a preservative/antimicrobial/bleaching agent. Sulfite is also produced internally/endogenously from the metabolism of sulfur-containing substances such as amino acids. Sulfite is well-known to trigger asthma and migraine headaches in some patients; of note, both asthma and migraine are complex disorders characterized in part by mitochondrial dysfunction. In 2004 Zhang and coworkers[1216] showed that the cellular toxicity of sulfite in brain cells is mediated (at least in part) by inhibition mitochondrial glutamate dehydrogenase, which converts the amino acid and neurotransmitter glutamate into the fuel source alpha-keto-glutarate (AKG); the addition of sulfite increased production of ROS and reduced production of ATP (ATP production was reduced by ~ 50%)—increased ROS and decreased ATP is the classic dyad of mitochondrial impairment. Therefore, sulfite is a mitochondrial toxin; this explains its ability to exacerbate asthma and migraine, two conditions strongly associated with preexisting mitochondrial dysfunction. Vitamin B-12 is available in several different forms—cyanocobalamin, hydroxocobalamin, adenosylcobalamin, methylcobalamin; of these, only the hydroxocobalamin form has been shown to bind to sulfite and neutralize or "detoxify" it in a clinically significant manner with benefits for patients with sulfite-induced asthma as well as migraines. Further, an indirect mechanism by which sulfur/sulfite-containing foods and drugs may trigger asthma is via the conversion of sulfur/sulfite to sulfur dioxide in the gastrointestinal tract by intestinal bacteria[1217]; the sulfur dioxide can then be either absorbed into the intestine and/or released from the gastrointestinal tract via regurgitation (i.e., "burping") to reach the lungs, where it may trigger asthma or be readily absorbed into the systemic circulation. Lastly and very importantly, sulfur-containing substances can be converted by some intestinal bacteria into the potent mitochondrial toxin hydrogen sulfide, which poisons the ETC more powerfully than does cyanide.

> **Vitamin B12 in the form of hydroxocobalamin can be used clinically to neutralize sulfite and hydrogen sulfide (H2S)**
>
> "Serum concentrations of sulfide before and after administration of hydroxocobalamin were 0.22 and 0.11 µg/mL, respectively; serum concentrations of thiosulfate before and after hydroxocobalamin administration were 0.34 and 0.04 µmol/mL, respectively. **Hydroxocobalamin is believed to form a complex with H2S in detoxification pathways of H2S.** …The decreased sulfide concentration suggests that hydroxocobalamin therapy may be effective for acute H2S poisoning. The decreased thiosulfate concentration seems to be associated with formation of a thiosulfate/hydroxocobalamin complex, because hydroxocobalamin can form a complex with thiosulfate. …Therefore, prompt administration of hydroxocobalamin after H2S exposure may be effective for H2S poisoning."
>
> Fujita et al. A fatal case of acute hydrogen sulfide poisoning caused by hydrogen sulfide: hydroxocobalamin therapy for acute H2S poisoning. *J Analytical Toxicol* 2011 Mar

- Mitochondrial mechanism(s): Sulfite is a mitochondrial toxin, especially in brain cells; therefore avoidance or neutralization of sulfite helps avoid interference with normal mitochondrial respiration. Hydrogen sulfide (H2S) poisons the mitochondrial ETC more powerfully than does cyanide. Sulfite and H2S are both chelated and neutralized by hydroxocobalamin.
- Clinical benefits: Sulfite avoidance helps some patients avoid exacerbations of asthma and migraine. Clinical trials have demonstrated that administration of the sulfite-binding nutrient vitamin B-12 in the form of hydroxocobalamin helps alleviate/prevent migraine and asthma in some patients. Oral administration of hydroxocobalamin 2,000-4,000 mcg per exposure (i.e., taken before exposure to sulfite-containing foods or medications) or daily doses of 4,000-8,000 mcg/day is reasonable; orally administered vitamin B12 at doses of 2,000 mcg/day can achieve higher serum levels than can routine medical protocol of intramuscular vitamin B12.

[1216] Zhang X, et al. A mechanism of sulfite neurotoxicity: direct inhibition of glutamate dehydrogenase. *J Biol Chem*. 2004 Oct 8;279(41):43035-45
[1217] "Inhalation of sulfur dioxide (SO2) generated in the stomach following ingestion of sulfite-containing foods or beverages..." Lester MR. Sulfite sensitivity: significance in human health. *J Am Coll Nutr*. 1995 Jun;14(3):229-32

PERSPECTIVES

Mitochondrial Medicine Arrives to Prime Time in Clinical Care: Nutritional Biochemistry and Mitochondrial Hyperpermeability ("Leaky Mitochondria") Meet Disease Pathogenesis and Clinical Interventions

Alex Vasquez, DC, ND, DO, FACN

Alex Vasquez, DC, ND, DO, FACN, is director of programs at the International College of Human Nutrition and Functional Medicine in Barcelona, Spain and online at ICHNFM.org. (Altern Ther Health Med. 2014;20(suppl 1):26-30.)

Corresponding author: Alex Vasquez, DC, ND, DO, FACN
E-mail address: ichnfm@gmail.com

MITOCHONDRIAL MEDICINE ARRIVES TO GENERAL PRACTICE AND ROUTINE PATIENT CARE

Mitochondrial disorders were once relegated to "orphan" status as topics for small paragraphs in pathology textbooks and the hospital-based practices of subspecialists. With the increasing appreciation of the high frequency and ease of treatment of mitochondrial dysfunction, this common cause and consequence of many conditions seen in both primary and specialty care deserves the attention of all practicing clinicians.

We all know that mitochondria are the intracellular organelles responsible for the production of the currency of cellular energy in the form of the molecule adenosine triphosphate (ATP); by this time, contemporary clinicians should be developing an awareness of the other roles that mitochondria play in (patho)physiology and clinical practice. Beyond being simple organelles that make ATP, mitochondria play clinically significant roles in autoimmunity, inflammation, cancer, insulin resistance, cardiometabolic disease such as hypertension and heart failure, and neurologic disorders such as Alzheimer's and Parkinson's diseases. As I stated during the recent International Conference on Human Nutrition and Functional Medicine[1] in Portland, Oregon, in September 2013, we have collectively arrived at a time when mitochondrial therapeutics and the contribution of mitochondrial dysfunction to clinical diseases must be considered on a routine basis in clinical practice. *Mitochondrial medicine* is no longer an orphan topic, nor is it a superfluous consideration relegated to boutique practices. Mitochondrial medicine is ready for prime time—now—both in the general practice of primary care as well as in specialty and subspecialty medicine. What I describe here as the "new" mitochondrial medicine is the application of assessments and treatments to routine clinical practice primarily for the treatment of secondary/acquired forms of mitochondrial impairment that contribute to common conditions such as fatigue, depression, fibromyalgia, diabetes mellitus, hypertension, neuropsychiatric and neurodegenerative conditions, and other inflammatory and dysmetabolic conditions such as allergy and autoimmunity.

BEYOND BIOCHEMISTRY

Structure and function are of course intimately related and must be appreciated before clinical implications can be understood and interventions thereafter applied with practical precision. The 4 main structures and spaces of the mitochondria are (1) intramitochondrial matrix—the innermost/interior aspect of the mitochondria containing various proteins, enzymes of the Krebs cycle, and mitochondrial DNA; (2) inner membrane—the largely impermeable lipid-rich convoluted/invaginated membrane that envelopes and defines the matrix and which is the structural home of many enzymes, transport systems, and important structures such as cardiolipin and the electron transport chain (ETC); (3) intermembrane space—contains noteworthy molecules: creatine-phosphokinase and cytochrome c; and (4) outer membrane—comparatively more permeable (to molecules <10 000 Dalton) and—like the inner membrane—very lipid-rich and with active and passive transport systems for select molecules that need to enter and exit the mitochondria. Clinicians need to appreciate that mitochondrial membrane integrity is of the highest importance; just as we have come to appreciate the

Food-Induced Activation of Toll-like Receptors, Endoplasmic Reticulum Stress, and the Unfolded Protein Response:
An Integrated Model for Understanding Metabolic Inflammation

Metabolic Inflammation: Diet-Induced Metabolic Impairment and Inflammation
In this section, I will describe and give structure to a model for understanding what I have previously described—albeit intuitively—as metabolic inflammation.

Introduction: In my model presented starting in 2012,[1218] I began differentiating/describing inflammatory conditions as existing along and within an *overlapping continuum* of ❶ metabolic inflammation, ❷ allergic inflammation, and ❸ autoimmune inflammation. The most basic definition/description of metabolic inflammation is simply that it is a pathophysiologic state of nonacute metabolic disruption/dysfunction combined with a state of chronic/sustained mild/nonacute inflammation. What I have also stated is that "chronic inflammation" as most of us were taught in our Pathology coursework does not—for the most part—exist; except for a few rare diseases, the body does not perpetuate clinically significant states of inflammation. So-called *chronic* inflammation only occurs via a *sustained* inflammatory response. Another newer—and perhaps more direct way—of shattering the outdated paradigm of "chronic disease" is to state that such *diseases* do not exist—only *responses* and *accumulated damage* exist. Clinicians should experiment with the possibilities and implications of exchanging their conception of "chronic diseases" in favor of "sustained responses"; I think they will find the experience to be more illuminating/empowering/engaging than resignation to the chronic disease model and its subsequent indefinite noncurative (poly)pharmacotherapy. The illustration below introduces and summarizes several key concepts.

Metabolic, microbial, and xenobiotic insults—often via TLR4—induce endoplasmic reticulum stress (ERS) and the subsequent unfolded protein response (UPR): Consequences include vicious cycles of inflammation, oxidative stress, mitochondrial dysfunction, insulin resistance and hyperphagia—all consistent with sustained sterile nonacute inflammation and metabolic dysfunction/impairment termed here as *metabolic inflammation*.

[1218] Vasquez A. *Functional Immunology and Nutritional Immunomodulation: Presentation Slides Part 1*. Publication Date: June 5, 2012, ISBN-13: 978-1477603857

Key components of metabolic inflammation: The following points serve to construct an understanding of the major components of metabolic inflammation, starting from the causative metabolic, microbial, and xenobiotic insults and resulting in sustained oxidative stress, inflammation, mitochondrial dysfunction, and insulin resistance.

> **Induction of metabolic inflammation as sequential socioeconomic stress → overeating → cellular fuel overload and intestinal microbial overgrowth → dysmetabolism via LPS, palmitate/ceramide, and xenobiotic accumulation**
>
> **The first manifestation of inflammation is metabolic disturbance.** In my model of sequential and overlapping forms of inflammation—metabolic, allergic, and autoimmune—**metabolic inflammation is generally the primary/first component** and—among most diseases seen in routine practice—is always a component of the other inflammatory states.
>
> "These signs [of inflammation] are typically more prominent in acute inflammation than **in chronic inflammation. A fifth clinical sign, loss of function (functio laesa)**, was added by Rudolf Virchow in the 19th century."
> Perkins JA. Chapter 2, "Acute and Chronic Inflammation" in *Pathologic Basis of Disease, Eighth Edition* 2010, p43-77

- Fuel overload promotes metabolic stress and inflammation via direct (palmitate, ceramide) and indirect (microbial, xenobiotic) effects—a compilation and review: Stated most simply, overconsumption of simple carbohydrates (e.g., wheat products, sucrose, potatoes) leads to hyperglycemia and hyperinsulinemia, which function synergistically in the formation of palmitate and ceramide, which lead to insulin resistance, inflammation, and metabolic impairment per mitochondrial dysfunction and endoplasmic reticulum stress. The situation is compounded by the fact that these sources of simple carbohydrates (e.g., wheat products, potatoes) also contain indigestible carbohydrates that promote microbial population growth, thereby increasing endotoxin (LPS) load. LPS, glucose, palmitate, and ceramide have additive/synergistic effects in promoting inflammation, mitochondrial dysfunction, and endoplasmic reticulum stress. Gut overgrowth of bacteria secondary to fermentable fuel overload—via LPS—impairs cytochrome p450 "phase 1" detoxification, thereby promoting drug and xenobiotic accumulation; xenobiotic accumulation activates the aryl hydrocarbon receptor to impair GLUT-4 receptor expression and also leads to mitochondrial impairment.[1219] In this manner, fuel overload from overconsumption of processed foods can cause inflammation, mitochondrial impairment, and the insulin resistance that causes type-2 diabetes purely by microbial and xenobiotic mechanisms independent from the content of "calories" and resultant adipogenesis. Obviously, the implications of the previous discussion of the AGE/RAGE and the polyol pathway apply here; as a reminder: Processed food + hyperglycemia → AGE → RAGE activation → inflammation

- Toll-like receptors (TLR, e.g., TLR2 and TLR4): Upregulated and activated by microbial motifs such as bacterial endotoxin/LPS as well as by glucose (hyperglycemia), long-chain saturated fatty acids, including palmitate.

- Endoplasmic reticulum (ER) and ER stress (ERS): The ER functions to synthesize and process proteins, whether used intracellularly, within the cell membrane, or secreted from the cell. In certain adverse situations—notably exposure to viruses, bacteria, hyperglycemia and hyper(long-chain saturated)lipidosis, disruption of ER function leads to accumulation of unfolded/misfolded proteins within the ER lumen; this "ER stress" leads to a complex adaptive cellular response termed the "unfolded protein response" (UPR), which increases production and release of proteins and cytokines needed for immune surveillance. Induction of ERS-UPR occurs following activation of the NFkB pathway and/or TLR2 or more potent TRL4 depicted as follows:

    Long-chain saturated fatty acids → TLR4 → NFkB → ERS+UPC → inflammation, orexia, insulin resistance

    ERS is obviously an adaptive mechanism, which most likely developed for sensing microbes, and which becomes maladaptive when chronically stimulated by overconsumption of carbohydrates and saturated fats; the sequel UPR is notably appropriate for response to microbes, and notably harmful when activated by habitual dietary excess. When ERS-UPR activation is sustained, the result is excess inflammation and immune system hypervigilance (e.g., pathophysiologic priming for disorders of metabolic/allergic/autoimmune inflammation); more extreme intensities of ERS-UPR activation may result in cell apoptosis.

- Unfolded protein response (UPR): Endoplasmic reticulum stress is somewhat analogous to a "traffic jam" inside the ER, and the unfolded protein response is a pro-inflammatory "public service announcement" in response. Without the metabolic insults of excess glucose and excess saturated fatty acids—both of which are overpresent

---

[1219] "Recently, much evidence has emerged showing that environmental toxins, including POPs, affect mitochondrial function and subsequently induce insulin resistance." Lim et al. Persistent organic pollutants, mitochondrial dysfunction, and metabolic syndrome. *Ann N Y Acad Sci.* 2010 Jul;1201:166-76 in Americanized/Westernized diets but which would have been absent for the vast majority of human history—the main expected stressors for induction of ERS would have been of microbial origin, and thus the resultant "sounding of the alarms" and amplification of immune responses would have clearly been a positive and meaningful response; now that industrialized societies have essentially codified hourly/daily hyperglycemia and higher intakes of saturated fat, this ERS-UPR pathway is maintained in a higher state (quantitatively more) of sustained activation (longer duration).

- <u>NFkB involvement in ERS-UPR inflammatory cytokine release</u>: Saturated long-chain fatty acids activate TLR4 and induce NFkB-mediated inflammation via ERS-UPR and routes that are independent from ERS-UPR. While the ERS-UPR pathway effects elaboration of pro-inflammatory cytokines in an NFkB-dependent manner, the opposite is also true: NFkB activation causes ERS-UPR. Therefore, one would reasonably expect that inhibitors/modulators of the NFkB pathway (detailed elsewhere in this chapter) would be of therapeutic value in conditions of ERS-UPR; however, the clinical focus should always remain on identifying and eliminating the *origin* of the ERS-UPR/NFkB activation.

The foundation of metabolic inflammation via confluence of diet, dysbiosis, and xenobiotics: Metabolic inflammation is best understood as a state of inflammation that has a metabolic origin rather than a "normal" origin from infection or injury. The clearest and most concrete examples of metabolic impairment that reciprocate with inflammation are mitochondrial dysfunction and endoplasmic reticulum stress; generally neither of these occur by spontaneous generation, but rather by identifiable and modifiable variables, the three most important of which are dietary excess, dysbiosis, and xenobiotic production/exposure/accumulation and each of which have been independently validated. In the real world—the world in which we live characterized by population-wide economic stress and public promotion and government subsidization of processed food overload, clinically epidemic dysbiosis, and pandemic global pollution—all of these factors converge to promote ==syndemic obesity, inflammation, cardiometabolic syndrome, and brain dysfunction==. Hyperglycemia and hyperinsulinemia upregulate production of palmitate, which is sufficient to promote oxidative and glycemic complications, and which leads to production of ceramide, which furthers the mitochondrial impairment and insulin resistance; these biochemical consequences also lead to brain inflammation which at the level of the hypothalamus reduces satiety and promotes insatiable food cravings while at the level of the cerebral cortex promotes cognitive impairment. Production of ceramide via the other two pathways of exohydrolases and sphingomyelinase appear to be less clinically relevant for most encounters in outpatient practice. Clinically notable is the alleviation of ceramide accumulation via L-carnitine's inhibition of sphingomyelinase[1220] and also—more importantly—via induction of ceramidase via adiponectin[1221] which is stimulated in humans by supplementation with acetyl-L-carnitine[1222], which was reviewed previously.

[1220] Andrieu-Abadie et al. L-carnitine prevents doxorubicin-induced apoptosis of cardiac myocytes: role of inhibition of ceramide generation. *FASEB J.* 1999 Sep;13(12):1501-10
[1221] Holland et al. Receptor-mediated activation of ceramidase activity initiates the pleiotropic actions of adiponectin. *Nat Med.* 2011 Jan;17(1):55-63
[1222] Ruggenenti et al. Ameliorating hypertension and insulin resistance in subjects at increased cardiovascular risk: effects of acetyl-L-carnitine. *Hypertension.* 2009 Sep;54:567-74

- Cytokine-induced and NFkB/inflammation-induced insulin resistance—a vicious cycle: Milanski et al note, "Cytokines, induced either by TLR activation and/or by ER stress, can play a pathogenetic role in the development of insulin resistance in peripheral tissues." Activation of the NFkB/inflammatory pathway inhibits insulin receptor function via several mechanisms, one of which is the serine phosphorylation of insulin receptor substrates (IRS) 1 and 2[1223]; the resultant insulin resistance and hyperinsulinemia obviously promote a sustained state of hyperglycemia and promotion of endogenous saturated fatty acid synthesis thereby creating a vicious cycle of hyperglycemia and hyperlipidosis which further promote inflammatory pathways and insulin resistance, via mechanisms including ERS-UPR, NFkB, mitochondrial dysfunction, and ceramide.
- ERS-UPR is triggered by xenobiotics and particulate pollution: Particulate pollution—such as air pollution particles <2.5 micrometers—triggers ERS-UPR in experimental models of lung injury, and these effects—which may become systemic via circulatory distribution of particulate matter—are mediated via oxidative stress.[1224] Drugs and nutrients that activate ERS-UPR cytopathology include several HIV-1 protease inhibitors (nelfinavir, atazanavir, ritonavir, lopinavir), the anti-cancer drug sorafenib, the NSAIDs/coxibs indomethacin and celecoxib, and the natural supplement resveratrol (possibly selective for cancer cells); flavonoids baicalein and apigenin and the nutritional supplement N-acetyl cysteine are protective against ERS-UPR.[1225]
- Connecting ERS with mitochondrial dysfunction (MitoDys): Given that both ER and mitochondria are nutrient-*sensing* organelles (not simply nutrient *processing* or *metabolizing*), we should reasonably anticipate some coordination between them; indeed per Hotamisligil, "Activation of the nutrient-responsive mTOR signaling pathway stimulates protein synthesis and folding in the ER." ER stress and mitochondrial dysfunction both serve adaptive roles and represent a conceptual point along a continuum spanning function and pathology. An interrelationship between ER stress and mitochondrial dysfunction clearly exists, and the relationship may be most powerful in the direction from mitochondria toward ER; given that mitochondrial mTOR is necessary for ER protein synthesis/folding, then dysfunction in mitochondria/mTOR would be anticipated to promote ER stress and the resultant UPR. ERS adversely impacts mitochondrial function via promotion of inflammation, but this—unlike the effect of mTOR on ER—is indirect and nonspecific. Conversely, correction of mitochondrial dysfunction and optimization of mitochondrial function would be expected to alleviate ER stress via enhanced "ER-Mito coordination"; with regard to the latter, I think this is likely but acknowledge that I am being (reasonably) speculative here. In living systems, and which is already apparent from the previous diagrams, insults against endoplasmic reticulum and mitochondria are often similar/identical, and—also as previously demonstrated—once activated the dysfunctions within ER and mitochondria tend to be self-perpetuating and mutually reinforcing; the cures for these problems are notably similar, namely avoiding the dietary/microbial/xenobiotic (DMX) insults while providing complete nutrition to repeat affected pathways and systems and restore/heal injured molecules/cells/tissues.
- Fuel overload (excess carbohydrate and saturated long-chain fatty acids) promotes ERS-UPR and mitochondrial dysfunction via oxidative and inflammatory mechanisms (e.g., 12/15-LOX induction) and by inhibition of mitochondrial biogenesis: The concept of *fuel overload* is highly important; *fuel overload* is the prototype and the major cause of *metabolic stress* to endoplasmic reticulum and mitochondria and which leads to metabolic inflammation.

Overeating → fuel overload → metabolic stress → ER stress & MitoDys → dysmetabolism & inflammation

Of note, when we discuss "fuel overload", we are discussing the biochemical and cellular consequences of overeating; in particular, we are specifying overconsumption of saturated (long-chain) fatty acids and of carbohydrates, which are converted to saturated fatty acids such as palmitate (which leads to induction of pro-inflammatory IL-6, which also promotes induction of TH-17 cells) and ceramide, which causes insulin resistance and mitochondrial dysfunction. Quite obviously, the epidemics of obesity, cardiometabolic disease, and other sustained/chronic diseases/responses are not initiated and maintained by overconsuming lean proteins, whole fruits, vegetables, and seeds. Therefore, overeating (OE) is the psychosocial behavior that leads

---

[1223] Hotamisligil GS. Endoplasmic reticulum stress and the inflammatory basis of metabolic disease. *Cell*. 2010 Mar 19;140(6):900-17
[1224] Velasco G. Endoplasmic reticulum stressed by pollution. *Am J Physiol Cell Physiol*. 2010 Oct;299(4):C727-8
[1225] Lafleur MA, Stevens JL, Lawrence JW. Xenobiotic perturbation of ER stress and the unfolded protein response. *Toxicol Pathol*. 2013 Feb;41(2):235-62

to the cellular and biochemical consequence of fuel overload (FO); since OE precedes and causes FO, the former should be foremost in the discussion. Further, to bring more clarity and specificity to OE, we can specify *acellular/refined/simple* carbohydrates (CHO) and the *harmful-when-overconsumed* fat(ty acid)s—the dietary fatty acids of consequence are saturated, hydrogenated, or the n6 PUFAs linoleic and arachidonic. Given these considerations, then **OverEating Carbohydrates** and dangerous **Fats** abbreviated as **OECF** is our best phrase for as the proximate cause of *fuel overload* (FO) which causes *metabolic stress* and the resultant *metabolic inflammation*; **OECF-FO** pairs overeating and fuel overload. The specific problem—already noted in the clinical drug protocols and pharmacodevelopment priorities—is the separation of FO from EOCF, so that OECF can be ignored while patients are kept drug-dependent to manage consequences of FO; this is pervasive in current DM2 guidelines.

- Food-induced hypothalamic inflammation: As described in an excellent article by Milanski et al[1226], ❶ long-chain saturated fatty acids produce an inflammatory response predominantly through the activation of TLR4 in hypothalamus with resultant local release of cytokines, and ❷ the physiologic consequences of diet-induced hypothalamic inflammation include local endoplasmic reticulum stress, systemic inflammation, adiposity, insulin resistance, and enhanced hunger, the latter via inhibited reception/function of anorexigenic (hunger-suppressing; the roots *orexi-, orex-, -orexia* are Greek with the denotation of hunger, desire, searching) hormones insulin and leptin. Inflammation in the hypothalamic region of the brain, which can occur following TLR activation secondary to glucose, saturated long-chain fatty acids, or exposure to microbial motifs (e.g., bacterial or viral). In the CNS, TLR4 are found in the microglia. Of additional note regarding brain inflammation, "…recent studies in the brain provide in vivo evidence supporting the model that both ER stress and inflammation are able to activate each other and to inhibit normal cellular metabolism."[1227] Thus, given that ERS-UPR and inflammation are self-perpetuating, the most logical targets for intervention are 1) blocking initiation of the cycle by reducing triggers, most common of which are dietary, microbial, xenobiotic (DMX), then 2) using safe and effective treatments to address *residual* inflammation and metabolic dysfunction; notice the importance of this sequence and how this approach differs from the "conventional allopathic approach" which usually ignores diet, dysbiosis, detoxification thereby allowing the causative problems to remain, fester, and expand, thereby *creating* the "**need**" for hard-hitting expensive hazardous pharmaceutical interventions.

Saturated fatty acids produce an inflammatory response through the activation of TLR4 in the hypothalamus
"In animal models of genetic and diet-induced obesity, the activation of an inflammatory response in the hypothalamus leads to the molecular and functional resistance to the adipostatic hormones, leptin and insulin, resulting in a defective control of food intake and energy expenditure. … In conclusion, saturated fatty acids activate TLR2 and TLR4 signaling and ER stress in hypothalamus. … The presence of a functional TLR4 signaling is required for the development of hyperlipidic dietary obesity." Milanski et al. *J Neurosci.* 2009 Jan

ER function, ER stress, UPR in a nutshell
- ER functions: Protein folding, maturation, quality control, trafficking; intracellular calcium homeodynamics; "…the ER should be viewed as an essential apparatus in the coordination of metabolic responses through its ability to control the synthetic and catabolic pathways of various nutrients."
- ER stress: Accumulation of newly synthesized unfolded proteins activates the UPR—unfolded protein response
- Three main triggers of ERS-UPR: The main molecular *final common pathways* are TLR4 and NFkB, which are themselves triggered by: ❶ Metabolic stress: Excess glucose, excess saturated long-chain fatty acids, metabolic demands of obesity and hyperglycemia/hyperinsulinemia ❷ Microbial exposure: Viruses and bacteria, especially Gram-negative bacteria ❸ Xenobiotic exposure: Chemical xenobiotics, particulate air pollution
- Five major *fingers* or *branches* of ERS-UPR effects: ❶ Pro-inflammatory: NFkB, JNK-AP1 ❷ Oxidative: Pro-oxidant pathways are activated along with Nrf2; despite the latter, ERS-UPR is pro-oxidative ❸ Metabolic: Altered metabolism/reception of glucose, lipids, insulin, leptin, and iron ❹ Catabolism: Reduction in protein synthesis and enhancement of protein degradation to alleviate ER stress ❺ Apoptosis: "All of these signals contribute to the triggering of apoptotic responses when ER stress is excessive, prolonged, or insufficiently neutralized." Hotamisligil, *Cell* 2010 Mar
- Main remedies to ERS-UPR: Avoid triggers, downmodulate TLR activation with fish oil and olive oil, suppress oxidative stress and NFkB as described in this textbook, supplementation with NAC and flavonoids baicalein (*Scutellaria baicalensis*) and apigenin (in many fruits and vegetables, especially parsley, celery and chamomile).

[1226] Milanski et al. Saturated fatty acids produce inflammatory response predominantly through activation of TLR4 signaling in hypothalamus. *J Neurosci* 2009 Jan;359-70
[1227] Hotamisligil GS. Endoplasmic reticulum stress and the inflammatory basis of metabolic disease. *Cell.* 2010 Mar 19;140(6):900-17

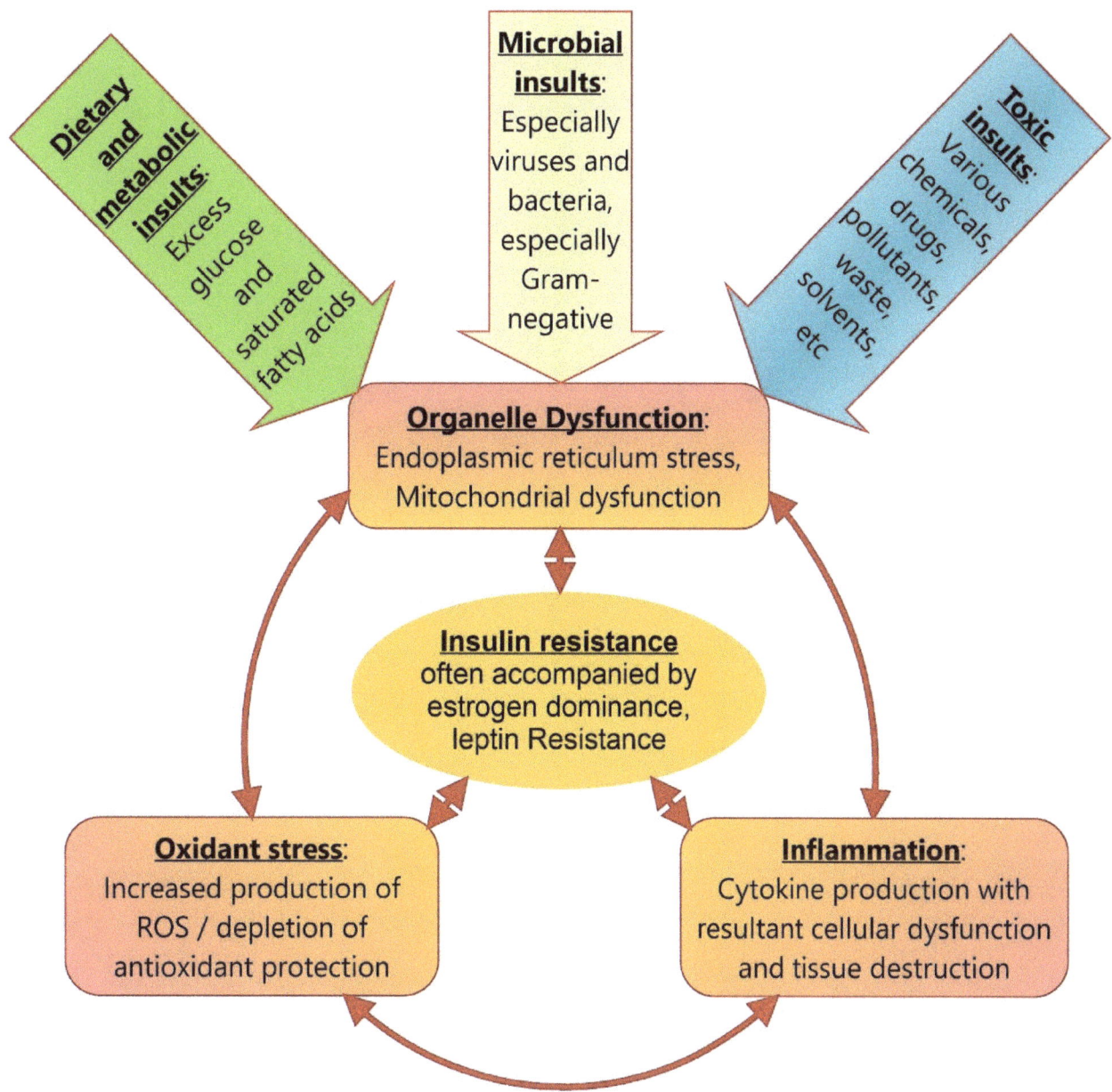

Genesis and consequences of organelle dysfunction—mitochondrial dysfunction (MitoDys) and endoplasmic reticulum stress (ERS): Common themes in organelle dysfunction include the causes—microbial insults, metabolic insults, xenobiotic insults—and consequences—vicious cycles of organelle dysfunction, inflammation, and oxidative stress. Attentive readers and those who want to master this material at a deeper level should take a few minutes to appreciate the number of vicious cycles represented in the diagram above: hint—ERS reciprocally causes mito-dys and therefore counts as one vicious cycle; each bidirectional arrow represents another vicious cycle, etc. Given that more components can be added to these interactions, these dynamic relationships have an additive tendency to be self-sustaining. The major exogenous triggers to organelle dysfunction (in this conversation: ER and mitochondria) are dietary excess (glucose and saturated fat), microbes (bacteria are quantitatively most important), and corporate-derived toxins such as pollution and pesticides.

❶ Food ❷ Infections ❸ Nutri-immunomod ❹ Dysmetab ❺ Stress/Sleep/Socio/Surg/Sup ❻ Endo ❼ Xeno

❺ Stress, Sleep, and Everything Else that starts "S": lifeStyle, Social and pSychological Influences, Self-Esteem, Somatic/Spinal Manipulation, Specialized Supplementation, Surgery,... Stamp Your Passport

> **Major Concepts in this Section**
> Initiated with stress modulation/reduction/mastery and sleep deprivation/optimization, this section has since expanded to include additional considerations, as described below, some of which have received additional details and citations, all of which are important.

- <u>Style of living—lifestyle</u>: Lifestyle includes many of the considerations below, as well as one's general approach to thinking, problem-solving, and living. Lifestyle is powerfully connected with culture (more accurately: *prevailing cultural morality*) and geography. Many of the relevant concepts and practical applications are included under the naturopathic profession's concept *reestablishing the foundation for health*.
- <u>Stress management/modulation/optimization</u>: Eustress is generally considered beneficial; but eventually even eustress can be detrimental if prolonged without respite. Dys-stress or distress impairs would healing, promotes nutrient loss, and promotes microbial pathogenicity via what is generally described as *microbial endocrinology*—the opportunistic enhancement of microbial pathogenicity following microbial reception of the host's elaboration of stress-related hormones/neurotransmitters such as norepinephrine.
    - <u>Microbial endocrinology—how stress influences susceptibility to infection (*Trends Microbiol* 2008 Feb[1228])</u>: Microbial endocrinology is the transdisciplinary field that represents the intersection of microbiology with mammalian endocrinology and neurophysiology; it is based on the tenet that microorganisms have evolved systems for using neurohormones, which are widely distributed throughout nature, as environmental cues to initiate growth and pathogenic processes.
- <u>Sleep</u>: Sleep deprivation/interruption promotes immune dysregulation and a pro-inflammatory response; accordingly, sleep deprivation/interruption is causatively associated with elevations in serum hsCRP and increased risks for obesity, diabetes mellitus and cardiometabolic syndrome.
    - <u>Sleep disturbance and older adults' inflammatory responses to acute stress (*Am J Geriatr Psychiatry* 2012 Sep[1229])</u>: "RESULTS: Participants categorized as poor sleepers on the basis of Pittsburgh Sleep Quality Index scores had significantly larger IL-6 responses to the cognitive stressors than good sleepers. The association between poor sleep and heightened IL-6 response to acute stress was not explained by other psychosocial factors previously linked to immune dysregulation, including depressive symptoms, perceived stress, and loneliness. CONCLUSIONS: Findings add to the growing evidence for poor sleep as an independent risk factor for poor mental and physical health. Older adults may be particularly vulnerable to effects of sleep disturbance due to significant age-related changes in sleep and inflammatory regulation."
- <u>pSychology</u>: One's mental outlook, self-perception, and psychoepistimology, etc. Some of the best contextualized conversations on these topics are by Bradshaw[1230], Bly[1231], and Branden.[1232]

[1228] Freestone PP, Sandrini SM, Haigh RD, Lyte M. Microbial endocrinology: how stress influences susceptibility to infection. *Trends Microbiol.* 2008 Feb;16(2):55-64
[1229] Heffner KL et al. Sleep disturbance and older adults' inflammatory responses to acute stress. *Am J Geriatr Psychiatry.* 2012 Sep;20(9):744-52
[1230] John Bradshaw's live performance recorded as *Healing the Shame that Binds You* (audio cassette version is different from the digital version and the book by the same name) is a very personal and yet very social and contextual journey and explanation of the personal issues that arise within the context of a fragmented society.
[1231] Robert Bly's *Iron John* is famous for having spawned the men's movement in America, but via Bly's knowledge of and sensitivity to historical facts and social trends, the book is also detailed and excellent accounting of the political and social changes that have promoted the degradation of society and which impact our personal self-perceptions and experiences of life; he followed this many years later with lectures titled *Where Have All the Parents Gone?* (audio cassette) related to his *Sibling Society*.
[1232] Nathaniel Branden discusses self-esteem and psychoepistimology in *Six Pillars of Self-Esteem* and *Psychology of Self-Esteem*, both in printed books and audiobooks.

- Self-esteem: Brilliantly articulated by Dr Nathaniel Branden to include the following: ❶ Living Consciously, ❷ Self-Acceptance, ❸ Self-Responsibility, ❹ Self-Assertiveness, ❺ Living Purposefully, ❻ Personal Integrity.
    - Branden N. The Six Pillars of Self-Esteem (paper book, audiobook, digital book): *I personally (DrV) consider this to be one of the most brilliant, practical, and important books/audios ever produced, despite what I perceive as a few imperfections; if the entire world (so to speak) read/understood/applied this book, our collective worldwide and lifetime reality would be improved for the better*: "There are realities we cannot avoid. One of them is the importance of self-esteem. Regardless of what we do or do not admit, we cannot be indifferent to our self-evaluation. However, we can run from this knowledge if it makes us uncomfortable. We can shrug it off, evade it, declare that we are only interested in "practical" matters, and escape into baseball or the evening news or the financial pages or a shopping spree or a sexual adventure or a drink. Yet self-esteem is a fundamental human need. ==Its impact requires neither our understanding nor our consent.== It works its way within us with or without our knowledge. We are free to seek to grasp the dynamics of self-esteem or to remain unconscious of them, but in the latter case we remain a mystery to ourselves and endure the consequences."
- Specialized supplementation: Atop the nutritional considerations discussed in this text, patients often benefit from additional custom-tailored supraphysiologic supplementation; beyond those already mentioned in this book, a few additional examples are provided in the table below. Many more examples provided within the context of clinical protocols are supported in *Chiropractic and Naturopathic Mastery of Common Clinical Disorders* (2009) and any succeeding updates to that work. As always throughout my books, doses listed are for adults unless otherwise specified.

Examples	Corresponding applications
Magnesium: 600 mg/d or to bowel tolerance	<ul><li>Constipation (assuming no bowel obstruction, renal insufficiency)</li><li>Headaches of most kinds, including post-traumatic headaches, tension headaches, migraine headaches</li></ul>
Pyridoxine: 250-800mg/d, always administered with magnesium, with food, within a context of dietary sufficiency, multivitamin/mineral supplementation, dietary alkalinization; pyridoxine HCL is generally sufficient while pyridoxal-5-phosphate is appreciated as the active form	<ul><li>Premenstrual problems, as pyridoxine has an impressive alterative/normalizing/balancing effect via lowering estrogen levels, raising progesterone levels, promoting diuresis[1233], and reducing excess glutaminergic neurotransmission which is consistently associated with depression/anxiety/moodiness</li><li>Excess glutaminergic neurotransmission, monosodium glutamate (MSG) sensitivity[1234]</li></ul>
Pyridoxine: 50-250 mg/d Methylfolate or folinic acid: 400 mcg-5 mg/d Cobalamin*: 2,000-6,000 mcg/d PO NAC: 1,500-4,500 mg/d Betaine: 3-6 g/d[1235] Soy lecithin for phosphatidylcholine: 2-10 tablespoons/d	<ul><li>Homocysteinemia, homocysteinuria</li><li>Methylation defects</li></ul>*Cobalamin should always be used in the form of hydroxocobalamin, methylcobalamin, or adenosylcobalamin—not cyanocobalamin, which contains cyanide, a mitochondrial toxin

- "Sweat" as metaphor for daily exercise and *exertion*—not simply *activity*.: For many people in industrialized societies, "work" is mostly intellectual/nonphysical/professional and therefore physically inactive; punctuating an inactive lifestyle and daily schedule with occasional spasms of activity (i.e., time-constrained ventures to the gym for "working out") is not the same as having a physically active lifestyle but—for many of us—it is the best

---

[1233] Abraham GE. Nutritional factors in the etiology of the premenstrual tension syndromes. *J Reprod Med*. 1983 Jul;28(7):446-64
[1234] Mousain-Bosc M, et al. Magnesium VitB6 intake reduces central nervous system hyperexcitability in children. *J Am Coll Nutr*. 2004;23(5):545S-548S
[1235] "Ten patients with cystathionine beta-synthase deficiency that was not responsive to pyridoxine and one patient with homocystinuria due to a defect in cobalamin metabolism were treated with 6 g daily of betaine added to conventional therapy, to improve homocysteine remethylation. All patients had a substantial decrease in plasma total homocysteine levels..." Wilcken et al. Homocystinuria—effects of betaine in the treatment of patients not responsive to pyridoxine. *N Engl J Med*. 1983;309:448-53

we can do. We should seek as much physical activity and engagement with the life experience as possible and reasonable per our individual needs and responsibilities. Life and its components have to be customized for an optimal personal experience and self-actualization; we might also appreciate that the vast majority of people in the world (presently and historically) have never had the luxury of time and freedom for such. Current guidelines[1236] encourage five 60-minute sessions per week emphasizing aerobic/endurance exercise and 2 sessions per week of resistance training *engaging all major muscle groups* (legs, hips, back, abdomen, chest, shoulders, arms)—such as calisthenics or weight-lifting; some activities such as hiking and yoga provide endurance and resistance training simultaneously.

- Surgery: Surgery is an important treatment consideration not simply for trauma and the removal of structural and gross pathologies, but also for more "functional" problems such as migraine headaches associated with patent foramen ovale and hypertension secondary to neurovascular compression of the ventrolateral medulla oblongata.
    - Surgery/procedure—Improving migraine by means of primary transcatheter patent foramen ovale (PFO) closure (*Am J Cardiovasc Dis* 2012 May[1237]): Obviously, migraine patients should be treated with the migraine protocol I have outlined in order to correct the primary (often accompanied by secondary contributions) mitochondrial dysfunction that is the fundamental cause of migraine.[1238] Following successful implementation of the mitochondrial protocol, for patients who continue to have symptoms, procedural correction of PFO closure can be considered. "RESULTS: 70/80 of patients (87.5%) reported improved migraine symptomatology (mean MIDAS score decreased 33 to10) whereas 12.5% reported no amelioration... Auras were definitively cured in 61/63 patients with migraine with aura (96.8%). CONCLUSIONS: Transcatheter PFO closure in a selected population of patients with severe migraine at high risk of paradoxical embolism resulted in a significant reduction in migraine over a long-term follow-up."
    - Surgery—Decrease of blood pressure by surgical ventrolateral medullary decompression in essential hypertension (*Lancet* 1998 Aug[1239]): "3 months after surgery, blood pressure and antihypertensive regimens had decreased substantially in three patients. ... No complications associated with decompression occurred. One patient experienced a transient vocal-cord paresis after the laryngeal part of the vagus nerve was maneuvered during surgery. We showed a direct causal relation between raised blood pressure and irritation of cranial nerves IX and X. A subgroup of patients with essential hypertension may exist who have secondary forms of hypertension related to neurovascular compression at the ventrolateral medulla and who may be successfully treated with [surgical] decompression."
- Spinal health and somatic dysfunction: Spinal manipulative therapy is remarkably effective for certain health problems for which no pharmaceutical/nutritional/botanical treatment is equally effective. Spinal health/function/manipulation/adjustment has obviously been the focus of the chiropractic profession, and "somatic dysfunction"—encompassing spinal health, fascia, ligaments, muscles as well as arterial, lymphatic, and venous flow—has been the focus (within its study of manipulative medicine) of the osteopathic profession.
    - Clinical trial: Chiropractic atlas vertebra realignment and achievement of arterial pressure goal in hypertensive patients (*J Hum Hypertens* 2007 May[1240]): "Using a double blind, placebo-controlled design at a single center, 50 drug naïve (n=26) or washed out (n=24) patients with Stage 1 hypertension were randomized to receive a National Upper Cervical Chiropractic (NUCCA) procedure or a sham procedure. ... At week 8, there were differences in systolic BP (-17 mm Hg, NUCCA versus -3 mm Hg, placebo; P<0.0001) and diastolic BP (-10 mm Hg, NUCCA versus -2 mm Hg; P=0.002). ... No adverse effects were recorded. We conclude that restoration of Atlas alignment is associated with marked and sustained reductions in BP similar to the use of two-drug combination therapy."

[1236] cdc.gov/physicalactivity/everyone/guidelines/adults.html Accessed 2014 Jun
[1237] Rigatelli et al. Improving migraine by means of primary transcatheter patent foramen ovale closure: long-term follow-up. *Am J Cardiovasc Dis*. 2012;2(2):89-95
[1238] My "migraine protocol" is detailed in *Integrative Orthopedics, Third Edition* (2012, text) and *Mitochondrial Medicine and Mitochondrial Nutrition for Primary Care Conditions* (2014, presentation slides) and will be updated again in Volume 2 of the Inflammation Mastery series described at InflammationMastery.com
[1239] Geiger et al. Decrease of blood pressure by ventrolateral medullary decompression in essential hypertension. *Lancet*. 1998 Aug 8;352(9126):446-9
[1240] Bakris et al. Atlas vertebra realignment and achievement of arterial pressure goal in hypertensive patients. *J Hum Hypertens*. 2007 May;21(5):347-52

- T4 syndrome (*J Manipulative Physiol Ther* 1995 Jan[1241]): "Upper extremity symptoms of nocturnal or early morning paresthesias, especially in a glove-like distribution, coupled with headaches and a stiff upper thoracic spine without neurological signs of disease may indicate a T4 syndrome. Manipulation of the dysfunctional upper thoracic segments may relieve these symptoms."
- A small example from the author's personal experience: I notice that I get a muscle twitch around my right eye when I carry—even very temporarily—a backpack on my right shoulder; this apparently results in a subluxated/dysfunctional right upper rib (approximately right posterior rib #2 or 3), manipulation/adjustment of which consistently and immediately resolves the eye twitch. *Without chiropractic-type manipulation of this rib, how would this problem be treated medically—muscle relaxant drugs, antianxiety drugs, with some lame excuse about how "it will go away on its own" which never happens?* I think it is analogous to the T4 syndrome described by DeFranca and Levine in *Journal of Manipulative and Physiological Therapeutics* in 1995; also noted here is the work of Gorman et al[1242,1243,1244,1245,1246,1247,1248,1249] documenting improved visual performance following manual manipulation of the cervical spine.

Examples of spinal manipulation and somatic manipulative medicine: *Photo left*: Cervical spine manipulation has been shown to be several-fold more safe than NSAIDs for the treatment of neck pain[1250] while being as least as effective or more effective (and likely more cost-effective) than drug treatment for HTN.[1251] *Photo right*: Dr Vasquez demonstrates his favorite manipulative procedure for dysfunctional costovertebral articulations and subluxated posterior ribs (i.e., the posterior aspect of the rib).

- Social influences and connections: Social influences on inflammatory and immune status are mediated via food, social connection vs isolation, xenobiotic pollution, and the level of sociopolitical chaos to which one is exposed.
  - The deafening silence: the near-complete absence of social perspectives in American medical schools): In medical school, we are taught to treat social problems of depression, anxiety, and isolation without any regard for their social context and political causes. As students and clinicians, we are taught to treat social problems with individual diagnoses and —essentially always— prescriptions for drugs (allopathic/osteopathic), or herbs or meditation (naturopathic), or nutritional supplements or exercise

---

[1241] DeFranca GG, Levine LJ. The T4 syndrome. *J Manipulative Physiol Ther*. 1995 Jan;18(1):34-7
[1242] Stephens D, Pollard H, Bilton D, Thomson P, Gorman F. Bilateral simultaneous optic nerve dysfunction after periorbital trauma: recovery of vision in association with chiropractic spinal manipulation therapy. *J Manipulative Physiol Ther*. 1999 Nov-Dec;22(9):615-21
[1243] Stephens D, Gorman F, Bilton D. The step phenomenon in the recovery of vision with spinal manipulation. *J Manipulative Physiol Ther*. 1997;20(9):628-33
[1244] Stephens D, Gorman F. The association between visual incompetence and spinal derangement. *J Manipulative Physiol Ther*. 1997 Jun;20(5):343-50.
[1245] Stephens D, Gorman RF. Does 'normal' vision improve with spinal manipulation? *J Manipulative Physiol Ther*. 1996 Jul-Aug;19(6):415-8
[1246] Gorman RF. Monocular scotomata and spinal manipulation: the step phenomenon. *J Manipulative Physiol Ther*. 1996 Jun;19(5):344-9
[1247] Gorman RF. Monocular visual loss after closed head trauma: immediate resolution associated with spinal manipulation. *J Manipulative Physiol Ther* 1995;18:308-14
[1248] Gorman RF. The treatment of presumptive optic nerve ischemia by spinal manipulation. *J Manipulative Physiol Ther*. 1995;18(3):172-7
[1249] Gorman RF. Automated static perimetry in chiropractic. *J Manipulative Physiol Ther*. 1993 Sep;16(7):481-7
[1250] "The best evidence indicates that cervical manipulation for neck pain is much safer than the use of NSAIDs, by as much as a factor of several hundred times. There is no evidence tha indicates NSAID use is any more effective than cervical manipulation for neck pain." Dabbs V, Lauretti WJ. A risk assessment of cervical manipulation vs. NSAIDs for the treatment of neck pain. *J Manipulative Physiol Ther*. 1995 Oct;18(8):530-6
[1251] Bakris et al. Atlas vertebra realignment and achievement of arterial pressure goal in hypertensive patients. *J Hum Hypertens*. 2007 May;21(5):347-52

(chiropractic). The dominant allopathic medical profession as a whole has failed miserably at maintaining public health via representation of the human needs and requirements for health.
- Social isolation in the USA (*American Sociological Review* 2006 Jun[1252]): In this very important paper, the authors follow-up on the 1985 General Social Survey (GSS) which collected the first nationally representative data on the confidants with whom Americans discuss important matters; the 2004 GSS replicated those questions to assess social change in core network structures. The findings show that American society is increasingly fragmented and isolationist. "Discussion networks are smaller in 2004 than in 1985. The number of people saying there is no one with whom they discuss important matters nearly tripled. The mean network size decreases by about a third (one confidant), from 2.94 in 1985 to 2.08 in 2004. The modal respondent now reports having no confidant; the modal respondent in 1985 had three confidants. Both kin and non-kin confidants were lost in the past two decades, but the greater decrease of non-kin ties leads to more confidant networks centered on spouses and parents, with fewer contacts through voluntary associations and neighborhoods. Most people have densely interconnected confidants similar to them. Some changes reflect the changing demographics of the U.S. population. Educational heterogeneity of social ties has decreased, racial heterogeneity has increased. The data may overestimate the number of social isolates, but these shrinking networks reflect an important social change in America."
- Relative deprivation—institutionalized inequality—makes people sick and "crazy" (*Soc Sci Med.* 2007 Nov[1253]): "… many problems associated with relative deprivation are more prevalent in more unequal societies. We summarize previously published evidence suggesting that this may be true of morbidity and mortality, obesity, teenage birth rates, mental illness, homicide, low trust, low social capital, hostility, and racism. To these we add new analyses which suggest that this is also true of poor educational performance among school children, the proportion of the population imprisoned, drug overdose mortality and low social mobility. That ill health and a wide range of other social problems associated with social status within societies are also more common in more unequal societies, may imply that income inequality is central to the creation of the apparently deep-seated social problems associated with poverty, relative deprivation or low social status."
- Social isolation, loneliness, and all-cause mortality in older men and women (*Proc Natl Acad Sci* 2013 Apr[1254]): "We found that mortality was higher among more socially isolated and more lonely participants. However, after adjusting statistically for demographic factors and baseline health, social isolation remained significantly associated with mortality (hazard ratio 1.26, 95% confidence interval, 1.08-1.48 for the top quintile of isolation), but loneliness did not (hazard ratio 0.92, 95% confidence interval, 0.78-1.09). ... Both social isolation and loneliness were associated with increased mortality. However, the effect of loneliness was not independent of demographic characteristics or health problems and did not contribute to the risk associated with social isolation. Although both isolation and loneliness impair quality of life and well-being, efforts to reduce isolation are likely to be more relevant to mortality."
- Economic inequality causes social harm (*TEDGlobal* 2011 Jul[1255]): Greater economic inequality correlates very strongly with the worst health/social outcomes. Adding more are more drugs to individual patients' treatment plans is not the solution; the solution to socially and politically fostered problems is meaningful social engagement and authentic political representation, both focused on the goal of optimizing education, *health*care, sustainability, working conditions, and the fabric (people, time, resources) of society.
- Social inequality is an underacknowledged source of mental illness/distress (*Br J Psychiatry* 2010 Dec[1256]): "Greater income inequality is associated with higher prevalence of mental illness and drug misuse in rich societies. There are threefold differences in the proportion of the population suffering from mental illness between more and less equal countries."

[1252] McPherson et al. Social Isolation in America: Changes in Core Discussion Networks over Two Decades. *Am Sociological Rev* 2006 June: 71;353-375
[1253] Wilkinson RG et al. The problems of relative deprivation: why some societies do better than others. *Soc Sci Med.* 2007 Nov;65(9):1965-78
[1254] Steptoe A, et al. Social isolation, loneliness, and all-cause mortality in older men and women. *Proc Natl Acad Sci U S A.* 2013 Apr 9;110(15):5797-801
[1255] https://ted.com/talks/richard_wilkinson/transcript
[1256] Pickett KE, Wilkinson RG. Inequality: an underacknowledged source of mental illness and distress. *Br J Psychiatry.* 2010 Dec;197(6):426-8

Gross social inequality increases physical and mental illness, and it cannot exist without government assistance
• Low-quality public education: Reduces opportunities for advancement among low-income persons, while higher-income persons are able to access better quality education through private institutions; increases likelihood that low-income persons will choose military as occupation, thus fragmenting lower-income parts of society (mostly by removing men and fathers), weakening lower-income sections financially, socially, and politically.
• Weak labor protection laws: Reduces fairness in the workplace, creating more of a master-slave relationship; generally increases profitability of the ownership while increasing poverty and work-related hazards among workers.
• No or very low minimum wage: Increases profitability of owners, increases poverty among workers, depletes government coffers via increased demand on government-sponsored social support (health, housing, food) programs; in this way, the government directly subsidizes corporate profitability by compensating for programmatic underpayment of employees while employees are kept at a financial and social level that barely provides for survival.
• Tax policies that protect high-income profitability and burden low-income survivability: The exemplar of government-imposed inequality.
• Institutionalized inequality causes physical and mental health problems (treated with drugs): These social problems are generally treated with drugs (or [privatized] imprisonment), increasing medical debts, profiting drug companies (and prison companies).
• International trade agreements that allow large-wealthy corporations to "off-shore" labor to countries that pay almost-slave wages to workers in horrid working conditions: This allows a few major corporations to make massive profit while forcing smaller local/domestic companies that pay fair wages to local workers to face bankruptcy; this results in corporate enrichment at the cost of domestic business-owner and worker—and thus lower/middle class—unemployment and disempowerment.
o The plain and simple fact is that American corporations such as Nike, McDonalds, WalMart, Target, HomeDepot, Sears, Apple and most electronics companies use the Chinese labor pool as a source almost-slave labor: a situation where the workers are so poor that they have no option other than to work long hours in horrid conditions with innumerable worker and human rights violations, where mistreatment and underpayment are deliberately concealed, and American corporations feign the appearance of concern but not to the extent that productivity and profitability are inconvenienced, nor that child labor is excluded, and where "employees at garment, electronics, and other export factories typically work more than 80 hours a week and make only 42 cents an hour" and are forced to work for consecutive weeks at a time without days off from work, according to the international business magazine *Business Week*. Many experts have claimed that this hurts the American economy by depleting the US of millions of jobs under the title of "free trade agreements" and designated agreements such as "permanent normal trade relations" (PNTR), formerly "most favored nation" (MFN). businessweek.com/stories/2006-11-26/secrets-lies-and-sweatshops
o "Most of what we buy from developing countries is grown or manufactured by workers whose rights are ignored in important ways. Cell-phone components from China, fruit grown in Mexico, and the Indian cotton in your shirt are commonly processed by workers who were not paid minimum wage, who were exposed to hazardous chemicals or dangerous machinery, who were forced to work overtime, or who were prevented from organizing to negotiate changes in such conditions." Viederman D. Overseas sweatshops are a US responsibility. *BusinessWeek*.com businessweek.com/debateroom/archives/2007/06/overseas_sweatshops_are_a_us_responsibility_1.html

- o Social inequality, systematic incarceration, and social-financial consequences (*Frontline* 2014 May[1257]): The United States now incarcerates more of its citizens per capita than any other country in the world. "The past 40 years have seen the United States become home to more prisoners than any other country in the world. Yet despite this dramatic boom in incarceration rates, a new report finds that the deterrent effect of tough-on-crime policies remain 'highly uncertain.' The report, published Wednesday by the National Research Council, describes the rise of incarceration in America as **"historically unprecedented and internationally unique."** It found that from 1973 to 2009, the prison population grew from about 200,000 to approximately 2.2 million. With this spike, the U.S. now holds close to a quarter of the world's prisoners, even though it accounts for just 5 percent of the global population. "We are concerned that the United States is past the point where the number of people in prison can be justified by social benefits," said Jeremy Travis, president of John Jay College of Criminal Justice and the chair of the committee behind the study." America's use of imprisonment does not reflect the rates of crime but rather political policies and campaigns such as "the war on drugs", which itself is impressively focused on the use of *Cannabis* (*sativa* and related variants), a plant with numerous well-documented medical benefits (e.g., alleviation of chronic and neuropathic pain, nausea, glaucoma, spasticity in multiple sclerosis[1258]), low cost, ease of cultivation, and many numerous nonmedical uses

---

[1257] pbs.org/wgbh/pages/frontline/criminal-justice/locked-up-in-america/new-report-slams-unprecedented-growth-in-us-prisons/
[1258] Leung L. Cannabis and its derivatives: review of medical use. *J Am Board Fam Med*. 2011 Jul-Aug;24(4):452-62

such as rapid growth of plant fiber for industrial uses such as clothing, rope, and paper manufacturing. NonCaucasians—Hispanics and African Americans specifically—are disproportionately affected by the "war on drugs" and the for-profit incarceration system of privatized prisons in America. According to the new report, the *purported social benefit* of such a system of incarceration does not appear to be offset by its *documented social harms*, most notably the decimation of human potential among those incarcerated and the impressively focal destruction of family systems and social cohesion especially among poor African American communities, wherein minor legal and behavioral issues (e.g., schoolyard fights, truancy) are treated with severe punishment (arrest, prison sentences) in ways that would not be *imposed within* nor *tolerated among* the more affluent and politically/financially advantaged sections of society.

Political genesis of the cycles of poverty, crime, imprisonment and blocked access to voting, housing, employment, and education

As a political-governmental creation, social inequality can be imposed directly (e.g., segregation, voting prohibitions) or—much more commonly—indirectly via substandard healthcare, substandard education, reduced opportunity for scholarship and higher education, higher per-percentage-of-income taxation, more frequent use of social-medical "labels" such as behavioral-psychiatric disorders and expedited imprisonment, which results in loss of voting and employment opportunities, and prohibited access to federal funding for education, low-cost housing, and food support. Pulling minorities into the military depletes these communities of men and fathers (and women and mothers to a lesser but growing extent), thus ensuring the fragmentation of families and the modeling of adult behavior and relationships for children. The consequences of **institutionalized social inequality** impact individual people, with outcomes including physical illness, mental illness and drug abuse; medical care is one of the leading causes of personal bankruptcy, and victimless crimes such as *Cannabis* possession are the most common causes of imprisonment.

The American Paradox: "land of the free" has 25% of world's prisoners yet only 5% of world population

"From 1973 to 2009, the [American] prison population grew from about 200,000 to approximately 2.2 million. With this spike, the U.S. now holds close to a quarter of the world's prisoners, even though it accounts for just 5 percent of the global population. ... In 2009, 62 percent of black children age 17 or younger, whose parents had not completed high school, had experienced a parent being sent to prison. Among white children, the rate was 15 percent."

New Report Slams "Unprecedented" Growth in US Prisons. May 1, 2014. pbs.org/wgbh/pages/frontline/criminal-justice/locked-up-in-america/new-report-slams-unprecedented-growth-in-us-prisons/

---

o Quantifying imprisonment—interview with Michelle Alexander (*Frontline* 2014 Apr[1259]): "The United States actually has a crime rate that is lower than the international norm, yet our incarceration rate is six to 10 times higher than other countries' around the world... Many people imagine that our explosion in incarceration was simply driven by crime and crime rates, but that's just not true... I think most Americans have no idea of the scale and scope of mass incarceration in the United States... But the reality is that today there are more African Americans under correctional control in prison or jail, on probation or parole, than were enslaved in 1850, a decade before the civil war began."

Institutionalized social fragmentation

"The impact that the system of mass incarceration has on entire communities, virtually decimating them, destroying the economic fabric and the social networks that exist there... The psychological impact, the emotional impact, the level of grief and suffering—it's beyond description."

Alexander M. Edited transcript of an interview conducted on 2013 Sep. pbs.org/wgbh/pages/frontline/criminal-justice/locked-up-in-america/michelle-alexander-a-system-of-racial-and-social-control/

---

o Xenobiotic pollution is a social phenomenon: Xenobiotic pollution could have only become a global, massive and inescapable problem if three essential components have likewise existed and persisted: ❶ a culture of corporate greed: Xenobiotic pollution results from failure of large-scale producers/polluters to fully consider and be accountable to the fate and consequences of their toxic products, ❷ failure of government accountability: Governments have failed to be accountable to maintaining the safety of their populations, and governments have failed to hold themselves accountable to the performance of

---

[1259] pbs.org/wgbh/pages/frontline/criminal-justice/locked-up-in-america/michelle-alexander-a-system-of-racial-and-social-control/

this duty, ❸ <u>failure of social engagement</u>: Populations worldwide have participated in their own marginalization by failing to engage effectively with whatever political structure they have; more often than not, populations are marginalized by their governments in such a way that popular political concern and activity (including "voting") really has no meaningful effect on the pervasive and largely invisible political-industrial infrastructure and core decisions and accountabilities that would promote preservation of our biological and social environments.

> **"The only thing necessary for the triumph of evil is for good men to do nothing."** Ed. Burke (1729-1797)
>
> "Probably the greatest responsibility for the cancer epidemic we're faced with lies with you. Your lack of interest in the past, your lack of involvement, your unwillingness to develop coherent strategies, your unwillingness to challenge authority—**these have created a vacuum in decision-making, that has been filled by professional groups with mindsets, with conflicts of interests, in some instances with close relationships with the chemical industries**—professional groups that are uninterested in [disease] prevention. By your quiescence and your acquiescence, you have allowed these situations to develop. ... **It is high time that empowerment and democracy and decision-making on these vital issues should be at least shared by you, if you should not indeed take a more prominent role."**
>
> Samuel Epstein, M.D. Professor of Occupational and Environmental Medicine at the School of Public Health, University of Illinois Medical Center Chicago. Excerpted from 1993 lecture converge.org.nz/pirm/pestican.htm

- <u>Spirituality</u>: Obviously "spirituality" and religion mean different things to different people; people generally feel good if they have some sense of connection with God(s)/god(s) and the Universe/universe and a story that makes sense to them and which assuages feelings of loneliness and existential angst and disorientation. Spirituality and religion are commonly used interchangeably or in connection with each other despite their clear distinctions, for example the former is a decidedly personal and therefore creative experience whereas the latter is culturally codified. Clearly, one can have *spirituality without religion, religion without meaningful spirituality, religion and spirituality together,* or *neither*[1260], but some type of "spiritual practice" and/or metaphysical ritual and renewal—even if it is a simple orienting mediation—is good, reasonable, and helpful; the transcultural work of the late Joseph Campbell is noteworthy (e.g., his *Power of Myth* series) and clearly extends beyond the overused soundbite "Follow your bliss" which is more intended to imply *fun and passion* rather than *irresponsibility*.

  > **"Spirituality" defined**
  > "Spirituality is defined as: that most human of experiences that seeks to transcend self and find meaning and purpose through connection with others, nature, and/or a Supreme Being, which may or may not involve religious structures or traditions."
  >
  > Buck HG. Spirituality: concept analysis and model development. *Holist Nurs Pract.* 2006 Nov-Dec;20:288-92

    o <u>Spirituality—the emperor's new clothes?</u> (*J Clin Nurs* 2004 Jan[1261]): "The paper concludes that: (i) 'Spirituality' is an elastic term not capable of universal definition as each person's spirituality is an individual matter for them and (ii) tools that are being developed for identifying a person's spirituality run the risk of making wrong presuppositions about what comprises spirituality."

    o <u>Use of spirituality for laziness/ease/comfort</u>: "Spirituality" can be used by patients and doctors as a means to circumvent harsh reality, the complexity of biochemistry, and predicted unfavorable outcomes. Spirituality should connect one with reality, not distance one from it; I am not in agreement with "spirituality" being (mis)used for ego-preserving escapism.

    o <u>Use of spirituality for maintenance of institutional and professional power</u>: My observation is that many hospitals provide "spiritual care" under the auspice of *complementary and alternative medicine* (CAM), and that this is done to decoy patients, to satiate them and discourage them from seeking truer and more effective "alternatives" to drugs that are often expensive, hazardous, and inefficacious. Most importantly, decoying/satiating patients with less potent "CAM" therapies reduces the likelihood of use of more highly potent "CAM" treatments such as interventional nutrition which are quite often

---

[1260] "A philosophy can serve either to satisfy those [religious, existential] needs or to set them aside." Nietzsche FW. *Human, all too human*. Section #27. Also contextualized brilliantly in Schacht R. *Giants of Philosophy: Nietzsche*. Knowledge Products, especially the longer audio cassette format
[1261] Bash A. Spirituality: the emperor's new clothes? *J Clin Nurs*. 2004 Jan;13(1):11-6

affordable, safe, and highly efficacious. In this manner, hospitals and insurance companies retain clients (i.e., patients paying for drugs and other medical treatments) via use of "spirituality" and "CAM", and the most clear examples of this are noted in medical cancer treatment centers where "spirituality" is encouraged but effective CAM treatments such as dietary interventions and enzyme therapy are eschewed as *unscientific* despite records of safety and efficacy.

> **Hospital-provided "spirituality services" are often a decoy from authentic and effective "CAM"**
>
> "We are oft to blame in this—it is too much proved: that with devotion's visage and pious action, we do sugar o'er the devil himself."
>
> William Shakespeare, *Hamlet*, Act 3, Scene 1

- o Spirituality (S) and religiosity (R) correlate with dietary practices, intake of fruits and vegetables (*Evid Based Complement Alternat Med* 2013[1262]): "Overall, the denominational studies showed that religious denomination is significantly related to fruit, vegetable, and fat intake. Specifically, the Adventists consumed more fruit and vegetable and less fat than non-Adventists. However, the relationship between the degree of R/S and dietary intake is mixed."

- <u>Stamp your passport</u>: Conscious and periodic implementation of *geographic cure* is reasonable and is a great way to renew, recharge, and see amazing things in the world that are inspiring for our lives. ==Importantly, vacation/travel allows us to get completely out of our ruts and *vicious cycles of thought and behavior* to see ourselves and life anew.==

Passports and fun: Utilize the passport; having fun on a tandem bike in Cartagena Colombia (2014 Apr)

> **Recreation is Re-creation: When was the last time you had real (healthy, health-promoting [not escapist, self-harmful, intoxicated]) fun?**
> - "Truth, however, must meet with opposition and be able to fight, and we must be able to rest from it at times in falsehood otherwise truth will grow tiresome, powerless, and insipid, and will render us equally so." *Friedrich Nietzsche, Daybreak, #507*
> - "Take a break from the work before the work breaks you." *Hernando Vasquez*
> - "I should mention that a purposeful, self-disciplined life does not mean a life without time or space for rest, relaxation, recreation, random or even frivolous activity. It merely means that such activities are chosen consciously, with the knowledge that it is safe and appropriate to engage in them. And in any event, the temporary abandonment of purpose also serves a purpose, whether consciously intended or not: that of regeneration." *Nathaniel Branden, Six Pillars of Self-Esteem*

[1262] Tan et al. Religiosity and Spirituality and the Intake of Fruit, Vegetable, and Fat: A Systematic Review. *Evid Based Complement Alternat Med.* 2013;2013:146214

<u>S</u>ustainability: This neighborhood sidewalk recycling center for small items is simple, and yet the implied sophistication of the accompanying forethought and infrastructure dwarfs what is commonly available in most other countries. One could reasonably be inconsolably baffled at the lack of international progress in sustainability, of which recycling is only one part, because it defies reason and is based on the synergism and interdependence of profiteering, politics, inertia. Many forces within society work directly against peace, progress, and sustainability; their goals are perpetual consumerism, international resource exploitation, and orchestration of public passivity to allow these.

❶ Food ❷ Infections ❸ Nutri-immunomod ❹ Dysmetab ❺ Stress/Sleep/Socio/Surg/Sup ❻ Endo ❼ Xeno

❻ Endocrine Imbalances (Dysendocrinism): Hormonal Evaluations and Interventions: Anti-inflammatory Orthoendocrinology

Major Concepts in this Section

Hormones affect and are affected by inflammatory status. In this section, I will focus on the seven hormones of greatest significance to inflammatory homeodynamics. Readers should mentally organize this information in the following way:

❶ Hormones that are commonly **elevated** and **need to be reduced** in inflammatory states: Prolactin, Insulin, Estrogen
❷ Hormones that are commonly **reduced** and **need to be elevated** in inflammatory states: Cortisol, DHEA, Testosterone
❸ Thyroid status is considered separately: See Chapter 1 for discussion of a novel way (contrasted to the standard allopathic viewpoint) of assessing and treating hypothyroidism in general and functional/peripheral/metabolic hypothyroidism in particular. Thyroid status is less potent as an influence on inflammatory balance when compared to the 6 other hormones listed above; however, occasionally a patient will have severe musculoskeletal inflammation (e.g., bilateral adhesive capsulitis, oligoarthritis, proximal myopathy[1263]) responsive solely to thyroid hormone monotherapy.

<u>Introduction</u>: Steroidal and peptide hormones have significant immunomodulating properties, and a characteristic pattern of disruption is commonly seen in patients with autoimmunity. Relatively simple natural and/or pharmacologic interventions can be used to safely and effectively correct hormonal disturbances with the dual benefits of improved overall health and the amelioration of autoimmunity. I have coined the term "orthoendocrinology"[1264] to describe this technique of addressing numerous disturbances in endocrine function by using the "right hormones" based on a similar conceptual model to Linus Pauling's suggestion that health might be optimized by the use of the "right molecules" (orthomolecular medicine, orthomolecular nutrition) rather than endless reliance on the cyclical prescriptions of what he called "toximolecular" substances. I will keep this overview and application straightforward, simple, and clinically relevant.

> **Hormones affect inflammation**
> "The altered hormonal status could result in relative immunological hyperactivity contributing to enhance tissue damage and disease severity."
>
> Mirone et al. Androgen and prolactin levels in systemic sclerosis: relationship to disease severity. *Ann N Y Acad Sci* 2006

The typical "inflammatory/autoimmune" hormonal pattern (partial is more common than complete):
- Low cortisol
- Low DHEA
- Low testosterone
- High prolactin
- High estrogen
- High insulin (surrogate marker for dietary CHO excess and insulin resistance, the latter of which is a marker of ERS and mitochondrial dysfunction, and thus also of microbial and xenobiotic loads)

Additional considerations:
- <u>Growth hormone</u>: Variable and apparently less important; can be assessed per patient.
- <u>Progesterone</u>: Variable and apparently less important; can be assessed per patient.
- <u>Pregnenolone</u>: Less potent with regard to inflammation than are prolactin, estrogen, cortisol, DHEA, and testosterone; can be measured by laboratory and treated per patient need. Earlier studies showed anti-inflammatory benefit with supplementation.
- <u>Thyroid</u>: Hypothyroidism and/or thyroid autoimmunity; see Chapter 1 for additional discussion, detailed review of assessments, case reports, and treatments.

[1263] Bowman CA, et al. Bilateral adhesive capsulitis, oligoarthritis and proximal myopathy as presentation of hypothyroidism. *Br J Rheumatol*. 1988 Feb;27(1):62-4
[1264] As of November 15, 2005 the word "orthoendocrinology" cannot be found either on Pubmed/Medline or Internet search using Google, Yahoo, or MSN search engines.

Testing and treatment hormonal status in patients with autoimmunity: Patients with autoimmune disorders commonly have deficiencies and imbalances in their hormones, particularly steroid and "sex" hormones, which are potent immunomodulators. The classic pattern which may be expressed incompletely in an individual patient, is that of excess prolactin and estrogen, and insufficient cortisol, testosterone, and DHEA. The role of progesterone seems less clear, with some patients showing normal, excess, or insufficient amounts; obviously, this can be tested in an individual patient (random serum test in men or 21st-day/midluteal serum sample from a premenopausal woman). All testing methods—via serum, saliva, or urine—have their individual advantages and disadvantages. Generally however, serum is considered the standard; following this I prefer polyhormonal assessment with 24-hour urine collections, and the last resort is saliva testing, which is the most controversial and least reliable. Thyroid autoimmunity and hypothyroidism are both common in autoimmune/inflammatory patients; comprehensive thyroid assessment with TSH, T4, and anti-TPO antibodies can be justified in nearly any rheumatic patient.

- **Hyperprolactinemia and latent hyperprolactinemia**: Besides its obvious role in lactation, prolactin is a polyfunctional hormone that, at the very least, stimulates the liver to produce excess sex-hormone-binding globulin (SHBG) which adsorbs sex hormones, rendering them less effective due to reduced bioavailability; the resultant *functional hypogonadism* deprives the immune system of the modulation/suppression normally effected by these hormones. Beyond these well-known physiologic roles, **prolactin is now known to be powerfully proinflammatory**.[1265] Patients with RA and SLE have higher basal and stress-induced levels of prolactin compared with normal controls.[1266,1267] Patients with scleroderma have relatively high prolactin[1268] and low DHEA.[1269] **Patients with polymyalgia rheumatica have elevated prolactin that correlates with increased symptomatology**.[1270] Elevated prolactin levels may further exacerbate immune dysfunction by increasing hepatic production of sex-hormone binding globulin and reducing bioavailability of testosterone, thus depriving cells and tissues of testosterone's potent anti-inflammatory and immunoregulatory properties. Prolactin is routinely measured in serum; high values should be reduced with effective treatment, whether nutritional, botanical, or pharmacologic.

> **Prolactin is pro-inflammatory, and anti-prolactin interventions provide an anti-inflammatory benefit**
>
> "Multiple lines of evidence support the concept that the anterior pituitary hormone **prolactin has a pathogenic role in rheumatic and autoimmune diseases** including, but not limited to, rheumatoid arthritis (RA), systemic lupus erythematosus (SLE), Reiter's syndrome, psoriatic arthritis, and uveitis."
>
> McMurray RW. *Semin Arthritis* Rheum. 2001

  - Thyroid hormone: **Hypothyroidism frequently causes hyperprolactinemia** that is reversible upon effective treatment of hypothyroidism. Conversely, due to its immunodysregulating effects, elevated prolactin appears capable of inducing hypothyroidism and autoimmune thyroiditis.[1271] Assessing hyperprolactinemic patients for thyroid disturbances with TSH, T4, T3, and anti-TPO antibodies is strongly advised. Thyroid status should be evaluated in all patients with hyperprolactinemia.
  - High-dose pyridoxine: B6 (250 mg qd-bid with food) is used by some doctors to lower prolactin despite the lack of consistently demonstrated benefit in the research literature.

[1265] "Multiple lines of evidence support the concept that the anterior pituitary hormone prolactin has a pathogenic role in rheumatic and autoimmune diseases including, but not limited to, rheumatoid arthritis (RA), systemic lupus erythematosus (SLE), Reiter's syndrome, psoriatic arthritis, and uveitis." McMurray RW. Bromocriptine in rheumatic and autoimmune diseases. *Semin Arthritis Rheum*. 2001 Aug;31(1):21-32

[1266] Dostal C, et al. Serum prolactin stress values in patients with systemic lupus erythematosus. *Ann Rheum Dis*. 2003 May;62(5):487-8

[1267] "RESULTS: A significantly higher rate of elevated PRL levels was found in SLE patients (40.0%) compared with the healthy controls (14.8%). No proof was found of association with the presence of anti-ds-DNA or with specific organ involvement. Similarly, elevated PRL levels were found in RA patients (39.3%)." Moszkorzova L, et al. Hyperprolactinaemia in patients with systemic lupus erythematosus. *Clin Exp Rheumatol*. 2002 Nov-Dec;20(6):807-12

[1268] Straub RH, Zeuner M, Lock G, Scholmerich J, Lang B. High prolactin and low dehydroepiandrosterone sulphate serum levels in patients with severe systemic sclerosis. *Br J Rheumatol*. 1997 Apr;36(4):426-32 rheumatology.oxfordjournals.org/cgi/reprint/36/4/426

[1269] "CONCLUSION: Our data show that, as in other autoimmune diseases, low serum DHEAS is a feature of premenopausal SSc patients. More extensive prospective studies are needed to define the exact role of DHEAS dysregulation in SSc." La Montagna G, Baruffo A, Buono G, Valentini G. Dehydroepiandrosterone sulphate serum levels in systemic sclerosis. *Clin Exp Rheumatol*. 2001 Jan-Feb;19(1):21-6

[1270] Straub RH, Georgi J, Helmke K, Vaith P, Lang B. In polymyalgia rheumatica serum prolactin is positively correlated with the number of typical symptoms but not with typical inflammatory markers. *Rheumatology* (Oxford). 2002 Apr;41(4):423-9 rheumatology.oxfordjournals.org/cgi/content/full/41/4/423

[1271] "...PRL level is higher in SLE patients and that in the presence of hyperPRL there is increased prevalence of antithyroid antibodies, evidencing the association of PRL and autoimmunity and pointing to the appropriateness of assessing and monitoring the progress of these markers in patients affected by these disorders." Kramer CK, Tourinho TF, de Castro WP, da Costa Oliveira M. Association between systemic lupus erythematosus, rheumatoid arthritis, hyperprolactinemia and thyroid autoantibodies. *Arch Med Res*. 2005 Jan-Feb;36(1):54-8

- *Vitex astus-cagnus* and other supporting botanicals and nutrients: **Vitex lowers serum prolactin in humans[1272,1273] via a dopaminergic effect.**[1274] Vitex is considered safe for clinical use; mild and reversible adverse effects possibly associated with Vitex include nausea, headache, gastrointestinal disturbances, menstrual disorders, acne, pruritus and erythematous rash. No drug interactions are known, but given the herb's dopaminergic effect it should probably be used with some caution in patients treated with dopamine antagonists such as the so-called antipsychotic drugs (most of which do not work very well and/or carry intolerable adverse effects[1275,1276]). In a recent review, Bone[1277] stated that daily doses can range from 500 mg to 2,000 mg DHE (dry herb equivalent) and can be tailored to the suppression of prolactin. Due at least in part to its content of L-dopa, *Mucuna pruriens* **shows clinical dopaminergic activity** as evidenced by its effectiveness in Parkinson's disease[1278]; up to 15-30 gm/d of mucuna has been used clinically but doses will be dependent on preparation and phytoconcentration. Triptolide and other **extracts from *Tripterygium wilfordii* Hook F** exert clinically significant anti-inflammatory action in patients with rheumatoid arthritis[1279,1280] and also offer protection to dopaminergic neurons.[1281,1282] Ironically, even though tyrosine is the nutritional precursor to dopamine with evidence of clinical effectiveness (e.g., narcolepsy[1283], enhancement of memory[1284] and cognition[1285]), **supplementation with tyrosine appears to actually increase rather than decrease prolactin levels[1286]; therefore tyrosine should be used cautiously if at all in patients with systemic inflammation.** Furthermore, the finding that **high-protein meals stimulate prolactin release**[1287] may partly explain the benefits of vegetarian diets in the treatment of systemic inflammation; since vegetarian diets are comparatively low in protein compared to omnivorous diets, they may lead to a relative reduction in prolactin production due to lack of stimulation.

[1272] "Since AC extracts were shown to have beneficial effects on premenstrual mastodynia serum prolactin levels in such patients were also studied in one double-blind, placebo-controlled clinical study. Serum prolactin levels were indeed reduced in the patients treated with the extract." Wuttke W, Jarry H, Christoffel V, Spengler B, Seidlova-Wuttke D. Chaste tree (Vitex agnus-castus)--pharmacology and clinical indications. *Phytomedicine*. 2003 May;10(4):348-57

[1273] German abstract from Medline: "The prolactin release was reduced after 3 months, shortened luteal phases were normalised and deficits in the luteal progesterone synthesis were eliminated." Milewicz A, Gejdel E, Sworen H, Sienkiewicz K, Jedrzejak J, Teucher T, Schmitz H. [Vitex agnus castus extract in the treatment of luteal phase defects due to latent hyperprolactinemia. Results of a randomized placebo-controlled double-blind study] *Arzneimittelforschung*. 1993 Jul;43(7):752-6

[1274] "Our results indicate a dopaminergic effect of Vitex agnus-castus extracts and suggest additional pharmacological actions via opioid receptors." Meier B, Berger D, Hoberg E, Sticher O, Schaffner W. Pharmacological activities of Vitex agnus-castus extracts in vitro. *Phytomedicine*. 2000 Oct;7(5):373-81

[1275] "The majority of patients in each group discontinued their assigned treatment owing to inefficacy or intolerable side effects or for other reasons." Lieberman JA, Stroup TS, McEvoy JP, Swartz MS, Rosenheck RA, Perkins DO, Keefe RS, Davis SM, Davis CE, Lebowitz BD, Severe J, Hsiao JK; Clinical Antipsychotic Trials of Intervention Effectiveness (CATIE) Investigators. Effectiveness of antipsychotic drugs in patients with chronic schizophrenia. *N Engl J Med*. 2005 Sep 22;353(12):1209-23

[1276] Whitaker R. The case against antipsychotic drugs: a 50-year record of doing more harm than good. *Med Hypotheses*. 2004;62(1):5-13

[1277] "In conditions such as endometriosis and fibroids, for which a significant estrogen antagonist effect is needed, doses of at least 2 g/day DHE may be required and typically are used by professional herbalists." Bone K. New Insights into Chaste Tree. *Nutritional Wellness* 2005 November nutritionalwellness.com/archives/2005/nov/11_bone.php

[1278] "CONCLUSIONS: The rapid onset of action and longer on time without concomitant increase in dyskinesias on mucuna seed powder formulation suggest that this natural source of L-dopa might possess advantages over conventional L-dopa preparations in the long term management of PD." Katzenschlager R, Evans A, Manson A, Patsalos PN, Ratnaraj N, Watt H, Timmermann L, Van der Giessen R, Lees AJ. Mucuna pruriens in Parkinson's disease: a double blind clinical and pharmacological study. *J Neurol Neurosurg Psychiatry*. 2004 Dec;75(12):1672-7

[1279] "The ethanol/ethyl acetate extract of TWHF shows therapeutic benefit in patients with treatment-refractory RA. At therapeutic dosages, the TWHF extract was well tolerated by most patients in this study." Tao X, Younger J, Fan FZ, Wang B, Lipsky PE. Benefit of an extract of Tripterygium Wilfordii Hook F in patients with rheumatoid arthritis: a double-blind, placebo-controlled study. *Arthritis Rheum*. 2002 Jul;46(7):1735-43

[1280] "CONCLUSION: The EA extract of TWHF at dosages up to 570 mg/day appeared to be safe, and doses > 360 mg/day were associated with clinical benefit in patients with RA." Tao X, Cush JJ, Garret M, Lipsky PE. A phase I study of ethyl acetate extract of the Chinese antirheumatic herb Tripterygium wilfordii hook F in rheumatoid arthritis. *J Rheumatol*. 2001 Oct;28(10):2160-7

[1281] "Our data suggests that triptolide may protect dopaminergic neurons from LPS-induced injury and its efficiency in inhibiting microglia activation may underlie the mechanism." Li FQ, Lu XZ, Liang XB, Zhou HF, Xue B, Liu XY, Niu DB, Han JS, Wang XM. Triptolide, a Chinese herbal extract, protects dopaminergic neurons from inflammation-mediated damage through inhibition of microglial activation. *J Neuroimmunol*. 2004 Mar;148(1-2):24-31

[1282] "Moreover, tripchlorolide markedly prevented the decrease in amount of dopamine in the striatum of model rats. Taken together, our data provide the first evidence that tripchlorolide acts as a neuroprotective molecule that rescues MPP+ or axotomy-induced degeneration of dopaminergic neurons, which may imply its therapeutic potential for Parkinson's disease." Li FQ, Cheng XX, Liang XB, Wang XH, Xue B, He QH, Wang XM, Han JS. Neurotrophic and neuroprotective effects of tripchlorolide, an extract of Chinese herb Tripterygium wilfordii Hook F, on dopaminergic neurons. *Exp Neurol*. 2003 Jan;179(1):28-37

[1283] "Of twenty-eight visual analogue scales rating mood and arousal, the subjects' ratings in the tyrosine treatment (9 g daily) and placebo periods differed significantly for only three (less tired, less drowsy, more alert)." Elwes RD, Crewes H, Chesterman LP, Summers R, Jenner P, Binnie CD, Parkes JD. Treatment of narcolepsy with L-tyrosine: double-blind placebo-controlled trial. *Lancet*. 1989 Nov 4;2(8671):1067-9

[1284] "Ten men and 10 women subjects underwent these batteries 1 h after ingesting 150 mg/kg of l-tyrosine or placebo. Administration of tyrosine significantly enhanced accuracy and decreased frequency of list retrieval on the working memory task during the multiple task battery compared with placebo." Thomas JR, Lockwood PA, Singh A, Deuster PA. Tyrosine improves working memory in a multitasking environment. *Pharmacol Biochem Behav*. 1999 Nov;64(3):495-500

[1285] "Ten subjects received five daily doses of a protein-rich drink containing 2 g tyrosine, and 11 subjects received a carbohydrate rich drink with the same amount of calories (255 kcal)." Deijen JB, Wientjes CJ, Vullinghs HF, Cloin PA, Langefeld JJ. Tyrosine improves cognitive performance and reduces blood pressure in cadets after one week of a combat training course. *Brain Res Bull*. 1999 Jan 15;48(2):203-9

[1286] "Tyrosine (when compared to placebo) had no effect on any sleep related measure, but it did stimulate prolactin release." Waters WF, et al. A comparison of tyrosine against placebo, phentermine, caffeine, and D-amphetamine during sleep deprivation. *Nutr Neurosci*. 2003;6(4):221-35

[1287] "Whereas carbohydrate meals had no discernible effects, high protein meals induced a large increase in both PRL and cortisol; high fat meals caused selective release of PRL."Ishizuka, et al. Pituitary hormone release in response to food ingestion. *J Clin Endocrinol Metab* 1983Dec;57:1111-6

- o   Bromocriptine: Bromocriptine has long been considered the pharmacologic treatment of choice for elevated prolactin.[1288] Typical dose is 2.5 mg per day (effective against lupus[1289]); gastrointestinal upset and sedation are common.[1290] **Clinical intervention with bromocriptine appears warranted in patients with RA, SLE, Reiter's syndrome, psoriatic arthritis, and probably multiple sclerosis and uveitis.**[1291]
- o   Cabergoline/Dostinex: Cabergoline/Dostinex is a newer dopamine agonist with few adverse effects; typical dose starts at 0.5 mg per week (0.25 mg twice per week).[1292] Several studies have indicated that cabergoline is safer and more effective than bromocriptine for reducing prolactin levels[1293] and the dose can often be reduced after successful prolactin reduction, allowing for reductions in cost and adverse effects.[1294] Although fewer studies have been published supporting the antirheumatic benefits of cabergoline than bromocriptine, the scientific rationale for its use is derived from the success of bromocriptine in various rheumatic/autoimmune diseases. Furthermore, clinicians need to appreciate that prolactin is an active proinflammatory signal within the immune system (functioning in an autocrine/paracrine manner among immunocytes) and that treatment can be implemented and is often effective regardless of serum prolactin levels; if a high serum prolactin is found then it should be treated, while a normal serum prolactin does not preclude use of antiprolactin treatment.
  - Case report: Control of unremitting rheumatoid arthritis by the prolactin antagonist cabergoline: Erb et al[1295] published a case report of a woman with unremitting rheumatoid arthritis who achieved remarkable clinical improvement and who was able to reduce her need for other antirheumatic drugs with the use of cabergoline 0.5 mg per day. They wrote, "The present case demonstrates a dramatic improvement of previously uncontrollable RA soon after treatment of coincidental hyperprolactinemia [serum prolactin 1623 mU/l (normal range 0–440 mU/l)] with the prolactin antagonist cabergoline. … Treatment with the prolactin antagonist cabergoline 500 μg daily was commenced. Within 2 months her menstrual cycle and prolactin levels were normal. She had no active synovitis in any of her joints, morning stiffness had declined to less than 30 min, and her ESR and CRP had almost normalized, at 25 mm in the first hour and 6 mg/l respectively. Her RA remains clinically and serologically controlled to the present day, despite gradual but continuous reduction of her anti-rheumatic medication."
  - Pilot randomized double-blind clinical trial: The effect of cabergoline on clinical and laboratory findings in active rheumatoid arthritis (*Iran Red Crescent Med J* 2011 Oct[1296]): "In this study, improvement of tender and swollen joint count, patient assessment of pain and patient global assessment of disease activity were significant when patients were treated by cabergoline [1 mg/week]. Prolactin is secreted not only by anterior pituitary gland, but also by immune cells that may have small effect on total serum prolactin level and a significant effect on immunomedulatory system, so cabergoline suppressed both kinds of

---

[1288] Beers MH, Berkow R (eds). *The Merck Manual. Seventeenth Edition*. Whitehouse Station; Merck Research Laboratories 1999 Page 77-78
[1289] "A prospective, double-blind, randomized, placebo-controlled study compared BRC at a fixed daily dosage of 2.5 mg with placebo... Long term treatment with a low dose of BRC appears to be a safe and effective means of decreasing SLE flares in SLE patients." Alvarez-Nemegyei J, Cobarrubias-Cobos A, Escalante-Triay F, Sosa-Munoz J, Miranda JM, Jara LJ. Bromcriptine in systemic lupus erythematosus: a double-blind, randomized, placebo-controlled study. *Lupus*. 1998;7(6):414-9
[1290] Serri O, Chik CL, Ur E, Ezzat S. Diagnosis and management of hyperprolactinemia. *CMAJ*. 2003 Sep 16;169(6):575-81 cmaj.ca/cgi/content/full/169/6/575
[1291] "...clinical observations and trials support the use of bromocriptine as a nonstandard primary or adjunctive therapy in the treatment of recalcitrant RA, SLE, Reiter's syndrome, and psoriatic arthritis and associated conditions unresponsive to traditional approaches." McMurray RW. Bromocriptine in rheumatic and autoimmune diseases. *Semin Arthritis Rheum*. 2001 Aug;31(1):21-32
[1292] Serri O, Chik CL, Ur E, Ezzat S. Diagnosis and management of hyperprolactinemia. *CMAJ*. 2003 Sep 16;169(6):575-81 cmaj.ca/cgi/content/full/169/6/575
[1293] "CONCLUSION: These data indicate that cabergoline is a very effective agent for lowering the prolactin levels in hyperprolactinemic patients and that it appears to offer considerable advantage over bromocriptine in terms of efficacy and tolerability." Sabuncu T, Arikan E, Tasan E, Hatemi H. Comparison of the effects of cabergoline and bromocriptine on prolactin levels in hyperprolactinemic patients. *Intern Med*. 2001 Sep;40(9):857-61
[1294] "Cabergoline also normalized PRL in the majority of patients with known bromocriptine intolerance or -resistance. Once PRL secretion was adequately controlled, the dose of cabergoline could often be significantly decreased, which further reduced costs of therapy." Verhelst J, Abs R, Maiter D, van den Bruel A, Vandeweghe M, Velkeniers B, Mockel J, Lamberigts G, Petrossians P, Coremans P, Mahler C, Stevenaert A, Verlooy J, Raftopoulos C, Beckers A. Cabergoline in the treatment of hyperprolactinemia: a study in 455 patients. *J Clin Endocrinol Metab*. 1999 Jul;84(7):2518-22 jcem.endojournals.org/cgi/content/full/84/7/2518
[1295] Erb N, et al. Control of unremitting rheumatoid arthritis by the prolactin antagonist cabergoline. *Rheumatology* (Oxford). 2001 Feb;40(2):237-9
[1296] Mobini M, et al. The effect of cabergoline on clinical and laboratory findings in active rheumatoid arthritis. *Iran Red Crescent Med J*. 2011 Oct;13(10):749-50

prolactin. The improvement in RA activity may be due to a significant suppression in secretion of prolactin by immune cells without a significant change in prolactin level."
- **Insulin, hyperinsulinemia:** As a marker for insulin resistance and perhaps xenobiotic exposure, fasting serum insulin is a surrogate marker for an inflammatory state. A challenge exists in determining the accurate pro- or anti-inflammatory effect of insulin itself, because the net effect of the hormone *in vivo* is inflammation-lowering via glucose-lowering. Although major medical labs such as LabCorp (website reviewed January 2014) use a reference range of 2.6-24.9 µIU/mL, such a range is clinically ridiculous except for screening for overt pathology and should be replaced with the following:
    - <u>Healthy fasting serum insulin</u>: <5 µIU/mL
    - <u>Mild-moderate insulin resistance fasting serum insulin</u>: 5-15 µIU/mL
    - <u>Marked-severe insulin resistance fasting serum insulin</u>: 15 µIU/mL

    The goal when considering serum insulin within the context of alleviating inflammation is not to lower serum insulin per se, but rather to alleviate the causative insulin resistance. Stated perhaps more plainly, an elevation in fasting serum insulin is indicative of insulin resistance (except in the exceedingly rare case of insulinoma or exogenous insulin administration which can be distinguished by concomitant measurement of C-peptide) which is itself a proinflammatory state; thus, our goal is to reduce fasting serum insulin not because we are targeting insulin per se but rather because we are measuring serum insulin as a marker for insulin resistance and thus a particular type of *metabolic inflammation*. First-line therapy for insulin resistance is carbohydrate restriction via plant-based low-carbohydrate Paleo diet, exercise and physical activity >60 minutes/day, vitamin and mineral supplementation, especially vitamin D3, chromium, magnesium, CoQ-10, and mixed tocopherols.

- **Estrogen:** Nearly all autoimmune disorders are more common in females than males, and occasionally a menstrual exacerbation is noted, suggesting a possible immunodysregulation by estrogen. Despite the complex and multifaceted nature of the endocrine system, we may safely generalize that the estrogens are immunostimulatory and immunodysregulatory while androgens are immunosuppressive and immunoregulatory[1297]; thus, elevated estrogen:androgen ratios promote/exacerbate autoimmunity. Furthermore, many chemical/pollutant xenobiotics have estrogen-like effects ("xenoestrogens") and are consistently associated with induction or exacerbation of autoimmunity. So-called **"estrogen-replacement therapy" used in postmenopausal women increases the risk for lupus and scleroderma.**[1298] **Men with rheumatoid arthritis show an excess of estradiol** and a decrease in DHEA, and the **excess estrogen is proportional to the degree of inflammation.**[1299] Estrogen(s) can be measured in serum and/or 24-hour urine samples. Beyond looking at estrogens from a *quantitative* standpoint, they can also be *qualitatively* analyzed with respect to the ratio of estrone:estradiol:estriol as well as the balance between the "good" 2-hydroxyestrone relative to the purportedly carcinogenic and proinflammatory 16-alpha-hydroxyestrone. Interventions to lower estrogen levels can include the following:

    > **Estrogen is pro-inflammatory, and anti-estrogen interventions provide an anti-inflammatory benefit**
    >
    > "Using **antiestrogen** medication [tamoxifen or **anastrozole**] in women with dermatomyositis may result in a significant improvement in their rash, possibly via the inhibition of TNF-alpha production by immune or other cells."
    >
    > Sereda and Werth. *Arch Dermatol.* 2006

    - <u>Weight loss and weight optimization</u>: Excess adiposity and obesity raise estrogen levels due to high levels of aromatase (the hormone that makes estrogens from androgens) in adipose tissue; weight optimization and loss of excess fat helps normalize hormone levels and reduce inflammation. In overweight patients, *weight loss* is the means to attaining the goal of *weight optimization*; the task is not complete until the body mass index is normalized/optimized.
    - <u>Avoidance of ethanol</u>: Ethanol stimulates estrogen production, particularly in men.

[1297] "In general, androgens seem to inhibit immune activity, while oestrogen seems to have a more powerful effect on immune cells and to stimulate immune activity." Tanriverdi F, Silveira LF, MacColl GS, Bouloux PM. The hypothalamic-pituitary-gonadal axis: immune function and autoimmunity. *J Endocrinol.* 2003 Mar;176(3):293-304 joe.endocrinology-journals.org/cgi/content/abstract/176/3/293

[1298] "These studies indicate that estrogen replacement therapy in postmenopausal women increases the risk of developing lupus, scleroderma, and Raynaud disease..." Mayes MD. Epidemiologic studies of environmental agents and systemic autoimmune diseases. *Environ Health Perspect.* 1999 Oct;107 Suppl 5:743-8

[1299] "RESULTS: DHEAS and estrone concentrations were lower and estradiol was higher in patients compared with healthy controls. DHEAS differed between RF positive and RF negative patients. Estrone did not correlate with any disease variable, whereas estradiol correlated strongly and positively with all measured indices of inflammation." Tengstrand B, Carlstrom K, Fellander-Tsai L, Hafstrom I. Abnormal levels of serum dehydroepiandrosterone, estrone, and estradiol in men with rheumatoid arthritis: high correlation between serum estradiol and current degree of inflammation. *J Rheumatol.* 2003 Nov;30(11):2338-43

- Surgical correction of varicocele in affected men: Men with varicocele have higher estrogen levels due to temperature-induced alterations in enzyme function in the testes; surgical correction of the varicocele lowers estrogen levels.
- "Anti-estrogen diet": Foods and supplements such as green tea, diindolylmethane (DIM), indole-3-carbinol (I3C), licorice, and a high-fiber crucifer-based "anti-estrogenic diet" can also be used; monitoring clinical status and serum estradiol will prove or disprove efficacy. Whereas **16-alpha-hydroxyestrone is pro-inflammatory and immunodysregulatory, 2-hydroxyestrone has anti-inflammatory action**[1300] and has been described as "the good estrogen"[1301] due to its anticancer and comparatively health-preserving qualities. **In a recent short-term study using I3C in patients with SLE, I3C supplementation at 375 mg per day was well tolerated and resulted in modest treatment-dependent clinical improvement as well as favorable modification of estrogen metabolism away from 16-alpha-hydroxyestrone and toward 2-hydroxyestrone.**[1302]
- Pharmacologic aromatase inhibition: In our office, we commonly measure serum estradiol in men and administer the aromatase inhibitor anastrozole/Arimidex 1 mg (≥2-3 doses per week) to men whose estradiol level is greater than 32 picogram/mL. The Life Extension Foundation[1303] advocates that the optimal serum estradiol level for a man is 10-30 picogram/mL. Clinical studies using anastrozole/Arimidex in men have shown that aromatase blockade lowers estradiol and raises testosterone[1304]; generally speaking, this is exactly the result that we want in patients with severe systemic autoimmunity. Whether using anastrozole/Arimidex, frequency of dosing is based on serum and clinical response. Letrozole/Femara is a newer pharmacologic aromatase inhibitor which appears to have slight superiority over anastrozole in terms of anti-estrogen efficacy; however, I am quite convinced that Letrozole/Femara is also an androgen receptor agonist and therefore I generally avoid this drug like the plague. Relatedly, the botanical *Rhodiola rosea* can elevate testosterone and estradiol, making the latter particularly difficult to control. On occasion, we have seen some men make so much testosterone→estradiol that they require both anastrozole/Arimidex *and* Letrozole/Femara along with licorice daily in order to control their testosterone and estradiol levels. Licorice lowers testosterone and thus the precursor to estradiol in both men and women within about four days of oral administration, whether by standardized capsules or by tea from the root. Of course, anastrozole/Arimidex can be administered to women in 1 mg doses ranging from once per week to 5-7 times per week depending on clinical and serologic response. **In two recent case reports, administration of anti-estrogen medication—either tamoxifen or anastrozole—resulted in clinical improvements in two women with dermatomyositis.**[1305]

The aromatase enzyme converts androgens to estrogens: If estrogens are high and androgens are low, then estrogens can be lowered and androgens raised via inhibition of aromatase. If androgens are low and estrogens are low, then administration of androgens will raise both the androgens and the estrogens, possibly necessitating coadministration of an aromatase inhibitor.

[1300] "Micromolar concentrations of beta-estradiol, estrone, 16-alpha-hydroxyestrone and estriol enhance the oxidative metabolism of activated human PMNL's. The corresponding 2-hydroxylated estrogens 2-OH-estradiol, 2-OH-estrone and 2-OH-estriol act on the contrary as powerful inhibitors of cell activity." Jansson G. Oestrogen-induced enhancement of myeloperoxidase activity in human polymorphonuclear leukocytes--a possible cause of oxidative stress in inflammatory cells. *Free Radic Res Commun*. 1991;14(3):195-208

[1301] "Even more dramatically, in the case of laryngeal papillomas induction of 2-hydroxylation with indole-3-carbinol (I3C) has resulted in inhibition of tumor growth during the time that the patients continue to take I3C or vegetables rich in this compound." Bradlow et al. 2-hydroxyestrone: the 'good' estrogen. *J Endocrinol*. 1996 Sep;150 Suppl:S259-65

[1302] "Women with SLE can manifest a metabolic response to I3C and might benefit from its antiestrogenic effects." McAlindon TE, Gulin J, Chen T, Klug T, Lahita R, Nuite M. Indole-3-carbinol in women with SLE: effect on estrogen metabolism and disease activity. *Lupus*. 2001;10(11):779-83

[1303] Male Hormone Modulation Therapy, Page 4 Of 7: lef.org/protocols/prtcl-130c.shtml Accessed October 30, 2005

[1304] "These data demonstrate that aromatase inhibition increases serum bioavailable and total testosterone levels to the youthful normal range in older men with mild hypogonadism." Leder et al. Effects of aromatase inhibition in elderly men with low or borderline-low serum testosterone levels. *J Clin Endocrinol Metab*. 2004 Mar;89:1174-80

[1305] "Using antiestrogen medication in women with DM may result in a significant improvement in their rash, possibly via the inhibition of TNF-alpha production by immune or other cells." Sereda D, Werth VP. Improvement in dermatomyositis rash associated with the use of antiestrogen medication. *Arch Dermatol*. 2006 Jan;142(1):70-2

- **Testosterone:** Androgen deficiencies predispose to, are exacerbated by, and contribute to autoimmune/inflammatory disorders. **A large proportion of men with lupus or RA have low testosterone**[1306] and suffer the effects of hypogonadism: fatigue, weakness, depression, slow healing, low libido, and difficulties with sexual performance. Particularly in men, blood samples should be drawn for *free* and *total* testosterone (fT and tT, respectively) along with serum estradiol. Since some labs accept ridiculously low levels of testosterone as "within normal limits" clinicians should not necessarily wait until the patient is pathologically hypogonadal before implementing treatment. Clinicians must appreciate the interrelationship of testosterone with estrogen in order to interpret the patient's status appropriately and implement proper treatment. Since testosterone is converted to estradiol by aromatase, a patient with low testosterone and high estradiol is properly treated with aromatase inhibition (e.g., Arimidex/anastrozole) rather than testosterone; administration of Arimidex/anastrozole to men simultaneously lowers estradiol and raises testosterone.[1307] Conversely, low testosterone along with low estrogen indicates the appropriateness of testosterone replacement and/or corrective treatment of the cause of the hypogonadism. The need for co-administration of testosterone and Arimidex/anastrozole is not uncommon in order to raise testosterone without leading to an iatrogenic increase in estrogen due to "estrogen shunting" by aromatase. Follow-up testing of testosterone and estradiol 4-8 weeks after the implementation of testosterone replacement is advised to ensure optimal hormone status and that the additional *immunoregulatory* testosterone is not being shunted into *immunodysregulatory* estradiol. For the purpose of gently but effectively modulating/lowering estrogen levels, Arimidex/anastrozole is typically administered as 1 mg administered 1-4 times *per week*; the drug appears to have a wide margin of safety, and doses of 1 mg *per day* (doses up to 10 mg/d have been used) are commonly and appropriately—as one of the safest and most effective treatments against breast cancer—used in women with estrogen-responsive breast cancer. As with any modulation/administration of testosterone and estrogen, follow-up testing of hormones and serum lipids is recommended to ensure the attainment of optimal status and the avoidance of complications, such as suppression of HDL synthesis which would be expected to have adverse cardiovascular consequences. Assessing serum PSA is a prerequisite to testosterone administration in men. **Testosterone therapy improves clinical status and wellbeing in women with rheumatoid arthritis.**[1308] Transdermal testosterone creams can be used with dose tailored to serum and clinical response.
- **Cortisol:** In physiologic doses cortisol is immunoregulatory and mildly yet significantly immunosuppressive ("*physiologic immunosuppression*"), while at higher doses *and particularly in its synthetic forms such as prednisone and prednisolone* the hormone becomes immunosuppressive ("*pharmacologic immunosuppression*") and brings additional adverse effects such as weight gain, truncal obesity, hypertension, glucose intolerance and increased susceptibility to infections—the classic manifestations of hypercortisolemia seen in Cushing's disease.[1309] Insufficiencies of cortisol production contribute to the development and perpetuation of allergies, fatigue, inflammation, and autoimmunity.[1310] The works of Drs. John Tintera and William Jefferies have remained important despite being ignored by most endocrinologists; Jefferies' books[1311] and articles[1312] are still widely available and provide concepts and

---

[1306] Karagiannis A, Harsoulis F. Gonadal dysfunction in systemic diseases. *Eur J Endocrinol*. 2005 Apr;152(4):501-13 eje-online.org/cgi/content/full/152/4/501
[1307] "These data demonstrate that aromatase inhibition increases serum bioavailable and total testosterone levels to the youthful normal range in older men with mild hypogonadism. Serum estradiol levels decrease modestly but remain within the normal male range." Leder BZ, Rohrer JL, Rubin SD, Gallo J, Longcope C. Effects of aromatase inhibition in elderly men with low or borderline-low serum testosterone levels. *J Clin Endocrinol Metab*. 2004 Mar;89(3):1174-80 jcem.endojournals.org/cgi/content/full/89/3/1174
[1308] "An improvement in ESR, Dutch health assessment questionnaire, and pain was noted. ...Testosterone may improve the general wellbeing of postmenopausal women with active rheumatoid arthritis." Booji A, Biewenga-Booji CM, Huber-Bruning O, Cornelis C, Jacobs JW, Bijlsma JW. Androgens as adjuvant treatment in postmenopausal female patients with rheumatoid arthritis. *Ann Rheum Dis*. 1996 Nov;55(11):811-5
[1309] Kirk LF Jr, Hash RB, Katner HP, Jones T. Cushing's disease: clinical manifestations and diagnostic evaluation. *Am Fam Physician*. 2000 Sep 1;62(5):1119-27, 1133-4 aafp.org/afp/20000901/1119.html
[1310] "Yet evidence that patients with rheumatoid arthritis improved with small, physiologic dosages of cortisol or cortisone acetate was reported over 25 years ago, and that patients with chronic allergic disorders or unexplained chronic fatigue also improved with administration of such small dosages was reported over 15 years ago..." Jefferies WM. Mild adrenocortical deficiency, chronic allergies, autoimmune disorders and the chronic fatigue syndrome: a continuation of the cortisone story. *Med Hypotheses*. 1994 Mar;42(3):183-9 thebuteykocentre.com/Irish_%20Buteykocenter_files/further_studies/med_hyp2.pdf and members.westnet.com.au/pkolb/med_hyp2.pdf
[1311] Jefferies WMcK. Safe Uses of Cortisol. Second Edition. Springfield, CC Thomas, 1996
[1312] "Yet evidence that patients with rheumatoid arthritis improved with small, physiologic dosages of cortisol or cortisone acetate was reported over 25 years ago, and that patients with chronic allergic disorders or unexplained chronic fatigue also improved with administration of such small dosages was reported over 15 years ago..." Jefferies WM. Mild adrenocortical deficiency, chronic allergies, autoimmune disorders and the chronic fatigue syndrome: a continuation of the cortisone story. *Med Hypotheses*. 1994 Mar;42(3):183-9 thebuteykocentre.com/Irish_%20Buteykocenter_files/further_studies/med_hyp2.pdf and members.westnet.com.au/pkolb/med_hyp2.pdf

clinically relevant applications. In a 1998 summary by Jefferies[1313] on the etiology of rheumatoid arthritis, he reviewed evidence suggesting that subacute hypoadrenalism results in insufficiencies of cortisol and DHEA, both of which are necessary for immunomodulation and immunocompetence; insufficiencies of these hormones leaves the body vulnerable to chronic infections (i.e., multifocal dysbiosis, as detailed previously) and the systemic proinflammatory sequelae that result in so-called "autoimmunity." Differential diagnoses in patients with low adrenal function include congenital adrenal hypoplasia, adrenoleukodystrophy, autoimmune Addison disease, and chronic hypopituarism. A small short-term randomized crossover clinical trial published in *The Lancet* showed benefit of 5-10 mg/day of cortisol in patients with chronic fatigue syndrome.[1314] Supplementation with up to 20 mg per day of cortisol/Cortef is physiologic; higher doses in the range of 40 mg per day may benefit patients, especially during times of stress, but are adrenosuppressive. My preference is to dose 10 mg first thing in the morning, then 5 mg in late morning and 5 mg in midafternoon in an attempt to replicate the diurnal variation and normal morning peak of cortisol levels. In patients with hypoadrenalism, administration of pregnenolone in doses of 10-60 mg in the morning may also be beneficial; DHEA supplementation is beneficial for patients with adrenal insufficiency.

Criteria for the diagnosis of adrenal insufficiency in children and adults

- <u>First-morning cortisol less than 8-10 mcg/dL</u>: An 8:00 am serum cortisol concentration less than 8-10 mcg/dL suggests adrenal insufficiency.
- <u>Serum cortisol less than 18 mcg/dL during illness or stress or with elevated ACTH</u>: Serum cortisol concentration less than 18 mcg/dL in a sick and stressed patient, or associated with an elevated ACTH, is highly suggestive of adrenal insufficiency.
- <u>Post-ACTH serum cortisol less than 18 mcg/dL</u>: Serum cortisol less than 18 mcg/dL obtained 30-60 minutes following ACTH injection is diagnostic of adrenal insufficiency.
- <u>Serum cortisol that fails to double within 30-60 minutes after ACTH injection</u>: This test involves three steps: 1) blood sample is taken for serum cortisol, 2) ACTH is injected, 3) blood sample for serum cortisol is taken again at 30-60 minutes. Cortisol production should double following injection of ACTH; this is a demonstration of adrenal reserve and the ability of the adrenal glands to respond to stress.
- <u>Low output of adrenal hormones measured in 24-hour urine samples</u>: This provides sufficient objective data to justify a clinical trial of cortisol replacement in patients with a suggestive clinical picture and lack of contraindications.
- <u>Proper dosing of cosyntropin/ACTH</u>: Injections of "ACTH" are generally performed with the intravenous or intramuscular injection of "Cosyntropin" which is a synthetic peptide fragment of ACTH used for adrenal stimulation. According to the review by Wilson, the **standard dose for adults is 250 mcg**. "For infants, the author suggests 50 mcg of cosyntropin (approximately 250 mg/m2)."

Jefferies WMcK. <u>Safe Uses of Cortisol. Second Edition</u>. Springfield, CC Thomas, 1996 page 39
medicinenet.com/cosyntropin-injectable/article.htm Accessed December 7, 2006
Wilson TA. Adrenal Hypoplasia. *eMedicine* emedicine.com/PED/topic45.htm Accessed November 18, 2005

- **DHEA (insufficiency and supraphysiologic supplementation):** Patients with autoimmunity should be tested for DHEA insufficiency by measurement of serum DHEA-sulfate; insufficiencies should generally be corrected except in cases of concomitant hormone-responsive cancer such as breast cancer or prostate cancer. Physiologic doses are approximately 15-25 mg for women and 25-50 mg for men. However, many patients with autoimmunity will respond favorably to supraphysiologic doses in the range of 200 mg per day. The rationale for using high-dose DHEA in patients with autoimmune diseases is supported by the following:
    1. DHEA is a natural metabolite/hormone of the human body made in the adrenal glands.
    2. Patients with autoimmune diseases are commonly treated with prednisone and other corticosteroids for months or years at a time. Use of prednisone causes adrenal suppression with resultant suppression of DHEA levels.[1315]

[1313] "The etiology of rheumatoid arthritis ...explained by a combination of three factors: (i) a relatively mild deficiency of cortisol, ..., (ii) a deficiency of DHEA, ...and (iii) infection by organisms such as mycoplasma,..." Jefferies WM. The etiology of rheumatoid arthritis. *Med Hypotheses*. 1998 Aug;51(2):111-4
[1314] "In some patients with chronic fatigue syndrome, low-dose hydrocortisone reduces fatigue levels in the short term." Cleare AJ, Heap E, Malhi GS, Wessely S, O'Keane V, Miell J. Low-dose hydrocortisone in chronic fatigue syndrome: a randomised crossover trial. *Lancet*. 1999 Feb 6;353(9151):455-8
[1315] "Basal serum DHEA and DHEAS concentrations were suppressed to a greater degree than was cortisol during both daily and alternate day prednisone treatments. ...Thus, adrenal androgen secretion was more easily suppressed than was cortisol secretion by this low dose of glucocorticoid, but there was no advantage to alternate day therapy." Rittmaster et al. Effect of daily and alternate day low dose prednisone on serum cortisol and adrenal androgens in hirsute women. *J Clin Endocrinol Metab*. 1988 Aug;67(2):400-3

3. As a consequence of prednisone treatment, many patients lose bone mass and develop osteoporosis. DHEA has been shown to reverse the osteoporosis and loss of bone mass induced by corticosteroid treatment.[1316]
4. DHEA shows no acute or subacute toxicity even when used in supraphysiologic doses, even when used in sick patients. For example, in a study of 32 patients with HIV, DHEA doses of 750 mg – 2,250 mg per day were well tolerated and produced no dose-limiting adverse effects.[1317] This lack of toxicity compares favorably with any and all so-called "antirheumatic" drugs, nearly all of which show alarming comparable toxicity.
5. DHEA is inexpensive. Even at the relatively high dose of 200 mg per day, the cost is less than $40 per month.
6. When used at doses of 200 mg per day, DHEA safely provides clinical benefit for patients with various autoimmune diseases, including ulcerative colitis, Crohn's disease[1318], and SLE.[1319]
7. 200 mg per day of DHEA allows SLE patients to reduce their dose of prednisone (thus avoiding its adverse effects) while achieving symptomatic improvement. In other words, it allows for improved health and reduced medication use and therefore fewer side effects.[1320]

Thus, based on these financial, safety, and effectiveness considerations, the administration of DHEA is reasonable for patients with moderate or severe autoimmune disease. Furthermore, since optimal clinical response appears to correlate with serum levels that are supraphysiologic[1321], treatment may be implemented with little regard for initial DHEA levels, particularly when 1) the dose of DHEA is kept as low as possible, 2) duration is kept as short as possible, 3) other interventions are used to address the underlying cause of the disease, 4) the patient is deriving benefit and the risk-to-benefit ratio is favorable.

- **Thyroid (insufficiency or autoimmunity):** Hypothyroidism is a common concomitant to many of the autoimmune diseases. Overt or imminent hypothyroidism is suggested by TSH greater than 2 mU/L[1322] or 3 mU/L[1323], low T4 or T3, and/or the presence of anti-thyroid peroxidase antibodies.[1324] Specific treatment considerations include the following:
  o <u>Selenium</u>: Supplementation with either selenomethonine[1325] or sodium selenite[1326,1327] can reduce thyroid autoimmunity and improve peripheral conversion of T4 to T3. Selenium may be started at 500-800 mcg per day (for 1-3 months) and tapered to 200-400 mcg per day for maintenance.[1328]
  o <u>L-thyroxine/levothyroxine/Synthroid—prescription synthetic T4</u>: 25-50 mcg per day is a common starting dose which can be adjusted based on clinical and laboratory response. Thyroid hormone supplements must be consumed separately from soy products (by at least 1-2 hours) and preferably

---

[1316] "CONCLUSION: Prasterone treatment prevented BMD loss and significantly increased BMD at both the lumbar spine and total hip in female patients with SLE receiving exogenous glucocorticoids." Mease PJ, Ginzler EM, Gluck OS, Schiff M, Goldman A, Greenwald M, Cohen S, Egan R, Quarles BJ, Schwartz KE. Effects of prasterone on bone mineral density in women with systemic lupus erythematosus receiving chronic glucocorticoid therapy. *J Rheumatol*. 2005 Apr;32(4):616-21

[1317] "Thirty-one subjects were evaluated and monitored for safety and tolerance. The oral drug was administered three times daily in doses ranging from 750 mg/day to 2,250 mg/day for 16 weeks. ... The drug was well tolerated and no dose-limiting side effects were noted." Dyner TS, Lang W, Geaga J, et al. An open-label dose-escalation trial of oral dehydroepiandrosterone tolerance and pharmacokinetics in patients with HIV disease. *J Acquir Immune Defic Syndr*. 1993 May;6(5):459-65

[1318] "CONCLUSIONS: In a pilot study, dehydroepiandrosterone was effective and safe in patients with refractory Crohn's disease or ulcerative colitis." Andus T, et al. Patients with refractory Crohn's disease or ulcerative colitis respond to dehydroepiandrosterone: a pilot study. *Aliment Pharmacol Ther*. 2003 Feb;17(3):409-14

[1319] "CONCLUSION: The overall results confirm that DHEA treatment was well-tolerated, significantly reduced the number of SLE flares, and improved patient's global assessment of disease activity." Chang DM, Lan JL, Lin HY, Luo SF. Dehydroepiandrosterone treatment of women with mild-to-moderate systemic lupus erythematosus: a multicenter randomized, double-blind, placebo-controlled trial. *Arthritis Rheum*. 2002 Nov;46(11):2924-7

[1320] "CONCLUSION: Among women with lupus disease activity, reducing the dosage of prednisone to < or = 7.5 mg/day for a sustained period of time while maintaining stabilization or a reduction of disease activity was possible in a significantly greater proportion of patients treated with oral prasterone, 200 mg once daily, compared with patients treated with placebo." Petri MA, Lahita RG, Van Vollenhoven RF, et al and GL601 Study Group. Effects of prasterone on corticosteroid requirements of women with systemic lupus erythematosus: a double-blind, randomized, placebo-controlled trial. *Arthritis Rheum*. 2002 Jul;46(7):1820-9

[1321] "CONCLUSION: The clinical response to DHEA was not clearly dose dependent. Serum levels of DHEA and DHEAS correlated only weakly with lupus outcomes, but suggested an optimum serum DHEAS of 1000 microg/dl." Barry NN, McGuire JL, van Vollenhoven RF. Dehydroepiandrosterone in systemic lupus erythematosus: relationship between dosage, serum levels, and clinical response. *J Rheumatol*. 1998 Dec;25(12):2352-6

[1322] Weetman AP. Hypothyroidism: screening and subclinical disease. *BMJ*. 1997 Apr 19;314(7088):1175-8 bmj.bmjjournals.com/cgi/content/full/314/7088/1175

[1323] "Now AACE encourages doctors to consider treatment for patients who test outside the boundaries of a narrower margin based on a target TSH level of 0.3 to 3.0. AACE believes the new range will result in proper diagnosis for millions of Americans who suffer from a mild thyroid disorder, but have gone untreated until now." American Association of Clinical Endocrinologists (AACE). 2003 Campaign Encourages Awareness of Mild Thyroid Failure, Importance of Routine Testing aace.com/pub/tam2003/press.php November 26, 2005

[1324] Beers MH, Berkow R (eds). <u>The Merck Manual. Seventeenth Edition</u>. Whitehouse Station; Merck Research Laboratories 1999 Page 96

[1325] Duntas et al. Effects of a six month treatment with selenomethionine in patients with autoimmune thyroiditis. *Eur J Endocrinol*. 2003 Apr;148(4):389-93

[1326] Gartner R, Gasnier BC, Dietrich JW, Krebs B, Angstwurm MW. Selenium supplementation in patients with autoimmune thyroiditis decreases thyroid peroxidase antibodies concentrations. *J Clin Endocrinol Metab*. 2002 Apr;87(4):1687-91 jcem.endojournals.org/cgi/content/full/87/4/1687

[1327] "We recently conducted a prospective, placebo-controlled clinical study, where we could demonstrate, that a substitution of 200 wg sodium selenite for three months in patients with autoimmune thyroiditis reduced thyroid peroxidase antibody (TPO-Ab) concentrations significantly." Gartner R, Gasnier BC. Selenium in the treatment of autoimmune thyroiditis. *Biofactors*. 2003;19(3-4):165-70

[1328] Bruns F, Micke O, Bremer M. Current status of selenium and other treatments for secondary lymphedema. *J Support Oncol*. 2003 Jul-Aug;1(2):121-30 supportiveoncology.net/journal/articles/0102121.pdf on an empty stomach to avoid absorption interference by food, fiber, and minerals, especially calcium. Doses are generally started at one-half of the daily dose for the first 10 days after which the full dose is used. Caution must be applied in patients with adrenal insufficiency and/or those with cardiovascular disease.

- o <u>Liothyronine, Cytomel®</u>: Cytomel is prescription synthetic T3. Except in patients with myxedema for whom the appropriate starting dose is 5 mcg per day, treatment generally starts with 25 mcg per day and can be increased to 75 mcg per day; dose is adjusted based on clinical and laboratory response. As stated previously, thyroid hormone supplements must be consumed separately from soy products (by at least 1-2 hours) and preferably on an empty stomach to avoid absorption interference by food, fiber, and minerals, especially calcium. Time-released T3 can be obtained from a compounding pharmacy.
- o <u>Armour thyroid—prescription natural T4 and T3 from cow/pig thyroid gland</u>: 60 mg (one grain) is a common starting and maintenance dose. Since administration of Armour thyroid frequently increases serum levels of anti-thyroid antibodies in patients with preexisting thyroid autoimmunity, **many doctors choose to not use Armour thyroid in patients with thyroid autoimmunity**. Some patients prefer to divide their daily dose to maintain constant serum levels of T3.
- o <u>Thyrolar/Liotrix—prescription synthetic T4 with T3</u>: Dosed incrementally as "1", "2", or "3." This product has been difficult to obtain for the past few years due to manufacturing problems (thyrolar.com/); previously it was my treatment of choice due to the combination of T4 and T3 and the lack of antigenicity compared to gland-derived products.
- o <u>Thyroid glandular—nonprescription T3</u>: Producers of nutritional products are able to distribute T3 because it is not listed by the FDA as a prescription item. Nutritional supplement companies may start with Armour thyroid, remove the T4, and sell the thyroid glandular with active T3 thereby providing a nonprescription source of active thyroid hormone. For many patients, one tablet per day is at least as effective as a prescription source of thyroid hormone. Since it is derived from a glandular and therefore potentially antigenic source, thyroid glandular is not used in patients with thyroid autoimmunity due to its ability to induce increased production of anti-thyroid antibodies.
- o <u>L-tyrosine and iodine</u>: Some patients with mild hypothyroidism respond to supplementation with L-tyrosine and iodine. Tyrosine is commonly used in doses of 4-9 grams per day in divided doses. According to Abraham and Wright[1329], doses of iodine may be as high as 12.5 milligrams (12,500 micrograms), which is slightly less than the average daily intake in Japan at 13.8 mg per day.

- **Pregnenolone:** Several reviews and clinical trials from the early 1950s showed moderate clinical effectiveness and absence of adverse effects from oral administration of pregnenolone in doses as high as 500-1,000 mg/d in patients with rheumatoid arthritis and other rheumatic conditions.[1330,1331,1332,1333] Following oral administration of pregnenolone in doses of approximately 500 mg/d, beneficial results are noted in approximately 50-80% of patients. Responders will show reduced pain, swelling, and objective reductions in inflammation measured by ESR and will have increased strength and mobility. No important adverse effects have been reported, particularly with regard to pulse rate, blood pressure, or glucose homeostasis. In contrast to the adverse withdrawal effects noted with prednisone/prednisolone, discontinuance of pregnenolone does not immediately result in exacerbation of inflammation and has never been reported to incite adrenal insufficiency. Oral administration of pregnenolone produces better clinical response than does intramuscular administration, apparently due to the relative insolubility of parenteral pregnenolone. The low cost and absence of adverse effects makes pregnenolone a reasonable therapeutic intervention in patients with rheumatic disease because the treatment may provide benefit and/or mitigate the need for treatments with greater toxicity and cost. However, this treatment should not

---

[1329] Wright JV. Why you need 83 times more of this essential, cancer-fighting nutrient than the "experts" say you do. *Nutrition and Healing* 2005; volume 12, issue 4.
[1330] Freeman H, Pincus G, Johnson CW, et al. Therapeutic efficacy of delta-5-pregnenolone in rheumatoid arthritis. *J American Medical Association* 1950; April 15: 1124-8
[1331] Stock JP, McClure EC. Pregnenolone in the treatment of rheumatoid arthritis. *Lancet* 1950 Jul 22;2(4):125-8
[1332] Dordick JR, Ehrlich ME, Alexander S, Kissin M. Pregnenolone in rheumatoid arthritis. *N Engl J Med*. 1951 Mar 1;244(9):324-6
[1333] Freeman H, Pincus G, Bachrach S, et al. Oral steroid medication in rheumatoid arthritis. *J Clin Endocrinol Metab*. 1950 Dec;10(12):1523-32

be relied upon as monotherapy and/or in patients with important inflammatory complications such as iritis, scleritis, or temporal arteritis. In contrast to the much higher doses of 500-1,000 mg/d reported in the studies cited above in this paragraph, I generally limit pregnenolone doses to 10-50 mg/d taken in the morning in patients who may derive benefit; some patients—generally those with hypoadrenalism—notice a marked improvement in energy (to the point of causing insomnia) with doses as low as 5-10 mg/d.

DrV's Summary and Practical Guide to Orthoendocrinology: Read preceding discussions

Assessments	Interventions and Notes
Serum prolactin	• Reduce elevations or treat empirically regardless of serum prolactin level; cabergoline 0.25-0.5 mg twice weekly; also consider using pyridoxine 250-500 mg/d, *Vitex* to effect. • Many studies have now demonstrated that empiric cabergoline is a reasonable, safe, and effective treatment for the more severe inflammatory disorders; cabergoline produces is anti-inflammatory benefit via blocking prolactin signaling within the immune system and not by primarily affecting pituitary output of prolactin.
Serum fasting insulin as a marker of insulin resistance and metabolic inflammation	• Improve insulin sensitivity by reducing carbohydrate intake and improving insulin secretion and reception. Insulin resistance most commonly results from 1) systemic inflammation, 2) xenobiotic down-regulation of GLUT receptors via the aryl-hydrocarbon receptor, 3) micronutrient deficiencies, 4) cortisol excess, 5) physiologic and protective insulin resistance secondary to ceramide accumulation as a result of cellular carbohydrate overload.
Serum estradiol	• Reduce serum estradiol with adipose loss, alcohol and caffeine avoidance, treatment for obesity, surgical correction of varicocele in men, anastrozole 1mg 2-3 times weekly is effective and safe in most cases, especially for men • Consider monitoring osteoporosis risk in cases of prolonged hypoestrogenemia, which should generally be avoided.
Serum DHEA sulfate	• Physiologic doses are 15 mg/d for women and 25 mg/d for men; supraphysiologic dosing up to 200mg/d is effective, safe, and well-represented in the rheumatology literature for the treatment of RA, SLE, and IBD.
Serum cortisol, preferably before and after ACTH	• See interpretive guide provided previously. • Physiologic doses of ≤ 10-20 mg/d orally administered cortisol can be used empirically under appropriate supervision, with the first dose of 10mg administered upon waking in the morning and optional additional doses of 5 mg each administered in the late morning and early afternoon to mimic physiologic secretion.
Serum free and total testosterone	• If total testosterone is low, evaluate for primary or secondary hypogonadism. • If testosterone is low and estrogen is low, consider transdermal testosterone therapy. • If free testosterone is low and total testosterone is normal, likely due to elevated SHBG, generally due to excess estrogen or excess prolactin. • If testosterone is low and estrogen is high, then use aromatase inhibition and/or correct the hypogonadism resulting from obesity/inflammation. • Always assess free and total testosterone in conjunction with serum estradiol.

Always use the lowest dose of hormonal intervention necessary to achieve the desired result based on dual consideration of laboratory results and the patient's response to treatment; lower doses of each intervention can be used when more interventions (e.g., nutritional, mitochondrial, antidysbiotic) are used.

❶ Food ❷ Infections ❸ Nutri-immunomod ❹ Dysmetab ❺ Stress/Sleep/Socio/Surg/Sup ❻ Endo ❼ Xeno

❼ Xenobiotic Immunotoxicity:
Exposure, Accumulation, Detoxification

> **Major Concepts in this Section**
> Exposure to "foreign substances" such as toxic chemicals and toxic metals is inescapable in our polluted world and modern lives; exposure invariably results in some level of accumulation. Accumulation of toxic metals and chemicals produces additive and synergistic toxic effects on the entire organism, notably via endocrine disruption, immune imbalance and suppression, oxidative stress, immunogenic modification of endogenous antigens via xenobiotic haptenization, and mitochondrial dysfunction, which then leads to systemic inflammation, reduced cell/tissue performance, and additional oxidative stress. Despite these facts and the obvious clinical implications, most doctorate-level physicians—except for naturopathic clinicians—receive no training in these topics and the clinical remediation via therapeutic detoxification. Thus, the naturopathic profession stands clearly preeminent in its profession-wide training in the appreciation, assessment and treatment of xenobiotic-induced illness.

Xenobiotic Immunotoxicity and Treatment by Therapeutic Detoxification: Ultracondensed Clinical Review
Chemicals such as pesticides, synthetic fertilizers, herbicides, fungicides, industrial pollution, car exhaust, solvents, and innumerable others are bioaccumulative and can alter immune function. The classic manifestation of xenobiotic immunotoxicity is the combination of reduced resistance to infections and increased allergic and autoimmune disorders. The subject of environmental medicine and detoxification is much too broad and complex to review completely in this textbook, and while naturopathic physicians are trained in these topics, other healthcare professionals are not unless they attend post-graduate training and take the time to read articles and textbooks on these topics. Readers for whom these topics are new are encouraged to access the following citations for additional information.[1334,1335,1336,1337,1338] What follows here will be an ultracondensed clinical review focusing on major concepts and problem-specific solutions.

- Chemical toxicity: Accumulation of xenobiotics can cause immune dysfunction and can contribute to the development of "autoimmunity." Examples of xenobiotic-induced autoimmunity include 1) the increased autoimmunity seen in farmers exposed to pesticides[1339], 2) the scleroderma-like disease that results from exposure to vinyl chloride[1340], 3) the association of mercury and pesticide exposure with lupus[1341], and 4) the well-recognized connection between drug and chemical exposure and various autoimmune syndromes such as drug-induced lupus.[1342] More than 40 pharmaceutical drugs are known to cause drug-induced

For the sake of simplicity and with recognition of the various nuances of different xenobiotics, I generalize toxicity into two categories, either *chemicals* or *heavy metals*. Most patients have an overlay of these two problems, so that the clinical manifestations and treatments have several commonalities.

[1334] "Caffeine enemas cause dilation of bile ducts, which facilitates excretion of toxic cancer breakdown products by the liver and dialysis of toxic products from blood across the colonic wall. The therapy must be used as an integrated whole." Gerson M. The cure of advanced cancer by diet therapy: a summary of 30 years of clinical experimentation. *Physiol Chem Phys*. 1978;10(5):449-64
[1335] "The writer has observed numerous cases suffering from such conditions as chronic arthritis, hypertension, coronary disease, chronic abdominal distention, constipation, and colitis, in which the element of constipation, auto-intoxication and possible colon infection seemed to play a prominent part, which responded very satisfactorily to colonic irrigations after failure to improve following the usual forms of medical treatment." Snyder RG. The value of colonic irrigations in countering auto-intoxication of intestinal origin. *Medical Clinics of North America* 1939; May: 781-788
[1336] Gonzalez et al. Evaluation of pancreatic proteolytic enzyme treatment of adenocarcinoma of pancreas, with nutrition and detoxification support. *Nutr Cancer* 1999;33:117-24
[1337] Crinnion WJ. Results of a decade of naturopathic treatment for environmental illness: a review of clinical records. *J Naturopathic Med* 1997;7:21-27
[1338] Sherman JD. *Chemical exposure and disease. Diagnostic and investigative techniques*. Princeton Scientific Publishing; 1994
[1339] "IgG levels decreased with increasing p,p'-DDE levels, with a statistically significant decrease of approximately 50% in the highest two categories of exposure. Sixteen (12%) were positive for antinuclear antibodies... These analyses provide evidence that p,p'-DDE modulates immune responses in humans." Cooper GS, et al. Associations between plasma DDE levels and immunologic measures in African-American farmers in North Carolina. *Environ Health Perspect*. 2004 Jul;112(10):1080-4
[1340] "Vinyl chloride (VC) monomer can induce a scleroderma-like syndrome in a proportion of workers exposed to it during production of polyvinyl chloride." Black CM, Welsh KI, Walker AE, et al. Genetic susceptibility to scleroderma-like syndrome induced by vinyl chloride. *Lancet*. 1983 Jan 1;1(8314-5):53-5
[1341] "...reported occupational exposure to mercury (OR 3.6), mixing pesticides for agricultural work (OR 7.4), and among dental workers (OR 7.1). ...these associations were fairly strong and statistically significant..." Cooper GS, et al. Occupational risk factors for development of systemic lupus erythematosus. *J Rheumatol*. 2004 Oct;31:1928-33
[1342] Hess EV. Environmental chemicals and autoimmune disease: cause and effect. *Toxicology*. 2002 Dec 27;181-182:65-70

lupus.[1343] Every one of us is exposed to toxic chemicals every day, and every one of us has chemical accumulation and the potential for xenobiotic-induced disease. Except for denial (shown to be clinically ineffective), we cannot escape from the chemical consequences of living in a world with tens of thousands of synthetic chemicals. According to limited analyses, the average American has accumulated at least 18 different chemicals[1344], and analyses that are more detailed show that even more chemicals and metals have been accumulated.[1345] Common sources of these chemicals include pesticides, synthetic fertilizers, herbicides, fungicides, industrial pollution, car exhaust, solvents, paints, perfumes, plastic food/drink containers, non-stick cookware, Styrofoam, trichloroethylene from dry cleaning, rubber, carpet, plastics, glues, propellants, petroleum fuels such as gasoline, detergents, and other "cleaners." Clinical consequences of chemical toxicity are diverse, can affect nearly every organ system, and may be predicted to some extent by the pattern of chemical exposure since some chemicals have characteristic sequelae. Most chemicals, especially those which are fat-soluble, can readily enter the body via respiratory, gastrointestinal, and transdermal routes. Once in the bloodstream, chemicals are either detoxified (inactivated and/or solubilized) by the liver and then excreted via urine or bile, or to a lesser extent exhaled from the lungs or excreted via sweat. Chemicals which are not excreted from the body are stored in the tissues, particularly lipid-rich organs such as the liver, adipose, and brain. Molecular turnover and recycling (particularly lipolysis) liberates fat-stored xenobiotics for another opportunity for either detoxification or additional toxicity. The main route for detoxification is the liver, which hydrosolubilizes xenobiotics via oxidation ("phase one") and conjugation ("phase two"). Generally speaking, oxidation reactions are dependent on the cytochrome P-450 system, which can be inhibited by various drugs (e.g., ketoconazole, erythromycin, ritonavir, cimetidine, omeprazole, ethanol), foods such as ethanol and grapefruit juice, bacterial endotoxin from bacterial overgrowth of the intestines, and/or by genetic defects known as single nucleotide polymorphisms ("SNiPs") which reduce xenobiotic clearance. Similarly, conjugation reactions can be inhibited by a low-vegetable diet, SNiPs, and insufficiencies of conjugation moieties such as glutathione, glycine, glutamine, taurine, ornithine, sulfur, and methyl groups. If oxidation is too slow, then xenobiotics are insufficiently detoxicated and insufficiently processed for conjugation, leading to xenobiotic accumulation. If oxidation is too fast relative to conjugation, then reactive intermediates are formed which are commonly more toxic than the original xenobiotic, and insufficient conjugation results in accumulation of reactive xenobiotics which are inherently prone to tissue haptenization (which can incite autoimmunity) and DNA intercalation (which promotes damage to DNA and the resultant mutation and oncogenesis). Optimally oxidized and conjugated xenobiotics are excreted in the urine (smaller molecules with molecular weight less than 400-600) or expelled in the bile (larger molecules with molecular weight greater than 400-600). Supranormal hydration and urinary alkalinization enhance renal clearance of weakly acidic xenobiotics and drugs, whereas dehydration and urinary acidity impair toxin excretion, generally speaking. Conjugated toxins expelled in the bile can be deconjugated by bacteria so that the toxin is reabsorbed, a phenomenon commonly referred to as "enterohepatic recycling"[1346] or "enterohepatic recirculation."[1347] Such recirculation is obviously less likely if gastrointestinal status and diet have been optimized to minimize the presence of deconjugating bacteria and to maximize fiber intake and laxation for the adsorption and expulsion of intraluminal toxins. Therapeutic colonics and enemas can be employed to stimulate bile flow from the liver[1348,1349] and to remove bile-secreted toxins from the gut before deconjugation and re-absorption occur. Bile formation and

---

[1343] "Drug-induced lupus has been reported as a side-effect of long-term therapy with over 40 medications... Several mechanisms for induction of autoimmunity will be discussed, including bystander activation of autoreactive lymphocytes due to drug-specific immunity or to non-specific activation of lymphocytes, direct cytotoxicity with release of autoantigens ..." Rubin RL. Drug-induced lupus. *Toxicology*. 2005;209(2):135-47
[1344] Kristin S. Schafer, Margaret Reeves, Skip Spitzer, Susan E. Kegley. Chemical Trespass: Pesticides in Our Bodies and Corporate Accountability. Pesticide Action Network North America. May 2004 panna.org/campaigns/docsTrespass/chemicalTrespass2004.dv.html
[1345] Body Burden: The Pollution in People. ewg.org/issues/siteindex/issues.php?issueid=5004
[1346] "Enterohepatic recycling occurs by biliary excretion and intestinal reabsorption of a solute, sometimes with hepatic conjugation and intestinal deconjugation. ... Of particular importance is the potential amplifying effect of enterohepatic variability in defining differences in the bioavailability, apparent volume of distribution and clearance of a given compound." Roberts MS, et al. Enterohepatic circulation: physiological, pharmacokinetic and clinical implications. *Clin Pharmacokinet*. 2002;41(10):751-90
[1347] Liska DJ. The detoxification enzyme systems. *Altern Med Rev*. 1998 Jun;3(3):187-98
[1348] Garbat, AL, Jacobi, HG: Secretion of Bile in Response to Rectal Installations. *Arch Intern Med* 1929; 44: 455-462
[1349] "Caffeine enemas cause dilation of bile ducts, which facilitates excretion of toxic cancer breakdown products by the liver and dialysis of toxic products from blood across the colonic wall. The therapy must be used as an integrated whole." Gerson M. The cure of advanced cancer by diet therapy: a summary of 30 years of clinical experimentation. *Physiol Chem Phys*. 1978;10(5):449-64

expulsion are further stimulated by botanical medicines such as beets, ginger[1350], curcumin/turmeric[1351], *Picrorhiza*[1352], milk thistle[1353], *Andrographis paniculata*[1354] and *Boerhaavia diffusa*.[1355] Respiratory exhalation of toxins is enhanced by deep breathing and exercise, and hyperventilation promotes respiratory alkalosis which elevates urine pH and promotes excretion of weakly acidic drugs and xenobiotics as previously mentioned. Dermal excretion of toxins via sweat and expedited lipolysis are stimulated via low-temperature saunas and regular aerobic exercise. Xenobiotic oxidation can be promoted (cautiously) by reducing endotoxins from the gut and by the use of botanicals such as *Hypericum perforatum* which induce several isoforms of cytochrome P-450 via activation of the pregane X receptor. Xenobiotic conjugation is likewise promoted via nutrigenomic induction stimulated by cruciferous vegetables and their derivatives such as indole-3-carbinol (I3C) and dimethylindolylemethane (DIM). The plant-based diet is employed to provide fiber for bowel cleansing and the urinary alkalinization that is necessary for optimal urinary excretion of toxins, the majority of which are weak acids and are thus excreted more efficiently in alkaline urine. Sodium bicarbonate can also be used to induce urinary alkalinization. The diet must contain high-quality protein and can be supplemented with amino acids to support amino acid and glutathione conjugation. Serum, urine, and adipose samples can be analyzed to determine the intensity and diversity of chemical accumulation; I tend reserve such testing for patients who have been exposed to a specific chemical, particularly in occupational settings. For most patients, their chemical accumulation is so diverse that they may not display abnormally high levels of a specific chemical; their clinical manifestations are rather a manifestation of a wide plethora of different chemicals, which individually may be only modestly increased. Detoxification genotype can be determined by genomic testing for SNPs in oxidation and conjugation enzymes. Phenotype can be assessed by serum and urine measurements of post-challenge detoxification of benzoate, caffeine, acetylsalicylic acid, and acetaminophen. Amino acid status can be quantified and qualified via serum or urine amino acid analysis. Stool testing assesses digestion, absorption, and microflora status. Clinical implementation follows a screening physical examination and basic laboratory assessment (minimally including CBC, metabolic panel, and urinalysis). Stool testing is always reasonable when working with patients with fatigue and/or autoimmunity; however, this and the other detoxification-related tests can often be deferred and/or used selectively. The Paleo-Mediterranean diet provides ample high-quality protein, alkalinization, fiber, and phytonutrients to which may be added supplements of protein, amino acids (especially NAC, glycine, and glutamine), and vitamins and minerals. Antioxidant teas and fresh fruit and vegetable juices are consumed to increase frequency of urination and promote urinary alkalinization, due primarily to the content of potassium citrate. Exercise and low-temperature saunas promote sweating and xenobiotic-mobilizing lipolysis. Colonics and enemas cleanse the bowel and stimulate bile flow.[1356,1357] Bile flow is further stimulated by consumption of beets, ginger, curcumin/turmeric, *Picrorhiza*, milk thistle, *Andrographis paniculata* and *Boerhaavia diffusa*. These interventions work in concert to enhance xenobiotic depuration ("The act or process of depurating or freeing from foreign or impure matter "[1358]) and cleanse the tissues of accumulated toxins. Intervention can be acute or periodic, but must be maintained for the long-term in order to resist the re-accumulation that is destined to result from the chemical onslaught that is inescapable in our polluted world.

[1350] "Further analyses for the active constituents of the acetone extracts through column chromatography indicated that [6]-gingerol and [10]-gingerol, which are the pungent principles, are mainly responsible for the cholagogic effect of ginger." Yamahara et al. Cholagogic effect of ginger and its active constituents. *J Ethnopharmacol*. 1985;13:217-25
[1351] "On the basis of the present findings, it appears that curcumin induces contraction of the human gall-bladder." Rasyid A, Lelo A. The effect of curcumin and placebo on human gall-bladder function: an ultrasound study. *Aliment Pharmacol Ther*. 1999 Feb;13(2):245-9
[1352] "Significant anticholestatic activity was also observed against carbon tetrachloride induced cholestasis in conscious rat, anaesthetized guinea pig and cat. Picroliv was more active than the known hepatoprotective drug silymarin." Saraswat B, Visen PK, Patnaik GK, Dhawan BN. Anticholestatic effect of picroliv, active hepatoprotective principle of Picrorhiza kurrooa, against carbon tetrachloride induced cholestasis. *Indian J Exp Biol*. 1993 Apr;31(4):316-8
[1353] "We conclude that SIL counteracts TLC-induced cholestasis by preventing the impairment in both the BS-dependent and -independent fractions of the bile flow." Crocenzi FA, et al. Preventive effect of silymarin against taurolithocholate-induced cholestasis in the rat. *Biochem Pharmacol*. 2003 Jul 15;66(2):355-64
[1354] "Andrographolide from the herb Andrographis paniculata (whole plant) per se produces a significant dose (1.5-12 mg/kg) dependent choleretic effect (4.8-73%) as evidenced by increase in bile flow, bile salt, and bile acids in conscious rats and anaesthetized guinea pigs." Shukla B, Visen PK, Patnaik GK, Dhawan BN. Choleretic effect of andrographolide in rats and guinea pigs. *Planta Med*. 1992 Apr;58(2):146-9
[1355] "The extract also produced an increase in normal bile flow in rats suggesting a strong choleretic activity." Chandan BK, Sharma AK, Anand KK. Boerhaavia diffusa: a study of its hepatoprotective activity. *J Ethnopharmacol*. 1991 Mar;31(3):299-307
[1356] Garbat, AL, Jacobi, HG: Secretion of Bile in Response to Rectal Installations. *Arch Intern Med* 1929; 44: 455-462
[1357] "Caffeine enemas cause dilation of bile ducts, which facilitates excretion of toxic cancer breakdown products by the liver and dialysis of toxic products from blood across the colonic wall. The therapy must be used as an integrated whole." Gerson M. The cure of advanced cancer by diet therapy. *Physiol Chem Phys*. 1978;10(5):449-64
[1358] "The act or process of depurating or freeing from foreign or impure matter." thefreedictionary.com/Depuration Verified March 11, 2007

- Heavy metal toxicity: In contrast to chemical toxicity for which a generalized non-specific cleansing protocol is appropriate, toxic metals more commonly require specific interventions; treatment is determined by the identity of the metal. Metals which are considered toxic or which are linked to the induction of human diseases include aluminum, arsenic, cadmium, lead, and mercury. Other metals and minerals such as manganese, lithium, copper, and iron can be toxic when present in high amounts. In this section I will limit the discussion to mercury since this metal is 1) commonly elevated in chronically toxic patients, and 2) because this metal can contribute to autoimmunity.
    - Mercury: Chronic mercury toxicity is commonly discovered in clinical practice in patients with chronic unwellness, and a recent study published in *JAMA* showed that 8% of American women of childbearing age have sufficient levels of mercury in their bodies to produce neurologic damage in their children.[1359] Accumulating evidence implicates mercury in the induction of immune dysfunction and the exacerbation of autoimmunity and allergy, and clinical trials indicate the benefit of mercury removal.
        - Mercury induces autoimmunity, immune complex formation and deposition, and the formation of antinuclear antibodies and antinucleolar antibodies in animal experiments.[1360,1361,1362]
        - In a case-control study of 265 recently diagnosed lupus patients, occupational exposure to mercury increased the risk of developing lupus by 360%, while working in a dental office increased the risk by 710%.[1363]
        - Patients with eczema have an increase body burden of mercury[1364], suggesting the probability that mercury accumulation induces immune dysfunction and contributes to the clinical picture of immune-induced skin inflammation, to which is affixed the label of "eczema."
        - Leukocytes from autistic patients produce autoantigens when exposed to ethyl mercury (Thimerosal), thus clearly implicating mercury in the incitement and perpetuation of autoimmunity.[1365]
        - A slight increase in risk for multiple sclerosis was noted among patients with many long-term mercury amalgam fillings.[1366]
        - It is highly probable that chronic mercury exposure, whether from diet or dental amalgams, alters gastrointestinal flora in favor of dysbiosis in general and antibiotic resistance in particular.[1367] Thus, mercury may indirectly contribute to autoimmunity by

---

[1359] "However, approximately 8% of women had concentrations higher than the US Environmental Protection Agency's recommended reference dose (5.8 microg/L), below which exposures are considered to be without adverse effects. Women who are pregnant or who intend to become pregnant should follow federal and state advisories on consumption of fish." Schober SE, et al. Blood mercury levels in US children and women of childbearing age, 1999-2000. *JAMA*. 2003 Apr 2;289(13):1667-74

[1360] "It is well established that in susceptible mouse strains, chronic treatment with subtoxic doses of mercuric chloride (HgCl2) induces a systemic autoimmune disease, which is characterized by increased serum levels of IgG1 and IgE antibodies, by the production of anti-nucleolar antibodies and by the development of immune complex-mediated glomerulonephritis." al-Balaghi S, Moller E, Moller G, Abedi-Valugerdi M. Mercury induces polyclonal B cell activation, autoantibody production and renal immune complex deposits in young (NZB x NZW)F1 hybrids. *Eur J Immunol*. 1996 Jul;26(7):1519-26

[1361] "It is well demonstrated that mercury induces a systemic autoimmune disease in susceptible mouse strains... The dominant antibody in the kidney eluate of mercury-injected mice was of IgG1 isotype and found to be directed against double-stranded DNA, collagen, cardiolipin, phosphatidylethanolamine, and the hapten trinitrophenol, but not against nucleolar antigens." Abedi-Valugerdi M, Hu H, Moller G. Mercury-induced renal immune complex deposits in young (NZB x NZW)F1 mice: characterization of antibodies/autoantibodies. *Clin Exp Immunol*. 1997 Oct;110(1):86-91

[1362] Abedi-Valugerdi et al. Mercury-induced anti-nucleolar autoantibodies can transgress the membrane of living cells in vivo and in vitro. *Int Immunol*. 1999 Apr;11(4):605-15

[1363] "...reported occupational exposure to mercury (OR 3.6), mixing pesticides for agricultural work (OR 7.4), and among dental workers (OR 7.1, 95% CI 2.2, 23.4). ...these associations were fairly strong and statistically significant..." Cooper GS, Parks CG, Treadwell EL, St Clair EW, Gilkeson GS, Dooley MA. Occupational risk factors for the development of systemic lupus erythematosus. *J Rheumatol*. 2004 Oct;31(10):1928-33

[1364] Weidinger et al. Body burden of mercury is associated with acute atopic eczema and total IgE in children from southern Germany. *J Allergy Clin Immunol* 2004;114:457-9

[1365] Vojdani A, Pangborn JB, Vojdani E, Cooper EL. Infections, toxic chemicals and dietary peptides binding to lymphocyte receptors and tissue enzymes are major instigators of autoimmunity in autism. *Int J Immunopathol Pharmacol*. 2003 Sep-Dec;16(3):189-99

[1366] "Although a suggestive elevated risk was found for those individuals with a large number of dental amalgams, and for a long period of time, the difference between cases and controls was not statistically significant." Bangsi D, Ghadirian P, Ducic S, Morisset R, Ciccocioppo S, McMullen E, Krewski D. Dental amalgam and multiple sclerosis: a case-control study in Montreal, Canada. *Int J Epidemiol*. 1998 Aug;27(4):667-71 ije.oxfordjournals.org/cgi/reprint/27/4/667

[1367] Pike R, Lucas V, Stapleton P, Gilthorpe MS, Roberts G, Rowbury R, Richards H, Mullany P, Wilson M. Prevalence and antibiotic resistance profile of mercury-resistant oral bacteria from children with and without mercury amalgam fillings. *J Antimicrob Chemother*. 2002 May;49(5):777-83 jac.oxfordjournals.org/cgi/content/full/49/5/777 This seems to be a rather tragic article insofar as the researchers' conclusions are inconsistent with their findings; they state that mercury does not contribute to increased prevalence or numbers of antibiotic resistant bacteria, yet their data in Table 4 clearly demonstrate that patients with dental amalgams have more drug-resistant isolates than do patients without such implants. Note also that the bacteria studied here were from the oral cavity, not the gastrointestinal tract. A much better article on this topic is the following: "Our findings indicate that mercury released from amalgam fillings can cause an enrichment of mercury resistance plasmids in the normal bacterial floras of primates. Many of these plasmids also carry antibiotic resistance, implicating the exposure to mercury from dental amalgams in an increased incidence of multiple antibiotic resistance plasmids in the normal floras of nonmedicated subjects." Summers AO, Wireman J, Vimy MJ, Lorscheider FL, Marshall B, Levy SB, Bennett S, Billard L. Mercury released from dental "silver" fillings provokes an increase in mercury- and antibiotic-resistant bacteria in oral and intestinal floras of primates. *Antimicrob Agents Chemother*. 1993 Apr;37(4):825-34 pubmedcentral.gov/articlerender.fcgi?tool=pubmed&pubmedid=8280208

promoting treatment-resistant dysbiosis, which then directly effects pro-inflammatory immune dysfunction.

- In a clinical trial with 35 patients, 71% experienced improvement in overall health following removal of mercury amalgams; the patients with the most improvement were patients with multiple sclerosis.[1368] Whether this was due to reducing autoimmunity or to reducing neurotoxicity is not clear; certainly both mechanisms may explain the improvement. Mercury is directly neurotoxic independently from its almost certain ability to contribute to neuroautoimmunity; this is visually demonstrated in a video of brain neuron degeneration following exposure to mercury, available on-line from the University of Calgary at commons.ucalgary.ca/mercury/.[1369]

Very interestingly, the patients most sensitive to mercury compounds appear to be those with a genotypic defect in phase-2 xenobiotic conjugation, specifically glutathione-S-transferase (GST).[1370] What makes this even more interesting is the finding that mercury compounds can inhibit GST and produce a GST-deficient phenotype even when the original genotype was GST-normal.[1371] Even though this latter finding was documented in *ex vivo* research with human erythrocytes, it correlates with the clinical experience of doctors who specialize in environmental medicine, namely that mercury accumulation appears to inhibit chemical xenobiotic detoxification. Thus mercury and chemical xenobiotics may work synergistically for the induction of immune dysfunction, with the former inhibiting the detoxification/conjugation of the latter. Regardless of the mechanisms involved, which are clearly numerous and synergistic, given that no safe level of mercury has been established, clinicians are justified in treating patients with evidence of mercury accumulation, chronic mercury toxicity. Based on numerous case reports documenting safety and efficacy of dimercaptosuccinic acid (DMSA), when used in children and adults[1372,1373,1374,1375,1376], it is my chelating agent of choice for most patients with lead and mercury toxicity as I review in the DMSA monograph in the pages that follow. Clinical implementation of metal detoxification can be performed simultaneously with the chemical detoxification program described previously and outlined in the pages that follow. The difference is the addition of DMSA first thing in the morning on an empty stomach at a dose of 10-30 mg per kg. Screening examination for overall health and kidney function should be performed before full-dose administration of DMSA, and sensitivity testing with <100 mg of DMSA is also reasonable to exclude allergy or idiosyncratic reactions to DMSA, which may indeed occur. DMSA is given in an "on and off" schedule, such as four days "on" and 3 days "off." Bile flow stimulation with botanicals and colonics for expulsion of mercury is the same as for xenobiotic detoxification. Two to four hours after consumption of DMSA, metal adsorbents such as phytochelatins and alginate can be used to bind metals in the gut and reduce enterohepatic recirculation. Antioxidants, especially selenium, are supplemented, and the diet is fresh, hypoallergenic, and Paleo-Mediterranean.

[1368] "Out of 35 patients, 25 patients (71%) showed improvement of health... The highest rate of improvement was observed in patients with multiple sclerosis... Mercury-containing amalgam may be an important risk factor for patients with autoimmune diseases." Prochazkova J, Sterzl I, Kucerova H, Bartova J, Stejskal VD. The beneficial effect of amalgam replacement on health in patients with autoimmunity. *Neuro Endocrinol Lett*. 2004 Jun;25(3):211-8

[1369] University of Calgary. How Mercury Causes Brain Neuron Degeneration. commons.ucalgary.ca/mercury/ Accessed November 24, 2005

[1370] "The combined deletion (GSTT1-/GSTM1-) was markedly more frequent among thimerosal-sensitized patients than in healthy controls (17.6% vs. 6.5%, P = 0.0093) and in the "para-compound" group (17.6% vs. 6.1%, P =0.014), revealing a synergistic effect of these enzyme deficiencies." Westphal GA, Schnuch A, Schulz TG, Reich K, Aberer W, Brasch J, Koch P, Wessbecher R, Szliska C, Bauer A, Hallier E. Homozygous gene deletions of the glutathione S-transferases M1 and T1 are associated with thimerosal sensitization. *Int Arch Occup Environ Health*. 2000 Aug;73(6):384-8

[1371] "Thus, sufficiently high doses of thimerosal may be able to change the phenotypic status of an individual--at least in vitro--by inhibition of the GST T1 enzyme." Muller M, et al. Inhibition of the human erythrocytic glutathione-S-transferase T1 (GST T1) by thimerosal. *Int J Hyg Environ Health*. 2001 Jul;203(5-6):479-81

[1372] Bradstreet J, Geier DA, Kartzinel JJ, Adams JB, Geier MR. A case-control study of mercury burden in children with autistic spectrum disorders. *Journal of American Physicians and Surgeons* 2003; 8: 76-79 jpands.org/vol8no3/geier.pdf

[1373] Crinnion WJ. Environmental medicine, part three: long-term effects of chronic low-dose mercury exposure. *Altern Med Rev*. 2000 Jun;5(3):209-23

[1374] Forman J, Moline J, Cernichiari E, et al. A cluster of pediatric metallic mercury exposure cases treated with meso-2,3-dimercaptosuccinic acid (DMSA). *Environ Health Perspect*. 2000 Jun;108(6):575-7 ehp.niehs.nih.gov/docs/2000/108p575-577forman/abstract.html

[1375] Miller AL. Dimercaptosuccinic acid (DMSA), a non-toxic, water-soluble treatment for heavy metal toxicity. *Altern Med Rev*. 1998 Jun;3(3):199-207

[1376] DMSA. *Altern Med Rev*. 2000 Jun;5(3):264-7 thorne.com/altmedrev/.fulltext/5/3/264.pdf

Problems and Solutions in Clinical Detoxification

Effects	Cause	Solutions
1) Toxicant exposure and accumulation	▪ Excess exposure in relation to genotypic/phenotypic detoxification capabilities	▪ Total load of all xenobiotics must be reduced because of the similar/identical pathways used for the elimination of chemicals. Avoid the following: paint fumes, perfume, varnish, new carpet, formaldehyde, food colors, food additives, artificial sweeteners, pesticides, herbicides, and industrial waste.[1377] ▪ Since the vast majority of toxicants originate from irresponsible corporations, social/political action is necessary to effect fundamental change.[1378]
2) Phase 1 Oxidation inhibited, too slow	▪ SNiPs and genotypic variations ▪ Certain drugs ▪ Certain food components: arachidonate and flavonoids such as bergapten (67%), quercetin (55%), naringenin (39%) naringin (6%) ▪ Viral infections ▪ Heavy metals ▪ Nutritional deficiencies ▪ Gut-derived LPS/endotoxin	▪ Reduce drug need by restoring health and addressing underlying problems ▪ Address viral infections and promote glutathione production, e.g., NAC[1379] and lipoic acid[1380] ▪ Vitamin/mineral supplements to correct common deficiencies in American diet[1381] and to induce activity of detoxifying enzymes[1382] ▪ Paleo[1383]/Mediterranean diet[1384] to provide foundational nutrition and improve health ▪ Avoidance of excess arachidonate and grapefruit ▪ Eliminate unfavorable microflora and reflorestate to reduce LPS/endotoxin load[1385] ▪ Chelate metals with chelating agent such as DMSA[1386]

[1377] Ross GH. Treatment options in multiple chemical sensitivity. *Toxicol Ind Health*. 1992 Jul-Aug;8(4):87-94
[1378] Kristin S. Schafer, Margaret Reeves, Skip Spitzer, Susan E. Kegley. Chemical Trespass: Pesticides in Our Bodies and Corporate Accountability. Pesticide Action Network North America. May 2004 Available at panna.org/campaigns/docsTrespass/chemicalTrespass2004.dv.html on August 1, 2004
[1379] "NAC treatment was well tolerated and resulted in a significant decrease in the frequency of influenza-like episodes, severity, and length of time confined to bed. Both local and systemic symptoms were sharply and significantly reduced in the NAC group." De Flora S, Grassi C, Carati L. Attenuation of influenza-like symptomatology and improvement of cell-mediated immunity with long-term N-acetylcysteine treatment. *Eur Respir J*. 1997 Jul;10(7):1535-41 Available on-line at erj.ersjournals.com/cgi/reprint/10/7/1535 on October 18, 2004
[1380] "These findings confirm the involvement of ROI in NFkB-mediated HIV gene expression as well as the efficacy of LA as a therapeutic regimen for HIV infection and acquired immunodeficiency syndrome (AIDS)." Merin JP, Matsuyama M, Kira T, Baba M, Okamoto T. Alpha-lipoic acid blocks HIV-1 LTR-dependent expression of hygromycin resistance in THP-1 stable transformants. *FEBS Lett*. 1996 Sep 23;394(1):9-13
[1381] Fletcher RH, Fairfield KM. Vitamins for chronic disease prevention in adults: clinical applications. *JAMA*. 2002 Jun 19;287(23):3127-9
[1382] Ames BN, Elson-Schwab I, Silver EA. High-dose vitamin therapy stimulates variant enzymes with decreased coenzyme binding affinity (increased K(m)): relevance to genetic disease and polymorphisms. *Am J Clin Nutr*. 2002 Apr;75(4):616-58
[1383] O'Keefe JH Jr, Cordain L. Cardiovascular disease resulting from a diet and lifestyle at odds with our Paleolithic genome: how to become a 21st-century hunter-gatherer. *Mayo Clin Proc*. 2004 Jan;79(1):101-8
[1384] Knoops KT, de Groot LC, Kromhout D, Perrin AE, Moreiras-Varela O, Menotti A, van Staveren WA. Mediterranean diet, lifestyle factors, and 10-year mortality in elderly European men and women: the HALE project. *JAMA*. 2004 Sep 22;292(12):1433-9
[1385] Shedlofsky SI, Israel BC, Tosheva R, Blouin RA. Endotoxin depresses hepatic cytochrome P450-mediated drug metabolism in women. *Br J Clin Pharmacol*. 1997 Jun;43(6):627-32
[1386] Miller AL. Dimercaptosuccinic Acid (DMSA), A Non-Toxic, Water-Soluble Treatment For Heavy Metal Toxicity. *Altern Med Rev* 1998;3(3):199-207

Problems and Solutions in Clinical Detoxification—*continued*

Effects	Cause	Solutions
3) Phase 1 Oxidation imbalanced, too fast relative to Phase 2	<ul><li>Certain drugs or other toxicant exposure from endogenous or exogenous sources leads to upregulation of Phase 1</li></ul>	<ul><li>Reduce drug need by restoring health and addressing underlying problems</li><li>Suspect excess enterohepatic recirculation (via excess fecal β-glucuronidase): assess and optimize gastrointestinal flora by eliminating harmful bacteria and using probiotics[1387]</li><li>Upregulate phase 2 with diet and botanicals, such as cruciferous vegetables[1388,1389]</li></ul>
4) Phase 2 Conjugation too slow	<ul><li>SNiPs: single nucleotide polymorphism defects in detoxification enzymes</li><li>Fluoridated water: inhibits glucuronidation in some patients with Gilbert's syndrome[1390]</li><li>Lack of stimulation with diet and botanicals (i.e., insufficient intake of cruciferous vegetables)</li></ul>	<ul><li>Avoid fluoridated water</li><li>Upregulate phase 2 with diet and botanicals (citations above)</li><li>Create balance by addressing the toxicant exposure that is upregulating phase 1</li></ul>
5) Phase 2 Conjugation Unsupported	<ul><li>Insufficient protein for amino acids and sulfur; insufficient vitamins/minerals</li><li>Poor digestion</li></ul>	<ul><li>Paleo-Mediterranean diet with plenty of protein (this is not the time to be a *junkitarian* or *breaditarian*)[1391]</li><li>Cofactor supplementation: NAC, glutamine, glycine, taurine, sulfur, whey[1392,1393]</li><li>Custom amino acid blend for recalcitrant cases[1394]</li></ul>

[1387] "Also they inhibited the harmful enzymes (beta-glucosidase, beta-glucuronidase, tryptophanase and urease) and ammonia production of intestinal microflora, and lowered pH of the culture media by increasing lactic acid bacteria of intestinal microflora." Park HY, Bae EA, Han MJ, Choi EC, Kim DH. Inhibitory effects of Bifidobacterium spp. isolated from a healthy Korean on harmful enzymes of human intestinal microflora. *Arch Pharm Res*. 1998 Feb;21(1):54-61

[1388] "In conclusion, consumption of glucosinolate-containing Brussels sprouts for 1 week results in increased rectal GST-alpha and -pi isozyme levels. We hypothesize that these enhanced detoxification enzyme levels may partly explain the epidemiological association between a high intake of glucosinolates (cruciferous vegetables) and a decreased risk of colorectal cancer." Nijhoff WA, Grubben MJ, Nagengast FM, Jansen JB, Verhagen H, van Poppel G, Peters WH. Effects of consumption of Brussels sprouts on intestinal and lymphocytic glutathione S-transferases in humans. *Carcinogenesis*. 1995 Sep;16(9):2125-8

[1389] "...human CYP1A2 and other CYP enzymes involved in oestrone 2-hydroxylation are induced by dietary broccoli." Kall MA, Vang O, Clausen J. Effects of dietary broccoli on human in vivo drug metabolizing enzymes: evaluation of caffeine, oestrone and chlorzoxazone metabolism. *Carcinogenesis*. 1996 Apr;17(4):793-9

[1390] Lee J. Gilbert's disease and fluoride intake. *Fluoride* 1983; 16: 139-45

[1391] O'Keefe JH Jr, Cordain L. Cardiovascular disease resulting from a diet and lifestyle at odds with our Paleolithic genome: how to become a 21st-century hunter-gatherer. *Mayo Clin Proc*. 2004 Jan;79(1):101-8 thepaleodiet.com/articles/Hunter-Gatherer%20Mayo.pdf

[1392] "CONCLUSION: Supplementation with whey proteins persistently increased plasma glutathione levels in patients with advanced HIV-infection. The treatment was well tolerated." Micke P, Beeh KM, Buhl R. Effects of long-term supplementation with whey proteins on plasma glutathione levels of HIV-infected patients. *Eur J Nutr*. 2002 Feb;41(1):12-8

[1393] "A significant increase in mononuclear cell glutathione was also observed in subjects receiving the WPI supplement following the 40 km simulated cycling trial." Middleton N, Jelen P, Bell G. Whole blood and mononuclear cell glutathione response to dietary whey protein supplementation in sedentary and trained male human subjects. *Int J Food Sci Nutr*. 2004 Mar;55(2):131-41

[1394] Bralley JA. Lord RS. Treatment of chronic fatigue syndrome with specific amino acid supplementation. *Journal of Applied Nutrition* 1994; 46(3): 74-78

Problems and Solutions in Clinical Detoxification—*continued*

Effects	Cause	Solutions
6) Insufficient bile flow	• "Normal" bile flow appears too slow to keep pace with supraphysiologic toxicant exposure	• Stimulate bile flow with rectal instillations[1395,1396] and botanical medicines such as *Picrorhiza kurroa*[1397] and *Andrographis paniculata*[1398]
7) Urinary excretion insufficient due to insufficient hydration	• Subclinical dehydration is common and is exacerbated by diuretics such as ethanol and caffeine	• Drink water and antioxidant-rich teas and juices
8) Renal pH too acidic for optimal toxicant excretion	• Western/American diet promotes an acidic renal pH[1399] which is known to reduce toxicant excretion[1400]	• Vegetarian or Paleo-Mediterranean diet to alkalinize renal pH • Fruit/vegetable juices provide potassium and citrate for effective alkalinization of urine[1401] • Use sodium bicarbonate[1402] and/or potassium citrate as needed
9) Enterohepatic recirculation	• Constipation • Excess microflora (quantitative or qualitative) producing β-glucuronidase • Leaky gut	• Promote generous laxation: magnesium, fiber, vegetables, fruit, nuts, seeds • Optimize gastrointestinal microflora • Assess and normalize mucosal integrity • Rectal instillations may be used to cleanse the bowel and to increase bile flow as previously documented radiographically[1403]; this appears to improve detoxification clinical results[1404,1405] presumably due to expedition of toxicant removal[1406]

[1395] Garbat, AL, Jacobi, HG: Secretion of Bile in Response to Rectal Installations. *Arch Intern Med* 1929; 44: 455-462

[1396] "Caffeine enemas cause dilation of bile ducts, which facilitates excretion of toxic cancer breakdown products by the liver and dialysis of toxic products from blood across the colonic wall. The therapy must be used as an integrated whole." Gerson M. The cure of advanced cancer by diet therapy: a summary of 30 years of clinical experimentation. *Physiol Chem Phys*. 1978;10(5):449-64

[1397] Vaidya AB, Antarkar DS, Doshi JC, Bhatt AD, Ramesh VV, Vora PV, Perissond DD, Baxi AJ, Kale PM. Picrorhiza kurroa (Kutaki) Royle ex Benth as a hepatoprotective agent--experimental & clinical studies. *J Postgrad Med* 1996;42:105-8 Available on October 18, 2004 at jpgmonline.com/article.asp?issn=0022-3859;year=1996;volume=42;issue=4;spage=105;epage=8;aulast=Vaidya

[1398] "Andrographolide from the herb Andrographis paniculata (whole plant) per se produces a significant dose (1.5-12 mg/kg) dependent choleretic effect (4.8-73%) as evidenced by increase in bile flow, bile salt, and bile acids in conscious rats and anaesthetized guinea pigs." Shukla B, Visen PK, Patnaik GK, Dhawan BN. Choleretic effect of andrographolide in rats and guinea pigs. *Planta Med* 1992 Apr;58(2):146-9

[1399] Cordain L: *The Paleo Diet: Lose weight and get healthy by eating the food you were designed to eat*. John Wiley & Sons Inc., New York 2002

[1400] Proudfoot AT, Krenzelok EP, Vale JA. Position Paper on urine alkalinization. *J Toxicol Clin Toxicol*. 2004;42(1):1-26

[1401] "New Guinean hunter-gatherer tribal group living in "the primitive feral condition"…urine pH of adults was usually between 7.5 and 9.0." Sebastian A, Frassetto LA, Sellmeyer DE, Merriam RL, Morris RC Jr. Estimation of the net acid load of the diet of ancestral preagricultural Homo sapiens and their hominid ancestors. *Am J Clin Nutr*. 2002 Dec;76(6):1308-16

[1402] "Urine alkalinization is a treatment regimen that increases poison elimination by the administration of intravenous sodium bicarbonate to produce urine with a pH > or = 7.5." Proudfoot AT, Krenzelok EP, Vale JA. Position Paper on urine alkalinization. *J Toxicol Clin Toxicol*. 2004;42(1):1-26

[1403] "Caffeine enemas cause dilation of bile ducts, which facilitates excretion of toxic cancer breakdown products by the liver and dialysis of toxic products from blood across the colonic wall. The therapy must be used as an integrated whole." Gerson M. The cure of advanced cancer by diet therapy: a summary of 30 years of clinical experimentation. *Physiol Chem Phys*. 1978;10(5):449-64

[1404] Snyder RG. The value of colonic irrigations in countering auto-intoxication of intestinal origin. *Medical Clinics of North America* 1939; May: 781-788

[1405] Gonzalez NJ, Isaacs LL. Evaluation of pancreatic proteolytic enzyme treatment of adenocarcinoma of the pancreas, with nutrition and detoxification support. *Nutr Cancer*. 1999;33(2):117-24

[1406] Crinnion WJ. Results of a decade of naturopathic treatment for environmental illness: a review of clinical records. *J Naturopathic Med* 1997;7:21-27

Problems and Solutions in Clinical Detoxification—*continued*

Effects	Cause	Solutions
10) Deconjugation by microflora	▪ Excess microflora (quantitative or qualitative) producing β-glucuronidase ▪ Constipation must be eliminated[1407]	▪ Botanical and/or pharmaceutical antimicrobials/antifungals to reduce bacterial load in the intestines, similar to the use of antibiotics in the treatment of hepatic encephalopathy ▪ Prebiotics and probiotics to optimize gut flora ▪ Dietary fiber may be used to promote laxation and excretion of toxicants before enterohepatic recirculation; cholestyramine may be used in selected cases to augment fecal elimination of toxicants such as pesticides[1408]
11) Heavy metal toxicity 12) Metal-induced alteration of detoxification (upregulation or downregulation of specific processes)	▪ Heavy metal exposure appears to inhibit Phase 1 oxidation (*in vitro*[1409])	▪ Reduce exposure to toxicants ▪ Chelation, such as with DMSA which appears effective for mercury[1410] and lead[1411] ▪ Promote generous laxation: magnesium, fiber, vegetables, fruit, nuts, seeds ▪ Optimize gastrointestinal microflora ▪ Fruit/vegetable juices provide potassium and citrate for effective urinary alkalinization
13) Disease promotion via toxicants stored in body tissues, particularly adipose and brain	▪ Chemical toxicants are inherently biologically persistent ▪ Defective detoxification	▪ Sauna, hyperthermia, exercise to promote sweating and lipolysis[1412,1413] ▪ "Fat exchange" via low-fat diet to effect weight loss followed by supplementation of health-promoting uncontaminated fatty acids[1414] ▪ Weight loss for obese patients only after detoxification program is well established

---

[1407] "Enemas and suppositories stimulate colonic contractions and soften stools. Water, saline, soap suds, hypertonic sodium phosphate, and mineral oil are used as enemas. Acute water intoxication can occur with water enemas, especially in infants, children, and the elderly, if they have difficulty evacuating the water." Dosh SA. Evaluation and treatment of constipation. *J Fam Pract*. 2002 Jun;51(6):555-9 Available at jfponline.com/content/2002/06/jfp_0602_00541.asp on October 18, 2004

[1408] "Output of chlordecone in bile was 10 to 20 times greater than in stool, suggesting that chlordecone is reabsorbed in the intestine. Cholestyramine, an anion-exchange resin that binds chlordecone, increased its fecal excretion by seven times." Cohn WJ, Boylan JJ, Blanke RV, Fariss MW, Howell JR, Guzelian PS. Treatment of chlordecone (Kepone) toxicity with cholestyramine. Results of a controlled clinical trial. *N Engl J Med*. 1978 Feb 2;298(5):243-8

[1409] "All four of the metals investigated decreased the extent of CYP1A1 induction in HepG2 cells by at least one of the five PAHs, in some cases decreases were marked. The same order of effectiveness of metal-mediated decreases in CYP1A1 were cadmium > arsenic > lead > mercury for all the PAHs." Vakharia DD, Liu N, Pause R, Fasco M, Bessette E, Zhang QY, Kaminsky LS. Polycyclic aromatic hydrocarbon/metal mixtures: effect on PAH induction of CYP1A1 in human HEPG2 cells. *Drug Metab Dispos*. 2001 Jul;29(7):999-1006 Available at dmd.aspetjournals.org/cgi/content/full/29/7/999 on October 18, 2004

[1410] "Thus, oral chelation with DMSA produced a significant mercury diuresis in these children. We observed no adverse side effects of treatment. DMSA appears to be an effective and safe chelating agent for treatment of pediatric overexposure to metallic mercury." Forman J, Moline J, Cernichiari E, Sayegh S, Torres JC, Landrigan MM, Hudson J, Adel HN, Landrigan PJ. A cluster of pediatric metallic mercury exposure cases treated with meso-2,3-dimercaptosuccinic acid (DMSA). *Environ Health Perspect*. 2000 Jun;108(6):575-7 Available at ehp.niehs.nih.gov/members/2000/108p575-577forman/108p575.pdf on October 18, 2004

[1411] "To conclude, awareness and early diagnosis of lead toxicity is important. Succimer is an effective chelator in patients for lead toxicity. It can be administered orally and hospitalization eliminated. However, chelation therapy should never be used as a substitute for environmental assessment and lead abatement for lead poisoned children." Kalra V, Dua T, Kumar V, Kaul B. Succimer in symptomatic lead poisoning. *Indian Pediatr*. 2002 Jun;39(6):580-5 Available at indianpediatrics.net/june2002/june-580-585.htm on October 18, 2004

[1412] Schnare DW, Ben M, Shields MG. Body Burden Reductions of PCBs, PBBs and Chlorinated Pesticide Residues in Human Subjects. *Ambio* 1984; 13 (5-6): 378-380

[1413] Krop J. Chemical sensitivity after intoxication at work with solvents: response to sauna therapy. *J Altern Complement Med* 1998 Spring;4(1):77-86

[1414] "Repeated fasting and refeeding with fish oil facilitated plasma exchange of n-3 for n-6 PUFA, improved BP, clinical metabolic parameters and lowered platelet reactivity in the vessel wall (primary hemostasis)." Yosefy C, Viskoper JR, Varon D, Ilan Z, Pilpel D, Lugassy G, Schneider R, Savyon N, Adan Y, Raz A. Repeated fasting and refeeding with 20:5, n-3 eicosapentaenoic acid (EPA): a novel approach for rapid fatty acid exchange and its effect on blood pressure, plasma lipids and hemostasis. *J Hum Hypertens* 1996 Sep;10 Suppl 3:S135-9

Toxicant Exposure: solvents, pesticides, herbicides, plastics, fire-proofing, dioxins, exhaust, PCB, mercury, lead, cadmium, and thousands of others; the ultimate causes and therefore solutions are found primarily in addressing corporate environmental policies and influence on government regulations, societal structure/expectations regarding materialism/independence/convenience/passivity

Biological Persistence: lipolysis/redistribution; detoxification/reabsorption

Promote lipolysis with diet, exercise, sauna

lipophilic chemicals are deposited in cell membranes/adipose

metals circulate and are deposited in tissues where they impair function and thereby contribute to 'disease'

some heavy metals may alter detoxification

treatment → DMSA chelation

Phase One: activation / oxidation
Rapidly inducible by toxicant exposure and some drugs; the main clinical problems here are
1) **inhibition** by SNiPs, nutrient deficiencies, drugs, LPS, heavy metals
2) **relative excess activity**: rapid phase one in relation to slow conjugation: the body is not making a mistake here; it is simply responding to exposure; the solutions are to reduce exposure and support conjugation

Clinical Solutions:
1) nutritional supplementation and diet improvement,
2) reduce exposure to drugs and other 'inducers' including enterohepatic recirculation (check increased permeability and fecal b-glucuronidase)
3) clean the gut to restore mucosal integrity and reduce LPS and b-glucuronidase

hydration/urination, bile formation/expulsion, maintenance of conjugation, botanical adsorbents, daily defecation

excretion in urine, excretion via bile flow and defecation

failure → enterohepatic recirculation

insufficient oxidation → **chemical toxicant accumulation**: increased disease risk: autoimmunity, Parkinson's disease, cancer, multiple chemical sensitivity, adverse drug reactions

sufficient oxidation → a few chemicals are excreted following Phase 1 (without Conjugation)

sufficient oxidation →

Phase Two: conjugation
Insufficiently induced by toxicant exposure; failure of conjugation following oxidation is highly problematic; the main clinical problems here are
1) **slow action**: phase 2 is commonly slower than phase 1; slow action can be caused by nutritional deficiencies, insufficient intake of vegetables/crucifers, and SNiPs, which are surprisingly common and are consistently associated with increased risk for disease;
2) **insufficient nutrient intake for conjugation**: recall that most conjugation factors are, of course, derived from foods: amino acids and sulphur

Clinical Solutions:
1) general nutritional supplementation and diet improvement,
2) reduce exposure to all endogenous and exogenous toxicants: drugs, chemicals, enterohepatic recirculation, hyperabsorption due to increased permeability and fecal b-glucuronidase
3) induce conjugation with cruciferous vegetables and specific botanicals
4) stimulate bile flow and bowel cleansing

insufficient conjugation

successful conjugation → Toxicant is solubilized for excretion in bile or urine

hydration, healthy renal function (and alkalosis) → excretion in urine

failure of bile formation, blockage in bile flow, dehydration, dysbiosis causing deconjugation, constipation promoting reabsorption, insufficient fiber

bile formation, bile expulsion, maintenance of conjugation, daily defecation → excretion via bile flow and defecation

enterohepatic recirculation

Overview of Toxicant Exposure and Detoxification/Depuration: Pathways and therapeutic implications

An Outline of the Use of Dimercaptosuccinic acid (DMSA)

Therapeutic: **Dimercaptosuccinic acid**
Common name: **DMSA**
Applications and mechanisms of action:

- DMSA is a well-documented chelating agent that is FDA-approved for the treatment of lead poisoning.[1415] It has been used safely and successfully in children and adults with lead and/or mercury toxicity, whether acute or chronic. The sulfur-containing moiety of the molecule binds to heavy metals, rendering them soluble, and then the metal-DMSA complex is excreted in urine or bile.

  A few of the better articles on this topic are listed here:
    - **DMSA-mercury testing in autistic children**: Two-hundred-twenty-one children with autism were challenged with 30 mg/kg of DMSA and showed significantly higher urinary mercury excretion compared to control subjects. The specific protocol is described as follows: "The Arizona State University Institutional Review Board approved our retrospective examination of cases and controls in this study. … Informed consent was obtained from both cases and controls for DMSA chelation treatment. Controls and cases were both challenged with a three-day oral treatment of **DMSA (10 mg/kg per dose given three times daily)**. After the ninth dose, the first voided morning urine was collected (when possible), or an overnight urine collection bag was worn. All laboratory analyses were performed by the Doctors Data, Inc., in Chicago, Ill."[1416] No adverse effects were reported.
    - **Mercury review by Dr. Walter Crinnion**: As one of the most experienced environmental medicine doctors in the US, Dr. Crinnion provides his perspective on the treatment of mercury toxicity, and states, "DMSA can be given to an adult at a dose of 500 mg tid… DMSA (30 mg/kg)… It is generally recommended that these agents be given in several day courses repeatedly, with rest periods in between."[1417]
    - **Nine cases of pediatric mercury poisoning safely treated with DMSA**: Nine mercury-poisoned children were treated with DMSA 30 mg/kg for 5 days followed by 20 mg/kg for 2 weeks; mercury levels declined in all children, and no adverse effects occurred.[1418]
    - **DMSA monographs**: monographs on the basic science and clinical applications of DMSA.[1419,1420]
    - **Acute poisoning review**: A "nutshell" review of the management of acute poisoning.[1421]

[1415] "The Food and Drug Administration has recently licensed the drug DMSA (succimer) for reduction of blood lead levels >/= 45 micrograms/dl. This decision was based on the demonstrated ability of DMSA to reduce blood lead levels. An advantage of this drug is that it can be given orally." Goyer RA, Cherian MG, Jones MM, Reigart JR. Role of chelating agents for prevention, intervention, and treatment of exposures to toxic metals. *Environ Health Perspect*. 1995 Nov;103(11):1048-52 ehp.niehs.nih.gov/docs/1995/103-11/meetingreport.html
[1416] Bradstreet J, Geier DA, Kartzinel JJ, Adams JB, Geier MR. A case-control study of mercury burden in children with autistic spectrum disorders. *Journal of American Physicians and Surgeons* 2003; 8: 76-79 jpands.org/vol8no3/geier.pdf
[1417] Crinnion WJ. Environmental medicine, part three: long-term effects of chronic low-dose mercury exposure. *Altern Med Rev*. 2000 Jun;5(3):209-23 thorne.com/altmedrev/.fulltext/5/3/209.pdf
[1418] Forman J, Moline J, Cernichiari E, Sayegh S, Torres JC, Landrigan MM, Hudson J, Adel HN, Landrigan PJ. A cluster of pediatric metallic mercury exposure cases treated with meso-2,3-dimercaptosuccinic acid (DMSA). *Environ Health Perspect*. 2000 Jun;108(6):575-7 ehp.niehs.nih.gov/docs/2000/108p575-577forman/abstract.html
[1419] Miller AL. Dimercaptosuccinic acid (DMSA), a non-toxic, water-soluble treatment for heavy metal toxicity. *Altern Med Rev*. 1998 Jun;3(3):199-207 thorne.com/altmedrev/.fulltext/3/3/199.pdf
[1420] DMSA. *Altern Med Rev*. 2000 Jun;5(3):264-7 thorne.com/altmedrev/.fulltext/5/3/264.pdf
[1421] Greene SL, Dargan PI, Jones AL. Acute poisoning: understanding 90% of cases in a nutshell. *Postgrad Med J*. 2005 Apr;81(954):204-16 pmj.bmjjournals.com/cgi/content/full/81/954/204

An Outline of the Use of Dimercaptosuccinic acid (DMSA) — *continued*

Toxicity:
- DMSA has a very favorable risk:benefit ratio when used in patients without renal/hepatic impairment and who are at average or greater-than-average risk for heavy metal accumulation/toxicity. Toxicity is very rare. Some articles make fleeting mention of bone marrow suppression, but this is almost never precipitated clinically and is practically never documented in the case reports and clinical studies using DMSA for the treatment of heavy metal toxicity. Patients should be tested for hematologic and metabolic status prior to DMSA administration; a CBC and metabolic/chemistry panel is sufficient.
- Allergic-type reactions to DMSA and/or the mobilization of heavy metals, especially mercury, are infrequent but not rare. To reduce the risk of precipitating such reactions, a trial dose of 100 mg (or less for children) should be used on a single occasion to ensure that IgE-mediated allergy or anaphylaxis does not occur with the higher doses used therapeutically. Like any drug, DMSA may precipitate idiosyncratic reactions, but these are by definition nearly impossible to predict. However, since idiosyncratic drug reactions appear to reflect imbalanced Phase 1 / Phase 2 detoxification, the likelihood of such a reaction can probably be reduced by ensuring that the patient is supplemented with antioxidants, fortified with sufficient protein for supporting Phase 2 conjugation reactions, and abstinent from other drugs which induce Phase 1 upregulation. Patients with adverse reactions to DMSA should either not use DMSA or should do so carefully, such as with a lower dose or after the underlying cause of the sensitivity has been addressed.

Dosage and administration:
- <u>Screening laboratory tests</u>: Urinalysis, CBC and chemistry panel with BUN, creatinine, and hepatic markers are sufficient for assessing renal, hepatic, and marrow status.
- <u>Empty stomach</u>: DMSA should be taken on an empty stomach, preferably 1-2 hours away from food. In particular, mineral supplements containing zinc and copper (etc) should be avoided for 4 hours before and after DMSA supplementation. Generally, first morning supplementation with a delayed or skipped breakfast is ideal.
- <u>The lowest therapeutic dose is generally 10 mg/kg per day, and the highest therapeutic dose is generally 30 mg/kg per day</u>. The 30 mg/kg dose is generally delivered in three divided doses (i.e., 10 mg/kg TID); however, a single-dose 30 mg/kg dose may be used provocatively for diagnostic purposes. Lower dosage schemes are appropriate for children or those with severe sensitivities. The highest scheme may also be appropriate for children but might otherwise be reserved for adult patients who are in otherwise good health. My clinical preference is to use 10mg/kg 3 days "on" and 4 days "off" with periodic monitoring of CBC and chemistry/metabolic parameters.

Body weight in lbs (kg)	10 mg/kg dose	30 mg/kg dose (bolus or divided)
40 lbs (18 kg)	180 mg	540 mg
80 lbs (36 kg)	360 mg	1080 mg
120 lbs (54 kg)	540 mg	1620 mg
160 lbs (72 kg)	720 mg	2,160 mg (limit to 2,000) mg
200 lbs (90 kg)	900 mg	2,700 (limit to 2,000) mg
240 lbs (108 kg)	1080 mg	3,240 (limit to 2,000) mg
280 lbs (126 kg)	1260 mg	3,780 (limit to 2,000) mg

An Outline of the Use of Dimercaptosuccinic acid (DMSA) — *continued*

Dosage and administration (continued):
- Cyclical dosing: DMSA is generally "cycled" which means that it is taken for a few days, the discontinued for a few days, then resumed, etc. This can be customized per patient for ease of compliance and variations in scheduling. For example, the patient might use DMSA for 5 days of the week, taking the weekends "off", or might use DMSA for 4 days on and 3 days off, etc. Every-other-day dosing is also reasonable. Treatment is generally continued for 1-2 months.
- Plenty of water: DMSA should be taken with 16 ounces of water. An additional 1-2 liters should be consumed over the next 2-4 hours.

Additional information:
- DMSA increases urinary excretion of copper in humans[1422]; if treatment were excessively prolonged then theoretically this might lead to copper deficiency. Additionally, DMSA might be useful for people with excess copper. These areas require more research.
- Co-supplementation with the following can increase urinary metal excretion and/or reduce enterohepatic recycling of toxic metals. These can be used during DMSA treatment but should not be taken within 2-4 hours of DMSA supplementation so as not to bind with or otherwise interfere with DMSA absorption and utilization.
  - *Fruit and vegetable juices*: Potassium citrate has been shown to significantly increase mercury excretion in humans when used alone and/or with DMSA.[1423,1424] Fruit and vegetable juices are rich sources of potassium citrate and should be consumed liberally by patients undergoing detoxification. Furthermore, since urinary alkalinization greatly increases the urinary excretion of chemical/xenobiotics toxicants[1425], essentially all patients undergoing detoxification programs should increase consumption of fruit and vegetable juices as well as fruits and vegetables.
  - *Phytochelatins*: Phytochelatins are metal-binding moieties from plants and algae.[1426] Clinically, doctors use phytochelatin supplementation to bind metals in the gut for enhanced excretion, i.e., to prevent re-absorption of metals that have been detoxified into the gut lumen via the bile. High-fiber plant-based diets are beneficial for the same purpose.
  - *Selenium*: Selenium (Se) has many important actions in the body, one of which is that of an antioxidant. It is generally dosed at 200 mcg per day, but doses up to 800-1,000 mcg per day are generally safe for most adults. The study by Seppanen et al[1427] showed 34% reduction in hair mercury following Se 100mcg/d.

[1422] "The Food and Drug Administration has recently licensed the drug DMSA (succimer) for reduction of blood lead levels >/= 45 micrograms/dl. This decision was based on the demonstrated ability of DMSA to reduce blood lead levels. An advantage of this drug is that it can be given orally." Goyer RA, Cherian MG, Jones MM, Reigart JR. Role of chelating agents for prevention, intervention, and treatment of exposures to toxic metals. *Environ Health Perspect*. 1995 Nov;103(11):1048-52 ehp.niehs.nih.gov/docs/1995/103-11/meetingreport.html

[1423] "Based on the increase in urinary Hg concentrations after single doses, compared with controls, the order of efficacy was: DMPS plus K Cit., NAC plus K Cit. and DMSA (each producing an increase of 163%), then in descending order, DMSA plus K Cit., DMPS, NAC and K Cit." Hibberd AR, Howard MA, Hunnisett AG. Mercury from dental amalgam fillings studies on oral chelating agents for assessing and reducing mercury burdens in humans. *J Nutr Environ Med* 1998;8:219-231

[1424] Crinnion WJ. Environmental medicine, part three: long-term effects of chronic low-dose mercury exposure. *Altern Med Rev*. 2000 Jun;5(3):209-23

[1425] Proudfoot AT, Krenzelok EP, Vale JA. Position Paper on urine alkalinization. *J Toxicol Clin Toxicol*. 2004;42(1):1-26. This is a very important paper. Posted by the European Association of Poisons Centres and Clinical Toxicologists at eapcct.org/publicfile.php?folder=congress&file=PS_UrineAlkalinization.pdf

[1426] Cobbett CS. Phytochelatins and their roles in heavy metal detoxification. *Plant Physiol*. 2000 Jul;123(3):825-32 plantphysiol.org/cgi/content/full/123/3/825 This is a basic science review with relevance for plant biology that discusses the use of phytochelatins to bind metals in the plant's environment. It does not discuss relevance of phytochelatins for the treatment of heavy metal exposure in humans.

[1427] "The selenium supplementation group received daily 100 micrograms of selenomethionine. Selenium supplementation reduced pubic hair mercury level by 34% (p = 0.005) and elevated serum selenium by 73% and blood selenium by 59% in the supplemented group (p < 0.001 for both). The study indicates that mercury accumulation in pubic hair can be reduced by dietary supplementation with small daily amounts of organic selenium in a short range of time." Seppanen K, et al. Effect of supplementation with organic selenium on mercury status as measured by mercury in pubic hair. *J Trace Elem Med Biol*. 2000 Jun;14(2):84-7

Outline the functional Inflammology protocol on this page to assess your ability to apply the information clinically:

> **Declarative knowledge:** If you truly know it, you can articulate it. If you don't know it, you cannot articulate it. Conceptual knowledge must ultimately be translated into applicable and communicable knowledge; otherwise, it is not much more than "nice ideas."
>
> "In order for a particular species to maintain itself and increase its power, its conception of reality must comprehend enough of the calculable and constant for it to base a scheme of behavior on it."
>
> Nietzsche FW. *The Will to Power*, 1901, #480

Chapter 5: Clinical Applications—Rheumatology

Introduction

- <u>Foundational belief in a rational universe</u>: Rheumatologic disorders are multifactorial, not idiopathic. The Functional Inflammology Protocol reviewed in Chapter 4 covers the most important concepts; in this chapter those concepts will encounter opportunities for clinical application in the management/comanagement of rheumatologic diseases, better described as rheumatologic/autoimmune disease *states*, with the latter added to imply their temporal and potentially escapable nature.
- <u>Comanagement and Risk Management</u>: A wise clinical strategy when managing any serious or potentially-life threatening condition is for the clinician to arrange for co-management with a specialist, and this is particularly true for conditions that might necessitate hospitalization or acute immunosuppression. Autoimmune diseases such as lupus are notorious for acute flares that can cause permanent damage (e.g., transverse myelitis resulting in paralysis); likewise, giant cell arteritis is notorious for causing rapid-onset visual loss, which is generally permanent and thus debilitating. Reviews of patient management, risk management, and common musculoskeletal emergencies are provided in Chapter 1—this information should be reviewed prior to the reading of this chapter and implementation of the clinical applications herein. Pharmaceuticalization of these patients offers no chance of cure but is useful for "controlling" inflammation, notably in the short term, with limited efficacy, and numerous adverse long-term effects; the best general approach is one that is etiotherapeutic/polyetiotherapeutic—directed at treating the cause(s) of the disorder while accessing pharmacoimmunosuppression on an "as needed" basis.
- <u>Video Presentations and Tutorials</u>: These are provided to help reinforce—*not replace*—the written material in this chapter, and these additional videos should be viewed *following* the videos corresponding to the overall protocol (Chapter 4), mitochondrial dysfunction (Chapter 4), the detailing of dysbiosis (Chapter 4 plus additional presentation slides—see presentation slides for video access). One of the major goals with these videos, in addition to simply providing more information and reinforcing the material in the text, is that these will promote learning of the material in a conversational style, because ultimately the material must be understood in words and communicable in words in order to be understood and applied: vimeo.com/album/3000884, password: DrV_Allergy_Rheum. Updates and sample syllabi: InflammationMastery.com/books/rheum/
- <u>Understanding autoimmunity as "patterns of inflammation"</u>: My perspective for years—supported by the phrase "patterns of inflammation" by WG Meggs MD PhD—is that autoimmune disorders as we appreciate them (phenomenonistically and diagnostically) are simply "variations on the theme" of the seven factors I've identified via the FINDSEX® acronym and functional inflammology protocol. As such, readers should note the consistency of the pattern, and also how research "specific" for one disease might well apply to a particular autoimmune/inflamed/autoinflammed patient even if he/she has a different diagnostic label; such is the rule, rather than the exception. As such, the information in this textbook needs to be appreciated and integrated in its entirety, not simply accessed for information on a specific topic without consideration of the provided—and synergistic—context.

Clinical Topics—following this introduction (above) and article reprint (following): Note that immediately before the start of the clinical topics is a summary outline of the **functional inflammology protocol** otherwise detailed in Chapter 4.

- Fibromyalgia
- Rheumatoid Arthritis
- Psoriasis and Psoriatic Arthritis
- Systemic Lupus Erythematosus
- Scleroderma & Systemic Sclerosis
- Vasculitic Diseases
- Spondyloarthropathies
- Sjögren Syndrome/Disease
- Raynaud's Syndrome/Phenomenon/Disorder

Layout of each section—listed once here to avoid unnecessary repetition at each section:

- Introduction and Overview
- Clinical Presentation
- Prevalence, Symptoms, and Clinical Findings
- Pathophysiology
- Differential Diagnosis
- Diagnosis
- Standard Medical Treatment
- Therapeutic Interventions—Clinical Application of the Functional Inflammology Protocol via FINDSEX™ acronym

Twilight of the Idiopathic Era and the Dawn of New Possibilities in Health and Healthcare

This article was originally published in *Naturopathy Digest* in 2006; minor edits were made in 2010 and 2014
naturopathydigest.com/archives/2006/mar/idiopathic.php

Among the perplexing paradoxes that exist in healthcare is coexistence of our adoration of allopathy for its "scientific method" along with the description of most chronic diseases as "idiopathic." If the allopathic use of the scientific method were so adroit, then why are so many conditions described as having "no known cause"? Is the scientific method inadequate, or is the allopathic lens incapable of bringing disease causation into focus? Perhaps a third option exists: that some groups—namely the allopaths and the pharmaceutical companies—benefit by convincing us that most diseases have "no known cause" and that therefore the best that doctors and patients can hope for is additive and endless pharmaceuticalization of all health problems. When the cause of our health problems is "unknown", we are disempowered, and we must depend on "experts" and those who have "the cure" to help us and save us. When the causes of our problems are known, we are empowered to take effective action. Certainly, some groups have financial and political interests in keeping us *as professionals* and *as patients* confused and disempowered.

The End of the Idiopathic Era: A stark contrast exists between primary research literature and the "facts" that are selectively reported in medical textbooks and which are used to buttress "conventional wisdom" and the resultant status quo. While I have been aware of this contrast for many years, the divergence was impressed upon me with renewed vigor during the preparation of a recent article[1] and the completion of my 2006 textbook *Integrative Rheumatology*.[2] Arthritis in general and autoimmune and rheumatic diseases in particular are frequently described as "idiopathic" and as having "no known cause" by most mainstream medical books like *The Merck Manual* and *Current Medical Diagnosis and Treatment*; these contentions are inconsistent with the abundant and diverse research showing that—rather than being *idiopathic*—most chronic musculoskeletal disorders are *multifactorial*. When a disease is codified as *idiopathic*, doctors lose their incentive to look for and treat the *causes* [plural] of the disease because the codified conventional wisdom has already stated that "The cause [singular] of the disease has not been identified." Similarly, patients are convinced to give up their hope of ever being *cured*; they chose what appears to be the second best option: lifelong medicalization. In these instances, acceptance of the codified conventional wisdom benefits doctors and patients by freeing them of the obligation to think, to mobilize their consciousness; the price paid for this exoneration from consciousness is perpetuated unconsciousness and drug dependence for doctors and patients. Being told by powerful institutions and ensconced authorities that "There's nothing else you can do, and nothing more to think about" lulls us all into apathy and conformity at the price of our individual and collective lives and consciousness.

Idiopathic, or Multifactorial?: Let's look at psoriasis and rheumatoid arthritis as two shining examples of *idiopathicity*. If one looks into a standard medical textbook, one sees that these conditions have *no known cause* and *therefore* the lifelong prescription of anti-inflammatory medications is presumptively justified. On the contrary, if one spends a few days in any medical library, one can find articles that point to the causes of these diseases and which then illuminate the path (and paths) by which doctors and patients can arrive at authentic improvement or permanent cure. Most patients can be cured of psoriasis, and a large percentage of rheumatoid arthritis patients can avoid the complications and medicalization associated with their disease, particularly if *the causes* of their condition are treated early. We now know that most autoimmune diseases are caused by and/or perpetuated by ~~chronic~~ sustained infections, phenotypic/epigenetic immune imbalances, a proinflammatory lifestyle, hormonal imbalances, and exposure to chemicals and metals that cause immune dysfunction/activation. When the cause(s) of the disease is treated, the disease has the potential to be cured, provided that it is treated comprehensively and hopefully before the onset of irreversible damage. When the disease is cured, lifelong medicalization becomes unnecessary, the patient is free to fully resume his/her life, and doctors are liberated from their roles as drug representatives and can resume their proper positions as healers and creative free-thinking individuals.

Asserting an empowered stance toward disease prevention and treatment carries implications beyond those for the doctor and the patient. These implications also point to new ways of living and stewarding the world. When we look at a disease like Parkinson's disease and then determine that it is *idiopathic*, then nothing happens to

---

[1] Vasquez A. Nutritional and Botanical Treatments against "Silent Infections" and Gastrointestinal Dysbiosis. *Nutritional Perspectives* 2006; January
[2] Vasquez A. *Integrative Rheumatology*. First Edition. 2006

change or shape our view of the world, our place in it, and the interconnected components of health and disease. Everyone agrees that that clinical manifestations of Parkinson's disease result from the death (or perhaps impairment?) of dopaminergic neurons. From the allopathic perspective, the disease is *idiopathic*, while from an integrative naturopathic perspective, we see Parkinson's disease as a *multifaceted disorder* associated with defective mitochondrial function, impaired xenobiotic detoxification, and occupational and/or recreational exposure to toxicants, particularly pesticides. These associations align to create a new model for the illness based on exposure to neurotoxicants such as pesticides[3] which are ineffectively detoxified[4] and then accumulate in the brain[5] and induce mitochondrial dysfunction[6] and resultant oxidative stress[7] which leads to impairment/death of dopaminergic neurons. Therefore, from the perspective of both prevention and treatment, the clinical approach to Parkinson's disease should include pesticide avoidance and optimization of detoxification to prevent the cellular accumulation of neurotoxic mitochondrial poisons. The plan must also include optimization of nutritional status, antioxidant capacity, and mitochondrial function.[8] Further, if our goal is to reduce the societal prevalence of Parkinson's disease, then we must begin living in better harmony with nature and thinking of ways to reduce our use of pesticides and herbicides, the chemicals that are consistently shown to cause premature neuronal death and which are increasingly pervasive in our home, work, and outdoor environments.

The Dawn of New Possibilities in Health and Healthcare: The time is now past when credible physicians can assert that most diseases are "of unknown origin." The truth is that we already have access to the information we need to help our patients. The truth is that we can often offer our patients the *probability of cure* rather than *lifelong and endless prescriptions for symptom-modifying drugs*. These truths imply that healthcare and our systems of healthcare delivery must change, because the pharmaceutical and medical icons that stand before us were built upon feet and legs of clay and interspersed lead. We stand at the dawn of a new era in healthcare—one in which patients with chronic diseases in general and autoimmune diseases in particular—have a tangible and authentic opportunity to regain their health.

Higher education

"Our real problem is to determine: *what is the goal of education?*

Are we forming children who are only capable of learning what is already known?

Or should we try to develop creative and innovative minds, capable of discovery from the preschool age onward, throughout life?"

Jean Piaget (1896-1980), Swiss developmental psychologist and philosopher known for his epistemological studies with children

---

[3] Ritz B, Yu F. Parkinson's disease mortality and pesticide exposure in California 1984-1994. *Int J Epidemiol*. 2000 Apr;29(2):323-9
[4] Menegon A, Board PG, Blackburn AC, et al. Parkinson's disease, pesticides, and glutathione transferase polymorphisms. *Lancet*. 1998;352(9137):1344-6
[5] Kamel F, Hoppin JA. Related Articles, Association of pesticide exposure with neurologic dysfunction and disease. *Environ Health Perspect*. 2004;112(9):950-8
[6] Parker WD Jr, Swerdlow RH. Mitochondrial dysfunction in idiopathic Parkinson disease. *Am J Hum Genet*. 1998;62(4):758-62
[7] Davey GP, Peuchen S, Clark JB. Energy thresholds in brain mitochondria. Potential involvement in neurodegeneration. *J Biol Chem*. 1998;273(21):12753-7
[8] Kidd PM. Parkinson's disease as multifactorial oxidative neurodegeneration: implications for integrative management. *Altern Med Rev*. 2000 Dec;5(6):502-29

Anonymous art-quality graffiti in Paris, France—photo by Dr Vasquez in 2013: This image reminds me of the (common, American) educational process, which is often stupefying and *stupidifying*. Throughout most of my educational experience—including 12 years of doctorate-level study—I've found that most schools have impressively little commitment to *instruction* (Latin: *instruere*: to pack in, to load) and even less to *education* (Latin: *educare*: to lead out); in fact, most "professional" academicians and so-called "administrators" do not appreciate these words or concepts for their meanings nor their implications. In my experience as a Professor and Director at various schools, I frequently found so-called "senior administrators" to be completely incompetent in their roles, and completely corrupt in their willingness to literally sell-out quality faculty for personal gain and financial advantage, even at major cost to students, programs, courses, and the institution—I have seen this in various schools in various professions, including professions and some schools which I previously cherished. The pervasiveness and high level of incompetence and corruption in healthcare professions and institutions is bewildering. What I strive for with my books and courses is to resist the "dumbing down" of students and the dehumanization and eunuchification of academia in general and intellectuality in particular.

Review of the Functional Inflammology Protocol and each of the FINDSEX® Components:
Summary to Reduce/Avoid Redundancy and Repeated Citations throughout the Clinical Application Subsections

The Functional Inflammology Protocol is reviewed and substantiated in Chapter 4; the protocol is reviewed/outlined here with the most important components cited. In the clinical application sections that follow, the protocol is applied, and its disease-specific implications are emphasized; the abbreviated overview/summary is included in each subsection with nuances noted and citations omitted to enhance safety/efficacy/applicability and space/time efficiency, respectively.

> **The Functional Inflammology Protocol is a decipherative clinical approach—"a scheme of behavior"—for the understanding and treatment of complex inflammatory disorders implemented via the FINDSEX® acronym**
>
> "In order for a particular species to maintain itself and increase its power, its conception of reality **must comprehend enough of the calculable and constant** for it to base a scheme of behavior on it."
> Nietzsche FW. *Will to Power*, 1901, #480
>
> **Factors that are "calculable and constant" in sustained inflammatory diseases**
> - **F**ood and nutritional variables
> - **I**nfections, dysbiosis
> - **N**utritional (deficiency) alternations in immune phenotype and function
> - **D**ysmetabolism of mitochondria, ER
> - **S**leep disturbance, social stressors, sweating deficiency (lack of exercise)
> - **E**ndocrine imbalances
> - **X**enobiotic immunotoxicity

- **FOOD & NUTRITION: 5-part "supplemented Paleo-Mediterranean diet" (SPMD, 5pSPMD)** The 5-part "supplemented Paleo-Mediterranean diet" (SPMD—reviewed in Chapter 4) consists of ❶ foundational plant-based low-carbohydrate diet of fruits, vegetables, nuts, seeds, berries and lean sources of protein: the plant-based diet optimizes antioxidant and phytonutrient intake[9] while promoting favorable modification of gastrointestinal flora for a systemic anti-inflammatory benefit[10]; carbohydrate intake is minimized and tailored per individual need for weight maintenance and exercise recovery/compensation; maintaining mild ketosis via low carbohydrate intake helps maintain optimal body weight, mitochondrial efficiency, bHB's antioxidant function and a rejuvenative phenotype via histone acetylation[11]; plant-based diets promote alkalinization and counteract the Western diet's promotion of diet-induced acidosis[12]; renal insufficiency mandates vigilance for hyperkalemia, especially when considering implementation of a potassium-rich diet ❷ multivitamin and multimineral supplementation: this component serves to correct pandemic nutritional deficiencies[13], prevent long-latency deficiency diseases[14], improve mood[15], reduce systemic inflammation[16], and provide some/partial/complete compensation for genotropic metabolic defects[17], ❸ physiologic doses of vitamin D3 (range 2,000-10,000 IU/d): vitamin D3 supplementation[18] alleviates pain, improves mood, reduces inflammation, enhances immunity, normalizes hypertension, ❹ combination fatty acid therapy (CFAT) with n3-ALA, n6-GLA, n3-EPA, n3-DHA, and phytochemical-rich olive oil which contains n9-oleate: anti-inflammatory, mood-enhancing, and cardioprotective benefits are conclusively documented, ❺ probiotics: probiotics promote immunotolerance via several mechanisms including induction of Treg; probiotic supplementation helps prevent and treat insufficiency dysbiosis, which causes 1) decreased colonization resistance, 2) increased bacterial translocation, and 3) failure of optimal Treg induction. Per "Expert consensus document: The International Scientific Association for Probiotics and Prebiotics consensus statement" published in *Nature Reviews Gastroenterology and Hepatology* 2014 Aug[19], probiotics—by definition—require administration of at least one billion (1,000,000,000 or 1x10^9) colony forming units (CFU); many probiotic nutritional supplements in the form of powders and

---

[9] Liu RH. Health benefits of fruit and vegetables are from additive and synergistic combinations of phytochemicals. *Am J Clin Nutr*. 2003 Sep;78(3 Suppl):517S-520S
[10] Peltonen R et al. Faecal microbial flora and disease activity in rheumatoid arthritis during a vegan diet. *Br J Rheumatol*. 1997 Jan;36(1):64-8
[11] Shimazu T, Hirschey MD, et al. Suppression of oxidative stress by β-hydroxybutyrate, an endogenous histone deacetylase inhibitor. *Science* 2013 Jan;339:211-4. To access more of Dr Matt Hirschey's work and video presentations, please see ichnfm.org/events/MitochondrialMedicine. For additional information on the rejuvenative effect of histone acetylation, see: Matuoka et al. Rapid reversion of aging phenotypes by nicotinamide through possible modulation of histone acetylation. *Cell Mol Life Sci*. 2001 Dec;58:2108-16
[12] Adeva et al. Diet-induced metabolic acidosis. *Clin Nutr*. 2011 Aug;30:416-21. Cordain et al. Origins and evolution of the Western diet. *Am J Clin Nutr*. 2005 Feb;81(2):341-54
[13] Fletcher RH, Fairfield KM. Vitamins for chronic disease prevention in adults: clinical applications. *JAMA*. 2002 Jun 19;287(23):3127-9
[14] Heaney RP. Long-latency deficiency disease: insights from calcium and vitamin D. *Am J Clin Nutr*. 2003 Nov;78(5):912-9
[15] Benton D, Haller J, Fordy J. Vitamin supplementation for 1 year improves mood. *Neuropsychobiology*. 1995;32(2):98-105
[16] Church TS, Earnest CP, Wood KA, Kampert JB. Reduction of C-reactive protein levels through use of a multivitamin. *Am J Med*. 2003 Dec 15;115(9):702-7
[17] Ames BN, et al. High-dose vitamin therapy stimulates variant enzymes with decreased coenzyme binding affinity (increased K(m)). *Am J Clin Nutr*. 2002 Apr;75(4):616-58
[18] See discussion and citaitons throughout Chapter 4. Vasquez A, Manso G, Cannell J. The clinical importance of vitamin D (cholecalciferol): a paradigm shift with implications for all healthcare providers. Altern Ther Health Med. 2004 Sep-Oct;10(5):28-36 inflammationmastery.com/reprints/
[19] Hill et al. Expert consensus document: The International Scientific Association for Probiotics and Prebiotics consensus statement on the scope and appropriate use of the term probiotic. *Nat Rev Gastroenterol Hepatol*. 2014 Aug;11(8):506-14

capsules contain 1-20 billion organisms yet not all organisms are viable at time of consumption and not all viable organisms become CFU. Importantly, some benefits of probiotic supplementation are not dependent on viable microorganisms but rather on the molecular signature of the microbe; other—and obviously more complete—benefits require microbial viability and are mediated via metabolites, which are themselves interdependent on microbes and the host's diet. Bertazzoni et al[20] extensively reviewed the issue of microbial/CFU count number and concluded that the appropriate dose is patient-dependent, disease-dependent, and strain-dependent and thus cannot be generalized; their review included several studies that safely and effectively used varying doses, e.g., 1, 30, 70, 300 billion CFU/d. Per expert clinical opinion, a clinician might use one billion [units = microbes or CFU] for a small or young child, and a starting dose of 10 billion scaling up to 90 billion per day for adults.[21]

- Additional details—implementation of the "low-carbohydrate (low fermentation) supplemented Paleo-Mediterranean diet ("low-carb SPMD")": The diet should be plant-based, but not necessarily vegan or vegetarian; I refer to this diet at "plant-based Paleo" since "the Paleo diet" as commonly discussed is simply a diet of whole natural foods which can generally be consumed without cooking or processing. For purposes of meeting physiologic expectations and attaining the highest satiety, weight optimization, and nutrient density with a phytonutrient-dense low-fermentation diet, the diet should primarily consist of fruits, vegetables, nuts, seeds, berries, and lean sources of protein; carbohydrate intake is modulated per caloric and carbohydrate needs while protein intake is tailored to lean body mass, exercise and healing/recuperation needs. Preferred sources of protein are grass-fed land animals as well as wild-caught cold-water fish, both of which are low in total fat and high in the anti-inflammatory and immunomodulatory omega-3 fatty acids, especially EPA and DHA. Whey protein isolate can also be used as it is an inexpensive convenient source of high-quality protein well-tolerated for most patients and as it also contains many functional components such as glutathione precursors, tryptophan, immunoglobulins, and growth factors anti-gastrin effects which help to heal/protect damaged intestinal mucosa. Plant-based diets, which can be further phyto-supplemented with food concentrates and fruit/vegetable smoothies/juices, provide the greatest dietary density and diversity of phytonutrients which generally have antioxidant and anti-inflammatory effects; also very important is the highly important modulation of gastrointestinal flora by plant-based diets which serves as a major mechanism by which such diets exert their clinically significant systemic anti-inflammatory benefits. I have detailed this diet—"the Supplemented Paleo-Mediterranean diet" as a combination of the "Paleolithic" or "Paleo diet" and the well-known "Mediterranean diet", both of which are well described in peer-reviewed journals and the lay press. (See Chapter 2 and my other publications[22,23] for details). This diet is the most nutrient-dense diet available, and its benefits are further enhanced by supplementation with vitamins, minerals, and the health-promoting fatty acids: ALA, GLA, EPA, DHA, and oleic acid. Vitamin and mineral supplementation is warranted in the general population and even more so among patients[24], who are more likely to be nutrient deficient due to their disease processes, mediations, and concomitant problems such as mild metabolic acidosis, malabsorption, and drug-induced nutrient depletions. Beyond routine vitamin-mineral supplementation, additional vitamin D3 supplementation is generally needed to meet the physiologic requirement of approximately 4,000 IU per day and to achieve the physiologic and clinical benefits including prevention/alleviation of depression, chronic pain, diabetes mellitus, hypertension, immunosuppression, immune activation, and cancer.[25] Likewise, absolute or relative deficiencies/insufficiencies of health-promoting anti-inflammatory fatty acids—namely: ALA, GLA, EPA, DHA, and oleic acid—are common and clinically consequential insofar as these deficiencies/insufficiencies promote chronic/sustained inflammation, pain, and neuroemotional

---

[20] Bertazzoni et al. Probiotics and clinical effects: is the number what counts? *J Chemother.* 2013 Aug;25(4):193-212
[21] Conversation and personal communication 2014 Aug with my friend and colleague Mike Ash DO ND, an international expert on probiotics and mucosal immunology, "But some studies suggest 1 billion is the number needed to generate an effect (of clinical relevance), and this may suit a small or young child. I tend to start at 10 billion and rarely ever exceed 90 billion in a day [for adults]."
[22] Vasquez A. A Five-Part Nutritional Protocol that Produces Consistently Positive Results. *Nutritional Wellness* 2005 September
[23] Vasquez A. Implementing the Five-Part Nutritional Wellness Protocol for the Treatment of Various Health Problems. *Nutritional Wellness* 2005 November
[24] "However, suboptimal intake of some vitamins, above levels causing classic vitamin deficiency, is a risk factor for chronic diseases and common in the general population, especially the elderly. ... Most people do not consume an optimal amount of all vitamins by diet alone. Pending strong evidence of effectiveness from randomized trials, it appears prudent for all adults to take vitamin supplements. ... Physicians should make specific efforts to learn about their patients' use of vitamins to ensure that they are taking vitamins they should, ..." Fletcher RH, Fairfield KM. Vitamins for chronic disease prevention in adults: clinical applications. *JAMA.* 2002 Jun 19;287(23):3127-9
[25] Vasquez et al. The clinical importance of vitamin D (cholecalciferol): a paradigm shift. *Altern Ther Health Med.* 2004 Sep-Oct;10(5):28-36 InflammationMastery.com/reprints

impairment; thus, combination fatty acid therapy/replacement/supplementation (CFAT) is indicated based on its physiological effects and clinical benefits. Probiotics, especially when consumed in conjunction with a plant-based diet which promotes an enhanced milieu for their growth and effect, provide clear clinical benefits which are both local to the gut (e.g., reduced incidence of opportunistic infections/colonizations, prevention/amelioration of increased intestinal permeability) and systemic via the anti-inflammatory benefits of enhanced induction of Treg cells at the reciprocal expense of Th-17 cells. This "supplemented Paleo-Mediterranean diet" obviates overconsumption of chemical preservatives, artificial sweeteners, and carbohydrate-dominant foods such as candies, pastries, breads, potatoes, grains, and other foods with a high glycemic load and high glycemic index (from a practical and conceptual standpoint: glycemic load x glycemic index = glycemic impact = more oxidative stress, antioxidant depletion, immunosuppression, and mitochondrial impairment).

- Supplemented Paleo-Mediterranean diet / Specific Carbohydrate Diet: The specifications of the *specific carbohydrate diet* (SCD) detailed by Gottschall[26] are met with adherence to the Paleo diet by Cordain.[27] The combination of both approaches and books will give patients an excellent combination of informational understanding and culinary versatility.
- The use of a low starch diet in the treatment of patients suffering from ankylosing spondylitis: alleviation of dysbiosis and immune complex formation via nutritional intervention (*Clin Rheumatol* 1996 Jan[28]): "The majority of ankylosing spondylitis (AS) patients not only possess HLA-B27, but during active phases of the disease have elevated levels of total serum IgA, suggesting that a microbe from the bowel flora is acting across the gut mucosa. .... Furthermore AS patients from 10 different countries have been found to have elevated levels of specific antibodies against Klebsiella bacteria. It has been suggested that these Klebsiella microbes, found in the bowel flora, might be the trigger factors in this disease and therefore reduction in the size of the bowel flora could be of benefit in the treatment of AS patients. Microbes from the bowel flora depend on dietary starch for their growth and therefore a reduction in starch intake might be beneficial in AS patients. A "low starch diet" involving a reduced intake of "bread, potatoes, cakes and pasta" has been devised and tested in healthy control subjects and AS patients. The "low starch diet" leads to a reduction of total serum IgA in both healthy controls as well as patients, and furthermore to a decrease in inflammation and symptoms in the AS patients."
  o Celiac disease and autoimmunity (*J Gastroenterol Hepatol* 2013 Jan[29]): 356 patients with CD participated in this study. "Autoimmune thyroiditis (10.6% vs 0.4%), insulin dependent diabetes mellitus (IDDM) (2.2% vs 1.7%), systemic lupus erythematosus (SLE) (1.1% vs 0), and psoriasis (12.9% vs 5.5%) occurred more frequently in CD patients."
  o Refractory immune thrombocytopenia successfully treated with high-dose vitamin D supplementation and hydroxychloroquine: two case reports (*J Med Case Rep.* 2013 Apr[30]): "In our two case reports, we found an association between vitamin D deficiency and immune thrombocytopenia where platelet levels responded to vitamin D treatment and hydroxychloroquine but not to prednisone. We believe there may be synergism between vitamin D supplementation and hydroxychloroquine."

- **INFECTIONS & DYSBIOSIS:** ❶ antimicrobial treatments, ❷ immunorestoration, ❸ immunotolerance via Treg induction   Essentially all autoimmune/rheumatic disorders are associated with microbial colonization and intolerance to same; the presence of persistent microbial colonization is *prima facie* evidence of immunosuppression, commonly due to nutritional deficiencies, psychoemotional stress, sleep deprivation, overconsumption of simple carbohydrates, or—most commonly since all of these are common—a combination of all of these. The eight areas of dysbiosis (multifocal)—listed here from head to toe and inside out—are: ❶ sinorespiratory, ❷ orodental, ❸ gastrointestinal, ❹ urogenital/genitourinary, ❺ parenchymal/tissue, ❻

---

[26] Gotschall E. *Breaking the Vicious Cycle: Intestinal health though diet*. Kirkton Press; Rev edition (August, 1994) scdiet.com/
[27] Cordain L. *The Paleo Diet*. John Wiley & Sons Inc., New York 2002 thepaleodiet.com/
[28] Ebringer A, Wilson C. The use of a low starch diet in the treatment of patients suffering from ankylosing spondylitis. *Clin Rheumatol*. 1996 Jan;15 Suppl 1:62-66
[29] Iqbal et al. Celiac disease arthropathy and autoimmunity study. *J Gastroenterol Hepatol*. 2013 Jan;28(1):99-105
[30] Bockow et al. Refractory immune thrombocytopenia successfully treated with high-dose vitamin D supplementation and hydroxychloroquine: two case reports. *J Med Case Rep*. 2013 Apr 4;7:91

microbial (dysbiosis within microbes, e.g., bacteriophages), ❼ dermal/cutaneous, and ❽ environmental. Patients with low mucosal sIgA levels, recurrent mucosal infections, or autoimmunity are candidates for serum IgA testing to evaluate for genotropic selective secretory IgA deficiency.

- o Interventions and antimicrobial agents for gastrointestinal dysbiosis:
  - *Saccharomyces boulardii*: A non-colonizing, non-pathogenic yeast that increases sIgA production and can aid in the elimination of pathogenic/dysbiotic yeast, bacteria, and parasites. It is particularly useful during antibiotic treatment to help prevent secondary *Candida* and *Clostridium difficile* infections. Common dose is 250 mg thrice daily for adults and twice daily for children.
  - Berberine (generally available as generic berberine hydrochloride or as a plant-based standardized extract with synergistic phytochemicals[31]) 1,000-1,500 mg/d in divided doses PO for up to 3 months: Berberine is a botanical alkaloid extracted from plants such as *Berberis vulgaris*, and *Hydrastis canadensis* with millennia of clinical use for various conditions and also specifically for the treatment of infectious diseases, such as those caused by *E coli*, *Giardia lamblia* (comparable to metronidazole), *Entamoeba histolytica*, *Streptococcus* and *Chlamydia trachomatis*.[32] Many clinicians use berberine as a standard treatment for gastrointestinal dysbiosis due to bacteria, yeast, and/or other microbes; it is very safe and has a wide range of antimicrobial action. Oral dose of 400 mg per day has been traditionally common for adults[33]; however newer clinical research has shown that berberine 1,000-1,5000 mg/d for three months provides major clinical benefits and is effective treatment for dyslipidemia, insulin resistance, diabetes mellitus type-2 (comparable to metformin), and overweight/obesity.[34,35,36,37] Berberine is available in a "generic" form from many nutraceutical companies.
  - Oregano oil (time-released emulsified preparation named "ADP" from Biotics Research Corporation) 600 mg/d generally given as 200 mg/d PO TID for 6 weeks: Oil of Mediterranean oregano *Oreganum vulgare* was orally administered to 14 adult patients whose stools tested positive for enteric parasites, *Blastocystis hominis*, *Entamoeba hartmanni* and *Endolimax nana*. Six weeks of supplementation with 600 mg emulsified oil of oregano daily resulted in complete disappearance of *Entamoeba hartmanni* (four cases), *Endolimax nana* (one case), and *Blastocystis hominis* in eight cases. *Blastocystis hominis* scores declined in three additional cases.[38] An *in vitro* study[39] and clinical experience support the use of emulsified oregano against *Candida albicans* and various gastrointestinal microbes. Many clinicians use ADP as a standard treatment for gastrointestinal

> **Emulsified time-released oil of oregano against gastrointestinal dysbiosis: one of the only agents (besides berberine) with human clinical data supporting efficacy and safety**
>
> "After 6 weeks of supplementation with 600 mg emulsified oil of oregano daily, there was complete disappearance of *Entamoeba hartmanni* (four cases), *Endolimax nana* (one case), and *Blastocystis hominis* in eight cases. Also, *Blastocystis hominis* scores declined in three additional cases. Gastrointestinal symptoms improved in seven of the 11 patients who had tested positive for *Blastocystis hominis*."
>
> Force et al. Inhibition of enteric parasites by emulsified oil of oregano in vivo. *Phytother Res.* 2000 May

---

[31] Stermitz FR, Lorenz P, Tawara JN, Zenewicz LA, Lewis K. Synergy in a medicinal plant: antimicrobial action of berberine potentiated by 5'-methoxyhydnocarpin, a multidrug pump inhibitor. *Proc Natl Acad Sci U S A*. 2000 Feb 15;97(4):1433-7
[32] [No authors listed]. Berberine. *Altern Med Rev.* 2000 Apr;5(2):175-7
[33] Berberine. Altern Med Rev. 2000 Apr;5(2):175-7 thorne.com/altmedrev/.fulltext/5/2/175.pdf
[34] Kong et al. Berberine is a novel cholesterol-lowering drug working through a unique mechanism distinct from statins. *Nat Med.* 2004 Dec;10(12):1344-51
[35] "...bese human subjects (Caucasian) were given 500 mg berberine orally 3 times a day for 12 weeks. Efficacy and safety of berberine treatment was determined by measurements of body weight, comprehensive metabolic panel, blood lipid and hormone levels, expression levels of inflammatory factors, complete blood count, and electrocardiograph. Sprague-Dawley rat experiment was also performed to identify anti-obesity effects of berberine treatment. Results demonstrate that berberine treatment produced mild weight loss (average 5 lb/subject) in obese human subjects. But more interestingly, treatment significantly reduced blood lipid levels (23% decrease of triglyceride and 12.2% decrease of cholesterol levels) in human subjects." Hu et al. Lipid-lowering effect of berberine in human subjects and rats. *Phytomedicine* 2012 Jul;19:861-7
[36] "In study A, 36 adults with newly diagnosed type 2 diabetes mellitus were randomly assigned to treatment with berberine or metformin (0.5 g 3 times a day) in a 3-month trial. The hypoglycemic effect of berberine was similar to that of metformin. Significant decreases in hemoglobin A1c (from 9.5%+/-0.5% to 7.5%+/-0.4%, P<.01), fasting blood glucose (from 10.6+/-0.9 mmol/L to 6.9+/-0.5 mmol/L, P<.01), postprandial blood glucose (from 19.8+/-1.7 to 11.1+/-0.9 mmol/L, P<.01), and plasma triglycerides (from 1.13+/-0.13 to 0.89+/-0.03 mmol/L, P<.05) were observed in the berberine group. In study B, 48 adults with poorly controlled type 2 diabetes mellitus were treated supplemented with berberine in a 3-month trial. Berberine acted by lowering fasting blood glucose and postprandial blood glucose from 1 week to the end of the trial. Hemoglobin A1c decreased from 8.1%+/-0.2% to 7.3%+/-0.3% (P<.001)." Yin J, Xing H, Ye J.Efficacy of berberine in patients with type 2 diabetes mellitus. *Metabolism.* 2008 May;57(5):712-7
[37] "One hundred sixteen patients with type 2 diabetes and dyslipidemia were randomly allocated to receive berberine (1.0 g daily) and the placebo for 3 months. ... In the berberine group, fasting and postload plasma glucose decreased from 7.0 +/- 0.8 to 5.6 +/- 0.9 and from 12.0 +/- 2.7 to 8.9 +/- 2.8 mm/liter, HbA1c from 7.5 +/- 1.0% to 6.6 +/- 0.7%, triglyceride from 2.51 +/- 2.04 to 1.61 +/- 1.10 mm/liter, total cholesterol from 5.31 +/- 0.98 to 4.35 +/- 0.96 mm/liter, and low-density lipoprotein-cholesterol from 3.23 +/- 0.81 to 2.55 +/- 0.77 mm/liter,..." Zhang et al. Treatment of type 2 diabetes and dyslipidemia with the natural plant alkaloid berberine. *J Clin Endocrinol Metab.* 2008 Jul;93(7):2559-65
[38] Force M, Sparks WS, Ronzio RA. Inhibition of enteric parasites by emulsified oil of oregano in vivo. *Phytother Res.* 2000 May;14(3):213-4
[39] Stiles JC, Sparks W, Ronzio RA. The inhibition of Candida albicans by oregano. *J Applied Nutr* 1995;47:96-102

dysbiosis due to bacteria, yeast, and/or other microbes; it is very safe and has a wide range of antimicrobial action.

- <u>Undecylenic acid (also known as 10-undecenoic acid, available as "Formula SF722" from Thorne Research, each gelcap contains 10-undecenoic acid 50 mg) dosed at "450-750 mg undecylenic acid daily in three divided doses"[40] equates to 10-15 capsules per day, or 5 capsules 2-3 times per day</u>: An eleven-carbon monounsaturated fatty acid found naturally in the body (occurring in sweat) and produced commercially by the vacuum distillation of castor bean oil, undecylenate shows laboratory and clinical human-trial effectiveness against *Herpes Simplex*, *Candida albicans*, and tinea pedis caused by *Trychophyton rubrumor* and *Trychophyton mentagrophytes*.

- <u>Combination botanical antimicrobials ("Tricycline" from Allergy Research Group)</u>: Contains black walnut, artemesinin, berberine, and citrus seed extract; in the early days of my clinical practice, I used this product routinely with a standard dosing of "2 capsules twice per day until the bottle [n=90] is empty."

- <u>DrV's (in)famous "vitamin C purge"—the author's perspective and rationale</u>: Generally when I lecture on the topic of dysbiosis to post-graduate audiences, I mention one of my preferred treatments for GI dysbiosis, for which I seem to be either famous or infamous, namely the "vitamin C purge." The application is essentially as straightforward as the underlying logic: the *per os* use of vitamin C (20-60 grams in 1 liter of water, preferably with two cups of coffee) for its osmotic laxative effect to rapidly reduce the quantity of bacteria/microorganisms throughout the gut by introduction of a cleansing water bolus; while the vitamin C and water serve as an osmotic nonstimulant laxative (perhaps with some antimicrobial effect), the coffee/caffeine serves as a bowel stimulant. I have used this treatment empirically with great success in achieving rapid quantitative reductions in gastrointestinal microbes. For many years plain ascorbic acid was used at doses of 20-60 grams 20,000-60,000 mg) to induce therapeutic laxation (occasionally described as "do-it-yourself top-to-bottom gastrointestinal lavage") with onset of action generally within 30-60 minutes following consumption of powered ascorbate in approximately one liter of water, preferably *and often necessarily* with a bowel peristalsis stimulant such as coffee. The goal and purpose are to achieve a cleansing water bolus that purges the bowels of dysbiotic microbes and their pro-inflammatory debris and mitochondria-impairing metabolites. The use of therapeutic laxatives for the treatment of intestinal parasitic disease is well represented in the Infectous Disease and Tropical Medicine literature; in this instance, we are using ascorbic acid as an osmotic laxative and the coffee as a bowel stimulant. In high concentrations, ascorbic acid is directly microbicidal, at least against *E coli* (per Gaby, c 1993). The vitamin C can be administered as ascorbic acid—perfectly fine but very acidic, Ca/Mg/K buffered ascorbate—same laxative effect with the additional nutritive or laxative effect of minerals, or as home-made buffered ascorbate by mixing—per my own use—one heaping teaspoon or tablespoon of ascorbic acid with 1/2-one teaspoon baking soda (sodium bicarbonate). Additional agents can be ingested simultaneously for additional antimicrobial effect (e.g., iodine-iodide 12-48 mg [given that the standard antimicrobial dose for systemic/dermal infections usually starts at 1,000mg/d]) or intraluminal adsorption (e.g., activated charcoal). Patient selection excludes those who are generally frail and those with renal impairment, cardiac arrhythmia, bowel obstruction, electrolyte imbalance, dementia/psychosis, postural instability and/or reduced mobility to attend the toilet promptly, etc; patients with iron overload are reasonably be excluded—thus serum ferritin should be tested as described in Chapter 1—given that oral vitamin C administration may lead to clinical deterioration in patients with hemochromatosis, per a single case report.[41] As a general rule, the vitamin C purge is initiated only in the morning 1-2 hours before the first meal and is followed later in the day—especially when used for several days consecutively—some effective form of electrolyte replacement, whether in supplemental pill/powder form or as salted vegetable juice;

---

[40] [No authors listed] Undecylenic acid. Monograph. *Altern Med Rev*. 2002 Feb;7(1):68-70
[41] "We describe rapidly fatal cardiomyopathy in a young man. He had for twelve months ingested large amounts of ascorbic acid and was admitted with severe heart failure having been symptomatic for two months. He died after eight days. Idiopathic haemochromatosis was diagnosed at autopsy." McLaran et al. Congestive cardiomyopathy and haemochromatosis--rapid progression possibly accelerated by excessive ingestion of ascorbic acid. *Aust N Z J Med*. 1982 Apr;12(2):187-8

patients can use this treatment PRN, at the beginning of antimicrobial therapy especially to break the vicious cycle of SIBO and resultant GI stasis resulting from microbial methane and H2S, or consecutively; when the latter, periodic assessment of serum electrolytes is reasonable, with one standard interval for monitoring dietary intervention being weekly.

Coffee as a gastrointestinal stimulant

"Coffee stimulates gastrin release and gastric acid secretion... Coffee induces cholecystokinin release and gallbladder contraction... **Coffee increases rectosigmoid motor activity within 4 min after ingestion** in some people. Its effects on the colon are found to be comparable to those of a 1000 kCal meal. ... Coffee promotes gastro-esophageal reflux, but is not associated with dyspepsia. Coffee stimulates gallbladder contraction and colonic motor activity.

Boekema et al. Coffee and gastrointestinal function: facts and fiction. *Scand J Gastroenterol.* 1999;230:35-9

"Caffeinated coffee, decaffeinated coffee and meal induced more activity in the colon with a greater area under the curve of pressure waves and a greater number of propagated contractions when compared with water. Caffeinated coffee, decaffeinated coffee and meal induced greater motor activity in the transverse/descending colon when compared with the rectosigmoid colon. ... **Caffeinated coffee stimulates colonic motor activity.** Its magnitude is similar to a meal, 60% stronger than water and 23% stronger than decaffeinated coffee."

Rao et al. Is coffee a colonic stimulant? *Eur J Gastroenterol Hepatol.* 1998 Feb;10(2):113-8

Laxatives promote eradication of intestinal microbes and are especially useful in patients with stasis/constipation

"Our case shows that although the dose of praziquantel is an important issue, **supportive care, including the optimal use of an oral laxative** and enemas to ensure smooth evacuation of the worm, is also important. This is especially true for young patients who are usually constipated or who cannot evacuate feces intentionally.

Fujita et al. A 2-year-old girl with Diphyllobothrium nihonkaiense infection treated with oral praziquantel and a laxative. *J Nippon Med Sch.* 2008 Aug;75:225-7

For irritable bowel syndrome with constipation: "Treatment with osmotic laxatives (milk of magnesia or polyethylene glycol) may increase stool frequency, improve stool consistency, and reduce straining."

Papadakis M, McPhee SJ, Rabow MW (eds). *Current Medical Diagnosis and Treatment 2014*

- *Artemisia annua*: Artemisinin has been safely used for centuries in Asia for the treatment of malaria, and it also has effectiveness against anaerobic bacteria due to the pro-oxidative sesquiterpene endoperoxide.[42,43] This author has commonly used artemisinin at 200 mg per day in divided doses for adults with dysbiosis. Given its pro-oxidative mechanism, treatment should probably be of limited duration, i.e., 1-2 months; concomitant neuroprotection with CoQ-10 (et al) would be reasonable.
- St. John's Wort (*Hypericum perforatum*): Hyperforin from *Hypericum perforatum* shows impressive antibacterial action *in vitro*, particularly against gram-positive bacteria such as *Staphylococcus aureus*, *Streptococcus pyogenes*, *Streptococcus agalactiae*[44] and perhaps gram-negative *Helicobacter pylori*.[45] Up to 600 mg three times per day of a 3% hyperforin standardized extract is customary in the treatment of depression.
- Bismuth: Bismuth is commonly used in the empiric treatment of diarrhea (e.g., "Pepto-Bismol") and is commonly combined with other antimicrobial agents to reduce drug resistance and increase antibiotic effectiveness.[46]
- Peppermint *(Mentha piperita)*: Peppermint shows antimicrobial and antispasmodic actions and has demonstrated clinical effectiveness in patients with bacterial overgrowth of the small bowel.

---

[42] Dien et al. Effect of food intake on pharmacokinetics of oral artemisinin in healthy Vietnamese subjects. *Antimicrob Agents Chemother.* 1997 May;41(5):1069-72
[43] Giao et al. Artemisinin for treatment of uncomplicated falciparum malaria: is there a place for monotherapy? *Am J Trop Med Hyg.* 2001 Dec;65(6):690-5
[44] Schempp CM, Pelz K, Wittmer A, Schopf E, Simon JC. Antibacterial activity of hyperforin from St John's wort, against multiresistant Staphylococcus aureus and gram-positive bacteria. *Lancet.* 1999 Jun 19;353(9170):2129
[45] "A butanol fraction of St. John's Wort revealed anti-Helicobacter pylori activity with MIC values ranging between 15.6 and 31.2 microg/ml." Reichling J, Weseler A, Saller R. A current review of the antimicrobial activity of Hypericum perforatum L. *Pharmacopsychiatry.* 2001 Jul;34 Suppl 1:S116-8
[46] Veldhuyzen van Zanten SJ, Sherman PM, Hunt RH. Helicobacter pylori: new developments and treatments. *CMAJ.* 1997;156(11):1565-74 cmaj.ca/cgi/reprint/156/11/1565.pdf

- Commonly used antibiotic/antifungal drugs: The most commonly employed drugs for intestinal bacterial overgrowth are described here.[47] Treatment duration is generally at least 2 weeks and up to 8 weeks, depending on clinical response and the severity and diversity of the intestinal overgrowth. With all anti*bacterial* treatments, use empiric anti*fungal* treatment to prevent yeast overgrowth; some patients benefit from antifungal treatment that is continued for *months* and occasionally *years*. Probiotic yeast and bacteria are generally appropriate except in patients with hypersensitivity, severe immunosuppression, or extreme or recalcitrant bacterial overgrowth of the intestines. Drugs can generally be co-administered with natural antibiotics/antifungals for improved efficacy. Treatment can be guided by identification of the dysbiotic microbes and the results of culture and sensitivity tests. Examples of doses are provided below, but clinicians must choose dose and duration per their judgment, experience, and the patient's situation, comorbidity, age, hepatic and renal function, and accompanying polypharmacy; the use of dosing and drug-interaction data (e.g., Epocrates) is strongly recommended.
  - Metronidazole: 250-500 mg BID-QID (generally limit to 1.5-2 g/d); metronidazole has systemic bioavailability and effectiveness against a wide range of dysbiotic microbes, including protozoans, amebas/Giardia, *H. pylori*, *Clostridium difficile* and most anaerobic gram-negative bacilli.[48] Adverse effects are generally limited to stomatitis, nausea, diarrhea, and—rarely and/or with long-term use—peripheral neuropathy, dizziness, and metallic taste; the drug must not be consumed with alcohol. Metronidazole resistance by *Blastocystis hominis* and other parasites has been noted.
  - Erythromycin: 250-500 mg TID-QID; this drug is a widely used antibiotic that also has intestinal promotility benefits (thus making it an ideal treatment for intestinal bacterial overgrowth associated with or caused by intestinal dysmotility/hypomotility such as seen in scleroderma[49,50]). Do not combine erythromycin with the promotility drug **cisapride** due to risk for serious cardiac arrhythmia.
  - Tetracycline: 250-500 mg QID
  - Ciprofloxacin: 500 mg BID, caution: tendonopathy and rupture can occur within 72 hours
  - Cephalexin/Keflex: 250 mg QID
  - Minocycline: Minocycline (200 mg/day)[51] has received the most attention in the treatment of rheumatoid arthritis due to its superior response (65%) over placebo (13%)[52]; in addition to its antibacterial action, the drug is also immunomodulatory and anti-inflammatory. Ironically, minocycline can cause drug-induced autoimmunity, especially lupus.[53,54]
  - **Nystatin:** Nystatin 500,000 units BID-TID with food; duration of treatment begins with a minimum duration of 2-4 weeks and may continue as long as the patient is deriving benefit.
- Antiviral (phyto)nutrition: Antiviral therapeutics should include those with the greatest safety, efficacy, synergistic/additive/collateral benefits, most obviously—per my antiviral protocol detailed in *Chiropractic and Naturopathic Mastery of Common Clinical Disorders*[55] appended to the end of this chapter— 1) 5pSPMD discussed previously, 2) vitamin D3 2,000-10,000 IU/d for its tolerogenic (via Treg) and antimicrobial (via AMP) benefits, 3) vitamin A 25,000 IU/d with discussion and monitoring for toxicity; particularly important given the high percentage of (female) patients who cannot effectively convert carotene to retinol, 4) selenium 600 mcg/d to retard viral mutagenesis and replication, 5) melatonin 2-20 mg nightly for antioxidant, immunostimulatory, antiinflammatory, and mitochondrial-protective

---

[47] Saltzman JR, Russell RM. Nutritional consequences of intestinal bacterial overgrowth. *Compr Ther*. 1994;20(9):523-30
[48] Tierney ML. McPhee SJ, Papadakis MA. *Current Medical Diagnosis and Treatment 2006. 45th edition*. New York; Lange Medical Books: 2006, pages 1578-1577
[49] "Prokinetic agents effective in pseudoobstruction include metoclopramide, domperidone, cisapride, octreotide, and erythromycin. ... The combination of octreotide and erythromycin may be particularly effective in systemic sclerosis." Sjogren RW. Gastrointestinal features of scleroderma. *Curr Opin Rheumatol*. 1996 Nov;8(6):569-75
[50] "Erythromycin accelerates gastric and gallbladder emptying in scleroderma patients and might be helpful in the treatment of gastrointestinal motor abnormalities in these patients." Fiorucci et al. Effect of erythromycin administration on upper gastrointestinal motility in scleroderma patients. *Scand J Gastroenterol* 1994 Sep:807-13
[51] "...48-week trial of oral minocycline (200 mg/d) or placebo." Tilley et al. Minocycline in rheumatoid arthritis. A 48-week, double-blind, placebo-controlled trial.. MIRA Trial Group. *Ann Intern Med*. 1995 Jan 15;122(2):81-9
[52] "In patients with early seropositive RA, therapy with minocycline is superior to placebo." O'Dell et al. Treatment of early rheumatoid arthritis with minocycline or placebo: results of a randomized, double-blind, placebo-controlled trial. *Arthritis Rheum*. 1997 May;40(5):842-8
[53] "...many cases of drug-induced lupus related to minocycline have been reported. Some of those reports included pulmonary lupus..." Christodoulou et al. Respiratory distress due to minocycline-induced pulmonary lupus. *Chest*. 1999 May;115(5):1471-3 chestjournal.org/cgi/content/full/115/5/1471
[54] Lawson TM, Amos N, Bulgen D, Williams BD. Minocycline-induced lupus: clinical features and response to rechallenge. *Rheumatology* (Oxford). 2001 Mar;40(3):329-35 rheumatology.oxfordjournals.org/cgi/content/full/40/3/329
[55] Vasquez A. *Chiropractic and Naturopathic Mastery of Common Clinical Disorders, 2009*, ISBN 1468113976. An update to this text is anticipated with the next few years but will certainly be published via a different title; see InflammationMastery.com for information.

benefits, 6) NAC 1,500 mg TID for antioxidant, GSH-promoting, anti-mTOR, anti-NFkB and antiviral benefits, to be used with 7) lipoic acid 400 mg TID for antioxidant, GSH-preserving, anti-IL-17, anti-NFkB and antiviral benefits, 8) zinc 20-50 mg/d for immunosupportive, pro-thymulin, anti-NFkB, and direct antiviral effects in its ionized form, 9) glycyrrhizin from licorice—doses of glycyrrhizin in the treatment of human viral diseases can be set at 40 mg per day, 5 mg/kg, or dosed reasonably from tea and supplements with periodic monitoring for hypokalemia and hypertension; the generally accepted safe daily dose of glycyrrhizin is 0.2 mg/kg[56], 10) lysine 2-3 g/d is effective and perhaps specific for HSV infections but may be generalizable for all herpes virus infections; generally, the treatment is administered along with a low-arginine diet but arginine itself is necessary for immunocompetence, 11) additional antiviral treatments include injectable adenosine monophosphate, oral/topical lemon balm (*Melissa officinalis*), and oral/topical lithium.

- **NUTRITIONAL IMMUNOMODULATION: Treg induction for modulation of Th-1/2/17 inflammation** Nutrients and therapeutic approaches that promote Treg or IL-10 induction and/or Th-17, IL-17 suppression include 1) mitochondrial optimization and mTOR suppression, 2) biotin, 3) vitamin E, 4) sodium avoidance, 5) transgenic/GMO food avoidance, 6) probiotics, 7) lipoic acid, 8) vitamin A, 9) inflammation reduction, 10) vitamin D, 11) fatty acid supplementation with GLA and n3, 12) infection and dysbiosis remediation, 13) green tea EGCG. Readers should recall the MiBESTPLAIDFIG acronym outlined in Chapter 4.
    - Altered Th17 cells and Th17/regulatory T-cell ratios indicate the subsequent conversion from undifferentiated connective tissue disease [UCTD] to definitive systemic autoimmune disorders (*Hum Immunol.* 2013 Dec[57]): "Th17-cells were increased in UCTD vs. controls, which further increased in those, whom developed SAIDs eventually. The Th17/nTreg ratio gradually increased from controls through UCTD patients, reaching the highest values in SAID-progressed patients. The derailed Th17/Treg balance may contribute to disease progression therefore could function as a prognostic marker."

- **DYSMETABOLISM & DYSFUNCTIONAL MITOCHONDRIA: MitoDys, ERS-UPR, AGE/RAGE, hyperglycemia and ceramide** The major clinical considerations in this section are mitochondrial dysfunction, endoplasmic reticulum stress, unfolded protein response, TLR activation, and the dysmetabolic effects of sustained hyperglycemia and hyperinsulinemia and resultant oxidative stress, inflammation, RAGE activation, and accumulation of AGE, palmitate and ceramide. The review of this information in Chapter 4 covered approximately 30 interventions relevant to dysmetabolism, mitochondrial dysfunction, ERS-UPR, etc; these will not be reviewed here except to mention those most commonly, easily, empirically, synergistically, and effectively used: 1) low-carbohydrate diet with 2) moderate exercise, 3) CoQ-10, 4) acetyl-carnitine with 5) lipoic acid, 6) NAC, 7) resveratrol, and 8) melatonin.

- **STYLE OF LIVING (LIFESTYLE) & SPECIAL CONSIDERATIONS: Sleep optimization, SocioPsychology, Stress management/avoidance, Somatic treatments, Special Supplementation, Sweat/exercise, Sauna/detoxification, Surgery, Stamp your passport and vacate current reality, Sensory deprivation therapy** This is a buffet of mostly lifestyle-based interventions yet also including considerations such as somatic treatments, additional supplementation, and surgery.

- **ENDOCRINE IMBALANCE & OPTIMIZATION: Prolactin, Insulin, Estrogen, DHEA, Cortisol, Testosterone, Thyroid** Common hormonal imbalances seen among autoimmune/inflammatory patients and which contribute to the genesis and perpetuation of these same autoimmune/inflammatory diseases are easily assessed with standard serum laboratory measurements; conveniently, three hormones tend to be elevated, and three tend to be reduced: ❶ *elevated* prolactin, ❷ *elevated* estrogen, ❸ *elevated* insulin—as a surrogate marker (insulin itself actually appears to have an anti-inflammatory effect, counteracting the effect of excess glucose; however the net effect of hyperglycemia-hyperinsulinemia is conclusively pathogenic) for excess carbohydrate intake, insufficient exercise, sarcopenia, mitochondrial dysfunction, nutrient deficiencies, xeobiotic exposure, palmitate and ceramide accumulation, etc, ❹ *reduced* DHEA, ❺ *reduced* cortisol, and ❻ *reduced* testosterone; see Chapter 4 for discussion of these hormones and respective interventions. Thyroid evaluation (patient + labs) should be comprehensive, as discussed in Chapter 1, with a low threshold for empiric treatment.

---

[56] Fiore et a. Antiviral effects of Glycyrrhiza species. *Phytother Res.* 2008 Feb;22(2):141-8
[57] Szodoray et al. Altered Th17 cells and Th17/regulatory T-cell ratios indicate the subsequent conversion from undifferentiated connective tissue disease to definitive systemic autoimmune disorders. *Hum Immunol.* 2013 Dec;74(12):1510-8

- **XENOBIOTIC ACCUMULATION & DETOXIFICATION: Chemical avoidance, nutritional support for detoxification pathways, urine alkalinization** The clinical relevance and pathogenic mechanisms of xenobiotic accumulation are irrefutably well documented and described. Population-wide toxin accumulation results from corporate irresponsibility and government collusion with industry via lax regulations; at times the situation is so grave that one might wonder if corporations and government are intentionally trying to poison the population (e.g., glyphosate application to water supply, rivers, and population-wide food despite consistently documented adverse effects[58]). These persistent organic pollutants (POPs) promote disease primarily via mitochondrial dysfunction and endoplasmic reticulum stress (thus directly promoting ATP production failure, oxidative injury, insulin resistance, antioxidant nutrient depletion, inflammation and promotion of Treg/Th-17 imbalance) and via additional immunogenic effects including bystander activation and haptenization—see discussion and review in Chapter 4. Clinical assessments include history, physical examination, and laboratory assessment (using serum, whole blood, urine or—rarely yet accurately—fat biopsy), and response to treatment. Treatments include nutritional support for Phases 1 and 2 of detoxification (e.g., oxidation and conjugation) and excretion via bile and urine; for the latter, urinary alkalinization is generally recommended. Chemical toxins can be bound in the gut using activated charcoal[59], cholestyramine[60], or Chlorella (6 g/d [2g TID cc] taken after breakfast, lunch, and dinner)[61]—all of these three treatments have documented safety and effectiveness; clinically and empirically, phytochelatin (plant-derived peptides that bind toxic metals[62]) concentrates appear safe and effective despite lack of conclusive published data supporting clinical use.

> **Corporate-derived government-enabled pollution: Now broadly acknowledged as a major contributor to adverse healthcare outcomes and rising healthcare expenses**
>
> Humans in the general population worldwide have become living repositories for industrial pollutants and environmental contaminants, generally referred to in contemporary literature as POPs—persistent organic pollutants. POP retention/accumulation is causatively associated with induction of insulin resistance and the resulting hyperinsulinemia and hyperglycemia via suppression of GLUT-4 receptor expression via xenobiotic-induced activation of the aryl hydrocarbon receptor. Additively or synergistically, POP-induced mitochondrial dysfunction retards insulin secretion from the pancreas and insulin reception in the periphery, thereby synergizing to create the essential pathophysiology that characterizes type-2 diabetes.
>
> "Health care spending in the U.S. has surged more than eightfold since the 1960s. Skyrocketing in that same time: Rates of chronic disease, use of synthetic chemicals, and evidence that many of these widely used substances may be wreaking havoc on human health. ... New research published on Wednesday offers an example of this financial burden, widely overlooked in the health care debate. The use of bisphenol A, or BPA, in food and beverage containers, according to the study, is responsible for an estimated $3 billion a year in costs associated with childhood obesity and adult heart disease."
>
> Peeples L. BPA among Toxic Chemicals Driving Up Health Care Costs. 2014 Jan huffingtonpost.com/2014/01/22/bpa-health-care-costs_n_4644372.html

  o <u>Chlorella (Chlorella pyrenoidosa) supplementation decreases dioxin and increases immunoglobulin a concentrations in breast milk (*J Med Food.* 2007 Mar[63])</u>: "The present results suggest that Chlorella supplementation not only reduces dioxin levels in breast milk, but may also have beneficial effects on nursing infants by increasing IgA levels in breast milk."
  o <u>Maternal-fetal distribution and transfer of dioxins in pregnant women in Japan, and attempts to reduce maternal transfer with Chlorella (Chlorella pyrenoidosa) supplements (*Chemosphere.* 2005 Dec[64])</u>: "Concentrations of 28 dioxin (polychlorinated dibenzo-p-dioxins, polychlorinated dibenzofurans, and

---

[58] Krüger et al. Detection of glyphosate residues in animals and humans. *J Environ Anal Toxicol* 2014, 4:2 omicsonline.org/open-access/detection-of-glyphosate-residues-in-animals-and-humans-2161-0525.1000210.pdf
[59] Goel et al. Pesticide poisoning. *Nat Med J India* 2007:20;182-191
[60] Cohn WJ et al. Treatment of chlordecone (Kepone) toxicity with cholestyramine. Results of a controlled clinical trial. *N Engl J Med.* 1978 Feb 2;298(5):243-8
[61] Nakano S, Takekoshi H, Nakano M. Chlorella (Chlorella pyrenoidosa) supplementation decreases dioxin and increases immunoglobulin a concentrations in breast milk. *J Med Food.* 2007 Mar;10(1):134-42. Nakano S, Noguchi T, Takekoshi H, Suzuki G, Nakano M. Maternal-fetal distribution and transfer of dioxins in pregnant women in Japan, and attempts to reduce maternal transfer with Chlorella (Chlorella pyrenoidosa) supplements. *Chemosphere.* 2005 Dec;61(9):1244-55
[62] Cobbett CS. Phytochelatin biosynthesis and function in heavy-metal detoxification. *Current Opinion in Plant Biology* 2000, 3:211–216. Cobbett CS. Phytochelatins and their roles in heavy metal detoxification. *Plant Physiology* 2000 Jul; 825–832. Readers should have noticed that these are plant physiology journals—not clinical journals. These articles substantiate that phytochelatins are plant-produced metal-binding peptides; in clinical practice, extracts from certain vegetables rich in phytochelatins are used to bind heavy metals in the gut to reduce absorption and enterohepatic recirculation and promote fecal excretion, in a manner analogous to that of cholestyramine and chlorella.
[63] Nakano et al. Chlorella (Chlorella pyrenoidosa) supplementation decreases dioxin and increases immunoglobulin a concentrations in breast milk. *J Med Food.* 2007 Mar;10(1):134-42
[64] Nakano et al. Maternal-fetal distribution and transfer of dioxins in pregnant women in Japan, and attempts to reduce maternal transfer with Chlorella (Chlorella pyrenoidosa) supplements. *Chemosphere.* 2005 Dec;61(9):1244-55

co-planar polychlorinated biphenyls) congeners in blood, adipose tissue, breast milk, cord blood and placenta collected from 44 pregnant Japanese women were measured. ... Correlations were observed between dioxin total toxic equivalents (total TEQ) in blood and total TEQ in adipose tissue (r=0.913, P<0.0001), breast milk (r=0.695, P=0.0007), and cord blood (r=0.759, P<0.0001). Dioxin levels transferred to fetuses and nursing infants reflect cumulative maternal concentrations of dioxins. ... Total TEQ in breast milk were approximately 30% lower in the Chlorella group than in controls (P=0.0113). This finding suggests that maternal transfer of dioxins can be reduced using dietary measures such as Chlorella supplements.

- Chlorella pyrenoidosa on fecal excretion and liver accumulation of polychlorinated dibenzo-p-dioxin in mice. (*Chemosphere.* 2005 Apr[65]): "Among mice fed the 10% C. pyrenoidosa diet, cumulative fecal excretion of H6CDD over the first week following administration was significantly greater (9.2-fold) than that observed among mice fed the basal diet. Moreover, excretion during the fifth week following administration of H6CDD was still significantly greater (3.1-fold) among mice fed the 10% C. pyrenoidosa diet than among mice fed the basal diet. Five weeks after administration of H6CDD, liver accumulation of H6CDD in mice fed the 10% C. pyrenoidosa diet was significantly less than that observed among mice fed either the basal diet and the Spinach diet (by 27.9% and 34.8%, respectively). These findings suggest that C. pyrenoidosa may be useful in inhibiting the absorption of dioxins via food and the reabsorption of dioxins stored already in the body in the intestinal tract, thus preventing accumulation of dioxins within the body."

---

[65] Takekoshi et al. Effect of Chlorella pyrenoidosa on fecal excretion and liver accumulation of polychlorinated dibenzo-p-dioxin in mice. *Chemosphere.* 2005 Apr;59(2):297-304

Clinical Applications: Rheumatology

Fibromyalgia: FM, FMS, FMD

> **Introduction:**
> Fibromyalgia—also referred to as fibromyalgia syndrome (FMS) but more properly referred to as fibromyalgia disease (FMD)—is an organic clinical entity that has remained enigmatic to the medical profession despite the consistent publication of research that delineates its cause and its effective treatments. This chapter summarizes clinical assessments, treatments, and essential background information that—when properly applied—should provide empowering knowledge for clinicians and for the patients suffering with this condition.

Introduction
- **Overview**: Fibromyalgia (FM) is commonly described as an "idiopathic" (of unknown origin) syndrome principally characterized by widespread body pain and numerous myofascial tender points at specific locations. FM is most common in women 20-50 years of age, and the condition often presents with associated complaints of fatigue, headaches, subjective numbness, altered sleep patterns, and gastrointestinal disturbances. FM in children and adolescents presents similarly to FM in adults except for the comparatively higher prevalence of sleep disturbance and the finding of fewer tender points in children.[66] Until recently, fibromyalgia was considered a *diagnosis of exclusion* after infection, autoimmunity, or other primary causes of widespread pain were excluded by clinical and laboratory assessment. However, current criteria base the diagnosis on positive findings of chronic, widespread musculoskeletal pain in characteristic locations; these criteria will be described below. Fibromyalgia shares several clinical, demographic, and pathologic features with chronic fatigue syndrome (CFS) and irritable bowel syndrome (IBS); the reason for these overlaps is not generally understood by most clinicians and researchers but will be made plain in this writing.
- **The common medical view—scientifically inaccurate, financially leveraged**: The prevailing medical view, expressed by most medical doctors and the authors of widely cited articles, is that fibromyalgia is idiopathic—*of unknown origin*—with strong neuropsychogenic (*neuro*=nerves and brain, *psyche*=mind, *genic*=origin) influences (in other words, "It's all in your head.") and that, since the underlying causes of the condition have not been identified, the best therapeutic approach is symptom suppression via perpetual pharmacotherapy with adjunctive use of psychotherapy and limited exercise.[67,68,69] This prevailing medical view is unscientific (not based on science) and counterscientific (ignores and contradicts published and validated research), unethical (fails to provide effective treatment when such treatment is available; condemns patients to medicalization and suffering), and commercially leveraged (diagnostic criteria revision and many review articles discussing treatment are sponsored by drug companies; medical profession benefits financially by having many long-term drug-dependent patients).
- **Fibromyalgia is a disease, not a syndrome**: The term *syndrome* connotes that a cluster of symptoms is of a nonorganic, psychogenic, or idiopathic nature, whereas *disease* validates the organic and pathophysiological nature of an illness. This author advocates the use of *disease* rather than *syndrome* when describing fibromyalgia in appreciation of the real, organic, biochemical, and histopathological (*histo*=cells and tissues, *pathological*=disease) findings which clearly indicate that fibromyalgia is a specific disease entity and not simply a psychogenic or enigmatic cluster of symptoms. If fibromyalgia is a real, organic clinical entity (as will be documented here), then the appropriate designation is *fibromyalgia disease* (FMD) rather than *fibromyalgia syndrome* (FMS). For consistency and clarity within this section, the general term "fibromyalgia" will be used. Relatedly, the term "irritable bowel syndrome" (IBS) is also a misnomer that confuses professionals as well as the general public into thinking that the condition does not have identified causes and (nonpharmaceutical) treatments; despite promulgations to the contrary, the cause of IBS is well-known[70], and effective treatment is readily available.

---

[66] Siegel DM, Janeway D, Baum J. Fibromyalgia syndrome in children and adolescents: clinical features at presentation and status at follow-up. *Pediatrics* 1998;101:377-82
[67] Chakrabarty S, Zoorob R. Fibromyalgia. *Am Fam Physician*. 2007 Jul 15;76(2):247-54
[68] Tierney ML. McPhee SJ, Papadakis MA (eds). *Current Medical Diagnosis and Treatment 2006, 45th Edition*. New York: Lange Medical Books, pages 820-821
[69] Simms RW. Nonarticular soft tissue disorders. In Andreoli TE, Carpenter CCJ, Griggs RC, and Benjamin IJ (eds). *Cecil Essentials of Medicine, 7th Edition*. Elsevier 2007:851-2
[70] Lin HC. Small intestinal bacterial overgrowth: a framework for understanding irritable bowel syndrome. *JAMA*. 2004 Aug 18;292(7):852-8

Clinical Presentation

- **Prevalence, symptoms, and clinical findings**: Fibromyalgia is one of the most common chronic pain conditions, affecting an estimated 10 million people in the U.S. and an estimated 3-6% of people world-wide.[71] Approximately 10% of affected patients have severe symptoms resulting in partial or total disability. Affected patients report chronic aches, pains, and stiffness with a proclivity for localization near the neck, shoulders, low back, and hips. Pain and fatigue are typically exacerbated following physical exertion or psychological stress. Associated manifestations include fatigue, sleep disorders (including insomnia, unrefreshing sleep, and objective abnormalities such as an increase in stage 1 sleep, a reduction in delta sleep, and alpha-delta sleep anomaly), subjective numbness, headaches, and gastrointestinal disturbances consistent with a clinical diagnosis of irritable bowel syndrome (IBS). Clinical findings shared between FM and IBS include abdominal pain and discomfort, changed frequency of stool, diarrhea and/or constipation, abdominal bloating/distention/gas and flatulence, dyspepsia/heartburn, headaches especially migraine-type headaches), fatigue, myalgias, restless leg syndrome, anxiety, and depression. The **high prevalence (>50%) of migraine-type headaches in FM patients** suggests an underlying pathogenesis shared between cephalgia (*ceph*=head, *algia*=pain) and widespread myalgia (*myo*=muscle, *algia*=pain); one of the established and most likely causative abnormalities shared between migraine and FM is impaired mitochondrial function, which will be explained in greater detail later in this publication. Cognitive symptoms such as "brain fog" ("fibro-fog") and difficulty with memory and word retrieval, as well as **environmental intolerance (EI) and multiple chemical sensitivity (MCS)**, are seen in both FM and CFS[72]; again, this overlap of shared symptoms suggests a common etiopathogenesis (*etio*=cause, *patho*=disease, *genesis*=initiation). Routine physical examination and laboratory findings are generally normal, with the exception the physical examination finding of fibromyalgia tender points (described and diagrammed below in the section on Diagnosis per the 1990 diagnostic criteria).

Pathophysiology

- **Abnormalities noted in muscle tissue of patients with FM**: Muscle biopsies from patients with fibromyalgia show numerous histological, ultrastructural, and biochemical abnormalities, including defects in mitochondrial structure and function, reduced numbers of capillaries in skeletal muscle (leading to reduced blood supply to muscles), thickened capillary endothelium (thicker vessel walls), and ragged red fibers consistent with the development of **mitochondrial myopathy** (*myo*=muscle, *pathos*=disease). The histological finding of "rubber-band morphology" with reticular threads connecting neighboring cells in muscle biopsies of FM patients is associated with prolonged contractions in adjacent/neighboring muscle fibers; these abnormalities result in and perpetuate a low-energy state within myocytes (*myo*=muscle, *cytes*=cells).[73] Other studies have shown disorganization of actin filaments, accumulation of lipofuscin (cellular debris) consistent with premature muscle aging, accumulation of glycogen and lipid accumulation consistent with **mitochondrial impairment**, increased DNA fragmentation, **significant reductions in the number of mitochondria**, and focal areas of chronic muscle contraction.[74] These histological abnormalities are important and establish the fact that **fibromyalgia is a *disease of metabolic dysfunction*** rather than an *emotional disorder of psychogenic origin*; therefore, attributing the pain and fatigue of fibromyalgia to a mental-psychological cause or a central nervous system disorder such as central sensitization is unscientific and illogical.
- **Biochemical abnormalities noted in patients with FM**: Ultrastructural and biochemical abnormalities appear to be more pathologically significant and clinically relevant than the noted histological changes in skeletal muscle biopsy samples. Importantly, **the biochemical abnormalities *are the cause* of the histologic/tissue abnormalities**. Numerous **mitochondrial enzyme defects are seen**, including reduced activity of 3-hydroxy-CoA dehydrogenase, citrate synthase, and cytochrome oxidase. Levels of free magnesium are reduced by 31%, and levels of complexed ATP-magnesium are reduced by 12% in muscle from FM patients compared with

---

[71] "Fibromyalgia is one of the most common chronic pain conditions. The disorder affects an estimated 10 million people in the U.S. and an estimated 3-6% of the world population." National Fibromyalgia Association. fmaware.org/PageServera6cc.html?pagename=fibromyalgia_affected Accessed Sept 2012.
[72] Brown MM, Jason LA. Functioning in individuals with chronic fatigue syndrome: increased impairment with co-occurring multiple chemical sensitivity and fibromyalgia. *Dyn Med*. 2007 May 31;6:6 dynamic-med.com/content/6/1/6
[73] Olsen NJ, Park JH. Skeletal muscle abnormalities in patients with fibromyalgia. *Am J Med Sci*. 1998 Jun;315(6):351-8
[74] Sprott H, Salemi S, Gay RE, et al. Increased DNA fragmentation and ultrastructural changes in fibromyalgic muscle fibres. *Ann Rheum Dis*. 2004 Mar;63(3):245-51

levels seen in healthy controls; these biochemical and bioenergetic defects contribute to rapid-onset fatigue and muscle pain. From a neurophysiological perspective, magnesium can promote hypersensitivity to pain due to a reduction in the partial blockade of N-methyl-D-aspartate (NMDA) neurotransmitter receptor sites.[75] Reduced perfusion of muscle tissue during exercise results in relative tissue hypoxia, reduced muscle healing after the microtrauma of exercise, and promotion of muscle soreness due to accumulation of L-lactate (lactic acid).[76] **Increased oxidative stress** is also seen in FM patients,[77] providing additional objective evidence of the systemic, organic, and non-psychogenic nature of the illness. Evidence of hypothalamic-pituitary-adrenal disturbance and **increased cytokine production (particularly interleukin-8, which promotes sympathetic pain, and interleukin-6, which induces hyperalgesia [increased perception of pain], fatigue, and depression**[78]) further characterize the systemic and organic nature of this condition and are well documented in the research literature. **The majority of fibromyalgia patients demonstrate laboratory evidence of bacterial overgrowth in the small bowel**[79], and the details and important implications of this will be discussed below. **Vitamin D deficiency**—a recognized cause of chronic widespread pain as well as depression, muscle fatigue, and chronic low-grade inflammation—is also common in fibromyalgia patients.[80,81] FM patients have **significantly elevated blood levels of pentosidine**, which is an advanced glycation end-product (AGE) and marker of oxidative stress and glycosylation (sugar-protein binding); AGEs promote chronic inflammation and nociceptive sensitization leading to chronic pain.[82] Another AGE very similar to pentosidine, **carboxy-methyl-lysine (CML) is found in higher levels in the blood and muscle of FM patients**[83]; both pentosidine and CML cause expedited "muscle aging" and promote chronic pain and inflammation. These objective abnormalities of

Objective "organic" abnormalities noted in patients with fibromyalgia
1. <u>Histologic and functional abnormalities in muscle tissue</u>: Disorganization of actin filaments, accumulation of lipofuscin bodies consistent with premature muscle aging, increased DNA fragmentation, and focal areas of chronic muscle contraction, reduced perfusion of muscle tissue during exercise (i.e., reduced blood flow to muscles).
2. <u>Mitochondrial defects</u>: Accumulation of glycogen (muscle sugar) and lipid (fat) indicate that intracellular energy production is impaired and that the cells are unable to efficiently convert fuel sources into energy in the form of ATP, adenosine triphosphate, which is the basic fuel source for cellular metabolism. Also noted are significant reductions in the number of mitochondria, reduced activity of important enzymes such as 3-hydroxy-CoA dehydrogenase, citrate synthase, and cytochrome oxidase. Nutritional deficiencies, such as CoQ-10 deficiency, promote mitochondrial dysfunction, thus leading to mitochondrial destruction (mitophagy) which ultimately results in reduced numbers of mitochondria and perpetuates and aggravates muscle fatigue, pain, and neurocognitive dysfunction (i.e., brain fog, difficulty thinking, depression).
3. <u>Oxidative stress</u>: Increased oxidative stress results from mitochondrial dysfunction and nutrient depletion.
4. <u>Neuroendocrine abnormalities</u>: Hypothalamic-pituitary-adrenal (HPA) disturbance indicates impaired function of the brain and endocrine system.
5. <u>Low-grade immune activation</u>: Increased cytokine production indicates a pro-inflammatory state.
6. <u>Bacterial overgrowth in the intestines</u>: FM patients nearly always have excess/overgrowth of bacteria in their intestines, referred to as SIBO—small intestine bacterial overgrowth.
7. <u>High prevalence of vitamin D deficiency</u>: Common in the general population but more common in patients with chronic pain; vitamin D deficiency causes chronic pain, depression/anxiety, and low-grade inflammation—all of these problems are seen in patients with fibromyalgia.
8. <u>Low blood levels of L-tryptophan</u>: FM patients have low levels of the amino acid tryptophan in their blood, despite adequate dietary intake. The most likely explanation for the deficiency of tryptophan is destruction of tryptophan by bacterial enzyme action. Several intestinal bacteria produce the enzyme tryptophanase, which destroys the amino acid tryptophan. Bacterial overgrowth results in more tryptophanase, resulting in tryptophan deficiency. Deficiency of tryptophan results in deficiencies of the hormones serotonin and melatonin, which result in anxiety, depression, food/sugar cravings, unrestful sleep, and mitochondrial dysfunction, since deficiency of melatonin causes reduced mitochondrial energy-production efficiency.

---

[75] Park JH, Niermann KJ, Olsen N. Evidence for metabolic abnormalities in the muscles of patients with fibromyalgia. *Curr Rheumatol Rep*. 2000 Apr;2(2):131-40
[76] Elvin et al. Decreased muscle blood flow in fibromyalgia patients during standardised muscle exercise. *Eur J Pain*. 2006 Feb;10(2):137-44
[77] Altindag O, Celik H. Total antioxidant capacity and the severity of the pain in patients with fibromyalgia. *Redox Rep*. 2006;11(3):131-5
[78] Wallace DJ, Linker-Israeli M, Hallegua D, et al. Cytokines play an aetiopathogenetic role in fibromyalgia. *Rheumatology* (Oxford). 2001 Jul;40(7):743-9
[79] Pimentel et al. A link between irritable bowel syndrome and fibromyalgia may be related to findings on lactulose breath testing. *Ann Rheum Dis*. 2004 Apr;63(4):450-2
[80] Huisman AM, White KP, Algra A, et al. Vitamin D levels in women with systemic lupus erythematosus and fibromyalgia. *J Rheumatol*. 2001 Nov;28(11):2535-9
[81] Armstrong DJ, Meenagh GK, Bickle I, et al. Vitamin D deficiency is associated with anxiety and depression in fibromyalgia. *Clin Rheumatol*. 2007 Apr;26(4):551-4
[82] Hein G, Franke S. Are advanced glycation end-product-modified proteins of pathogenetic importance in fibromyalgia? *Rheumatology* (Oxford). 2002 Oct;41(10):1163-7
[83] "In the interstitial connective tissue of fibromyalgic muscles we found a more intensive staining of the AGE CML, activated NF-kappaB, and also higher CML levels in the serum of these patients compared to the controls. RAGE was only present in FM muscle." Rüster M, Franke S, Späth M, Pongratz DE, Stein G, Hein GE. Detection of elevated N epsilon-carboxymethyllysine levels in muscular tissue and in serum of patients with fibromyalgia. *Scand J Rheumatol*. 2005 Nov-Dec;34(6):460-3

biochemical, histological, nutritional, and microbiological/gastrointestinal status force clinicians to appreciate the valid and organic nature of fibromyalgia. As previously stated, this evidence refutes promulgations espoused within standard allopathic/pharmaceutical medicine that fibromyalgia is an idiopathic condition warranting lifelong medicalization with expensive and potentially hazardous analgesic and antidepressant drugs; the focus on drug treatment to mask/suppress the pain of fibromyalgia detours doctors and patients away from focusing on the legitimate and validated causes of fibromyalgia and physiology-based (rather than pharmacology-based) means for alleviating the suffering and pain that these patients experience.

CONTROL

PATIENT

Blood cells in FM patients show mitochondrial destruction (mitophagy), smaller size and lower number of mitochondria: Structure of blood mononuclear cells (BMCs, cells of the immune system) from FM patients. The healthy/control BMCs show mitochondria with a normal structure. Autophagosomes (indicated by arrows), where mitochondria are destroyed (the process of mitophagy [*mito*=mitochondria, *phagy*=consumption], are noted in the BMCs of patients with FM. [Bar = 1 micrometer]. This open-access image is respectfully attributed to the brilliant research published by these researchers Cordero MD, De Miguel M, Moreno Fernández AM, Carmona López IM, Garrido Maraver J, Cotán D, Gómez Izquierdo L, Bonal P, Campa F, Bullon P, Navas P, Sánchez Alcázar JA. Mitochondrial dysfunction and mitophagy activation in blood mononuclear cells of fibromyalgia patients. *Arthritis Res Ther*. 2010;12(1):R17 arthritis-research.com/content/12/1/R17

Mitophagy: The body's inherent mechanism for the destruction of dysfunctional mitochondria

Concept: Autophagic destruction of mitochondria is termed "mitophagy" and is the body's inherent mechanism for eliminating superfluous or dysfunctional mitochondria; this generally has a protective and life-sustaining effect. However, in the case of fibromyalgia wherein the mitochondrial dysfunction is persistent, prolonged mitophagy contributes to failure of adequate energy production and thereby contributes to clinical manifestations of fatigue, dyscognition, and impaired exercise/activity performance. Further, the consistent documentation of significant mitophagy in patients with fibromyalgia proves the biological/organic/real/pathophysiologic character of the illness and refutes the pharmacocentric paradigm which holds that the condition is of psychogenic or neurologic origin and thus to be treated with so-called "antidepressants" and/or analgesic drugs, respectively.

- "The removal of damaged mitochondria that could contribute to cellular dysfunction or death is achieved through process of mitochondrial autophagy, i.e. mitophagy." Novak I. *Antioxid Redox Signal*. 2011
- "Mitochondrial number and health are regulated by mitophagy, a process by which excessive or damaged mitochondria are subjected to autophagic degradation." Rambold. *Cell Cycle*. 2011
- **"Autophagy can be beneficial for the cells by eliminating dysfunctional mitochondria, but massive autophagy can promote cell injury and may contribute to the pathophysiology of FM (fibromyalgia)."** Cordero. *Arthritis Res Ther*. 2010

Diagnosis

- **Clinical criteria—description and contrast of the 1990 criteria and the 2010 criteria**: Per guidelines published in 1990 by the American College of Rheumatology (ACR), a diagnosis of fibromyalgia can be made in a patient with inexplicable, widespread myofascial pain of at least 3 months' duration; *inexplicable* denotes normalcy of routine laboratory and physical examination findings and failure to find an alternate explanation or diagnosis, while *widespread* denotes bilateral pain above and below the waist not attributable to trauma or rheumatic disease and with pain at 11 of 18 classic tender point locations (see illustration below). FM tender points are assessed bilaterally at 9 paired sites: (sub)occiput (below the head at the neckline), low cervical spine (lower neck), trapezius and supraspinatus (two of the shoulder muscles), second rib (anterior, near costosternal [rib-breastbone] junction), lateral epicondyle, gluteal region, greater trochanter, and medial fat pad of the knees. Tender points are provoked by the clinician's application of approximately 9 pounds of fingertip pressure, which is sufficient to cause blanching of the clinician's nail bed. The tender points of fibromyalgia are distinguished from myofascial trigger points (MFTP, described by Travell[84]) and strain-counterstrain tender points (described in the osteopathic literature by Jones[85]). In contrast to MFTP, which are located toward the center of the muscle fiber and which refer pain and show spontaneous electrocontractile activity[86], tender points of fibromyalgia are located near the tendinous insertions of muscle to bone and cause local pain only, without pain referral or contractile activity.

Clinical findings: Pain, on digital palpation, must be present in at least 11 of the following 18 tender point sites:
1. Occiput: at the suboccipital muscle insertions.
2. Low cervical: at the anterior aspects of the intertransverse spaces at C5-C7.
3. Trapezius: at the midpoint of the upper border.
4. Supraspinatus: at origins, above the scapula spine near the medial border.
5. Second rib: upper lateral to the second costochondral junction.
6. Lateral epicondyle: 2 cm distal to the epicondyles.
7. Gluteal: in upper outer quadrants of buttocks in anterior fold of muscle.
8. Greater trochanter: posterior to the trochanteric prominence.
9. Knee: at the medial fat pad proximal to the joint line.

Illustration of the 9 paired locations of FM tender points: Per 1990 ACR guidelines, the diagnosis of FM is supported when at least 11 out of 18 of these locations are painful. Digital palpation should be performed with an approximate force of 4 kg (9 lbs). A tender point has to be painful at palpation, not just "tender."[87]

The new 2010 ACR guidelines for the diagnosis and assessment of FM[88] are significantly different from the 1990 guidelines. These new guidelines are mostly illogical and appear to have been structured to broaden the definition of fibromyalgia, to allow patients and nonphysicians to make the diagnosis, and generally to increase the patient population available for a diagnosis of fibromyalgia, thereby increasing the sales of drugs.

---

[84] Simons DG, Travell JG, Simons LS. *Travell & Simons' Myofascial Pain and Dysfunction. The Trigger Point Manual*. Baltimore: Lippincott Williams & Wilkins; 1999
[85] Jones L, Kusunose R, Goering E. *Jones Strain-Counterstrain*. Carlsbad, Jones Strain Counterstrain Incorporated, 1995. [ISBN 0964513544]
[86] Hubbard DR, Berkoff GM. Myofascial trigger points show spontaneous needle EMG activity. *Spine*. 1993 Oct 1;18(13):1803-7
[87] The American College of Rheumatology 1990 Criteria for the Classification of Fibromyalgia. nfra.net/Diagnost.htm Accessed Nov 2011
[88] Wolfe F, et al. The ACR preliminary diagnostic criteria for fibromyalgia and measurement of symptom severity. *Arthritis Care Res*. 2010;62(5):600-10

Widespread pain index (WPI): Each positive location receives one point (max = 19)

1. Shoulder girdle, left	7. Hip (buttock/trochanter), left	13. Jaw, left
2. Shoulder girdle, right	8. Hip (buttock/trochanter), right	14. Jaw, right
3. Upper arm, left	9. Upper leg, left	15. Chest (sternum area)
4. Upper arm, right	10. Upper leg, right	16. Abdomen
5. Lower arm, left	11. Lower leg, left	17. Neck
6. Lower arm, right	12. Lower leg, right	18. Upper back
		19. Lower back

Symptom severity (SS)—part 1: Each of the following three problems is quantified with the following scale (max = 9):

0 none: no problem **1 mild**: intermittent or mild problems
2 moderate: often present, considerable problems **3 severe**: continuous, life-disturbing problems

0 1 2 3 Fatigue   0 1 2 3 Waking unrefreshed   0 1 2 3 Cognitive symptoms

Symptom severity (SS)—part 2: The clinician considers the patient's "somatic symptoms in general" (listed below) and applies the following scale (max = 3):
0 no symptoms 1 few symptoms
2 a moderate number of symptoms 3 a great deal of symptoms

0 1 2 3 muscle pain	0 1 2 3 itching
0 1 2 3 irritable bowel syndrome	0 1 2 3 wheezing
0 1 2 3 fatigue/tiredness	0 1 2 3 Raynaud's phenomenon
0 1 2 3 thinking or remembering problems	0 1 2 3 hives/welts
0 1 2 3 muscle weakness	0 1 2 3 ringing in ears
0 1 2 3 headache	0 1 2 3 vomiting
0 1 2 3 pain/cramps in the abdomen	0 1 2 3 heartburn
0 1 2 3 numbness/tingling	0 1 2 3 oral ulcers
0 1 2 3 dizziness	0 1 2 3 loss of/change in taste
0 1 2 3 insomnia	0 1 2 3 seizures
0 1 2 3 depression	0 1 2 3 dry eyes
0 1 2 3 constipation	0 1 2 3 shortness of breath
0 1 2 3 pain in the upper abdomen	0 1 2 3 loss of appetite
0 1 2 3 nausea	0 1 2 3 skin rash
0 1 2 3 nervousness	0 1 2 3 sun sensitivity
0 1 2 3 chest pain	0 1 2 3 hearing difficulties
0 1 2 3 blurred vision	0 1 2 3 easy bruising
0 1 2 3 fever	0 1 2 3 hair loss
0 1 2 3 diarrhea	0 1 2 3 frequent urination
0 1 2 3 dry mouth	0 1 2 3 painful urination
	0 1 2 3 bladder spasms

Tally points from above; patients may be diagnosed with FM if **"WPI >7 and SS >5"** or **"WPI 3–6 and SS >9"**.
WPI = ____
SS1 + SS2 = ____

2010 Fibromyalgia diagnostic criteria—summary, chart for clinical use, discussion: Per the 2010 diagnostic criteria[89], patients may be diagnosed with fibromyalgia if "WPI >7 and SS >5" or "WPI 3–6 and SS >9". Of note, these new criteria reflect a major departure from the former criteria published and codified in 1990; of additional note, publication of these new criteria received sponsorship from a drug company which has an FDA-approved drug for this condition—this represents a massive conflict of interest, full manifestation of which would have the same for-profit entity influencing the criteria used by doctors for the diagnosis and then providing (i.e., selling for profit) one of the only approved drug treatment options. I have discussed these conundrums in video format at Vimeo.com/ICHNFM and Vimeo.com/DrVasquez.

Very curiously, the authors state that one of their objectives was to create criteria that "do not require a tender point examination"; at first, this seems odd and clinically inconsistent considering that the tender point examination ❶ takes only about 60 seconds to perform, ❷ is noninvasive, ❸ was previously the standard by which the diagnosis was made, and ❹ is reasonable and responsible—physical examination of patients with pain is a reasonable standard of care. Oddly, the authors of the new guidelines note several "important problems" with the 1990 ACR criteria, such as "Patients who improved or whose symptoms and tender points

---

[89] Wolfe F, et al. The ACR preliminary diagnostic criteria for fibromyalgia and measurement of symptom severity. *Arthritis Care Res.* 2010;62(5):600-10

decreased could fail to satisfy the ACR 1990 classification definition" and "there was little variation in symptoms among fibromyalgia patients." Clinicians should note that these so-called "problems" *are not problems at all* because patients who improve and thus no longer meet diagnostic criteria should not be considered to have an active disease/diagnosis, and that high-quality clinical criteria should indeed result in the specific definition of clinical disorder and thus in a well-defined cohort of patients; correcting these "problems" results in patients being diagnosed for longer periods of time (more *long-term* patients) and also results in more patients being diagnosed with fibromyalgia (more *total* patients). Perhaps even more curious is the fact that development of these new guidelines was sponsored by Lilly Research Laboratories—the front page of the article states "these criteria were developed with support from the study sponsor, Lilly Research Laboratories", which is the "research" section of Eli Lilly and Company, one of the world's largest drug companies and the manufacturer of duloxetine/Cymbalta® which is one of the only drugs approved by the US Food and Drug Administration (FDA) for the treatment of fibromyalgia.[90] Among patients labeled with fibromyalgia, the new criteria increase the percentage of patients diagnosable by criteria from 75% to 88%; whether the motivation to expand the patient population diagnosed with fibromyalgia is altruistic or financially motivated is subject to debate. The new criteria rely on a summation of two tallies—"widespread pain index" (WPI) and "symptom severity" (SS, parts 1 and 2)—with the diagnosis being supported by either **"WPI >7 and SS >5"** or **"WPI 3–6 and SS >9"**. Pain must have been consistent for at least three months and must not be attributable to another (obvious) cause.

- **Clinical profile and findings on common laboratory tests**: New-onset fibromyalgia is unlikely over age 50, and the condition never causes fever, significant weight loss, or other objective signs of acute or subacute illness. Hypothyroidism is common and can produce widespread myofascial pain along with depression and other complaints, resulting in a clinical picture that closely resembles FM; thus, a complete thyroid evaluation (detailed later) is essential during the initial evaluation of any fibromyalgia-like condition. Common rheumatic conditions such as rheumatoid arthritis (RA) and systemic lupus erythematosus (SLE) are excluded by the lack of other clinical manifestations (e.g., joint pain and swelling) and the lack of positive laboratory findings such as anti-cyclic citrullinated protein (CCP) antibodies and antinuclear antibodies (ANA), respectively. C-reactive protein (CRP) and erythrocyte sedimentation rate (ESR) are normal in FM patients; abnormalities with these or other common laboratory assessments suggest inflammatory disease, infection, or other concomitant illness. Hypophosphatemia (a low level of the electrolyte phosphate in the blood) can cause bone pain and muscle weakness; this condition is easily excluded by demonstration of normal serum phosphate level.

Standard Medical Treatment for Fibromyalgia
- **Overview**: Mild exercise, "patient education", and the use of pain-relieving drugs are mainstays of standard medical treatment delivered by most allopathic medical doctors (MDs), and osteopathic medical doctors (DOs) may add manual musculoskeletal treatments to enhance the benefits of drugs.[91] These interventions are only partially effective and offer no hope of actually curing the disease; thus, medical treatment relegates patients to a future of drug dependency, potential adverse effects (some of which can be fatal), and therapeutic inefficacy insofar as none of these treatments addresses the underlying cause of the disorder.
    - **Amitriptyline**: For many years, the most widely used drug for symptomatic treatment of fibromyalgia was amitriptyline (a tricyclic antidepressant), which has been used "off label"—without approval from the FDA—for this application. In the treatment of FM, the drug has low efficacy and high potential for adverse effects; up to 20% of patients suffer from weight gain, constipation, orthostatic hypotension, and/or agitation as a side-effect of the drug. Only 25% to 30% of fibromyalgia patients experience clinically significant improvement with amitriptyline.[92] According to recent research in rats, administration of amitriptyline causes deficiency of CoQ-10, impaired mitochondrial function, reduced ATP/energy

---

[90] lilly.com/research/Pages/research.aspx and newsroom.lilly.com/ReleaseDetail.cfm?releaseid=316740 Accessed January 2012
[91] Gamber RG, Shores JH, Russo DP, Jimenez C, Rubin BR. Osteopathic manipulative treatment in conjunction with medication relieves pain associated with fibromyalgia syndrome: results of a randomized clinical pilot project. *J Am Osteopath Assoc.* 2002 Jun;102(6):321-5 jaoa.org/content/102/6/321.full.pdf
[92] Leventhal LJ. Management of fibromyalgia. *Ann Intern Med.* 1999 Dec 7;131(11):850-8

production, and increased oxidative stress and free radical damage[93]; all of these drug-induced problems (discussed in detail later in this paper) are expected to worsen the pain and suffering experienced by FM patients. Thus, the use of amitriptyline cannot be considered to be consistent with the practice of good medicine due to its low efficacy and unacceptable risks for adverse effects.

- **Pregabalin**: In 2007, the United States Food and Drug Administration (US FDA) approved pregabalin (Lyrica® sold/marketed by Pfizer) for symptomatic treatment of fibromyalgia[94]; however, because the drug does not address the primary cause(s) of the disease, patients must continue treatment indefinitely. Adverse effects of pregabalin include dizziness, sleepiness, blurred vision, **weight gain**, dry mouth, swelling of hands and feet, impairment of motor function, and problems with concentration and attention. Pregabalin when given at the recommended dose of 150-225 mg twice per day for fibromyalgia costs $94-190 per month (pricing in 2013).

  > **Suicide and depression risk warning for pregabalin/Lyrica from the US FDA**
  >
  > "Antiepileptic drugs (AEDs), including Lyrica, increase the risk of suicidal thoughts or behavior in patients taking these drugs for any indication. Patients treated with any AED for any indication should be monitored for the emergence or worsening of depression, suicidal thoughts or behavior, and/or any unusual changes in mood or behavior."
  >
  > fda.gov/Safety/MedWatch/SafetyInformation/Safety-RelatedDrugLabelingChanges/ucm154524.htm

- **Duloxetine**: In 2008, the FDA announced duloxetine (Cymbalta® sold/marketed by Lilly) as the second approved drug for the treatment of fibromyalgia. Ironically, many physicians consider any "approved" drug to have scientific substantiation; however, in the case of duloxetine (as well as pregabalin) the exact mechanism of action is unknown[95] although duloxetine appears to inhibit reuptake of norepinephrine and serotonin, thereby increasing the action of these neurotransmitters in the synaptic cleft. Adverse effects from duloxetine include nausea, dry mouth, sleepiness, constipation, decreased appetite, and increased sweating; **duloxetine can also increase the risk of suicidal thinking and behavior and for this reason the drug carries a black box warning on the container**. Duloxetine can cause serious and fatal adverse effects including the following: worsening depression and suicidality, serotonin syndrome, neuroleptic malignant syndrome, seizures, and Stevens-Johnson syndrome. Duloxetine given at the recommended dose of 60 mg per day for FM costs $170 per month (pricing in 2013).

  > **Suicide and depression risk warning for duloxetine/Cymbalta**
  >
  > "WARNING: Suicidality and Antidepressant Drugs: Antidepressants increased the risk compared to placebo of suicidal thinking and behavior (suicidality) in children, adolescents, and young adults in short-term studies of major depressive disorder (MDD) and other psychiatric disorders. Anyone considering the use of Cymbalta or any other antidepressant in a child, adolescent, or young adult must balance this risk with the clinical need. Short-term studies did not show an increase in the risk of suicidality with antidepressants compared to placebo in adults beyond age 24; there was a reduction in risk with antidepressants compared to placebo in adults aged 65 and older. Depression and certain other psychiatric disorders are themselves associated with increases in the risk of suicide. Patients of all ages who are started on antidepressant therapy should be monitored appropriately and observed closely for clinical worsening, suicidality, or unusual changes in behavior. Families and caregivers should be advised of the need for close observation and communication with the prescriber. Cymbalta is not approved for use in pediatric patients."
  >
  > pi.lilly.com/us/cymbalta-pi.pdf

- **Milnacipran**: Approved for the treatment of FM by the US FDA in 2009, milnacipran (Savella® sold/marketed by Forest Pharmaceuticals) inhibits norepinephrine and serotonin reuptake, i.e., it potentiates (increases the effect of) the neurotransmitters norepinephrine and serotonin, both of which decrease the experience of pain and elevate mood. Of course, other non-drug treatments (such as nutrients and dietary optimization) can have the same effect, but most medical doctors have no training in nondrug

---

[93] "Amitriptyline is a tricyclic antidepressant commonly prescribed for the treatment of several neuropathic and inflammatory illnesses. We have already reported that amitriptyline has cytotoxic effect in human cell cultures, increasing oxidative stress, and decreasing growth rate and mitochondrial activity." Bautista-Ferrufino MR, Cordero MD, Sánchez-Alcázar JA, et al. Amitriptyline induces coenzyme Q deficiency and oxidative damage in mouse lung and liver. *Toxicol Lett.* 2011 Jul 4;204(1):32-7
[94] FDA Approves First Drug for Treating Fibromyalgia. fda.gov/bbs/topics/NEWS/2007/NEW01656.html
[95] "exact mechanism of action unknown; inhibits norepinephrine and serotonin reuptake" https://online.epocrates.com; "Both Lyrica and Cymbalta reduce pain and improve function in people with fibromyalgia. While those with fibromyalgia have been shown to experience pain differently from other people, the mechanism by which these drugs produce their effects is unknown. fda.gov/ForConsumers/ConsumerUpdates/ucm107802.htm. Accessed January 2012

treatments[96,97,98,99] and thus habitually turn to drugs as the one-and-only answer to the patients' problems[100], especially when these are sanctified by FDA/government approval. Nondrug treatments that enhance serotonergic and noradrenergic neurotransmission include exercise, relaxation, massage, and nutritional supplementation with omega-3 fatty acids (as found in fish oil), nutritional supplementation in general and vitamin D supplementation in particular. Adverse effects associated with use of

> **Suicide and depression risk warning for milnacipran/Savella**
>
> "Savella is a selective serotonin and norepinephrine reuptake inhibitor (SNRI), similar to some drugs used for the treatment of depression and other psychiatric disorders. Antidepressants increased the risk compared to placebo of suicidal thinking and behavior (suicidality) in children, adolescents, and young adults in short-term studies of major depressive disorder (MDD) and other psychiatric disorders."
>
> frx.com/pi/Savella_pi.pdf, linked as "Full Prescribing Information" from savella.com/important-risk-information.aspx

milnacipran include seizures, suicidality, depression, worsening hypomania/mania, Stevens-Johnson syndrome (which is a medical emergency that can be fatal), serotonin syndrome, neuroleptic malignant syndrome, hypertensive (elevated blood pressure) crisis, tachycardia (rapid heart rate), hyponatremia (low sodium in the blood, which can occasionally result in permanent brain damage), abnormal bleeding (due to abnormal platelet function), glaucoma, and liver toxicity.[101] Treatment of fibromyalgia is the only FDA-approved use of this medication, which when used at the recommended dose of 50 mg twice daily costs $144 per month (pricing in April 2013). This drug is accompanied by a "black box warning" alerting physicians and patients to an increase in risk of suicide.

- **Cyclobenzaprine, Tramadol, and acetaminophen**: Cyclobenzaprine (a muscle-relaxing drug), Tramadol (a non-typical opioid, centrally-acting narcotic analgesic) and acetaminophen (centrally acting analgesic), show low efficacy and have little research supporting their use in the treatment of FM; these drugs also carry important risks for adverse effects, and they do not favorably alter the course of the disease over the long-term.[102] Per recent information from the American College of Rheumatology (ACR), treatment of FM with opioid drugs "may cause greater pain sensitivity or make pain persist."[103]
- **Exercise**: Low-intensity aerobic exercise may initially exacerbate symptoms but can result in very modest mental and physical improvement. Exercise alone cannot cure FM.
- **Cognitive-behavioral therapy (CBT)**: Cognitive-behavioral therapy helps patients deal with and adapt to the impact of the illness. Therapy alone cannot cure FM.
- **Patient (mis)education in standard medicine**: "Patient education" from a *medical* perspective generally means telling patients that ❶ they will probably have the condition forever, ❷ they will not immediately die from it, ❸ they need to take it seriously (i.e., comply with medical treatment), and ❹ they need to rely on drugs for alleviation of symptoms since no cause of the condition is known and therefore no direct treatment is available. From the medial perspective, these communications are considered "helpful" and "reassuring"; however, part of the effect that is created is **dependency** ("You need these drugs from me."), **passivity** ("There's nothing you can do about this, so don't even try to think for yourself or seek 'alternative' treatments."), and **co-victimization** ("We are both victims of our ignorance; I am in this with you in that we are both blind and dependent on drug management."). In the examples that follow, I will review and summarize patient educational materials from major medical journals; for efficiency, I will use quotes followed by my comments in *italics*:

---

[96] "Internal medicine interns' perceive nutrition counseling as a priority, but lack the confidence and knowledge to effectively provide adequate nutrition education." Vetter ML, Herring SJ, Sood M, Shah NR, Kalet AL. What do resident physicians know about nutrition? An evaluation of attitudes, self-perceived proficiency and knowledge. *J Am Coll Nutr*. 2008 Apr;27(2):287-98 ncbi.nlm.nih.gov/pmc/articles/PMC2779722/
[97] "The amount of nutrition education that medical students receive continues to be inadequate." Adams KM, Kohlmeier M, Zeisel SH. Nutrition education in U.S. medical schools: latest update of a national survey. *Acad Med*. 2010 Sep;85(9):1537-42
[98] "Scientific advances on the relationship of dietary substances to the cellular mechanisms of disease occur with regularity and frequency. Yet, despite the prevalence of nutritional disorders in clinical medicine and increasing scientific evidence on the significance of dietary modification to disease prevention, present day practitioners of medicine are typically untrained in the relationship of diet to health and disease." Halsted CH. The relevance of clinical nutrition education and role models to the practice of medicine. *Eur J Clin Nutr*. 1999 May;53 Suppl 2:S29-34
[99] Vasquez A. Interventions need to be consistent with osteopathic philosophy. *J Am Osteopath Assoc*. 2006 Sep;106(9):528-9 jaoa.org/content/106/9/528.full.pdf
[100] Ely et al. Analysis of questions asked by family doctors regarding patient care. *BMJ*. 1999 Aug 7;319(7206):358-61 ncbi.nlm.nih.gov/pmc/articles/PMC28191/
[101] https://online.epocrates.com/noFrame/showPage.do?method=drugs&MonographId=4950 Accessed April 2012.
[102] Goldenberg DL, Burckhardt C, Crofford L. Management of fibromyalgia syndrome. *JAMA*. 2004 Nov 17;292(19):2388-95
[103] rheumatology.org/practice/clinical/patients/diseases_and_conditions/fibromyalgia.asp Accessed April 2012

- Patient education from American Academy of Family Physicians accessed April 2012 from the website FamilyDoctor.org[104]:
    - "…your muscles and organs are not being damaged." — *This is false/inaccurate information. Several primary research studies have demonstrated consistently pathologic and biochemical abnormalities in muscle tissue from patients with fibromyalgia; this research has been published in widely available peer-reviewed medical journals.*
    - "This condition is not life-threatening, but it is chronic (ongoing). Although there is no cure,..." — *This is false information (the condition is curable); the statement as it reads produces patient passivity and drug-dependency, which is exactly what the medical profession and the drug industry wants.*
    - "There isn't currently a cure for fibromyalgia. Your care will focus on helping you minimize the impact of fibromyalgia on your life and treating your symptoms. Your doctor can prescribe medicine to help with your pain,... The treatment recommendations your doctor makes won't do any good unless you follow them." — *Again, false information that promotes passivity and medical-drug dependency.*
    - Weak recommendations under the guise of "taking an active role in your healthcare" include 1) maintaining a healthy outlook, 2) support groups, 3) **take medicines exactly as prescribed**, 4) moderate exercise, 5) stress management, 6) "establish healthy sleep habits", 7) make a routine daily schedule, 8) "make healthy lifestyle choices." *Most of these recommendations are blatantly passive, vague, and ineffective while fostering drug-dependency.*
- "Patient Education—Fibromyalgia" from the American College of Rheumatology accessed in April 2012 from the website Rheumatology.org[105]:
    - "Though there is no cure, medications can relieve symptoms." — *This is a commonly used statement within the medical community from doctors to patients to create passivity and drug/medical dependency.*
    - "There likely are certain genes that can make people more prone to getting fibromyalgia and the other health problems that can occur with it. Genes alone, though, do not cause fibromyalgia." — *These are common statements in the medical community, basically summed as "We don't know what we are doing but your only hope is to depend on us."*
    - "For the person with fibromyalgia, it is as though the "volume control" is turned up too high in the brain's pain processing centers." — *This promotes the concept of "primary central sensitization" (i.e., the brain has defied normal physiology and has somehow [without known cause, by itself] become too sensitive to pain); this "blame the brain" concept is used to leverage drug sales for pain-relieving and anti-depressant drugs as I have recently reviewed in video: youtube.com/watch?v=41opevN87qs*
    - "There is no cure for fibromyalgia. However, symptoms can be treated with both medication and non-drug treatments." — *This is the standard "party line" for the medical profession, whose chief goal is not to cure diseases but rather to drug them indefinitely, thereby creating a perpetual audience for their services and prescriptions. Honorable mention (more accurately: dishonorable mention) is generally given to "lifestyle modification" but is generally done so in a way that provides vague advice for ineffective interventions, thereby **creating the illusion of options** while undercutting any potential for these "options" to actually work.*
    - Non-drug treatments reviewed: relaxation, deep breathing, meditation, sleep, avoidance of nicotine and caffeine, exercise including such revelations as "take the stairs instead of the elevator, or park further [sic] away from the store", and "education" from other medical and special interest groups. *These are all essentially worthless suggestions, but they are effective distractions for patients and doctors so that effective treatments are marginalized and drug/medical dependency is fostered.*
    - Prescription drugs are given the primary emphasis in the treatment section. *Whether drugs are effective or not, the medical profession relies on drugs for its position in society and will therefore advocate their use.*

---

[104] American Academy of Family Physicians. familydoctor.org/familydoctor/en/diseases-conditions/fibromyalgia.html Accessed March 31, 2012
[105] rheumatology.org/practice/clinical/patients/diseases_and_conditions/fibromyalgia.asp Accessed March 31, 2012

	The most common pattern in medical books and articles: components of the medical paradigm
1.	Diseases are describable yet incomprehensible: The condition generally is described as a complex interplay of genetic factors with numerous environmental factors; generally little or no intellectually worthwhile effort is made to understand these environmental factors, so the ultimate view that medical physicians are taught is the disease is not understood and that drug therapy is the best available treatment.
2.	Characteristics and diagnostic criteria are reviewed: The medical profession is very good at defining and diagnosing problems, but the reliance on drugs often detours from the more effective nondrug treatments.
3.	Nondrug treatments are marginalized: Brief mention is made of diet and lifestyle and other non-drug treatments, but the information is nonspecific, very general, and almost always diluted to the point of inefficacy.
4.	Authentic integrative and functional medicine approaches are essentially never mentioned: Generally, the only nondrug treatments that are mentioned are weak or are mentioned so casually that no action can be taken from the information presented.
5.	Nearly always the disease is described as chronic and incurable: Even if a cure is known and published in available peer-reviewed research, most medical books and articles conclude that the causes are unknown and that drug treatment is warranted.
6.	Drug treatments are emphasized: Drug benefits are inflated and adverse effects are minimized if mentioned at all. Many review articles published in clinical journals are authored by consultants to the drug industry who profit from the sale of the drugs used to treat the condition about which they write; the general conclusion of these articles is that "Medical research is making considerable advances in our understanding of Disease X, which results from a complex interplay of genetic and environmental factors. The appropriate treatment for Disease X is Drug X, then others.
7.	Hope for the future is always placed back in the hands of "more research" and "drug development": Often some mention of "hope for the future" is made, generally in the guise of "medical research" and "drug development"; all the while, safe and effective non-drug treatment approaches that go far beyond diet and lifestyle are virtually never mentioned.

Functional/Naturopathic Considerations, Assessments, and Interventions

- **Foundational perspectives**: Two fundamental premises of are: (1) ~~chronic~~ sustained *diseases* are manifestations of ~~chronic~~ sustained *dysfunctions*, and (2) dysfunction can result from a wide range of interconnected genotropic (gene-influenced), metabolic, nutritional, microbial, inflammatory, toxic, environmental, and psychological and social influences. **Many of these dysfunctions lie outside the narrow, pathology-based, pharmacocentric (drug-centered) view of standard allopathic medicine**. The functional/naturopathic medicine approach to each individual fibromyalgia patient is based firstly on the presumption that the condition has an underlying primary cause (or several interconnected causes) and that the cause(s) can be identified and addressed—in this manner, the clinical approach is one of positive psychoepistimology (ie, affirmative that we can understand this situation), rather than pathodefetism (ie, "we can't understand this disease") resulting pharmacodependency. The cause(s) may be manifold and multifaceted and may differ among patients with the same diagnostic label. This approach includes the diagnostic and therapeutic considerations of standard medicine but extends far beyond these in assessment, treatment, and understanding. Clinicians should appreciate that as a diagnostic label, fibromyalgia is commonly applied to any patient with chronic, widespread pain and that the current trend to limit diagnostic evaluation in such patients will clearly result in failure to identify and address readily diagnosable and treatable problems that can result in a clinical picture that resembles FM. Clinicians must consider chronic infections (such as with hepatitis C virus, *Borrelia burgdorferi* [the bacteria strongly associated with Lyme disease], *Chlamydia/Chlamydophila pneumoniae*, and the protozoan parasite *Babesia*, which is also associated with Lyme disease and co-infection with *Borrelia burgdorferi*), cancerous conditions such as multiple myeloma and lymphoma, and autoimmune/rheumatic diseases such as polymyositis and polymyalgia rheumatica. A few of the other more exemplary conditions to consider in patients with widespread pain are vitamin D deficiency, hypothyroidism, iron overload, and chronic exposure to and accumulation of xenobiotics—perhaps most importantly mercury and lead.

Common differential diagnoses

- **Vitamin D deficiency**: A clinical picture nearly identical to fibromyalgia—chronic widespread pain, mental depression/anxiety, headaches, low-grade systemic inflammation—can result from vitamin D deficiency.[106] Fibromyalgia patients are commonly deficient in vitamin D, and indeed, **vitamin D deficiency—with its**

---

[106] Plotnikoff GA, Quigley JM. Prevalence of severe hypovitaminosis D in patients with persistent, nonspecific musculoskeletal pain. *Mayo Clin Proc*. 2003;78(12):1463-70

attendant pain, anxiety/depression, and normal lab values on routine laboratory testing—is often **misdiagnosed as fibromyalgia**, as reported by Holick.[107] Increased severity of the deficiency correlates with worsening depression and anxiety in these patients.[108] Correction of vitamin D deficiency by administration of vitamin D3 (cholecalciferol) in doses of 5,000-10,000 IU (international units) per day for several months has resulted in a dramatic alleviation of pain; such intervention among patients with low back pain has resulted in cure rates greater than 95%.[109] Other studies with vitamin D3 using doses 400-4,000 IU/day have shown that vitamin D3 supplementation for the correction of vitamin D deficiency alleviates depression and enhances sense of well-being. Vitamin D3 supplementation—or adequate endogenous production from ultraviolet light exposure (approximately 10-30 minutes per day of full-body exposure at midday, near the equator)—to meet physiological requirements of approximately 4,000 IU/day is safe and results in numerous major health benefits.[110,111,112] The only risk associated with vitamin D supplementation is hypercalcemia—too much calcium in the blood, mostly as a result of increased gastrointestinal absorption of calcium; hypercalcemia can cause abdominal pain, bone pain, fatigue, constipation, abnormal heart rhythm (arrhythmia), kidney stones, increased thirst and urination [additional details[113]]. Hypercalcemia caused solely by vitamin D3 supplementation is extremely rare; vitamin D supplementation in the range of 2,000 – 10,000 IU per day for adults is remarkably safe.[114,115] The main drug-nutrient interaction of relevance to vitamin D supplementation is with the drug hydrochlorothiazide, which is a diuretic drug used for the treatment of high blood pressure; this drug causes calcium retention by the kidney and when combined with vitamin D supplementation may lead to high levels of calcium in the blood (hypercalcemia). *Note from Dr Vasquez: I have only seen this occur one time in my clinical practice in a hypertensive patient taking hydrochlorothiazide who was vitamin D deficient; vitamin D supplementation at 2,000 IU/d caused a mild hypercalcemia within 10 days which was treated simply by discontinuing the vitamin D supplementation (also note that discontinuation of appropriate nutritional supplementation in favor of continuing a symptom-suppressing drug is generally not my preference but in this particular situation it was the best choice).* A group of conditions called granulomatous diseases—which can include lymphoma, sarcoidosis, and Crohn's disease—increase the risk for hypercalcemia; caution and more frequent laboratory monitoring must be employed when using physiological doses of vitamin D3 in patients with these conditions. Diagnosis of vitamin D3 deficiency is simple and is based upon measurement of serum 25-hydroxy vitamin D3 (25[OH]D) levels. Supplementation effectiveness and safety are monitored by measuring 25(OH)D levels and serum calcium, respectively. The two goals with supplementation of vitamin D3 are ❶ safety—avoidance of hypercalcemia or any calcium-related complications, and ❷ efficacy—serum 25[OH]D levels should enter into the optimal range of 50 – 100 ng/mL (125 - 250 nmol/L) per Vasquez[116,117] and Vasquez et al[118,119,120] as discussed in Chapters 1 and 4.

- **Functional/metabolic hypothyroidism**: Insufficient levels of thyroid hormone lead to an associated clinical condition called hypothyroidism (*hypo*=low, *thyroidism*=thyroid condition). Both mild and overt hypothyroidism are well known in the rheumatology literature as causes of diffuse body pain. As a cause of diffuse muscle pain, mild-moderate hypothyroidism can mimic fibromyalgia; more severe cases of hypothyroidism cause "hypothyroid myopathy" which typically manifests as polymyositis-like disease with proximal muscle weakness and an increased serum level of the enzyme creatine kinase, indicating muscle damage. In its most extreme, hypothyroid myopathy presents as muscle enlargement (pseudohypertrophy); in

---

[107] Holick MF. Vitamin D: importance in the prevention of cancers, type 1 diabetes, heart disease, and osteoporosis. *Am J Clin Nutr*. 2004 Mar;79(3):362-71
[108] Armstrong DJ, et al. Vitamin D deficiency is associated with anxiety and depression in fibromyalgia. *Clin Rheumatol*. 2007 Apr;26(4):551-4
[109] Al Faraj S, Al Mutairi K. Vitamin D deficiency and chronic low back pain in Saudi Arabia. *Spine*. 2003;28:177-9
[110] Holick MF. Vitamin D: importance in the prevention of cancers, type 1 diabetes, heart disease, and osteoporosis. *Am J Clin Nutr*. 2004 Mar;79(3):362-71
[111] Vieth R. Vitamin D supplementation, 25-hydroxyvitamin D concentrations, and safety. *Am J Clin Nutr*. 1999 May;69(5):842-56
[112] Zittermann A. Vitamin D in preventive medicine: are we ignoring the evidence? *Br J Nutr*. 2003 May;89(5):552-72
[113] Mild hypercalcemia is not necessarily a problem by itself and must be evaluated within the patient's clinical context. When blood levels of calcium (normal range: 8.7-10.4 mg/dL) reach approximately 12.0 mg/dL, patients will start to develop symptoms; with levels of 14 mg/dL or higher, the patient is generally experiencing symptoms and complications and is in need of treatment (initially with administration of intravenous fluids and a loop diuretic such as furosemide).
[114] Vieth R. Vitamin D supplementation, 25-hydroxyvitamin D concentrations, and safety. *Am J Clin Nutr*. 1999 May;69(5):842-56
[115] Vasquez A, Manso G, Cannell J. The Clinical Importance of Vitamin D (Cholecalciferol): A Paradigm Shift with Implications for All Healthcare Providers. *Alternative Therapies in Health and Medicine* 2004; 10: 28-37 InflammationMastery.com/reprints
[116] Vasquez A. *Musculoskeletal Pain: Expanded Clinical Strategies*. Institute for Functional Medicine. 2008
[117] Vasquez A. Revisiting the Five-Part Nutritional Wellness Protocol: The Supplemented Paleo-Mediterranean Diet. *Nutritional Perspectives* 2011 Jan
[118] Vasquez A, Manso G, Cannell J. Clinical Importance of Vitamin D (Cholecalciferol): Paradigm Shift with Implications for All Healthcare Providers. *Alternative Therapies in Health and Medicine* 2004; 10: 28-37 InflammationMastery.com/reprints
[119] Vasquez A, Cannell J. Calcium and vitamin D in preventing fractures: data are not sufficient to show inefficacy. [letter] *BMJ: British Medical Journal* 2005;331:108-9
[120] Vasquez A. Subphysiologic Doses of Vitamin D are Subtherapeutic. *The Lancet* 2005 May 6 InflammationMastery.com/reprints

adults, this condition is called Hoffmann syndrome while in children it is known as Kocher-Debré-Sémélaigne syndrome.[121] Hypothyroidism is well known to cause depression and low-grade systemic inflammation; these are two findings common in FM. Another related problem commonly seen with both FM and hypothyroidism is IBS and small intestinal bacterial overgrowth (SIBO); hypothyroidism causes a slowing of intestinal motility, promoting stasis in the gastrointestinal tract which leads to an overgrowth of bacteria.[122] Detailed thyroid assessment should include measurements of thyroid stimulating hormone (TSH), free T4, free T3, total T3, reverse T3 (rT3), and antithyroid peroxidase (anti-TPO) and antithyroglobulin antibodies.

> **Terminology related to thyroid hormone production and metabolism—see Chapter 1 for complete review**
> - TSH—thyroid stimulating hormone: Hormone secreted from the anterior pituitary gland to stimulate T4 and T3 production from the thyroid gland.
> - T4: The inactive form of thyroid hormone, accounting for about 80% of thyroid gland output.
> - T3: The active form of thyroid hormone produced from conversion of T4, accounts for about 20% of thyroid gland output. This is the form of thyroid hormone that is most important, because it is active and ready to stimulate metabolic processes.
> - rT3—reverse T3: During times of stress and also as a result of some drugs, T4 is preferentially converted to rT3, which is inactive and may actually impair the utilization of active T3. In some people, especially after a period of severe emotional stress, their thyroid hormone metabolism becomes skewed toward rT3 production, perhaps as an adaptive mechanism to conserve energy. However, increased rT3 production results in impaired thyroid hormone function and thereby promotes a clinical picture of hypothyroidism (low function of the thyroid gland) even when gland function is adequate; the problem is the hormone's peripheral metabolism, not its production from the gland.

- **Occult infections, especially with *Mycoplasma* species and *Chlamydia/Chlamydophila pneumoniae*:** Clinicians are increasingly appreciating the role of occult intracellular infections in the genesis and/or perpetuation of chronic health problems, including some previously perplexing problems such as chronic fatigue syndrome (CFS), inflammatory arthritis, and multiple sclerosis (MS). For chronic *Chlamydophila* (previously *Chlamydia*) *pneumoniae* infection, testing for serum levels of antibodies is useful followed by treatment with antibacterial drugs such as azithromycin and nutritional supplements such as N-acetyl-cysteine (NAC) in appropriately selected patients; for chronic *Mycoplasma* infections, because of the various subspecies involved, polymerase chain reaction (PCR) testing appears to be preferred followed by treatment with doxycycline in adults.
  - Clinical investigation: Prevalence of antibodies to *Chlamydophila pneumoniae* in persons without clinical evidence of respiratory infection (*Journal of Clinical Pathology* 2002 May[123]): The authors note that "Because there is as yet no standardization of serological criteria for persistent infection, we considered antibody titers of > 1/20 in the IgA fraction, together with **IgG titers of 1/64 to 1/256, to be indicative of persistent infection.**" This article supports clinical experience and post-graduate presentations[124] showing that in persons with fatigue and various other chronic health disorders characterized by pain and inflammation (such as chronic inflammatory arthritis[125] or spine[126] inflammation), the finding of IgG antibody levels >1:64 suggests that the patient has a persistent *Chlamydophila pneumoniae* infection which may be alleviated by the administration of—for example—the antibiotic **azithromycin** (adult dose 250 mg every other day due to the drug's long half-life, given for several weeks or months until symptoms are resolved and/or antibody titers are normalized) and **N-acetyl-cysteine** (NAC: 500-1,200 mg 1-3 times per day by mouth between

---

[121] Kedlaya D. Hypothyroid Myopathy. emedicine.medscape.com/article/313915-overview Accessed April 2012
[122] Lauritano EC, Bilotta AL, Gabrielli M, et al. Association between hypothyroidism and small intestinal bacterial overgrowth. *J Clin Endocrinol Metab*. 2007 Nov;92(11):4180-4
[123] Ben-Yaakov M, Eshel G, Zaksonski L, Lazarovich Z, Boldur I. Prevalence of antibodies to Chlamydia pneumoniae in an Israeli population without clinical evidence of respiratory infection. *J Clin Pathol*. 2002 May;55(5):355-8 jcp.bmj.com/content/55/5/355.long
[124] Stratton C. The Role of Chlamydophila in Autoimmune Disease. 2011 International Symposium. "The Challenge of Emerging Infections in the 21st Century: Terrain, Tolerance, and Susceptibility" hosted by Institute for Functional Medicine in Seattle, Washington in May 2011
[125] "This study was a 9-month, prospective, double-blind, triple-placebo trial assessing a 6-month course of combination antibiotics as a treatment for Chlamydia-induced ReA. Groups received 1) doxycycline and rifampin plus placebo instead of azithromycin; 2) azithromycin and rifampin plus placebo instead of doxycycline; or 3) placebos instead of azithromycin, doxycycline, and rifampin. ... These data suggest that a 6-month course of combination antibiotics is an effective treatment for chronic Chlamydia-induced ReA." Carter JD, Espinoza LR, Inman RD, et al. Combination antibiotics as a treatment for chronic Chlamydia-induced reactive arthritis: a double-blind, placebo-controlled, prospective trial. *Arthritis Rheum*. 2010 May;62(5):1298-307
[126] "The frequency of Chlamydia-positive ST samples, as determined by PCR, was found to be significantly higher in patients with uSpA than in patients with OA. Our results suggest that in many patients with uSpA, chlamydial infection, which is often occult, may be the cause." Carter JD, et al. Chlamydiae as etiologic agents in chronic undifferentiated spondylarthritis. *Arthritis Rheum*. 2009 May;60(5):1311-6

meals). Positive antibody titers (levels) are common because the infection itself is common *as a transient condition*; the issue here is the determination of which patients have a *chronic* and *persistent* low-grade infection. The finding of an elevated antibody titer—that is a level greater than 1:64—indicates the need to consider long-term antimicrobial intervention.

```
Chlamydia pneumoniae IgG      >1:256    High         Neg:<1:16
Chlamydia pneumoniae IgM      <1:10                  Neg:<1:10
```

Elevated titers to *Chlamydia/Chlamydophila pneumoniae* suggesting chronic persistent infection in a 40yo male physician *without pulmonary symptoms* but with a positive history of chronic sinus congestion and low-grade fatigue—improvement with azithromycin and NAC: This patient experienced years of severe psychologic and physiologic stress during a doctorate program and then had an acute upper respiratory illness onset in September 2010 while working in hospital emergency rooms and urgent care clinics; recurrent bouts of upper respiratory illness—attributed to viral infections—persisted for five months until February 2011. By the summer of 2011, the patient was relatively asymptomatic except for persistent sinus congestion and low-grade fatigue. No pulmonary symptoms such as shortness of breath were ever present. Following detection of the elevated antibody titer, the patient started on azithromycin and NAC as described above, which resulted in a short-term (12-hour) exacerbation of symptoms followed by complete and sustained resolution of sinus congestion and improved energy levels and exercise endurance.[127]

- Review: *Mycoplasma* blood infection in chronic fatigue and **fibromyalgia** syndromes (*Rheumatology International* 2003 Sep[128]): The author notes that "**Chronic fatigue syndrome (CFS) and fibromyalgia syndrome (FMS)** are characterized by a lack of consistent laboratory and clinical abnormalities. Although they are distinguishable as separate syndromes based on established criteria, a great number of patients are diagnosed with both." He goes on to say, "In studies using **polymerase chain reaction [PCR] methods, mycoplasma blood infection has been detected in about 50% of patients with CFS and/or FMS**, including patients with Gulf War illnesses and symptoms that overlap with one or both syndromes. **Such infection is detected in only about 10% of healthy individuals**, significantly less than in patients. Most patients with CFS/FMS who have mycoplasma infection appear to recover and reach their pre-illness state after **long-term antibiotic therapy with doxycycline**, and the infection cannot be detected after recovery. ... It is not clear whether mycoplasmas are associated with CFS/FMS as causal agents, cofactors, or opportunistic infections in patients with immune disturbances."
- Clinical investigation: High prevalence of Mycoplasmal infections in symptomatic (chronic fatigue syndrome) family members of *Mycoplasma*-positive Gulf War illness patients (*Journal of Chronic Fatigue Syndrome* 2003[129]): The authors state, "…a relatively common finding in Gulf War Illness patients is a bacterial infection due to *Mycoplasma* species, we examined military families (149 patients: 42 veterans, 40 spouses, 32 other relatives and 35 children with at least one family complaint of illness) selected from a **group of 110 veterans with Gulf War Illness who tested positive (~41%) for at least one of four *Mycoplasma* species**: *M. fermentans, M. hominis, M. pneumoniae* or *M. genitalium*. Consistent with previous results, over 80% of Gulf War Illness patients who were positive for blood mycoplasmal infections had **only one *Mycoplasma* species, in particular *M. fermentans*** (Odds ratio = 17.9, P <0.001). In healthy control subjects the incidence of mycoplasmal infection was ~8.5% and none were found to have multiple mycoplasmal species."
- **Hemochromatosis and iron overload:** Genetic hemochromatosis is a common iron-accumulation disease that causes chronic persistent musculoskeletal pain, even while most routine laboratory tests are normal; thus, the clinical presentation of iron overload may be confused with that of fibromyalgia—both are common conditions commonly presenting with inexplicable (i.e., normal values of routine laboratory tests) nontraumatic musculoskeletal pain. Hemochromatosis is one of the most common hereditary disorders among Caucasians, with a homozygote (two of the same genes, results in more severe disease) frequency of approximately 1 in 200 to 250 persons and a heterozygote (only one affected gene, less severe disease) frequency of approximately 1 in

---

[127] Appreciation is given to Bill Beakey DOM of Professional Co-Op Services professionalcoop.com for provision of this laboratory assessment.
[128] Endresen GK. Mycoplasma blood infection in chronic fatigue and fibromyalgia syndromes. *Rheumatol Int*. 2003 Sep;23(5):211-5
[129] Nicolson GL, Nasralla MY, Nicolson NL. High prevalence of Mycoplasmal infections in symptomatic (chronic fatigue syndrome) family members of *Mycoplasma*-positive Gulf War illness patients. *Journal of Chronic Fatigue Syndrome* 2003; 11(2): 21-36 immed.org/GulfWarIllness/10.01.11update/GWIfamilyJCFS_.pdf

7 persons. Various other hereditary iron overload disorders affect all races, with the highest prevalence in persons of African descent (as high as 1 in 80 according to some small studies among hospitalized African-American patients).[130,131] Eighty percent of hemochromatosis patients have chronic musculoskeletal pain, which is commonly the earliest or only presenting complaint.[132] In contrast to the clinical presentation of FM, the musculoskeletal manifestations of iron overload are classically arthritic (i.e., in the joints) rather than muscular, with the joints of the hands, wrists, hips, and knees most commonly affected. However, due to the widespread distribution of pain and the normalcy of routine laboratory results, iron overload can mimic fibromyalgia. Given the high population prevalence of iron overload and the high frequency with which it presents with musculoskeletal manifestations, **all patients with chronic, nontraumatic musculoskeletal pain must be tested for iron overload.** Serum ferritin, which can be used alone or with transferrin saturation, is the best single laboratory test; confirmed results greater than 200 mcg/L in women and 300 mcg/L in men necessitate treatment with diagnostic and therapeutic phlebotomy (frequent "blood donation" is the most effective treatment for chronic iron overload).[133]

- **Accumulation of xenobiotics (including mercury and lead):** Xenobiotic (foreign chemical) accumulation may occasionally cause widespread pain resembling fibromyalgia, and xenobiotic detoxification (depuration) can alleviate pain in affected patients. Toxic chemical and toxic metal accumulation is common in humans worldwide and has been well-documented in Americans. Eight percent (8%) of American women of childbearing age have sufficiently high levels of mercury in their blood to increase the risk of health problems such as neurological damage in their children.[134] Americans in general show alarmingly high concentrations and combinations of neurotoxic (nerve-damaging), carcinogenic (cancer-causing), diabetogenic (diabetes-causing), and immunotoxic (immune-poisoning) xenobiotics/toxins.[135] Adverse effects of toxic chemicals (e.g., pesticides, herbicides, solvents, plastics, formaldehyde, petroleum byproducts) and heavy metals (especially lead and mercury) are well described throughout the biomedical literature and have been clinically reviewed by Crinnion.[136,137,138,139] Among toxins with the ability to produce chronic muscle pain, mercury may deserve special recognition given its ubiquitous distribution in the human population and the scientific evidence detailing its numerous adverse effects.[140,141] Whether by metabolic, neurological, or endocrinologic means, occult mercury toxicity may manifest as a syndrome of widespread muscle pain that resembles fibromyalgia.[142] Acrodynia is a subacute peripheral pain syndrome due to mercury toxicity classically seen in children.[143] Acute mercury intoxication can result in severe skeletal muscle damage (rhabdomyolysis).[144] Mercury in organic and inorganic forms interferes with acetylcholine reception and several crucial aspects of the sarcoplasmic reticulum, including calcium-magnesium-ATPase and calcium transport; these adverse effects establish a molecular basis for a *mercurial myopathy* (mercury-induced muscle disease).[145,146] The toxicity of mercury is greatly increased by

> **Potential benefits of reducing the body burden of mercury in patients with chronic pain and fatigue**
>
> "We suggest that **metal-driven inflammation** may affect the hypothalamic-pituitary-adrenal axis (HPA axis) and indirectly trigger psychosomatic multisymptoms characterizing **chronic fatigue syndrome, fibromyalgia**, and other diseases of unknown etiology."
>
> Sterzl et al. Mercury and nickel allergy: risk factors in fatigue and autoimmunity. *Neuro Endocrinol Lett.* 1999

---

[130] Wurapa RK, Gordeuk VR, Brittenham GM, Khiyami A, Schechter GP, Edwards CQ. Primary iron overload in African Americans. *Am J Med.* 1996 Jul;101(1):9-18
[131] Barton JC, Edwards CQ, Bertoli LF, Shroyer TW, Hudson SL. Iron overload in African Americans. *Am J Med.* 1995 Dec;99(6):616-23
[132] Vasquez A. Musculoskeletal disorders and iron overload disease: comment on the American College of Rheumatology guidelines for the initial evaluation of the adult patient with acute musculoskeletal symptoms. *Arthritis Rheum.* 1996 Oct;39(10):1767-8 InflammationMastery.com/reprints
[133] Barton JC, McDonnell SM, Adams PC, et al. Management of hemochromatosis. Hemochromatosis Management Working Group. *Ann Intern Med.* 1998 Dec 1;129(11):932-9
[134] "However, approximately 8% of women had concentrations higher than US Environmental Protection Agency's recommended reference dose (5.8 μg/L), below which exposures are considered to be without adverse effects." Schober et al. Blood mercury levels in US children and women of childbearing age,1999-2000. *JAMA* 2003;289:1667-74
[135] Kristin S. Schafer, Margaret Reeves, Skip Spitzer, Susan E. Kegley. Chemical Trespass: Pesticides in Our Bodies and Corporate Accountability. Pesticide Action Network North America. May 2004 Available at panna.org/ on August 1, 2004 See also: Body Burden: The Pollution in People. ewg.org/ 2006 Feb
[136] Crinnion WJ. Environmental medicine, part 1: the human burden of environmental toxins and their common health effects. *Altern Med Rev.* 2000 Feb;5(1):52-63
[137] Crinnion WJ. Environmental medicine, part 2: health effects of and protection from ubiquitous airborne solvent exposure. *Altern Med Rev.* 2000 Apr;5(2):133-43
[138] Crinnion WJ. Environmental medicine, part 3: long-term effects of chronic low-dose mercury exposure. *Altern Med Rev.* 2000 Jun;5(3):209-23
[139] Crinnion WJ. Environmental medicine, part 4: pesticides - biologically persistent and ubiquitous toxins. *Altern Med Rev.* 2000 Oct;5(5):432-47
[140] Elemental Mercury Vapor Poisoning -- North Carolina, 1988. cdc.gov/mmwr/preview/mmwrhtml/00001499.htm
[141] Shih H, Gartner JC Jr. Weight loss, hypertension, weakness, and limb pain in an 11-year-old boy. *J Pediatr.* 2001 Apr;138(4):566-9
[142] Sterzl I, Prochazkova J, Hrda P, et al. Mercury and nickel allergy: risk factors in fatigue and autoimmunity. *Neuro Endocrinol Lett.* 1999;20:221-8
[143] Padlewska KK. Acrodynia. Last Updated: February 15, 2007 eMedicine emedicine.com/derm/topic592.htm Accessed October 25, 2007
[144] Chugh KS, Singhal PC, Uberoi HS. Rhabdomyolysis and renal failure in acute mercuric chloride poisoning. *Med J Aust.* 1978 Jul 29;2(3):125-6
[145] Chiu VC, Mouring D, Haynes DH. Action of mercurials on the active and passive transport properties of sarcoplasmic reticulum. *J Bioenerg Biomembr.* 1983 Feb;15(1):13-25
[146] Shamoo AE, Maclennan DH, Elderfrawi ME. Differential effects of mercurial compounds on excitable tissues. *Chem Biol Interact.* 1976 Jan;12(1):41-52

simultaneous accumulation of lead, elevated levels of which are also common in the U.S. population. Demonstration of high mercury and lead levels in urine following administration of a chelating agent such as dimercaptosuccinic acid (DMSA) can be used to diagnose chronic mercury or lead overload, and orally administered DMSA is also used for treatment.[147,148,149,150] Failure to preadminister a chelating agent prior to measurement of urine mercury renders the test insensitive for chronic accumulation and can thus give the false impression that mercury is not contributory to fibromyalgia, as concluded by Kotter et al.[151] Orally administered selenium, phytochelatins (metal-binding peptides from plants[152]), a high-fiber diet, and potassium citrate can be used to augment mercury excretion.[153]

- Case report: Therapeutic detoxification to reduce the body burden of toxic metals (lead and mercury) in a woman diagnosed with FM leads to complete relief of FM symptoms: This 54-year-old athletic female with healthy diet, lifestyle, and supportive relationship presented with chronic diffuse musculoskeletal pain. Health history was significant for decades of environmental illness/intolerance (EI) also known as multiple chemical sensitivity (MCS). Family history was positive for maternal temporal (giant cell) arteritis, an autoimmune disease characterized by inflamed arteries in the neck, head, and shoulders. Physical examination revealed numerous tender points consistent with fibromyalgia. The patient's history and stool analysis (comprehensive bacteriology and parasitology, tests for intestinal "infections") were unremarkable and unsupportive of either identifiable infection or nonspecific bacterial overgrowth. Laboratory investigations revealed normal results for hsCRP (high-sensitivity c-reactive protein, a marker for inflammation), CK (creatine kinase, a marker of muscle damage and myositis), ANA (anti-nuclear antibodies, elevated in many autoimmune diseases such as lupus/SLE), vitamin D, calcium, phosphorus, and comprehensive thyroid evaluation. The patient was then (defensively) referred to an excellent osteopathic medical internist who diagnosed the patient with fibromyalgia. The patient was unsatisfied with the diagnosis of FM and returned to the current author, who then performed urine heavy metal testing provoked with 10 mg per kilogram of dimercaptosuccinic acid (DMSA). Results revealed the highest levels of lead and mercury encountered in the author's practice at that time. As in the accompanying lab results, lead levels were 6x above the reference range and mercury levels were 7x above the reference range. The patient was commenced on DMSA 10 mg/kg/d three days "on" and 4 days "off" (cyclic dosing is used to avoid toxicity in general and bone marrow toxicity [neutropenia] in particular), selenium 800 mcg/d to promote excretion of toxic metals and to support renal and antioxidant protection, vegetable juices to provide potassium and citrate for urinary alkalinization and enhanced excretion of xenobiotics[154], and a proprietary phytochelatin (metal-binding peptides from plants) concentrate to bind toxic metals in the gut and thereby promote their fecal excretion by blocking enterohepatic recycling/recirculation. DMSA chelation is approved by the US Food and Drug Administration (FDA) for the treatment of lead toxicity in children.[155] The use of DMSA for children and adults is supported by peer-reviewed literature.[156,157,158,159,160] After approximately 8 months of treatment, the patient was completely free of pain, and the clinical improvement was associated with a reduction in both lead and mercury of approximately 50% as demonstrated by follow-up laboratory testing. This case was published in peer-reviewed literature for continuing education credits for physicians.[161]

---

[147] Kalra V, et al. Succimer in Symptomatic Lead Poisoning. *Indian Pediatrics* 2002; 39:580-585 indianpediatrics.net/june2002/june-580-585.htm
[148] Bradstreet et al. Case-control study of mercury burden in children with autistic spectrum disorders. *J Am Physicians Surgeons* 2003; 8: 76-79 jpands.org/vol8no3/geier.pdf
[149] Forman J, Moline J, Cernichiari E, et al. A cluster of pediatric metallic mercury exposure cases treated with meso-2,3-dimercaptosuccinic acid (DMSA). *Environ Health Perspect*. 2000 Jun;108(6):575-7 ehp.niehs.nih.gov/docs/2000/108p575-577forman/abstract.html
[150] Miller AL. Dimercaptosuccinic acid (DMSA), a non-toxic, water-soluble treatment for heavy metal toxicity. *Altern Med Rev*. 1998 Jun;3(3):199-207
[151] Kotter I, Durk H, Saal JG, et al. Mercury exposure from dental amalgam fillings in the etiology of primary fibromyalgia. *J Rheumatol*. 1995;22:2194-5
[152] Cobbett CS. Phytochelatins and their roles in heavy metal detoxification. *Plant Physiol*. 2000;123:825-32 plantphysiol.org/content/123/3/825
[153] Vasquez A. *Musculoskeletal Pain: Expanded Clinical Strategies*. Institute for Functional Medicine, 2008
[154] Crinnion WJ. Environmental medicine, part3:long-term effects of chronic low-dose mercury exposure. *Altern Med Rev* 2000 Jun;5:209-23
[155] "The Food and Drug Administration has recently licensed the drug DMSA (succimer) for reduction of blood lead levels >/= 45 micrograms/dl. This decision was based on the demonstrated ability of DMSA to reduce blood lead levels. An advantage of this drug is that it can be given orally." Goyer RA, Cherian MG, Jones MM, Reigart JR. Role of chelating agents for prevention, intervention, and treatment of exposures to toxic metals. *Environ Health Perspect*. 1995 Nov;103(11):1048-52
[156] Bradstreet et al. A case-control study of mercury burden in children with autistic spectrum disorders. *Journal of American Physicians and Surgeons* 2003; 8: 76-79
[157] Crinnion WJ. Environmental medicine, part three: long-term effects of chronic low-dose mercury exposure. *Altern Med Rev*. 2000 Jun;5(3):209-23
[158] Forman J, Moline J, Cernichiari E, et al. A cluster of pediatric metallic mercury exposure cases treated with meso-2,3-dimercaptosuccinic acid (DMSA). *Environ Health Perspect*. 2000 Jun;108(6):575-7 ehp.niehs.nih.gov/docs/2000/108p575-577forman/abstract.html
[159] Miller AL. Dimercaptosuccinic acid (DMSA), a non-toxic, water-soluble treatment for heavy metal toxicity. *Altern Med Rev*. 1998 Jun;3(3):199-207
[160] DMSA. *Altern Med Rev*. 2000 Jun;5(3):264-7 thorne.com/altmedrev/.fulltext/5/3/264.pdf
[161] Vasquez A. *Musculoskeletal Pain: Expanded Clinical Strategies*. Institute for Functional Medicine. 2008

Marked accumulation of lead and mercury in a patient diagnosed with FM—complete elimination of pain and stiffness following identification and reduction in the body burden of lead and mercury: *Presentation*: 54yo woman presents with nontraumatic widespread pain consistent with a diagnosis of fibromyalgia; the diagnosis of FM is confirmed by two clinicians. All laboratory test results were normal except for urine toxic metal testing which showed 6x elevations of lead and 7x elevations of mercury. Treatment for lead and mercury toxicity was started as described above and the patient experienced safe and effective alleviation of all pain after 8 months of treatment; reductions in pain correlated directly with reductions in body burden of lead and mercury.

Small intestine bacterial overgrowth (SIBO) is the ultimate cause of and most logical explanation for FM:

- Small intestine bacterial overgrowth (SIBO)—also referred to as "intestinal bacterial overgrowth" or simply "bacterial overgrowth"—provides the single best model for explaining the clinical and pathophysiological manifestations of fibromyalgia. Although commonly underappreciated by many clinicians, SIBO is common in clinical practice, affecting for example approximately 40% of patients with rheumatoid arthritis, 84% of patients with IBS, and 90% to 100% of patients with fibromyalgia. **In a study of 42 fibromyalgia patients, all 42 FM patients showed laboratory evidence of SIBO, and the severity of the intestinal bacterial overgrowth correlated positively with the severity of the fibromyalgia**, thus indicating the plausibility of a causal relationship.[162] The links between fibromyalgia and IBS are also strong; **most IBS patients meet strict diagnostic criteria for fibromyalgia, and most fibromyalgia patients meet strict criteria for IBS**. Lubrano et al[163] showed that fibromyalgia severity correlated with IBS severity among patients who met strict diagnostic criteria for both conditions. The high degree of overlap between these two diagnostic labels suggests that these conditions are two variations of a common pathophysiological process—SIBO.[164] SIBO causes altered bowel function, immune activation, and visceral hypersensitivity, and it is the best causative explanation for the clinical and pathophysiological manifestations of IBS; for more details and citations, see the excellent review by Lin published in *Journal of the American Medical Association* in 2004.[165] IBS is characterized by *visceral* hyperalgesia (hypersensitivity to pain), just as fibromyalgia is characterized by *skeletal muscle* hyperalgesia. Given that strong evidence indicates that IBS is caused by SIBO and that IBS and fibromyalgia are variations of the same pathophysiological process, then fibromyalgia may therefore be caused by SIBO. However, these links and interconnections require substantiation, as provided below.

What is the evidence linking fibromyalgia with SIBO? What are the molecular mechanisms by which absorbed toxins and metabolites from SIBO can contribute to muscle pain and the mitochondrial/ATP/energy defects and the muscle tissue abnormalities seen in fibromyalgia patients?

1. <u>Small intestine bacterial overgrowth is highly prevalent in fibromyalgia</u>: Several studies have shown that 90% to 100% of fibromyalgia patients have evidence of SIBO; such a strong correlation and the dose-response relationship imply causality and must be integrated into any science-based model of fibromyalgia.

---

[162] Pimentel et al. A link between irritable bowel syndrome and fibromyalgia may be related to findings on lactulose breath testing. *Ann Rheum Dis*. 2004 Apr;63(4):450-2
[163] Lubrano E, et al. Fibromyalgia in patients with irritable bowel syndrome. An association with the severity of the intestinal disorder. *Int J Colorectal Dis*. 2001 Aug;16(4):211-5
[164] Veale et al. Primary fibromyalgia and the irritable bowel syndrome: different expressions of a common pathogenetic process. *Br J Rheumatol*. 1991 Jun;30(3):220-2
[165] Lin HC. Small intestinal bacterial overgrowth: a framework for understanding irritable bowel syndrome. *JAMA*. 2004 Aug 18;292(7):852-8

- Clinical study: Patients with FM have evidence of frequent and severe bacterial overgrowth in the intestines (*Annals of the Rheumatic Diseases* 2004 Apr[166]): The **breath hydrogen test** is used for the detection of SIBO and involves orally administering a carbohydrate (such as lactulose, a source of sugar for bacteria) which is converted to hydrogen through bacterial fermentation; the exhaled hydrogen in the breath is measured as an indirect quantification of the amount of bacteria in the intestines. In this study, 20% of "healthy" control patients were found to have intestinal bacterial overgrowth via an abnormal hydrogen breath test compared with 93/111 (84%) subjects with IBS and **42/42 (100%) with fibromyalgia**. Subjects with fibromyalgia had higher hydrogen production (indicating more severe SIBO), peak hydrogen, and area under the curve than subjects with IBS. **The degree of somatic pain in fibromyalgia correlates significantly with the hydrogen level seen on the breath test**.

2. Fibromyalgia is tightly correlated with irritable bowel syndrome, a condition caused by small intestine bacterial overgrowth: Fibromyalgia and IBS are strongly convergent, and the evidence indicates that IBS is caused largely or completely by SIBO; again, for more details and citations, see the brilliant article by Lin, cited previously.

3. Small intestine bacterial overgrowth leads to systemic absorption of toxins that impair brain/nerve and muscle/mitochondrial function: SIBO is associated with overproduction and absorption of bacterial cellular debris (e.g., lipopolysaccharide [LPS], bacterial DNA, peptidoglycans, teichoic acid, exotoxins) and antimetabolites—substances which are directly toxic to cellular energy/ATP production and muscle and nerve function—such as D-lactic acid, tyramine, tartaric acid, hydrogen sulfide. Intestinal gram-negative bacteria produce endotoxin (also known as lipopolysaccharide, LPS), which impairs skeletal muscle energy/ATP production (by stimulating skeletal muscle sodium-potassium-ATPase). Endotoxin also raises blood lactate (indicating impaired cellular energy production) under aerobic conditions in humans.[167] **Thus, via direct and indirect effects on cellular metabolism, chronic low-dose bacterial LPS/endotoxin exposure can result in impaired muscle metabolism and reduced ATP synthesis via impairment of mitochondrial function.** Intestinal bacteria also produce D-lactate, a well-known metabolic toxin in humans; SIBO often results in variable levels of D-lactate acidosis, severe cases of which can progress from fatigue and malaise to encephalopathy (e.g., confusion, ataxia, slurred speech, altered mental status) and death.[168] Supporting the proposal that bacterial overgrowth with D-lactate-producing bacteria is a contributor to the chronic fatigue syndromes including fibromyalgia is an excellent study published in 2009 showing that **patients with chronic fatigue syndrome have intestinal overgrowth of bacteria that produce the cellular toxin D-lactate**; specifically the research showed that these chronic fatigue patients have **a 7-fold increase in D-lactate producing *Enterococcus* and 1,100-fold increase in D-lactate producing *Streptococcus***. Energy/ATP underproduction and lactate overproduction cause muscle fatigue and muscle pain. An additional cellular toxin produced by intestinal bacteria is hydrogen sulfide (H2S),

> **Patients with "chronic fatigue syndrome" and the associated neurologic dysfunction and muscle dysfunction have intestinal overgrowth of bacteria that produce D-lactic acid, a known neurotoxin and metabolic poison**
>
> In 2007 and 2008, the current author (AV) wrote and published *Musculoskeletal Pain: Expanded Clinical Strategies** with the Institute for Functional Medicine; this chapter on fibromyalgia is derived and updated from that work. In that publication, I reviewed evidence that fibromyalgia—at that time considered mysterious, idiopathic, chronic, relentless, and treatable only by pain-relieving drugs—was most likely caused by small intestine bacterial overgrowth (SIBO) and the resultant absorption of metabolic toxins and immunogenic debris. This perspective has been supported by numerous publications, particularly the article published by Sheedy et al** in 2009, which showed for the first time that patients with chronic fatigue syndrome—a condition tightly correlated with and which often overlaps with fibromyalgia—have SIBO with various bacteria that are high-output producers of D-lactic acid, a known neurotoxin and metabolic poison which potentially contributes to many of the main clinical, biochemical, and histologic manifestations of FM, namely mental fatigue and dyscognition (difficulty thinking), muscle fatigue and pain, biochemical evidence of mitochondrial impairment, and histologic evidence of mitochondrial myopathy.
>
> *Vasquez A. *Musculoskeletal Pain: Expanded Clinical Strategies*. Institute for Functional Medicine, 2008.
> **Sheedy, et al. Increased d-lactic acid intestinal bacteria in patients with chronic fatigue syndrome. *In Vivo*. 2009 Jul

---

[166] Pimentel et al. A link between irritable bowel syndrome and fibromyalgia may be related to findings on lactulose breath testing. *Ann Rheum Dis*. 2004 Apr;63(4):450-2
[167] Bundgaard H, et al. Endotoxemia stimulates skeletal muscle Na+-K+-ATPase and raises blood lactate under aerobic conditions in humans. *Am J Physiol Heart Circ Physiol*. 2003 Mar;284(3):H1028-34
[168] Vella A, Farrugia G. D-lactic acidosis: pathologic consequence of saprophytism. *Mayo Clin Proc*. 1998 May;73(5):451-6

which causes DNA damage[169] (noted previously to be increased in fibromyalgia patients) and which impairs cellular energy production, a finding relevant to *but not necessarily limited to* the pathogenesis of ulcerative colitis.[170,171] Bacteria and yeast in the intestines produce H2S, which can bind to the mitochondrial enzyme cytochrome c oxidase (part of Complex IV of the electron transport chain), thereby impairing oxidative phosphorylation and ATP production; this may partly explain the association of gastrointestinal dysbiosis and small intestine bacterial overgrowth (SIBO) with conditions such as chronic fatigue syndrome (CFS) and fibromyalgia.[172]

> **Exposure to the bacterial endotoxin lipopolysaccharide (LPS) causes increased sensitivity to painful stimuli (hyperalgesia) and a reduction in opioid analgesia (anti-analgesia)**
>
> "Intraperitoneal injection of toxins, such as the bacterial endotoxin lipopolysaccharide (LPS), is associated with a well-characterized increase in sensitivity to painful stimuli (hyperalgesia) and a longer-lasting reduction in opioid analgesia (anti-analgesia) when pain sensitivity returns to basal levels."
>
> Johnston et al. Inhibition of morphine analgesia by LPS. *Behav Brain Res* 2005 Jan

- Experimental study: Effect of *E. coli* endotoxin on mitochondrial form and function (*Annals of Surgery* 1971 Dec[173]): Authors of this paper show that treatment of normal rat liver mitochondria with *E. coli* endotoxin results in mitochondrial impairment. They note previous research showing that animal exposure to *E. coli* endotoxin causes inhibition of mitochondrial respiration and uncoupling of oxidative phosphorylation. Near their conclusion, the authors write, "Thus we have evidence to show that topical **E. coli endotoxin has pathologic effects on both membrane integrity and internal mechanochemical systems of isolated mitochondria**." Readers should appreciate that *E. coli* is a common inhabitant of the gastrointestinal tract of humans and that its population is quantitatively increased during states of bacterial overgrowth of the small bowel, as is commonly seen in most patients with fibromyalgia. More recently, research has shown that impairment of mitochondrial function (noted in patients with fibromyalgia) can lead to destruction of mitochondria by a process termed "mitophagy" (noted in patients with fibromyalgia); over time, loss of mitochondria via mitophagy leads to reduced numbers of mitochondria in muscle and other tissues (noted in patients with fibromyalgia) and contributes to the fatigue and other symptoms which characterize FM.

- Clinical study: Increased D-lactic acid intestinal bacteria in patients with chronic fatigue syndrome (*In Vivo* 2009 Jul-Aug[174]): This excellent clinical research fully supports the pathoetiologic (disease causation) model presented in this chapter, which is derived and updated from a previous publication by this author: Vasquez A. *Musculoskeletal Pain: Expanded Clinical Strategies* published by the Institute for Functional Medicine in 2008. The authors of this 2009 study state in the summary of their research, "Patients with chronic fatigue syndrome (CFS) are affected by symptoms of cognitive dysfunction and neurological impairment, the cause of which has yet to be elucidated. However, these symptoms are strikingly similar to those of patients presented with D-lactic acidosis. A significant increase of Gram-positive facultative anaerobic fecal microorganisms in 108 CFS patients as compared to 177 control subjects is presented in this report. The viable count of D-lactic acid producing *Enterococcus* and *Streptococcus* spp. in the fecal samples from the CFS group (3.5 x 10(7) cfu [colony forming units]/L and 9.8 x 10(7) cfu/L respectively) were significantly higher than those for the control group (5.0 x 10(6) cfu/L and 8.9 x 10(4) cfu/L respectively). **[Note: This is approximately a 7x increase in D-lactate producing *Enterococcus* and 1,100x increase in D-lactate producing *Streptococcus*.]** Analysis of exometabolic profiles of *Enterococcus faecalis* and *Streptococcus sanguinis*, representatives of *Enterococcus* and *Streptococcus* spp. respectively, by NMR and HPLC showed that these organisms produced significantly more lactic acid from (13)C-labeled glucose, than the Gram negative *Escherichia coli*. Further, **both *E. faecalis* and *S. sanguinis* secrete more D-lactic acid than *E. coli*.** This study suggests a probable link between intestinal colonization of Gram-positive facultative anaerobic D-lactic acid bacteria and symptom expressions in a subgroup of patients with CFS. Given the fact that **this**

---

[169] Attene-Ramos MS, Wagner ED, Gaskins HR, Plewa MJ. Hydrogen sulfide induces direct radical-associated DNA damage. *Mol Cancer Res*. 2007 May;5(5):455-9
[170] Magee et al. Contribution of dietary protein to sulfide production in large intestine: in vitro and controlled feeding study in humans. *Am J Clin Nutr*. 2000 Dec;72(6):1488-94
[171] Babidge W, Millard S, Roediger W. Sulfides impair short chain fatty acid beta-oxidation at acyl-CoA dehydrogenase level in colonocytes: implications for ulcerative colitis. *Mol Cell Biochem*. 1998 Apr;181(1-2):117-24
[172] Lemle MD. Hypothesis: chronic fatigue syndrome is caused by dysregulation of hydrogen sulfide metabolism. *Med Hypotheses*. 2009 Jan;72(1):108-9
[173] White et al. Effect of E. coli endotoxin on mitochondrial form and function. *Ann Surg*. 1971 Dec;174(6):983-90
[174] Sheedy JR, Wettenhall RE, Scanlon D, et al. Increased d-lactic acid intestinal bacteria in patients with chronic fatigue syndrome. *In Vivo*. 2009 Jul-Aug;23(4):621-8

might explain not only neurocognitive dysfunction in CFS patients but also mitochondrial dysfunction, these findings may have important clinical implications."

4. <u>Bacterial LPS and other antigens absorbed from the intestine during SIBO contribute to a subclinical inflammatory state that results in pain hypersensitivity and increased cytokine release, both of which are characteristics of fibromyalgia</u>: In animal models and in human research studies, exposure to bacterial endotoxin/LPS has been shown to increase the brain's sensitivity to and perception of pain. Immune-mediated and inflammation-mediated pathways that promote pain sensitivity and pain perception include ❶ reduced production of nitric oxide with ❷ increased production of prostaglandins and cytokines, resulting in ❸ the sensitization of peripheral and/or central neurons to pain perception/transmission. In support of this concept, Lin[175] wrote in 2004, "**The immune response to bacterial antigen in SIBO provides a framework for understanding the hypersensitivity in both fibromyalgia and IBS.**" A later paper by Othmanm, Agüero, and Lin[176] in 2008 stated, "…a recent animal study demonstrated that exposure to endotoxin increased the production of prostaglandins and simultaneously decreased nitrous oxide production, resulting in inflammatory hyperalgesia" and "These observations suggest that SIBO is a common feature in both [IBS and FM] disorders and that altered gut microbiota in SIBO may play a role in the induction of somatic or visceral hypersensitivity, with affected patients meeting the diagnostic criteria for IBS, fibromyalgia or both disorders."

Mitochondrial dysfunction promotes central sensitization via oxidative stress and cytokine release: Mitochondrial dysfunction increases free radical production, which promotes "neurologic hypersensitivity" to pain, i.e., the pain in fibromyalgia is not simply due to muscle fatigue due to mitochondrial dysfunction although that is clearly a major component. The mitochondrial dysfunction also promotes central sensitization, which should be treated directly via alleviating the mitochondrial dysfunction and the causative dysbiosis, in addition to patient-specific factors.

---

[175] Lin HC. Small intestinal bacterial overgrowth: a framework for understanding irritable bowel syndrome. *JAMA*. 2004 Aug 18;292(7):852-8
[176] Othman M, Agüero R, Lin HC. Alterations in intestinal microbial flora and human disease. *Curr Opin Gastroenterol*. 2008 Jan;24(1):11-6

5. Central sensitization (enhanced and autonomous pain hypersensitivity) seen in FM can be caused by bacterial LPS: Somewhat independent from the immune/inflammation-mediated hyperalgesia induced by LPS is the hyperalgesia mediated by central nervous system responses. The central sensitization seen with fibromyalgia[177] might be explained as being caused by intestinally-derived bacterial toxins. **Bacterial LPS/endotoxin promotes central sensitization via direct activation of NMDA receptors and by inducing hyperalgesia (elevated pain perception) and anti-analgesia (reduced response to pain inhibition)**.[178] Accumulated evidence suggests that fibromyalgia may be a disorder of somatic hypersensitivity induced by bacterial toxins derived from quantitative excess or qualitative abnormalities in gut bacteria.[179]

6. SIBO commonly causes nutrient malabsorption and thus predisposes to subclinical selective malnutrition, specifically micronutrient deficiency: SIBO causes nutrient malabsorption[180] and can thereby contribute to the vitamin D and magnesium deficiencies that promote pain and mitochondrial dysfunction, respectively, and which are common in fibromyalgia. Intestinal bacterial overgrowth causes nutrient malabsorption via intestinal inflammation and villus atrophy (anatomic impairment) and impairment of digestion, specifically the enzymatic degradation of mucosal peptidases and disaccharidases by bacterial proteases (biochemical impairment). As reported by McEvoy and colleagues[181], bacterial contamination [overgrowth] of the small intestine is an important cause of occult malabsorption and malnutrition, especially in the elderly.

7. SIBO can be triggered or exacerbated by emotional stress: SIBO can be triggered in humans by reduced mucosal immunity following stressful life events, and this helps explain the link between psychoemotional stress and the SIBO-related conditions IBS and FM. Chronic mental-emotional stress causes reduced production of the antibody secretory IgA (sIgA) which is the primary line of defense against bacteria and other microorganisms in the gastrointestinal tract; thus, mental-emotional stress can reduce intestinal immunity and thereby promote SIBO. Further, stress in humans triggers enhanced microbial pathogenicity via microbial endocrinology.

8. Oxidative stress triggers exaggerated pain perception—hyperalgesia (hypersensitivity to pain) and allodynia (perception of pain from normal stimuli): Patients with fibromyalgia show evidence of increased free radical (oxidant) production and reduced antioxidant defenses. Increased oxidative stress can be caused by immune activation and mitochondrial dysfunction; immune activation and mitochondrial dysfunction also promote oxidative stress and depletion of antioxidants, resulting in a vicious cycle, as illustrated. In the excellent review by Cordero et al[182], the authors note that recent studies have shown that oxidative stress causes peripheral and central sensitization and alters nerve sensitivity to pain (nociception), resulting in hyperalgesia—hypersensitivity to normal stimuli. The free radical (oxidant) superoxide promotes the development of pain through direct peripheral sensitization and the release of various cytokines (such as TNF-α, IL-1β, and IL-6), the formation of peroxynitrite (ONOO-), and PARP activation. PARP—poly-ADP-ribose-polymerase—is a nuclear enzyme activated by superoxide/peroxynitrite radicals; activation of PARP promotes the development of pain syndromes, including the components of small sensory fiber neuropathy, thermal and mechanical hyperalgesia, tactile allodynia, and exaggerated pain behavior in animal models of diabetic neuropathy.[183,184]

9. Low plasma levels of L-tryptophan seen in fibromyalgia patients can be caused by degradation of dietary tryptophan by the bacterial enzyme tryptophanase: Patients with fibromyalgia have low blood levels of the amino acid L-tryptophan[185], which is used in the body to make serotonin (important for mood maintenance and pain alleviation) and melatonin (important for normal sleep and for support of mitochondrial function and antioxidant protection). Bacteria such as *Escherichia coli, Proteus vulgaris,* and *Bacteroides* produce the enzyme

---

[177] Meeus et al. Central sensitization: biopsychosocial explanation for chronic widespread pain in patients with fibromyalgia and chronic fatigue syndrome. *Clin Rheumatol*. 2007 Apr;26(4):465-73
[178] Johnston IN, Westbrook RF. Inhibition of morphine analgesia by LPS: role of opioid and NMDA receptors and spinal glia. *Behav Brain Res*. 2005;156(1):75-83
[179] Othman M, Agüero R, Lin HC. Alterations in intestinal microbial flora and human disease. *Curr Opin Gastroenterol*. 2008 Jan;24(1):11-6
[180] Elphick HL, Elphick DA, Sanders DS. Small bowel bacterial overgrowth. An underrecognized cause of malnutrition in older adults. Geriatrics. 2006 Sep;61(9):21-6
[181] McEvoy A, Dutton J, James OF. Bacterial contamination of the small intestine is an important cause of occult malabsorption in the elderly. *Br Med J* (Clin Res Ed). 1983 Sep 17;287(6395):789-93 ncbi.nlm.nih.gov/pmc/articles/PMC1549133/
[182] Cordero MD, et al. Mitochondrial dysfunction and mitophagy activation in blood mononuclear cells of fibromyalgia patients. *Arthritis Res Ther*. 2010;12(1):R17
[183] Wang ZQ, Porreca F, Cuzzocrea S et al. A newly identified role for superoxide in inflammatory pain. *J Pharmacol Exp Ther*. 2004 Jun;309(3):869-78
[184] Ilnytska O, et al. Poly(ADP-ribose) polymerase inhibition alleviates experimental diabetic sensory neuropathy. *Diabetes* 2006 Jun;55:1686-94
[185] "Plasma-free tryptophan is inversely related to the severity of subjective pain in 8 patients who fulfilled criteria for a variety of non-articular rheumatism, the "fibrositis syndrome". The observation is consistent with animal and human studies suggesting a relationship between reduced brain serotonin metabolism and pain reactivity." Moldofsky H, Warsh JJ. Plasma tryptophan and musculoskeletal pain in non-articular rheumatism ("fibrositis syndrome"). *Pain*. 1978 Jun;5(1):65-71

tryptophanase[186], which destroys L-tryptophan in the gut before it is absorbed from ingested foods; thus, generalized bacterial overgrowth of the small intestine could reasonably be expected to exacerbate this phenomenon. In patients with fibromyalgia, higher tryptophan levels correlate positively with serotonin levels and with less pain and better sleep, while lower tryptophan levels are associated with sleep impairment, reduced serotonin levels, and higher levels of substance P, a neurotransmitter that promotes inflammation and pain perception.[187] Fibromyalgia patients produce 31% less melatonin than do healthy controls, and "this may contribute to impaired sleep at night, fatigue during the day, and changed pain perception."[188] Thus, a likely sequence of events is that, for example, a period of stressful life events can cause impair gastrointestinal immunity leading to intestinal bacterial overgrowth, which itself causes tryptophan degradation via elaboration of bacterial tryptophanase, causing tryptophan deficiency and resultant deficiencies of serotonin (leading to pain, depression, anxiety, and food/carbohydrate craving) and melatonin (leading to sleep disturbance, impaired antioxidant defense and mitochondrial function, and impaired immune responsiveness).

10. <u>The therapies that help fibromyalgia share mechanisms of action consistent with the model presented here</u>: As will be reviewed below under *Therapeutic Interventions*, essentially all of the most successful therapies for fibromyalgia have effects on intestinal flora, muscle perfusion/contractility, or mitochondrial bioenergetics (biological production of cellular energy/ATP). This is true for vegetarian diets (which favorably alter gut flora and improve antioxidant defenses), supplementation with tryptophan/melatonin (which preserve mitochondrial function during bacterial LPS/endotoxin exposure), physical treatments such as acupuncture (which improves tissue perfusion), and the use of nutrients such as magnesium, acetyl-L-carnitine, D-ribose, creatine, and coenzyme Q-10—all of which support or improve mitochondrial function.

11. <u>Restless leg syndrome and fibromyalgia commonly co-exist, and restless leg syndrome can be alleviated by eradication of SIBO</u>: Restless leg syndrome (RLS) occurs in approximately 30% of FM patients and can be effectively treated by addressing SIBO with a combination of antibiotics (drugs or botanical medicines that eradicate bacteria) and probiotics (products containing beneficial bacteria, which help restore "microbial balance" in the gastrointestinal tract).[189]

12. <u>Antimicrobial/antibiotic treatment alleviates fibromyalgia in most FM patients, just as it also alleviates gastrointestinal symptoms in patients with irritable bowel syndrome (IBS)</u>: Finally and most importantly, **antimicrobial therapy alleviates FM (and IBS) symptoms in direct proportion to the success of bacterial overgrowth eradication**, thus adding strong direct evidence in support of SIBO as a main cause of FM.[190,191] Recent clinical trials have shown that treatment of the fibromyalgia-related conditions IBS and SIBO by use of the nonabsorbed oral antibiotic rifaximin results in significant diminution of IBS-SIBO symptomatology with benefits lasting after the discontinuation of therapy.[192,193]

- Clinical trial: Rifaximin therapy for patients with irritable bowel syndrome without constipation (*New England Journal of Medicine* 2011 Jan[194]): Authors of this study evaluated rifaximin, a minimally absorbed antibiotic, as treatment for IBS. Subjects were given rifaximin at a dose of 550 mg or placebo, three times daily for 2 weeks and were followed for 10 weeks thereafter. "Significantly more patients in the rifaximin group than in the placebo group had adequate relief of global IBS symptoms during the first 4 weeks after treatment (40.8% vs. 31.2%). Similarly, more patients in the rifaximin group than in the placebo group had adequate relief of bloating (39.5% vs. 28.7%). In addition, significantly more patients in the rifaximin group had a response to treatment as assessed by daily ratings of IBS symptoms, bloating, abdominal pain, and stool consistency. The incidence of adverse events was similar in the two groups." Thus, among patients who had IBS without constipation, treatment with rifaximin for 2 weeks provided significant relief of IBS

---

[186] Demoss RD, Moser K. Tryptophanase in Diverse Bacterial Species. *Journal of Bacteriology* 1969; 98: 167-171

[187] "A strong negative correlation between SP and 5-HIAA (P = .000) as well as between SP and TRP (P = .009) could be demonstrated. High serum concentrations of 5-HIAA and TRP showed a significant relation to low pain scores (5-HIAA: P = .030; TRP: P = .014). Moreover, 5-HIAA was strongly related to good quality of sleep (P = .000), while SP was related to sleep disturbance (P = .005)." Schwarz MJ, Späth M, Müller-Bardorff H, Pongratz DE, Bondy B, Ackenheil M. Relationship of substance P, 5-hydroxyindole acetic acid and tryptophan in serum of fibromyalgia patients. *Neurosci Lett.* 1999 Jan 15;259(3):196-8

[188] "The FMS patients had a 31% lower MT secretion than healthy subjects during the hours of darkness... Patients with fibromyalgic syndrome have a lower melatonin secretion during the hours of darkness than healthy subjects. This may contribute to impaired sleep at night, fatigue during the day, and changed pain perception." Wikner J, Hirsch U, Wetterberg L, Röjdmark S. Fibromyalgia--a syndrome associated with decreased nocturnal melatonin secretion. *Clin Endocrinol* (Oxf). 1998 Aug;49:179-83

[189] Weinstock et al. Restless Legs Syndrome in Patients with Irritable Bowel Syndrome: Response to Small Intestinal Bacterial Overgrowth Therapy. *Dig Dis Sci* 2007 May:1252-6

[190] Wallace DJ, Hallegua DS. Fibromyalgia: the gastrointestinal link. *Curr Pain Headache Rep.* 2004 Oct;8(5):364-8

[191] Pimentel et al. Improvement of symptoms by eradication of small intestinal overgrowth in FM: a double-blind study. [Abstract] *Arthritis Rheum* 1999, 42:S343

[192] Pimentel et al. The effect of a nonabsorbed oral antibiotic (rifaximin) on the symptoms of the irritable bowel syndrome. *Ann Intern Med.* 2006 Oct 17;145(8):557-63

[193] Sharara et al. A randomized double-blind placebo-controlled trial of rifaximin in patients with abdominal bloating and flatulence. *Am J Gastroenterol.* 2006 Feb;101(2):326-33

[194] Pimentel M, Lembo A, Chey WD, et al. Rifaximin therapy for patients with irritable bowel syndrome without constipation. *N Engl J Med.* 2011 Jan 6;364(1):22-32

symptoms, bloating, abdominal pain, and loose or watery stools. *Comments by Dr Vasquez: Shortcomings of the intervention used in this IBS-rifaximin study include* ❶ *failure to use long-term treatment, which is often necessary in the treatment of chronic SIBO,* ❷ *failure to co-administer an antifungal agent to avert fungal growth in the intestines which commonly occurs as a result of antimicrobial/antibacterial drug treatment,* ❸ *failure to administer probiotics to re-establish beneficial flora, and* ❹ *failure to implement dietary modification to sustain the beneficial eradication of excess bacteria—allowing patients to continue their unhealthy diets and lifestyles is the most assured way to ensure that the condition (SIBO-IBS) will return.*

- Review of clinical trials: Rifaximin as treatment for SIBO and IBS (*Expert Opinion on Investigational Drugs* 2009 Mar[195]): A recognized expert in the treatment of SIBO-related conditions, Dr Pimentel writes, "**Rifaximin is a broad-range, gastrointestinal-specific antibiotic that demonstrates no clinically relevant bacterial resistance.** Therefore, rifaximin may be useful in the treatment of gastrointestinal disorders associated with altered bacterial flora, including irritable bowel syndrome (IBS) and small intestinal bacterial overgrowth (SIBO)." He also notes regarding the use of rifaximin in the treatment of IBS, "Rifaximin improved global symptoms in 33 - 92% of patients and eradicated SIBO in up to 84% of patients with IBS, with results sustained up to 10 weeks post-treatment. Rifaximin caused a lower number of adverse events compared with metronidazole or levofloxacin and may have a more favorable adverse event profile than systemic antibiotics, without clinically relevant antibiotic resistance."

- Results of two clinical trials of antibiotics in the treatment of fibromyalgia: Fibromyalgia—the gastrointestinal link (*Current Pain and Headache Reports* 2004 Oct[196]): This article discusses the results of two experiments using antibiotics in the treatment of FM: ❶ 96 patients with SIBO diagnosed by lactulose hydrogen breath testing (LHBT) were offered antibiotic treatment for the reduction of gastrointestinal bacteria; 25 of the 96 patients returned for a follow-up LHBT. Neomycin was the most commonly used antibiotic. Eleven of the 25 patients achieved complete transient eradication of SIBO after antibiotic treatment and experienced better improvement in more of their FM symptom scores when compared with the patients who did not achieve complete eradication. This indicates that **a direct relationship exists between the presence of SIBO and intestinal and extraintestinal symptoms in fibromyalgia, and that FM can be alleviated by effective antimicrobial/antibiotic treatment.** ❷ In this double-blind trial of eradication of SIBO in fibromyalgia, 46 patients fulfilling the established criteria for FM were tested for SIBO using LHBT. Forty-two of the 46 patients (91.3%) were positive for SIBO and were randomized to receive placebo or 500 mg of liquid neomycin (a minimally-absorbed gastrointestinal-specific antibiotic drug) twice daily for 10 days. Only six of the 20 patients (30%) in the neomycin group achieved eradication (indicating inefficacy of treatment); thus, no statistically significant difference between groups was available for analysis. Thereafter, 28 patients in the double-blind study testing positive for SIBO went on to receive open-label antibiotic treatment to eradicate SIBO, and this time 17 of the 28 patients (60.7%) achieved eradication of SIBO. When these 23 patients were compared with the 15 patients who failed to eradicate or did not undergo open-label treatment, significant improvement attributable to antibiotic treatment in the FM scores was detected. **Results show that eradication of bacterial overgrowth results in a clinically significant alleviation of FM symptoms.**

Thus, overall and when integrated together, the research literature provides compelling evidence linking intestinal bacterial overgrowth with the genesis and perpetuation of fibromyalgia. Chronic low-dose exposure to bacterial debris such as lipopolysaccharide/endotoxin and metabolic toxins such as hydrogen sulfide and D-lactic acid from SIBO is a plausible cause of impaired cellular energy production that results in chronic, widespread muscle fatigue and soreness and which may culminate in the clinical presentation of fibromyalgia. The individual components of this model have been substantiated by mechanistic studies in animals and/or research studies in humans. CFS also shares many epidemiological and clinical similarities with FM, and a similar pathophysiology is highly probable.

A consistent report from many CFS and fibromyalgia patients is that of environmental intolerance (EI) and multiple chemical sensitivity (MCS), often grouped together as EI-MCS; these are complex disorders that the medical

---

[195] Pimentel M. Review of rifaximin as treatment for SIBO and IBS. *Expert Opin Investig Drugs.* 2009 Mar;18(3):349-58
[196] Wallace DJ, Hallegua DS. Fibromyalgia: the gastrointestinal link. *Curr Pain Headache Rep.* 2004 Oct;8(5):364-8

profession has failed to appreciate and which are characterized by adverse physiological responses to ambient levels of toxic chemicals and other environmental exposures. EI-MCS can be plausibly explained by SIBO because bacterial LPS/endotoxin impairs hepatic cytochrome P450 detoxification enzymes, resulting in reduced drug metabolism and impaired clearance of xenobiotics/toxins.[197] Accumulation of xenobiotics in CFS patients[198] might therefore be explained in part by LPS-induced inhibition of xenobiotic clearance secondary to SIBO. Further, the metabolic and immunologic effects of LPS can also account for the immune activation, neurological dysfunction, and musculoskeletal complaints noted in patients with CFS, IBS, and FM. A simplified yet accurate model of fibromyalgia which accounts for the major clinical and objective abnormalities seen with this condition is presented in the diagram that follows. Following the exclusion of diagnosable and treatable conditions that can contribute to or mimic fibromyalgia, and by using an integrated model, clinicians can design treatment plans based on the previously reviewed pathogenesis and on the therapeutic considerations detailed in the following section.

How small intestine bacterial overgrowth (SIBO) causes fibromyalgia: Bacterial overgrowth of the small bowel leads to chronic low-grade tryptophan insufficiency resulting in reduced endogenous production of serotonin (important for positive mood and relief from anxiety pain) and of melatonin (important for restful sleep and protection of mitochondria from oxidative stress). Bacterial mitochondrial toxins such as endotoxin, H2S, D-lactate cause impaired mitochondrial energy production, which leads to mitophagy, muscle fatigue, pain, and cognitive impairment.

Therapeutic Interventions
- **Overview**: Treatments for FM should be ❶ science-based and should ❷ directly address the cause(s) of the disorder; treatments should be ❹ safe (generally) and ❺ effective and ❻ without potential for serious adverse effects. Drug treatment of FM does not meet these criteria; the integrative, nutritional, and functional medicine approaches outlined below can—when properly employed by a skilled clinician—address the cause(s) of FM

---
[197] Shedlofsky et al. Endotoxin administration to humans inhibits hepatic cytochrome P450-mediated drug metabolism. *J Clin Invest*. 1994 Dec;94(6):2209-14
[198] Dunstan et al. A preliminary investigation of chlorinated hydrocarbons and chronic fatigue syndrome. *Med J Aust*. 1995 Sep 18;163(6):294-7

in a way that is scientific, direct, safe, effective, and well tolerated by essentially all patients. **Treatments for FM must emphasize eradication of SIBO, prevention of SIBO recurrence, the restoration/establishment of optimal nutritional status, and specific support for optimal mitochondrial function; anything less than this will fail to be effective.** Clinical interventions for the treatment of SIBO include dietary carbohydrate restriction, normalization of slow gastrointestinal transit time (e.g., correction of hypothyroidism), selective use of probiotic supplements to normalize intestinal flora, support of mucosal immunity (with nutrients such as vitamin A, zinc, and L-glutamine), and eradication of bacterial overgrowth with drugs (such as ciprofloxacin, rifaximin, amoxicillin/Augmentin[199], metronidazole) and/or natural products (such as berberine[200], *Artemisia annua*, peppermint oil[201], and emulsified time-released oil of oregano[202])—each of these have been reviewed in greater detail elsewhere by this author.[203] Failure of any monotherapeutic approach to immediately resolve the clinical manifestations of FM can explained by the secondary metabolic, immune, and neurophysiological effects that have generally persisted over periods ranging from years to decades for most patients; in other words, the treatment program must be multifaceted in order to address the numerous major problems that cause FM, and the treatment plan must also be sustained long enough to correct the abnormal physiologic patterns that have been established by the body's response/adaptation to the disease process. The treatment program (examples provided) must be complete in order to facilitate correction of systemic oxidative damage (broad-spectrum antioxidant support), resultant nutritional deficiencies (diet optimization, vitamin and mineral supplementation), immune sensitization and induction of proinflammatory cycles (anti-inflammatory nutrition), alterations in neurotransmission and membrane receptor function (amino acid and fatty acid supplementation), and the inflammation-induced disturbances in pain reception and hypothalamic-pituitary-endocrine function (assess/correct hormonal imbalances; supplement with n-3 fatty acids and olive oil to reduce hypothalamic inflammation[204], etc.). Further, patients treated for SIBO who do not positively change their diets and lifestyles (which probably promoted the genesis and perpetuation of the disease-causing SIBO in the first place) are subject to continual recurrence until such changes are implemented and faithfully maintained.

- **FOOD & NUTRITION** As with many rheumatologic/painful/inflammatory conditions with a strong component of gastrointestinal dysbiosis, the single best diet is a vegan or pesco-vegetarian diet free of gluten and most grains (judicious use of brown rice excepted); clearly the diet must emphasize vegetable intake and avoidance of fermentable substrate to induce quantitative reductions and qualitative improvements in microbial populations and metabolic activity. Beyond the gut, the benefits of minimized carbohydrate intake include weight loss (generally beneficial in this patient population), alleviation of physiologic and psychologic dependence on carbohydrate (over)consumption, and increased endogenous production of beta-hydroxy-butyrate which stimulates the terminal complexes of the mitochondrial electron transport chain while also promoting histone acetylation (via inhibition of histone deacetylase) for enhanced DNA transcription resulting in what has been referred to as a rejuvenative phenotype. My foundational diet-nutritional program—the 5-part "supplemented Paleo-Mediterranean Diet"—can easily be modified to pesco-vegetarian or lacto-pesco-vegetarian variants to enhance high-quality protein intake while continuing to emphasize vegetable, nut, and seed intake to maximize fiber and micronutrient intake. In particular, whey protein isolate is attractive in this patient population due to the high content of tryptophan (to correct the common tryptophan deficiency), the glutathione precursors (to alleviate oxidative stress and enhance mitochondrial function), immunoglobulins (to

> **Patients with migraine headaches—noted in 50% of patients with fibromyalgia—often have food allergies/sensitivities/intolerances**
>
> "The commonest foods causing reactions were wheat (78%), orange (65%), eggs (45%), tea and coffee (40% each), chocolate and milk (37% each), beef (35%), and corn, cane sugar, and yeast (33% each). When an average of ten common foods were avoided there was a dramatic fall in the number of headaches per month, 85% of patients becoming headache-free."
>
> Grant EC. Food allergies and migraine. *Lancet*. 1979 May

---

[199] Malik BA, Xie YY, Wine E, Huynh HQ. Diagnosis and pharmacological management of small intestinal bacterial overgrowth in children with intestinal failure. *Can J Gastroenterol*. 2011 Jan;25(1):41-5. This is a remarkable article and probably one of the most brilliant articles on the treatment of SIBO with drugs.
[200] [No authors listed] Berberine. *Altern Med Rev*. 2000 Apr;5(2):175-7
[201] "A case report of a patient with SIBO who showed marked subjective improvement in IBS-like symptoms and significant reductions in hydrogen production after treatment with ECPO is presented. While further investigation is necessary, results in this case suggest one of mechanisms by which ECPO improves IBS symptoms is antimicrobial activity in small intestine." Logan et al. Treatment of small intestinal bacterial overgrowth with enteric-coated peppermint oil: a case report. *Altern Med Rev*. 2002 Oct;7(5):410-7
[202] Force M, Sparks WS, Ronzio RA. Inhibition of enteric parasites by emulsified oil of oregano in vivo. *Phytother Res*. 2000 May;14(3):213-4
[203] Vasquez A. Nutritional and Botanical Treatments Against "Silent Infections" and Gastrointestinal Dysbiosis. *Nutr Perspect* 2006; Jan: 5-21
[204] Milanski et al. Saturated fatty acids produce inflammatory response predominantly through activation of TLR4 signaling in hypothalamus. *J Neurosci*. 2009 Jan;29(2):359-70

support mucosal defenses against bacterial overgrowth), and growth factors including whey's insulotrophic effect to promote anabolism with resultant improvements in muscle function and gut mucosal integrity. Systemic alkalinization supported by plant-based potassium citrate promotes xenobiotic excretion (reduction in total load of persistent organic pollutants and toxic metals such as lead and mercury) and endogenous production of endorphins (enhanced mood, pain relief). The increased intake of vitamins (including physiologic doses of vitamin D3), minerals, ALA, GLA, EPA, DHA, and probiotics all synergize to alleviate SIBO, oxidative stress, pain and inflammation while also promoting optimal immune and mitochondrial functions. Allergy identification and avoidance is easily achieved via the very practical and no-cost elimination-and-challenge technique. In particular for patients with fibromyalgia, magnesium intake is increased via consumption of dark green vegetables and nutritional supplements while magnesium absorption is promoted by optimized vitamin D status while renal retention of magnesium is promoted with urinary alkalinization. The consistent and pathologic secondary tryptophan deficiency is foremost corrected by eradicating the causative SIBO and the resultant intraintestinal bacterial tryptophanase-catalyzed degradation of ingested tryptophan and via dietary supplementation with L-tryptophan, 5-hydroxytryptophan, and/or whey protein isolate.

- Diet optimization with the five-part "supplemented Paleo-Mediterranean Diet" (*Nutr Perspect* 2011 Jan[205]): The "supplemented Paleo-Mediterranean Diet" (SPMD)—the 5-part nutritional wellness protocol—as described in most of my textbooks in "chapter 2" and also in my articles available on-line at optimalhealthresearch.com/protocol.html should be implemented for most FM patients; exceptions to this general rule might include patients with renal insufficiency due to the risk for potassium excess (hyperkalemia [Note 206]). Because any patient might have an allergy or intolerance to any food (even a healthy food like citrus fruit, chicken or eggs), patients and doctors must be aware of the potential for food allergies and will therefore have to customize the Paleo-Mediterranean diet *for each individual patient* to exclude foods to which the patient might be allergic or sensitive/intolerant. Otherwise, this 5-part nutrition protocol is based on ❶ vegetables, nuts, seeds, (berries, fruits, and juices generally have to be avoided during treatment for SIBO due to the high content of sugars and—with juice—the rapid passage through the gastrointestinal tract) and lean sources of protein, ❷ high-potency multivitamin and multimineral supplementation, ❸ physiologic doses of vitamin D3 to optimize blood levels of vitamin D3 (measured as 25-OH-vitamin D), ❹ combination fatty acid supplementation (with flax oil [for ALA], fish oil [for EPA and DHA], and borage oil [for GLA] with oleic acid from olive oil incorporated into the diet), and ❺ probiotics—foods or supplements that contain living bacteria with beneficial qualities. The diet should emphasize strict avoidance of grains in general and gluten-containing grains *especially wheat* in particular. This diet is essential for the provision of sufficient protein, fiber, phytonutrients, and alkalinization—potassium citrate is most concentrated in vegetables and helps the body maintain proper acid-alkaline balance.[207] The diet should be low in carbohydrates to reduce fermentable substrate to intestinal bacteria. The most important books for patients to read in support of this diet are *The Paleo Diet* by Dr Loren Cordain and *Breaking the Vicious Cycle* by Elaine Gottschall; an open-access summary of the diet plan is available at OptimalHealthResearch.com/spmd.html.

- Vegetarian diet: Fibromyalgia syndrome improved using a mostly raw vegetarian diet (*BMC Complementary and Alternative Medicine* 2001 Sep[208]): Diets high in fruits, vegetables, nuts, berries, and seeds provide ample fiber to promote laxation and can be useful as adjunctive treatment for gastrointestinal dysbiosis in general and SIBO in particular (i.e., *quantitative* reduction in GI dysbiosis). Perhaps more importantly, plant-based diets result in *qualitative* benefits by changing microbial behavior and reducing production of irritants, toxins, and bacterial metabolites, including the mitochondrial poisons D-lactate and

---

[205] Vasquez A. Revisiting the Five-Part Nutritional Wellness Protocol: Supplemented Paleo-Mediterranean Diet. *Nutr Perspect* 2011 Jan InflammationMastery.com/reprints

[206] Because the kidneys are responsible for excreting potassium, reduced kidney function (kidney failure, renal insufficiency) implies that the kidneys may not be able to perform the function of excreting potassium; thus, consumption of a potassium-rich diet could contribute to a dangerous situation of excess potassium in the blood known as hyperkalemia (*hyper*=too much, *kal*=potassium, *emia*=blood disorder). For patients with renal insufficiency, consumption of an otherwise health-promoting diet rich in fruits and vegetables might cause a problem if potassium accumulates in the blood due to impaired excretion. Blood tests can assess renal function as well as the blood potassium level. This is one example of why a clinician/doctor should be employed by patients before implementing diet modification and nutritional supplementation.

[207] "The modern Western-type diet is deficient in fruits and vegetables and contains excessive animal products, generating the accumulation of non-metabolizable anions and a lifespan state of overlooked metabolic acidosis, whose magnitude increases progressively with aging due to the physiological decline in kidney function." Adeva MM, Souto G. Diet-induced metabolic acidosis. *Clin Nutr*. 2011 Aug;30(4):416-21

[208] Donaldson et al. Fibromyalgia syndrome improved using a mostly raw vegetarian diet. *BMC Complement Altern Med*. 2001;1:7 biomedcentral.com/1472-6882/1/7

hydrogen sulfide. Fibromyalgia patients who consume a mostly vegetarian diet have experienced significant improvements in function and reductions in FM symptomatology. Poorly designed dietary interventions that allow abundant intake of whole-grain bread, pasta, rice, and fruit juice[209] would be expected to fail because such high-carbohydrate diets feed intestinal bacteria with an abundance of substrate and would therefore be expected to sustain or exacerbate SIBO. Another advantage to a plant-based mostly-raw diet is the avoidance of dietary advanced glycation end-products (AGEs) which are inflammation-promoting chemical combinations of proteins with sugars, which can be consumed in the diet (e.g., baked deserts) or formed endogenously/internally as a result of oxidative stress and elevated blood sugar levels (e.g., diabetes mellitus). As discussed previously, FM patients show higher levels of AGEs in blood cells and muscle tissue; AGEs promote chronic pain and inflammation[210], and therefore dietary and nutritional strategies that reduce AGE intake and/or AGE formation are 1) without risk, and 2) likely to provide manifold health benefits, including but not limited to reductions in pain and inflammation.

Dr Vasquez's Five-part Nutrition Protocol: The "Supplemented Paleo-Mediterranean Diet"

1. **Diet: Emphasize vegetables, nuts, seeds, berries, and lean sources of protein** (fish, grass-fed lamb/beef). Minimize fruit intake due to higher sugar content while treating SIBO; the goal is to deprive the bacteria and yeast in the intestines of their preferred food source (carbohydrates, sugars). Make modifications for patient-specific food allergies and sensitivities; this is especially important for patients with known allergy-related conditions such as migraine headaches. Patients with kidney disease should use caution when consuming a potassium-rich diet. (Vasquez A. Revisiting the Five-Part Nutritional Wellness Protocol: The Supplemented Paleo-Mediterranean Diet. *Nutritional Perspectives* 2011 Jan)
2. **Multivitamin and multimineral supplement**: Nutrient deficiencies are common and are easily treated with nutritional supplementation. (Fletcher and Fairfield. Vitamins for chronic disease prevention in adults. *JAMA* 2002 Jun)
3. **Vitamin D dosed at 2,000-10,000 IU per day**: The adult requirement for vitamin D3 is approximately 4,000 IU per day; some patients may achieve optimal blood levels with lower doses, but generally daily doses of 4,000-10,000 IU are necessary. (Vasquez A, et al. The Clinical Importance of Vitamin D. *Alternative Therapies in Health and Medicine* 2004 Sep)
4. **Combination fatty acid supplementation**: A combination of flax oil, borage oil, and fish oil provides the health-promoting fatty acids (ALA, GLA, EPA, DHA). Patients should consume organic virgin olive oil liberally with foods. (Vasquez A. New Insights into Fatty Acid Supplementation and Its Effect on Eicosanoid Production and Genetic Expression. *Nutritional Perspectives* 2005; Jan)
5. **Probiotics**: Health-promoting bacteria can be consumed in the form of powders, pills, and fermented foods such as yogurt and kefir.

- **Tryptophan and 5-hydroxytryptophan (5-HTP):** Tryptophan is an amino acid found in many foods and is essential for human health and survival. Tryptophan is available as a nutritional supplement only by a doctor's prescription; it is available over-the-counter in a nonprescription supplement in the form of 5-hydroxytryptophan (5-HTP), which is commonly sourced from the seeds of *Griffonia simplicifolia*, a woody climbing shrub native to West and Central Africa. Tryptophan is the precursor to the neurotransmitter serotonin, which has antidepressant, anti-anxiety, and analgesic properties. Patients with FM are known to have low blood levels (i.e., functional nutritional insufficiency) of tryptophan, and the severity of the deficiency correlates with the severity of pain.[211,212,213] Blood levels of serotonin are often below normal in FM patients.[214] The accepted *medical-pharmacological* use of selective serotonin reuptake inhibitors (SSRI) drugs to treat the pain, depression, and anxiety associated with FM supports the use of 5-HTP to raise serotonin levels *naturally* by correcting the underlying nutritional insufficiency. As an over-the-counter

---

[209] Michalsen et al. Mediterranean diet or extended fasting's influence on changing the intestinal microflora, immunoglobulin A secretion and clinical outcome in patients with rheumatoid arthritis and fibromyalgia: an observational study. *BMC Complement Altern Med.* 2005 Dec 22;5:22
[210] "In the interstitial connective tissue of fibromyalgic muscles we found a more intensive staining of the AGE CML, activated NF-kappaB, and also higher CML levels in the serum of these patients compared to the controls. RAGE was only present in FM muscle." Rüster et al. Detection of elevated N epsilon-carboxymethyllysine levels in muscular tissue and in serum of patients with fibromyalgia. *Scand J Rheumatol.* 2005 Nov-Dec;34(6):460-3
[211] Moldofsky H, Warsh JJ. Plasma tryptophan and musculoskeletal pain in non-articular rheumatism ("fibrositis syndrome"). *Pain.* 1978 Jun;5(1):65-71
[212] Yunus MB, Dailey JW, Aldag JC, Masi AT, Jobe PC. Plasma tryptophan and other amino acids in primary fibromyalgia: a controlled study. *J Rheumatol.* 1992 Jan;19(1):90-4
[213] Russell IJ, Michalek JE, Vipraio GA, Fletcher EM, Wall K. Serum amino acids in fibrositis/fibromyalgia syndrome. *J Rheumatol* Suppl. 1989 Nov;19:158-63
[214] Wolfe F, Russell IJ, Vipraio G, Ross K, Anderson J. Serotonin levels, pain threshold, and fibromyalgia symptoms in the general population. *J Rheumatol.* 1997;24(3):555-9

nutritional supplement, the 5-hydroxylated form of tryptophan (5-HTP) has been used clinically and in numerous research studies. **Supplementation with 5-HTP has been shown to significantly alleviate symptoms of fibromyalgia.**[215] Commonly used doses range from 50 to 300 mg/d, with larger doses divided throughout the day. If tryptophan rather than 5-HTP is used, results are improved when taken on an empty stomach with carbohydrate (such as honey or fruit juice) to induce insulin secretion, which preferentially promotes uptake of tryptophan into the brain. Deficiency of either magnesium or vitamin B6 impairs conversion of 5-HTP into serotonin, and therefore the interventional program must ensure nutritional supra-sufficiency.

- Primary fibromyalgia syndrome and 5-hydroxy-L-tryptophan: a 90-day open study (*Journal of Internal Medicine Research* 1992 Apr[216]): An open 90-day study in 50 fibromyalgia patients showed significant improvement in all measured parameters (number of tender points, anxiety, pain intensity, quality of sleep, fatigue) after treatment with 5-HTP; global clinical improvement assessed by the patient and the investigator indicated a "good" or "fair" response in nearly 50% of the patients during the treatment period.
- Double-blind study of 5-hydroxytryptophan versus placebo in the treatment of primary fibromyalgia syndrome (*Journal of Internal Medicine Research* 1990 May-Jun[217]): A double-blind, placebo-controlled study using 5-HTP in 50 fibromyalgia patients showed significant improvement in all measured parameters, with only mild and transient side effects. *Note by DrV: Again, the common dose range for 5-HTP is 50 to 300 mg per day with doses greater than 100 mg generally best divided throughout the day (e.g., 50 mg thrice per day). I generally recommend starting with 50-100 mg about one hour before bedtime, then adding incremental additions of 50 mg throughout the day for a maximum daily dose of 300 mg. Effectiveness is increased with additional supplementation with magnesium, vitamin B6 (pyridoxine), and the fatty acids found in fish oil (EPA and DHA).*

- **Magnesium:** Magnesium deficiency is epidemic in industrialized societies due to insufficient dietary intake (e.g., from mineral water and leafy green vegetables) and concomitant metabolic-urinary acidosis, which increases urinary magnesium loss.[218,219] Additional causes of magnesium deficiency in fibromyalgia patients include vitamin D deficiency, malabsorption due to SIBO, and the stress of chronic illness. Magnesium deficiency exacerbates the symptoms of fibromyalgia by contributing to impairment of energy/ATP production in skeletal muscle, increased muscle tone and spasms (hypomagnesemic tetany), and anxiety and increased pain sensitivity—hyperalgesia via NMDA receptor overstimulation and neurocortical hyperexcitability. Magnesium deficiency also promotes constipation and intestinal stasis, which exacerbates SIBO. Magnesium supplementation (600 mg or to bowel tolerance to a limit of 1,500 mg in divided doses [bowel tolerance is defined as the dose—commonly of magnesium or vitamin C—that produces slightly loose stools due to the osmotic laxative effect]) should be used routinely in fibromyalgia patients; the primary cautions with magnesium use are renal insufficiency and the use of magnesium-sparing drugs such as the diuretic drug spironolactone. Modest benefits demonstrated in clinical trials with magnesium and malic acid[220] can easily be exceeded with concomitant interventions to address vitamin D deficiency, SIBO, and mitochondrial dysfunction.

- **S-adenosylmethionine (SAMe):** Studies using oral or intravenous administration of the nutritional supplement SAMe have reported conflicting results; however, the overall trend seems to indicate that SAMe (800 mg/d orally) is safe and beneficial in the treatment of fibromyalgia.[221] SAMe helps maintain mitochondrial function by preserving glutathione, and its contribution of methyl groups is important for the regulation of gene expression and neurotransmitter synthesis. *Comment by Dr Vasquez: I do not regularly use this supplement, and I would only use it as a last resort if nothing else had worked or if a particular patient had a specific indication for this supplement.*

---

[215] Caruso I, et al. Double-blind study of 5-hydroxytryptophan versus placebo in the treatment of primary fibromyalgia syndrome. *J Int Med Res*. 1990 May-Jun;18(3):201-9
[216] Sarzi Puttini P, Caruso I. Primary fibromyalgia syndrome and 5-hydroxy-L-tryptophan: a 90-day open study. *J Int Med Res*. 1992 Apr;20(2):182-9
[217] Caruso I et al. Double-blind study of 5-hydroxytryptophan versus placebo in the treatment of primary fibromyalgia syndrome. *J Int Med Res*. 1990 May-Jun;18(3):201-9
[218] Cordain L, et al. Origins and evolution of the Western diet: health implications for the 21st century. *Am J Clin Nutr*. 2005 Feb;81(2):341-54
[219] Rylander R, Remer T, Berkemeyer S, Vormann J. Acid-base status affects renal magnesium losses in healthy, elderly persons. *J Nutr*. 2006 Sep;136(9):2374-7
[220] Russell et al. Treatment of fibromyalgia syndrome with Super Malic: randomized, double blind, placebo controlled, crossover pilot study. *J Rheumatol*. 1995 May;22(5):953-8
[221] Leventhal LJ. Management of fibromyalgia. *Ann Intern Med*. 1999 Dec 7;131(11):850-8

- **INFECTIONS & DYSBIOSIS** As reviewed in a previous section, fibromyalgia patients have a remarkably high prevalence of occult SIBO, the severity of which directly correlates with the severity of FM symptomatology and the eradication of which directly correlates with alleviation of FM. SIBO is the single primary pathoetiologic mechanism that explains each and every abnormality seen in this condition; the response of fibromyalgia patients to gastrointestinal-specific nonabsorbable antimicrobial treatments such as rifaximin provides diagnostic proof of effective treatment of the causative SIBO. Jejunal aspiration is expensive, inconvenient, cumbersome, invasive, and not completely sensitive, while breath hydrogen and methane testing is also cumbersome and relatively expensive (especially when compared to making a clinical diagnosis and confirmatory treatment) and is likewise not completely reliable. Post-prandial gas and bloating is a reliable clinical indicator of SIBO, and empiric treatment of SIBO with a low-carbohydrate diet (LCD) and antimicrobial agents that results in clinical improvement (which may include alleviation of musculoskeletal pain, improved cognition, alleviation of fatigue, and—especially in elderly patients—alleviation of malabsorption and malnutrition) confirms the diagnosis. Stated more plainly, effective implementation of LCD with antimicrobial treatment is both diagnostic and therapeutic; this allows the diagnosis to be made efficiently and with high specificity, (sensitivity depends upon efficacy) and bypassing expensive/insensitive/nontherapeutic/cumbersome diagnostic methods expedites physicians' efficacy and patients' relief in a manner that is safe and cost-effective, especially when compared to perpetual nontherapeutic symptomatic polypharmacy.
    - <u>Low-carbohydrate diet, specific-carbohydrate diet</u>: Patients can follow a diet that emphasizes consumption of low-carbohydrate vegetables, nuts, and seeds and excludes grains (especially wheat, which is very highly fermentable), starches from foods such as potatoes, and disaccharides such as lactose and sucrose; most of the characteristics of a competent low-carbohydrate diet can be achieved within a "Paleo diet" such as described and popularized by Cordain. Alternatively or additionally, patients can follow the specific-carbohydrate diet described and popularized by Gottschall.
    - <u>Probiotics</u>: Probiotics are beneficial bacteria that can be consumed in foods or as nutritional supplements to populate the gut, particularly following antibiotic use or long-term dietary neglect. In addition to their availability in capsules and powders, probiotics are widely consumed in the form of yogurt, kefir, and other cultured foods, and they have an excellent record of safety. Probiotic supplements are available in different strengths (quantity), potencies (viability), and combinations of bacteria (diversity). Some probiotics also contain fermentable carbohydrates (prebiotics) such as fructooligosaccharides (FOS) and inulin, which are substrates to nourish the beneficial bacteria. From a practical clinical perspective, the clinician can choose probiotic foods and supplements and instruct the patient to use these on an ongoing, periodic, or rotational basis. Probiotics (i.e., bacteria only) may have a therapeutic advantage over prebiotics or synbiotics (probiotics+prebiotics) when treating SIBO because the fermentable carbohydrate in prebiotics and synbiotics may exacerbate the preexisting bacterial overgrowth by providing already overpopulated bacteria with additional substrate. The benefits of probiotic supplementation have been demonstrated in patients with IBS, rotavirus infection, eczema and increased intestinal permeability, and SIBO associated with renal failure. To date, no studies using probiotics in the treatment of fibromyalgia have been published.
    - <u>Antimicrobial agents</u>: Antimicrobial agents can be categorized as either natural or pharmaceutical, and as absorbable and systemic or nonabsorbable and gastrointestinal-specific. These can be used empirically, as such treatment for suspected SIBO is well documented in the peer-reviewed clinical medicine literature; however, clinicians must always consider risk-to-benefit ratios especially when using the pharmaceutical antimicrobials which can induce systemic adverse effects (e.g., drug allergy or Stevens-Johnson syndrome or quinolone tendonopathy) or gastrointestinal adverse effects (e.g., nonspecific diarrhea, yeast overgrowth, *Clostridium difficile* diarrhea). Clinicians must always determine the proper choice and dose of therapeutic agents per patient. Two of the best and most important articles on the subject of SIBO are "Lin HC. Small intestinal bacterial overgrowth: a framework for understanding irritable bowel syndrome. *JAMA* 2004 Aug" (concepts and system-wide pathophysiology) and "Malik et al. Diagnosis and pharmacological management of small intestinal bacterial overgrowth in children with intestinal failure. *Can J Gastroenterol*

2011 Jan" (excellent sections on clinical diagnosis and pharmacologic management emphasizing rotational implementation of gut-specific antimicrobials). I prefer to use natural antimicrobial agents continuously for an extended period of time either alone or in conjunction with pharmaceutical antibacterial drugs, which I tend to use on a rotating basis of 7-14 days. Occasionally I will use a short course of an antiparasitic drug such as metronidazole or tinidazole, and I nearly always implement an extended course of antifungal treatment—either oregano oil or nystatin as nonabsorbable agents—punctuated by fluconazole/Diflucan if I suspect treatment resistant gastrointestinal yeast or any dermatologic or sinorespiratory yeast. Clinicians should appreciate that *yeast* colonization of the intestines promotes *bacterial* colonization of the intestines via—for example—elaboration by *Candida albicans* of a sIgA-protease and gliotoxin, an appreciated immunosuppressant. The following list emphasizes the antimicrobial agents I most commonly utilize, always in conjunction with nutritional supplementation (to restore immune function and mucosal defenses) and reduction in dietary carbohydrate intake (to reduce fermentable substrate and thereby "starve the microbes"). Although some dosage and duration suggestions are provided, the clinical reality is that patients need to be treated with *"dose and duration to effect"* or *"titrate to effect"*—meaning that the milligram dose per day and the duration of treatment can and should be customized per the patient's response to treatment. Combination therapy (i.e., more than one treatment at a time), prolonged therapy (treatment of chronic [poly]dysbiosis generally requires longer duration of treatment than does treatment of acute monomicrobial infections), and periodic/punctual treatment (for exacerbations and recurrences).

- Clinical support favoring "open label" empiric antimicrobial treatment of SIBO in patients with fibromyalgia (*Current Pain and Headache Reports* 2004 Oct[222]): This article discusses the results of two experiments using antibiotics in the treatment of FM: ❶ 96 patients with SIBO diagnosed by lactulose hydrogen breath testing (LHBT) were offered **antibiotic treatment** for the reduction

> **A practical summary of SIBO: small intestine bacterial overgrowth**
>
> 1. Definition: Generalized nonspecific overpopulation of bacteria (commonly with other microbes such as yeast) in the small intestine (and large intestine, too).
> 2. Frequency: Very common in clinical practice and the general population.
> 3. Primary symptoms: Gas and bloating, especially after carbohydrate consumption; may also have constipation and/or diarrhea.
> 4. Secondary symptoms: Fatigue, muscle aches, difficulty with concentration and cognition ("brain fog"), nutritional deficiencies due to malabsorption, immune activation due to absorption of microbial debris and metabolites, muscle pain due to dysbiotic mitochondriopathy and LPS- and cytokine-induced central sensitization.
> 5. Diagnosis: ❶ Based on the symptoms above, ❷ jejunal aspiration is the gold standard but is expensive, cumbersome, and potentially hazardous, ❸ measurement of fermentation products (hydrogen and methane) in breath following consumption of a carbohydrate such as glucose, sucrose, or lactulose; the amount of "gas" produced is proportional to the bacterial population, ❹ may find elevated short chain fatty acids (SCFA) in stool or elevated folate in blood, but not all cases of SIBO produce high levels of SCFA or folate, ❺ clinical response to low-carbohydrate diet and/or antibiotic drugs or antimicrobial herbs. The current author (AV) uses #1 in conjunction with #5 most commonly.
> 6. Treatments: Low-carbohydrate diet with antibiotic drugs (e.g., Xifaxan/Rifaximin (200 or 550 mg each) 400-550 mg tid po [1,200-1,650 mg daily] for 10-30 days) or antimicrobial herbs (e.g., time-released emulsified oregano oil 600 mg daily for 4-6 weeks, and/or berberine 400-1,500 mg daily for 4 weeks).

of gastrointestinal bacteria; 25 of the 96 patients returned for a follow-up LHBT. **Neomycin** was the most commonly used antibiotic. Eleven of the 25 patients achieved complete transient eradication of SIBO after antibiotic treatment and experienced better improvement in more of their FM symptom scores when compared with the patients who did not achieve complete eradication. This indicates that a direct relationship exists between the presence of SIBO and intestinal and extraintestinal symptoms in fibromyalgia, and that FM can be alleviated by effective antimicrobial/antibiotic treatment. ❷ In this double-blind trial of eradication of SIBO in fibromyalgia, 46 patients fulfilling the established criteria for FM were tested for SIBO using LHBT. Forty-two of the 46 patients (91.3%) were positive for SIBO and were randomized to receive placebo or 500 mg of **liquid neomycin** (a minimally-absorbed gastrointestinal-specific antibiotic drug) twice daily for 10 days. Only six of the 20 patients (30%) in the

---

[222] Wallace DJ, Hallegua DS. Fibromyalgia: the gastrointestinal link. *Curr Pain Headache Rep.* 2004 Oct;8(5):364-8

neomycin group achieved eradication (indicating inefficacy of treatment); thus, no statistically significant difference between groups was available for analysis. Thereafter, 28 patients in the double-blind study testing positive for SIBO went on to receive **open-label antibiotic treatment** to eradicate SIBO, and this time 17 of the 28 patients (60.7%) achieved eradication of SIBO. When these 23 patients were compared with the 15 patients who failed to eradicate or did not undergo open-label treatment, significant improvement attributable to antibiotic treatment in the FM scores was detected. Results suggest that eradication of bacterial overgrowth results in a statistically and clinically significant alleviation of FM symptoms.
- Nonprescription antimicrobial agents—examples: Most of the agents listed below have their primary or exclusive area of effectiveness within the lumen of the gastrointestinal tract. These agents are generally broad-spectrum and nonspecific, which is perfectly appropriate when treating nonspecific SIBO.
    - See summary at the start of this chapter; not repeated to save space and to reduce redundancy.
- Prescription-restricted antimicrobial agents—examples: In this section specific for the SIBO of fibromyalgia, nonabsorbable agents (rifaximin, vancomycin, nystatin) are appropriate; agents with systemic absorption (Augmentin and fluconazole) are listed here due to their high efficacy and frequent clinical utilization.
    - Rifaximin/Xifaxan: Rifaximin (gut-specific antibacterial drug) should not be confused with rifampin (systemic antibacterial drug, often used in the treatment of mycobacterium infections such as tuberculosis but also used for other bacterial infections); remember to "get your **facts/fax** right by using ri**fax**imin/Xi**fax**an" while you "use ri**famp**in to **amp**lify the effectiveness of systemic antibiotics in the treatment of chronic infections but it also **amps up** cytochrome p450 and adverse drug effects."
    - Vancomycin orally administered: Clinicians should consider this non/poorly-absorbed antibiotic which is effective against Gram-positive bacteria. Human studies have shown effectiveness in the treatment of IBS, constipation, and primary sclerosing cholangitis. In one particularly remarkable case of a patient with rheumatoid arthritis, I prescribed 125mg/d with great success with the intention to target Gram-positive Th17-inducing segmented filamentous bacteria.
    - Augmentin 1-2g BID: This combination of amoxicillin and clavulanate shows efficacy against more than 90% of gastrointestinal bacteria which contribute to SIBO.
    - Nystatin 500,000 units BID-TID PO duration as needed (e.g., 1-6 months empirically or with any use of antibacterial drugs): Nystatin is a safe nonabsorbable gentle and commonly effective antifungal agent originally derived from a natural source of soil microorganisms. Its lack of significant intestinal absorption reduces the incidence of adverse effects while also prohibiting systemic antifungal effectiveness, except for reducing the total microbial load (TML) by reducing gastrointestinal fungal population. Nystatin is safe for long-term use, is inexpensive, and should generally be used anytime that antibiotic/antibacterial drugs are employed.
    - Fluconazole/Diflucan 100-150-200 mg every other day for 4-5 doses over 8-10 days: The long half-life of 30 hours allows discontinuous alternate-day dosing without loss of efficacy for most routine outpatient applications. This drug is absorbed systemically with excellent tissue penetration for the delivery of multifocal antifungal effectiveness (e.g., alleviation of sinus and genitourinary fungal infections/colonization)

- **NUTRITIONAL IMMUNOMODULATION** My coinage of the term and technique "nutritional immunomodulation" refers to a specific protocol designed to induce epigenetic modifications in undifferentiated Th-0 cells for their preferential promotion into the T-regulatory (Treg) FOXp3+ phenotype while shifting immune (im)balance away from the proinflammatory Th-1, Th-2, and Th-17 phenotypes. The primary components of this protocol can be safely implemented in essentially any and all patients without adverse effect; these fundamental components include low-carbohydrate plant-based diet to promote a systemic anti-inflammatory state, vitamin D3, combination fatty acid supplementation for n-3 fatty acids and GLA, probiotics (note that the first four components of the protocol are already represented in the foundational five-part nutritional protocol), vitamin A, lipoic acid, green tea, and a low-sodium diet. More assertive antidysbiotic interventions to promote healthy microbial balance in the gastrointestinal lumen may include botanical/nutritional/pharmacologic antimicrobial interventions, with some preferential utilization of orally administered vancomycin based on research supporting its effectiveness against segmented filamentous bacteria which are specific inducers of the Th-17 phenotype. Since fibromyalgia in its pure form is not directly due to an immune imbalance in the way considered here, this component of the functional inflammology protocol is not specifically relevant; however, for the many patients with concomitant diagnoses of fibromyalgia with another systemic/inflammatory/autoimmune disease (such as diabetes mellitus, rheumatoid arthritis, multiple sclerosis, or psoriasis) then of course this nutritional immunomodulation protocol should be implemented.

- **DYSFUNCTIONAL MITOCHONDRIA** The basic view that mitochondria are the "powerhouses" of the cell responsible for the formation of cellular energy in the form of ATP is what most people learn in high school biology, and little if any additional knowledge is added to medical physicians' appreciation of the diversity of mitchondria's biologic roles in medical school. Lack of appreciation of the importance of the role of mitochondrial in general and mitochondrial dysfunction in particular in health and disease has left a huge blind spot in the therapeutic vision of most clinicians; by failing to appreciate and correct mitochondrial dysfunction, clinicians have missed a valuable component to the treatment plans of many and probably most of their patients. In addition to the well-known role that mitochondria have in the formation of energy-ATP, mitochondria also play major roles in pancreatic insulin secretion, peripheral insulin reception, microbial surveillance, and maintenance of inflammatory balance, insofar as mitochondrial dysfunction clearly contributes to a pro-diabetic and insulin-insulin resistant state, as well as enhanced pro-inflammatory responsiveness to microbial (including viral) stimuli. Fibromyalgia is clearly identified with mitochondrial dysfunction, and while the secondary mitochondrial dysfunction is one of the major causes of fibromyalgic muscle pain and fatigue, the mitochondrial dysfunction does not itself cause fibromyalgia, the primary cause of which is SIBO. Thus, SIBO's generation of LPS, D-lactate, and other mitochondrial toxins is the primary/direct cause of the mitochondrial dysfunction; effective treatment must emphasize SIBO eradication and mitochondrial resuscitation. We can compartmentalize major components of mitochondrial structure and function into these three main components: ❶ citric acid cycle, ❷ electron transport chain, ❸ and the structural integrity of the inner and outer mitochondrial membranes. The main area of clinical importance can be discussed within a conversation of the electron transport chain (ETC) since this is fed by the citric acid cycle and is structurally interwoven into the inner mitochondrial membrane and fully dependent upon the nonpermeability of the outer mitochondrial membrane for the maintenance of the electromechanical proton gradient. Primary treatment must always be directed at the primary cause of any disease—not its secondary complications; in the case of FM, the SIBO must always be treated. Among mitochondria-specific treatments for fibromyalgia, supplementation with CoQ-10, melatonin, and acetyl-carnitine (preferably with lipoic acid) are the best studied and most efficacious.
  - **Coenzyme Q10 (CoQ-10):** An endogenous antioxidant, vitamin-like substance, and essential component of the mitochondrial electron transport chain, oral supplementation with CoQ-10 has been used therapeutically in numerous studies for the successful treatment of migraine, heart failure, hypertension, and renal failure. Additional data have shown immunomodulatory roles for CoQ-10, and many clinicians employ it as adjunctive treatment for viral infections, cancer, and allergies.[223,224] The electron transport chain is the terminal step in mitochondrial energy/ATP production; as readers can see in the following diagram, each step or "complex" of the electron transport chain requires nutrients, without which energy/ATP production will be impaired, and provision of which (via supplementation) will generally enhance mitochondrial energy/ATP production. Per Cordero et al[225] in 2012, **CoQ-10 levels are 40% lower in blood cells of patients with FM compared with levels in healthy persons**, and reduced levels of CoQ-10 correlate with markers associated with expedited destruction of mitochondria (mitophagy).

---

[223] Gaby AR. The role of Coenzyme Q10 in clinical medicine: Part 1. *Altern Med Rev* 1996;1:11-17
[224] Gaby AR. The role of Coenzyme Q10 in clinical medicine: Part 2. *Altern Med Rev* 1996;1:168-175
[225] Cordero MD, De Miguel M, Moreno Fernández AM, et al. Mitochondrial dysfunction and mitophagy activation in blood mononuclear cells of fibromyalgia patients: implications in the pathogenesis of the disease. *Arthritis Res Ther.* 2010;12(1):R17

- Clinical investigation: Mitochondrial dysfunction and mitophagy activation in blood mononuclear cells of fibromyalgia patients (*Arthritis Research Therapy* 2010 Jan[226]): The authors studied 2 male and 18 female FM patients and 10 healthy controls. They evaluated mitochondrial function in blood mononuclear cells from FM patients measuring CoQ-10 levels with high-performance liquid chromatography (HPLC) and measuring mitochondrial membrane potential with flow cytometry. Oxidative stress was determined by measuring mitochondrial superoxide production and lipid peroxidation in blood mononuclear cells and plasma from FM patients. Autophagy activation was evaluated in blood mononuclear cells; mitophagy was confirmed by measuring citrate synthase activity and electron microscopy examination of blood mononuclear cells. The authors **found reduced levels of CoQ-10, decreased mitochondrial membrane potential, increased levels of mitochondrial superoxide in blood mononuclear cells (indicating increased oxidative stress and reduced antioxidant defense),** and increased levels of lipid peroxidation in both blood mononuclear cells and plasma from FM patients. Importantly, the authors note that "mitochondrial dysfunction was also associated with increased expression of autophagic genes and the elimination of dysfunctional mitochondria with mitophagy." *Comment by Dr Vasquez: What this means in practical terms is that the biochemical aberrations that cause mitochondrial dysfunction lead to destruction of mitochondria via "mitophagy" which literally means "mitochondrial consumption", a process by which dysfunctional mitochondria are eliminated by degradative processes.*

- Clinical trial using a combination of *Ginkgo biloba* and CoQ-10 (*Journal of Internal Medicine Research* 2002 Mar[227]): In an open trial of 23 fibromyalgia patients, the combination of 200 mg CoQ-10 and 200 mg *Ginkgo biloba* (for a total dose of 48 mg flavone glycosides and 12 mg terpene lactones) daily for 84 days was shown to provide clinical benefit in 64% of patients. CoQ-10 is often deficient in FM patients, and this deficiency both *causes* and *results from* mitochondrial dysfunction; stated differently, CoQ-10 depletion and mitochondrial dysfunction form a vicious cycle, a relationship of reciprocal causality. *Ginkgo biloba* extract is an extensively researched botanical medicine with a long history of safe and effective clinical use for various conditions, especially those associated with reduced blood flow and impaired mitochondrial function. *Ginkgo biloba* is a botanical/herbal medicine with a long history of human use; the three most important physiologic effects of *Ginkgo biloba* are ❶ vasodilation—improves blood circulation (which is often compromised in FM patients), ❷ improves mitochondrial function and ATP/energy production, and ❸ antioxidant benefits—quenches/absorbs free radicals, which are oxygen-containing molecules that cause damage to cell structures and body tissues. Given these therapeutic benefits, *Ginkgo* would appear to be a reasonable therapeutic agent to address the secondary pathophysiology in fibromyalgia. *Ginkgo biloba* products are generally standardized for the content of flavone glycosides (approximately 24%) and terpene lactones (approximately 6%) with adult doses ranging from 60-240 mg/d and generally 120 mg/d. *Comment by Dr Vasquez: Ginkgo biloba and CoQ-10 are very safe and appropriate for use by nearly all FM patients.*

- Case series of FM patients treated with CoQ-10 (*Mitochondrion* 2011 Jul[228]): The authors note that CoQ-10 is an essential electron carrier in the mitochondrial respiratory chain and a strong antioxidant and that **low CoQ-10 levels have been detected in patients with FM**. The authors found that **"FM patients with CoQ-10 deficiency showed a statistically significant reduction in symptoms after CoQ-10 treatment during 9 months (300 mg/day)**. Determination of deficiency and consequent supplementation in FM may result in clinical improvement." *Comment by Dr Vasquez: This is a small but important study documenting 1) that CoQ-10 deficiency is common in FM patients, and 2) that CoQ-10 supplementation alleviates the clinical manifestations/symptoms of FM, consistent with the integrated model of FM presented in this book, which includes the components of nutrient deficiency and mitochondrial dysfunction. Although standardized blood testing for CoQ-10 levels is widely available, testing for and documentation of CoQ-10 deficiency is not necessary before the use of CoQ-10 supplementation.*

---

[226] Cordero et al. Mitochondrial dysfunction and mitophagy activation in blood mononuclear cells of fibromyalgia patients. *Arthritis Res Ther*. 2010;12(1):R17
[227] Lister. Open, pilot study to evaluate potential benefits of coenzyme Q10 combined with Ginkgo biloba extract in fibromyalgia syndrome. *J Int Med Res* 2002 Mar-Apr;30:195-9
[228] Cordero MD et al. Coenzyme Q(10): a novel therapeutic approach for Fibromyalgia? case series with 5 patients. *Mitochondrion*. 2011 Jul;11(4):623-5

Reduce mitochondrial protein synthesis: Tetracyclines, chloramphenicol
Cause mtDNA depletion: Adriamycin/doxorubicin, zidovudine, herpes simplex virus
Damage mitochondrial inner membrane: Roundup ® (mixture of glyphosate and solvent/inert chemicals) per *Environ Toxicol Pharmacol* 2012 Sep, *Toxicol In Vitro* 2013 Feb, *Toxicology* 2013 Nov

Each step of the mitochondrial electron transport chain requires specific nutrients, without which energy/ATP production cannot proceed: Complex 1 requires vitamin B2 (riboflavin), vitamin B3 (niacin), and CoQ-10. Complex 2 requires vitamin B2 (riboflavin), iron, CoQ-10, and the fatty acid DHA for the function of succinate dehydrogenase. Complex 3 requires iron. Complex 4 requires vitamin C and copper. Step 4 is the enzyme ATP synthase, which produces cellular energy in the form of ATP.

- Clinical investigation and clinical trial: Oxidative stress, headache symptoms in fibromyalgia and the role of CoQ-10 in clinical improvement (*PLoS One* 2012 Apr[229]): The authors introduce this study by noting that FM is a chronic pain syndrome with "unknown etiology" and a wide spectrum of symptoms such as allodynia (perception of pain from stimuli that are not normally painful), debilitating fatigue, joint stiffness, and migraine headaches. The authors note a link between oxidative stress and the clinical symptoms in FM. In this study, the researchers examined oxidative stress and bioenergetic status in blood mononuclear cells (BMCs) and the association with headache symptoms in FM patients. Following this correlative analysis, the authors assessed the effects of oral CoQ-10 supplementation on biochemical markers and clinical improvements. In 20 FM patients and 15 healthy controls, a variety of validated clinical and biochemical parameters was assessed; specifically for the biochemical component, measurements were performed for serum CoQ-10, catalase, lipid peroxidation (LPO) levels and ATP levels in BMCs. In patients with FM, the authors found lower CoQ-10 (CoQ-10 deficiency), lower catalase (reduced antioxidant defenses) and lower ATP levels (reduced energy production) in BMCs while FM patients also showed elevated LPO (evidence of free-radical damage) in BMCs. Lower levels of CoQ-10 and catalase levels in BMCs correlated with greater severity-frequency of headache. **In this clinical trial using CoQ-10 300 mg/d for 3 months, CoQ-10 supplementation caused significant reductions in pain and tender points, significant reductions in headache impact, significant elevations in cellular levels of CoQ-10, a reduction in malondialdehyde (marker of lipid peroxidation) from 30nmol to 5 nmol (normal 6 nmol), an increase in catalase levels from 35 U/mg to 85 U/mg (normal 96 U/mg), and an increase in BMC production of ATP/energy from 61 nmol/mg to 191 nmol/mg (normal 202 nmol/mg).** Supplementation with CoQ-10 300 mg/day divided in three doses for 3 months "restored biochemical parameters and induced a significant improvement in clinical and headache symptoms." *Note by Dr Vasquez: The dose of CoQ-10 used clinically is generally approximately 100 mg per day, and occasionally a patient or doctor might decide to use a higher dose, which might be up to 300 mg per day.*
- **Melatonin:** Melatonin is a hormone produced in the pineal gland of the brain; melatonin is synthesized from the neurotransmitter serotonin, and production of both serotonin and melatonin are dependent on the nutritional availability of tryptophan and/or 5-HTP as discussed above. Patients with FM show

---

[229] Cordero et al. Oxidative stress correlates with headache symptoms in fibromyalgia: coenzyme Q$_{10}$ effect on clinical improvement. *PLoS One*. 2012;7(4):e35677 ncbi.nlm.nih.gov/pmc/articles/PMC3330812/

decreased nocturnal secretion of melatonin.[230] Melatonin benefits FM patients through a wide range of mechanisms, including promotion of restful sleep and reduction in LPS-induced mitochondrial impairment. As a powerful antioxidant, melatonin scavenges oxygen and nitrogen-based reactants generated in mitochondria and thereby limits the loss of intramitochondrial glutathione, the most important component of antioxidant defense; this prevents damage to mitochondrial protein and DNA. **Melatonin increases the activity of Complexes 1 and 4 of the mitochondrial electron transport chain, improving mitochondrial respiration and increasing ATP synthesis** under various physiological and experimental conditions.[231] Successful treatment with melatonin or its precursor tryptophan/5-HTP should not deter the clinician from addressing other contributing or causative problems such as vitamin D deficiency, gastrointestinal dysbiosis including SIBO, magnesium deficiency, and chronic psychoemotional stress. The adult physiologic dose which mimics natural internal (endogenous) production is approximately 200-500 mcg [micrograms] nightly. In adults, supplementation with melatonin has a wide therapeutic index and has been used safely and effectively in doses up to 20 to 40 mg [milligrams] nightly.

- Case series (n=4): Melatonin therapy in fibromyalgia (*Journal of Pineal Research* 2006 Jan[232]): Melatonin (3–6 mg per night, administered orally 1 hour before bedtime) has been reported to normalize sleep, alleviate pain and fatigue, and resolve many other clinical manifestations of FM. The authors report, "After 15 days of treatment with melatonin, all patients developed a sleep/wake cycle that was considered normal. They also mentioned a significant reduction of pain. At this time, the patients were taken off hypnotics. Thirty days after the initiation of melatonin, other medications were withdrawn and thereafter they only took melatonin." *Comment by Dr Vasquez: These results are impressive, but—again—the other components of FM such as SIBO and CoQ-10 deficiency should also be treated assertively to reduce the risk of relapse and to treat the underlying problems; good healthcare and good self-care should extend beyond mere symptom alleviation.*

- Clinical trial (n=101): Adjuvant use of melatonin for treatment of fibromyalgia (*Journal of Pineal Research.* 2011 Apr[233]): group A (24 patients) treated with 20 mg/day fluoxetine alone; group B (27 patients) treated with melatonin 5 mg alone; group C (27 patients) treated with 20 mg fluoxetine plus 3 mg melatonin; group D (23 patients) treated with 20 mg fluoxetine plus 5 mg melatonin for 8 weeks. "Using melatonin (3 mg or 5 mg/day) in combination with 20 mg/day fluoxetine resulted in significant reduction in both total and different components of Fibromyalgia Impact Questionnaire score compared to the pretreatment values. In conclusion, **administration of melatonin, alone or in a combination with fluoxetine, was effective in the treatment of patients with FMS**."

- **Acetyl-L-carnitine (ALC):** Acetyl-L-carnitine is a form of the amino acid L-carnitine, most notable for its critical role in supporting mitochondrial energy/ATP production by supporting the metabolism (beta oxidation) of fatty acids in the mitochondria. A large study with 102 patients showed that ALC (administered by oral and parenteral routes, 1500 mg/d) was beneficial in patients with fibromyalgia.[234] Given the role of ALC in supporting and improving mitochondrial function, this supplement probably benefits fibromyalgia patients by compensating for LPS-induced skeletal muscle dysfunction.

- **D-ribose:** D-ribose is a naturally occurring pentose carbohydrate available as a dietary supplement. When administered orally (5 g thrice daily), it safely provides numerous benefits to fibromyalgia patients, according to a recent pilot study with 41 patients.[235] Improvements are seen in energy, sleep, mental clarity, pain intensity, and well-being, as well as global assessment. Among its beneficial mechanisms of action is enhancement of mitochondrial ATP production. Thus, the benefits of D-ribose supplementation may be mediated by restoration or preservation of mitochondrial impairment caused by LPS in fibromyalgia patients.

- **Creatine monohydrate:** Skeletal muscle levels of phosphocreatine and ATP are reduced in patients with fibromyalgia compared with normal controls; thus, oral supplementation with creatine would appear to

---

[230] Wikner J, et al. Fibromyalgia--a syndrome associated with decreased nocturnal melatonin secretion. *Clin Endocrinol* (Oxf). 1998 Aug;49(2):179-83
[231] León J, Acuña-Castroviejo D, Escames G, Tan DX, Reiter RJ. Melatonin mitigates mitochondrial malfunction. *J Pineal Res*. 2005 Jan;38(1):1-9
[232] Acuna-Castroviejo D, Escames G, Reiter RJ. Melatonin therapy in fibromyalgia. *J Pineal Res*. 2006 Jan;40(1):98-9
[233] Hussain SA, Al-Khalifa II, Jasim NA, Gorial FI. Adjuvant use of melatonin for treatment of fibromyalgia. *J Pineal Res*. 2011 Apr;50(3):267-71
[234] Rossini M, et al. Double-blind, multicenter trial comparing acetyl l-carnitine with placebo in treatment of fibromyalgia patients. *Clin Exp Rheumatol*. 2007 Mar-Apr;25:182-8
[235] Teitelbaum JE, Johnson C, St Cyr J. The use of D-ribose in chronic fatigue syndrome and fibromyalgia: a pilot study. *J Altern Complement Med*. 2006 Nov;12:857-62

be an obvious intervention to restore these depressed levels to normal. Although no formal trials have been conducted, Artimal et al[236] reported that a patient with severe refractory fibromyalgia attained sustained alleviation of depression and pain, as well as improvements in sleep and quality of life, following oral administration of creatine monohydrate for 4 weeks (3 grams daily in the first week, then 5 grams daily). Creatine supplementation has been shown to improve ATP production and oxygen utilization in brain and skeletal muscle in humans.[237]

- **SOCIOLOGY, SLEEP, STRESS, SOMATIC TREATMENTS, SWEAT** Common clinical and lifestyle considerations are listed in the following sections.
  - **Sociology/psychology, and stress management/reduction**: Everyone—patients as well as clinicians—can benefit from developing self-awareness, emotional intelligence, and other core life skill and insights; since much of our perception of stress has a psycho-epistemological basis, enhanced self-awareness in this key area can help to deconstruct the phenomenon of stress and its secondary consequences. Because this consideration is self-evident in terms of safety, efficacy, broad applicability, and life-enhancement, specific literature will not be reviewed here.
  - **Sleep**: Sleep deprivation induces immune suppression, enhanced sensitivity to pain, and an objectively documentable proinflammatory state evidenced by increases in serum hsCRP. Patients should be encouraged to optimize sleep by avoiding late-in-the-day exercise, overstimulation, caffeine (which generally has a half-life of six hours), and overuse of bright lights following nightfall; items that are conducive to sleep are having a dark and quiet room, relaxing music or reading, and using melatonin. Enhancement of sleep quality and duration have been shown to alleviate systemic inflammation, tendency toward insulin resistance, and pain perception/sensitivity.
  - **Sweating and exercise**: Obesity/overweight and physical inactivity are consistently associated with elevated risk for and experience of depression, low self-esteem, social isolation, systemic inflammation, cardiometabolic disease and diabetes mellitus type-2, cancers of various types, and inflammatory disorders such as asthma and psoriasis. Weight optimization and physical activity promote enhanced self-confidence, self-efficacy, skill-building, social interaction, and reductions in cause-specific and all-cause mortality. Mechanistically, exercise—defined here as physical activity of sustained duration and intensity to promote diaphoresis/sweating—promotes lipolysis (for mobilization of adipose-stored toxins, weight reduction, and enhanced BHB production for induction of histone acetylation and ECT stimulation), promotes glycolysis (to promote induction of enhanced mitochondrial function and insulin sensitivity), and hyperventilation which results in respiratory alkalosis and secondary urinary alkalinization (which promotes mineral retention, xenobiotic excretion, endorphin elevation, and cortisol reduction). Commonly accepted international guidelines as well as common sense advocate 30-60 minutes of daily exercise that should globally include components such as aerobic training, resistance training, skill-building, balance, and flexibility; intensity, duration, and variety are tailored to patient needs and preferences. Because this consideration is self-evident in terms of safety, efficacy, broad applicability, and life-enhancement, specific literature will not be reviewed here.
  - **Somatic treatments (chiropractic, acupuncture, osteopathic manipulation, qigong, balneotherapy)**: Chiropractic treatment (including spinal manipulation, stretching, soft tissue treatments, and therapeutic ultrasound) has shown benefit in several fibromyalgia case series and clinical trials.[238,239] Acupuncture (including traditional, nontraditional, and electrical stimulation) also has been found beneficial for fibromyalgia patients.[240,241,242] Acupuncture may relieve fibromyalgia pain by improving regional blood flow, in addition to other mechanisms.[243,244] Because specific needle placement does not appear to be

---

[236] Amital D, Vishne T, Rubinow A, Levine J. Observed effects of creatine monohydrate in a patient with depression and fibromyalgia. *Am J Psychiatry*. 2006 Oct;163(10):1840-1
[237] Watanabe A, Kato N, Kato T. Effects of creatine on mental fatigue and cerebral hemoglobin oxygenation. *Neurosci Res*. 2002 Apr;42(4):279-85
[238] Citak-Karakaya I, et al. Short and long-term results of connective tissue manipulation and combined ultrasound therapy in patients with fibromyalgia. *J Manipulative Physiol Ther*. 2006 Sep;29(7):524-8
[239] Blunt KL, et al. The effectiveness of chiropractic management of fibromyalgia patients: a pilot study. *J Manipulative Physiol Ther*. 1997 Jul-Aug;20(6):389-99
[240] Martin DP, et al. Improvement in fibromyalgia symptoms with acupuncture: results of a randomized controlled trial. *Mayo Clin Proc*. 2006 Jun;81(6):749-57
[241] Singh BB, et al. Effectiveness of acupuncture in the treatment of fibromyalgia. *Altern Ther Health Med*. 2006 Mar-Apr;12(2):34-41
[242] Deluze C, Bosia L, Zirbs A, Chantraine A, Vischer TL. Electroacupuncture in fibromyalgia: results of a controlled trial. *BMJ*. 1992 Nov 21;305(6864):1249-52
[243] Sandberg M, Larsson B, Lindberg LG, Gerdle B. Different patterns of blood flow response in the trapezius muscle following needle stimulation (acupuncture) between healthy subjects and patients with fibromyalgia and work-related trapezius myalgia. *Eur J Pain*. 2005 Oct;9(5):497-510
[244] Sandberg M, Lindberg LG, Gerdle B. Peripheral effects of needle stimulation (acupuncture) on skin and muscle blood flow in fibromyalgia. *Eur J Pain*. 2004 Apr;8(2):163-71

important[245], the conclusion that true acupuncture is ineffective because it may not differ markedly from the results obtained by sham acupuncture[246] may not be logical. A similar conundrum is seen in other clinical trials involving physical interventions such as manual osseous manipulation, wherein authentic treatments and sham treatments may both be effective by virtue of common physiological responses.[247] A short-term trial showed that osteopathic manipulative therapy with standard medical care was superior to medical care alone for FM patients.[248] Qigong was found helpful for 10 fibromyalgia patients, and benefits were still apparent at 3 months' follow-up.[249] In a randomized, controlled clinical trial among 24 female fibromyalgia patients, balneotherapy (bath therapy) in daily 20-minute sessions 5 days per week for 3 weeks (total of 15 sessions; water temperature: 96.8°F = 36°C), resulted in statistically significant reductions in measured inflammatory mediators (PGE2, interleukin-1, LTB4) and amelioration of clinical symptoms among treated FM patients.[250] The symptomatic benefits of balneotherapy for FM patients have been corroborated in other trials.[251,252,253]

- **ENDOCRINE IMBALANCE & OPTIMIZATION** Peptide-based and steroid-based hormones have wide-ranging effects beyond those with which they are classically and thus simplistically associated. The "main" hormones that we consider in most chronic inflammatory disorders are the three pro-inflammatory hormones (prolactin, estradiol, and insulin) and the three anti-inflammatory hormones (DHEA, cortisol, and testosterone); each of these hormones can be objectively assessed with serologic testing and modulated with therapeutic intervention. A full thyroid evaluation—including history, physical examination (with particular scrutiny for cold extremities [DDX: hypothyroidism, hypogonadism, vasoconstriction/vaso-obstruction, Raynaud's disorder, peripheral vascular disease, H2S-producing GI dysbiosis], relative bradycardia [DDX, hypothyroidism, heart block, beta-blocker medications], and delayed Achilles reflex return [considered diagnostic of hypothyroidism]), and laboratory evaluation (including TSH, free T4, total or free T3, rT3, and antithyroid antibodies) is warranted in any patient whose concerns include fatigue, depression, systemic inflammation and chronic pain; musculoskeletal manifestations of hypothyroidism include muscle pain, weakness, myopathy, and adhesive capsulitis. The pineal hormone melatonin was discussed in a previous section.

- **XENOBIOTIC ACCUMULATION & DETOXIFICATION** The term "xenobiotics" is generally used to refer to carbon-based foreign chemicals such as persistent organic pollutants (POPs) including herbicides, pesticides, phthalates, parabens, dioxin-related chemicals, and many others; used more casually, the term may also be used to include noncarbon-based foreign substances such as toxic metals like lead, mercury, cadmium, and arsenic. Thus, "xenobiotics" has become somewhat synonymous with "toxins" in both professional-level and vernacular conversations. Laboratory assessments for chemical and metal toxins are commercially available through specialized medical laboratories and are based on analysis of blood and urine. The many biochemical and physiologic components of detoxification/depuration have been reviewed in chapter 4 of this book. Essentially everyone—all humans on the planet worldwide—have biochemical evidence of xenobiotic chemical/metal accumulation, generally with numerous xenobiotics, which have additive and synergistic adverse effects on physiology and health. Thus, scientifically, since xenobiotic accumulation is pandemic, consideration of and treatment for xenobiotic accumulation via therapeutic detoxification programs and lifestyle interventions should be routine. Easy and effective means for promoting detoxification of chemicals and metals include plant-based diet to promote bowel and renal excretion of toxins (via reduced enterohepatic recycling [better microflora, more fiber for adsorption, more frequent fecal excretion] and reduced renal resorption [urinary alkalinization], respectively), NAC for arsenic chelation and GSH production,

---

[245] Harris RE, Tian X, Williams DA, Tian TX, Cupps TR, Petzke F, Groner KH, Biswas P, Gracely RH, Clauw DJ. Treatment of fibromyalgia with formula acupuncture: investigation of needle placement, needle stimulation, and treatment frequency. *J Altern Complement Med.* 2005 Aug;11(4):663-71
[246] Assefi NP, et al. A randomized clinical trial of acupuncture compared with sham acupuncture in fibromyalgia. *Ann Intern Med.* 2005 Jul 5;143(1):10-9
[247] Mein EA, et al. Manual medicine diversity: research pitfalls and the emerging medical paradigm. *J Am Osteopath Assoc.* 2001 Aug;101(8):441-4
[248] Gamber RG, Shores JH, Russo DP, Jimenez C, Rubin BR. Osteopathic manipulative treatment in conjunction with medication relieves pain associated with fibromyalgia syndrome: results of a randomized clinical pilot project. *J Am Osteopath Assoc.* 2002 Jun;102(6):321-5
[249] Chen KW, Hassett AL, Hou F, et al. A pilot study of external qigong therapy for patients with fibromyalgia. *J Altern Complement Med.* 2006 Nov;12(9):851-6
[250] Ardiç F, Ozgen M, Aybek H, et al. Effects of balneotherapy on serum IL-1, PGE2 and LTB4 levels in fibromyalgia patients. *Rheumatol Int.* 2007 Mar;27(5):441-6
[251] Evcik D, Kizilay B, Gökçen E. The effects of balneotherapy on fibromyalgia patients. *Rheumatol Int.* 2002 Jun;22(2):56-9
[252] Fioravanti A, Perpignano G, Tirri G, et al. Effects of mud-bath treatment on fibromyalgia patients: a randomized clinical trial. *Rheumatol Int.* 2007 Oct;27(12):1157-61
[253] Dönmez A, Karagülle MZ, Tercan N, et al. SPA therapy in fibromyalgia: a randomised controlled clinic study. *Rheumatol Int.* 2005 Dec;26(2):168-72

sweating/exercise (lipolysis promotes mobilization of lipophilic toxins from adipose tissue, diaphoresis promotes direct toxin excretion), sufficient micronutrient and protein intake supports phase 1 and phase 2 of the oxidation and conjugation processes in the liver. Chemical xenobiotics can be bound in the gut during the normal process of enterohepatic recycling/recirculation with periodic or rotational use of activated charcoal, cholestyramine, and chlorella; anecdotal reports from clinical practices support the use of phytochelatin (metal-binding peptides from plants, used by plants for protection from metal toxicity) in the prevention/treatment of metal toxicity in humans but no formal clinical studies have been performed to document the effectiveness of this approach although its safety is clinically appreciated.

- Pilot study: *Chlorella pyrenoidosa* for patients with fibromyalgia syndrome (*Phytother Res* 2000 May[254]): *Chlorella pyrenoidosa* is a unicellular green alga that grows in fresh water. It is a dense source of nutrients, particularly vitamin D (500 IU vitamin D per 1.35 g *Chlorella*). *Chlorella* may have value in treating some fibromyalgia patients, but overall the efficacy is low. Thus, *Chlorella* should not be used as monotherapy for fibromyalgia, although it may be a useful adjunct either as a source of vitamin D, as a means to help modify gut flora, or as an aid in the detoxification of xenobiotics due to its ability to bind ingested and bile-excreted toxins and prevent their absorption and reabsorption in a manner similar to that of cholestyramine, a drug used to bind cholesterol in the gut, promote its excretion, and thereby lower blood cholesterol levels.[255,256,257] This "detoxifying" effect of *Chlorella* in humans is supported by 2 clinical trials showing that nursing mothers who supplement with *Chlorella* during lactation transfer less dioxin in their breast milk compared to nursing mothers who do not consume *Chlorella*.[258,259]

- Clinical investigation: Reduced exposure to xenobiotics (cosmetics) alleviates fibromyalgia (*Journal of Women's Health* 2004 Mar[260]): Women use more cosmetic products than do men, and fibromyalgia is more common in women. Cosmetic products generally contain skin-absorbable xenobiotics with potentially adverse effects; therefore this study was conducted to determine if avoidance of cosmetics would alleviate symptoms of FM. The author of this report describes a prospective, randomized, controlled trial of 48 women with FM (some of whom had a rheumatic condition) who were regular users of cosmetics was carried out to investigate if a reduced use of cosmetics would reduce the symptoms. The patients were told to avoid or completely abstain from using all ointments, creams, skin lotions, pain-relieving liniments, cleaning lotions, oil treatments, hair-coloring chemicals, and tanning lotion; they were also advised to reduce their use of soap and shampoo, both of which—like skin creams—are generally formulated with perfumes and other chemicals and applied to large regions of the body. This research showed that, after 2 years, FM patients who reduced their exposure to chemicals/xenobiotics/cosmetics experienced significant reductions in pain, sleep disturbances, and musculoskeletal stiffness ($p < 0.02$), together with better physical function and improved sense of well-being as measured by the Fibromyalgia Impact Questionnaire (FIQ). Thus, avoiding chemical exposure appears to provide no-cost no-risk therapeutic benefit to FM patients by alleviating pain and improving several indicators of overall health.

Conclusions

- In sum, current research indicates that fibromyalgia results from impairment of cellular energy/ATP production (mitochondrial dysfunction) and induction of pain hypersensitivity (peripheral and central sensitization) due to absorbed metabolic toxins from bacterial/microbial overgrowth of the gastrointestinal tract; this is complicated by induction of tryptophan deficiency which is most likely caused by tryptophan degradation by bacterial tryptophanase activity and which leads to serotonin and melatonin insufficiencies, which lead to associated biochemical and clinical consequences, discussed previously. Available studies have shown that SIBO is ubiquitous among fibromyalgia patients and that antimicrobial interventions—whether pharmaceutical or nutritional—are efficacious. Secondary physiological effects such as mitochondrial

---

[254] Merchant RE, et al. Nutritional supplementation with Chlorella pyrenoidosa for patients with fibromyalgia syndrome: a pilot study. *Phytother Res* 2000 May;14:167-73
[255] Pore RS. Detoxification of chlordecone poisoned rats with chlorella and chlorella derived sporopollenin. *Drug Chem Toxicol*. 1984;7(1):57-71
[256] Morita K, Ogata M, Hasegawa T. Chlorophyll derived from Chlorella inhibits dioxin absorption from the gastrointestinal tract and accelerates dioxin excretion in rats. *Environ Health Perspect*. 2001 Mar;109(3):289-94
[257] Morita K, Matsueda T, Iida T, Hasegawa T. Chlorella accelerates dioxin excretion in rats. *J Nutr*. 1999 Sep;129(9):1731-6
[258] Nakano S, Noguchi T, Takekoshi H, Suzuki G, Nakano M. Maternal-fetal distribution and transfer of dioxins in pregnant women in Japan, and attempts to reduce maternal transfer with Chlorella (Chlorella pyrenoidosa) supplements. *Chemosphere*. 2005 Dec;61(9):1244-55
[259] Nakano et al. Chlorella (Chlorella pyrenoidosa) supplementation decreases dioxin and increases immunoglobulin a concentrations in breast milk. *J Med Food*. 2007 Mar:134-42
[260] Sverdrup B. Use less cosmetics—suffer less from fibromyalgia? *J Womens Health* (Larchmt). 2004 Mar;13(2):187-94

impairment, pain sensitization, nutritional deficiencies, oxidative stress, and reduced tissue perfusion are treated with combined use of select therapeutics as reviewed previously. Patients presenting with widespread pain should be screened for causative underlying disease; if no other explanation can be found, then the diagnosis of fibromyalgia should be made, and the condition should be treated with the nondrug therapeutics discussed above. The first visit can include history, physical examination, and laboratory tests; initial laboratory assessment should include complete blood count (CBC), metabolic/chemistry panel, serum 25-hydroxyvitamin D, C-reactive protein (CRP), anti-nuclear antibodies (ANA), antibodies against cyclic citrullinated proteins (anti-CCP antibodies), ferritin, muscle enzymes aldolase and creatine kinase, and a complete thyroid assessment including TSH, free T4, free T3, total T3, reverse T3 (rT3), and antithyroid peroxidase and antithyroglobulin antibodies. First-day interventions can include dietary optimization, multivitamin-multimineral supplementation (including vitamin D3 and magnesium), tryptophan/5-HTP, CoQ10, mixed tocopherols, and combination fatty acids including gamma-linolenic acid (GLA), eicosapentaenoic acid (EPA) and docosahexaenoic acid (DHA). SIBO can be treated empirically, or it can be objectively assessed with breath hydrogen and methane testing, stool analysis, culture, microscopy, and parasitology. At follow-up visits, additional assessments and interventions (such as for toxic metals and chronic occult infections) can be used to fine-tune the diagnosis and further discover and define its contributors in order to maximize the patient's response to treatment and promote optimal recovery and health.

MIGRAINE HEADACHES, HYPOTHYROIDISM, AND FIBROMYALGIA:

ASSESSMENTS AND THERAPEUTIC APPROACHES USING INTEGRATIVE CHIROPRACTIC, NATUROPATHIC, OSTEOPATHIC, AND FUNCTIONAL MEDICINE

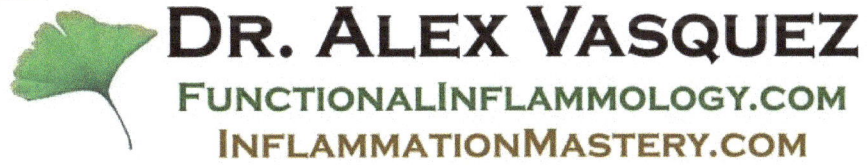
Is "central sensitization" in fibromyalgia a bunch of c.r.a.p. (Commercial Rationalization Advocating Pharmaceuticals)?

DR. ALEX VASQUEZ
FUNCTIONALINFLAMMOLOGY.COM
INFLAMMATIONMASTERY.COM

Video reviews by Dr Vasquez: Please see vimeo.com/DrVasquez and vimeo.com/ICHNFM for many videos by Dr Vasquez and colleagues.

Rheumatoid Arthritis, RA

Introduction:

Rheumatoid arthritis (RA) is one of the most common and "most classic" systemic autoimmune diseases. Despite its name, RA affects much more than the musculoskeletal system: rheumatoid lung, rheumatoid kidney disease, and other systemic, vasculitic, and (sub)cutaneous complications are not uncommon. Readers should begin to recognize the "patterns of inflammation" that result in distinct diagnostic labels are simply "variations on a theme" based on a finite number of identifiable and modifiable factors, which are largely amenable to nonpharmacologic interventions.

Rheumatoid arthritis and psoriasis are very similar conditions—different patterns of inflammation—and these conditions and their respective assessments and treatments should be viewed as prototypical for other conditions; as such, and especially considering that these conditions are very common in clinical practice, a reasonable assumption will be made that readers will have studied these sections so that some facts and concepts will not have to be unnecessarily repeated throughout the book for each condition that follows a similar pattern of pathogenesis and resolution.

Description/pathophysiology:

- <u>Description in a nutshell</u>: RA is a relatively common, persistent, symmetric, destructive, systemic inflammatory "autoimmune" disease chiefly characterized by peripheral arthritis but which may also affect the proximal joints (e.g., hips and shoulders), the axial skeleton (e.g., spine—notably the atlantoaxial joint—as well as the sacroiliac joints), and internal organs (e.g., "rheumatoid lung") and vascular system (e.g., rheumatoid vasculitis).
- <u>Basic pathology</u>: A pathogenic hallmark of the disease is immune complex formation and intra-articular deposition with resultant release of cytokines and other pro-inflammatory mediators. Immune complexes are important instigators of rheumatoid arthritis and vasculitis, and rheumatoid factor (RF) antibodies are important contributors to these immune complexes.[261,262] The chronic/sustained inflammation leads to synovial thickening, villous hypertrophy (pannus formation), and intraarticular colonization with activated lymphocytes and plasma cells. The localized immunocytes cause inflammation and tissue destruction via elaboration of matrix metalloproteinases (including collagenases), prostaglandins, and cytokines such as IL-1.
- <u>Prevalence</u>: Affects 0.8-1% of all populations: considered the second most common rheumatic diagnosis[263] after "osteoarthritis", many cases of which are actually genetic hemochromatosis, one of the most common hereditary conditions in humans (heterozygote frequency: 1:7; homozygote frequency 1:200-250).
    - <u>Musculoskeletal disorders and iron overload disease</u> (*Arthritis Rheum* 1996 Oct[264]—full text provided within this textbook): "Arthropathy affects up to 80% of iron-overloaded patients and is often the only manifestation of the disease. ... Thus, since iron overload affects such a large portion of the population and arthropathy is a common manifestation of this disorder, patients with musculoskeletal symptoms should be screened for iron overload."
- <u>Introduction to standard allopathic medical perspective and treatment</u>: From the allopathic perspective, RA is seen as a chronic "idiopathic" inflammatory disorder primarily affecting the peripheral joints but also affecting the axial skeleton and internal organs; it is generally treated with NSAIDs and other "anti-inflammatory" and immunosuppressive drugs, which are palliative and have no chance of providing cure. The standard sequential protocol is as follows: NAIDs and acetaminophen, prednisone, methotrexate, (perhaps sulfasalazine and hydroxychloroquine), then—ever more commonly prescribed—the "biologics", which may be followed by newer experimental and immunoparalytic drugs; this routine protocol has value in the acute suppression of inflammation, but it is notoriously expensive, wrought with adverse effects, and ineffective for the authentic treatment of rheumatoid arthritis, as noted in the landmark 2012 article cited here:
    - <u>Sustained rheumatoid arthritis remission is uncommon in clinical practice</u> (*Arthritis Res Ther* 2012 Mar[265]): "This study shows that in clinical practice, a minority of RA patients are in sustained remission. ... Other

---

[261] Beers MH, Berkow R (eds). *The Merck Manual. Seventeenth Edition*. Whitehouse Station; Merck Research Laboratories: 1999, page 416
[262] Jonsson T, Valdimarsson H. What about IgA rheumatoid factor in rheumatoid arthritis? *Ann Rheum Dis*. 1998 Jan;57(1):63-4 ard.bmjjournals.com/cgi/content/full/57/1/63
[263] Hardin JG, Waterman J, Labson LH. Rheumatic disease: Which diagnostic tests are useful? *Patient Care* 1999; March 15: 83-102
[264] Vasquez A. Musculoskeletal disorders and iron overload disease: comment on the American College of Rheumatology guidelines for the initial evaluation of the adult patient with acute musculoskeletal symptoms. *Arthritis Rheum*. 1996 Oct;39(10):1767-8
[265] Prince et al. Sustained rheumatoid arthritis remission is uncommon in clinical practice. *Arthritis Res Ther*. 2012 Mar 19;14(2):R68 arthritis-research.com/content/14/2/R68

studies have described sustained remission in daily practice as uncommon, being reached by only 17% to 36% of RA patients for up to 6 months. These studies did not evaluate time in remission beyond 6 months. A recent study investigated the probability of remaining in remission up to 24 months, according to the ACR/EULAR, SDAI, and CDAI remission criteria in two different cohorts. They also concluded that long-term remission is rare, considering that probability of a remission lasting 2 years was 6-14%."

- Introduction to naturopathic medicine and functional medicine perspective and treatment: From the perspective of naturopathic medicine and functional medicine, the condition is considered highly amenable to treatment provided that such treatment is multifaceted and addresses the allergic, dysbiotic, nutritional, mitochondrial, endocrinologic, and immunophenotypic components of this multifaceted phenomenon.
- Etiological considerations include:
    - Genetic predisposition and HLA-DR: HLA-DR4 is positive in 70% of RA patients, compared to 28% of control patients. "Genetic risk factors do not fully account for the incidence of RA, suggesting that environmental factors also play a role in the etiology of the disease. ...[C]limate and urbanization have a major impact on the incidence and severity of RA in groups of similar genetic background."[266]
    - Urbanization / Western lifestyle: Urbanization is a risk factor for the development of rheumatic disease.[267,268] Urbanization is associated with increased risk of vitamin D deficiency and increased exposure to nutritionally-depleted multiallergenic genetically-modified AGE-laden phytonutrient-deficient prohyperglycemic "convenience foods", sleep disturbances, and exposure to particulate debris (i.e., pollution from diesel and other petrochemical combustion); each of these factors has been shown in animal models or human trials to promote systemic inflammation.
    - Female gender / estrogen: Women are affected 2-3x more often than men. Male RA patients tend to have relative reductions in DHEA and testosterone and relative excess of estrogen and prolactin. Predisposing factors for women include vitamin D deficiency, dysestrogenism, and the anatomically shorter urethra which predisposes the female urinary tract to recurrent microbial colonization.
    - Tobacco/cigarette smoke: Habitual tobacco/cigarette smoking increases exposure to reactive oxygen species, vasoactive/vasoconstrictive substances, carcinogens, and bacterial endotoxin. Tobacco leaves are noted for their high surface area which—unfortunately for smokers—serves as a deposition reservoir for both ambient radioactive particles[269,270] as well as Gram-negative bacteria, Gram-positive bacteria, and fungi[271]; thereby, tobacco smoking increases exposure to radioactive particles as well as microbial debris (e.g., endotoxin, exotoxin, and bacterial DNA). Thus, the finding that tobacco smoking—particularly from cigarette smoke which is inhaled deeply into the lungs in contrast with cigar smoke which is generally inhaled only into the mouth and pharynx—is a major risk factor for the development of rheumatoid arthritis and other systemic inflammatory/autoimmune/autoinflammatory disorders is consistent with the microbial/dysbiotic model discussed later in this section.
        - Cigarette smoking and inflammation (J Dent Res 2012 Feb[272]): "**CS [cigarette smoking] impairs innate defenses against pathogens, modulates antigen presentation, and promotes autoimmunity.** ... Potential mechanisms by which CS promotes rheumatoid arthritis include the release of intracellular proteins from ROS-activated or injured cells, augmentation of auto-reactive

---

[266] Fauci AS, Braunwald E, Isselbacher KJ, et al., eds. *Harrison's Principles of Internal Medicine. 14th ed*. New York, NY: McGraw-Hill; 1998, page 1881
[267] "In particular, a significantly lower prevalence of RA in rural areas compared with urban cohorts has led to the hypothesis that environmental factors associated with urbanization may be involved in disease pathogenesis." Adebajo A, Davis P. Rheumatic diseases in African blacks. *Semin Arthritis Rheum*. 1994 Oct;24(2):139-53
[268] "The general impression is that rheumatoid arthritis (RA) has a lower prevalence and a milder course in developing countries. Epidemiological studies from different regions show that varying prevalence is possibly related to urbanization." Kalla AA, Tikly M. Rheumatoid arthritis in the developing world. *Best Pract Res Clin Rheumatol*. 2003 Oct;17(5):863-75
[269] "Tobacco leaves are large and have sticky exudates that retain the radon decay products once they deposit on the leaves." Savidou A, Kehagia K, Eleftheriadis K. Concentration levels of 210Pb and 210Po in dry tobacco leaves in Greece. *J Environ Radioact*. 2006;85(1):94-102
[270] "Leaf tobacco contains minute amounts of lead 210 (210Pb) and polonium 210 (210Po), both of which are radioactive carcinogens and both of which can be found in smoke from burning tobacco. Tobacco smoke also contains carcinogens that are nonradioactive. People who inhale tobacco smoke are exposed to higher concentrations of radioactivity than nonsmokers. Deposits of 210Pb and alpha particle-emitting 210Po form in the lungs of smokers, generating localized radiation doses far greater than the radiation exposures humans experience from natural sources. This radiation exposure, delivered to sensitive tissues for long periods of time, may induce cancer both alone and synergistically with nonradioactive carcinogens." Kilthau GF. Cancer risk in relation to radioactivity in tobacco. *Radiol Technol*. 1996 Jan-Feb;67(3):217-22
[271] "Cured tobacco in diverse types of cigarettes is known to harbor a plethora of bacteria (Gram-positive and Gram-negative), fungi (mold, yeast), spores, and is rich in endotoxin (lipopolysaccharide). Reviewed herein are recent observations of the authors' team and other investigators that support the hypothesis that lung inflammation of long-term smokers may be attributed in part to tobacco-associated bacterial and fungal components that have been identified in tobacco and tobacco smoke." Pauly JL, Smith LA, Rickert MH, Hutson A, Paszkiewicz GM. Review: Is lung inflammation associated with microbes and microbial toxins in cigarette tobacco smoke? *Immunol Res*. 2010 Mar;46(1-3):127-36
[272] Lee et al. Cigarette smoking and inflammation: cellular and molecular mechanisms. *J Dent Res*. 2012 Feb;91(2):142-9 ncbi.nlm.nih.gov/pmc/articles/PMC3261116/

B-cell function, altered presentation of antigens by CS-impaired antigen-presenting cells, altered regulatory T-cell functions, and T-cell activation by antigens found in CS."
- Occult viral, bacterial or parasitic infections:
    - Viral: "**Cytomegalovirus and rubella viruses have been cultured from the synovium in patients with rheumatoid arthritis...**" "Some evidence suggests hepatitis C virus as a possible trigger to rheumatoid arthritis."[273] The implications of this data are unclear; however, possibilities include: 1) virus *directly* provoking joint destruction, 2) virus *indirectly* provoking joint destruction, such as via immune complexes, 3) noncausal, coincidental finding, 4) inability of RA patients to clear this infection due to immunologic deficits which accompany immune dysfunction. Remember, "Unhealthy people are unhealthy", and an *associated* abnormality does not imply a *causal* relationship. Sick people tend to get sicker and enter vicious cycles that can amplify the original illness and lead to the genesis of new, additive health problems. Additionally, given that nutritional deficiencies—pandemic in the general population and even more common in patients with chronic illness (due to malabsorption, hypermetabolism of immune activation, and nutrient losses and malabsorption due to pharmaceutical drugs, etc)—promote viral mutagenesis and replication, the possibility exists that enhanced viral replication in patients with RA/autoimmunity is a surrogate marker for nutritional deficiency; relatedly, enhanced viral replication might be a surrogate marker for enhanced activity of the NFkB pathway, which is upregulated in inflammatory responses and which promotes viral replication. More likely from this author's perspective is the probability that increased viral replication/presence is—regardless of primary etiology—a likely contributor to the total microbial load (TML) and total inflammatory/antigenic load (TIL, TAL) that perpetuates chronic/sustained immune activation and which thus drives systemic inflammation and the clinical manifestation of autoimmunity.
    - Bacterial (specific species and generalized SIBO—small intestine bacterial overgrowth): RA is associated with gastrointestinal and genitourinary colonization with *Proteus mirabilis*.[274,275] Approximately 40% of patients with rheumatoid arthritis have bacterial overgrowth of the small bowel, and the severity of bacterial overgrowth correlates positively with the severity of the musculoskeletal inflammation, suggesting the probability of a causal relationship.[276] Relatedly, clinicians should recall that peptidoglycans, bacterial cell wall debris, endotoxins, indole, skatole and numerous other gut-derived "toxins" can promote joint inflammation.[277,278] **Animal models have demonstrated that gut-derived metabolites can cause inflammatory degenerative arthritis that resembles rheumatoid arthritis.**[279,280] **The dysbiotic contribution to rheumatoid arthritis is likely to be both *qualitative* (related to specific inciting microbes) and *quantitative* (related to total, nonspecific bacterial overgrowth of the gut and multifocal mucosal colonization).** Accordingly, research published in 2007 showed that dietary modification was comparable in benefit to prednisolone, supporting the model that gastrointestinal dysfunction—namely, food allergic reactions (and probably intestinal dysbiosis)—is a major etiologic component of rheumatoid arthritis, at least in its initial stages; the authors concluded, "**This study supports the concept that rheumatoid arthritis may be a reaction to a food antigen(s) and that the disease process starts within the intestine.**"[281]

> **Prototypic multifocal dysbiosis in RA**
> - Nasopharynx: *Streptococcus pyogenes*
> - Gastrointestinal: *Eubacterium aerofaciens*
> - Genitourinary: *Proteus mirabilis*

---

[273] Siegel LB, Gall EP. Viral infection as a cause of arthritis. *Am Fam Physician* 1996 Nov 1;54(6):2009-15
[274] Ebringer A, Rashid T, Wilson C. Rheumatoid arthritis: proposal for the use of anti-microbial therapy in early cases. *Scand J Rheumatol* 2003;32(1):2-11
[275] Rashid T, Darlington G, Kjeldsen-Kragh J, Forre O, Collado A, Ebringer A. Proteus IgG antibodies and C-reactive protein in English, Norwegian and Spanish patients with rheumatoid arthritis. *Clin Rheumatol* 1999;18(3):190-5
[276] "Eight (32%) of the patients with RA had hypochlorhydria or achlorhydria... A high frequency of small intestinal bacterial overgrowth was found in patients with RA; it was associated with a high disease activity and observed in patients with hypochlorhydria or achlorhydria and in those with normal acid secretion." Henriksson AE, Blomquist L, Nord CE, Midtvedt T, Uribe A. Small intestinal bacterial overgrowth in patients with rheumatoid arthritis. *Ann Rheum Dis*. 1993 Jul;52(7):503-10
[277] Simelyte E, Rimpilainen M, Lehtonen L, Zhang X, Toivanen P. Bacterial cell wall-induced arthritis: chemical composition and tissue distribution of four Lactobacillus strains. *Infect Immun*. 2000 Jun;68(6):3535-40 iai.asm.org/cgi/reprint/68/6/3535
[278] Toivanen P. Normal intestinal microbiota in the aetiopathogenesis of rheumatoid arthritis. *Ann Rheum Dis*. 2003 Sep;62(9):807-11 ard.bmjjournals.com/cgi/reprint/62/9/807
[279] Nakoneczna I, Forbes JC, Rogers KS. The arthritogenic effect of indole, skatole and other tryptophan metabolites in rabbits. *Am J Pathol*. 1969 Dec;57(3):523-38
[280] Rogers KS, Forbes JC, Nakoneczna I. Arthritogenic properties of lipophilic, aryl molecules. *Proc Soc Exp Biol Med*. 1969 Jun;131(2):670-2
[281] Podas et al. Is rheumatoid arthritis a disease that starts in intestine? Pilot study comparing an elemental diet with oral prednisolone. *Postgrad Med J*. 2007 Feb;83(976):128-31

- **Parasitic**: Gastrointestinal parasite infections, such as with *Endolimax nana*[282] and other microbes such a *Giardia lamblia*, can induce a systemic inflammatory response that mimics rheumatoid arthritis and is cured with parasite eradication.

Clinical presentations:
- Course: Variable course with exacerbations and remissions; the general trend is one of progressive joint destruction and systemic inflammation-induced damage.
- Presentation: The disease begins slowly in 2/3 of patients and can be slow to reach a diagnostic threshold—generally takes 9 months between initial onset and diagnosis; may affect only one joint initially. 10% have acute-onset polyarthritis. RA can affect any age, either gender, and clinical presentations will vary.
    - 2-3x more common in women than men.
    - Age of onset is typically 25-50 years of age.
    - "Peripheral symmetric polyarthropathy" is a classic description for RA; but this same description can be applied to many cases of hemochromatosis and SLE as well.
    - Palpable joint swelling with synovitis and effusion.
    - Morning stiffness > 1 hour.
    - Typical autoimmune systemic manifestations: fatigue, malaise, low-grade fever, anorexia, and weight loss—note that all of these clinical presentations are manifestations of immune activation in general and increased cytokine production in particular.
- Musculoskeletal:
    - The joints most commonly affected are the wrists, MCP, PIP, MTP (metatarsophalangeal) joints, and knees (Baker's cyst is common). In severe or advanced disease, essentially any joint in the body—including the TMJ and upper cervical spine—can be involved.
    - Most common at PIP, MCP joints, wrists (i.e., "knuckles and wrists").
    - Upper cervical spine involvement can lead to atlantoaxial instability—upper cervical spine manipulation is contraindicated until atlantoaxial instability has been excluded clinically or radiographically.
    - Periarticular muscle atrophy and osteoporosis—due to inflammation and disuse.
    - Generalized osteoporosis is common due to inflammation, disuse/deconditioning, hypogonadism, and drug effects.
    - Advanced complications include radial deviation of the wrists and ulnar deviation of the fingers, swan neck deformity (PIP hyperextension with DIP hyperflexion), and boutonniere deformity (PIP hyperflexion with DIP hyperextension).
- Skin: Rheumatoid nodules (subcutaneous inflammatory granulomas) are seen in up to 30% of patients. These are also rarely seen in patients with hemochromatoic arthropathy mimicking RA.[283]
- Arteries and vessels: Rheumatoid vasculitis leads to impaired circulation, causing necrosis of affected tissues/organs: fingers, skin, internal organs, and nerves (peripheral neuropathy).
- Pulmonary manifestations: Dyspnea, pulmonary nodules, fibrosis; more common in men.
- Eye: Complications are seen in 1% of patients but can lead to rapid blindness.
- Other autoimmune diseases: Up to 20% of patients with RA develop Sjogren's syndrome. SLE, MS, Hashimoto's thyroiditis, and mixed connective tissue disease can easily co-exist beside a primary clinical presentation of RA.

Major differential diagnoses:
- Osteoarthritis (OA): OA tends to be monoarticular or oligoarticular rather than polyarticular; OA is generally only minimally inflammatory (except after the progression of joint destruction) whereas RA is clearly more inflammatory as assessed clinically and serologically (with ESR or CRP). OA is more likely to be asymmetric whereas RA is nearly always symmetric (except in cases of stroke, paralysis, or peripheral nerve lesion due to

---

[282] "Endolimax nana grew on stool culture. Both the patient's diarrhea and arthritis responded effectively to therapy with metronidazole. The diagnosis of parasitic rheumatism was made in retrospect." Burnstein SL, Liakos S. Parasitic rheumatism presenting as rheumatoid arthritis. *J Rheumatol*. 1983 Jun;10(3):514-5
[283] "These manifestations which are common to rheumatoid arthritis may be seen in hemochromatotic arthropathy." Bensen WG, Laskin CA, Little HA, Fam AG. Hemochromatotic arthropathy mimicking rheumatoid arthritis. A case with subcutaneous nodules, tenosynovitis, and bursitis. *Arthritis Rheum*. 1978 Sep-Oct;21(7):844-8

interference with neurogenic inflammation). Lab tests such as ANA, RF, and CCP antibodies are expected to be normal in OA; CRP and ESR may be moderately elevated in severe OA but inflammatory markers are generally much lower than the levels seen in RA.
- SLE: Differentiated by nonerosive arthritis, anti-DS-DNA antibodies, anti-Smith antibodies, low serum complement, the classic "butterfly rash", and an earlier and more frequent development of mucosal, serosal, vasculitic and renal complications.
- Septic arthritis: Differentiated by monoarthritis, fever, and purulent joint aspiration.
    - **Septic arthritis may complicate pre-existing rheumatoid arthritis, and patients with RA appear to be predisposed to septic arthritis**: Reasons for this septic predisposition include immune dysfunction, use of prednisone or other immunosuppressant medications, and concomitant obesity and/or diabetes. **Patients may lack the classic systemic manifestations of septic arthritis (fever, chills, leukocytosis) due to age, disease, or pharmaceutical immunosuppression.**[284,285] Patients may have concomitant respiratory or urinary tract infections, which makes the clinical presentation even more unclear. Treatment may require systemic antibiotics (oral or intravenous) and joint lavage with antibiotics.[286] **Failure to diagnose and treat septic arthritis promptly may result in deformity, disability, or death.**
- Hemochromatosis and iron overload: Given its high frequency and multifarious clinical presentations, iron overload is an essential diagnostic consideration in patients with rheumatic disease.[287,288] Doctors must test serum ferritin and transferrin saturation (along with CRP) as discussed in Chapter 1.
- Reactive arthritis: Differentiated by the recent history of infection, greatly increased prevalence of HLA-B27, and the presence of uveitis/iritis, sacroiliac and lumbar involvement, predominant acute/subacute-onset inflammation of the heels, knees, hips. *Perspective from DrV*: I think rheumatoid arthritis should be considered a variant of reactive arthritis, with RA being triggered by multifocal dysbiosis (several subclinical infections) whereas the latter is triggered by a single true infection.
- Gout and other crystal-induced arthropathy: Asymmetric arthritis, negatively birefringent crystals demonstrated with joint aspiration.
- Arthritis related to viral infection: Such as parvovirus and hepatitis C[289]; clinical correlation with appropriate serologies are warranted.
- Psoriatic arthritis: Skin lesions, nail pitting, asymmetric arthritis, negative RF and CCP. Rarely, the joint inflammation of psoriatic arthritis precedes the expected dermatologic lesions: well-demarcated erythematous patches covered with silvery scales.
- Adult Still's disease: Diagnosis relies on *all of the following*: high fevers (>102.2°F), arthralgia/arthritis, RF<80, ANA<1:100, *plus two of the following*: skin rash (generalized and confluent red papules and plaques), pleuritis/pericarditis, WBC count >15,000 cells/mm^3, and hepatomegaly/spenomegaly/lymphadenopathy.
- Ewing's sarcoma: An aggressive bone malignancy that typically presents in children and young adults with periarticular bone pain and fever which can mimic inflammatory monoarthritis.

Clinical assessment:
- **History/subjective**:
    - Systemic manifestations with symmetric peripheral polyarthropathy.
    - Morning stiffness lasting more than 30-60 minutes is common.

---

[284] "Many patients lacked distinctive features of joint sepsis (fever, chills) and only one half had leukocytosis." Blackburn WD Jr, Dunn TL, Alarcon GS. Infection versus disease activity in rheumatoid arthritis: eight years' experience. *South Med J*. 1986 Oct;79(10):1238-41

[285] "Pain and loss of motion in the affected joint were prominent, but toxic features of pyogenic infections--hectic fever, chills, sweats, local warmth, or erythema--were conspicuously absent. Two patients had moderate fever and three patients had mild leukocytosis." Kraft SM, Panush RS, Longley S. Unrecognized staphylococcal pyarthrosis with rheumatoid arthritis. *Semin Arthritis Rheum*. 1985 Feb;14(3):196-201

[286] Septic arthritis complicating rheumatoid arthritis was due to Staphylococcus aureus (12 cases) and Escherichia coli (1 case). Recommended treatment: "The authors recommend as the treatment of choice: systemic antibiotic therapy and immediate arthrotomy followed by through-and-through irrigation with fluid containing the appropriate antibiotics." Gristina AG, Rovere GD, Shoji H. Spontaneous septic arthritis complicating rheumatoid arthritis. *J Bone Joint Surg Am*. 1974 Sep;56(6):1180-4

[287] Vasquez A. Musculoskeletal disorders and iron overload disease: comment on the American College of Rheumatology guidelines for the initial evaluation of the adult patient with acute musculoskeletal symptoms. *Arthritis Rheum*. 1996 Oct;39(10):1767-8

[288] "These manifestations which are common to rheumatoid arthritis may be seen in hemochromatotic arthropathy." Bensen WG, Laskin CA, Little HA, Fam AG. Hemochromatotic arthropathy mimicking rheumatoid arthritis. A case with subcutaneous nodules, tenosynovitis, and bursitis. *Arthritis Rheum*. 1978 Sep-Oct;21(7):844-8

[289] Siegel LB, Gall EP. Viral infection as a cause of arthritis. *Am Fam Physician* 1996 Nov 1;54(6):2009-15

- **Physical examination/objective**:
    - Assess joints, especially the distal/peripheral joints of the wrists/hands and ankles/feet. Remember that the initial manifestation of RA, like all inflammatory arthropathies, can affect any joint in the body, including the atlantoaxial joint. Flexion contractures and ulnar deviation of the fingers are common, classic findings of developed disease.
    - Clinically assess patient for exclusion of other diseases. Some patients with RA will develop other autoimmune diseases, especially hypothyroidism and Sjogren's syndrome.
- **Laboratory assessments**: Goals of laboratory testing are 1) exclude serious life-threatening conditions (e.g., septic arthritis), 2) quantitatively and qualitatively assess patient's health status, 3) determine nature and severity of underlying diseases and disorders for which correction can contribute to an overall improvement in immune function and reduction in total inflammatory load.
    - **CCP: Cyclic citrullinated protein antibody; Citrullinated protein antibodies (CPA); anti-CCP antibodies: anti-cyclic citrullinated peptide antibody**: Anti-CCP antibodies have 95-98% specificity for RA[290] and has become the laboratory standard for evaluating the diagnosis and prognosis of RA.[291] The best current data indicates that anti-CCP antibodies are sensitive and specific for RA[292], and clinicians should use this test in the diagnosis of RA.[293] Anti-CCP antibodies with a positive rheumatoid factor (RF) is termed "composite/conjugate seropositivity" and appears to be more specific than isolated anti-CCP or RF positivity.[294]
    - **C-reactive protein**: CRP can be used to support the diagnosis (as it indicates inflammation) and can be used to monitor the disease and the response to treatment.[295]
    - **Erythrocyte sedimentation rate**: ESR is elevated in 90% of patients and can be used to support the diagnosis (as it indicates inflammation) and can be used to monitor the disease and the response to treatment.[296]
    - **Complete blood count**: CBC may reveal anemia of chronic disease, anemia due to NSAID-related gastrointestinal bleeding, or suggest nutritional deficiencies (namely B12 and folic acid as discussed in Chapter 1); elevated WBC suggests infection and requires clinical correlation.
    - **Ferritin**: As an acute phase reactant, serum ferritin is elevated by inflammation; as a marker for iron status, serum ferritin is elevated by iron overload and lowered by iron deficiency. Transferrin saturation and serum iron should be low in RA due to inflammation, whereas they are commonly elevated in patients with iron overload. In order to determine the acute phase contribution to an elevated ferritin level, an independent marker of inflammation such as CRP or ESR should be tested simultaneously. When in doubt, iron overload can be excluded with diagnostic phlebotomy, liver MRI, liver biopsy (especially if liver enzymes are elevated), or the response to therapeutic phlebotomy.[297]
    - **Rheumatoid factor**: RF is positive in 70-80% of patients with RA but is not specific and is not necessary for the diagnosis of RA. RF provides "supportive evidence" for the diagnosis of RA only in the presence of corresponding

> **CCP antibodies: the single best laboratory test for the early detection, diagnosis, and monitoring of RA**
>
> "The anti-CCP test is more specific than the commonly used RF test (95% versus less than 90%) and has a comparable sensitivity (more than 70%). ... In conclusion, testing for anti-CCP autoantibodies is widely accepted as an indispensable tool for diagnosis and early treatment in the management of rheumatoid arthritis patients."
>
> van Venrooij et al. *Ann N Y Acad Sci* 2008 Nov

---

[290] Hill J, Cairns E, Bell DA. The joy of citrulline: new insights into the diagnosis, pathogenesis, and treatment of rheumatoid arthritis. *J Rheumatol*. 2004 Aug;31(8):1471-3
[291] "We conclude that, at present, the antibody response directed to citrullinated antigens has the most valuable diagnostic and prognostic potential for RA." van Boekel MA, et al. Autoantibody systems in rheumatoid arthritis: specificity, sensitivity and diagnostic value. *Arthritis Res*. 2002;4(2):87-93 arthritis-research.com/content/4/2/87
[292] "Serum antibodies reactive with citrullinated proteins/peptides are a very sensitive and specific marker for rheumatoid arthritis." Migliorini P, Pratesi F, Tommasi C, Anzilotti C. The immune response to citrullinated antigens in autoimmune diseases. *Autoimmun Rev*. 2005 Nov;4(8):561-4
[293] "The anti-CCP test is more specific than the commonly used RF test (95% versus less than 90%) and has a comparable sensitivity (more than 70%). ... In conclusion, testing for anti-CCP autoantibodies is widely accepted as an indispensable tool for diagnosis and early treatment in the management of rheumatoid arthritis patients." van Venrooij WJ, van Beers JJ, Pruijn GJ. Anti-CCP Antibody, a Marker for the Early Detection of Rheumatoid Arthritis. *Ann N Y Acad Sci*. 2008 Nov;1143:268-85
[294] "...our findings suggest that a positive anti-CCP antibody result does not necessarily exclude SLE in African American patients presenting with inflammatory arthritis. In such patients, the additional assessment of IgA-RF or IgM-RF isotypes may be of added value since composite seropositivity appears to be nearly exclusive to patients with RA." Mikuls et al. Anti-cyclic citrullinated peptide antibody and rheumatoid factor isotypes in African Americans with early rheumatoid arthritis. *Arthritis Rheum*. 2006 Sep;54:3057-9
[295] Gabay C, Kushner I. Acute-phase proteins and other systemic responses to inflammation. *N Engl J Med*. 1999 Feb 11;340(6):448-54
[296] Klippel JH (ed). *Primer on the Rheumatic Diseases. 11th Edition*. Atlanta: Arthritis Foundation. 1997 page 94
[297] "Therapeutic phlebotomy is used to remove excess iron and maintain low normal body iron stores, and it should be initiated in men with serum ferritin levels of 300 microg/L or more and in women with serum ferritin levels of 200 microg/L or more, regardless of the presence or absence of symptoms." Barton et al. Management of hemochromatosis. Hemochromatosis Management Working Group. *Ann Intern Med*. 1998 Dec 1;129(11):932-9

clinical manifestations. High RF levels indicate more severe disease and worse prognosis. IgA-RF appears to have clinical superiority over other forms of RF.[298] RF is seen in 5% of apparently healthy people, and it is present in some patients with iron overload, thus making the distinction between RA and hemochromatoic arthropathy all the more difficult.[299] Diseases (other than RA) associated with RF positivity include iron overload, chronic infections, hepatitis, sarcoidosis, and bacterial endocarditis.

- Thyroid assessment: Hypothyroidism can mimic systemic rheumatic disease by causing an inflammatory oligoarthropathy and myopathy, complete with elevations of CRP and ESR.[300] Overt or imminent hypothyroidism is suggested by TSH greater than 2 mU/L[301] or 3 mU/L[302], low T4 or T3, and/or the presence of anti-thyroid peroxidase antibodies (anti-TPO).[303] This author's current practice is—for the laboratory evaluation of hypothyroidism—to assess the full spectrum of thyroid indexes: THS, free T4, free or total T3, reverse T3 (rT3), and the antithyroid antibodies anti-thyroglobulin and anti-thyroid peroxidase (anti-TPO).

- Complete hormone assessment: Patients with RA commonly show elevations of prolactin and estradiol along with insufficiencies of testosterone, cortisol, and DHEA. These can be tested in serum, and early-morning serum cortisol is more accurate than late-day cortisol. Other options and details are provided in the following section under *Treatments* and in the section in Chapter 4 on *Orthoendocrinology*.

- Lactulose-mannitol assay for "leaky gut": Increased intestinal permeability (IP) is a common contributor to and complication of many inflammatory/rheumatic/chronic diseases including psoriasis[304], Behcet's disease[305], ankylosing spondylitis[306] and seronegative spondyloarthritis[307], enteropathic spondyloarthropathy and oligoarticular juvenile idiopathic arthritis[308], lupus[309], and chronic congestive heart failure.[310] This test may be used for the evaluation of gastrointestinal mucosal integrity, which simultaneously serves as a barometer of overall health and when elevated can indicate the presence of a variety of intestinal disorders, including celiac disease, food allergies, and GI dysbiosis. Thus, an elevated lactulose:mannitol ratio is *sensitive* but not *specific* for the presence of intestinal disorders. An elevated lactulose:mannitol ratio correlates with ❶ malnutrition, ❷ inflammatory bowel disease, ❸ NSAID or ethanol enterotoxicity, ❹ food allergies including celiac disease, and/or ❺ gastrointestinal dysbiosis, the latter of which then needs to be characterized with comprehensive stool testing and comprehensive parasitology; astute clinicians can generally exclude items 1-3 with appropriate history, physical examination, and routine laboratory assessments, thus leaving an abnormal IP test to be attributed to food allergies or GI parasites/dysbiosis, the former of which is assessed serologically or with elimination-challenge protocol (reviewed in Chapter 4) while the latter is assessed with comprehensive stool testing (including fecal sIgA and inflammatory markers such as lactoferrin and lysozyme) and comprehensive parasitology, which includes microscopic, culture, and antigen/toxin detection techniques.

- Comprehensive stool analysis and comprehensive parasitology with bacterial and fungal culture and sensitivity: All patients with rheumatoid arthritis should be considered to have gastrointestinal dysbiosis until proven otherwise by ❶ dysbiosis laboratory assessment (including comprehensive stool testing with parasitology *performed by a specialty laboratory*), and ❷ response to anti-dysbiosis treatment which minimally includes the combination of anti-dysbiosis dietary modification (nutritional supplementation,

---

[298] Jonsson T, Valdimarsson H. What about IgA rheumatoid factor in rheumatoid arthritis? *Ann Rheum Dis*. 1998 Jan;57(1):63-4 ard.bmjjournals.com/cgi/content/full/57/1/63
[299] "These manifestations which are common to rheumatoid arthritis may be seen in hemochromatotic arthropathy." Bensen WG, Laskin CA, Little HA, Fam AG. Hemochromatotic arthropathy mimicking rheumatoid arthritis. A case with subcutaneous nodules, tenosynovitis, and bursitis. *Arthritis Rheum*. 1978;21(7):844-8
[300] Bowman et al. Bilateral adhesive capsulitis, oligoarthritis and proximal myopathy as presentation of hypothyroidism. *Br J Rheumatol*. 1988;27(1):62-4
[301] Weetman AP. Hypothyroidism: screening and subclinical disease. *BMJ*. 1997 Apr 19;314(7088):1175-8 bmj.bmjjournals.com/cgi/content/full/314/7088/1175
[302] "Now AACE encourages doctors to consider treatment for patients who test outside the boundaries of a narrower margin based on a target TSH level of 0.3 to 3.0. AACE believes the new range will result in proper diagnosis for millions of Americans who suffer from a mild thyroid disorder, but have gone untreated until now." American Association of Clinical Endocrinologists (AACE). 2003 Campaign Encourages Awareness of Mild Thyroid Failure, Importance of Routine Testing aace.com/pub/tam2003/press.php November 26, 2005
[303] Beers MH, Berkow R (eds). *Merck Manual. Seventeenth Edition*. Whitehouse Station; Merck Research Laboratories 1999 Page 96
[304] Humbert P, Bidet A, Treffel P, Drobacheff C, Agache P. Intestinal permeability in patients with psoriasis. *J Dermatol Sci*. 1991 Jul;2(4):324-6
[305] Fresko I, et al. Intestinal permeability in Behcet's syndrome. *Ann Rheum Dis*. 2001 Jan;60(1):65-6
[306] Vaile et al. Bowel permeability and CD45RO expression on circulating CD20+ B cells in patients with ankylosing spondylitis and their relatives. *J Rheumatol* 1999 Jan:128-35
[307] Di Leo et al. Effect of Helicobacter pylori and eradication therapy on gastrointestinal permeability. Implications for patients with seronegative spondyloarthritis. *J Rheumatol*. 2005 Feb;32(2):295-300
[308] Picco P, et al. Increased gut permeability in juvenile chronic arthritides. A multivariate analysis of the diagnostic parameters. *Clin Exp Rheumatol*. 2000 Nov-Dec;18(6):773-8
[309] "Fourteen cases of primary lupus-associated protein-losing enteropathy have now been reported in the English-language literature." Perednia DA, Curosh NA. Lupus-associated protein-losing enteropathy. *Arch Intern Med*. 1990 Sep;150(9):1806-10
[310] "Chronic heart failure patients had a 35% increase of small intestinal permeability (lactulose/mannitol ratio: 0.023 vs. 0.017 ..., p = 0.006), a 210% increase of large intestinal permeability (sucralose excretion: 0.62 ... vs. 0.20), and a 29% decrease of D-xylose absorption, indicating bowel ischemia (26.7% vs. 37.4%, p = 0.003)." Sandek A, Bauditz J, Swidsinski A, et al. Altered intestinal function in patients with chronic heart failure. *J Am Coll Cardiol*. 2007 Oct 16;50(16):1561-9

plant-based diet, low-fermentation, high-fiber, superadequate protein and phytonutrients) <u>with antimicrobial drugs or botanicals</u>, commonly including berberine (500mg BID-TID for 3 months), emulsified time-released oil of oregano (200mg TID for 6 weeks[311]), Augmentin (2,000mg BID for variable durations of days to months to years—supportively, note successful use of long-term penicillin in the treatment of psoriasis[312]), azithromycin (500mg every other day for variable durations of days to months to years[313]), ciprofloxacin (short course only to avoid exacerbation/induction of tendonopathy), and metronidazole. Recently, I've become impressed by the efficacy of low-dose oral vancomycin 125-250mg PO QD; as a nonabsorbed antibiotic, the drug remains in the gut and is effective against segmented filamentous bacteria (SFB) which have been shown in several animal experiments to induce Th-17 effector cells which promote chronic arthritis/autoimmunity. A **three-sample comprehensive stool analysis and parasitology examination** performed by a **specialty laboratory** is strongly recommended as a minimal component of basic care. In lieu of *or preferably in addition to* a comprehensive parasitology test, patients can be treated for 4-8 weeks with broad-spectrum antimicrobial treatment (including an anti-dysbiosis diet) that is effective against gram-positive and gram-negative bacteria, aerobes and anaerobes, yeast, protozoa and amebas. For additional details, see the Section on *Multifocal Dysbiosis* in Chapter 4.

- **Imaging**:
    - Radiographic changes are not seen in early disease and only have utility for clarifying diagnostic uncertainty later in the disease, screening for complications such as atlantoaxial instability, or for pre-operative assessment in patients who are candidates for joint repair or replacement.
    - Radiographic findings when clustered are relatively specific in developed disease: soft tissue swelling, periarticular osteoporosis, joint space narrowing due to loss of cartilage, **marginal erosions**, ulnar/lateral deviation of the fingers, and subluxation and dislocation may occur.
- **Establishing the diagnosis**:
    - The diagnosis is established by pattern recognition of the typical clinical manifestations and laboratory abnormalities and reasonable exclusion of protean diseases such as hepatitis C, SLE, and iron overload.

Complications:
- Disease complications are common and range from the inconveniences of pain and inflammation for patients with milder disease to the major complications of joint deformity, occupational and social disability, serious cardiovascular/renal/pulmonary/cerebral complications (due mostly to inflammation, fibrosis, and vasculitis), infections (especially septic arthritis), depression, and suicide. Adding drug side-effects

---

2010 American College of Rheumatology/European League against Rheumatism classification criteria

Screening: Patients with at least 1 joint and definite clinical synovitis which is not explained by another disease.

A score of ≥6 is needed for classification of definite RA:
- Score 1 large joint: 0
- 2–10 large joints: 1
- 1–3 small joints (with or without large joints): 2
- 4–10 small joints (with or without large joints): 3
- >10 joints (at least 1 small joint): 5

Serology: At least 1 test is needed:
- Negative RF (rheumatoid factor) and negative ACPA (anticitrullinated protein antibody): 0
- Low positive RF or low positive ACPA: 2
- High positive RF or high positive ACPA: 3

Acute phase reactants: At least 1 result is needed.
- Normal CRP (C-reactive protein) and normal ESR: 0
- Abnormal CRP or ESR: 1

Duration of symptoms: (self-reported)
- <6 weeks: 0
- ≥6 weeks: 1

Although patients with a score <6/10 are not classifiable as having RA, their status can be reassessed and the criteria might be fulfilled cumulatively over time.

onlinelibrary.wiley.com/doi/10.1002/art.27580/pdf
ncbi.nlm.nih.gov/pmc/articles/PMC3077961/pdf/nihms266537.pdf
unboundmedicine.com/5minute/view/5-Minute-Clinical-Consult/116053/all/Arthritis_Rheumatoid__RA

---

[311] "Oil of Mediterranean oregano *Oreganum vulgare* was orally administered to 14 adult patients whose stools tested positive for enteric parasites, *Blastocystis hominis*, *Entamoeba hartmanni* and *Endolimax nana*. After 6 weeks of supplementation with 600 mg emulsified oil of oregano daily, there was complete disappearance of *Entamoeba hartmanni* (four cases), *Endolimax nana* (one case), and *Blastocystis hominis* in eight cases. Also, *Blastocystis hominis* scores declined in three additional cases. Gastrointestinal symptoms improved in seven of the 11 patients who had tested positive for *Blastocystis hominis*." Force M, Sparks WS, Ronzio RA. Inhibition of enteric parasites by emulsified oil of oregano in vivo. *Phytother Res*. 2000 May;14(3):213-4
[312] Saxena VN, Dogra J. Long-term use of penicillin for the treatment of chronic plaque psoriasis. *Eur J Dermatol*. 2005 Sep-Oct;15(5):359-6
[313] Saxena VN, Dogra J. Long-term oral azithromycin in chronic plaque psoriasis: a controlled trial. *Eur J Dermatol*. 2010 May-Jun;20(3):329-33

atop these manifold disease complications makes managing the disease more difficult for doctors, and enduring the disease more difficult for patients.
- Mild disease results in mild symptoms and manageable impact on ADL (activities of daily living) and QOL (quality of life). Severe disease is painful, less responsive to treatment, disfiguring and generally devastating. Treatments that are inefficacious, unavailable, prohibitively expensive, or complicated by significant side effects contribute to despair. **RA patients are at increased risk for social isolation, depression, and suicide**[314]; these sociopsychiatric complications can be attributed to chronic pain, neuropsychiatric effects of inflammatory cytokines, therapeutic nihilism, adverse drug effects (e.g., NSAID- and steroid-induced psychosis), cerebral vasculitis, and nutritional deficiencies (e.g., EPA, DHA, vitamin D, zinc) in patients not cared for by competent integrative clinicians.
- Decreased life expectancy by 3-7 years, mostly due to infection, gastrointestinal bleeding, and cardiorenal complications.
- Patients with systemic inflammatory diseases are at increased risk for cardiovascular disorders (including hypertension, accelerated atherosclerosis, vasculitis) and renal complications (secondary to hypertension, vasculitis, immune complex deposition, NSAIDs and other drugs).

<u>Clinical management</u>:
- <u>Routine assessment, surveillance for complications, compliance, consultation, laboratory follow-up, access to treatments</u>: Clinical visits should include surveillance for subjective and objective indicators of disease progression/remission, treatment compliance (including overzealous compliance with its risk of adverse toxic effects or unnecessary expense, or undercompliance with attendant hazards of inefficacy and disease exacerbation), and overall health status. Questions are answered, and problems addressed. Necessary consultations are scheduled as needed; the referring provider sends a narrative letter and ensures that the patient has a scheduled appointment. Review and anticipatory scheduling of laboratory tests should be performed. Access to treatments should be verified. Appropriate documentation is mandatory.
- <u>Standard medical treatments</u>:
    - <u>Discouraging the discouragement of "nutritional quackery"</u>: According to the *Merck Manual (1999)*, "Food and diet quackery is common and should be discouraged."[315] In contrast to this allopathic rhetoric, the biomedical literature strongly supports the use of nutritional interventions for **direct benefits** (e.g., anti-inflammatory, analgesic, immunomodulatory, and drug-sparing effects) and **indirect benefits** (e.g., cardiorenal protection, alleviation of depression).
    - <u>NSAIDs as first-line treatment</u>: NSAIDS provide temporary pain relief while contributing to increased intestinal permeability, gastrointestinal hemorrhage, liver toxicity (dose-response relationship), renal toxicity (dose-response relationship) possible exacerbation of food allergies[316], and accelerated destruction of articular structures (especially indomethacin).[317,318,319]
    - <u>Immunosuppression with prednisone, methotrexate, or other DMARD (disease-modifying antirheumatic drugs)</u>: **Despite the clinical drawbacks, philosophical inadequacies, and steep financial consequences, pharmacologic immunosuppression has a role in the management of patients with autoimmunity when their disease flares and threatens vital structures, particularly the heart, kidneys, and nervous system.** A common sequence of medicalization used by rheumatologists is:

---

[314] "Rheumatoid arthritis (RA) is a somatic disorder, which is known to be associated with major depression, and prevalences exceeding even 40% have been reported [5, 6]. Recently, Treharne et al. [7] showed that 11% of hospital out-patients with RA had experienced suicidal ideation." Timonen M, Viilo K, Hakko H, Särkioja T, Ylikulju M, Meyer-Rochow VB, Väisänen E, Räsänen P. Suicides in persons suffering from rheumatoid arthritis. *Rheumatology* (Oxford). 2003 Feb;42(2):287-91
[315] Beers MH, Berkow R (eds). *The Merck Manual. Seventeenth Edition*. Whitehouse Station; Merck Research Laboratories: 1999, page 419
[316] Abbreviations: cow's milk beta-lactoglobulin absorption (BLG), acetylsalicylic acid (ASA), disodium chromoglycate (DSCG). "ASA administration strongly increased BLG absorption, not prevented by DSCG pretreatment. ... Our results suggest that prolonged treatment with nonsteroidal anti-inflammatory drugs induces an increase of food antigen absorption, apparently not related to anaphylaxis mediator release, with possible clinical effects." Fagiolo U, Paganelli R, Ossi E, Quinti I, Cancian M, D'Offizi GP, Fiocco U. Intestinal permeability and antigen absorption in rheumatoid arthritis. Effects of acetylsalicylic acid and sodium chromogycate. *Int Arch Allergy Appl Immunol*. 1989;89(1):98-102
[317] "At...concentrations comparable to those... in the synovial fluid of patients treated with the drug, several NSAIDs suppress proteoglycan synthesis... These NSAID-related effects on chondrocyte metabolism ... are much more profound in osteoarthritic cartilage than in normal cartilage, due to enhanced uptake of NSAIDs by the osteoarthritic cartilage." Brandt KD. Effects of nonsteroidal anti-inflammatory drugs on chondrocyte metabolism in vitro and in vivo. *Am J Med*. 1987 Nov 20; 83: 29-34
[318] "The case of a young healthy man, who developed avascular necrosis of head of femur after prolonged administration of indomethacin, is reported here." Prathapkumar KR, Smith I, Attara GA. Indomethacin induced avascular necrosis of head of femur. *Postgrad Med J*. 2000 Sep; 76(899): 574-5
[319] "This highly significant association between NSAID use and acetabular destruction gives cause for concern, not least because of the difficulty in achieving satisfactory hip replacements in patients with severely damaged acetabula." Newman et al. Acetabular bone destruction related to non-steroidal anti-inflammatory drugs. *Lancet*. 1985; 2: 11-4

- Begin first-visit treatment with daily/PRN low-dose prednisone (5-7.5 mg/day) and weekly methotrexate (7.5-15 mg/week, with daily folic acid to improve efficacy and reduce toxicity),
- Eventually add hydroxychloroquine and/or sulfasalazine as disease progresses,
- When the patient becomes "resistant to treatment" add either an oral immunosuppressant or one of the "biologics" such as the parenterally-administered TNF/cytokine blockers: etanercept, infliximab, adalimumab, etc.

Such a drug protocol might easily cost $50,000 per year and carry complications such as increased risk and severity of opportunistic infections (especially tuberculosis), exacerbation of heart failure, and increased risk for lymphoma and—less commonly—SLE and CNS demyelination similar to multiple sclerosis. Immunosuppression with corticosteroids/prednisone promotes bacterial overgrowth of the small bowel in humans[320], and animal studies have demonstrated increased bacterial translocation following prednisone administration[321]; recall that intestinal bacterial overgrowth/translocation are both pro-inflammatory and arthritogenic. Prednisone also causes mitochondrial dysfunction, which exacerbates fatigue and inflammation.

o Surgery: Surgery is used for deformities and other orthopedic complications, including atlantoaxial instability and protrusio acetabuli.

- **FOOD & NUTRITION: 5-part "supplemented Paleo-Mediterranean diet" (SPMD)** The 5-part "supplemented Paleo-Mediterranean diet" (SPMD—reviewed in Chapter 4) consists of ❶ foundational plant-based low-carbohydrate diet of fruits, vegetables, nuts, seeds, berries and lean sources of protein, ❷ multivitamin and multimineral supplementation, ❸ physiologic doses of vitamin D3 (range 2,000-10,000 IU/d), ❹ combination fatty acid therapy (CFAT) with n3-ALA, n6-GLA, n3-EPA, n3-DHA, and phytochemical-rich olive oil which contains n9-oleate, and ❺ probiotics.

o Avoidance of pro-inflammatory foods: Pro-inflammatory foods act *directly* and *indirectly* to promote and exacerbate systemic inflammation. *Direct* mechanisms include the activation of Toll-like receptors and NF-kappaB, while *indirect* mechanisms include depleting the body of anti-inflammatory nutrients and dietary displacement of more nutrient-dense anti-inflammatory foods. Arachidonic acid (found in cow's milk, beef, liver, pork, and lamb) is the direct precursor to pro-inflammatory prostaglandins and leukotrienes[322] and pain-promoting isoprostanes.[323] Saturated fats promote inflammation by activating/enabling pro-inflammatory Toll-like receptors, which are otherwise "specific" for inducing pro-inflammatory responses to microorganisms.[324] Consumption of saturated fat in the form of cream creates marked oxidative stress and lipid peroxidation that lasts for at least 3 hours postprandially.[325] Corn oil rapidly activates NF-kappaB (in hepatic Kupffer cells) for a pro-inflammatory effect[326]; similarly, consumption of PUFA and linoleic acid promotes antioxidant depletion and may thus promote oxidation-mediated inflammation via activation of NF-kappaB. Linoleic acid causes intracellular oxidative stress and calcium influx and results in increased NF-kappaB-stimulated transcription of pro-inflammatory genes.[327] High glycemic foods cause oxidative stress[328,329] and inflammation via activation

---

[320] "A 63-year-old man with systemic lupus erythematosus and selective IgA deficiency developed intractable diarrhoea the day after treatment with prednisone, 50 mg daily, was started. The diarrhoea was considered to be caused by bacterial overgrowth and was later successfully treated with doxycycline." Denison H, Wallerstedt S. Bacterial overgrowth after high-dose corticosteroid treatment. *Scand J Gastroenterol*. 1989 Jun;24(5):561-4
[321] "These bacteria also translocated to the mesenteric lymph nodes in mice injected with cyclophosphamide or prednisone." Berg RD, Wommack E, Deitch EA. Immunosuppression and intestinal bacterial overgrowth synergistically promote bacterial translocation. *Arch Surg*. 1988 Nov;123(11):1359-64
[322] Vasquez A. New Insights into Fatty Acid Supplementation and Its Effect on Eicosanoid Production and Genetic Expression. *Nutritional Perspectives* 2005; Jan: 5-16
[323] Evans AR, Junger H, Southall MD, Nicol GD, Sorkin LS, Broome JT, Bailey TW, Vasko MR. Isoprostanes, novel eicosanoids that produce nociception and sensitize rat sensory neurons. *J Pharmacol Exp Ther*. 2000 Jun;293(3):912-20
[324] Lee et al. Saturated fatty acids not unsaturated fatty acids induce expression of cyclooxygenase-2 mediated through Toll-like receptor 4. *J Biol Chem* 2001 May;276:16683-9
[325] "The increase in ROS generation lasted 3 h after cream intake and 1 h after protein intake." Mohanty et al. Both lipid and protein intakes stimulate increased generation of reactive oxygen species by polymorphonuclear leukocytes and mononuclear cells. *Am J Clin Nutr*. 2002 Apr;75(4):767-72
[326] Rusyn et al. Corn oil rapidly activates nuclear factor-kappaB in hepatic Kupffer cells by oxidant-dependent mechanisms. *Carcinogenesis*. 1999 Nov;20(11):2095-100
[327] "Exposing endothelial cells to 90 micromol linoleic acid/L for 6 h resulted in a significant increase in lipid hydroperoxides that coincided wih an increase in intracellular calcium concentrations." Hennig B, et al. Linoleic acid activates nuclear transcription factor-kappa B (NF-kappa B) and induces NF-kappa B-dependent transcription in cultured endothelial cells. *Am J Clin Nutr*. 1996 Mar;63(3):322-8 ajcn.org/cgi/reprint/63/3/322
[328] Mohanty et al. Glucose challenge stimulates reactive oxygen species (ROS) generation by leucocytes. *J Clin Endocrinol Metab*. 2000 Aug;85(8):2970-3 Glucose/carbohydrate and saturated fat consumption appear to be the two biggest offenders in the food-stimulated production of oxidative stress. The effect by protein is much less. "CONCLUSIONS: Both fat and protein intakes stimulate ROS generation. The increase in ROS generation lasted 3 h after cream intake and 1 h after protein intake. Cream intake also caused a significant and prolonged increase in lipid peroxidation." Mohanty et al. Both lipid and protein intakes stimulate increased generation of reactive oxygen species by polymorphonuclear leukocytes and mononuclear cells. *Am J Clin Nutr*. 2002 Apr;75(4):767-72
[329] Koska et al. Insulin, catecholamines, glucose and antioxidant enzymes in oxidative damage during different loads in healthy humans. *Physiol Res*. 2000;49 Suppl 1:S95-100

of NF-kappaB and other mechanisms—e.g., *white bread causes inflammation*[330] as does *a high-fat high-carbohydrate fast-food-style breakfast*.[331] High glycemic foods suppress immune function[332,333] and thus promote the perpetuation of microbial colonization and dysbiosis. Delivery of a high carbohydrate load to the gastrointestinal lumen promotes bacterial overgrowth[334,335], which is inherently pro-inflammatory[336,337] and which appears to be myalgenic in humans[338] at least in part due to the ability of endotoxin to impair muscle function.[339] Overconsumption of high-carbohydrate low-phytonutrient grains, potatoes, and manufactured foods displaces phytonutrient-dense foods such as fruits, vegetables, nuts, seeds, and berries which contain more than 8,000 phytonutrients, many of which have antioxidant and thus anti-inflammatory actions.[340,341]

> **Systemic inflammatory diseases almost always have a major gastrointestinal component**
>
> "This study supports the concept that rheumatoid arthritis may be a reaction to a food antigen(s) and that the disease process starts within the intestine."
>
> Podas et al. Is rheumatoid arthritis a disease that starts in the intestine? A pilot study comparing an elemental diet with oral prednisolone. *Postgrad Med J.* 2007 Feb

- Avoidance of allergenic foods: **Gluten-free vegetarian diets benefit patients with rheumatoid arthritis.**[342] Any patient may be allergic to any food, even if the food is generally considered a health-promoting food. Generally speaking, the most notorious allergens are wheat, citrus (especially citrus *juice* due to the industrial use of fungal hemicellulases), cow's milk, eggs, peanuts, chocolate, and yeast-containing foods. According to a study in patients with migraine, some patients will have to avoid as many as 10 specific foods in order to become symptom-free.[343] **Celiac disease can present with inflammatory oligoarthritis that resembles rheumatoid arthritis and which remits with avoidance of wheat/gluten.** The inflammatory arthropathy of celiac disease has preceded bowel symptoms and/or an accurate diagnosis by as many as 3-15 years.[344,345] Clinicians must explain to their patients that celiac disease and wheat allergy are two different clinical entities and that exclusion of one does not exclude the other, and in neither case does mutual exclusion obviate the promotion of intestinal bacterial overgrowth (i.e., pro-inflammatory dysbiosis) by indigestible wheat oligosaccharides.
- Gluten-free vegetarian/vegan diet: **Gluten-free vegetarian diets benefit patients with rheumatoid arthritis.**[346] Vegetarian/vegan diets have a place in the treatment plan of all patients with

---

[330] "Conclusion - The present study shows that high GI carbohydrate, but not low GI carbohydrate, mediates an acute proinflammatory process as measured by NF-kappaB activity." Dickinson S, Hancock DP, Petocz P, Brand-Miller JC. High glycemic index carbohydrate mediates an acute proinflammatory process as measured by NF-kappaB activation. *Asia Pac J Clin Nutr.* 2005;14 Suppl:S120
[331] Aljada et al. Increase in intranuclear nuclear factor kappaB and decrease in inhibitor kappaB in mononuclear cells after a mixed meal. *Am J Clin Nutr.* 2004 Apr;79(4):682-90
[332] Sanchez A, Reeser JL, Lau HS, et al. Role of sugars in human neutrophilic phagocytosis. *Am J Clin Nutr.* 1973 Nov;26(11):1180-4
[333] "Postoperative infusion of carbohydrate solution leads to moderate fall in the serum concentration of inorganic phosphate. ... The hypophosphatemia was associated with significant reduction of neutrophil phagocytosis, intracellular killing, consumption of oxygen and generation of superoxide during phagocytosis." Rasmussen A, Segel E, Hessov I, Borregaard N. Reduced function of neutrophils during routine postoperative glucose infusion. *Acta Chir Scand.* 1988 Jul-Aug;154(7-8):429-33
[334] Ramakrishnan T, Stokes P. Beneficial effects of fasting and low carbohydrate diet in D-lactic acidosis associated with short-bowel syndrome. *JPEN J Parenter Enteral Nutr.* 1985 May-Jun;9(3):361-3
[335] Gottschall E. *Breaking the Vicious Cycle: Intestinal Health through Diet.* Kirkton Press; Rev edition (August 1, 1994)
[336] Lin HC. Small intestinal bacterial overgrowth: a framework for understanding irritable bowel syndrome. *JAMA.* 2004 Aug 18;292(7):852-8
[337] Lichtman et al. Reactivation of arthritis induced by small bowel bacterial overgrowth in rats. *Infect Immun.* 1995 Jun;63(6):2295-301
[338] Pimentel M, et al. A link between irritable bowel syndrome and fibromyalgia may be related to findings on lactulose breath testing. *Ann Rheum Dis.* 2004 Apr;63:450-2
[339] Bundgaard H, et al. Endotoxemia stimulates skeletal muscle Na+-K+-ATPase and raises blood lactate under aerobic conditions in humans. *Am J Physiol Heart Circ Physiol.* 2003 Mar;284(3):H1028-34 ajpheart.physiology.org/cgi/reprint/284/3/H1028
[340] "We propose that the additive and synergistic effects of phytochemicals in fruit and vegetables are responsible for their potent antioxidant and anticancer activities, and that the benefit of a diet rich in fruit and vegetables is attributed to the complex mixture of phytochemicals present in whole foods." Liu RH. Health benefits of fruit and vegetables are from additive and synergistic combinations of phytochemicals. *Am J Clin Nutr.* 2003 Sep;78(3 Suppl):517S-520S
[341] Seaman DR. The diet-induced proinflammatory state: a cause of chronic pain and other degenerative diseases? *J Manipulative Physiol Ther.* 2002;25(3):168-79
[342] "The immunoglobulin G (IgG) antibody levels against gliadin and beta-lactoglobulin decreased in the responder subgroup in the vegan diet-treated patients, but not in the other analysed groups." Hafstrom I, et al. A vegan diet free of gluten improves the signs and symptoms of rheumatoid arthritis: the effects on arthritis correlate with a reduction in antibodies to food antigens. *Rheumatology* (Oxford). 2001 Oct;40(10):1175-9 rheumatology.oxfordjournals.org/cgi/content/abstract/40/10/1175
[343] Grant EC. Food allergies and migraine. *Lancet.* 1979 May 5;1(8123):966-9
[344] "We report six patients with coeliac disease in whom arthritis was prominent at diagnosis and who improved with dietary therapy. Joint pain preceded diagnosis by up to three years in five patients and 15 years in one patient." Bourne et al. Arthritis and coeliac disease. *Ann Rheum Dis.* 1985 Sep;44(9):592-8
[345] "A 15-year-old girl, with synovitis of the knees and ankles for 3 years before a diagnosis of gluten-sensitive enteropathy, is described." Pinals RS. Arthritis associated with gluten-sensitive enteropathy. *J Rheumatol.* 1986 Feb;13(1):201-4
[346] "The immunoglobulin G (IgG) antibody levels against gliadin and beta-lactoglobulin decreased in the responder subgroup in the vegan diet-treated patients, but not in the other analysed groups." Hafstrom I, et al. A vegan diet free of gluten improves the signs and symptoms of rheumatoid arthritis: the effects on arthritis correlate with a reduction in antibodies to food antigens. *Rheumatology* (Oxford). 2001 Oct;40(10):1175-9 rheumatology.oxfordjournals.org/cgi/content/abstract/40/10/1175

autoimmune/inflammatory disorders[347,348,349]; this is also true for patients for whom long-term exclusive reliance on a meat-free vegetarian diet is either not appropriate or not appealing. No scientist or clinician familiar with the research literature doubts the antirheumatic power and anti-inflammatory advantages of vegetarian diets, whether used short-term or long term.[350] The benefits of gluten-free vegetarian diets are well documented, and the mechanisms of action are well elucidated, including reduced intake of pro-inflammatory linoleic[351] and arachidonic acids[352], iron[353], common food antigens[354], gluten[355] and gliadin[356,357], pro-inflammatory sugars[358] and increased intake of omega-3 fatty acids, micronutrients[359], and anti-inflammatory and antioxidant phytonutrients.[360] Vegetarian diets also effect subtle yet biologically and clinically important changes—both *qualitative* and *quantitative*—in intestinal flora[361,362] that correlate with clinical improvement.[363] Patients who rely on the Paleo-Mediterranean diet (which is inherently omnivorous) can use vegetarian *meals* on a daily basis or for days at a time—for example, by having a daily vegetarian meal, or one week per month of vegetarianism. Some (not all) patients can use a purely vegetarian diet long-term provided that nutritional needs (especially protein and cobalamin) are consistently met.

o <u>Routine carbohydrate restriction, periodic short-term fasting</u>: Whether the foundational diet is Paleo-Mediterranean, vegetarian, vegan, or a combination of all of these, autoimmune/inflammatory patients will still benefit from periodic fasting, whether on a weekly (e.g., every Saturday), monthly (every first week or weekend of the month, or every other month), or yearly (1-2 weeks of the year) basis. The diet should generally be low in carbohydrates in order to promote ketogenesis and to retard SIBO. Since consumption of food—particularly "unhealthy" (i.e., high-fat, high-sugar, allergenic, nutritionally depleted, AGE-laden) foods—induces an inflammatory effect[364], abstinence from food provides a relative anti-inflammatory effect. Fasting indeed provides a distinct anti-inflammatory benefit and may help "re-calibrate" metabolic and homeostatic mechanisms by breaking self-perpetuating "vicious cycles"[365] that autonomously promote inflammation independent of pro-inflammatory stimuli. Water-only fasting is completely hypoallergenic (assuming that the patient is not sensitive to chlorine, fluoride, or other contaminants), and subsequent re-introduction of foods provides the ideal opportunity to identify

---

[347] "After four weeks at the health farm the diet group showed a significant improvement in number of tender joints, Ritchie's articular index, number of swollen joints, pain score, duration of morning stiffness, grip strength, erythrocyte sedimentation rate, C-reactive protein, white blood cell count, and a health assessment questionnaire score." Kjeldsen-Kragh J, et al. Controlled trial of fasting and one-year vegetarian diet in rheumatoid arthritis. *Lancet*. 1991 Oct 12;338(8772):899-902

[348] "During fasting, arthralgia was less intense in many subjects. In some types of skin diseases (pustulosis palmaris et plantaris and atopic eczema) an improvement could be demonstrated during the fast. During the vegan diet, both signs and symptoms returned in most patients, with the exception of some patients with psoriasis who experienced an improvement." Lithell H, Bruce A, et al. A fasting and vegetarian diet treatment trial on chronic inflammatory disorders. *Acta Derm Venereol*. 1983;63(5):397-403

[349] Tanaka T, Kouda K, Kotani M, et al. Vegetarian diet ameliorates symptoms of atopic dermatitis through reduction of the number of peripheral eosinophils and of PGE2 synthesis by monocytes. *J Physiol Anthropol Appl Human Sci*. 2001 Nov;20(6):353-61 jstage.jst.go.jp/article/jpa/20/6/20_353/_article/-char/en

[350] "For the patients who were randomised to the vegetarian diet there was a significant decrease in platelet count, leukocyte count, calprotectin, total IgG, IgM rheumatoid factor (RF), C3-activation products, and the complement components C3 and C4 after one month of treatment." Kjeldsen-Kragh J, Mellbye OJ, Haugen M, Mollnes TE, Hammer HB, Sioud M, Forre O. Changes in laboratory variables in rheumatoid arthritis patients during a trial of fasting and one-year vegetarian diet. *Scand J Rheumatol*. 1995;24(2):85-93

[351] Rusyn I, Bradham CA, Cohn L, Schoonhoven R, Swenberg JA, Brenner DA, Thurman RG. Corn oil rapidly activates nuclear factor-kappaB in hepatic Kupffer cells by oxidant-dependent mechanisms. *Carcinogenesis*. 1999 Nov;20(11):2095-100 carcin.oxfordjournals.org/cgi/content/full/20/11/2095

[352] Vasquez A. New Insights into Fatty Acid Supplementation and Its Effect on Eicosanoid Production and Genetic Expression. *Nutritional Perspectives* 2005; January: 5-16

[353] Dabbagh AJ, Trenam CW, Morris CJ, Blake DR. Iron in joint inflammation. *Ann Rheum Dis*. 1993 Jan;52(1):67-73

[354] Hafstrom I, et al. A vegan diet free of gluten improves the signs and symptoms of rheumatoid arthritis: the effects on arthritis correlate with a reduction in antibodies to food antigens. *Rheumatology* (Oxford). 2001 Oct;40(10):1175-9 rheumatology.oxfordjournals.org/cgi/reprint/40/10/1175

[355] "The data provide evidence that dietary modification may be of clinical benefit for certain RA patients, and that this benefit may be related to a reduction in immunoreactivity to food antigens eliminated by the change in diet." Hafstrom I, Ringertz B, et al. A vegan diet free of gluten improves the signs and symptoms of rheumatoid arthritis: the effects on arthritis correlate with a reduction in antibodies to food antigens. *Rheumatology* (Oxford). 2001 Oct;40(10):1175-9

[356] "Despite the increased AGA [antigliadin antibodies] positivity found distinctively in patients with recent-onset RA, none of the RA patients showed clear evidence of coeliac disease." Paimela L, Kurki P, Leirisalo-Repo M, Piirainen H. Gliadin immune reactivity in patients with rheumatoid arthritis. Clin Exp Rheumatol. 1995 Sep-Oct;13(5):603-7

[357] "The median IgA antigliadin ELISA index was 7.1 (range 2.1-22.4) for the RA group and 3.1 (range 0.3-34.9) for the controls (p = 0.0001)." Koot et al. Elevated level of IgA gliadin antibodies in patients with rheumatoid arthritis. *Clin Exp Rheumatol*. 1989 Nov-Dec;7(6):623-6

[358] Seaman DR. The diet-induced proinflammatory state: a cause of chronic pain and other degenerative diseases? *J Manipulative Physiol Ther*. 2002 Mar-Apr;25(3):168-79

[359] Hagfors L, Nilsson I, Skoldstam L, Johansson G. Fat intake and composition of fatty acids in serum phospholipids in a randomized, controlled, Mediterranean dietary intervention study on patients with rheumatoid arthritis. *Nutr Metab* (Lond). 2005 Oct 10;2:26 nutritionandmetabolism.com/content/2/1/26

[360] Liu. Health benefits of fruit and vegetables from additive and synergistic combinations of phytochemicals. *Am J Clin Nutr* 2003:517S-520S ajcn.org/cgi/content/full/78/3/517S

[361] "Significant alteration in the intestinal flora was observed when the patients changed from omnivorous to vegan diet. ... This finding of an association between intestinal flora and disease activity may have implications for our understanding of how diet can affect RA." Peltonen et al. Changes of faecal flora in rheumatoid arthritis during fasting and one-year vegetarian diet. *Br J Rheumatol*. 1994 Jul;33(7):638-43

[362] Toivanen P, Eerola E. A vegan diet changes the intestinal flora. *Rheumatology* (Oxford). 2002 Aug;41(8):950-1 rheumatology.oxfordjournals.org/cgi/reprint/41/8/950

[363] "We conclude that a vegan diet changes the faecal microbial flora in RA patients, and changes in the faecal flora are associated with improvement in RA activity." Peltonen et al. Faecal microbial flora and disease activity in rheumatoid arthritis during a vegan diet. *Br J Rheumatol*. 1997 Jan;36(1):64-8 rheumatology.oxfordjournals.org/cgi/reprint/36/1/64

[364] Aljada et al. Increase in intranuclear nuclear factor kappaB and decrease in inhibitor kappaB in mononuclear cells after a mixed meal. *Am J Clin Nutr*. 2004 Apr;79(4):682-90

[365] "The ability of therapeutic fasts to break metabolic vicious cycles may also contribute to the efficacy of fasting in the treatment of type 2 diabetes and autoimmune disorders." McCarty MF. A preliminary fast may potentiate response to a subsequent low-salt, low-fat vegan diet in the management of hypertension - fasting as a strategy for breaking metabolic vicious cycles. *Med Hypotheses*. 2003 May;60(5):624-33

offending foods. Fasting deprives intestinal microbes of substrate[366], stimulates intestinal B-cell immunity[367], improves the bactericidal action of neutrophils[368], reduces lysozyme release and leukotriene formation[369], and ameliorates intestinal hyperpermeability.[370] Fasting and carbohydrate avoidance also promote endogenous production of beta-hydroxybutyrate (bHB) which promotes histone acetylation for induction of a rejuvenative phenotype while bHB also stimulates complexes 3 and 4 of the mitochondrial electron transport chain (mETC) for enhanced mitochondrial function and efficiency. **In case reports and clinical trials, short-term fasting (or protein-sparing fasting) has been documented as safe and effective treatment for SLE[371], RA[372], and non-rheumatic diseases such as chronic severe hypertension[373], moderate hypertension[374], obesity[375,376], type-2 diabetes[377], and epilepsy.[378]**

- o <u>Broad-spectrum fatty acid therapy with ALA, EPA, DHA, GLA and oleic acid</u>: Fatty acid supplementation should be delivered in the form of combination therapy with ALA, GLA, DHA, and EPA. Given at doses of 3,000 – 9,000 mg per day, ALA from flaxseed oil has impressive anti-inflammatory benefits demonstrated by its ability to halve prostaglandin production in humans.[379] **Numerous studies have demonstrated the benefit of GLA in the treatment of rheumatoid arthritis when used at doses between 500 mg – 4,000 mg per day.**[380,381] **Fish oil provides EPA and DHA which have well-proven anti-inflammatory benefits in rheumatoid arthritis**[382,383,384] **and lupus.**[385,386] ALA, EPA, DHA, and GLA need to be provided in the form of supplements; when using high doses of therapeutic oils, *liquid* supplements that can be mixed in juice or a smoothie are generally more convenient and palatable than are *capsules*. For example, at the upper end of oral fatty acid administration, the patient may be consuming as much as one-quarter cup per day of fatty acid supplementation; this same dose administered in the form of pills would require at least 72 capsules to attain the equivalent doses of ALA, EPA, DHA, and GLA. Therapeutic amounts of oleic acid can be obtained from generous use of olive oil, preferably on fresh vegetables. Supplementation with polyunsaturated fatty acids warrants increased intake of antioxidants from diet, from fruit and vegetable juices, and from properly formulated supplements. Since patients with systemic inflammation are generally in a pro-oxidative state, consideration must be given to the timing and starting dose of fatty acid supplementation and the need for antioxidant protection; some

---

[366] Ramakrishnan et al. Beneficial effects of fasting and low carbohydrate diet in D-lactic acidosis associated with short-bowel syndrome. *JPEN J Parenter Enteral Nutr.* 1985 May-Jun;9(3):361-3

[367] Trollmo C, Verdrengh M, Tarkowski A. Fasting enhances mucosal antigen specific B cell responses in rheumatoid arthritis. *Ann Rheum Dis.* 1997 Feb;56(2):130-4 ard.bmjjournals.com/cgi/content/full/56/2/130

[368] "An association was found between improvement in inflammatory activity of the joints and enhancement of neutrophil bactericidal capacity. Fasting appears to improve the clinical status of patients with RA." Uden AM, Trang L, Venizelos N, Palmblad J. Neutrophil functions and clinical performance after total fasting in patients with rheumatoid arthritis. *Ann Rheum Dis.* 1983 Feb;42(1):45-51

[369] "We thus conclude that a reduced ability to generate cytotaxins, reduced release of enzyme, and reduced leukotriene formation from RA neutrophils, together with an altered fatty acid composition of membrane phospholipids, may be mechanisms for the decrease of inflammatory symptoms that results from fasting." Hafstrom et al. Effects of fasting on disease activity, neutrophil function, fatty acid composition, and leukotriene biosynthesis in patients with rheumatoid arthritis. *Arthritis Rheum.* 1988 May;31(5):585-92

[370] "The results indicate that, unlike lactovegetarian diet, fasting may ameliorate the disease activity and reduce both the intestinal and the non-intestinal permeability in rheumatoid arthritis." Sundqvist T, et al. Influence of fasting on intestinal permeability and disease activity in patients with rheumatoid arthritis. *Scand J Rheumatol.* 1982;11(1):33-8

[371] Fuhrman et al. Brief case reports of medically supervised water-only fasting associated with remission of autoimmune disease. *Altern Ther Health Med* 2002 Jul-Aug;1 12,110-1

[372] "An association was found between improvement in inflammatory activity of the joints and enhancement of neutrophil bactericidal capacity. Fasting appears to improve the clinical status of patients with RA." Uden AM, Trang L, Venizelos N, Palmblad J. Neutrophil functions and clinical performance after total fasting in patients with rheumatoid arthritis. *Ann Rheum Dis.* 1983 Feb;42(1):45-51

[373] "The average reduction in blood pressure was 37/13 mm Hg, with the greatest decrease being observed for subjects with the most severe hypertension. Patients with stage 3 hypertension (those with systolic blood pressure greater than 180 mg Hg, diastolic blood pressure greater than 110 mg Hg, or both) had an average reduction of 60/17 mm Hg at the conclusion of treatment." Goldhamer A, Lisle D, Parpia B, Anderson SV, Campbell TC. Medically supervised water-only fasting in the treatment of hypertension. *J Manipulative Physiol Ther.* 2001 Jun;24(5):335-9 healthpromoting.com/335-339Goldhamer115263.QXD.pdf

[374] "RESULTS: Approximately 82% of the subjects achieved BP at or below 120/80 mm Hg by the end of the treatment program. The mean BP reduction was 20/7 mm Hg, with the greatest decrease being observed for subjects with the highest baseline BP." Goldhamer A et al. Medically supervised water-only fasting in the treatment of borderline hypertension. *J Altern Complement Med.* 2002 Oct;8(5):643-50 healthpromoting.com/Articles/articles/study%202/acmpaper5.pdf

[375] Vertes V, Genuth SM, Hazelton IM. Supplemented fasting as a large-scale outpatient program. *JAMA.* 1977 Nov 14;238(20):2151-3

[376] Bauman WA, et al. Early and long-term effects of acute caloric deprivation in obese diabetic patients. *Am J Med.* 1988 Jul;85(1):38-46

[377] Goldhamer AC. Initial cost of care results in medically supervised water-only fasting for treating high blood pressure and diabetes. *J Altern Complement Med.* 2002 Dec;8(6):696-7 healthpromoting.com/Articles/pdf/Study%2032.pdf

[378] "The ketogenic diet should be considered as alternative therapy for children with difficult-to-control seizures. It is more effective than many of the new anticonvulsant medications and is well tolerated by children and families when it is effective." Freeman JM, Vining EP, Pillas DJ, Pyzik PL, Casey JC, Kelly LM. The efficacy of the ketogenic diet-1998: a prospective evaluation of intervention in 150 children. *Pediatrics.* 1998 Dec;102(6):1358-63 pediatrics.aappublications.org/cgi/reprint/102/6/1358

[379] Adam et al. Effect of alpha-linolenic acid in human diet on linoleic acid metabolism and prostaglandin biosynthesis. *J Lipid Res.* 1986 Apr;27:421-6 jlr.org/cgi/reprint/27/4/421

[380] "Other results showed a significant reduction in morning stiffness with gamma-linolenic acid at 3 months and reduction in pain and articular index at 6 months with olive oil." Brzeski et al. Evening primrose oil in patients with rheumatoid arthritis and side-effects of non-steroidal anti-inflammatory drugs. *Br J Rheumatol.* 1991 Oct;30(5):370-2

[381] Rothman D, DeLuca P, Zurier RB. Botanical lipids: effects on inflammation, immune responses, and rheumatoid arthritis. *Semin Arthritis Rheum.* 1995 Oct;25(2):87-96

[382] Adam O, et al. Anti-inflammatory effects of a low arachidonic acid diet and fish oil in patients with rheumatoid arthritis. *Rheumatol Int.* 2003 Jan;23(1):27-36

[383] Lau CS, Morley KD, Belch JJ. Effects of fish oil supplementation on non-steroidal anti-inflammatory drug requirement in patients with mild rheumatoid arthritis--a double-blind placebo controlled study. *Br J Rheumatol.* 1993 Nov;32(11):982-9

[384] Kremer et al. Fish-oil fatty acid supplementation in active rheumatoid arthritis. A double-blinded, controlled, crossover study. *Ann Intern Med.* 1987 Apr;106(4):497-503

[385] Walton AJ, et al. Dietary fish oil and the severity of symptoms in patients with systemic lupus erythematosus. *Ann Rheum Dis.* 1991 Jul;50(7):463-6

[386] Duffy et al. The clinical effect of dietary supplementation with omega-3 fish oils and/or copper in systemic lupus erythematosus. *J Rheumatol.* 2004 Aug;31(8):1551-6

patients should start with a low dose of fatty acid supplementation until inflammation and the hyperoxidative state have been reduced. Clinicians must realize that fatty acids are not clinically or biochemically interchangeable and that one fatty acid does not substitute for another; each of the health-promoting fatty acids—ALA, GLA, EPA, DHA, and oleic acid—must be supplied in order for its benefits to be obtained; imbalanced supplementation causes or exacerbates biochemical imbalances and produces suboptimal results.[387]

- Vitamin D3 supplementation with physiologic doses and/or tailored to serum 25(OH)D levels: Vitamin D deficiency is common in the general population and is even more common in patients with chronic illness and chronic musculoskeletal pain.[388] Correction of vitamin D deficiency supports normal immune function against infection and provides a clinically significant anti-inflammatory[389] and analgesic benefit in patients with back pain[390] and limb pain.[391] Reasonable daily doses for children and adults are 1,000-2,000 and 4,000 IU, respectively.[392] Deficiency and response to treatment are monitored with serum 25(OH)vitamin D while safety is monitored with serum calcium; inflammatory granulomatous diseases and certain drugs such as hydrochlorothiazide greatly increase the propensity for hypercalcemia and warrant increment dosing and frequent monitoring of serum calcium. Vitamin D2 (ergocalciferol) is not a human nutrient and should not be used in clinical practice.

- **INFECTIONS & DYSBIOSIS: ❶ antimicrobial treatments, ❷ immunorestoration, ❸ immunotolerance via Treg induction** Essentially all autoimmune/rheumatic disorders are associated with microbial colonization and intolerance to same; the presence of persistent microbial colonization is *prima facie* evidence of immunosuppression. The eight areas of dysbiosis (multifocal) are: ❶ sinorespiratory, ❷ orodental, ❸ gastrointestinal, ❹ urogenital/genitourinary, ❺ parenchymal/tissue, ❻ microbial, ❼ dermal/cutaneous, and ❽ environmental.
  - Gastrointestinal dysbiosis: **All patients with rheumatoid arthritis have gastrointestinal dysbiosis until proven otherwise by the combination of 1) three-sample comprehensive parasitology examinations performed by a specialty laboratory and 2) clinical response to at least two 2-4 week courses of broad-spectrum antimicrobial treatment.** Yeast, bacteria, and parasites are treated as indicated based on identification and sensitivity results from comprehensive parasitology assessments. Patients taking immunosuppressant drugs such as corticosteroids/prednisone have increased risk of intestinal bacterial overgrowth and translocation.[393,394] Other dysbiotic loci should be investigated as discussed in Chapter 4 in the section on *Multifocal Dysbiosis*.
    - Cell wall fragments from major residents of the human intestinal flora induce chronic arthritis in rats (*J Rheumatol* 1989 Aug[395]): "A single intraperitoneal injection of cell wall fragments from ***Eubacterium aerofaciens*** or *Bifidobacterium* species induced persistent chronic arthritis, in contrast to those from *Eubacterium rectale, Clostridium species* and *Lactobacillus leichmanii*. The results show that cell wall fragments of major residents from the human fecal flora can induce chronic arthritis in the rat and support the hypothesis that normal human intestinal flora plays a role in the induction of arthritis in man."
    - Normal intestinal microbiota in the etiopathogenesis of rheumatoid arthritis (*Ann Rheum Dis* 2003 Sep[396]): The ability of bacterial cell walls to induce chronic, erosive arthritis was first described in the rat by using *Streptococcus pyogenes*. Self-perpetuating arthritis, closely resembling human

---

[387] Vasquez A. New Insights into Fatty Acid Supplementation and Its Effect on Eicosanoid Production and Genetic Expression. *Nutritional Perspectives* 2005; January: 5-16
[388] Plotnikoff GA, Quigley JM. Prevalence of severe hypovitaminosis D in patients with persistent, nonspecific musculoskeletal pain. *Mayo Clin Proc*. 2003 Dec;78(12):1463-70
[389] Timms PM, Mannan N, Hitman GA, Noonan K, Mills PG, Syndercombe-Court D, Aganna E, Price CP, Boucher BJ. Circulating MMP9, vitamin D and variation in the TIMP-1 response with VDR genotype: mechanisms for inflammatory damage in chronic disorders? *QJM*. 2002 Dec;95(12):787-96 qjmed.oxfordjournals.org/cgi/content/full/95/12/787
[390] Al Faraj S, Al Mutairi K. Vitamin D deficiency and chronic low back pain in Saudi Arabia. *Spine*. 2003 Jan 15;28(2):177-9
[391] Masood et al. Persistent limb pain and raised serum alkaline phosphatase the earliest markers of subclinical hypovitaminosis D in Kashmir. *Indian J Physiol Pharmacol*. 1989 Oct-Dec;33(4):259-61
[392] Vasquez et al. Clinical importance of vitamin D (cholecalciferol): a paradigm shift for all healthcare providers. *Altern Ther Health Med*. 2004 Sep-Oct;10(5):28-36
[393] "A 63-year-old man with systemic lupus erythematosus and selective IgA deficiency developed intractable diarrhoea the day after treatment with prednisone, 50 mg daily, was started. The diarrhoea was considered to be caused by bacterial overgrowth and was later successfully treated with doxycycline." Denison H, Wallerstedt S. Bacterial overgrowth after high-dose corticosteroid treatment. *Scand J Gastroenterol*. 1989 Jun;24(5):561-4
[394] "These bacteria also translocated to the mesenteric lymph nodes in mice injected with cyclophosphamide or prednisone." Berg RD, Wommack E, Deitch EA. Immunosuppression and intestinal bacterial overgrowth synergistically promote bacterial translocation. *Arch Surg*. 1988 Nov;123(11):1359-64
[395] Severijnen AJ, et al. Cell wall fragments from major residents of the human intestinal flora induce chronic arthritis in rats. *J Rheumatol*. 1989 Aug;16(8):1061-8
[396] Toivanen P. Normal intestinal microbiota in the aetiopathogenesis of rheumatoid arthritis. *Ann Rheum Dis*. 2003 Sep;62(9):807-11

rheumatoid arthritis by histological criteria, develops in susceptible rat strains after a single intraperitoneal injection of the bacterial cell wall. In addition to *Streptococcus pyogenes*, several bacterial species representing *Lactobacillus, Bifidobacterium, Eubacterium, Collinsella,* and *Clostridium* have been observed to have a similar ability.

- Orodental dysbiosis: The systemic inflammatory response triggered by subclinical oral/dental "infections" is now believed to exacerbate conditions associated with inflammation, such as cardiovascular disease and diabetes mellitus.[397] Patients with RA have heightened antibody levels against common oral bacteria. IgG levels against *Porphyromonas gingivalis, Prevotella melaninogenica, Bacteroides forsythus,* and *Prevotella intermedia* were found to be significantly higher in RA patients when compared with those of controls.[398] In the first human clinical trial to test the hypothesis that treatment of orodental dysbiosis would provide subjective and objective clinical benefits for patients with RA, AlKatma et al[399] showed that **periodontal treatment consisting of scaling/root planing and oral hygiene instruction reduced symptom scores and ESR levels in patients with RA**.
- Genitourinary dysbiosis: Microbial contamination of the genitourinary tract can cause a systemic pro-inflammatory arthritogenic response in susceptible individuals; **in a study of 234 patients with inflammatory arthritis, 44% of patients had subclinical genitourinary colonization, mostly due to *Chlamydia, Mycoplasma,* or *Ureaplasma*.**[400]

- **NUTRITIONAL IMMUNOMODULATION: Treg induction for modulation of Th-1/2/17 inflammation**
Nutrients and therapeutic approaches that promote Treg or IL-10 induction and/or Th-17, IL-17 suppression include 1) mitochondrial optimization and mTOR suppression, 2) biotin, 3) vitamin E, 4) sodium avoidance, 5) transgenic/GMO food avoidance, 6) probiotics, 7) lipoic acid, 8) vitamin A, 9) inflammation reduction, 10) vitamin D, 11) fatty acid supplementation with GLA and n3, 12) infection and dysbiosis remediation, 13) green tea EGCG. Acronym: MiBESTPLAIDFIG, as detailed and substantiated in Chapter 4.

- **DYSMETABOLISM & DYSFUNCTIONAL MITOCHONDRIA: MitoDys, ERS-UPR, AGE/RAGE, hyperglycemia and ceramide** The major clinical considerations in this section are mitochondrial dysfunction, endoplasmic reticulum stress, unfolded protein response, TLR activation, and the dysmetabolic effects of sustained hyperglycemia and hyperinsulinemia and resultant oxidative stress, inflammation, RAGE activation, and accumulation of AGE, palmitate and ceramide. The review of this information in Chapter 4 covered approximately 30 interventions relevant to dysmetabolism, mitochondrial dysfunction, ERS-UPR, etc; these will not be reviewed here except to mention those most commonly, easily, empirically, synergistically, and effectively used: 1) low-carbohydrate diet with 2) moderate exercise, 3) CoQ-10, 4) acetyl-carnitine with 5) lipoic acid, 6) NAC, 7) resveratrol, and 8) melatonin.

- **STYLE OF LIVING (LIFESTYLE) & SPECIAL CONSIDERATIONS: Sleep optimization, SocioPsychology, Stress management/avoidance, Somatic treatments, Special Supplementation, Sweat/exercise, Sauna/detoxification, Surgery, Stamp your passport and vacate current reality, Sensory deprivation therapy**
This is a buffet of mostly lifestyle-based interventions yet also including considerations such as somatic treatments, additional supplementation, and surgery.
  - Self-expression and therapeutic writing: Limited evidence indicates that self-expressive writing can significantly reduce symptomatology in patients with RA.[401]

- **ENDOCRINE IMBALANCE & OPTIMIZATION: Prolactin, Insulin, Estrogen, DHEA, Cortisol, Testosterone, Thyroid** Common hormonal imbalances seen among autoimmune/inflammatory patients are: ❶ *elevated* prolactin, ❷ *elevated* estrogen, ❸ *elevated* insulin, and ❹ *reduced* DHEA, ❺ *reduced* cortisol, and ❻ *reduced* testosterone; see Chapter 4 for discussion of these hormones and respective interventions. Thyroid

---

[397] Amar S, Han X. The impact of periodontal infection on systemic diseases. *Med Sci Monit*. 2003 Dec;9(12):RA291-9 medscimonit.com/pub/vol_9/no_12/3776.pdf
[398] Ogrendik M, Kokino S, Ozdemir F, Bird PS, Hamlet S. Serum antibodies to oral anaerobic bacteria in patients with rheumatoid arthritis. *MedGenMed*. 2005 Jun 16;7(2):2
[399] "There was a statistically significant difference in DAS28 (4.3 +/- 1.6 vs. 5.1 +/- 1.2) and erythrocyte sedimentation rate (31.4 +/- 24.3 vs. 42.7 +/- 22) between the treatment and the control groups." Al-Katma MK, et al. Control of periodontal infection reduces the severity of active rheumatoid arthritis. *J Clin Rheumatol*. 2007 Jun;13(3):134-7
[400] "Urogenital swab cultures showed a microbial infection in 44% of the patients with oligoarthritis (15% Chlamydia, 14% Mycoplasma, 28% Ureaplasma), whereas in the control group only 26% had a positive result (4% Chlamydia, 7% Mycoplasma, 21% Ureaplasma)." Erlacher L, Wintersberger W, Menschik M, Benke-Studnicka A, Machold K, Stanek G, Soltz-Szots J, Smolen J, Graninger W. Reactive arthritis: urogenital swab culture is the only useful diagnostic method for the detection of the arthritogenic infection in extra-articularly asymptomatic patients with undifferentiated oligoarthritis. *Br J Rheumatol*. 1995 Sep;34(9):838-42 rheumatology.oxfordjournals.org/cgi/content/abstract/34/9/838
[401] "Rheumatoid arthritis patients in the experimental group showed improvements in overall disease activity (a mean reduction in disease severity from 1.65 to 1.19 [28%] on a scale of 0 [asymptomatic] to 4 [very severe]) at the 4-month follow-up; P=.001), whereas control group patients did not change." Smyth JM, Stone AA, Hurewitz A, Kaell A. Effects of writing about stressful experiences on symptom reduction in patients with asthma or rheumatoid arthritis: a randomized trial. *JAMA*. 1999 Apr 14;281(14):1304-9

evaluation (patient + labs) should be comprehensive, as discussed in Chapter 1, with a low threshold for empiric treatment.
- Estradiol: Men with rheumatoid arthritis show an excess of estradiol and a decrease in DHEA, and the excess estrogen is proportional to the degree of inflammation.[402]
- Testosterone (insufficiency): Androgen deficiencies predispose to, are exacerbated by, and contribute to autoimmune/inflammatory disorders. **A large proportion of men with SLE or RA have low testosterone**[403,404] and suffer the effects of hypogonadism: fatigue, weakness, depression, slow healing, low libido, and difficulties with sexual performance. Testosterone levels may rise following DHEA supplementation (especially in women) and can be elevated in men by the use of anastrozole/Arimidex. Otherwise, transdermal testosterone such as Androgel, Testim, or custom-compounded formula can be applied as indicated.
- DHEA (insufficiency / supraphysiologic supplementation): DHEA is an anti-inflammatory and immunoregulatory hormone that is commonly deficient in patients with autoimmunity and inflammatory arthritis.[405] DHEA levels are suppressed by prednisone[406], and DHEA supplementation has been shown to reverse the osteoporosis and loss of bone mass induced by corticosteroid treatment.[407] DHEA shows no acute or subacute toxicity even when used in supraphysiologic doses, even when used in sick patients. For example, in a study of 32 patients with HIV, DHEA doses of 750 mg – 2,250 mg per day were well-tolerated and produced no dose-limiting adverse effects.[408] This lack of toxicity compares favorably with any and all so-called "antirheumatic" drugs, nearly all of which show impressive comparable toxicity. **When used at doses of 200 mg per day, DHEA safely provides clinical benefit for patients with various autoimmune diseases, including ulcerative colitis, Crohn's disease**[409], **and SLE.**[410] In patients with SLE, DHEA supplementation allows for reduced dosing of prednisone (thus avoiding its adverse effects) while providing symptomatic improvement.[411] Optimal clinical response appears to correlate with serum levels that are supraphysiologic[412], and therefore treatment may be implemented with little regard for initial/baseline DHEA levels provided that the patient is free of contraindications, particularly high risk for sex-hormone-dependent malignancy. Other than mild adverse effects predictable with any androgen (namely voice deepening, transient acne, and increased facial hair), DHEA supplementation does not cause serious adverse effects[413], and it is appropriate for routine clinical use particularly when 1) the dose of DHEA is kept as low as possible, 2) duration is kept as short as possible, 3) other interventions are used to address the underlying cause of the disease, 4) the patient is

---

[402] "RESULTS: DHEAS and estrone concentrations were lower and estradiol was higher in patients compared with healthy controls. DHEAS differed between RF positive and RF negative patients. Estrone did not correlate with any disease variable, whereas estradiol correlated strongly and positively with all measured indices of inflammation." Tengstrand B, Carlstrom K, Fellander-Tsai L, Hafstrom I. Abnormal levels of serum dehydroepiandrosterone, estrone, and estradiol in men with rheumatoid arthritis: high correlation between serum estradiol and current degree of inflammation. *J Rheumatol.* 2003 Nov;30(11):2338-43

[403] Karagiannis A, Harsoulis F. Gonadal dysfunction in systemic diseases. *Eur J Endocrinol.* 2005 Apr;152(4):501-13 eje-online.org/cgi/content/full/152/4/501

[404] "Using analysis of covariance, patients with rheumatoid arthritis showed significantly lower serum testosterone (p less than 0.05) and derived free testosterone (p less than 0.01) concentrations and significantly higher serum LH and FSH concentrations (p less than 0.05) compared with controls." Gordon D, Beastall GH, Thomson JA, Sturrock RD. Androgenic status and sexual function in males with rheumatoid arthritis and ankylosing spondylitis. *Q J Med.* 1986 Jul;60(231):671-9

[405] "DHEAS concentrations were significantly decreased in both women and men with inflammatory arthritis (IA) (P < 0.001)." Dessein et al. Hyposecretion of the adrenal androgen dehydroepiandrosterone sulfate and its relation to clinical variables in inflammatory arthritis. *Arthritis Res.* 2001;3(3):183-8 arthritis-research.com/content/3/3/183

[406] "Basal serum DHEA and DHEAS concentrations were suppressed to a greater degree than was cortisol during both daily and alternate day prednisone treatments. ...Thus, adrenal androgen secretion was more easily suppressed than was cortisol secretion by this low dose of glucocorticoid, but there was no advantage to alternate day therapy." Rittmaster et al. Effect of daily and alternate day low dose prednisone on serum cortisol and adrenal androgens in hirsute women. *J Clin Endocrinol Metab.* 1988 Aug;67(2):400-3

[407] "CONCLUSION: Prasterone treatment prevented BMD loss and significantly increased BMD at both the lumbar spine and total hip in female patients with SLE receiving exogenous glucocorticoids." Mease PJ, Ginzler EM, Gluck OS, Schiff M, Goldman A, Greenwald M, Cohen S, Egan R, Quarles BJ, Schwartz KE. Effects of prasterone on bone mineral density in women with systemic lupus erythematosus receiving chronic glucocorticoid therapy. *J Rheumatol.* 2005 Apr;32(4):616-21

[408] "Thirty-one subjects were evaluated and monitored for safety and tolerance. The oral drug was administered three times daily in doses ranging from 750 mg/day to 2,250 mg/day for 16 weeks. ... The drug was well tolerated and no dose-limiting side effects were noted." Dyner TS, Lang W, Geaga J, et al. An open-label dose-escalation trial of oral dehydroepiandrosterone tolerance and pharmacokinetics in patients with HIV disease. *J Acquir Immune Defic Syndr.* 1993 May;6(5):459-65

[409] "CONCLUSIONS: In a pilot study, dehydroepiandrosterone was effective and safe in patients with refractory Crohn's disease or ulcerative colitis." Andus T, et al. Patients with refractory Crohn's disease or ulcerative colitis respond to dehydroepiandrosterone: a pilot study. *Aliment Pharmacol Ther.* 2003 Feb;17(3):409-14

[410] "CONCLUSION: The overall results confirm that DHEA treatment was well-tolerated, significantly reduced the number of SLE flares, and improved patient's global assessment of disease activity." Chang DM, Lan JL, Lin HY, Luo SF. Dehydroepiandrosterone treatment of women with mild-to-moderate systemic lupus erythematosus: a multicenter randomized, double-blind, placebo-controlled trial. *Arthritis Rheum.* 2002 Nov;46(11):2924-7

[411] "CONCLUSION: Among women with lupus disease activity, reducing the dosage of prednisone to < or = 7.5 mg/day for a sustained period of time while maintaining stabilization or a reduction of disease activity was possible in a significantly greater proportion of patients treated with oral prasterone, 200 mg once daily, compared with patients treated with placebo." Petri MA, et al; GL601 Study Group. Effects of prasterone on corticosteroid requirements of women with systemic lupus erythematosus: a double-blind, randomized, placebo-controlled trial. *Arthritis Rheum.* 2002 Jul;46(7):1820-9

[412] "CONCLUSION: The clinical response to DHEA was not clearly dose dependent. Serum levels of DHEA and DHEAS correlated only weakly with lupus outcomes, but suggested an optimum serum DHEAS of 1000 microg/dl." Barry NN, McGuire JL, van Vollenhoven RF. Dehydroepiandrosterone in systemic lupus erythematosus: relationship between dosage, serum levels, and clinical response. *J Rheumatol.* 1998 Dec;25(12):2352-6

[413] Tierney ML. McPhee SJ, Papadakis MA. *Current Medical Diagnosis and Treatment 2006. 45th edition.* New York; Lange Medical Books: 2006, page 1721

deriving benefit, and 5) the risk-to-benefit ratio is favorable. Astute clinicians should anticipate that DHEA supplementation can increase testosterone and estradiol levels—the former with benefit and the latter with detriment in patients with autoimmunity; thus, serum levels of DHEA, testosterone, and estradiol (and potentially other estrogen metabolites) need to be reevaluated if DHEA is added to the daily regimen. Commonly, rheumatic patients will show an increase in estradiol following use of DHEA, and these over-producers of estrogen ("rapid converters") should be co-treated with an aromatase inhibitor if DHEA supplementation elevates estrogen levels, especially if testosterone levels are low.

- Prolactin and antiprolactin treatments: Patients with RA and SLE have higher basal and stress-induced levels of prolactin compared with normal controls.[414,415] Men with RA have higher serum levels of prolactin, and these levels correlate with the severity and duration of the disorder.[416,417] Serum prolactin is the standard assessment of prolactin status. Since elevated prolactin may be a sign of pituitary tumor, assessment for headaches, visual deficits, and other abnormalities of pituitary hormones (e.g., GH and TSH) should be performed; CT or MRI must be considered. Patients with prolactin levels less than 100 ng/mL and normal CT/MRI findings can be managed conservatively with effective prolactin-lowering treatment and annual radiologic assessment (less necessary with favorable serum response).[418, see review 419] Specific treatment options include the following:
  - Thyroid hormone: Hypothyroidism frequently causes hyperprolactinemia which is reversible upon effective treatment of hypothyroidism. Obviously therefore, thyroid status should be evaluated in all patients with hyperprolactinemia. Thyroid assessment and treatment is reviewed in Chapter 4 and later in this section.
  - *Vitex astus-cagnus* and other supporting botanicals and nutrients: **Vitex lowers serum prolactin in humans**[420,421] **via a dopaminergic effect.**[422] Vitex is considered safe for clinical use; mild and reversible adverse effects possibly associated with Vitex include nausea, headache, gastrointestinal disturbances, menstrual disorders, acne, pruritus and erythematous rash. No drug interactions are known, but given the herb's dopaminergic effect it should probably be used with some caution in patients treated with dopamine antagonists such as the so-called antipsychotic drugs.[423,424] Bone[425] stated that daily doses can range from 500 mg to 2,000 mg DHE (dry herb equivalent) and can be tailored to the suppression of prolactin. Due at least in part to its content of L-dopa, ***Mucuna pruriens* shows clinical dopaminergic activity** as evidenced by its effectiveness in Parkinson's disease[426]; up to 15-30 gm/d of mucuna has been used clinically but doses will be dependent on preparation and phytoconcentration. **Triptolide and other extracts from *Tripterygium wilfordii* Hook F exert**

---

[414] Dostal et al. Serum prolactin stress values in patients with systemic lupus erythematosus. *Ann Rheum Dis*. 2003 May;62(5):487-8 ard.bmjjournals.com/cgi/content/full/62/5/487
[415] "RESULTS: A significantly higher rate of elevated PRL levels was found in SLE patients (40.0%) compared with the healthy controls (14.8%). No proof was found of association with the presence of anti-ds-DNA or with specific organ involvement. Similarly, elevated PRL levels were found in RA patients (39.3%)." Moszkorzova L, Lacinova Z, Marek J, Musilova L, Dohnalova A, Dostal C. Hyperprolactinaemia in patients with systemic lupus erythematosus. *Clin Exp Rheumatol*. 2002 Nov-Dec;20(6):807-12
[416] "CONCLUSION: Men with RA have high serum PRL levels and concentrations increase with longer disease evolution and worse functional stage." Mateo L, Nolla JM, Bonnin MR, Navarro MA, Roig-Escofet D. High serum prolactin levels in men with rheumatoid arthritis. *J Rheumatol*. 1998 Nov;25(11):2077-82
[417] "Male patients affected by RA showed high serum PRL levels. The serum PRL concentration was found to be increased in relation to the duration and the activity of the disease. Serum PRL levels do not seem to have any relationship with the BMD, at least in RA." Seriolo B, Ferretti V, Sulli A, Fasciolo D, Cutolo M. Serum prolactin concentrations in male patients with rheumatoid arthritis. *Ann N Y Acad Sci*. 2002 Jun;966:258-62
[418] Beers MH, Berkow R (eds). *The Merck Manual. Seventeenth Edition*. Whitehouse Station; Merck Research Laboratories 1999 Page 77-78
[419] Serri O, Chik CL, Ur E, Ezzat S. Diagnosis and management of hyperprolactinemia. *CMAJ*. 2003 Sep 16;169(6):575-81 cmaj.ca/cgi/content/full/169/6/575
[420] "Since AC extracts were shown to have beneficial effects on premenstrual mastodynia serum prolactin levels in such patients were also studied in one double-blind, placebo-controlled clinical study. Serum prolactin levels were indeed reduced in the patients treated with the extract." Wuttke W, Jarry H, Christoffel V, Spengler B, Seidlova-Wuttke D. Chaste tree (Vitex agnus-castus)--pharmacology and clinical indications. *Phytomedicine*. 2003 May;10(4):348-57
[421] German abstract from Medline: "The prolactin release was reduced after 3 months, shortened luteal phases were normalised and deficits in the luteal progesterone synthesis were eliminated." Milewicz A, Gejdel E, Sworen H, Sienkiewicz K, Jedrzejak J, Teucher T, Schmitz H. [Vitex agnus castus extract in the treatment of luteal phase defects due to latent hyperprolactinemia. Results of a randomized placebo-controlled double-blind study] *Arzneimittelforschung*. 1993 Jul;43(7):752-6
[422] "Our results indicate a dopaminergic effect of Vitex agnus-castus extracts and suggest additional pharmacological actions via opioid receptors." Meier B, Berger D, Hoberg E, Sticher O, Schaffner W. Pharmacological activities of Vitex agnus-castus extracts in vitro. *Phytomedicine*. 2000 Oct;7(5):373-81
[423] "The majority of patients in each group discontinued their assigned treatment owing to inefficacy or intolerable side effects or for other reasons." Lieberman JA, Stroup TS, McEvoy JP, Swartz MS, Rosenheck RA, Perkins DO, Keefe RS, Davis SM, Davis CE, Lebowitz BD, Severe J, Hsiao JK; Clinical Antipsychotic Trials of Intervention Effectiveness (CATIE) Investigators. Effectiveness of antipsychotic drugs in patients with chronic schizophrenia. *N Engl J Med*. 2005 Sep 22;353(12):1209-23
[424] Whitaker R. The case against antipsychotic drugs: a 50-year record of doing more harm than good. *Med Hypotheses*. 2004;62(1):5-13
[425] "In conditions such as endometriosis and fibroids, for which a significant estrogen antagonist effect is needed, doses of at least 2 g/day DHE may be required and typically are used by professional herbalists." Bone K. New Insights Into Chaste Tree. *Nutritional Wellness* 2005 November nutritionalwellness.com/archives/2005/nov/11_bone.php
[426] "CONCLUSIONS: The rapid onset of action and longer on time without concomitant increase in dyskinesias on mucuna seed powder formulation suggest that this natural source of L-dopa might possess advantages over conventional L-dopa preparations in the long term management of PD." Katzenschlager R, et al. Mucuna pruriens in Parkinson's disease: a double blind clinical and pharmacological study. *J Neurol Neurosurg Psychiatry*. 2004 Dec;75(12):1672-7

clinically significant anti-inflammatory action in patients with rheumatoid arthritis[427,428] and also offer protection to dopaminergic neurons.[429,430] Ironically, even though tyrosine is the nutritional precursor to dopamine with evidence of clinical effectiveness (e.g., narcolepsy[431], enhancement of memory[432] and cognition[433]), **supplementation with tyrosine appears to actually increase rather than decrease prolactin levels[434]; therefore tyrosine should be used cautiously (if at all) in patients with systemic inflammation and elevated prolactin.** Furthermore, the finding that **high-protein meals stimulate prolactin release**[435] may partly explain the benefits of vegetarian diets in the treatment of systemic inflammation; since vegetarian diets are comparatively low in protein compared to omnivorous diets, they may lead to a relative reduction in prolactin production due to lack of protein-induced prolactin stimulation.

- <u>Bromocriptine</u>: Bromocriptine has long been considered the pharmacologic treatment of choice for elevated prolactin.[436] Typical dose is 2.5 mg per day (effective against lupus[437]); gastrointestinal upset and sedation are common.[438] Clinical intervention with bromocriptine appears warranted in patients with RA, SLE, reactive arthritis, psoriatic arthritis, and probably multiple sclerosis and uveitis.[439]

- <u>Cabergoline/Dostinex</u>: Cabergoline/Dostinex is a newer dopamine agonist with few adverse effects; typical dose starts at 0.5 mg per week (0.25 mg twice per week).[440] Several studies have indicated that cabergoline is safer and more effective than bromocriptine for reducing prolactin levels[441] and the dose can often be reduced after successful prolactin reduction, allowing for reductions in cost and adverse effects.[442] Although fewer studies have been published supporting the antirheumatic benefits of cabergoline than bromocriptine, its antirheumatic benefits have been documented in a case report of a patient with unremitting RA.[443]

---

[427] "The ethanol/ethyl acetate extract of TWHF shows therapeutic benefit in patients with treatment-refractory RA. At therapeutic dosages, the TWHF extract was well tolerated by most patients in this study." Tao X, Younger J, Fan FZ, Wang B, Lipsky PE. Benefit of an extract of Tripterygium Wilfordii Hook F in patients with rheumatoid arthritis: a double-blind, placebo-controlled study. *Arthritis Rheum*. 2002 Jul;46(7):1735-43

[428] "The EA extract of TWHF at dosages up to 570 mg/day appeared to be safe, and doses > 360 mg/day were associated with clinical benefit in patients with RA." Tao et al. A phase I study of ethyl acetate extract of the chinese antirheumatic herb Tripterygium wilfordii hook F in rheumatoid arthritis. *J Rheumatol*. 2001 Oct;28(10):2160-7

[429] "Our data suggests that triptolide may protect dopaminergic neurons from LPS-induced injury and its efficiency in inhibiting microglia activation may underlie the mechanism." Li FQ, Lu XZ, Liang XB, Zhou HF, Xue B, Liu XY, Niu DB, Han JS, Wang XM. Triptolide, a Chinese herbal extract, protects dopaminergic neurons from inflammation-mediated damage through inhibition of microglial activation. *J Neuroimmunol*. 2004 Mar;148(1-2):24-31

[430] "Moreover, tripchlorolide markedly prevented the decrease in amount of dopamine in the striatum of model rats. Taken together, our data provide the first evidence that tripchlorolide acts as a neuroprotective molecule that rescues MPP+ or axotomy-induced degeneration of dopaminergic neurons, which may imply its therapeutic potential for Parkinson's disease." Li FQ, Cheng XX, Liang XB, Wang XH, Xue B, He QH, Wang XM, Han JS. Neurotrophic and neuroprotective effects of tripchlorolide, an extract of Chinese herb Tripterygium wilfordii Hook F, on dopaminergic neurons. *Exp Neurol*. 2003 Jan;179(1):28-37

[431] "Of twenty-eight visual analogue scales rating mood and arousal, the subjects' ratings in the tyrosine treatment (9 g daily) and placebo periods differed significantly for only three (less tired, less drowsy, more alert)." Elwes RD, Crewes H, Chesterman LP, Summers B, Jenner P, Binnie CD, Parkes JD. Treatment of narcolepsy with L-tyrosine: double-blind placebo-controlled trial. *Lancet*. 1989 Nov 4;2(8671):1067-9

[432] "Ten men and 10 women subjects underwent these batteries 1 h after ingesting 150 mg/kg of l-tyrosine or placebo. Administration of tyrosine significantly enhanced accuracy and decreased frequency of list retrieval on the working memory task during the multiple task battery compared with placebo." Thomas JR, Lockwood PA, Singh A, Deuster PA. Tyrosine improves working memory in a multitasking environment. *Pharmacol Biochem Behav*. 1999 Nov;64(3):495-500

[433] "Ten subjects received five daily doses of a protein-rich drink containing 2 g tyrosine, and 11 subjects received a carbohydrate rich drink with the same amount of calories (255 kcal)." Deijen JB, Wientjes CJ, Vullinghs HF, Cloin PA, Langefeld JJ. Tyrosine improves cognitive performance and reduces blood pressure in cadets after one week of a combat training course. *Brain Res Bull*. 1999 Jan 15;48(2):203-9

[434] "Tyrosine (when compared to placebo) had no effect on any sleep related measure, but it did stimulate prolactin release." Waters WF, et al. A comparison of tyrosine against placebo, phentermine, caffeine, and D-amphetamine during sleep deprivation. *Nutr Neurosci*. 2003;6(4):221-35

[435] "Whereas carbohydrate meals had no discernible effects, high protein meals induced a large increase in both PRL and cortisol; high fat meals caused selective release of PRL." Ishizuka et al. Pituitary hormone release in response to food ingestion: evidence for neuroendocrine signals from gut to brain. *J Clin Endocrinol Metab*. 1983 Dec;57(6):1111-6

[436] Beers MH, Berkow R (eds): *Merck Manual. Seventeenth Edition*. Whitehouse Station; Merck Research Laboratories 1999 Page 77-78

[437] "A prospective, double-blind, randomized, placebo-controlled study compared BRC at a fixed daily dosage of 2.5 mg with placebo... Long term treatment with a low dose of BRC appears to be a safe and effective means of decreasing SLE flares in SLE patients." Alvarez-Nemegyei J, Cobarrubias-Cobos A, Escalante-Triay F, Sosa-Munoz J, Miranda JM, Jara LJ. Bromocriptine in systemic lupus erythematosus: a double-blind, randomized, placebo-controlled study. *Lupus*. 1998;7(6):414-9

[438] Serri O, Chik CL, Ur E, Ezzat S. Diagnosis and management of hyperprolactinemia. *CMAJ*. 2003 Sep 16;169(6):575-81 cmaj.ca/cgi/content/full/169/6/575

[439] "...clinical observations and trials support the use of bromocriptine as a nonstandard primary or adjunctive therapy in the treatment of recalcitrant RA, SLE, Reiter's syndrome, and psoriatic arthritis and associated conditions unresponsive to traditional approaches." McMurray RW. Bromocriptine in rheumatic and autoimmune diseases. *Semin Arthritis Rheum*. 2001 Aug;31(1):21-32

[440] Serri O, Chik CL, Ur E, Ezzat S. Diagnosis and management of hyperprolactinemia. *CMAJ*. 2003 Sep 16;169(6):575-81 cmaj.ca/cgi/content/full/169/6/575

[441] "CONCLUSION: These data indicate that cabergoline is a very effective agent for lowering the prolactin levels in hyperprolactinemic patients and that it appears to offer considerable advantage over bromocriptine in terms of efficacy and tolerability." Sabuncu T, Arikan E, Tasan E, Hatemi H. Comparison of the effects of cabergoline and bromocriptine on prolactin levels in hyperprolactinemic patients. *Intern Med*. 2001 Sep;40(9):857-61

[442] "Cabergoline also normalized PRL in the majority of patients with known bromocriptine intolerance or -resistance. Once PRL secretion was adequately controlled, the dose of cabergoline could often be significantly decreased, which further reduced costs of therapy." Verhelst J, Abs R, Maiter D, van den Bruel A, Vandeweghe M, Velkeniers B, Mockel J, Lamberigts G, Petrossians P, Coremans P, Mahler C, Stevenaert A, Verlooy J, Raftopoulos C, Beckers A. Cabergoline in the treatment of hyperprolactinemia: a study in 455 patients. *J Clin Endocrinol Metab*. 1999 Jul;84(7):2518-22 jcem.endojournals.org/cgi/content/full/84/7/2518

[443] Erb N, Pace AV, Delamere JP, Kitas GD. Control of unremitting rheumatoid arthritis by the prolactin antagonist cabergoline. *Rheumatology* (Oxford). 2001 Feb;40(2):237-9 rheumatology.oxfordjournals.org/cgi/content/full/40/2/237

- **XENOBIOTIC ACCUMULATION & DETOXIFICATION: Chemical avoidance, nutritional support for detoxification pathways, urine alkalinization** The clinical relevance and pathogenic mechanisms of xenobiotic accumulation are irrefutably well documented and described. Clinical assessments include history, physical examination, and laboratory assessment (using serum, whole blood, urine or—rarely yet accurately—fat biopsy), and response to treatment. Treatments include nutritional support for Phases 1 and 2 of detoxification (e.g., oxidation and conjugation) and excretion via bile and urine; for the latter, urinary alkalinization is generally recommended. Chemical toxins can be bound in the gut using activated charcoal, cholestyramine, or *Chlorella*—all of these three treatments have documented safety and effectiveness; clinically and empirically, phytochelatin (plant-derived peptides that bind toxic metals) concentrates appear safe and effective despite lack of conclusive published data supporting clinical use.

Clinical Case Exemplary case of clinical and laboratory evidence of reversal of "severe, aggressive, drug-resistant" rheumatoid arthritis in a 51yoWF following implementation of the Functional Inflammology Protocol: This summarizes the 13-month clinical outcome of the first patient treated with the updated functional inflammology protocol after its revision and expansion in March 2012.[444] After being diagnosed accurately by a rheumatologist—for this patient very clearly met diagnostic criteria—this patient presented for care following notably inefficacious treatment with the full medicopharmaceutical antirheumatic protocol comprised of NSAIDs, prednisone (she had only minimal response to prednisone >60mg/d), methotrexate, hydroxychloroquine, and "biologics" including etanercept/Enbrel; she was now being recommended to start newer "experimental" drugs. Following the failure of medical treatment, the patient was treated at the teaching clinic of a naturopathic college where her treatments included a clinician-supervised 26-day water-only fast, which resulted in the loss of 30 pounds (13.6 kilograms) but provided no clinical benefit for the rheumatoid arthritis. [Note: I/Dr Vasquez treat this patient at no charge. Dr William J Beakey of Professional Co-Op Services (Professionalco-op.com) generously donated these laboratory tests for collaborative/research purposes. Biotics Research Corporation (BioticsResearch.com) generously donated nutritional supplements for this patient.]

March 2012—severe symptoms and CCP >250: Patient reports suffering significantly with joint pain and lower extremity edema; foundational nutritional protocol[445] is implemented with antidysbiotic/antimicrobial intervention limited to emulsified oregano oil 600mg/d, mitochondrial support and the nutritional immunomodulation protocol. CCP level at this time is beyond laboratory testing limits, measured simply as "greater than" 250 units.

```
CCP Antibodies IgG/IgA      >250   High      units              0 - 19
                                          Negative              <20
                                          Weak positive         20 - 39
                                          Moderate positive     40 - 59
                                          Strong positive       >59
```

January 2013—mild symptoms and CCP 195: Few modifications are made for the first 9 months and patient feels progressively better, but wants to "move to the next level of improvement" because—despite feeling and functioning significantly better solely with dietary and nutritional interventions—patient still notes exacerbations of pain, particularly following extended manual farm labor. At this time, labs are drawn showing an impressive reduction in CCP levels from "greater than" 250 units to 195 units, correlating with a reduction of at least 22%. At this time, patient was commenced on additional treatments including cabergoline, oral vancomycin, and azithromycin.

```
CCP Antibodies IgG/IgA      195    High      units              0 - 19
                                          Negative              <20
                                          Weak positive         20 - 39
                                          Moderate positive     40 - 59
                                          Strong positive       >59
```

April 2013—virtually normal, CCP 54: Patient continues to improve clinically; her subjective and objective clinical improvements (including additional loss of 30 pounds [13.6 kilograms] and reduction in hand swelling necessitating resizing of wedding ring) correlate nicely with the reduction in CCP levels, which have reduced from >250 units to 54 units, for a reduction of more than 78%. Thus, by objective physical and laboratory criteria, this patient appears to be experiencing authentic reversal—cure—of her disease due to the functional inflammology protocol.

```
CCP Antibodies IgG/IgA      54     High      units              0 - 19
                                          Negative              <20
                                          Weak positive         20 - 39
                                          Moderate positive     40 - 59
                                          Strong positive       >59
```

---

[444] Vasquez A. *Functional Immunology and Nutritional Immunomodulation*. 2012 createspace.com/3899760 and updated as *F.I.N.D. S.E.X® The Easily Remembered Acronym for the Functional Inflammology Protocol*. 2013 createspace.com/4234627
[445] Vasquez A. Revisiting the Five-Part Nutritional Wellness Protocol: Supplemented Paleo-Mediterranean Diet. *Nutr Perspect* 2011 Jan ichnfm.org/faculty/vasquez/profile.html

Psoriasis & Psoriatic Arthritis

Introduction:
Psoriasis is my favorite condition to treat; successful implementation of the Functional Inflammology protocol can lead to such rapid resolution of long-term skin lesions that objective improvement is clearly and objectively demonstrable—providing irrefutable proof of efficacy while immediately improving the patient's quality of life, sense of efficacy, and self-esteem.

From this chapter onward, readers should use the information in Chapter 4—detailing the concepts and implementation of the Functional Inflammology protocol—and apply those concepts and interventions to the clinical conditions in the book and encountered in clinical practice.

Description/pathophysiology:
- Psoriatic arthritis is an inflammatory arthropathy seen in patients with psoriasis that can have both peripheral (e.g., hands and feet) and axial (i.e., spine and sacroiliac joints) manifestations. This condition has frequently been referred to as *psoriatic rheumatism* or *rheumatic psoriasis*.
- Similar to reactive arthritis and rheumatoid arthritis; strongly associated with streptococcal infections as well as staphylococcal infections.[446] Although many researchers have contributed to the literature which establishes psoriasis as a disease of multifocal dysbiosis, to the best of my knowledge the work of Patricia W. Noah PhD is exceptionally noteworthy; her 1990 review published in *Seminars in Dermatology*[447] is required reading for doctors wishing to gain independent *peer-reviewed* confirmation that **multifocal dysbiosis is the major initiator and perpetuator of this systemic autoimmune inflammatory disorder.** In this particular article, Dr Noah documents the experience of her group at the College of Medicine at the University of Tennessee, their anti-dysbiosis protocol, and its success in the treatment of psoriasis.
- **Psoriasis and psoriatic arthritis must be considered an autoimmune diseases** based on the findings of autoantibodies directed against dermal structures—stratum corneum[448] and keratinocytes[449]—and antibody-dependent and antibody-independent immune-mediated tissue destruction. Although stratum corneum antibodies are found in healthy patients without consequence, what makes them uniquely pathogenic in psoriasis is their tissue penetration in lesioned skin, their ability to bind with autoantigens, and their activation of complement.[450,451]

Commentary: Given the **overwhelming basic science and clinical research** implicating multifocal dysbiosis as the primary initiator of psoriasis—and by extension, psoriatic arthritis—it seems impossible that major allopathic textbooks such as *The Merck Manual*[452] and the widely read *Principles of Dermatology*[453] and *Current Medical Diagnosis and Treatment*[454] would perpetuate the myth that the condition is "idiopathic" so that no cure can be hoped for other than additive, endless, and perpetually "new" medicalization. This is clearly an example of medical practice being incongruent with biomedical research—at the patient's expense.

---

[446] Klippel JH (ed). *Primer on the Rheumatic Diseases. 11th Edition*. Atlanta: Arthritis Foundation. 1997 page 176
[447] Noah PW. The role of microorganisms in psoriasis. *Semin Dermatol*. 1990 Dec;9(4):269-76
[448] "... titers of IgG anti-SC autoantibodies in psoriatic patients were not specifically higher than in normal controls but were more variable, indicating that their circulating levels are dependent on a delicate balance between consumption at inflammatory sites and a secondary increase due to SC-antigen release following inflammation." Tagami H, Iwatsuki K, Yamada M. Profile of anti-stratum corneum autoantibodies in psoriatic patients. *Arch Dermatol Res*. 1983;275(2):71-5
[449] "It seems that autoantibodies, although they do not appear to participate in the pathogenesis of psoriasis, are an important feature, and that skin antigens, which appear in lesional immature keratinocytes, cross-react with S. pyogenes and contribute to the autoimmune process in psoriasis." Perez-Lorenzo R, Zambrano-Zaragoza JF, Saul A, Jimenez-Zamudio L, Reyes-Maldonado E, Garcia-Latorre E. Autoantibodies to autologous skin in guttate and plaque forms of psoriasis and cross-reaction of skin antigens with streptococcal antigens. *Int J Dermatol*. 1998 Jul;37(7):524-31. The authors found that all psoriasis patients had dermal autoantibodies and that these antibodies reacted specifically with endogenous dermal antigens; thus their finding that "Deposits of immunoglobulin G (IgG) were not detected in the lesions" is unexpected and inexplicable. This statement from their research is inconsistent with the findings of other research groups, and—specifically—must be placed in a context of other articles, most notably "... titers of IgG anti-SC autoantibodies in psoriatic patients were not specifically higher than in normal controls but were more variable, indicating that their circulating levels are dependent on a delicate balance between consumption at inflammatory sites and a secondary increase due to SC-antigen release following inflammation." Tagami H, Iwatsuki K, Yamada M. Profile of anti-stratum corneum autoantibodies in psoriatic patients. *Arch Dermatol Res*. 1983;275(2):71-5.
[450] "The stratum corneum (SC) antibodies are present in all human sera as seen by indirect immunofluorescence (IF) staining... IF tests with proper controls showed that the SC antigen in psoriatic scales is coated not only with IgG but in a majority of the lesions also with complement." Beutner EH, Jarzabek-Chorzelska M, Jablonska S, Chorzelski TP, Rzesa G. Autoimmunity in psoriasis. A complement immunofluorescence study. *Arch Dermatol Res*. 1978 Apr 7;261(2):123-34
[451] "Indirect immunofluorescent (IF) tests on sections of normal human skin reveal the presence of antibodies to the stratum corneum in most normal human sera. ...Direct IF tests of psoriatic lesions revealed the presence of in vivo bound IgG as well as other immunoglobulins and complement in the stratum corneum." Beutner EH, Jablonska S, Jarzabek-Chorzelska M, Marciejowska E, Rzesa G, Chorzelski TP. Studies in immunodermatology. VI. IF studies of autoantibodies to the stratum corneum and of in vivo fixed IgG in stratum corneum of psoriatic lesions. *Int Arch Allergy Appl Immunol*. 1975;48(3):301-23
[452] Beers MH, Berkow R (eds). *The Merck Manual. Seventeenth Edition*. Whitehouse Station; Merck Research Laboratories 1999 pages 448 and 816
[453] Lookingbill DP, Marks JG, eds. *Principles of dermatology*. Philadelphia: W.B. Saunders, 1986: 138
[454] Tierney LM, McPhee SJ Papadakis MA (eds). *Current Medical Diagnosis and Treatment. 35th edition*. New York: Lange; 1996, page 101

Clinical presentations:
- Dermal lesions are generally described as well demarcated erythematous patches with silvery scales. Lesions may be widespread or comparatively minor. Patients may have *hidden* dermal lesions on scalp or in gluteal cleft; clinical examination in patients with oligoarthritis can search for dermal psoriatic lesions while assessing for cutaneous dysbiosis. Rarely, nail pitting is the only cutaneous lesion.
- Chronologic association of *dermal psoriasis* with *psoriatic arthritis*:
    o 7-30% of patients with (dermal) psoriasis develop psoriatic arthritis
    o In 70% of patients, *dermal psoriasis* precedes *psoriatic arthritis* by several years
    o In 15% of patients, *dermal psoriasis* and *psoriatic arthritis* occur at the same time
    o In 15% of patients, *psoriatic arthritis* precedes *dermal psoriasis*—this 'reverse presentation' is particularly common in children
- Onset may be gradual (70%) or acute (30%)
- In some patients the onset and disease can be of such severity that hospitalization is required.
- Peripheral joint involvement is more common in women; spinal involvement is more common in men, particularly in association with HLA-B27
- Peak onset age 30-55 years
- Musculoskeletal manifestations: prevalence: hands > feet > sacroiliac > spine
    o Oligoarticular peripheral arthropathy—distal interphalangeal (DIP) joints are notably affected
    o Peripheral polyarthritis: distribution may be symmetric or asymmetric
    o Arthritis mutilans: total destruction of the phalanges and meta-tarsals/carpals
    o Spinal and sacroiliac involvement: may affect any portion of the spine in a random fashion—lumbar spondylitis and sacroiliitis are more common than atlantoaxial instability; spinal involvement is more common in patients positive for HLA-B27
    o Enthesitis: inflammation at the junction of tendons to bones, classically noted at the Achilles tendon
- Systemic manifestations and complications
    o Conjunctivitis, uveitis: seen in 30%
    o Nail pitting may or may not be present; other findings may include transverse ridging, thickening, flaking and brittleness
    o Aortic insufficiency
    o Pulmonary fibrosis
    o Swelling of the fingers and hands

Major differential diagnoses:
- <u>Ankylosing spondylitis</u>: does not occur with dermal psoriatic lesions
- <u>Rheumatoid arthritis</u>: differentiated from rheumatoid arthritis by 1) skin lesions, 2) absence of rheumatoid nodules, 3) negative rheumatoid factor
- <u>Hemochromatosis</u>: non-inflammatory peripheral arthropathy
- <u>Reactive arthritis</u>: does not classically occur with dermal psoriatic lesions
- <u>Septic arthritis</u>: e.g., infected psoriatic skin lesion predisposing to septicemia with resultant joint infection
- <u>HIV infection</u>: increased prevalence of psoriasis[455] especially associated with "an explosive onset of psoriasis and psoriatic arthritis" [456]

Clinical assessments:
- **History/subjective**:
    o Inquire about the clinical presentations listed above
    o Family and personal history of psoriasis is often positive

---
[455] Beers MH, Berkow R (eds). *The Merck Manual. Seventeenth Edition*. Whitehouse Station; Merck Research Laboratories 1999 page 448
[456] Klippel JH (ed). *Primer on the Rheumatic Diseases. 11th Edition*. Atlanta: Arthritis Foundation. 1997 page 176

- o Historical risk factors for psoriasis include bacterial pharyngitis and stressful life events[457]
- **Physical examination/objective**:
  - o Psoriasis—sharply demarcated erythematous plaque with silver scales
  - o Neuromusculoskeletal examination as indicated—see *Integrative Orthopedics*[458]
  - o Assess blood pressure and perform screening physical examination
- **Laboratory assessments**:
  - o <u>ANA</u>: Antinuclear antibodies are present in 47% of patients with psoriatic arthritis, further supporting the "autoimmune" description of this disease.[459]
  - o <u>Rheumatoid factor</u>: RF is negative: positive RF suggests concomitant RA along with psoriasis.
  - o <u>Chemistry/metabolic panel with uric acid</u>: Assess for overall status and elevated uric acid, the latter may be increased due to rapid skin turnover.
  - o <u>Ferritin</u>: Assess ferritin preferably with transferrin saturation and CRP to exclude iron overload.
  - o <u>CRP</u>: Generally elevated; can be used to track progression/remission of the disease
  - o <u>HLA-B27</u>: Present in 40% of patients with psoriatic arthritis; correlates with increased severity of disease, including increased CRP, increased propensity for sacroiliitis, and more extensive joint destruction.[460]
  - o <u>HIV serologic testing</u>: Especially for patients with severe disease and/or sudden onset.
  - o <u>Lactulose/mannitol assay for "leaky gut"</u>: Patients with psoriasis have increased intestinal permeability.[461]
  - o <u>Dysbiosis assessments</u>
    - <u>Gastrointestinal dysbiosis</u>: Comprehensive stool and parasitology testing must include bacterial/yeast culture; antigen or antibody testing for *H. pylori* is recommended; patients with psoriasis have shown a greatly increased prevalence of *H. pylori* compared with controls[462], and the authors of this study suggested a causal association; likewise intestinal colonization with yeasts including *Candida albicans* and *Geotrichum candidum* are found much more commonly in psoriatics than controls.[463] Stressing the importance of this association, Waldman et al[464] wrote, "Our results reinforce the hypothesis that *C. albicans* is one of the triggers to both exacerbation and persistence of psoriasis. We propose that in psoriatics with a significant quantity of *Candida* in feces, an antifungal treatment should be considered as an adjuvant treatment of psoriasis."
    - <u>Dermal dysbiosis</u>: Skin/nail culture, Giemsa staining, culture lesioned skin on blood agar, MacConkey agar, Sabouraud plates.[465]
    - <u>Sinorespiratory dysbiosis</u>: Nasal swab and culture, throat culture for bacteria and yeasts.[466]
    - <u>Genitourinary dysbiosis</u>: Culture and sensitivity testing for all organisms from clean catch specimens; assessment of sexual partners is advised.[467]

> **Microbial colonization contributes to psoriasis**
>
> "We have repeatedly observed psoriatic flares associated with microbial infection, sequestered antigen, and colonization. **Removal of these microbial foci results in clearing of the disease.**"
>
> Noah P. The role of microorganisms in psoriasis. *Semin Dermatol*. 1990 Dec

---

[457] "The study confirmed that recent pharyngeal infection is a risk factor for guttate psoriasis… Finally, the study added evidence to the belief that stressful life events may represent risk factors for the onset of psoriasis." Naldi et al; Psoriasis Study Group of Italian Group for Epidemiological Research in Dermatology. Family history of psoriasis, stressful life events, and recent infectious disease are risk factors for first episode of acute guttate psoriasis: results of a case-control study. *J Am Acad Dermatol*. 2001 Mar:433-8
[458] Vasquez A. *Integrative Orthopedics*: InflammationMastery.com
[459] "RESULTS: 44/94 (47%) patients with PsA were ANA positive (>/=1/40); 13/94 (14%) had a clinically significant titre of >/=1/80. Three per cent had dsDNA antibodies, 2% had RF and anti-Ro antibodies, 1% had anti-RNP antibodies, and none had anti-La or anti-Smith antibodies." Johnson SR, Schentag CT, Gladman DD. Autoantibodies in biological agent naive patients with psoriatic arthritis. *Ann Rheum Dis*. 2005 May;64(5):770-2
[460] Tsai YG, Chang DM, Kuo SY, Wang WM, Chen YC, Lai JH. Relationship between human lymphocyte antigen-B27 and clinical features of psoriatic arthritis. *J Microbiol Immunol Infect*. 2003 Jun;36(2):101-4 jmii.org/content/abstracts/v36n2p101.php
[461] "The 24-h urine excretion of 51Cr-EDTA from psoriatic patients was 2.46 +/- 0.81%. These results differed significantly from controls (1.95 +/- 0.36%; P less than 0.05)." Humbert P, Bidet A, Treffel P, Drobacheff C, Agache P. Intestinal permeability in patients with psoriasis. *J Dermatol Sci*. 1991 Jul;2:324-6
[462] "In the current study, 20 (40%), psoriatic patients and 5 (10%) patients of control group demonstrated H. pylori antibodies… Although our study supports a causal role of H. pylori in the pathogenesis of psoriasis, a large scale study is needed to confirm the findings." Qayoom S, Ahmad QM. Psoriasis and helicobacter pylori. *Indian J Dermatol Venereol Leprol* 2003;69:133-134 ijdvl.com/
[463] Candida albicans (and other yeasts) was detected in 68% of psoriatics, 70% of eczematics, 54% of the controls. Qualitative analysis revealed a predominance of Candida albicans. Geotrichum candidum occurred in 22% of psoriatics, 10% of eczematics, and 3% of controls. Buslau M, Menzel I, Holzmann H. Fungal flora of human faeces in psoriasis and atopic dermatitis. *Mycoses*. 1990 Feb;33(2):90-4
[464] "Our results reinforce the hypothesis that C. albicans is one of the triggers to both exacerbation and persistence of psoriasis. We propose that in psoriatics with a significant quantity of Candida in faeces, an antifungal treatment should be considered as an adjuvant treatment of psoriasis." Waldman A, Gilhar A, Duek L, Berdicevsky I. Incidence of Candida in psoriasis--a study on the fungal flora of psoriatic patients. *Mycoses*. 2001 May;44(3-4):77-8
[465] Noah PW. The role of microorganisms in psoriasis. *Semin Dermatol*. 1990 Dec;9(4):269-76
[466] Noah PW. The role of microorganisms in psoriasis. *Semin Dermatol*. 1990 Dec;9(4):269-76
[467] Noah PW. The role of microorganisms in psoriasis. *Semin Dermatol*. 1990 Dec;9(4):269-76

- **Orodental dysbiosis**: Culture of dentures and oral cavity for yeast and bacteria.
- **Environmental dysbiosis**: Examination, culture, and/or thorough cleaning of wigs, shoes, furniture, whirlpool/pool water.[468]
- **Imaging**:
  o Radiographic findings are characteristic and can aid in differential diagnosis; findings such as the osteolytic "pencil-in-cup" and "marginal erosions" are characteristic and differentiate psoriatic arthropathy from other conditions.
  o Radiographic changes in the spine may be severe even when the patient has mild or no symptoms—assess the spine radiographically before initiating spinal manipulative therapy. Note that inflammatory changes such as facet ankylosis and atlantoaxial instability may occur and could potentially complicate manipulative therapy.[469] Myelocompressive atlantoaxial subluxation has been reported as the presenting manifestation of psoriatic arthropathy.[470] Remarkably, Lee and Lui[471] published that, "...atlantoaxial subluxation without high cervical myelopathy has been reported in 45% of cases of psoriatic spondylitis."
- **Establishing the diagnosis**:
  o Pattern recognition: psoriasis with arthritis after the exclusion of RA, iron overload, AS, and HIV

Complications:
- Infection of skin lesions, may progress to septicemia or septic arthritis
- Atlantoaxial instability
- Cosmetic and functional deformity
- Pain
- Destructive and crippling arthritis
- Depression, social isolation, pain, reduced quality of life: **"Patients with psoriasis reported reduction in physical functioning and mental functioning comparable to that seen in cancer, arthritis, hypertension, heart disease, diabetes, and depression."**[472]

Clinical management:
- Referral if clinical outcome is unsatisfactory or if serious complications are evident.

Treatments:
- **Medical treatments**: The goal of medical treatment is to suppress inflammation and dermal proliferation; no consideration is given to searching for and addressing the underlying cause(s) of the disorder because the disease is considered idiopathic.[473] Medical textbooks describe the treatment as merely targeted toward the symptoms, e.g., "Treatment [of psoriatic arthritis] is symptomatic."[474]
  o *For dermal psoriasis*:
    - Prescription topical steroids
    - Topical coal tars and hydrocarbons: carcinogenic
    - UV-B radiation: kills active lymphocytes in skin and results in short-term superficial disappearance of psoriatic skin lesions
    - PUVA: psoralen with UV-A radiation; may result in cataracts and skin cancer
    - Methotrexate
    - Etretinate: a severely teratogenic retinoid

---

[468] Noah PW. The role of microorganisms in psoriasis. *Semin Dermatol*. 1990 Dec;9(4):269-76
[469] Laiho K, Kauppi M. The cervical spine in patients with psoriatic arthritis. *Ann Rheum Dis*. 2002 Jul;6:650-2 ard.bmjjournals.com/cgi/content/full/61/7/650
[470] "We report severe upward axial dislocation and acquired basilar impression as a presenting manifestation of psoriatic arthropathy." Kaplan JG, Rosenberg RS, DeSouza T, Post KD, Freilich MD, Salamon O, Lantos G, Reinitz E. Atlantoaxial subluxation in psoriatic arthropathy. *Ann Neurol*. 1988 May;23(5):522-4
[471] "...atlantoaxial subluxation without high cervical myelopathy has been reported in 45% of cases of psoriatic spondylitis." Lee ST, Lui TN. Psoriatic arthritis with C-1-C-2 subluxation as a neurosurgical complication. *Surg Neurol*. 1986 Nov;26(5):428-30
[472] "Patients with psoriasis reported reduction in physical functioning and mental functioning comparable to that seen in cancer, arthritis, hypertension, heart disease, diabetes, and depression." Rapp et al. Psoriasis causes as much disability as other major medical diseases. *J Am Acad Dermatol* 1999 Sep;41(3 Pt 1):401-7
[473] Lookingbill DP, Marks JG, eds. *Principles of dermatology*. Philadelphia: W.B. Saunders, 1986: 138
[474] Tierney ML. McPhee SJ, Papadakis MA. *Current Medical Diagnosis and Treatment 2006. 45th edition*. New York; Lange Medical: 2006, pages 851-855

- *For psoriatic arthritis*: Medical treatments for psoriatic arthritis are essentially the same as for rheumatoid arthritis[475] and are generally noncurative and "symptomatic."[476]
    - Etretinate: a severely teratogenic retinoid
    - PUVA: psoralen with UV-A radiation; may result in cataracts and skin cancer
    - Corticosteroids are not highly effective
    - Antimalarial drugs (commonly used against systemic lupus erythematosus) frequently exacerbate psoriasis
    - Methotrexate: Used for recalcitrant psoriatic arthritis.[477]
    - TNF inhibitors: Etanercept 25 mg subcutaneously twice weekly, or infliximab 5 mg/kg every other month. These drugs are clinically effective from the perspective of anti-inflammation, but they are associated with increased risks for lymphoma, infections, congestive heart failure, demyelinating diseases, and systemic lupus erythematosus.

- **FOOD & NUTRITION: 5-part "supplemented Paleo-Mediterranean diet" (SPMD)** The 5-part "supplemented Paleo-Mediterranean diet" (SPMD—reviewed in Chapter 4) consists of ❶ foundational plant-based low-carbohydrate diet of fruits, vegetables, nuts, seeds, berries and lean sources of protein, ❷ multivitamin and multimineral supplementation, ❸ physiologic doses of vitamin D3 (range 2,000-10,000 IU/d), ❹ combination fatty acid therapy (CFAT) with n3-ALA, n6-GLA, n3-EPA, n3-DHA, and phytochemical-rich olive oil which contains n9-oleate, and ❺ probiotics.
    - Vitamin D3 supplementation with physiologic doses and/or tailored to serum 25(OH)D levels: Vitamin D deficiency is common in the general population and is even more common in patients with chronic illness and chronic musculoskeletal pain.[478] Vitamin D3 can be applied topically and is about as effective as topical steroids in the treatment of psoriatic skin lesions.[479] Correction of vitamin D deficiency supports normal immune function against infection and provides a clinically significant anti-inflammatory[480] and analgesic benefit in patients with back pain[481] and limb pain.[482] Reasonable daily doses for children and adults are 2,000 and 4,000 IU, respectively, as defined by Vasquez, et al.[483] Deficiency and response to treatment are monitored with serum 25(OH)vitamin D while safety is monitored with serum calcium; inflammatory granulomatous diseases and certain drugs such as hydrochlorothiazide greatly increase the propensity for hypercalcemia and warrant increment dosing and frequent monitoring of serum calcium.
    - Alcohol/ethanol avoidance: Consumption of alcoholic beverages—even in low doses—increases intestinal permeability and exacerbates psoriasis. Psoriatics should avoid ethanol consumption[484]; wheat/grain antigens are immunogenic, ethanol exacerbates intestinal hyperpermeability, and some patients are sensitive to brewer's yeast.
    - Gluten-free vegetarian diet: Vegetarian/vegan diets have a place in the treatment plan of all patients with autoimmune/inflammatory disorders[485], including psoriasis and psoriatic arthritis[486]; this is also true for patients for whom long-term exclusive reliance on a meat-free vegetarian diet is either not appropriate or not appealing. No legitimate scientist or literate clinician doubts the antirheumatic power and anti-inflammatory advantages of vegetarian diets, whether used short-term or long term.[487] The benefits of gluten-free vegetarian diets are well documented, and the mechanisms of action are well elucidated,

---

[475] Beers MH, Berkow R (eds). *The Merck Manual. Seventeenth Edition*. Whitehouse Station; Merck Research Laboratories 1999 page 448
[476] Tierney ML. McPhee SJ, Papadakis MA. *Current Medical Diagnosis and Treatment 2006. 45th edition*. New York; Lange Medical: 2006, pages 851-855
[477] Tierney ML. McPhee SJ, Papadakis MA. *Current Medical Diagnosis and Treatment 2006. 45th edition*. New York; Lange Medical: 2006, pages 851-855
[478] Plotnikoff GA, Quigley JM. Prevalence of severe hypovitaminosis D in patients with persistent, nonspecific musculoskeletal pain. *Mayo Clin Proc*. 2003 Dec;78(12):1463-70
[479] Lookingbill DP, Marks JG, eds. *Principles of dermatology*. Philadelphia: W.B. Saunders, 1986: 141
[480] Timms et al. Circulating MMP9, vitamin D and variation in TIMP-1 response with VDR genotype. *QJM*. 2002 Dec;95(12):787-96
[481] Al Faraj S, Al Mutairi K. Vitamin D deficiency and chronic low back pain in Saudi Arabia. *Spine*. 2003 Jan 15;28(2):177-9
[482] Masood et al. Persistent limb pain and raised serum alkaline phosphatase earliest markers of subclinical hypovitaminosis D. *Indian J Physiol Pharmacol* 1989 Oct:259-61
[483] Vasquez et al. The clinical importance of vitamin D (cholecalciferol): a paradigm shift for all healthcare providers. *Altern Ther Health Med*. 2004 Sep-Oct;10(5):28-36
[484] "We recommend that clinicians discourage patients with psoriasis from consuming alcohol, especially during periods of disease exacerbation." Behnam SM, Behnam SE, Koo JY. Alcohol as a risk factor for plaque-type psoriasis. *Cutis*. 2005 Sep;76(3):181-5
[485] "After four weeks at the health farm the diet group showed a significant improvement in number of tender joints, Ritchie's articular index, number of swollen joints, pain score, duration of morning stiffness, grip strength, erythrocyte sedimentation rate, C-reactive protein, white blood cell count, and a health assessment questionnaire score." Kjeldsen-Kragh J, et al. Controlled trial of fasting and one-year vegetarian diet in rheumatoid arthritis. *Lancet*. 1991 Oct 12;338(8772):899-902
[486] "During the vegan diet, both signs and symptoms returned in most patients, with the exception of some patients with psoriasis who experienced an improvement." Lithell H, Bruce A, Gustafsson IB, et al. A fasting and vegetarian diet treatment trial on chronic inflammatory disorders. *Acta Derm Venereol*. 1983;63(5):397-403
[487] "For the patients who were randomised to the vegetarian diet there was a significant decrease in platelet count, leukocyte count, calprotectin, total IgG, IgM rheumatoid factor (RF), C3-activation products, and the complement components C3 and C4 after one month of treatment." Kjeldsen-Kragh J, Mellbye OJ, Haugen M, Mollnes TE, Hammer HB, Sioud M, Forre O. Changes in laboratory variables in rheumatoid arthritis patients during a trial of fasting and one-year vegetarian diet. *Scand J Rheumatol*. 1995;24(2):85-93

including reduced intake of proinflammatory linoleic[488] and arachidonic acids[489], iron[490], common food antigens[491], gluten[492] and gliadin[493,494], proinflammatory sugars[495] and increased intake of omega-3 fatty acids and micronutrients[496], and anti-inflammatory and anti-oxidant phytonutrients[497]; vegetarian diets also effect profound changes—both *qualitative* and *quantitative*—in intestinal flora[498,499] that correlate with clinical improvement.[500] Patients who rely on the Paleo-Mediterranean Diet can use vegetarian meals, on a daily basis or for days at a time, for example, by having a daily vegetarian meal, or one week per month of vegetarianism. Of course, some (not all) patients can use a purely vegetarian diet long-term provided that nutritional needs (especially protein and cobalamin) are consistently met. One particular advantage to low-protein diets in psoriasis is that the relative reduction in amino acid availability should serve to reduce polyamine formation. Formed from amino acids via ornithine decarboxylase and other enzymes, polyamines stimulate dermal hyperproliferation and are elevated in patients with psoriasis.[501] Effective psoriasis treatments are associated with a reduction in dermal/urinary polyamine levels, and, conversely, reducing polyamine formation—via either dietary manipulation or antibiologic/pharmaceutical drugs—is associated with clinical improvements in patients with psoriasis.

- **INFECTIONS & DYSBIOSIS:** ❶ antimicrobial treatments, ❷ immunorestoration, ❸ immunotolerance via Treg induction Essentially all autoimmune/rheumatic disorders are associated with microbial colonization and intolerance to same; the presence of persistent microbial colonization is *prima facie* evidence of immunosuppression. The eight areas of dysbiosis (multifocal) are: ❶ sinorespiratory, ❷ orodental, ❸ gastrointestinal, ❹ urogenital/genitourinary, ❺ parenchymal/tissue, ❻ microbial, ❼ dermal/cutaneous, and ❽ environmental.
  - Psoriatogenic multifocal dysbiosis—overview of and homage to the work of Patricia Noah PhD: In a very intensive investigation into the role of bacteria, yeast/fungi, and viruses in the pathogenesis of psoriasis, Noah[502] assessed microflora of 297 psoriasis patients by culture and serologic tests. Culture samples for aerobic bacteria, yeast, and dermatophytes were taken from the throat, urine, and skin surfaces from scalp, ears, chest, face,

Microorganisms causally associated with psoriasis:

1. Streptococcal groups A (including *Streptococcus pyogenes*), B, C, D, F, G, *S viridans*, *S pneumoniae*
2. *Klebsiella pneumoniae, oxytoca*
3. *Escherichia coli*
4. *Enterobacter cloacae, E aerogenes, E agglomerans*
5. *Proteus mirabilis, P vulgaris*
6. *Citrobacter freundii, C diversus*
7. *Morganella morganii*
8. *Pseudomonas aeruginosa, P maltiphilia, P putida*
9. *Serratia marcescens*
10. *Acinetobacter calbio aceticus, A luoffi*
11. *Flavobacterium* species
12. CDC groups Ve-1, Ve-2, E-o2
13. *Bacillus subtilis, B cereus*
14. *Staphylococcus aureus*
15. *Candida albicans, C parapsilosis*
16. *Torulopsis/Candida glabrata*
17. *Rhodotorula* spp.
18. *H. pylori**

See Noah P. The role of microorganisms in psoriasis. *Semin Dermatol.* 1990;9:269
* Qayoom S, Ahmad QM. Psoriasis and helicobacter pylori. *Indian J Dermatol Venereol Leprol* 2003;69:133-134

---

[488] Rusyn I, Bradham CA, Cohn L, Schoonhoven R, Swenberg JA, Brenner DA, Thurman RG. Corn oil rapidly activates nuclear factor-kappaB in hepatic Kupffer cells by oxidant-dependent mechanisms. *Carcinogenesis.* 1999 Nov;20(11):2095-100 carcin.oxfordjournals.org/cgi/content/full/20/11/2095
[489] Vasquez A. New Insights into Fatty Acid Supplementation and Its Effect on Eicosanoid Production and Genetic Expression. *Nutritional Perspectives* 2005; January: 5-16
[490] Dabbagh AJ, Trenam CW, Morris CJ, Blake DR. Iron in joint inflammation. *Ann Rheum Dis.* 1993 Jan;52(1):67-73
[491] Hafstrom I, et al. A vegan diet free of gluten improves the signs and symptoms of rheumatoid arthritis: the effects on arthritis correlate with a reduction in antibodies to food antigens. *Rheumatology* (Oxford). 2001 Oct;40(10):1175-9 rheumatology.oxfordjournals.org/cgi/reprint/40/10/1175
[492] "The data provide evidence that dietary modification may be of clinical benefit for certain RA patients, and that this benefit may be related to a reduction in immunoreactivity to food antigens eliminated by the change in diet." Hafstrom I, et al. A vegan diet free of gluten improves the signs and symptoms of rheumatoid arthritis: the effects on arthritis correlate with a reduction in antibodies to food antigens. *Rheumatology* (Oxford). 2001 Oct;40(10):1175-9
[493] "Despite the increased AGA [antigliadin antibodies] positivity found distinctively in patients with recent-onset RA, none of the RA patients showed clear evidence of coeliac disease." Paimela L, Kurki P, Leirisalo-Repo M, Piirainen H. Gliadin immune reactivity in patients with rheumatoid arthritis. Clin Exp Rheumatol. 1995 Sep-Oct;13(5):603-7
[494] "The median IgA antigliadin ELISA index was 7.1 (range 2.1-22.4) for the RA group and 3.1 (range 0.3-34.9) for the controls (p = 0.0001)." Koot VC, Van Straaten M, Hekkens WT, Collee G, Dijkmans BA. Elevated level of IgA gliadin antibodies in patients with rheumatoid arthritis. *Clin Exp Rheumatol.* 1989 Nov-Dec;7(6):623-6
[495] Seaman DR. The diet-induced proinflammatory state: a cause of chronic pain and other degenerative diseases? *J Manipulative Physiol Ther.* 2002 Mar-Apr;25(3):168-79
[496] Hagfors L, Nilsson I, Skoldstam L, Johansson G. Fat intake and composition of fatty acids in serum phospholipids in a randomized, controlled, Mediterranean dietary intervention study on patients with rheumatoid arthritis. *Nutr Metab* (Lond). 2005 Oct 10;2:26 nutritionandmetabolism.com/content/2/1/26
[497] Liu RH. Health benefits of fruit and vegetables are from additive and synergistic combinations of phytochemicals. *Am J Clin Nutr* 2003;78(3 Suppl):517S-520S
[498] "Significant alteration in the intestinal flora was observed when the patients changed from omnivorous to vegan diet. ... This finding of an association between intestinal flora and disease activity may have implications for our understanding of how diet can affect RA." Peltonen R, Kjeldsen-Kragh J, Haugen M, Tuominen J, Toivanen P, Forre O, Eerola E. Changes of faecal flora in rheumatoid arthritis during fasting and one-year vegetarian diet. *Br J Rheumatol.* 1994 Jul;33(7):638-43
[499] Toivanen P, Eerola E. A vegan diet changes the intestinal flora. *Rheumatology* (Oxford). 2002 Aug;41(8):950-1 rheumatology.oxfordjournals.org/cgi/reprint/41/8/950
[500] "We conclude that a vegan diet changes the faecal microbial flora in RA patients, and changes in the faecal flora are associated with improvement in RA activity." Peltonen R, Nenonen M, Helve T, Hanninen O, Toivanen P, Eerola E. Faecal microbial flora and disease activity during a vegan diet. *Br J Rheumatol.* 1997 Jan;36(1):64-8 rheumatology.oxfordjournals.org/cgi/reprint/36/1/64
[501] "Psoriasis lesions showed increased ornithine decarboxylase activity compared with uninvolved skin." Lowe NJ, Breeding J, Russell D. Cutaneous polyamines in psoriasis. *Br J Dermatol.* 1982 Jul;107(1):21-5
[502] Noah PW. The role of microorganisms in psoriasis. *Semin Dermatol.* 1990 Dec;9(4):269-76

axillary, submammary, umbilical, upper back, inguinal crease, gluteal-fold, perirectal, vaginal, pubis, penis, scrotal, leg, hands, feet, finger, and toenail areas. More than 15 different microbes were causatively associated with exacerbation of psoriasis; this finding is entirely logical and is consistent with the 'idiopathic' nature of the illness and why Koch-indoctrinated researchers and clinicians have failed to understand the microbial contribution to autoimmune/inflammatory diseases. Given that each of the microbes listed (see shaded box on upcoming page) is a *common—* but not necessarily *optimal*—inhabitant of human surfaces and orifices, it is possible to see how their synergism *particularly in a genetically susceptible patient with hormonal imbalances and a proinflammatory lifestyle/diet* could tip the scales in favor of systemic inflammation and the picture/illusion of autoimmunity.

> **Microbial antigens evoke psoriasis and autoimmunity**
> "RESULTS: The predicted microbial product appeared heavily in lesional epidermis, but unexpectedly also as a thin deposit along the skin basement membrane zone (SBMZ) of apparently unaffected skin. Staining was negative for nonpsoriatic subjects.
> CONCLUSIONS: The findings support a direct effect of microbial antigen in psoriasis."
>
> Noah et al. Skin basement membrane zone: a depository for circulating microbial antigen evoking psoriasis and autoimmunity. *Skinmed*. 2006 Mar-Apr

Of the more than 15 categories/subspecies listed as causative microbes, what if only seven of these common "commensals" were present in a systemically-genetically-nutritionally-hormonally-emotionally predisposed patient, and each contributed only 5% to the pathophysiology of a patient's psoriasis? We would have already arrived at 35% of the psoriatic pathogenesis, leaving 10% each for hormones, diet, allergy, nutrition, xenobiotic accumulation (present in everyone[503,504]). While these numbers and percentages are purely speculative, I left 15% for "idiopathic" to keep researchers and clinicians alert to new possibilities and to placate the therapeutic and epidemiologic nihilists that have so far dominated the field of rheumatology with their "unknown cause" rhetoric. Each cause—each contributor to disease—may in itself be "clinically insignificant" but when additive and synergistic influences coalesce, we find ourselves confronted with an "idiopathic disease" and the decision to choose between the only two available options: 1) despair in the failure of our "one cause, one disease, one drug" paradigm, or 2) appreciate that numerous influences work together to disrupt physiologic function and produce the biologic dysfunction that we experience as disease.

o <u>Gastrointestinal dysbiosis</u>: Patients with psoriasis have shown a greatly increased prevalence of *H. pylori*[505] and *Candida albicans*[506] and *Geotrichum candidum*.[507]
o <u>Sinorespiratory and dermal dysbiosis</u>: Sinorespiratory and dermal dysbiosis in patients with
o is *qualitatively* (increased prevalence in psoriatics compared with healthy controls) and *quantitatively* (increased prevalence of toxin-producing strains compared to those found in controls) associated with the severity of the disease.[508] Patients with psoriasis show an increased rate of nasal/dermal colonization with *Staphylococcus aureus*[509,510], a microbe known to produce several powerfully inflammatory antigens, toxins, and superantigens, and nasal colonization with which appears causally associated with the

---

[503] "Although the use of HCB as a fungicide has virtually been eliminated, detectable levels of HCB are still found in nearly all people in the USA." Robinson PE, et al. An evaluation of hexachlorobenzene body-burden levels in the general population of the USA. *IARC Sci Publ* 1986;77:183-92
[504] "Many U.S. residents carry toxic pesticides in their bodies above government assessed "acceptable" levels." Pesticide Action Network North America (PANNA). Chemical Trespass: Pesticides in Our Bodies and Corporate Accountability. panna.org/campaigns/docsTrespass/chemicalTrespass2004.dv.html
[505] "In the current study, 20 (40%), psoriatic patients and 5 (10%) patients of control group demonstrated H. pylori antibodies... Although our study supports a causal role of H. pylori in the pathogenesis of psoriasis, a large scale study is needed to confirm the findings." Qayoom S, Ahmad QM. Psoriasis and helicobacter pylori. *Indian J Dermatol Venereol Leprol* 2003;69:133-134 ijdvl.com/
[506] "Our results reinforce the hypothesis that C. albicans is one of the triggers to both exacerbation and persistence of psoriasis. We propose that in psoriatics with a significant quantity of Candida in faeces, an antifungal treatment should be considered as an adjuvant treatment of psoriasis." Waldman A, Gilhar A, Duek L, Berdicevsky I. Incidence of Candida in psoriasis--a study on the fungal flora of psoriatic patients. *Mycoses*. 2001 May;44(3-4):77-8
[507] Candida albicans (and other yeasts) was detected in 68% of psoriatics, 70% of eczematics, 54% of the controls. Qualitative analysis revealed a predominance of Candida albicans. Geotrichum candidum occurred in 22% of psoriatics, 10% of eczematics, and 3% of controls. Buslau M, Menzel I, Holzmann H. Fungal flora of human faeces in psoriasis and atopic dermatitis. *Mycoses*. 1990 Feb;33(2):90-4
[508] "In this study, S aureus was present in more than 50% of patients with AD and PS. We found that the severity of AD and PS significantly correlated to enterotoxin production of the isolated S aureus strains." Tomi NS, Kranke B, Aberer E. Staphylococcal toxins in patients with psoriasis, atopic dermatitis, and erythroderma, and in healthy control subjects. *J Am Acad Dermatol*. 2005 Jul;53(1):67-72
[509] "In this study, S aureus was present in more than 50% of patients with AD and PS. We found that the severity of AD and PS significantly correlated to enterotoxin production of the isolated S aureus strains." Tomi NS, Kranke B, Aberer E. Staphylococcal toxins in patients with psoriasis, atopic dermatitis, and erythroderma, and in healthy control subjects. *J Am Acad Dermatol*. 2005 Jul;53(1):67-72
[510] "The nasal carriage rate of Staphylococcus aureus in psoriatics was higher than the control groups." Singh et al. Bacteriology of psoriatic plaques. *Dermatologica*. 1978:21-7

inflammatory/autoimmune disorder Wegener's granulomatosis.[511,512] A study by Bartenjev et al[513] showed that subclinical streptococcal/staphylococcal infections were detected in 68% of psoriasis patients and in only 11 % of the control group; these authors encouraged searching for and eliminating microbial infections as an important aspect of the management of psoriasis. Supportively, other researchers[514] have found that infection with *S pyogenes* can initiate and/or exacerbate guttate psoriasis; therefore streptococcal throat infections should be treated assertively and early to avoid triggering an exacerbation of psoriasis.[515] *Streptococcus pyogenes* is a very likely trigger of psoriasis[516]; chronic penicillin treatment leads to clinical improvement of recalcitrant psoriasis.[517] Patients with guttate psoriasis have increased oropharyngeal colonization with *Streptococcus hemolyticus* compared with controls.[518] Similar to Behcet's disease[519], the dermal lesions of psoriasis are commonly colonized by proinflammatory microbes including *Staphylococcus aureus*.[520] More conclusively, research by Villeda-Gabriel et al[521] and Perez-Lorenzo et al[522] has clearly shown that antibodies against *Streptococcus pyogenes* cross-react (perhaps via molecular mimicry or epitope spreading) with dermal antigens; additionally, the work of Muto et al[523] showed that antibodies against streptococcal cell wall proteins could bind with nuclei and cytoplasm of cells from skin and synovium. Thus, psoriasis is indeed a microbe-induced autoimmune disease by virtue of these cross-reacting endogenous antibodies that bind with nuclear, dermal, and articular antigens. Patients with psoriasis have elevated serum levels of antibodies against streptococcal M12 protein[524], and patients with psoriatic arthritis have a heightened inflammatory response to staphylococcal superantigens.[525]

- o <u>Antimicrobial treatments for (gastrointestinal) dysbiosis commonly include but are not limited to the following</u>: Doses listed are for adults. Combination therapy generally allows for lower doses of each intervention to be used. Severe dysbiosis often requires weeks or months of treatment. Drugs are not

---

[511] Brons RH, Bakker HI, Van Wijk RT, et al. Staphylococcal acid phosphatase binds to endothelial cells via charge interaction; a pathogenic role in Wegener's granulomatosis? *Clin Exp Immunol.* 2000 Mar;119(3):566-73 blackwell-synergy.com/doi/abs/10.1046/j.1365-2249.2000.01172.x

[512] Popa et al. Staphylococcus aureus and Wegener's granulomatosis. *Arthritis Res.* 2002;4(2):77-9 arthritis-research.com/content/4/2/77

[513] "Subclinical streptococcal and/or staphylococcal infections were detected in 68 % of tested patients and in only 11 % of the control group. The results of this study indicate that subclinical bacterial infections of the upper respiratory tract may be an important factor in provoking a new relapse of chronic plaque psoriasis. Searching for, and eliminating, microbial infections could be of importance in the treatment of psoriasis." Bartenjev I, Rogl Butina M, Potocnik M. Subclinical microbial infection in patients with chronic plaque psoriasis. *Acta Derm Venereol Suppl* (Stockh). 2000;(211):17-8

[514] "This study confirms the strong association between prior infection with S pyogenes and guttate psoriasis but suggests that the ability to trigger guttate psoriasis is not serotype specific." Telfer et al. The role of streptococcal infection in the initiation of guttate psoriasis. *Arch Dermatol.* 1992 Jan;128(1):39-42

[515] "CONCLUSIONS: This study confirms anecdotal and retrospective reports that streptococcal throat infections can cause exacerbation of chronic plaque psoriasis." Gudjonsson JE, Thorarinsson AM, Sigurgeirsson B, Kristinsson KG, Valdimarsson H. Streptococcal throat infections and exacerbation of chronic plaque psoriasis: a prospective study. *Br J Dermatol.* 2003 Sep;149(3):530-4

[516] "These findings justify the hypothesis that S pyogenes infections are more important in the pathogenesis of chronic plaque psoriasis than has previously been recognized, and indicate the need for further controlled therapeutic trials of antibacterial measures in this common skin disease." El-Rachkidy RG, et al. Increased Blood Levels of IgG Reactive with Secreted Streptococcus pyogenes Proteins in Chronic Plaque Psoriasis. *J Invest Dermatol.* 2007 Mar 8

[517] "Total duration of the study was two years. Initially benzathine penicillin 1.2 million units, was given I.M. AST fortnightly. After 24 weeks benzathine penicillin was reduced to 1.2 million units once a month... Significant improvement in the PASI score was noted from 12 weeks onwards. All patients showed excellent improvement at 2 years." Saxena VN, Dogra J. Long-term use of penicillin for the treatment of chronic plaque psoriasis. *Eur J Dermatol.* 2005 Sep-Oct;15(5):359-62

[518] "A high incidence of Streptococcus hemolyticus culture was observed in the guttate psoriatic group compared with the plaque psoriasis and control groups." Zhao et al. Acute guttate psoriasis patients have positive streptococcus hemolyticus throat cultures and elevated antistreptococcal M6 protein titers. *J Dermatol.* 2005;32(2):91-6

[519] "At least one type of microorganism was grown from each pustule. Staphylococcus aureus (41/70, 58.6%, p = 0.008) and Prevotella spp (17/70, 24.3%, p = 0.002) were significantly more common in pustules from BS patients, and coagulase negative staphylococci (17/37, 45.9%, p = 0.007) in pustules from acne patients. CONCLUSIONS: The pustular lesions of BS are not usually sterile." Hatemi G, et al. The pustular skin lesions in Behcet's syndrome are not sterile. *Ann Rheum Dis.* 2004 Nov;63(11):1450-2

[520] "In this study, S aureus was present in more than 50% of patients with AD and PS. We found that the severity of AD and PS significantly correlated to enterotoxin production of the isolated S aureus strains." Tomi NS, Kranke B, Aberer E. Staphylococcal toxins in patients with psoriasis, atopic dermatitis, and erythroderma, and in healthy control subjects. *J Am Acad Dermatol.* 2005 Jul;53(1):67-72

[521] "The recognition by immunoblot of streptococcal antigens by serum of guttate psoriasis patients, the presence of autoantibodies against their own skin, and recognition of the same skin antigens by anti-streptococcal rabbit antibodies confirm the participation of the immune system and of streptococcal infections in guttate psoriasis." Villeda-Gabriel G, et al. Recognition of Streptococcus pyogenes and skin autoantigens in guttate psoriasis. *Arch Med Res.* 1998 Summer;29(2):143-8

[522] "It seems that autoantibodies, although they do not appear to participate in the pathogenesis of psoriasis, are an important feature, and that skin antigens, which appear in lesional immature keratinocytes, cross-react with S. pyogenes and contribute to the autoimmune process in psoriasis." Perez-Lorenzo R, Zambrano-Zaragoza JF, Saul A, Jimenez-Zamudio L, Reyes-Maldonado E, Garcia-Latorre E. Autoantibodies to autologous skin in guttate and plaque forms of psoriasis and cross-reaction of skin antigens with streptococcal antigens. *Int J Dermatol.* 1998 Jul;37(7):524-31. The authors found that all psoriais paitents had dermal autoantiboes and that these antibodies reacted specifically with endogenous dermal antigens; thus their finding that "Deposits of immunoglobulin G (IgG) were not detected in the lesions" is unexpected and inexplicable. This statement from their research is inconsistent with the findings of other research groups, and—specifically—must be placed in a context of other articles, most notably "… titers of IgG anti-SC autoantibodies in psoriatic patients were not specifically higher than in normal controls but were more variable, indicating that their circulating levels are dependent on a delicate balance between consumption at inflammatory sites and a secondary increase due to SC-antigen release following inflammation." Tagami H, Iwatsuki K, Yamada M. Profile of anti-stratum corneum autoantibodies in psoriatic patients. *Arch Dermatol Res.* 1983;275(2):71-5

[523] "Monoclonal antibodies directed against type 12 Group A streptococcal cell wall antigens cross-react with nuclei and cytoplasm of cells from skin and synovium from controls, uninvolved skin of psoriatics and psoriatic plaques." Muto M, Fujikura Y, Hamamoto Y, Ichimiya M, Ohmura A, Sasazuki T, Fukumoto T, Asagami C. Immune response to Streptococcus pyogenes and the susceptibility to psoriasis. *Australas J Dermatol.* 1996 May;37 Suppl 1:S54-5

[524] "Patients with psoriasis had high serum titres of antibody against the M12 (C-region) streptococcal antigen compared to controls." Muto M, et al. Immune response to Streptococcus pyogenes and the susceptibility to psoriasis. *Australas J Dermatol.* 1996 May;37 Suppl 1:S54-5

[525] "Our data raised the possibility that staphylococcal superantigens may also play an exacerbating role in PA." Yamamoto T, Katayama I, Nishioka K. Peripheral blood mononuclear cell proliferative response against staphylococcal superantigens in patients with psoriasis arthropathy. *Eur J Dermatol.* 1999 Jan-Feb;9(1):17-21

necessarily more effective than natural treatments; in fact, often the botanicals work when the pharmaceuticals do not. See introductory review at the start of this chapter as well as details provided in Chapter 4 for details on anti-dysbiotic treatments.

- **St. John's Wort (*Hypericum perforatum*)**: *Hypericum* may prove to be a useful botanical for the treatment of psoriasis due to the combination of its antidepressant and antimicrobial benefits. Hyperforin from *Hypericum perforatum* also shows impressive antibacterial action, particularly against gram-positive bacteria such as *Staphylococcus aureus, Streptococcus pyogenes, Streptococcus agalactiae*[526] and perhaps *Helicobacter pylori*.[527] Up to 600 mg three times per day of a 3% hyperforin standardized extract is customary in the treatment of depression.
- **Topical antimicrobials**: Treating the dermal lesions of psoriatic arthritis may help break the vicious cycles of (super)antigen absorption which perpetuates immune dysfunction. A variety of botanical and pharmaceutical creams are available. *In vitro* evidence supports the use of equal parts honey, olive oil, and beeswax against *Staph aureus* and *Candida albicans*.[528] As mentioned previously, topical *Mahonia/Berberis* is effective for dermal psoriasis.[529] A topical gel containing artemesinin is also available for clinical use, and animal studies have demonstrated systemic absorption from topical application[530]; its use in humans with psoriasis has not been studied. Topical honey is better than acyclovir against oral and genital herpes; apply *qid* for 15 minutes.[531]
- **Sarsaparilla (*Smilax* spp)**: A clinical trial published in the *New England Journal of Medicine* in 1942 documented benefit of a sarsaparilla compound in psoriasis.[532] The proposed mechanism of action includes the binding of bacterial endotoxins and preventing their local action and systemic absorption.

o **Commonly used antibiotic/antifungal drugs:** The most commonly employed drugs for intestinal bacterial overgrowth are described here.[533] Treatment duration is generally at least 2 weeks and up to 8 weeks, depending on clinical response and the severity and diversity of the intestinal overgrowth. With all anti*bacterial* treatments, use empiric anti*fungal* treatment to prevent yeast overgrowth; some patients benefit from antifungal treatment that is continued for *months* and occasionally *years*. Drugs can generally be coadministered with natural antibiotics/antifungals for improved efficacy. Treatment can be guided by identification of the dysbiotic microbes and the results of culture and sensitivity tests.

- **Penicillin**: Chronic penicillin treatment leads to clinical improvement of recalcitrant psoriasis; benefits are seen when treatment is continued for at least 12 weeks, according to a clinical trial of treatment lasting for two years.[534]
- **Metronidazole**: 250-500 mg BID-QID (generally limit to 1.5 g/d); metronidazole has systemic bioavailability and effectiveness against a wide range of dysbiotic microbes, including protozoans, amebas/Giardia, *H. pylori, Clostridium difficile* and most anaerobic gram-negative bacilli.[535] Adverse effects are generally limited to stomatitis, nausea, diarrhea, and—rarely and/or with long-term use—peripheral neuropathy, dizziness, and metallic taste; the drug must not be consumed with alcohol. Metronidazole resistance by *Blastocystis hominis* and other parasites has been noted.

---

[526] Schempp et al. Antibacterial activity of hyperforin from St John's wort against multiresistant Staphylococcus aureus and gram-positive bacteria. *Lancet*. 1999 Jun;353:2129

[527] "A butanol fraction of St. John's Wort revealed anti-Helicobacter pylori activity with MIC values ranging between 15.6 and 31.2 microg/ml." Reichling J, Weseler A, Saller R. A current review of the antimicrobial activity of Hypericum perforatum L. *Pharmacopsychiatry*. 2001 Jul;34 Suppl 1:S116-8

[528] "Honey, beeswax and olive oil mixture (1:1:1, v/v) is useful in the treatment of diaper dermatitis, psoriasis and eczema... CONCLUSIONS: Honey and honey mixture apparently could inhibit growth of S. aureus or C. albicans." Al-Waili NS. Mixture of honey, beeswax and olive oil inhibits growth of Staphylococcus aureus and Candida albicans. *Arch Med Res*. 2005 Jan-Feb;36(1):10-3

[529] "Taken together, these clinical studies conducted by several investigators in several countries indicate that Mahonia aquifolium is a safe and effective treatment of patients with mild to moderate psoriasis." Gulliver WP, Donsky HJ. A report on three recent clinical trials using Mahonia aquifolium 10% topical cream and a review of the worldwide clinical experience with Mahonia aquifolium for the treatment of plaque psoriasis. *Am J Ther*. 2005 Sep-Oct;12:398-406

[530] "This paper reports results of pharmacokinetic studies of this preparation when applied onto a fixed area of the shaved skin of mice and rabbits. ...The drug was found to be easily absorbed from the skin." Zhao KC, Xuan WY, Zhao Y, Song ZY. [The pharmacokinetics of a transdermal preparation of artesunate in mice and rabbits] [Article in Chinese] Yao Xue Xue Bao. 1989;24(11):813-6

[531] Al-Waili NS. Topical honey application vs. acyclovir for the treatment of recurrent herpes simplex lesions. *Med Sci Monit*. 2004 Aug;10(8):MT94-8 medscimonit.com/pub/vol_10/no_8/4431.pdf

[532] Thurmon FM. The treatment of psoriasis with a sarsaparilla compound. *N Engl J Med* 1942; 227 (4): 128-33

[533] Saltzman JR, Russell RM. Nutritional consequences of intestinal bacterial overgrowth. *Compr Ther*. 1994;20(9):523-30

[534] "Total duration of the study was two years. Initially benzathine penicillin 1.2 million units, was given I.M. AST fortnightly. After 24 weeks benzathine penicillin was reduced to 1.2 million units once a month... Significant improvement in the PASI score was noted from 12 weeks onwards. All patients showed excellent improvement at 2 years." Saxena VN, Dogra J. Long-term use of penicillin for the treatment of chronic plaque psoriasis. *Eur J Dermatol*. 2005 Sep-Oct;15(5):359-62

[535] Tierney ML. McPhee SJ, Papadakis MA. *Current Medical Diagnosis and Treatment 2006. 45th edition*. New York; Lange Medical: 2006, pages 1578-1577

- **Erythromycin**: 250-500 mg TID-QID; this drug is a widely used antibiotic that also has intestinal promotility benefits (thus making it an ideal treatment for intestinal bacterial overgrowth associated with or caused by intestinal dysmotility/hypomotility such as seen in scleroderma[536,537]). Do not combine erythromycin with the promotility drug cisapride due to risk for serious cardiac arrhythmia.

Antimicrobial treatment for psoriasis

"Patients are questioned, examined, and subjected to microbiologic laboratory investigations in an attempt to identify possibly relevant microorganisms, and then are treated with antibiotics. ... Results obtained with this approach compare favorably with those achieved with more usual anti-psoriasis treatments. We recommend that a microbiologic investigation and a trial of antimicrobial treatment should precede any plan to treat psoriasis patients with anything more than the simplest topical agents."

Rosenberg EW, Noah PW, Skinner RB Jr. Microorganisms and psoriasis. *J Natl Med Assoc*. 1994 Apr;86(4):305-10

Long-term penicillin for psoriasis

"Significant improvement in the PASI score was noted from 12 weeks onwards. All patients showed excellent improvement at 2 years. Patients tolerated the therapy well. Controlled studies are needed to further confirm the benefits of long-term use of benzathine penicillin in the treatment of psoriasis."

Saxena VN, Dogra J. Long-term use of penicillin for treatment of chronic plaque psoriasis. *Eur J Dermatol*. 2005 Sep

---

Long-term azithromycin for psoriasis

"30 randomly selected patients with moderate to severe chronic plaque psoriasis received azithromycin for 48 weeks as a single oral 500 mg daily dose for 4 days with a gap of 10 days (total 24 such courses). ... Though the trial concluded at 48 weeks, patients in the azithromycin-arm were followed for another year to observe any relapse. A significant improvement in PASI score was noted from 12 weeks in the majority of patients in the azithromycin group. At the end of 48 weeks, 18 patients (60%) showed excellent improvement, while 6 patients (20%) showed good improvement and 4 patients (13.33%) showed mild improvement. ... An exacerbation in lesions was reported in 5 cases (16.66%) in the group receiving azithromycin. These exacerbations also responded by continuing the same treatment. ... Patients tolerated the therapy well."

Saxena VN, Dogra J. Long-term oral azithromycin in chronic plaque psoriasis. *Eur J Dermatol*. 2010 May

---

- **NUTRITIONAL IMMUNOMODULATION: Treg induction for modulation of Th-1/2/17 inflammation**
  Nutrients and therapeutic approaches that promote Treg or IL-10 induction and/or Th-17, IL-17 suppression include 1) mitochondrial optimization and mTOR suppression, 2) biotin, 3) vitamin E, 4) sodium avoidance, 5) transgenic/GMO food avoidance, 6) probiotics, 7) lipoic acid, 8) vitamin A, 9) inflammation reduction, 10) vitamin D, 11) fatty acid supplementation with GLA and n3, 12) infection and dysbiosis remediation, 13) green tea EGCG. Acronym: MiBESTPLAIDFIG.

- **DYSMETABOLISM & DYSFUNCTIONAL MITOCHONDRIA: MitoDys, ERS-UPR, AGE/RAGE, hyperglycemia and ceramide** The major clinical considerations in this section are mitochondrial dysfunction, endoplasmic reticulum stress, unfolded protein response, TLR activation, and the dysmetabolic effects of sustained hyperglycemia and hyperinsulinemia and resultant oxidative stress, inflammation, RAGE activation, and accumulation of AGE, palmitate and ceramide. The review of this information in Chapter 4 covered approximately 30 interventions relevant to dysmetabolism, mitochondrial dysfunction, ERS-UPR, etc; these will not be reviewed here except to mention those most commonly, easily, empirically, synergistically, and effectively used: 1) low-carbohydrate diet with 2) moderate exercise, 3) CoQ-10, 4) acetyl-carnitine with 5) lipoic acid, 6) NAC, 7) resveratrol, and 8) melatonin.
  - Carnitine / fumarate: Fumaric acid 250-500 mg 3 times a day was advocated by Wright and Gaby[538], who advised beginning with a low dose and slowly increasing the dose over a period of weeks. Flushing and hypoglycemia may occur; serial measurements of liver and kidney function tests are mandatory since

---

[536] "Prokinetic agents effective in pseudoobstruction include metoclopramide, domperidone, cisapride, octreotide, and erythromycin. ... The combination of octreotide and erythromycin may be particularly effective in systemic sclerosis." Sjogren RW. Gastrointestinal features of scleroderma. *Curr Opin Rheumatol*. 1996 Nov;8(6):569-75
[537] "Erythromycin accelerates gastric and gallbladder emptying in scleroderma patients and might be helpful in the treatment of gastrointestinal motor abnormalities in these patients." Fiorucci et al. Effect of erythromycin administration on upper gastrointestinal motility in scleroderma patients. *Scand J Gastroenterol*. 1994 Sep;29(9):807-13
[538] Gaby A, Wright JV. *Nutritional Protocols*. 1998 by Nutrition Seminars

fumarate has been reported to cause liver and/or renal damage. Carnitine appears to have anti-inflammatory action via its corticosteroid receptor agonist properties[539,540] and has been reported as beneficial in a case of psoriatic arthritis.[541]

- **STYLE OF LIVING (LIFESTYLE) & SPECIAL CONSIDERATIONS: Sleep optimization, SocioPsychology, Stress management/avoidance, Somatic treatments, Special Supplementation, Sweat/exercise, Sauna/detoxification, Surgery, Stamp your passport and vacate current reality, Sensory deprivation therapy**
  This is a buffet of mostly lifestyle-based interventions yet also including considerations such as somatic treatments, additional supplementation, and surgery.
    o Folinic acid or methylfolate 5-20 mg per day: Patients with psoriasis have reduced folate status and elevated homocysteine levels.[542] Wright and Gaby recommended 50-150 mg per day of folic acid for psoriatics.[543] Folic acid has antiproliferative and anti-inflammatory effects mediated by nutrigenomic mechanisms. Folic acid, along with other vitamins and nutrients, may also help alleviate the biochemical aspect of the depression that is common in patients with psoriasis. Always supplement with vitamin B-12 in form of hydroxocobalamin or methylcobalamin (e.g., 2,000 mcg per day) when using high-dose folic acid. Most clinicians no longer use folic acid due to is causation of intracellular oxidative stress and association with malignancy; instead, folinic acid and methylated folate are preferred.
    o Topical *Berberis/Mahonia*: Topical *Berberis/Mahonia* is effective for dermal psoriasis.[544] Very obviously, topical treatments do not address the underlying problems in psoriasis and should therefore only be used for symptomatic/cosmetic improvement within the context of an overall treatment plan designed to correct the underlying/internal imbalances.
    o Topical *Capsicum annuum, Capsicum frutescens* (Cayenne pepper, hot chili pepper): Topical capsaicin has proven beneficial for alleviating the pruritus of psoriasis, presumably by depleting cutaneous neurons of substance P.[545] Very obviously, topical treatments do not address the underlying problems in psoriasis and should therefore only be used for symptomatic/cosmetic improvement within the context of an overall treatment plan designed to correct the underlying/internal imbalances.
    o Spinal manipulation: Many years ago I read a published case report of a female patient who experienced acute onset of psoriasis following trauma received during a skiing accident. Her psoriasis resolved promptly following a series of treatments of chiropractic spinal manipulative therapy.
    o Hydrotherapy, local hyperthermia: Hot bath hyperthermia (or heating pads[546]) improves skin lesions and lessens pruritus in the majority of patients with psoriasis.[547] The dermatologic improvements following hyperthermia can be objectively documented clinically and histologically/microscopically.[548]

- **ENDOCRINE IMBALANCE & OPTIMIZATION: Prolactin, Insulin, Estrogen, DHEA, Cortisol, Testosterone, Thyroid** Common hormonal imbalances seen among autoimmune/inflammatory patients are: ❶ *elevated* prolactin, ❷ *elevated* estrogen, ❸ *elevated* insulin, and ❹ *reduced* DHEA, ❺ *reduced* cortisol, and ❻ *reduced* testosterone; see Chapter 4 for discussion of these hormones and respective interventions. Thyroid evaluation (patient + labs) should be comprehensive, as discussed in Chapter 1, with a low threshold for empiric treatment.
    o Melatonin: Melatonin is a pineal hormone with well-known sleep-inducing and immunomodulatory properties, and it is commonly administered in doses of 1-40 mg in the evening, before bedtime. Its

---

[539] "Accumulating evidence from both animal and human studies indicates that pharmacologic doses of L-carnitine (LCAR) have immunomodulatory effects resembling those of glucocorticoids (GC)." Manoli I, et al. Modulatory effects of L-carnitine on glucocorticoid receptor activity. *Ann N Y Acad Sci*. 2004 Nov;1033:147-57
[540] "Taken together, our results suggest that pharmacological doses of L-carnitine can activate GRalpha and, through this mechanism, regulate glucocorticoid-responsive genes, potentially sharing some of the biological and therapeutic properties of glucocorticoids."Alesci S, De Martino MU, Mirani M, Benvenga S, Trimarchi F, Kino T, Chrousos GP. L-carnitine: A nutritional modulator of glucocorticoid receptor functions. *FASEB J*. 2003 Aug;17(11):1553-5. Epub 2003 Jun 17 fasebj.org/cgi/reprint/02-1024fjev1
[541] Afeltra et al. Clinical improvement in psoriatic arthritis symptoms during treatment for infertility with carnitine. *Clin Exp Rheumatol*. 2004 Jan-Feb;22(1):138
[542] "The mean levels of serum tHcy, fibrinogen, fibronectin, sICAM, PAI-1 and AuAb-oxLDL were increased in patients whereas tPA, vitamin B(12) and folate levels were decreased significantly." Vanizor Kural et al. Plasma homocysteine and its relationships with atherothrombotic markers in psoriatic patients. *Clin Chim Acta*. 2003 Jun;332:23-30
[543] Gaby A, Wright JV. *Nutritional Protocols*. 1998 Nutrition Seminars
[544] "Taken together, these clinical studies conducted by several investigators in several countries indicate that Mahonia aquifolium is a safe and effective treatment of patients with mild to moderate psoriasis." Gulliver WP, Donsky HJ. A report on three recent clinical trials using Mahonia aquifolium 10% topical cream and a review of the worldwide clinical experience with Mahonia aquifolium for the treatment of plaque psoriasis. *Am J Ther*. 2005 Sep-Oct;12:398-406
[545] "CONCLUSION: Topically applied capsaicin effectively treats pruritic psoriasis, a finding that supports a role for substance P in this disorder." Ellis CN, et al. A double-blind evaluation of topical capsaicin in pruritic psoriasis. *J Am Acad Dermatol* 1993 Sep;29(3):438-42
[546] Urabe H, Nishitani K, Kohda H. Hyperthermia in the treatment of psoriasis. *Arch Dermatol*. 1981 Dec;117(12):770-4
[547] "These results indicate that simple repetitive water bath hyperthermia alone is effective in the treatment of psoriatic lesions in heatable locations." Boreham DR, Gasmann HC, Mitchel RE. Water bath hyperthermia is a simple therapy for psoriasis and also stimulates skin tanning in response to sunlight. *Int J Hyperthermia*. 1995 Nov-Dec;11(6):745-54
[548] "Electron microscopy of psoriatic skin prior to and after local hyperthermia revealed both temporary and gradual changes following treatment." Imayama S, Urabe H. Human psoriatic skin lesions improve with local hyperthermia: an ultrastructural study. *J Cutan Pathol*. 1984 Feb;11(1):45-52

exceptional safety is well documented. Although psoriatic patients appear to have lost the physiologic nocturnal peak of melatonin[549], the role of supplemental melatonin in the treatment of patients with psoriasis has not been researched; however clinicians may reasonably decide to add this to their patients' treatment plan as appropriate. In contrast to implementing treatment with high doses of 20-40 mg, starting with a relatively low dose (e.g., 1-5 mg) and increasing as tolerated is recommended. Melatonin (20 mg hs) appears to have cured two patients with drug-resistant sarcoidosis[550] and 3 mg provided immediate short-term benefit to a patient with multiple sclerosis.[551] Immunostimulatory anti-infective action of melatonin was demonstrated in a clinical trial wherein septic newborns administered 20 mg melatonin showed significantly increased survival over nontreated controls[552]; given that psoriasis is associated with many subclinical infections, melatonin may provide therapeutic benefit by virtue of its anti-infective properties.

- o Prolactin (excess): According to clinical trials with small numbers of patients, whether prolactin levels are high or not, treatment with prolactin-lowering treatment (such as bromocriptine[553]) appears beneficial in patients with psoriatic arthritis. Serum prolactin is the standard assessment of prolactin status. Since elevated prolactin may be a sign of pituitary tumor, assessment for headaches, visual deficits, other abnormalities of pituitary hormones (e.g., GH and TSH) should be performed and CT or MRI must be considered. Patients with prolactin levels less than 100 ng/mL and normal CT/MRI findings can be managed conservatively with effective prolactin-lowering treatment and annual radiologic assessment (less necessary with favorable serum response).[554, see review 555] Patients with RA and SLE have higher basal and stress-induced levels of prolactin compared with normal controls.[556,557] A normal serum prolactin level does not necessarily exclude the use of prolactin-lowering intervention, especially since many autoimmune patients have latent hyperprolactinemia which may not be detected with random serum measurement of prolactin. Bromocriptine has long been considered the pharmacologic treatment of choice for elevated prolactin.[558] Bromocriptine appears to benefit most patients with psoriasis/psoriatic arthritis, according to a small Italian study[559] and three case reports in the French literature.[560] Typical dose is 2.5 mg per day (effective against lupus[561]); gastrointestinal upset and sedation are common.[562] Clinical intervention with bromocriptine appears warranted in patients with RA, SLE, Reiter's syndrome, psoriatic arthritis, and probably multiple sclerosis and uveitis.[563] A normal serum prolactin level does not necessarily exclude the use of prolactin-lowering intervention, especially since many autoimmune patients have latent hyperprolactinemia which may not be detected with random serum measurement of prolactin. Cabergoline/Dostinex is a newer dopamine agonist with few adverse effects; typical dose

---

[549] "Our results show that psoriatic patients had lost the nocturnal peak and usual circadian rhythm of melatonin secretion. Levels of melatonin were significantly lower than in controls at 2 a.m., and higher at 6 and 8 a.m. and at 12 noon." Mozzanica et al. Plasma melatonin levels in psoriasis. *Acta Derm Venereol*. 1988;68(4):312-6

[550] Cagnoni ML, Lombardi A, Cerinic MC, Dedola GL, Pignone A. Melatonin for treatment of chronic refractory sarcoidosis. *Lancet*. 1995 Nov 4;346(8984):1229-30

[551] "...administration of melatonin (3 mg, orally) at 2:00 p.m., when the patient experienced severe blurring of vision, resulted within 15 minutes in a dramatic improvement in visual acuity and in normalization of the visual evoked potential latency after stimulation of the left eye." Sandyk R. Diurnal variations in vision and relations to circadian melatonin secretion in multiple sclerosis. *Int J Neurosci*. 1995 Nov;83(1-2):1-6

[552] Gittoet al. Effects of melatonin treatment in septic newborns. *Pediatr Res*. 2001 Dec;50(6):756-60 pedresearch.org/cgi/content/full/50/6/756

[553] "In 2 cases of psoriatic arthritis, adding bromocriptine to gold salts and nonsteroidal anti-inflammatory drug was followed by a drastic efficacy with spectacular improvement in clinical, biological and occupational status. Because none of the cases had hyperprolactinaemia, bromocriptine acted probably had an intrinic anti-inflammatory effect independent of its antiproclactinic effect." Eulry F, Mayaudon H, Bauduceau B, Lechevalier D, Crozes P, Magnin J, Claude-Berthelot C. [Blood prolactin under the effect of protirelin in spondylarthropathies. Treatment trial of 4 cases of reactive arthritis and 2 cases of psoriatic arthritis with bromocriptine] *Ann Med Interne* (Paris). 1996;147(1):15-9. French.

[554] Beers MH, Berkow R (eds). *The Merck Manual. Seventeenth Edition*. Whitehouse Station; Merck Research Laboratories 1999 Page 77-78

[555] Serri O, Chik CL, Ur E, Ezzat S. Diagnosis and management of hyperprolactinemia. *CMAJ*. 2003 Sep 16;169(6):575-81 cmaj.ca/cgi/content/full/169/6/575

[556] Dostal C, et al. Serum prolactin stress values in patients with systemic lupus erythematosus. *Ann Rheum Dis*. 2003 May;62(5):487-8

[557] "RESULTS: A significantly higher rate of elevated PRL levels was found in SLE patients (40.0%) compared with the healthy controls (14.8%). No proof was found of association with the presence of anti-ds-DNA or with specific organ involvement. Similarly, elevated PRL levels were found in RA patients (39.3%)." Moszkorzova L, Lacinova Z, Marek J, Musilova L, Dohnalova A, Dostal C. Hyperprolactinaemia in patients with systemic lupus erythematosus. *Clin Exp Rheumatol*. 2002 Nov-Dec;20(6):807-12

[558] Beers MH, Berkow R (eds). *The Merck Manual. Seventeenth Edition.* Whitehouse Station; Merck Research Laboratories 1999 Page 77-78

[559] "Bromocriptin was shown to be effective in 13 of our 18 psoriatic patients." Valentino A, Fimiani M, Bilenchi R, Castelli A, Francini G, Gonnelli S, Gennari C, Andreassi L. [Therapy with bromocriptine and behavior of various hormones in psoriasis patients] *Boll Soc Ital Biol Sper*. 1984 Oct 30;60(10):1841-4. Italian.

[560] "All three were treated with bromocriptine (5 mg/d in 2 doses) after verification of normal baseline and protirelin-stimulation prolactin levels. There was a beneficial effect in nocturnal pain relief, morning stiffness, the Lee and Ritchie scores and biological markers of inflammation." Eulry F, Mayaudon H, Lechevalier D, Bauduceau B, Ariche L, Ouakil H, Crozes P, Magnin J. [Treatment of rheumatoid psoriasis with bromocriptine] *Presse Med*. 1995 Nov 18;24(35):1642-4. French.

[561] "A prospective, double-blind, randomized, placebo-controlled study compared BRC at a fixed daily dosage of 2.5 mg with placebo... Long term treatment with a low dose of BRC appears to be a safe and effective means of decreasing SLE flares in SLE patients." Alvarez-Nemegyei J, Cobarrubias-Cobos A, Escalante-Triay F, Sosa-Munoz J, Miranda JM, Jara LJ. Bromocriptine in systemic lupus erythematosus: a double-blind, randomized, placebo-controlled study. *Lupus*. 1998;7(6):414-9

[562] Serri O, Chik CL, Ur E, Ezzat S. Diagnosis and management of hyperprolactinemia. *CMAJ*. 2003 Sep 16;169(6):575-81 cmaj.ca/cgi/content/full/169/6/575

[563] "...clinical observations and trials support the use of bromocriptine as a nonstandard primary or adjunctive therapy in the treatment of recalcitrant RA, SLE, Reiter's syndrome, and psoriatic arthritis and associated conditions unresponsive to traditional approaches." McMurray RW. Bromocriptine in rheumatic and autoimmune diseases. *Semin Arthritis Rheum*. 2001 Aug;31(1):21-32

starts at 0.5 mg per week (0.25 mg twice per week).[564] Several studies have indicated that cabergoline is safer and more effective than bromocriptine for reducing prolactin levels[565] and the dose can often be reduced after successful prolactin reduction, allowing for reductions in cost and adverse effects.[566] Although fewer studies have been published supporting the antirheumatic benefits of cabergoline than those supporting bromocriptine; its antirheumatic benefits have indeed been documented.[567]

- o Estrogen (excess): Although the classic pattern in patients with autoimmunity is elevated estrogen (generally considered immunodysregulatory) and reduced testosterone (generally considered anti-inflammatory and immunoregulatory), data in patients with psoriatic arthritis is inadequate to extend this otherwise consistent and successful generalization to this group. On the contrary, Stevens et al[568] published a case report of a woman with recalcitrant psoriasis and psoriatic arthritis who responded very well to anti-estrogen treatment. The small amount of data available actually suggests that estrogen may be beneficial (reduction in skin lesions with pregnancy) and that testosterone (in one woman who developed psoriasis following a testosterone-containing hormonal implant following oophorectomy) could exacerbate the disease.

> **Estrogen promotes inflammation**
> "We report a patient with severe psoriatic arthritis in whom the severity of both the arthritis and psoriasis fluctuated with the menstrual cycle. These features failed to improve with standard therapy, but there was a prompt response to treatment which suppressed estrogen secretion."
>
> Stevens HP, et al. Cyclical psoriatic arthritis responding to anti-oestrogen therapy. *Br J Dermatol*. 1993 Oct

- o Testosterone (insufficiency): Androgen deficiencies predispose to, are exacerbated by, and contribute to autoimmune/inflammatory disorders. Female patients with psoriasis have lower levels of testosterone compared to those seen in healthy controls.[569] A large proportion of men with lupus or RA have low testosterone[570] and suffer the effects of hypogonadism: fatigue, weakness, depression, slow healing, low libido, and difficulties with sexual performance. Testosterone levels may rise following DHEA supplementation (especially in women) and can be elevated in men by the use of anastrozole/Arimidex. Otherwise, transdermal testosterone such as Androgel or Testim can be applied as indicated.

- o DHEA: DHEA is an anti-inflammatory and immunoregulatory hormone that is commonly deficient in patients with autoimmunity and inflammatory arthritis.[571] However, the role of DHEA in psoriatic arthritis *en masse* is unclear due to conflicting data. One study showed that patients with psoriasis did not show evidence of DHEA insufficiency[572], while other studies—especially in the German literature—have consistently documented low serum and intracellular levels of DHEA.[573] DHEA levels should be measured in these patients—especially those with severe disease, deficiencies should be treated unless contraindicated, and therapeutic trials are not unreasonable.

- **XENOBIOTIC ACCUMULATION & DETOXIFICATION: Chemical avoidance, nutritional support for detoxification pathways, urine alkalinization** The clinical relevance and pathogenic mechanisms of xenobiotic accumulation are irrefutably well documented and described. Clinical assessments include history, physical examination, and laboratory assessment (using serum, whole blood, urine or—rarely yet accurately—fat biopsy), and response to treatment. Treatments include nutritional support for Phases 1 and 2 of

---

[564] Serri O, Chik CL, Ur E, Ezzat S. Diagnosis and management of hyperprolactinemia. *CMAJ*. 2003 Sep 16;169(6):575-81

[565] "CONCLUSION: These data indicate that cabergoline is a very effective agent for lowering the prolactin levels in hyperprolactinemic patients and that it appears to offer considerable advantage over bromocriptine in terms of efficacy and tolerability." Sabuncu T, Arikan E, Tasan E, Hatemi H. Comparison of the effects of cabergoline and bromocriptine on prolactin levels in hyperprolactinemic patients. *Intern Med*. 2001 Sep;40(9):857-61

[566] "Cabergoline also normalized PRL in the majority of patients with known bromocriptine intolerance or -resistance. Once PRL secretion was adequately controlled, the dose of cabergoline could often be significantly decreased, which further reduced costs of therapy." Verhelst et al. Cabergoline in the treatment of hyperprolactinemia: a study in 455 patients. *J Clin Endocrinol Metab*. 1999 Jul;84(7):2518-22 jcem.endojournals.org/cgi/content/full/84/7/2518

[567] Erb N, Pace AV, Delamere JP, Kitas GD. Control of unremitting rheumatoid arthritis by the prolactin antagonist cabergoline. *Rheumatology* (Oxford). 2001 Feb;40(2):237-9 rheumatology.oxfordjournals.org/cgi/content/full/40/2/237

[568] "We report a patient with severe psoriatic arthritis in whom the severity of both the arthritis and psoriasis fluctuated with the menstrual cycle. These features failed to improve with standard therapy, but there was a prompt response to treatment which suppressed oestrogen secretion." Stevens HP, Ostlere LS, Black CM, Jacobs HS, Rustin MH. Cyclical psoriatic arthritis responding to anti-oestrogen therapy. *Br J Dermatol*. 1993 Oct;129(4):458-60

[569] "The testosterone levels and LH/FSH ratio were significantly lower in the psoriatic group." Pietrzak A, Lecewicz-Torun B, Jakimiuk A. Lipid and hormone profile in psoriatic females. *Ann Univ Mariae Curie Sklodowska* [Med]. 2002;57(2):478-83

[570] Karagiannis A, Harsoulis F. Gonadal dysfunction in systemic diseases. *Eur J Endocrinol*. 2005 Apr;152(4):501-13 eje-online.org/cgi/content/full/152/4/501

[571] "DHEAS concentrations were significantly decreased in both women and men with inflammatory arthritis (IA) (P < 0.001)." Dessein PH, et al. Hyposecretion of the adrenal androgen dehydroepiandrosterone sulfate and its relation to clinical variables in inflammatory arthritis. *Arthritis Res*. 2001;3(3):183-8 arthritis-research.com/content/3/3/183

[572] "Assessing the patients by group, the mean DHEAS level was markedly lower in the pemphigoid/pemphigus than in the psoriasis and OA patients (geometric mean 600 vs. 2130 and 2100 nmol/l, respectively; p < 0.001)." de la Torre B, Fransson J, Scheynius A. Blood dehydroepiandrosterone sulphate (DHEAS) levels in pemphigoid/pemphigus and psoriasis. *Clin Exp Rheumatol*. 1995 May-Jun;13(3):345-8

[573] "The effects of this dehydroepiandrosterone deficiency are changes in the humoral regulation of events in growth and proliferation in patients with psoriasis." Holzmann H, Benes P, Morsches B. [Dehydroepiandrosterone deficiency in psoriasis. Hypothesis on the etiopathogenesis of this disease] *Hautarzt*. 1980 Feb;31(2):71-5. Review. German.

detoxification (e.g., oxidation and conjugation) and excretion via bile and urine; for the latter, urinary alkalinization is generally recommended. Chemical toxins can be bound in the gut using activated charcoal, cholestyramine, or *Chlorella*—all of these three treatments have documented safety and effectiveness; clinically and empirically, phytochelatin (plant-derived peptides that bind toxic metals) concentrates appear safe and effective despite lack of conclusive published data supporting clinical use.

- Detoxification support: Cytochrome P450 (Cyp450) defects (phenotypic—not genotropic—in this research) have been noted in patients with psoriasis and correlate with the severity of the disease.[574] Assuming a causal relationship, one can speculate as to the nature and direction of that relationship:
  - Cause of disease: Perhaps the detoxification defects lead to xenobiotic accumulation which alters immune function in favor of xenobiotic immunotoxicity: resulting in immune impairment and exaggerated inflammatory response.
  - Effect of disease: Perhaps the inflammation or oxidative stress or nutritional deficiencies of psoriasis is/are the cause of the detoxification defects.
  - Shared causality: Perhaps the increased total bacterial load impairs Cyp450 via LPS and also causes the inflammatory dysfunction that precipitates psoriasis.
  - Nonexclusivity, additive/synergistic effects: All of the above.

---

[574] "Low CYP2C activity was associated with severe psoriasis, poor metaboliser status occurring in 50% of the severe group, but in none of the mild cases, p < 0.01." Helsby NA, et al. Hepatic cytochrome P450 CYP2C activity in psoriasis: studies using proguanil as a probe compound. *Acta Derm Venereol* 1998 Mar;78(2):81-3

Systemic Lupus Erythematosus: "SLE" or "Lupus"

> **Introduction:**
> As was said to me once by a Vice President of one of the largest hospital systems in Texas, SLE is a "big league" disease with numerous and potentially fatal complications; it is not to be taken lightly. Best interests of both doctor and patient are served by having a rheumatologist and/or internist as part of the care team. SLE is the prototype of multiorgan autoimmunity, mediated by a combination of cellular and humoral factors especially including immune-complex deposition and localized inflammation in the vascular system (vasculitis), skin (dermatitis), joints (arthritis) and kidneys (nephritis).

Description/pathophysiology:

- SLE as the prototype of multisystem autoimmune disease: SLE is the prototype of multisystem autoimmune disease, characterized by a chronic progressive course with remissions and relapses; as the prototype of multiorgan "idiopathic" autoimmunity, SLE will serve to model facts and concepts that are applicable to other conditions. The skin, joints, kidneys, serosal membranes (pleura, pericardium, peritoneum), and vascular system are the most prominent targets of inflammatory attack; however, any cell and tissue may be damaged, either directly or indirectly. Autoantibodies (and resultant immune complexes) against a wide range of endogenous/self targets are pathogenic in SLE; however, **the current pathologic paradigm places ultimate responsibility on CD4+ helper T-cells—i.e., e.g., the Th1, Th2, Th17, and Treg cells discussed in Chapter 4—** rather than the antibody-producing B-cells/plasma cells. Tissue damage in SLE is largely mediated by autoantibodies—particularly anti-nuclear antibodies (ANA)—and the resulting immune complexes, cryoglobulins, and the subsequent inflammatory cascade.[575,576,577,578] **Patients with SLE have impaired ability to clear immune complexes via hepatic and splenic routes**[579,580]; therapeutic implications are discussed below. **SLE is considered a type-3 hypersensitivity disease because it is largely mediated by immune complex deposition** and secondary activation of the complement cascade and other inflammatory pathways.

  > **Immune complex pathophysiology**
  > Consecutive linking of antigen and antibody results in formation of immune complexes which are predisposed for deposition in joints, skin, kidneys, and vasculature. Immune complex deposition results in focal and atopic (distant from site of antigen exposure) inflammatory damage of surrounding tissue via local activation of complement pathway and local inflammation, including recruitment of neutrophils and monocytes which release free radicals and autolytic lysosomal enzymes.

- Allopathic perspective = "idiopathic": This condition is generally considered "idiopathic" in most cases, though in some patients the disease is induced by pharmaceutical drugs (especially hydralazine, procainamide, D-penicillamine) and is then generally reversible upon discontinuation of the drug. Most people with complement deficiencies (a group of congenital immune defects) develop SLE. Other precipitating/contributing factors include ultraviolet light exposure, chemical exposure, and possibly consumption of alfalfa sprouts (based on animal data[581] and very little human data). Abnormal hormone metabolism has also been noted and may play a role in the pathogenesis as described in the section on *Orthoendocrinology*.

- Integrative/functional/naturopathic perspective = multifactorial: Numerous—not innumerable—factors contribute to SLE pathogenesis; these are well represented within the FINDSEX™ of the functional inflammology protocol.

- The role of microbes, especially viral infections: The cytokine pattern and many of the pathogenic features of SLE have pointed toward "a viral etiology" for many years; one is simultaneously challenged with the paradox of wanting to accept this as plausible and wanting to reject it as yet another *undefined* and therefore *useless* and

---

[575] Tierney ML. McPhee SJ, Papadakis MA (eds). *Current Medical Diagnosis and Treatment 2006. 45th edition*. New York; Lange Medical Books: 2006, pages 833-837
[576] Suzuki et al. Development of pathogenic anti-DNA antibodies in patients with systemic lupus erythematosus. *FASEB J*. 1997 Oct;11:1033-8 fasebj.org/cgi/reprint/11/12/1033
[577] "Pisetsky DS. Antibody responses to DNA in normal immunity and aberrant immunity. *Clin Diagn Lab Immunol*. 1998 Jan;5(1):1-6 cvi.asm.org/cgi/reprint/5/1/1
[578] Sikander FF, Salgaonkar DS, Joshi VR. Cryoglobulin studies in systemic lupus erythematosus. *J Postgrad Med* [serial online] 1989 [cited 2005 Nov 2];35:139-43
[579] "These observations support the hypothesis that IC handling is abnormal in SLE." Davies KA, Peters AM, Beynon HL, Walport MJ. Immune complex processing in patients with systemic lupus erythematosus. In vivo imaging and clearance studies. *J Clin Invest*. 1992 Nov;90(5):2075-83
[580] "These results indicate that Fc-mediated clearance of ICs is defective in patients with SLE and suggest that ligation of ICs by Fc receptors is critical for their efficient binding and retention by the fixed MPS in the liver." Davies KA, Robson MG, Peters AM, Norsworthy P, Nash JT, Walport MJ. Defective Fc-dependent processing of immune complexes in patients with systemic lupus erythematosus. *Arthritis Rheum*. 2002 Apr;46(4):1028-38
[581] "L-Canavanine sulfate, a constituent of alfalfa sprouts, was incorporated into the diet and reactivated the syndrome in monkeys in which an SLE-like syndrome had previously been induced by the ingestion of alfalfa seeds or sprouts." Malinow MR, Bardana EJ Jr, Pirofsky B, Craig S, McLaughlin P. Systemic lupus erythematosus-like syndrome in monkeys fed alfalfa sprouts: role of a nonprotein amino acid. *Science*. 1982 Apr 23;216(4544):415-7

therefore *idiopathic* allopathic description of disease pathogenesis. With more currently available research however, I think the viral hypothesis—or more accurately the *poly*viral and polymicrobial model—is gaining credible and clinically usable merit. I will outline this territory as I see it:

- Increased and/or altered total microbial load (TML): Some evidence has shown that SLE patients have evidence of increased microbial loads—both bacterial and viral. For example, patients with SLE, psoriasis, Wegener's, and eczema have all shown increased nasal carriage of *Staphylococcus aureus*. Even if no immune abnormalities were present, increased antigenic exposure would be expected to result in increased humor antibody response and the formation of more—perhaps a pathogenic "excess" of—immune complexes; if the immune system were hyperresponsive, say due to vitamin D deficiency and the resulting lack of Treg induction, then the situation would only get worse as the causes of immune hyperresponsiveness become additive or synergistic. Obviously, the TML contributes directly and powerfully to the TIL—total inflammatory load.

- Impaired immune complex clearance: Impaired clearance of immune complexes would—of course—complicate the aforementioned problems associated with increased TML and TIL; in fact, the result would be a positive/upward dissociation of the TIL from the TML as the inflammatory consequences become greater than normal/proportionate.

The total viral load (TVL): TVL contributes to TML (total microbial load) and thus to the TIL (total inflammatory load), to which are added the TCL (total carbohydrate load) and TXL (total xenobiotic load).

- Viruses, part 1—Known/popular "epigenomic" viruses: I categorize as "known" and/or "popular" those viruses that we commonly consider, such as Epstein-Bar virus (EBV), parvovirus B-19 (PvB19), cytomegalovirus (CMV), human papilloma virus (HPV) and other such viruses as we generally consider clinically and/or studied in whatever medical school we as clinicians attended. These have been described as epigenomic and/or exogenous viruses because they are close to but not part of the human genome— "epi" is a Greek-derived prefix denoting "above, on, over, nearby, upon"; these *epigenomic* viruses are contrasted with the *endogenous* viruses that are integrally "built in" to the human DNA. All four viruses mentioned in the previous sentence have been associated with autoimmunity; more recently has arrived the data supporting our new appreciation that "autoimmune patients" *may well be* and *generally are* "actively infected" with many of these viruses simultaneously—this is well-documented now in scleroderma, patients with which show active and "ectopic" (unusual locations) infections simultaneously with EBV, PvB19, and CMV. *Helicobacter pylori* may play a powerful role as a synergistic bioagent via its ability to *simultaneously* and *paradoxically* cause immunosuppression (thereby allowing other microbes to flourish) and systemic inflammation[582]; in this manner, the bacterial infection is permissive to and perhaps necessary for the autoimmune-inducing vasculopathic and fibrogenic viral infections (see section on Scleroderma for pathology details). An important concept to remember is that viral infections promote other viral infections—transactivation—via direct genomic enhancement of viral replication, by promoting a favorable cytokine environment for viral replication, and/or by stimulating

---

[582] "Infectious agents such as Helicobacter pylori (Hp) may cause chronic inflammation and autoimmune reactivity in susceptible subjects. The results of in vitro experiments performed with lymphocytes from Hp infected patients indicate that Hp can cause immunosuppression which might be eliminated by successful eradication therapy." Hybenova et al. The role of environmental factors in autoimmune thyroiditis. *Neuro Endocrinol Lett.* 2010;31(3):283-9

NFkB which is commonly "hijacked" by viruses to promote viral replication; therefore activation or suppression of any virus can be said to contribute *indirectly* to the activation or suppression, respectively, of other viral populations.[583] Relatedly and as will be discussed in the following section on endogenous viruses, replication of exogenous/epigenomic viruses—such as influenza virus and herpes simplex type-1—increases expression of endogenous viruses.

> **Rationale for anti-viral therapy for treating autoimmunity**
>
> "Cited epidemiologic and experimental evidence suggests that increased replication of epigenomic viral pathogens such as Epstein-Barr Virus (EBV) in chronic human autoimmune diseases such as rheumatoid arthritis (RA), systemic lupus erythematosus (SLE), and multiple sclerosis (MS) may activate endogenous human retroviruses (HERV) as a pathologic mechanism."
>
> Dreyfus DH. Autoimmune disease: A role for new anti-viral therapies? *Autoimmun Rev.* 2011 Dec

- Epstein-Barr virus in the pathogenesis of some autoimmune disorders (*Eur J Microbiol Immunol* 2011 Dec[584]): "Moreover, many observations indicate that EBV contributes also to the pathomechanism of SLE. However, this contribution differs from the relationship between EBV and MS, as shown by the lack of any increase in the risk of SLE after IM [infectious mononucleosis]. In SLE, EBV serology is quantitatively and qualitatively different from the normal response - that is, EBV viral load is higher and a strong cross-reaction can be detected between certain EBV antigens and autoantigens of pathological importance."

- Lupus and Epstein-Barr (*Curr Opin Rheumatol* 2012 Jul[585]): "SLE patients have a dysregulated immune response against EBV. EBV antigens exhibit structural molecular mimicry with common SLE antigens and functional molecular mimicry with critical immune-regulatory components. SLE patients, from a number of unique geographic regions, are shown to have higher rates of EBV seroconversion, especially against early EBV antigens, suggesting frequent viral reactivation. SLE patients also have increased EBV viral loads and impaired EBV-specific CD8 cytotoxic T cells, with impaired cytokine responses to EBV in lupus patients. ... Recent advances demonstrate SLE-specific serologic responses, gene expression, viral load, T-cell responses, humoral fine specificity, and molecular mimicry with EBV, further supporting potential roles for EBV in lupus etiology and pathogenesis."

- HTLV (human T-lymphotropic virus) in SLE (*Clin Immunol.* 2002 Feb[586]): "SLE patients produce high titer antibodies to various retroviral proteins, including Gag, Env, and Nef of HIV and HTLV (human T-lymphotropic virus), in the absence of overt retroviral infection. ... In particular, we consider the role of HTLV-1-related endogenous sequence (HRES-1) in SLE. We propose that molecular mimicry between HRES-1 and the small ribonucleoprotein complex initiates the production of autoantibodies, leading to immune complex formation, complement fixation, and pathological tissue deposition."

o Viruses, part 2—Human endogenous retroviruses (endoretroviruses, HERVs or ERVs): Human DNA is "pre-loaded" with remnants of viral infections that have coursed through and been transmitted from parents to offspring for millions of years; these endogenous viral genomes implanted into human DNA are now known to undergo reactivation with the production of immunogenic viral remnants and the anticipated inflammatory immune response. As mentioned previously related to exogenous viral transactivation, replication of exogenous/epigenomic viruses—such as influenza virus and herpes simplex type-1—increases expression of endogenous viruses[587]; as such, one method to reduce/control activation of HERVs is to suppress replication of exogenous viruses. HERV activation is inhibited by

---

[583] White et al. Reciprocal transactivation between HIV-1 and other human viruses. *Virology.* 2006 Aug 15;352(1):1-13
[584] Füst G. The role of the Epstein-Barr virus in the pathogenesis of some autoimmune disorders - Similarities and differences. *Eur J Microbiol Immunol* (Bp). 2011 Dec;1:267-78
[585] James JA, Robertson JM. Lupus and Epstein-Barr. *Curr Opin Rheumatol.* 2012 Jul;24(4):383-8
[586] Adelman MK, Marchalonis JJ. Endogenous retroviruses in systemic lupus erythematosus: candidate lupus viruses. *Clin Immunol.* 2002 Feb;102(2):107-16
[587] "Since viral infections have previously been reported to transactivate retroviral long terminal repeat regions we examined the basal expression of HERV-W elements and following infections by influenza A/WSN/33 and Herpes simplex 1 viruses in human cell-lines. ... Subsets of HERV-W elements were transactivated by viral infection in the different cell-lines. Transcriptional activation of these elements, including that encoding syncytin, was dependent on viral replication and was not induced by antiviral responses." Nellaker et al. Transactivation of elements in the human endogenous retrovirus W family by viral infection. *Retrovirology.* 2006 Jul 6;3:44

DNA methylation; conversely, DNA hypomethylation is consistently associated with SLE in humans and animals.[588,589]

- Human endogenous retroviruses in the development of autoimmune diseases (*Int Rev Immunol* 2010 Aug[590]): In 2010, Balada et al provided a succinct and authoritative summary of HERVs and their relationship to the pathogenesis of autoimmunity: "Retroviruses can exist in an endogenous form, in which viral sequences are integrated into the human germ line and are vertically transmitted in a Mendelian fashion. Human endogenous retroviruses (HERVs), probably representing footprints of ancient germ-cell retroviral infections, occupy about 1% of the human genome. ... Although some of these elements show mutations and deletions, some HERVs are transcriptionally active and produce functional proteins. Some medical conditions, such as cancer and autoimmune diseases, are linked to the transcription of some of the HERVs genes, to the expression of HERVs proteins (that may act as superantigens, for example), and/or to the development of antibodies against them that might cross-react with our own proteins. Their genetic sequences may also be, totally or partially, integrated into genes that regulate the immune response. These mechanisms could give rise to autoimmune diseases, such as lupus erythematosus, insulin-dependent diabetes mellitus, multiple sclerosis, Sjögren's syndrome, and rheumatoid arthritis, among others."

> **HERV-autoimmunity associations**
> - **Rheumatoid arthritis**: expression of multiple ERVs detected in RA patients; HERV-K10 shows molecular mimicry
> - **Juvenile RA**: HERV-K10
> - **Multiple sclerosis**: MS-associated retroviral element (MRSV)-type HERV-W; increased expression of the env RNA and protein expression in the blood and brain cells of MS patients; also clear increase in HERV-H/F family HERV-Fc1 activity and RNA production; HERV-K18 on chromosome 1 is a risk factor for MS
> - **Psoriasis**: Increased expression of HERV-W, K, E, and variant ERV-9/HERV-W
> - **Lupus**: Hypomethylation of HERV-E and HERV-K
>
> **Mechanisms for HERV-induced autoimmune diseases**:
> - Molecular mimicry (HERV-K10)
> - Superantigen production (HERV-K)
> - LTR (long terminal repeat)-mediated alterations of gene expression
> - Antigenicity and immune complex formation
>
> **Activation of HERVs**:
> - DNA hypomethylation
> - Transactivation

Clear and complete as that is, readers might reasonably want additional sources of support, and I have provided samples of such here:

- Human endogenous retroviruses in the pathogenesis of autoimmune diseases (*Med Sci Monit.* 2012 Jun[591]): "This theory takes into account the existence in the human genome, since approximately 40 million years, of so-called human endogenous retroviruses (HERVs), which are transmitted to descendants vertically by the germ cells. It was recently established that these generally silent sequences perform some physiological roles, but occasionally become active and influence the development of some chronic diseases like diabetes, some neoplasms, chronic diseases of the nervous system (e.g., sclerosis multiplex), schizophrenia and autoimmune diseases."
- Endogenous retroviral pathogenesis in lupus (*Curr Opin Rheumatol.* 2010 Sep[592]): "ERV proteins may trigger lupus through structural and functional molecular mimicry, whereas the accumulation of ERV-derived nucleic acids stimulates interferon and anti-DNA antibody production in SLE."
- Autoimmune disease treatment with anti-viral therapies (*Autoimmun Rev* 2011 Dec[593]): "Cited epidemiologic and experimental evidence suggests that increased replication of epigenomic viral pathogens such as Epstein-Barr Virus (EBV) in chronic human autoimmune diseases such as rheumatoid arthritis (RA), systemic lupus Erythematosus (SLE), and multiple sclerosis (MS) may activate endogenous human retroviruses (HERV) as a pathologic mechanism. ... Other [drug] anti-

---

[588] "This raises the possibility that HERV demethylation participates in the pathogenesis of SLE." Renaudineau et al. Epigenetics and autoimmunity, with special emphasis on methylation. *Keio J Med.* 2011;60(1):10-6
[589] "Hypomethylation of HERV-E and HERV-K was also observed in SLE patients." Katoh et al. Association of endogenous retroviruses and long terminal repeats with human disorders. *Front Oncol.* 2013 Sep 11;3:234
[590] Balada E et al. Implication of human endogenous retroviruses in the development of autoimmune diseases. *Int Rev Immunol.* 2010 Aug;29(4):351-70
[591] Brodziak et al. The role of human endogenous retroviruses in the pathogenesis of autoimmune diseases. *Med Sci Monit.* 2012 Jun;18(6):RA80-8
[592] Perl et al. Endogenous retroviral pathogenesis in lupus. *Curr Opin Rheumatol.* 2010 Sep;22(5):483-92
[593] Dreyfus DH. Autoimmune disease: A role for new anti-viral therapies? *Autoimmun Rev.* 2011 Dec;11(2):88-97

viral therapies of chronic autoimmune diseases, such as retroviral integrase inhibitors, could be effective, although not without risk." This article provides support and rationale for using antiviral therapies in the treatment of autoimmunity; since anti-viral drugs nearly always have limited effectiveness and an excess of adverse effects and high cost while natural antiviral agents are safer and more broadly effective, the therapeutic choice is very clear.

- Role of endogenous retroviruses in murine SLE—an established animal model of human SLE[594] (*Autoimmun Rev.* 2010 Nov[595]): "Among the principal targets of the autoantibodies produced in murine SLE are nucleic acid-protein complexes and the envelope glycoprotein gp-70 of endogenous retroviruses. Recent studies have revealed that the innate receptor TLR-7 plays a pivotal role in the development of a wide variety of autoimmune responses against DNA- and RNA-containing nuclear antigens… Moreover, the demonstration that TLR-7 is involved in the acute phase expression of serum gp70 uncovers an additional pathogenic role of TLR7 in murine lupus nephritis by promoting the expression of nephritogenic gp-70 autoantigen." Thus this animal model proves with molecular detail the cause-and-effect relationship between ERVs and SLE and further points to TLR-7 as a necessary byway for nephritogenic autoantigen expression; parallels to human SLE and according therapeutic interventions are likely. While most readers should already appreciate that TLRs recognize pathogen-associated molecular patterns (PAMPs) expressed on infectious agents (and saturated fatty acids for TLR-4, as discussed in Chapter 4) and mediate the specific PAMP-TLR expression of inflammatory cytokines for immune defense responses, what is important to note here is that TLR-7 recognizes single-stranded RNA in endosomes, a common feature of viral genomes internalized within macrophages and dendritic cells; in this manner, TLR-7 is poised to be the mediator of virus-induced HERV transactivation with resultant production of pathogenic autoantigens.

- Selective antibody reactivity with peptides from human endogenous retroviruses—HERVs—and nonviral poly(amino acids) in patients with systemic lupus erythematosus (*Arthritis Rheum* 1996 Oct[596]): "Measurement by immunoassay revealed increased frequencies of antiretroviral antibodies against 2 peptides derived from the env gene of the type C-like class, which includes ERV-9 and HERV-H, and against 2 peptides from the gag region of human T-lymphotropic virus type I-related endogenous sequence 1, in patients with SLE. Antibodies to 2 nonviral peptides, polyhistidine and polyproline, were also overrepresented in patient sera. In 1 patient, longitudinal data obtained over a period of 12 years indicated that the concentrations of certain antiretroviral antibodies varied according to disease activity. CONCLUSION: Reactivity to certain type C HERV-derived antigens was found among patients with SLE. This reactivity could be explained by increased exposure to cross-reactive epitopes from essentially complete type C HERVs."

- Endogenous retroviruses in systemic lupus erythematosus: candidate lupus viruses (*Clin Immunol.* 2002 Feb[597]): "SLE patients produce high titer antibodies to various retroviral proteins, including Gag, Env, and Nef of HIV and HTLV (human T-lymphotropic virus), in the absence of overt retroviral infection. … In particular, we consider the role of HTLV-1-related endogenous sequence (HRES-1) in SLE. We propose that molecular mimicry between HRES-1 and the small ribonucleoprotein complex initiates the production of autoantibodies, leading to immune complex formation, complement fixation, and pathological tissue deposition."

Thus given that HERVs are 100% pervasive among humans and give rise to active transcription to HERV proteins, superantigens and the resulting antibodies—noting that microbial proteins + superantigens + antibodies = the perfect recipe for immune complex disease, made even worse among persons (e.g., lupus patients) with an inability to clear immune complexes—the most important question then becomes *what steps can be taken to suppress/repress/hamper HERV replication? Can we use the same effective antiviral treatments which already have available (in the previously listed antiviral protocol)?* Obviously, since

---

[594] "Murine models are useful tools for the study of the etiology of lupus. A multitude of models exist, each sharing a subset of attributes with SLE observed in humans. In addition, each model affords the study of different aspects of lupus pathogenesis." Perry et al. Murine Models of Systemic Lupus Erythematosus. *J Biomed Biotech* 2011; 271694
[595] Baudino et al. Role of endogenous retroviruses in murine SLE. *Autoimmun Rev*. 2010 Nov;10(1):27-34
[596] Bengtsson et al. Selective antibody reactivity with peptides from human endogenous retroviruses and nonviral poly(amino acids) in patients with systemic lupus erythematosus. *Arthritis Rheum*. 1996 Oct;39(10):1654-63
[597] Adelman MK, Marchalonis JJ. Endogenous retroviruses in systemic lupus erythematosus: candidate lupus viruses. *Clin Immunol*. 2002 Feb;102(2):107-16

we are not dealing with free viral particles, some of the previously mentioned antiviral treatments will have no effect because the mechanisms are irrelevant (such as selenium's prevention of immune-escape by reducing viral mutagenesis) or cannot reach within the nucleus to have effect (such as the virucidal activity of zinc ions, or the binding-inactivating effect of glycyrrhetinic acid to HSV particles). Given that "the virus" is already and permanently embedded/encoded within the human genome, the most immediate and obvious solutions would be those of promoting DNA methylation to silence HERV long terminal repeats (LTR, not to be confused with TLR for Toll-like receptors) and to prevent/reduce active transcription of those HERV LTR via transcription factors like NFkB and/or a pro-inflammatory cytokine milieu. This is to say, the means would most likely have to be ❶ *contra* DNA transcription, most notably via the promotion of DNA methylation, ❷ reducing any contribution of viral transactivation, ❸ reducing any contribution of inflammatory (e.g., TLR-7 pathway) and stress-induced (trans)activation.

> **Managing the simplicities of complexity is the best way to manage complexity**
>
> "The general approach I am taking seems to me rather simple-minded and unsophisticated, but nevertheless correct."
>
> Noam Chomsky, in presentation to Jean Piaget, in Royaumont, France 1975. (See *Manufacturing Consent* documentary film)

- Blocking HERV transcription by promoting DNA methylation: "There has been a reasonable prediction that aberrant LTR activation could trigger malignant disorders and autoimmune responses if epigenetic changes including DNA hypomethylation occur in somatic cells. ... Hypomethylation of HERV-E and HERV-K was also observed in SLE patients."[598]
    - Clinical implementation of optimal DNA methylation: For optimization of DNA methylation, methyl-donating/transferring nutrients such as folate (used clinically as folinic acid and/or methylfolate), betaine, and (methyl)cobalamin are necessary but not sufficient. Other nutrients—particularly vitamin D3—play critical and complex roles, promoting methylation of some DNA regions and demethylation of others[599]; in the case of vitamin D, we note consistent epidemiologic and clinical experimental research showing that vitamin D3 protects against and treats inflammatory/autoimmune diseases. The complexity of nutrients, in this case vitamin D3, is demonstrated by the observation that vitamin D causes complex changes in gene expression at different locations and likely under different circumstances; vitamin D and activation of its receptor correlate with DNA methylation and the *conceptual opposite* DNA demethylation (occurring at different DNA sites), while also promoting histone acetylation of some regions and histone deacetylation of others.[600] Lastly and very importantly, clinicians have to think beyond nutrients and methylating nutrients to fully appreciate and optimize DNA methylation, given that this process is potently impacted by numerous environmental factors, including xenobiotic/toxin exposure, ultraviolet (UV) light exposure, and drug exposure (e.g., procainamide, hydralazine); again noted is the fact that SLE patients show global hypomethylation of DNA[601] therefore suggesting that the patients need a combination of nutritional optimization (adding methyl-active nutrients such as folinic acid, cobalamin, and cholecalciferol) and environmental optimization (subtracting injurious agents such as UV light, xenobiotics and drugs) in order to optimize DNA methylation patterns and balance.
- Blocking HERV transcription by blocking exogenous virus replication—Rationale for autoimmune disease treatment with anti-viral therapies: "Cited epidemiologic and experimental evidence suggests that increased replication of epigenomic viral pathogens such as Epstein-Barr Virus (EBV)

---

[598] Katoh et al. Association of endogenous retroviruses and long terminal repeats with human disorders. *Front Oncol*. 2013 Sep 11;3:234
[599] "In summary, alterations in DNA methylation lead to aberrant gene expression and disruptions of genomic integrity, which contribute to development and progression of diseases. Vitamin D can regulate these processes; the mechanisms behind need further investigations." Fetahu et al. Vitamin D and the epigenome. *Front Physiol*. 2014 Apr 29;5:164
[600] "These changes involve the methylation of genomic DNA and/or reversible post-translational modifications of histone proteins, such as acetylation or deacetylation at exposed lysine residues." Carlberg C. Genome-wide (over)view on the actions of vitamin D. *Front Physiol*. 2014 Apr 29;5:167
[601] "The mechanisms causing altered DNA methylation in autoimmunity, aging and carcinogenesis are incompletely characterized but include exposure to environmental agents and drugs, diet, altered signaling in pathways regulating DNA methyltransferase expression and changes in endogenous regulatory mechanisms. ... Initial studies demonstrated that T cells from patients with active lupus had globally hypomethylated DNA. ... Treating normal T cells with DNA methylation inhibitors is sufficient to cause a lupus-like disease in animal models, so exposure to exogenous DNA methylation inhibitors might similarly contribute to the development of autoimmunity. In support of this, the two drugs most frequently implicated in causing a lupus-like disease, procainamide and hydralazine, have been reported to inhibit DNA methylation...and induce autoreactivity in human and murine T lymphocytes." Richardson BC. Role of DNA methylation in the regulation of cell function: autoimmunity, aging and cancer. *J Nutr*. 2002 Aug;132(8 Sup):2401S-2405S

in chronic human autoimmune diseases such as rheumatoid arthritis (RA), systemic lupus Erythematosus (SLE), and multiple sclerosis (MS) may activate endogenous human retroviruses (HERV) as a pathologic mechanism."[602]

- Blocking HERV transcription by blocking exogenous virus replication: "Herpes simplex viruses are known to transactivate retroviral regulatory LTR regions of both exogenous and endogenous human retroviruses..."[603]
- Blocking HERV transcription by blocking nonspecific cellular stress and inflammation: "Induction of cellular stress responses through serum deprivation did however, to some extent, mimic the effects of virus infection in terms of transcription of HERV-W elements. ... Environmental stressors can modulate the transcriptional activities of certain HERV-W elements which could thereby be markers for such insults." [604]

o Viruses, part 3— Bacteriophages, especially of the gastrointestinal bacteria: The fact that the lumen of the gastrointestinal tract is loaded with bacteria is well known; progressively, all healthcare providers and researchers are appreciating that bacterial imbalances (quantitative) and metabolic/behavioral disturbances (qualitative) contribute to various disease via multiple mechanisms, as reviewed in the section on dysbiosis in Chapter 4. The next step in our understanding of dysbiosis is what I have referred to previously as microbial dysbiosis—infections within microbes. Bacteriophages are viruses that infect bacteria, and the gastrointestinal bacteria, which are themselves susceptible to innumerable quantitative and qualitative imbalances, are susceptible to viral infections. Thus, any complete understanding of dysbiosis must also consider

Bacteriophages (also called "phages" or "virus-like particles" or VLP): mechanisms of contribution to dysbiosis, inflammation, and autoimmunity

- Bacteriophages ("viruses that infect bacteria") are the most abundant biological entities on earth; they outnumber bacteria by 10x; more than 1,200 genotypes found within the human gastrointestinal tract
- The gut virome is dominated by these prokaryotic viruses that prey on gut bacteria; since the reproductive capability of all phage particles is unknown, describing them as "viruses" is discouraged in preference for "virus-like particles" (VLP)
- Bacteriophages influence bacterial diversity and "population structure" via "destabilization of bacterial communities"; the infectious and lytic nature of bacteriophages will obviously influence survival and death of specific populations of bacteria while the effects of lysogeny result directly in more viral particles and death of bacteria with release of bacterial and viral immunogens. Conversely, human gut bacteriophage populations do not change impressively with the corresponding bacterial colonizations (exception seen with *Faecalibacterium prausnitzii* which has a proportionate phage population) within physiologic norms (longitudinal stability); the majority of phages seem to correspond (34-41%) to the *Firmicutes* phylum of bacteria.
- Bacteriophages participate in gene transfer and genome reorganization; they also carry numerous antibiotic resistance genes: multidrug efflux transporters (n = 355), vancomycin resistance genes (n = 129), tetracycline resistance genes (n = 18), and beta-lactamases (n = 16).
- VLP sequences represent 4% to 17% of the total DNA from human stool; this quantitative minority of DNA material could have profound pathological implications for conditions characterized by anti-nuclear antibodies and the resulting immune complexes. Viral particles from intestinal bacteriophages are certainly absorbed and would thereafter contribute to 1) primary inflammation, and almost certainly to 2) transactivation of HERVs, 3) cross-reactivity to DNA (e.g., ANA), and 4) immune complex deposition.
- Patients with the "autoimmune disease" Crohn's disease harbor many more bacteriophages per biopsy sample (2.1-4.1 billion) than do healthy controls (1.2 billion).
- Phage populations are modified via dietary change (*Genome Res* 2012 Oct); but the implications are not clear.

the role of bacteriophages; these will be reviewed via the following survey of the literature.

- Dysbiosis in inflammatory bowel disease via bacteriophages (*Gut*. 2008 Mar[605]): In this excellent and brief report by Lepage et al, the authors propose that bacteriophage-mediated or bacteriophage-induced inflammatory dysbiosis may play a role in inflammatory bowel disease; and they note that bacteriophages outnumber bacteria 10-fold "in many natural ecosystems." Bacteriophages are diverse, with more than 1,200 genotypes found within the human gastrointestinal tract; per biopsy

---

[602] Dreyfus DH. Autoimmune disease: A role for new anti-viral therapies? *Autoimmun Rev*. 2011 Dec;11(2):88-97
[603] Nellaker et al. Transactivation of elements in the human endogenous retrovirus W family by viral infection. *Retrovirology*. 2006 Jul 6;3:44
[604] Nellaker et al. Transactivation of elements in the human endogenous retrovirus W family by viral infection. *Retrovirology*. 2006 Jul 6;3:44
[605] Lepage et al. Dysbiosis in inflammatory bowel disease: a role for bacteriophages? *Gut*. 2008 Mar;57(3):424-5

sample from the human gastrointestinal tract, an average of 1.2 billion (1.2x10⁹) virus-like particles (VLP) are quantifiable and dominated by the families *Siphoviridae*, *Myoviridae* and *Podoviridae*. Patients with the "autoimmune disease" Crohn's disease (CD) harbor many more VLP per biopsy sample (2.1-4.1 billion) than do healthy controls (1.2 billion).
- Human gut virome: inter-individual variation and response to diet (*Genome Res*. 2011 Oct[606]): "VLP sequences represent a minority of the total DNA from stool, in the range of from 4% to 17%"; while this may be a *numerical* minority the physiologic and immunogenic significance could be massive. This article provides technical information and demonstrates phage response to diet, but the clinical implications and the authors' presentation of data are not clear.
  o Viruses, part 4—Bacterial synergism via NFkB activation and immunosuppression:
    - Bacterial promotion of viral replication via inflammatory pathways: Bacterial debris such as DNA and LPS are known to trigger inflammatory responses via TLR and NFkB; activation of NFkB—the proinflammatory transcription factor often "hijacked" by viruses to promote their own replication—promotes viral replication. Thus, increased total bacterial load (TBL, such as SIBO) would be expected to promote viral replication.
    - Bacterial promotion of viral replication via immunosuppression: As a specific example, *Helicobacter pylori* may play a powerful role as a synergistic bioagent for the microbial promotion of autoimmunity via its ability to *simultaneously* and *paradoxically* cause immunosuppression (thereby allowing other microbes to flourish) and systemic inflammation[607]; in this manner, the bacterial infection is permissive to and perhaps necessary for the autoimmune-inducing vasculopathic and fibrogenic viral infections (see section on Scleroderma for pathology details).

Clinical presentations:
- Subtypes and overlapping presentations: As shown in the diagram below, SLE has several subtypes which can present exclusively or in combination, ie, a patient may have classic SLE with no skin lesions, skin lesions without fulminant SLE, or classic SLE with one or more types of skin lesions.

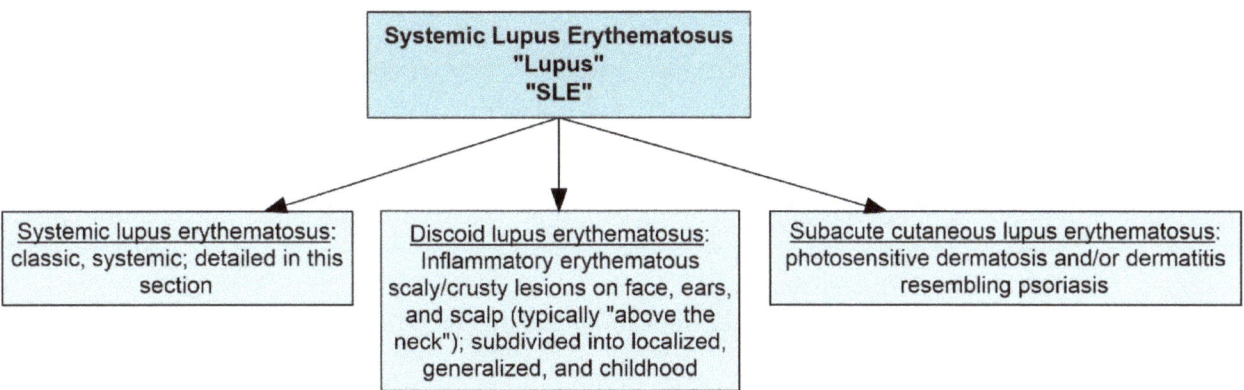

SLE has several subtypes which can present exclusively or in combination

- Gender: 85-90% of new patients are women in their childbearing years (frequency: 1 per 700 women); the ratio of women to men is 9:1 except among prepubertal children and older/postmenopausal men and women in which the ratio is 2:1.[608] The much higher prevalence of the disorder among women of childbearing age compared to men of the same age (11:1) implicates sex hormones and hormonal fluctuations as causative factors that predispose young women to this disorder.

---

[606] Minot et al. The human gut virome: inter-individual variation and dynamic response to diet. *Genome Res*. 2011 Oct;21(10):1616-25
[607] "Infectious agents such as Helicobacter pylori (Hp) may cause chronic inflammation and autoimmune reactivity in susceptible subjects. The results of in vitro experiments performed with lymphocytes from Hp infected patients indicate that Hp can cause immunosuppression which might be eliminated by successful eradication therapy." Hybenova et al. The role of environmental factors in autoimmune thyroiditis. *Neuro Endocrinol Lett*. 2010;31(3):283-9
[608] Manzi S. Epidemiology of systemic lupus erythematosus. *Am J Manag Care*. 2001 Oct;7(16 Suppl):S474-9 ajmc.com/files/articlefiles/A01_131_2001octManziS474_9.pdf

- 4x more common in women of African descent (1 per 250) than Caucasian women (1 per 1000).[609] The increased prevalence of SLE in dark-skinned women may be due at least in part to their higher prevalence of vitamin D deficiency, which unquestionably predisposes to inflammation, immune dysfunction, and the clinical manifestation of autoimmunity.[610] Although administration of vitamin D3 to cholecalciferol-deficient adults clearly has anti-inflammatory action[611,612], important windows of opportunity appear to occur *in utero* and within the first few postnatal months and years; for example, administration of vitamin D to **infants** reduces the subsequent incidence of type-1 *autoimmune-mediated* diabetes by 78%.[613] Vitamin D sufficiency appears to support immune function and thereby reduce the acquisition of infectious diseases[614]; thus, vitamin D may exert an anti-*rheumatic* benefit by exerting an anti-*infectious* benefit; i.e., by preventing the dysbiotic infections that may serve to trigger autoimmunity. Given the strength of evidence supporting the routine use of vitamin D3 supplementation in infants, children, and adults, healthcare providers should ensure adequate vitamin D status in their patients[615,616,617] for the treatment and prevention of long-latency deficiency diseases[618] and alleviation of systemic inflammation.[619]
- Positive family history of the disease is common: daughters of a mother with SLE have a 1 in 40 prevalence of SLE, whereas sons have a 1 in 250 prevalence
- Clinical course may be slow or acute, involving many organ systems or only one, and is characterized by exacerbations and remissions
- **Classic autoimmune systemic manifestations: fatigue, malaise, low-grade fever, anorexia, weight loss, peripheral polyarthritis**. Septicemia and septic arthritis should always be considered in patients with SLE, especially those taking immunosuppressive drugs and those experiencing what appears to be an exacerbation of the disease.
    - Skin:
        - Malar "butterfly" rash over the cheeks and bridge of the nose: this is a classic manifestation of the disease but is seen in less than half of SLE patients
        - Photosensitivity: erythematous skin rash develops readily on sun-exposed areas
        - Hair loss
        - Nail infarcts, periungual erythema, splinter hemorrhages
        - Purpura
    - Musculoskeletal:
        - 90% of patients have polyarthralgia—most commonly affecting the peripheral joints of the hands, wrists, knees, feet
        - Polymyalgia, myositis, and myopathy; avascular necrosis due to corticosteroids
    - Renal/kidney:
        - Immune complex-mediated glomerulonephritis: 50% of patients have clinical nephritis, hematuria, and proteinuria; renal function commonly declines during exacerbation of disease and then improves with disease remission
        - **Renal failure is a leading cause of death in patients with SLE**[620]
    - CNS:
        - 70% have EEG abnormalities
        - **Neuropsychiatric lupus is a medical emergency**[621]: characteristics include psychosis, seizures, transient ischemic attacks, severe depression, delirium, confusion. Exclude adverse drug effect (especially corticosteroid psychosis), infection, and hyponatremia.

---

[609] Tierney ML. McPhee SJ, Papadakis MA. *Current Medical Diagnosis and Treatment 2006. 45th edition*. New York; Lange Medical Books: 2006, pages 833-837
[610] Cantorna MT. Vitamin D and autoimmunity: is vitamin D status an environmental factor affecting autoimmune disease prevalence? *Proc Soc Exp Biol Med*. 2000;223:230-3
[611] Timms et al. Circulating MMP9, vitamin D and variation in TIMP-1 response with VDR genotype: mechanisms for inflammatory damage chronic disorders? *QJM* 2002:787-96
[612] Van den Berghe G, et al. Bone turnover in prolonged critical illness: effect of vitamin D. *J Clin Endocrinol Metab*. 2003;88(10):4623-32
[613] "Children who regularly took recommended dose of vitamin D (2000 IU daily) had a RR of 0.22 (0.05-0.89) compared with those who regularly received less than recommended amount." Hypponen et al. Intake of vitamin D and risk of type 1 diabetes: birth-cohort study. *Lancet* 2001;358:1500-3: very important article
[614] Wayse V, et al. Association of subclinical vitamin D deficiency with severe acute lower respiratory infection in Indian children under 5 y. *Eur J Clin Nutr*. 2004;58(4):563-7
[615] Vasquez A, Manso G, Cannell J. The clinical importance of vitamin D (cholecalciferol). *Altern Ther Health Med*. 2004 Sep-Oct;10(5):28-36
[616] Heaney RP. Vitamin D, nutritional deficiency, and the medical paradigm. *J Clin Endocrinol Metab*. 2003 Nov;88(11):5107-8
[617] Hollis BW, Wagner CL. Assessment of dietary vitamin D requirements during pregnancy and lactation. *Am J Clin Nutr*. 2004 May;79:717-26
[618] Heaney RP. Long-latency deficiency disease: insights from calcium and vitamin D. *Am J Clin Nutr*. 2003;78(5):912-9 jcem.endojournals.org/cgi/content/full/88/11/5107
[619] Timms et al. Circulating MMP9, vitamin D and variation in the TIMP-1 response with VDR genotype. *QJM*. 2002;95:787-96
[620] Suzuki et al. Development of pathogenic anti-DNA antibodies in patients with systemic lupus erythematosus. *FASEB J* 1997 Oct;11:1033-8
[621] McInnes I, Sturrock R. Rheumatological emergencies. *Practitioner*. 1994 Mar;238(1536):220-4

- Headaches, migraine, stroke
- Peripheral and cranial neuropathies, transverse myelitis
- Increased risk for meningitis when immunosuppressive therapy is used.
    o Cardiovascular and circulation:
- Vasculitis
- Thrombosis and **increased risk for myocardial infarction**
- Pericarditis, myocarditis: may result in sudden death, heart failure, arrhythmias
- Hypertension due to renal injury
- Raynaud's phenomenon—periodic vasospasm affecting the hands and fingers
- Antiphospholipid antibody syndrome—a major cause of complications
    o Lungs/pulmonary:
- Pneumonitis: presents with fever, cough, dyspnea—important to **assess with radiographs and exclude infection**
- Pleurisy, pleural effusion; **alveolar hemorrhage can be life-threatening**
    o Hematologic/CBC abnormalities:
- Leukopenia, lymphopenia, thrombocytopenia, anemia
- Immune complexes: Immune complexes are elevated in patients with active SLE[622]
    o Gastrointestinal:
- Nausea
- Diarrhea
- **Intestinal/mesenteric vasculitis and infarct—surgical emergency**—postprandial abdominal pain, cramps, vomiting, diarrhea
- Pancreatitis
- Increased intestinal permeability, occasionally protein-losing enteropathy results[623]
    o Eyes:
- **Retinal vasculitis** (look for exudates with fundoscopic examination) can cause blindness in days—**treat as an emergency**
- Other manifestations include conjunctivitis, photophobia, blurred vision
    o Other:
- Edema—may be seen with cardiac or renal damage
- Lymphadenopathy
- Mucocutaneous ulcerations
- Increased risk of miscarriage and congenital heart block

Major differential diagnoses:
- Infection
- Cancer, lymphoma
- RA or other autoimmune disease such as scleroderma, vasculitis, sarcoidosis
- Iron overload
- Fibromyalgia
- Porphyria cutanea tarda
- Drug hypersensitivity and drug-induced lupus: SLE is differentiated from drug-induced lupus by the following characteristics of drug-induced lupus: 1) temporal association with drug/medication use; remission of disease following drug discontinuation, and 2) lack of fully characteristic pattern of clinical and laboratory manifestations: lack of renal and CNS involvement, lack of hypocomplementemia and anti-native DNA antibodies. Clinicians must exclude drug-induced lupus before making diagnosis of SLE.

---

[622] Suzuki N, Mihara S, Sakane T. Development of pathogenic anti-DNA antibodies in patients with systemic lupus erythematosus. *FASEB J*. 1997 Oct;11(12):1033-8
[623] "Fourteen cases of primary lupus-associated protein-losing enteropathy have now been reported in the English-language literature." Perednia DA, Curosh NA. Lupus-associated protein-losing enteropathy. *Arch Intern Med*. 1990 Sep;150(9):1806-10

Algorithm for use of initial laboratory testing for SLE: This diagram is to be used in conjunction with other information presented in this book and any new published guidelines; however, this information will likely always remain clinically relevant and reasonably useful.

Clinical assessments:
- **History and physical examination**: consistent with the clinical presentations listed previously
- **Laboratory assessments**:
  o Comprehensive laboratory evaluation: Use other tests (e.g. and especially, metabolic/chemistry panel, UA, CBC, etc.) to assess for complications and concomitant disease.

- ANA—anti-nuclear antibodies: ANA is the best screening test and has been described as positive in 100% of SLE patients[624] despite the acknowledged existence of ANA-negative SLE. ANA levels correlate with disease activity. Previous editions of standard medical textbooks reported that this test was less than 100% sensitive for SLE; it may be that improvements in laboratory analysis now account for the 100% sensitivity. A positive ANA test result—even with a high titer—does not necessarily indicate that the patient has SLE, especially if no other signs or symptoms are present. ANA are directed against the following four targets: ❶ DNA, ❷ histones, ❸ non-histone proteins bound to RNA, ❹ nucleolar antigens.
    - Anti-double stranded (DS, native) DNA antibodies (anti-dsDNA): Positive in ~60% of patients; specific (not sensitive) for SLE; when positive, anti-dsDNA levels correlate with disease activity.
    - Anti-Sm (anti-Smith) antibodies: Positive in ~30% of patients; specific (not sensitive) for SLE.[625]
    - Anti-histone antibodies: Seen in drug-induced lupus.
    - Anti-Ro antibodies (SSA: Sjogren's syndrome antibodies): Seen with cutaneous SLE, Sjogren's syndrome, and neonatal lupus.[626]
- CRP: Sensitive indicator of inflammation, *except in SLE* where CRP levels can be normal even with severe active disease.[627,628]
- ESR: Not useful in all patients with SLE.[629]
- Complement levels (CH50): Complement levels are lowered in accord with complement pathway activation by immune complexes; levels tend to normalize when disease is in remission.
- Inherited complement deficiencies: 6% of SLE patients has an inherited/genetic deficiency in one or more complement proteins. Deficiency of C1q, C2, or **C4** appears to result in inability to clear immune complexes and thus results in exacerbation of disease manifestations due to immune complex deposition. C1q deficiency may impair clearance of apoptotic cells and thus promote antigenicity toward nuclear debris via—for example—activation of DAMP (damage-associated molecular pattern) receptors.
- HLA-DR2 and HLA-DR3: These are more common in patients with SLE than in the general population.
- Serologic testing for syphilis (VDRL): A false-positive test for syphilis is characteristic of SLE and is a reflection of antiphospholipid antibodies.
- Antiphospholipid and Anticardiolipin antibodies: Antiphospholipid antibodies (directed against plasma proteins complexed to phospholipids) are seen in 40-50% of SLE patients. Antiphospholipid antibodies are associated with significantly increased risk for venous and arterial thrombosis. In SLE patients with antiphospholipid antibodies, treatment with anticoagulants such as warfarin/coumadin are commonly used (see INR below):
    - Anticardiolipin antibodies: This is one of several types of antiphospholipid antibodies; also used in syphilis serologic testing, and therefore SLE patients with anticardiolipin antibodies may have false positive result for syphilis. Anticardiolipin antibodies interfere with the PT (partial thromboplastin) test and are thus occasionally called "lupus anticoagulant"—this factitious anticoagulation is purely an *in vitro* phenomenon and is misleading since these same patients actually have a hypercoagulable state that predisposes them to arterial and venous thromboses. Readers attentive to the information on mitochondrial will have also noted that the phospholipid cardiolipin is located on the mitochondrial inner membrane, where it serves as an anchor for the enzyme succinate dehydrogenase; this data suggests an important role for mitochondrial dysfunction in SLE: a fact which is now very well proven, although not widely known by many practicing clinicians.
    - INR: International Normalized Ratio is a standardized quantification of Prothrombin Time (PT), which is a measure of clotting/bleeding tendency. INR is used to monitor dosing of warfarin/coumadin; generally the INR should be kept between 2.0-3.0.[630]

---

[624] Tierney ML. McPhee SJ, Papadakis MA. *Current Medical Diagnosis and Treatment 2006. 45th edition*. New York; Lange Medical Books: 2006, pages 833-837
[625] Shojania K. Rheumatology: 2. What laboratory tests are needed? *CMAJ*. 2000 Apr 18;162(8):1157-63 cmaj.ca/cgi/content/full/162/8/1157
[626] Shojania K. Rheumatology: 2. What laboratory tests are needed? *CMAJ*. 2000 Apr 18;162(8):1157-63
[627] Deodhar SD. C-reactive protein: the best laboratory indicator available for monitoring disease activity. *Cleve Clin J Med* 1989 Mar-Apr;56(2):126-30
[628] Gabay C, Kushner I. Acute-phase proteins and other systemic responses to inflammation. *N Engl J Med*. 1999 Feb 11;340(6):448-54
[629] Klippel JH (ed). *Primer on the Rheumatic Diseases. 11th Edition*. Atlanta: Arthritis Foundation. 1997 page 94
[630] Tierney ML. McPhee SJ, Papadakis MA. *Current Medical Diagnosis and Treatment 2006. 45th edition*. New York; Lange Medical Books: 2006, pages 833-837

- Comprehensive testing for celiac disease and wheat allergy: Some patients diagnosed with "systemic lupus erythematosus" actually have autoimmunity and systemic inflammation due to occult celiac disease. These patients achieve clinical remission after avoiding gluten/gliadin-containing grains such as wheat.[631,632] More than 23% of patients with SLE have anti-gliadin antibodies.[633] In addition to IgA and IgG anti-gliadin antibodies, serologic testing for celiac disease includes IgA and IgG antiendomysial and anti-transglutaminase antibodies which should be interpreted along with a test for total serum IgA to identify those patients with selective IgA deficiency.

- **Imaging**:
    - Imaging is used to in the assessment of complications and exclusion of concomitant diseases.
    - The arthritis of SLE is typically mild (compared to rheumatoid arthritis) and is nondeforming.

Establishing the diagnosis:
- Clinical presentation and lab tests; more positives = more confident diagnosis.

Qualification for a diagnosis of SLE requires quantification of at least four of these eleven criteria:
1. Malar/cheek rash
2. Discoid rash
3. Photosensitivity
4. Ulcerations of oral mucosa
5. Joint pain and inflammation not attributable to other disease or trauma
6. Serositis: Inflammation of the serous tissues, which line the lungs (pleura), heart (pericardium), and the inner lining of the abdomen (peritoneum) and associated organs
7. Renal disease (any of the following): >3+ proteinuria measured by dipstick; cellular casts; proteinuria >0.5 grams per day
8. CNS involvement: seizures or psychosis without other cause
9. Hematologic abnormalities (any of the following): hemolytic anemia, leucopenia (45%), lymphopenia, thrombocytopenia (30%), anemia of chronic disease
10. Positive ANA
11. Additional serologic tests (any of the following):
○ Positive LE cell prep
○ Anti-native DNA antibody (50%)
○ Anti-Sm antibody (20%)
○ False-positive test for syphilis (25%)

Life-threatening complications and medical emergencies:
- **Infection** — Infections are now the leading cause of death in patients with SLE[634]
- **SLE complications: renal failure and CNS involvement**
- **Stroke, myocardial infarction** — Increased risk with male gender and antiphospholipid antibodies
- **Septic arthritis**
- **Thromboembolism**
- **10-year survival is >85%**[635]

Overview of clinical management:
- The clinical course of the disease is variable, marked by exacerbations and remissions. Life-threatening complications can develop rapidly and must be managed effectively to prevent patient morbidity and practitioner liability.

---

[631] "The immunological profile of IgA deficiency and/or raised double stranded DNA in the absence of antinuclear factor together with raised inflammatory markers and symptoms suggestive of an immune diathesis should alert the physician to the possibility of gluten sensitivity." Hadjivassiliou M, Sanders DS, Grunewald RA, Akil M. Gluten sensitivity masquerading as systemic lupus erythematosus. *Ann Rheum Dis*. 2004 Nov;63(11):1501-3 ard.bmjjournals.com/cgi/content/full/63/11/1501
[632] "Villous atrophy on duodenal biopsy specimens with a favorable response to a gluten-free diet was noted in all five patients." Zitouni M, Daoud W, Kallel M, Makni S. Systemic lupus erythematosus with celiac disease: a report of five cases. *Joint Bone Spine*. 2004 Jul;71(4):344-6
[633] "Twenty-four of 103 (23.3%) systemic lupus erythematosus patients tested positive for either antigliadin antibody, whereas none of the 103 patients tested positive for antiendomysial antibody." Rensch et al. The prevalence of celiac disease autoantibodies in patients with systemic lupus erythematosus. *Am J Gastroenterol*. 2001 Apr;96(4):1113-5 For the authors to state that these patients did not have celiac disease simply because their intestinal biopsies were normal is inconsistent with the modern paradigm of celiac disease which acknowledges that the disease can be present in the absence of gastrointestinal lesions.
[634] Tierney ML. McPhee SJ, Papadakis MA. *Current Medical Diagnosis and Treatment 2006. 45th edition*. New York; Lange Medical Books: 2006, pages 833-837
[635] Tierney ML. McPhee SJ, Papadakis MA. *Current Medical Diagnosis and Treatment 2006. 45th edition*. New York; Lange Medical Books: 2006, pages 833-837

- Treat patient safely and effectively. If you cannot get good results, refer them to someone who can. Refer if clinical outcome is unsatisfactory or if serious complications are possible. Stable patients are seen every 3-6 months for monitoring of disease activity, re-examination, and treatment recalibration.[636] Patients must understand that acute exacerbations and/or new symptoms—especially fever—must be evaluated promptly.
- Treatment must be customized to the patient and must be flexible to accommodate the natural exacerbations and remissions of the disease.
- To the extent possible, discourage use of NSAIDs since these drugs exacerbate joint destruction, renal impairment, and increased intestinal permeability which increases exposure to dietary and microbial antigens.

Treatments: The standard medical protocol centers on and starts with (new drugs are always being developed and added): prednisone, Plaquenil and immunoparalytic and immunosuppressive drugs.
- Drug treatments:
  - **NSAIDs**: For joint pain[637] despite adverse effects on the gut[638], joints[639,640,641] and kidneys.
  - **Antimalarial drug: hydroxychloroquine/Plaquenil**): Adverse effects include retinal damage, neuropathy, myopathy. As with anticonvulsant drugs, hydroxychloroquine/Plaquenil interferes with conversion of 25-hydroxycholecalciferol to the more active 1-25-dihydroxycholecalciferol[642]; this would be expected to exacerbate immune dysfunction, inflammation, hypertension, and depression.
  - **Danazol is an androgenic corticosteroid:** particularly used against thrombocytopenia
  - **Immunosuppression** with prednisone (promotes bacterial overgrowth and osteoporosis), cyclophosphamide (especially for renal involvement), mycophenolate mofetil, azathioprine, or other DMARD (disease-modifying antirheumatic drugs) is commonly used, particularly for the more serious complications of the disease such as those affecting the brain, heart, lungs, and kidneys. **Despite the clinical drawbacks and philosophical inadequacies, pharmacologic immunosuppression has a role in the management of patients with autoimmunity when their disease flares and threatens vital structures, particularly the heart, brain, and kidneys.**
  - **Anticoagulant drugs such as warfarin** are used for patients with antiphospholipid antibodies and resultant thrombotic complications.
- **FOOD & NUTRITION: 5-part "supplemented Paleo-Mediterranean diet" (SPMD)** The 5-part "supplemented Paleo-Mediterranean diet" (SPMD—reviewed in Chapter 4) consists of ❶ foundational plant-based low-carbohydrate diet of fruits, vegetables, nuts, seeds, berries and lean sources of protein, ❷ multivitamin and multimineral supplementation, ❸ physiologic doses of vitamin D3 (range 2,000-10,000 IU/d), ❹ combination fatty acid therapy (CFAT) with n3-ALA, n6-GLA, n3-EPA, n3-DHA, and phytochemical-rich olive oil which contains n9-oleate, and ❺ probiotics.
  - Gluten avoidance: Celiac disease can present with inflammatory oligoarthritis that resembles rheumatoid arthritis and which remits with avoidance of wheat/gluten; the inflammatory arthropathy of celiac disease has preceded bowel symptoms and/or an accurate diagnosis by as many as 3-15 years.[643,644] Some patients diagnosed with "systemic lupus erythematosus" actually have autoimmunity and systemic

---

[636] Manzi S. Epidemiology of systemic lupus erythematosus. *Am J Manag Care* 2001 Oct;7(16Sup):S474-9 ajmc.com/files/articlefiles/A01_131_2001octManziS474_9.pdf
[637] Tierney ML. McPhee SJ, Papadakis MA. Current Medical Diagnosis and Treatment 2006. 45th edition. New York; Lange Medical Books: 2006, pages 833-837
[638] Abbreviations: cow's milk beta-lactoglobulin absorption (BLG), acetylsalicylic acid (ASA), disodium chromoglycate (DSCG). "ASA administration strongly increased BLG absorption, not prevented by DSCG pretreatment. In normal controls treated with a single dose of ASA we obtained similar results. Our results suggest that prolonged treatment with nonsteroidal anti-inflammatory drugs induces an increase of food antigen absorption, apparently not related to anaphylaxis mediator release, with possible clinical effects." Fagiolo U, Paganelli R, Ossi E, Quinti I, Cancian M, D'Offizi GP, Fiocco U. Intestinal permeability and antigen absorption in rheumatoid arthritis. Effects of acetylsalicylic acid and sodium chromoglycate. *Int Arch Allergy Appl Immunol.* 1989;89(1):98-102
[639] "At...concentrations comparable to those... in the synovial fluid of patients treated with the drug, several NSAIDs suppress proteoglycan synthesis...." Brandt KD. Effects of nonsteroidal anti-inflammatory drugs on chondrocyte metabolism in vitro and in vivo. *Am J Med.* 1987 Nov 20; 83(5A): 29-34
[640] "This highly significant association between NSAID use and acetabular destruction gives cause for concern, not least because of the difficulty in achieving satisfactory hip replacements in patients with severely damaged acetabula." Newman NM, Ling RS. Acetabular bone destruction related to non-steroidal anti-inflammatory drugs. *Lancet.* 1985 Jul 6; 2(8445): 11-4
[641] Vidal y Plana et al. Articular cartilage pharmacology: In vitro studies on glucosamine and non steroidal anti-inflammatory drugs. *Pharmacol Res Commun.* 1978 Jun;10:557-69
[642] "Half the SLE and FM patients had 25(OH)-vitamin D levels < 50 nmol/l, a level at which PTH stimulation occurs. Our data suggest that in SLE patients HCQ might inhibit conversion of 25(OH)-vitamin D to 1,25(OH)2-vitamin D." Huisman et al. Vitamin D levels in women with systemic lupus erythematosus and fibromyalgia. *J Rheumatol.* 2001 Nov;28(11):2535-9
[643] "We report six patients with coeliac disease in whom arthritis was prominent at diagnosis and who improved with dietary therapy. Joint pain preceded diagnosis by up to three years in five patients and 15 years in one patient." Bourne JT, et al. Arthritis and coeliac disease. *Ann Rheum Dis.* 1985 Sep;44(9):592-8
[644] "A 15-year-old girl, with synovitis of the knees and ankles for 3 years before a diagnosis of gluten-sensitive enteropathy, is described." Pinals RS. Arthritis associated with gluten-sensitive enteropathy. *J Rheumatol.* 1986 Feb;13(1):201-4

inflammation due to occult celiac disease, and they achieve remarkable improvement—complete remission of systemic inflammation and the ability to discontinue all anti-inflammatory drugs—after avoiding gluten/gliadin-containing grains, most notoriously, wheat.[645] In a study of 103 SLE patients, more than 23% of SLE patients had anti-gliadin antibodies.[646]

- o <u>Short-term fasting</u>: In case reports and clinical trials, short-term fasting (or protein-sparing fasting) has been documented as safe and effective treatment for SLE[647], RA[648], and non-rheumatic diseases such as chronic severe hypertension[649], moderate hypertension[650], obesity[651,652], type-2 diabetes[653], and epilepsy.[654] The combination of energy restriction and fish oil supplementation was shown highly beneficial in an animal model of SLE.[655]

- o <u>Broad-spectrum fatty acid therapy with ALA, EPA, DHA, GLA and oleic acid</u>: Fish oil provides EPA and DHA which have well-proven anti-inflammatory benefits when used in the treatment of SLE.[656,657,658] Fatty acid supplementation should be delivered in the form of combination therapy with ALA, GLA, DHA, and EPA. Given at doses of 3,000 – 9,000 mg per day, ALA from flax oil has impressive anti-inflammatory benefits demonstrated by its ability to halve prostaglandin production in humans.[659] Numerous studies have demonstrated the benefit of GLA in the treatment of rheumatoid arthritis when used at doses between 500 mg – 4,000 mg per day.[660,661] Fish oil provides EPA and DHA which have well-proven anti-inflammatory benefits in RA[662,663,664] and SLE.[665,666]

- o <u>Vitamin D3 supplementation with physiologic doses and/or tailored to serum 25(OH)D levels</u>: Vitamin D deficiency is common in the general population and is even more common in patients with chronic illness and chronic musculoskeletal pain.[667] **At least 50% of patients with SLE are deficient in vitamin D**[668], and even more would be found deficient if stricter and more appropriate criteria are used.

---

[645] "The immunological profile of IgA deficiency and/or raised double stranded DNA in the absence of antinuclear factor together with raised inflammatory markers and symptoms suggestive of an immune diathesis should alert the physician to the possibility of gluten sensitivity." Hadjivassiliou M, Sanders DS, Grunewald RA, Akil M. Gluten sensitivity masquerading as systemic lupus erythematosus. *Ann Rheum Dis.* 2004 Nov;63(11):1501-3 ard.bmjjournals.com/cgi/content/full/63/11/1501

[646] "Twenty-four of 103 (23.3%) systemic lupus erythematosus patients tested positive for either antigliadin antibody, whereas none of the 103 patients tested positive for antiendomysial antibody." Rensch MJ, Szyjkowski R, Shaffer RT, Fink S, Kopecky C, Grissmer L, Enzenhauer R, Kadakia S. The prevalence of celiac disease autoantibodies in patients with systemic lupus erythematosus. *Am J Gastroenterol.* 2001 Apr;96(4):1113-5. For the authors to state that these patients did not have celiac disease simply because their intestinal biopsies were normal seems to indicate that the authors were ignorant of the modern paradigm of celiac disease which acknowledges that the disease can be present in the absence of gastrointestinal lesions.

[647] Fuhrman J, Sarter B, Calabro DJ. Brief case reports of medically supervised, water-only fasting associated with remission of autoimmune disease. *Altern Ther Health Med.* 2002 Jul-Aug;8(4):112, 110-1

[648] "An association was found between improvement in inflammatory activity of the joints and enhancement of neutrophil bactericidal capacity. Fasting appears to improve the clinical status of patients with RA." Uden AM, Trang L, Venizelos N, Palmblad J. Neutrophil functions and clinical performance after total fasting in patients with rheumatoid arthritis. *Ann Rheum Dis.* 1983 Feb;42(1):45-51

[649] "The average reduction in blood pressure was 37/13 mm Hg, with the greatest decrease being observed for subjects with the most severe hypertension. Patients with stage 3 hypertension (those with systolic blood pressure greater than 180 mg Hg, diastolic blood pressure greater than 110 mg Hg, or both) had an average reduction of 60/17 mm Hg at the conclusion of treatment." Goldhamer et al. Medically supervised water-only fasting in the treatment of hypertension. *J Manipulative Physiol Ther.* 2001 Jun;24(5):335-9

[650] "RESULTS: Approximately 82% of the subjects achieved BP at or below 120/80 mm Hg by the end of the treatment program. The mean BP reduction was 20/7 mm Hg, with the greatest decrease being observed for subjects with the highest baseline BP." Goldhamer AC, Lisle DJ, Sultana P, Anderson SV, Parpia B, Hughes B, Campbell TC. Medically supervised water-only fasting in the treatment of borderline hypertension. *J Altern Complement Med.* 2002 Oct;8(5):643-50

[651] Vertes V, Genuth SM, Hazelton IM. Supplemented fasting as a large-scale outpatient program. *JAMA.* 1977 Nov 14;238(20):2151-3

[652] Bauman WA, Schwartz E, Rose HG, et al. Early and long-term effects of acute caloric deprivation in obese diabetic patients. *Am J Med.* 1988 Jul;85(1):38-46

[653] Goldhamer AC. Initial cost of care results in medically supervised water-only fasting for treating high blood pressure and diabetes. *J Altern Complement Med.* 2002 Dec;8(6):696-7

[654] "The ketogenic diet should be considered as alternative therapy for children with difficult-to-control seizures. It is more effective than many of the new anticonvulsant medications and is well tolerated by children and families when it is effective." Freeman JM, et al. The efficacy of the ketogenic diet-1998: a prospective evaluation of intervention in 150 children. *Pediatrics.* 1998 Dec;102(6):1358-63 pediatrics.aappublications.org/cgi/reprint/102/6/1358

[655] "In conclusion, our data strongly indicate that ER and FO maintain antioxidant status and GSH:GSSG ratio, thereby protecting against renal deterioration from oxidative insults during ageing." Kelley VE, Ferretti A, Izui S, Strom TB. A fish oil diet rich in eicosapentaenoic acid reduces cyclooxygenase metabolites, and suppresses lupus in MRL-lpr mice. *J Immunol.* 1985 Mar;134(3):1914-9

[656] "No major side effects were noted, and it is suggested that dietary modification with additional marine oil may be a useful way of modifying disease activity in systemic lupus erythematosus." Walton et al. Dietary fish oil and the severity of symptoms in patients with systemic lupus erythematosus. *Ann Rheum Dis.* 1991 Jul;50(7):463-6

[657] "CONCLUSION: In the management of SLE, dietary supplementation with fish oil may be beneficial in modifying symptomatic disease activity." Duffy et al. The clinical effect of dietary supplementation with omega-3 fish oils and/or copper in systemic lupus erythematosus. *J Rheumatol.* 2004 Aug;31(8):1551-6

[658] "Oral supplementation of EPA and DHA induced prolonged remission of SLE in 10 consecutive patients without any side-effects. These results suggest that n-3 fatty acids, EPA and DHA, are useful in the management of SLE and possibly, other similar collagen vascular diseases." Das UN. Beneficial effect of eicosapentaenoic and docosahexaenoic acids in the management of systemic lupus erythematosus and its relationship to the cytokine network. *Prostaglandins Leukot Essent Fatty Acids.* 1994 Sep;51(3):207-13

[659] Adam O, Wolfram G, Zollner N. Effect of alpha-linolenic acid in the human diet on linoleic acid metabolism and prostaglandin biosynthesis. *J Lipid Res.* 1986 Apr;27(4):421-6

[660] "Other results showed a significant reduction in morning stiffness with gamma-linolenic acid at 3 months and reduction in pain and articular index at 6 months with olive oil." Brzeski et al. Evening primrose oil in patients with rheumatoid arthritis and side-effects of non-steroidal anti-inflammatory drugs. *Br J Rheumatol.* 1991 Oct;30(5):370-2

[661] Rothman D, DeLuca P, Zurier RB. Botanical lipids: effects on inflammation, immune responses, and rheumatoid arthritis. *Semin Arthritis Rheum.* 1995 Oct;25(2):87-96

[662] Adam et al. Anti-inflammatory effects of a low arachidonic acid diet and fish oil in patients with rheumatoid arthritis. *Rheumatol Int.* 2003 Jan;23(1):27-36

[663] Lau et al. Effects of fish oil supplementation on non-steroidal anti-inflammatory drug requirement in patients with mild rheumatoid arthritis. *Br J Rheumatol* 1993 Nov:982-9

[664] Kremer et al. Fish-oil fatty acid supplementation in active rheumatoid arthritis. A double-blinded, controlled, crossover study. *Ann Intern Med.* 1987 Apr;106(4):497-503

[665] Walton et al. Dietary fish oil and the severity of symptoms in patients with systemic lupus erythematosus. *Ann Rheum Dis.* 1991 Jul;50(7):463-6

[666] Duffy et al. The clinical effect of dietary supplementation with omega-3 fish oils and/or copper in systemic lupus erythematosus. *J Rheumatol.* 2004 Aug;31(8):1551-6

[667] Plotnikoff GA, Quigley JM. Prevalence of severe hypovitaminosis D in patients with persistent, nonspecific musculoskeletal pain. *Mayo Clin Proc.* 2003 Dec;78(12):1463-70

[668] "Half the SLE and FM patients had 25(OH)-vitamin D levels < 50 nmol/l, a level at which PTH stimulation occurs. Our data suggest that in SLE patients HCQ might inhibit conversion of 25(OH)-vitamin D to 1,25(OH)2-vitamin D." Huisman et al. Vitamin D levels in women with systemic lupus erythematosus and fibromyalgia. *J Rheumatol.* 2001 Nov;28(11):2535-9

Clinical Applications: Rheumatology

- **INFECTIONS & DYSBIOSIS: ❶ antimicrobial treatments, ❷ immunorestoration, ❸ immunotolerance via Treg induction** Essentially all autoimmune/rheumatic disorders are associated with microbial colonization and intolerance to same; the presence of persistent microbial colonization is *prima facie* evidence of immunosuppression. The eight areas of dysbiosis (multifocal) are: ❶ sinorespiratory, ❷ orodental, ❸ gastrointestinal, ❹ urogenital/genitourinary, ❺ parenchymal/tissue, ❻ microbial, ❼ dermal/cutaneous, and ❽ environmental. Dysbiotic loci should be investigated as discussed previously in Chapter 4. Recall that patients with lupus have abnormal gastrointestinal bacteria (decreased colonization resistance[669]), and some evidence suggests that gastrointestinal bacteria in these patients may translocate into the systemic circulation to induce formation of antibodies that cross-react with double-stranded DNA to produce the clinical manifestations of the disease.[670,671] Each cause—each contributor to disease—may in itself be "clinically insignificant" but when numerous "insignificant" additive and synergistic influences coalesce, we find ourselves confronted with an "idiopathic disease." We must then decide between the only two available options: 1) despair in the failure of our "one cause, one disease, one drug" paradigm, or 2) appreciate that numerous influences work together to disrupt physiologic function and produce the biologic dysfunction that we experience as disease. Experimental evidence shows that exposure to single-stranded bacterial DNA can provoke formation of antibodies to single-stranded mammalian DNA. Human patients with SLE have a reduced ability to bind bacterial DNA with antibodies, thus allowing normal/ambient levels of bacterial DNA to provoke an ongoing inflammatory response.[672] Recall from Chapter 4 that stimulation of inflammation by bacterial DNA is one of the 17 pathomechanisms of autoimmune/inflammation induction by multifocal dysbiosis
    - Sinorespiratory/nasopharyngeal and dermal dysbiosis: **Increased nasal colonization with *Staphylococcus aureus* has been noted in patients with SLE.**[673]
    - Gastrointestinal dysbiosis: Yeast, bacteria, and parasites are treated as indicated based on identification and sensitivity results from comprehensive parasitology assessments.
- **NUTRITIONAL IMMUNOMODULATION: Treg induction for modulation of Th-1/2/17 inflammation** Nutrients and therapeutic approaches that promote Treg or IL-10 induction and/or Th-17, IL-17 suppression include 1) mitochondrial optimization and mTOR suppression, 2) biotin, 3) vitamin E, 4) sodium avoidance, 5) transgenic/GMO food avoidance, 6) probiotics, 7) lipoic acid, 8) vitamin A, 9) inflammation reduction, 10) vitamin D, 11) fatty acid supplementation with GLA and n3, 12) infection and dysbiosis remediation, 13) green tea EGCG. Acronym: MiBESTPLAIDFIG as reviewed in Chapter 4.
- **DYSMETABOLISM & DYSFUNCTIONAL MITOCHONDRIA: MitoDys, ERS-UPR, AGE/RAGE, hyperglycemia and ceramide** The major clinical considerations in this section are mitochondrial dysfunction, endoplasmic reticulum stress, unfolded protein response, TLR activation, and the dysmetabolic effects of sustained hyperglycemia and hyperinsulinemia and resultant oxidative stress, inflammation, RAGE activation, and accumulation of AGE, palmitate and ceramide. The review of this information in Chapter 4 covered approximately 30 interventions relevant to dysmetabolism, mitochondrial dysfunction, ERS-UPR, etc; these will not be reviewed here except to mention those most commonly, easily, empirically, synergistically, and effectively used: 1) low-carbohydrate diet with 2) moderate exercise, 3) CoQ-10, 4) acetyl-carnitine with 5) lipoic acid, 6) NAC, 7) resveratrol, and 8) melatonin.
    - Mitochondrial hyperpolarization and ATP depletion in patients with systemic lupus erythematosus (*Arthritis Rheum* 2002 Jan[674]): **"Mitochondrial hyperpolarization and the resultant ATP depletion sensitize T cells for necrosis, which may significantly contribute to inflammation in patients with SLE."**

---

[669] "Colonization Resistance (CR)...tended to be lower in active SLE patients than in healthy individuals. This could indicate that in SLE more and different bacteria translocate across the gut wall due to a lower CR. Some of these may serve as polyclonal B cell activators or as antigens cross-reacting with DNA." Apperloo-Renkema HZ, et al. Host-microflora interaction in systemic lupus erythematosus (SLE): colonization resistance of the indigenous bacteria of the intestinal tract. *Epidemiol Infect*. 1994;112(2):367-73
[670] "The lower IgG antibacterial antibody titres in active SLE might possibly result from sequestration of these IgG antibodies in immune complexes, indicating a possible role for antibacterial antibodies in exacerbations of SLE." Apperloo-Renkema HZ, Bootsma H, Mulder BI, Kallenberg CG, van der Waaij D. Host-microflora interaction in systemic lupus erythematosus (SLE): circulating antibodies to the indigenous bacteria of the intestinal tract. *Epidemiol Infect*. 1995 Feb;114(1):133-41
[671] Pisetsky DS. Antibody responses to DNA in normal immunity and aberrant immunity. *Clin Diagn Lab Immunol*. 1998 Jan;5(1):1-6 cdli.asm.org/cgi/content/full/5/1/1
[672] Pisetsky DS. Antibody responses to DNA in normal immunity and aberrant immunity. *Clin Diagn Lab Immunol*. 1998 Jan;5(1):1-6 cdli.asm.org/cgi/content/full/5/1/1
[673] Medline abstract from Polish research: "In 9 from 14 patients with (64.3%) a.b. very massive growth of Staphylococcus aureus in culture from vestibulae of the nose swab was, in other cultures very massive growth of physiological flora was seen. ...clinical significance of asymptomatic bacteriuria and pathogenic bacteria colonisation of nostrils as a precedence to symptomatic infections needs further investigations." Koseda-Dragan M, Hebanowski M, Galinski J, Krzywinska E, Bakowska A. [Asymptomatic bacteriuria in women diagnosed with systemic lupus erythematosus (SLE)] *Pol Arch Med Wewn*. 1998 Oct;100(4):321-30.
[674] Gergely et al. Mitochondrial hyperpolarization and ATP depletion in patients with systemic lupus erythematosus. *Arthritis Rheum*. 2002 Jan;46(1):175-90

- **STYLE OF LIVING (LIFESTYLE) & SPECIAL CONSIDERATIONS: S**leep optimization, **S**ocioPsychology, **S**tress management/avoidance, **S**omatic treatments, **S**pecial **S**upplementation, **S**weat/exercise, **S**auna/detoxification, **S**urgery, **S**tamp your passport and vacate current reality, **S**ensory deprivation therapy

  This is a buffet of mostly lifestyle-based interventions yet also including considerations such as somatic treatments, additional supplementation, and surgery.

  - Cardiovascular disease (CVD) risk reduction: Patients with SLE have an increased risk of cardiovascular disease due to the synergistic effects of inflammation, oxidative stress, antiphospholipid antibodies, and elevated homocysteine. Obviously, the risk for CVD will be exacerbated if the SLE patient has other risk factors such as tobacco use, diabetes, obesity, hypertension, or physical inactivity. Therapeutic and interventional considerations specific to the prevention of cardiovascular disease include but are not limited to the following:
    - Cardioprotective diet: Paleo-Mediterranean diet
    - Fatty acid supplementation: Combination fatty acid supplementation with ALA, GLA, EPA, DHA[675,676]
    - Magnesium supplementation: > 200 mg up to bowel tolerance
  - Treatments to lower homocysteine: Doses given here for various treatments are for adults:
    - Folic acid: 5-10 mg, should be used with high-dose vitamin B-12
    - Hydroxocobalamin: 2,000-6,000 mcg/d orally, or 1,000-4,000 mcg/wk by injection
    - Pyridoxine: 250 mg/day with meals, co-administered with magnesium (e.g., >200 mg/d)
    - NAC: 600 mg tid
    - Betaine/ trimethylglycine: 1-2 grams tid (>6 grams daily when used alone)
    - Lecithin: 2.6 g choline/d (as phosphatidylcholine) decreased mean fasting plasma homocysteine by 18%.[677] Attaining this high dose might require as many as 45 capsules of commercially available supplements; an equivalent dose in the form of powdered lecithin granules delivered in a smoothie may be better tolerated than the capsules.
  - **N-Acetyl-Cysteine (NAC) for antioxidant, antiviral, and mitochondrial-protective benefits**: NAC provides cysteine for GSH production. NAC also inhibits NFkB. NAC inhibits viral replication (e.g., HIV) more effectively than and independently from its conversion to GSH. Recently, NAC at relatively high doses of 4,800mg/d in divided doses was shown to modulate mitochondrial hyperpolarization (by dissociating the generally resultant mTOR activation) and lead to very important clinical and immunological improvements in patients with SLE; NAC was shown to be safe and well-tolerated by all SLE patients up to 2.4g/d with reversible nausea in 33% of patients receiving 4.8g/d. This study by Lai, Hanczko, Bonilla, et al[678] is truly a landmark contribution and advance in the field of rheumatology and immunology because it proves 1) that mitochondrial dysfunction directly leads to an autoimmune phenotype, and 2) that inhibition of mTOR by NAC is safe and effective in patients with SLE; important insights from this remarkable work are as follows:

    > **Mechanistic and clinical proof of anti-rheumatic benefit of NAC**
    >
    > "Similar to the effect of rapamycin, **suppression of mTOR by NAC was accompanied by increased FoxP3 expression in CD4+/CD25+ T cells**. These results suggest that the effect of NAC on the immune system is 1) cell type-specific and 2) it occurs through disconnecting the activation of mTOR from the elevation of Δψm in lupus T cells, similar to the effect of rapamycin."
    >
    > Lai et al. N-acetylcysteine reduces disease activity by blocking mammalian target of rapamycin in T cells from systemic lupus erythematosus patients. *Arthritis Rheum*. 2012 Sep

    - NAC 4,800mg/d proved safe and clinically beneficial in patients with SLE, leading to reductions in disease activity and ANA levels.
    - Mitochondrial hyperpolarization (MHP) causes mTOR activation which in turn suppresses the expression of the FoxP3 transcription factor necessary for induction of T-regulatory cells. Note that

---

[675] Vasquez A. New Insights into Fatty Acid Supplementation and Its Effect on Eicosanoid Production and Genetic Expression. *Nutritional Perspectives* 2005; January: 5-16
[676] Laidlaw M, Holub BJ. Effects of supplementation with fish oil-derived n-3 fatty acids and gamma-linolenic acid on circulating plasma lipids and fatty acid profiles in women. *Am J Clin Nutr*. 2003 Jan;77(1):37-42 ajcn.org/cgi/content/full/77/1/37
[677] Olthof MR, Brink EJ, Katan MB, Verhoef P. Choline supplemented as phosphatidylcholine decreases fasting and postmethionine-loading plasma homocysteine concentrations in healthy men. *Am J Clin Nutr*. 2005 Jul;82(1):111-7
[678] Lai et al. NAC reduces disease activity by blocking mammalian target of rapamycin in T cells from systemic lupus erythematosus patients. *Arthritis Rheum* 2012 Sep:2937-46

the mTOR activation is the cause of the FoxP3 suppression; ironically, NAC actually increases MHP but dissociates it from mTOR by having a greater effect on and via mTOR suppression. The nutritional supplement NAC works in a similar manner as does the immunosuppressive drug rapamycin, with a mechanism of suppression of mTOR and the effect of enhancing endogenous anti-inflammatory immunomodulation via CD4+ CD25+ FoxP3+ T-regulatory cells. Stated again and differently, NAC paradoxically worsens mitochondrial hyperpolarization in patients with SLE but does so at the same time that it has a more significant impact on mTOR; NAC's rapamycin-like targeting of mTOR dissociates mitochondrial hyperpolarization from mTOR activation. The reduction in mTOR activity (which is of greater consequence than the increase in MIM polarization) allows enhanced expression of FoxP3 for increased elaboration of T-regulatory cells, thereby providing endogenous immunoregulation.

- "MHP of lupus T cells, which most prominently affects DN [double-negative, autoimmunity-promoting] T cells, was associated with resistance to activation-induced apoptosis. In 27 SLE patients receiving daily NAC doses of 1.2 g, 2.4 g, and 4.8 g considered together, both **spontaneous and CD3/CD28-induced apoptosis of DN T cells were markedly increased** and the **expansion of these cells was effectively reversed**. The **elimination of DN T cells, which are known promote anti-DNA autoantibody production by B cells**, is likely to contribute to reduced anti-DNA titers and to the efficacy of NAC.

- "The therapeutic importance of NAC for SLE is reflected by: 1) achieving clinical improvement in two validated disease activity scores within 3 months; 2) diminishing fatigue (21), which is considered the most disabling symptom in a majority of SLE patients (22); 3) absence of significant side-effects; and 4) affordability of this medication. A monthly supply of 600-mg NAC capsules (120–240 capsules) costs $15–$30 on the retail market. This sharply contrasts with average annual direct medical costs estimated to be ~$22,580 per patient in 2009.Thus, the cost of NAC at $180–$360/year would be negligible in comparison to the overall expenditures to society and the expected benefit in reducing the need for vastly more expensive medications burdened with potentially serious side-effects."

o <u>Oral enzyme therapy with proteolytic/pancreatic enzymes</u>: Polyenzyme supplementation is used to ameliorate the pathophysiology induced by immune complexes, such as the related condition rheumatoid arthritis.[679]

o <u>CoQ10 (antihypertensive, renoprotective, and probably immunomodulatory)</u>: CoQ10 is a powerful antioxidant with a wide margin of safety and excellent clinical tolerability. At least four studies have documented its powerful blood-pressure-lowering ability, which often surpasses the clinical effectiveness of antihypertensive drugs.[680,681,682,683] Furthermore, at least two published papers[684,685] and one case report[686] advocate that CoQ10 has powerful renoprotective benefits. CoQ10 levels are low in patients with allergies[687], and the symptomatic relief that many allergic patients experience following supplementation with CoQ10 suggests that CoQ10 has an immunomodulatory effect. Common doses start at > 100 mg per day with food; doses of 200 mg per day are not uncommon, and doses up to 1,000 mg per day are clinically well tolerated though the high financial toll resembles that of many pharmaceutical drugs.

---

[679] Galebskaya et al. Human complement system state after wobenzyme intake. *Vestnik Moskovskogo Universiteta (Seriya 2: Khimiya)*. 2000. Vol. 41, No. 6. Supp 148-149
[680] Burke et al. Randomized, double-blind, placebo-controlled trial of coenzyme Q10 in isolated systolic hypertension. *South Med J*. 2001 Nov;94(11):1112-7
[681] Singh et al. Effect of hydrosoluble coenzyme Q10 on blood pressures and insulin resistance in hypertensive patients coronary artery disease. *J Hum Hypertens* 1999 Mar:203-8
[682] Digiesi et al. Coenzyme Q10 in essential hypertension. *Mol Aspects Med*. 1994;15 Suppl:s257-63
[683] Langsjoen P, Langsjoen P, Willis R, Folkers K. Treatment of essential hypertension with coenzyme Q10. *Mol Aspects Med*. 1994;15 Suppl:S265-72
[684] Singh et al. Randomized, double-blind placebo-controlled trial of coenzyme Q10 in chronic renal failure: discovery of a new role. *J Nutr Environ Med* 2000;10:281-8
[685] Singh et al. Randomized, Double-blind, Placebo-controlled Trial of Coenzyme Q10 in Patients with End-stage Renal Failure. *J Nutr Environ Med* 2003;13: 13–22
[686] Singh RB, Singh MM. Effects of CoQ10 in new indications with antioxidant vitamin deficiency. *J Nutr Environ Med* 1999; 9:223-228
[687] Ye CQ, Folkers K, et al. A modified determination of coenzyme Q10 in human blood and CoQ10 blood levels in diverse patients with allergies. *Biofactors*. 1988 Dec;1:303-6

- Anti-autoantibody interventions: Patients with SLE have impaired ability to clear immune complexes via hepatic and splenic routes.[688,689] Given that anti-DNA and related immune complexes and cryoglobulins are considered the most fundamental abnormalities in the pathogenesis of this disorder, we can explore at least three routes of clinical intervention based on this limited focus. First, therapeutic interventions might be used that inhibit the *de novo* formation of autoantibodies, particularly those that are directed against double-stranded DNA. This could be accomplished via bio-logical immunomodulation, pharmacologic/anti-biological immunosuppression, or by removing the underlying stimuli and predisposing factors ("etiologic approach"). Second, treatments might be implemented to nullify or diminish the adverse effects of these antibodies. Third, we might use interventions that remove the autoantibodies that are formed so that they are not significantly available to contribute to disease pathogenesis. As discussed previously in the section on treatments for multifocal dysbiosis, at least two primary mechanisms exist for the removal of autoantibody-containing immune complexes, namely 1) phagocytosis and proteolytic degradation by macrophages embedded in the liver and spleen, and 2) transport via hepatocytes directly into the bile for excretion. IgG double-stranded DNA antibodies are consumed and proteolytically/oxidatively/enzymatically degraded by monocytes/phagocytes[690] while IgA-containing immune complexes are preferentially consumed by hepatocytes and exported intact into the bile for excretion.

- **ENDOCRINE IMBALANCE & OPTIMIZATION: Prolactin, Insulin, Estrogen, DHEA, Cortisol, Testosterone, Thyroid** Hormonal imbalances seen among autoimmune/inflammatory patients are: ❶ *elevated prolactin*, ❷ *elevated estrogen*, ❸ *elevated insulin*, and ❹ *reduced DHEA*, ❺ *reduced cortisol*, and ❻ *reduced testosterone*; see Chapter 4 for discussion of these hormones and respective interventions. Thyroid evaluation (patient + labs) should be comprehensive, as discussed in Chapter 1, with a low threshold for empiric treatment.
    - Melatonin: Melatonin is a pineal hormone with well-known sleep-inducing and immunomodulatory properties, and it is commonly administered in doses of 1-40 mg in the evening, before bedtime. Starting with a relatively low dose (e.g., 1-5 mg) and increasing as tolerated is recommended. Melatonin (20 mg hs) appears to have cured two patients with drug-resistant sarcoidosis[691] and 3 mg provided immediate short-term benefit to a patient with multiple sclerosis.[692]
    - Prolactin (excess): **Prolactin has proinflammatory and immunodysregulatory actions and is commonly elevated—either overtly or latently—in patients with inflammatory/autoimmune disease.** Accordingly prolactin-lowering treatment shows safety and effectiveness in the treatment of numerous inflammatory/autoimmune diseases; often these results are noted even when the patient's prolactin level was not initially elevated, suggesting the alleviation of latent hyperprolactinemia and/or an inherent anti-inflammatory action of the prolactin-lowering treatment. According to clinical trials with small numbers of patients, whether prolactin levels are high or not, prolactin-lowering treatment (such as bromocriptine) appears highly beneficial when used with other anti-rheumatic treatments ("…drastic efficacy with spectacular improvement in clinical, biological and occupational status…"[693]) in patients with psoriatic arthritis. Serum prolactin is the standard assessment of prolactin status. Since elevated prolactin may be a sign of pituitary tumor, assessment for headaches, visual deficits, other abnormalities of pituitary hormones (e.g., GH and TSH) should be performed and CT or MRI must be considered. Patients with prolactin levels less than 100 ng/mL and normal CT/MRI findings can be managed conservatively with effective prolactin-lowering treatment and annual radiologic assessment (less necessary with favorable

---

[688] "These observations support the hypothesis that IC handling is abnormal in SLE." Davies KA, Peters AM, Beynon HL, Walport MJ. Immune complex processing in patients with systemic lupus erythematosus. *J Clin Invest*. 1992 Nov;90(5):2075-83
[689] "These results indicate that Fc-mediated clearance of ICs is defective in patients with SLE and suggest that ligation of ICs by Fc receptors is critical for their efficient binding and retention by the fixed MPS in the liver." Davies et al. Defective Fc-dependent processing of immune complexes in patients with systemic lupus erythematosus. *Arthritis Rheum*. 2002 Apr;46(4):1028-38
[690] "In the presence of U937 [monocytic] cells, both the AHP-anti-dsDNA and C3b-opsonized ICs were rapidly removed from the erythrocytes; at 37 degrees C, more than half of the complexes were removed in 2 minutes." Craig ML, Bankovich AJ, McElhenny JL, Taylor RP. Clearance of anti-double-stranded DNA antibodies: the natural immune complex clearance mechanism. *Arthritis Rheum*. 2000 Oct;43(10):2265-75
[691] Cagnoni ML, Lombardi A, Cerinic MC, Dedola GL, Pignone A. Melatonin for treatment of chronic refractory sarcoidosis. *Lancet*. 1995 Nov 4;346(8984):1229-30
[692] "…administration of melatonin (3 mg, orally) at 2:00 p.m., when the patient experienced severe blurring of vision, resulted within 15 minutes in a dramatic improvement in visual acuity and in normalization of the visual evoked potential latency after stimulation of the left eye." Sandyk R. Diurnal variations in vision and relations to circadian melatonin secretion in multiple sclerosis. *Int J Neurosci*. 1995 Nov;83(1-2):1-6
[693] Abstract from article in French: "In 2 cases of psoriatic arthritis, adding bromocriptine to gold salts and nonsteroidal anti-inflammatory drug was followed by a drastic efficacy with spectacular improvement in clinical, biological and occupational status. Because none of the cases had hyperprolactinaemia, bromocriptine acted probably had an intrinsic anti-inflammatory effect independent of its antiprolactinic effect." Eulry et al. [Blood prolactin under the effect of protirelin in spondylarthropathies. Treatment trial of 4 cases of reactive arthritis and 2 cases of psoriatic arthritis with bromocriptine] *Ann Med Interne* (Paris). 1996;147(1):15-9. French

serum response).[694, see review 695] **Patients with RA and SLE have higher basal and stress-induced levels of prolactin compared with normal controls.**[696,697] A normal serum prolactin level does not necessarily exclude the use of prolactin-lowering intervention, especially since many autoimmune patients have **latent hyperprolactinemia** which may not be detected with random serum measurement of prolactin. Vitex lowers serum prolactin in humans[698,699] via a dopaminergic effect.[700] Due at least in part to its content of L-dopa, *Mucuna pruriens* shows clinical dopaminergic activity as evidenced by its effectiveness in Parkinson's disease[701]; up to 15-30 gm/d of mucuna has been used clinically but doses will be dependent on preparation and phytoconcentration. Clinical intervention with bromocriptine appears warranted in patients with RA, SLE, Reiter's syndrome, psoriatic arthritis, and probably multiple sclerosis and uveitis.[702] A normal serum prolactin level does not necessarily exclude the use of prolactin-lowering intervention, especially since many autoimmune patients have latent hyperprolactinemia which may not be detected with random serum measurement of prolactin. Cabergoline/Dostinex is a newer dopamine agonist with few adverse effects; typical dose starts at 0.5 mg per week (0.25 mg twice per week).[703] Several studies have indicated that cabergoline is safer and more effective than bromocriptine for reducing prolactin levels[704] and the dose can often be reduced after successful prolactin reduction, allowing for reductions in cost and adverse effects.[705] Although fewer studies have been published supporting the antirheumatic benefits of cabergoline than those supporting bromocriptine; its antirheumatic benefits have indeed been documented.[706]

- <u>Cruciferous vegetables, DIM, I3C</u>: In a short-term study using I3C in patients with SLE, I3C supplementation at 375 mg per day was well tolerated and resulted in modest treatment-dependent clinical improvement as well as favorable modification of estrogen metabolism away from 16-alpha-hydroxyestrone and toward 2-hydroxyestrone.[707]
- <u>DHEA</u>: DHEA is an anti-inflammatory and immunoregulatory hormone that is commonly deficient in patients with autoimmunity, including polymyalgia rheumatica, SLE, RA, and inflammatory arthritis.[708,709] DHEA levels are suppressed by prednisone[710], and DHEA has been shown to reverse the

---

[694] Beers MH, Berkow R (eds). *The Merck Manual. Seventeenth Edition*. Whitehouse Station; Merck Research Laboratories 1999 Page 77-78
[695] Serri O, Chik CL, Ur E, Ezzat S. Diagnosis and management of hyperprolactinemia. *CMAJ*. 2003 Sep 16;169(6):575-81 cmaj.ca/cgi/content/full/169/6/575
[696] Dostal C, Moszkorzova L, Musilova L, Lacinova Z, Marek J, Zvarova J. Serum prolactin stress values in patients with systemic lupus erythematosus. *Ann Rheum Dis*. 2003 May;62(5):487-8 ard.bmjjournals.com/cgi/content/full/62/5/487
[697] "RESULTS: A significantly higher rate of elevated PRL levels was found in SLE patients (40.0%) compared with the healthy controls (14.8%). No proof was found of association with the presence of anti-ds-DNA or with specific organ involvement. Similarly, elevated PRL levels were found in RA patients (39.3%)." Moszkorzova L, Lacinova Z, Marek J, et al. Hyperprolactinaemia in patients with systemic lupus erythematosus. *Clin Exp Rheumatol*. 2002 Nov-Dec;20(6):807-12
[698] "Since AC extracts were shown to have beneficial effects on premenstrual mastodynia serum prolactin levels in such patients were also studied in one double-blind, placebo-controlled clinical study. Serum prolactin levels were indeed reduced in the patients treated with the extract." Wuttke W, Jarry H, Christoffel V, Spengler B, Seidlova-Wuttke D. Chaste tree, Vitex agnus-castus—pharmacology and clinical indications. *Phytomedicine*. 2003 May;10(4):348-57
[699] German abstract from Medline: "The prolactin release was reduced after 3 months, shortened luteal phases were normalised and deficits in the luteal progesterone synthesis were eliminated." Milewicz A, Gejdel E, Sworen H, Sienkiewicz K, Jedrzejak J, Teucher T, Schmitz H. [Vitex agnus castus extract in the treatment of luteal phase defects due to latent hyperprolactinemia. Results of a randomized placebo-controlled double-blind study] *Arzneimittelforschung*. 1993 Jul;43(7):752-6
[700] "Our results indicate a dopaminergic effect of Vitex agnus-castus extracts and suggest additional pharmacological actions via opioid receptors." Meier B, Berger D, Hoberg E, Sticher O, Schaffner W. Pharmacological activities of Vitex agnus-castus extracts in vitro. *Phytomedicine*. 2000 Oct;7(5):373-81
[701] "CONCLUSIONS: The rapid onset of action and longer on time without concomitant increase in dyskinesias on mucuna seed powder formulation suggest that this natural source of L-dopa might possess advantages over conventional L-dopa preparations in the long term management of PD." Katzenschlager et al. Mucuna pruriens in Parkinson's disease: a double blind clinical and pharmacological study. *J Neurol Neurosurg Psychiatry*. 2004 Dec;75(12):1672-7
[702] "...clinical observations and trials support the use of bromocriptine as a nonstandard primary or adjunctive therapy in the treatment of recalcitrant RA, SLE, Reiter's syndrome, and psoriatic arthritis and associated conditions unresponsive to traditional approaches." McMurray RW. Bromocriptine in rheumatic and autoimmune diseases. *Semin Arthritis Rheum*. 2001 Aug;31(1):21-32
[703] Serri O, Chik CL, Ur E, Ezzat S. Diagnosis and management of hyperprolactinemia. *CMAJ*. 2003 Sep 16;169(6):575-81 cmaj.ca/cgi/content/full/169/6/575
[704] "CONCLUSION: These data indicate that cabergoline is a very effective agent for lowering the prolactin levels in hyperprolactinemic patients and that it appears to offer considerable advantage over bromocriptine in terms of efficacy and tolerability." Sabuncu T, Arikan E, Tasan E, Hatemi H. Comparison of the effects of cabergoline and bromocriptine on prolactin levels in hyperprolactinemic patients. *Intern Med*. 2001 Sep;40(9):857-61
[705] "Cabergoline also normalized PRL in the majority of patients with known bromocriptine intolerance or -resistance. Once PRL secretion was adequately controlled, the dose of cabergoline could often be significantly decreased, which further reduced costs of therapy." Verhelst et al. Cabergoline in the treatment of hyperprolactinemia: a study in 455 patients. *J Clin Endocrinol Metab*. 1999 Jul;84(7):2518-22 jcem.endojournals.org/cgi/content/full/84/7/2518
[706] Erb N, Pace AV, Delamere JP, Kitas GD. Control of unremitting rheumatoid arthritis by the prolactin antagonist cabergoline. *Rheumatology* (Oxford). 2001 Feb;40(2):237-9 rheumatology.oxfordjournals.org/cgi/content/full/40/2/237
[707] "Women with SLE can manifest a metabolic response to I3C and might benefit from its antiestrogenic effects." McAlindon TE, Gulin J, Chen T, Klug T, Lahita R, Nuite M. Indole-3-carbinol in women with SLE: effect on estrogen metabolism and disease activity. *Lupus*. 2001;10(11):779-83
[708] "The low levels found in patients with PM:TA are in accordance with those previously reported in immune-mediated diseases such as systemic lupus erythematosus (SLE) and rheumatoid arthritis, suggesting that diminution of DHEAS is a constant endocrinologic feature in these categories of patients." Nilsson et al. Blood dehydroepiandrosterone sulphate (DHEAS) levels in polymyalgia rheumatica/giant cell arteritis and primary fibromyalgia. *Clin Exp Rheumatol*. 1994 Jul-Aug;12(4):415-7
[709] "DHEAS concentrations were significantly decreased in both women and men with inflammatory arthritis (IA) (P < 0.001)." Dessein et al. Hyposecretion of the adrenal androgen dehydroepiandrosterone sulfate and its relation to clinical variables in inflammatory arthritis. *Arthritis Res*. 2001;3(3):183-8 arthritis-research.com/content/3/3/183
[710] "Basal serum DHEA and DHEAS concentrations were suppressed to a greater degree than was cortisol during both daily and alternate day prednisone treatments. ...Thus, adrenal androgen secretion was more easily suppressed than was cortisol secretion by this low dose of glucocorticoid, but there was no advantage to alternate day therapy." Rittmaster et al. Effect of daily and alternate day low dose prednisone on serum cortisol and adrenal androgens in hirsute women. *J Clin Endocrinol Metab*. 1988 Aug;67(2):400-3

osteoporosis and loss of bone mass induced by corticosteroid treatment.[711] DHEA shows no acute or subacute toxicity even when used in supraphysiologic doses, even when used in sick patients. For example, in a study of 32 patients with HIV, DHEA doses of 750 mg – 2,250 mg per day were well-tolerated and produced no dose-limiting adverse effects.[712] This lack of toxicity compares favorably with any and all so-called "antirheumatic" drugs, nearly all of which show impressive comparable toxicity. High-dose supplemental DHEA has benefits in the treatment of SLE that are comparable to those obtained with antimalarial drugs.[713] When used at doses of 200 mg per day, DHEA safely provides clinical benefit for patients with various autoimmune diseases, including ulcerative colitis, Crohn's disease[714], and SLE.[715] In patients with SLE, DHEA supplementation allows for reduced dosing of prednisone (thus avoiding its adverse effects) while providing symptomatic improvement.[716] Optimal clinical response appears to correlate with serum levels that are supraphysiologic[717], and therefore treatment may be implemented with little regard for initial/baseline DHEA levels provided that the patient is free of contraindications, particularly high risk for sex-hormone-dependent malignancy. Other than mild adverse effects predictable with any androgen (namely voice deepening, transient acne, and increased facial hair), DHEA supplementation does not cause serious adverse effects[718], and it is appropriate for routine clinical use particularly when 1) the dose of DHEA is kept as low as possible, 2) duration is kept as short as possible, 3) other interventions are used to address the underlying cause of the disease, 4) the patient is deriving benefit, and 5) the risk-to-benefit ratio is favorable.

- **XENOBIOTIC ACCUMULATION & DETOXIFICATION: Chemical avoidance, nutritional support for detoxification pathways, urine alkalinization** The clinical relevance and pathogenic mechanisms of xenobiotic accumulation are irrefutably well documented and described. Clinical assessments include history, physical examination, and laboratory assessment (using serum, whole blood, urine or—rarely yet accurately—fat biopsy), and response to treatment. Treatments include nutritional support for Phases 1 and 2 of detoxification (e.g., oxidation and conjugation) and excretion via bile and urine; for the latter, urinary alkalinization is generally recommended. Chemical toxins can be bound in the gut using activated charcoal, cholestyramine, or *Chlorella*—all of these three treatments have documented safety and effectiveness; clinically and empirically, phytochelatin (plant-derived peptides that bind toxic metals) concentrates appear safe and effective despite lack of conclusive published data supporting clinical use. Mercury exposure via working in a dental office is one of the greatest occupational risks ever identified for the development of SLE in humans.

---

[711] "CONCLUSION: Prasterone treatment prevented BMD loss and significantly increased BMD at both the lumbar spine and total hip in female patients with SLE receiving exogenous glucocorticoids." Mease PJ, Ginzler EM, Gluck OS, Schiff M, Goldman A, Greenwald M, Cohen S, Egan R, Quarles BJ, Schwartz KE. Effects of prasterone on bone mineral density in women with systemic lupus erythematosus receiving chronic glucocorticoid therapy. *J Rheumatol*. 2005 Apr;32(4):616-21

[712] "Thirty-one subjects were evaluated and monitored for safety and tolerance. The oral drug was administered three times daily in doses ranging from 750 mg/day to 2,250 mg/day for 16 weeks. ... The drug was well tolerated and no dose-limiting side effects were noted." Dyner et al. An open-label dose-escalation trial of oral dehydroepiandrosterone tolerance and pharmacokinetics in patients with HIV disease. *J Acquir Immune Defic Syndr*. 1993 May;6(5):459-65

[713] Tierney ML. McPhee SJ, Papadakis MA. Current Medical Diagnosis and Treatment 2006. 45th edition. New York; Lange Medical Books: 2006, pages 833-837

[714] "CONCLUSIONS: In a pilot study, dehydroepiandrosterone was effective and safe in patients with refractory Crohn's disease or ulcerative colitis." Andus et al. Patients with refractory Crohn's disease or ulcerative colitis respond to dehydroepiandrosterone: a pilot study. *Aliment Pharmacol Ther*. 2003 Feb;17(3):409-14

[715] "CONCLUSION: The overall results confirm that DHEA treatment was well-tolerated, significantly reduced the number of SLE flares, and improved patient's global assessment of disease activity." Chang DM, Lan JL, Lin HY, Luo SF. Dehydroepiandrosterone treatment of women with mild-to-moderate systemic lupus erythematosus: a multicenter randomized, double-blind, placebo-controlled trial. *Arthritis Rheum*. 2002 Nov;46(11):2924-7

[716] "CONCLUSION: Among women with lupus disease activity, reducing the dosage of prednisone to < or = 7.5 mg/day for a sustained period of time while maintaining stabilization or a reduction of disease activity was possible in a significantly greater proportion of patients treated with oral prasterone, 200 mg once daily, compared with patients treated with placebo." Petri et al; GL601 Study Group. Effects of prasterone on corticosteroid requirements of women with systemic lupus erythematosus: a double-blind, randomized, placebo-controlled trial. *Arthritis Rheum*. 2002 Jul;46(7):1820-9

[717] "CONCLUSION: The clinical response to DHEA was not clearly dose dependent. Serum levels of DHEA and DHEAS correlated only weakly with lupus outcomes, but suggested an optimum serum DHEAS of 1000 microg/dl." Barry NN, McGuire JL, van Vollenhoven RF. Dehydroepiandrosterone in systemic lupus erythematosus: relationship between dosage, serum levels, and clinical response. *J Rheumatol*. 1998 Dec;25(12):2352-6

[718] Tierney ML. McPhee SJ, Papadakis MA. *Current Medical Diagnosis and Treatment 2006. 45th edition*. New York; Lange Medical Books: 2006, page 1721

Scleroderma & Systemic Sclerosis

> **Introduction:**
> Scleroderma and systemic sclerosis are related conditions of either dermal or dermal+systemic fibrosis, respectively. A reasonable conceptualization is that of an inflammation/ROS-driven fibrotic response; the solution then—of course—is to address the disease-specific and patient-specific causes of excess inflammation and immune imbalance. The vicious cycles of nutritional deficiency, gastrointestinal dysbiosis, and persistent active viral infections must be addressed.

Description/pathophysiology:
- Overview: Generally considered "idiopathic" from the allopathic medical perspective; for example, a 2008 article published by the American Academy of Family Physicians introduces the topic in this manner, providing a brief description along with undermining any possible desire to treat the cause of the illness via the promulgation that the cause is officially declared to be unknown: "Systemic sclerosis (systemic scleroderma) is a chronic connective tissue disease of unknown etiology that causes widespread microvascular damage and excessive deposition of collagen in the skin and internal organs."[719] The terms *scleroderma* and *systemic sclerosis* are used somewhat interchangeably; yet, as these terms suggest, *scleroderma* is properly assigned to disease that is limited to the skin, while *systemic sclerosis* denotes visceral involvement in addition to skin changes. *Scleroderma* will be the default term in this section for linguistic expediency; because the initials "SS" can equally suggest Sjogren's syndrome as well as systemic sclerosis, the initials *SSc* will be used to denote systemic sclerosis—again interchangeably with *scleroderma*.
- **Characterized by fibrosis of the skin and internal organs, including the esophagus, intestines, lung, heart, and kidneys.** The condition can be mild and limited to the skin only, or it can be systemic and rapidly fatal due to internal organ involvement.
- Main subtypes:
  1. Limited, cutaneous scleroderma—60% of cases: Primarily affecting the skin, especially of the fingers and face; distribution often described as distal to the neck, elbows and knees; major complications are GERD, Raynaud's, and pulmonary hypertension, notably "Patients with limited cutaneous systemic sclerosis have the greatest risk of pulmonary arterial hypertension."[720]
     - CREST syndrome—variant of limited/cutaneous scleroderma: Calcinosis, Raynaud's phenomenon, esophageal dysmotility/dysfunction, sclerodactyly, telangiectasia
  2. Diffuse, systemic sclerosis—35% of cases: Characterized by systemic fibrosis of skin and internal organs, especially interstitial lung disease; may rapidly progress to death via scleroderma renal crisis.
  3. Systemic sclerosis sine scleroderma—approximately 5 percent of patients with systemic sclerosis): Characteristic internal organ manifestations of the disease without skin thickening.
  4. Localized/linear scleroderma and morphea: Primarily affects children, not associated with Raynaud phenomenon or significant internal organ involvement.
  5. Mixed connective tissue disease and "overlap syndromes"—less common: Combination of scleroderma with another autoimmune disease, such as dermatomyositis (sclerodermatomyositis) or RA, SLE, etc.
  6. Scleroderma secondary to xenobiotic immunotoxicity—rare: Scleroderma can result from exposure to vinyl chloride, silicone, petroleum products, toxic oil syndrome, solvents, cocaine, and pesticides.
- Patients with scleroderma have evidence of **increased oxidative stress** demonstrated by a doubling of urinary isoprostane excretion.[721] Oxidative stress *results from* and *contributes to* systemic inflammation because 1) increased immune activity results in elaboration of oxidants, and 2) oxidative stress upregulates NFkB (and other pathways) for additive immune activation; oxidative stress and inflammation both contribute to tissue fibrosis.

---
[719] Hinchcliff M, Varga J. Systemic sclerosis/scleroderma: a treatable multisystem disease. *Am Fam Physician*. 2008 Oct 15;78(8):961-8
[720] Hinchcliff M, Varga J. Systemic sclerosis/scleroderma: a treatable multisystem disease. *Am Fam Physician*. 2008 Oct 15;78(8):961-8
[721] "CONCLUSION: This study provides evidence of enhanced lipid peroxidation in both SSc and UCTD, and suggests a rationale for antioxidant treatment of SSc." Cracowski JL, Marpeau C, Carpentier PH, et al. Enhanced in vivo lipid peroxidation in scleroderma spectrum disorders. *Arthritis Rheum* 2001 May;44(5):1143-8

Clinical presentations:
- **Classic presentation**: "The typical patient is a young or middle-age woman with a history of Raynaud phenomenon who presents with skin induration and internal organ dysfunction."[722] 4x more common in women, general age of onset is 20-40 years. More than 95% of scleroderma/SSc patients have Raynaud's phenomenon, thereby giving this clinical manifestation a considerable degree of importance in the initial/historical assessment.
- **Skin changes**: Hyperpigmentation, tightness, tightness and thickening of the face results in "mask-like face", telangiectasia, may also have depigmentation; dermal pitting (mild) and ulceration (more severe) of fingertips; swelling and thickening of the fingers is termed sclerodactyly.
- **Soft tissue calcification**: Especially in the hands; systemic calcification is also seen.
- **Polyarthralgia**: Affects 90% of patients; flexion contractures of the joints due to fibrosis is also common.
- **Autonomic dysfunction: Raynaud's phenomenon**: Seen in 90% of patients and often precedes sclerodermatous manifestations by a period of up to 5 years; the high level of overlap among these two conditions suggests a common etiology—the factor most strongly associated with both conditions and especially Raynaud's is *H pylori* infection, discussed later in this section on SSc and also in the section on Raynaud's.
- **Pulmonary**: Dyspnea, pulmonary hypertension.
- **Cardiac**: Arrhythmias, CHF, hypertension, ECG abnormalities—may be fatal.
- **Renal**: Renal failure is a leading cause of death—see renal assessments in Chapter 1. "Scleroderma renal crisis develops in 3 to 10 percent of all patients with systemic sclerosis and in 10 to 20 percent of those with rapidly progressive diffuse cutaneous systemic sclerosis; the greatest risk occurs within the first three years of the disease. ... Patients with scleroderma renal crisis characteristically present with sudden-onset accelerated hypertension that is often associated with progressive oliguric renal failure with proteinuria, microangiopathic anemia, and microscopic hematuria. Ten to 15 percent of patients with scleroderma renal crisis are normotensive, but hypertensive when compared with their baseline blood pressure measurements."[723]
- **GI disturbances**:
    - Esophageal dysfunction and dysphagia eventually occur in most patients; histologic/biopsy examination reveals degeneration of intestinal nerves, vessels, and smooth muscle.[724]
    - Greatly increased risk for Barrett's esophagus (33% of all scleroderma patients) with a notably low risk of esophageal adenocarcinoma.
    - Slow intestinal transit—intestinal hypomotility in scleroderma promotes bacterial overgrowth of the small bowel, which probably contributes to the pathogenesis of the disease via the pro-inflammatory and immune activating effects discussed in Chapter 4. Treatment of bacterial overgrowth with antibiotics (ciprofloxacin 500 mg bid[725]) or promotility drugs (octreotide[726]) is effective treatment for scleroderma according to published case reports; **such research supports the hypothesis that intestinal dysbiosis—namely bacterial overgrowth—is an important contributor to the perpetuation of scleroderma.**

Major differential diagnoses:
- **Parkinson's disease**: Mask-like face
- **Other autoimmune disorders**: Overlap syndromes, mixed connective tissue diseases
- **Amyloidosis**: Primary or secondary forms; often leads to skin thickening due to amyloid deposition however skin generally remains soft and more edematous-like than induration-like
- **Nephrogenic systemic fibrosis**: "Nephrogenic systemic fibrosis (NSF) is a fibrosing disorder, recently described in patients with advanced chronic kidney disease, usually after exposure to gadolinium (Gd)-based contrast agents, characterized by progressive fibrotic involvement mainly of the skin. At clinical examination, the cutaneous findings of NSF may partly resemble those of systemic sclerosis. However, the different topographic

---

[722] Hinchcliff M, Varga J. Systemic sclerosis/scleroderma: a treatable multisystem disease. *Am Fam Physician*. 2008 Oct 15;78(8):961-8
[723] Hinchcliff M, Varga J. Systemic sclerosis/scleroderma: a treatable multisystem disease. *Am Fam Physician*. 2008 Oct 15;78(8):961-8
[724] "We found ultrastructural signs of axonal degeneration and cytoskeletal abnormalities in the bundles of unmyelinated fibers. There was also focal degeneration of smooth muscle cells, often in association with the presence of partially degranulated mast cells." Malandrini A, Selvi E, Villanova M, et al. Autonomic nervous system and smooth muscle cell involvement in systemic sclerosis: ultrastructural study of 3 cases. *J Rheumatol*. 2000 May;27(5):1203-6
[725] Over KE, Bucknall RC. Regression of skin changes in a patient with systemic sclerosis following treatment for bacterial overgrowth with ciprofloxacin. *Br J Rheumatol*. 1998 Jun;37(6):696 rheumatology.oxfordjournals.org/cgi/reprint/37/6/696a
[726] "After 8 months of treatment, normal weight was obtained and skin induration was spectacularly reduced and pigmentation returned to a normal state." Descamps V, et al. Global improvement of systemic scleroderma under long-term administration of octreotide. *Eur J Dermatol* 1999 Sep;9(6):446-8

distribution of the skin thickening and hardening, usually involving the limbs and trunk, whilst sparing the face, the lack of serologic abnormalities and the distinctive histopathological findings allow this new disease entity to be distinguished from systemic sclerosis and other scleroderma-like fibrosing disorders (scleromyxedema, scleredema, eosinophilic fasciitis, etc.)."[727]

- <u>Vinyl chloride disease</u>: exposure to vinyl chloride (VC) monomer, a volatile substance mostly used for polyvinyl chloride (PVC) synthesis produces a scleroderma-like disorder that may be complicated by vasculitic and neurologic sequelae.[728,729,730]
- <u>Dermal infections and other diseases</u>: Zygomycosis, sporotrichosis, cutaneous lymphoma
- <u>Toxic oil syndrome</u>: A syndrome of incapacitating myalgias, marked peripheral eosinophilia, pulmonary infiltrates, and increased prevalence of scleroderma and neurologic disorders following consumption of contaminated oil.[731]

Clinical assessments:
- **History/subjective**:
  - Symptoms and complications from dermal induration/hardening and fibrosis
  - Intestinal and digestive complaints
  - Areas affected, ROM, ADL, QOL
  - <u>Xenobiotic exposure</u>: Occupational exposure to silica is associated with scleroderma; some cases appear to be linked to silicone breast implants[732] (controversial[733]) and anti-silicate antibodies may be valuable for documenting humoral response to silicone.[734] Clinicians should ask about any history of iatrogenic, occupational, recreational or domestic xenobiotic exposure, such as to organic solvents[735], pesticides, epoxy resins[736], and other immunotoxins.[737] Use of cocaine may cause or exacerbate scleroderma.[738]
- **Physical examination/objective**: routine, including the following:
  - <u>Dermal exam, including nailfold capillaroscopy</u>: Symptoms and complications from dermal induration/hardening, swelling, fibrosis, and calcium deposition: swollen fingers, tight skin on face and hands, dermal ulcerations and hypopigmentation. The "colors of Raynaud's phenomenon" are white (vasospasm), blue-purple (ischemia), and red (hyperemia).
    - <u>Nailfold capillaroscopy—viewed clinically with magnifying lens</u>: Reveals microvascular changes consistent with autoimmunity and autoimmune-expedited cardiovascular disease. Per Cutolo et al[739], "Raynaud's phenomenon (RP) represents the most frequent clinical aspect of cardio/microvascular involvement and is a key feature of several autoimmune rheumatic diseases. Moreover, RP is associated in a statistically significant manner with many coronary diseases. In

---

[727] Rota et al. Nephrogenic systemic fibrosis: an unusual scleroderma-like fibrosing disorder. *Rheumatol Int*. 2010 Aug;30(10):1389-91

[728] "Occupational exposure to vinyl chloride monomers is known to induce Raynaud's phenomenon, periportal fibrosis, liver angiosarcoma and scleroderma-like syndrome." Serratrice et al. A case of polymyositis with anti-histidyl-t-RNA synthetase (Jo-1) antibody syndrome following extensive vinyl chloride exposure. *Clin Rheumatol* 2001;20:379-82

[729] "An unusual case of systemic sclerosis occurring in a patient exposed to the vinyl chloride monomer (VCM) is presented." Ostlere et al. Atypical systemic sclerosis following exposure to vinyl chloride monomer. A case report and review of the cutaneous aspects of vinyl chloride disease. *Clin Exp Dermatol*. 1992 May;17(3):208-10

[730] "Angiosarcoma of the liver, Raynaud's phenomenon, scleroderma-like lesions, acroosteolysis and neuritis are known to be typical vinyl chloride-associated manifestations (VC disease)." Magnavita N, Bergamaschi A, Garcovich A, Giuliano G. Vasculitic purpura in vinyl chloride disease: a case report. *Angiology*. 1986 May;37(5):382-8

[731] "In 1981, in Spain, the ingestion of an oil fraudulently sold as olive oil caused an outbreak of a previously unrecorded condition, later known as toxic oil syndrome (TOS), clinically characterized by intense incapacitating myalgias, marked peripheral eosinophilia, and pulmonary infiltrates." Gelpi et al; WHO/CISAT Scientific Committee for the Toxic Oil Syndrome. The Spanish toxic oil syndrome 20 years after its onset: multidisciplinary review of scientific knowledge. *Environ Health Perspect*. 2002 May;110(5):457-64

[732] "...idiopathic form of scleroderma and related conditions. CONCLUSION. These findings suggest that ANA positivity is relatively common in individuals with silicone breast implants, and may support the existence of autoimmune mechanisms in the pathogenesis of the clinical manifestations seen in this population." Cuellar ML, Scopelitis E, Tenenbaum SA, et al. Serum antinuclear antibodies in women with silicone breast implants. *J Rheumatol*. 1995 Feb;22(2):236-40

[733] "Neither the case-control studies nor the other epidemiologic data support the hypothesis that scleroderma is associated with or causally related to breast implants." Whorton D, Wong O. Scleroderma and silicone breast implants. *West J Med* 1997 Sep;167(3):159-65

[734] Shen GQ, Ojo-Amaize EA, Agopian MS, Peter JB. Silicate antibodies in women with silicone breast implants: development of an assay for detection of humoral immunity. *Clin Diagn Lab Immunol*. 1996 Mar;3(2):162-6 cdli.asm.org/cgi/reprint/3/2/162?view=reprint&pmid=8991630

[735] "We describe a sclerodermatous syndrome in a middle-aged man who had worked with a wide variety of organic solvents over a prolonged period." Bottomley WW, et al. A sclerodermatous syndrome with unusual features following prolonged occupational exposure to organic solvents. *Br J Dermatol* 1993 Feb;128(2):203-6

[736] "A new occupational disorder characterized by skin sclerosis is described. This disease developed acutely in workmen exposed to the vapor of epoxy resins." Yamakage A, et al. Occupational scleroderma-like disorder occurring in men engaged in the polymerization of epoxy resins. *Dermatologica*. 1980;161(1):33-44

[737] "There is growing concern about the association between systemic sclerosis and certain environmental and occupational risk factors, including exposures to vinyl chloride, adulterated cooking oils, L-tryptophan, silica, silicone breast implants, organic solvents, and other agents such as epoxy resins, pesticides, and hand/arm vibration." Nietert PJ, Silver RM. Systemic sclerosis: environmental and occupational risk factors. *Curr Opin Rheumatol* 2000 Nov;12(6):520-6

[738] "It has been reported that cocaine may initiate scleroderma in an already susceptible individual or unmask it at an earlier age in subclinical disease." Attoussi S, Faulkner ML, Oso A, Umoru B. Cocaine-induced scleroderma and scleroderma renal crisis. *South Med J* 1998 Oct;91(10):961-3

[739] Cutolo M, Sulli A, Secchi ME, Paolino S, Pizzorni C. Nailfold capillaroscopy is useful for the diagnosis and follow-up of autoimmune rheumatic diseases. A future tool for the analysis of microvascular heart involvement? *Rheumatology* (Oxford). 2006 Oct;45 Suppl 4:iv43-6 rheumatology.oxfordjournals.org/content/45/suppl_4/iv43.full.pdf

normal conditions or in primary RP (excluding during the cold-exposure test), the normal nailfold capillaroscopic pattern shows a regular disposition of the capillary loops along with the nailbed. On the contrary, in subjects suffering from secondary RP, one or more alterations of the capillaroscopic findings should alert the physician of the possibility of a connective tissue disease not yet detected. ==Nailfold capillaroscopy (NV) represents the best method to analyze microvascular abnormalities in autoimmune rheumatic diseases. Architectural disorganization, giant capillaries, hemorrhages, loss of capillaries, angiogenesis and avascular areas characterize >95% of patients with overt scleroderma (SSc)."==
- Range of motion (ROM): Limited range of motion is characteristic secondary to a "straight jacket" effect secondary to tightened and fibrotic skin; reduced neck extension is termed "platysma sign"
- Abdominal exam: Abdominal exam, gastrointestinal motility
- Pulmonary exam: Pulmonary examination and auscultation; needs to be complemented by additional diagnostic testing. "Dyspnea is a late manifestation of systemic sclerosis–related lung disease; however, lung involvement is common and is the leading cause of death in patients with systemic sclerosis. … Thus, routine screening with pulmonary function tests and Doppler echocardiography in all patients is essential for the early detection of interstitial lung disease and pulmonary arterial hypertension, respectively."[740]
- Cardiovascular exam: Assessment for hypertension is mandatory

- **Laboratory assessments**: *lab assessments are only minimally supportive for the diagnosis, but are helpful to monitor for complications*
  - Urinalysis: Screen for renal compromise as previously detailed
  - Chemistry panel: Assess for renal and liver status, electrolytes, etc.
  - CBC: May reveal anemia due to malabsorption-induced deficiencies of B12, folate, iron, hypoproliferation due to inflammation (i.e., the anemia of chronic disease).
  - Rheumatoid factor: positive in 33%
  - Breath hydrogen/methane for SIBO: This test is used to assess for bacterial overgrowth; it is not a perfect test and it delays treatment (dietary, antimicrobial) that should generally be implemented regardless of the results of this test.
  - Lactulose and mannitol assay for "leaky gut" and malabsorption: Abnormal results are likely due to bacterial overgrowth and/or celiac disease with resultant malabsorption and increased intestinal permeability.[741]
  - Fecal calprotectin—assessment for gastrointestinal involvement: "Fecal calprotectin (F-calprotectin) is increased in a majority of patients with SSc. It correlates with objective and clinically important features of GI disease, and fecal concentrations do not vary with plasma concentrations. We suggest that F-calprotectin is a promising objective non-invasive biomarker of GI involvement in SSc."[742]
  - Leukocyte antigens: Increased prevalence of HLA-DR5 and HLA-DR1
  - *Helicobacter pylori* detection: Given the increased prevalence of *Helicobacter pylori* infection[743,744], the addition of antigen testing onto a comprehensive stool analysis and comprehensive parasitology examination is recommended.
  - Comprehensive stool analysis and comprehensive parasitology: essential
  - ==**ANA (nucleolar): Positive in up to 96% of patients with scleroderma;** nucleolar pattern is most specific==
  - ==**Anticentromere antibody**: Positive in 50% with CREST; generally—relatively speaking—portends disease course more limited to dermal involvement[745]; correlates with and requires monitoring for pulmonary arterial hypertension==

---

[740] Hinchcliff M, Varga J. Systemic sclerosis/scleroderma: a treatable multisystem disease. *Am Fam Physician*. 2008 Oct 15;78(8):961-8
[741] "Coeliac disease may account for malabsorption in scleroderma patients even when test suggest bacterial overgrowth." Marguerie C, Kaye S, Vyse T, Mackworth-Young C, Walport MJ, Black C. Malabsorption caused by coeliac disease in patients who have scleroderma. *Br J Rheumatol*. 1995 Sep;34(9):858-61
[742] Andréasson et al. Faecal calprotectin: a biomarker of gastrointestinal disease in systemic sclerosis. *J Intern Med*. 2011 Jul;270(1):50-7
[743] "Thus, risk for gastric diseases caused by HP infection is enhanced in patients with systemic sclerosis compared with white healthy, asymptomatic persons examined in other studies." Reinauer et al. Helicobacter pylori in patients with systemic sclerosis: detection with the 13C-urea breath test and eradication. *Acta Derm Venereol*. 1994 Sep;74(5):361-3
[744] "Patients with SSc have H. pylori infection at a higher prevalence than the general population." Yazawa N, Fujimoto M, Kikuchi K, et al. High seroprevalence of Helicobacter pylori infection in patients with systemic sclerosis: association with esophageal involvement. *J Rheumatol*. 1998 Apr;25(4):650-3
[745] Ho KT, Reveille JD. The clinical relevance of autoantibodies in scleroderma. Arthritis Res Ther. 2003;5(2):80-93 arthritis-research.com/content/5/2/80

- **Anti-SCL-70 antibodies = anti-topoisomerase-1 antibodies**: Positive in 20-30% of patients; specific for scleroderma; portends disease course with internal organ involvement, particularly of the lungs; correlates with rapidly progressive skin thickening, scleroderma renal crisis, pulmonary fibrosis
- Antifibrillarin antibodies: seen in a small portion (~4%) of patients with scleroderma and correlates with internal organ involvement[746]
- Antimitochondrial antibodies, assessment for primary biliary cirrhosis: 225 Japanese SSc patients were retrospectively examined for PBC-associated autoantibodies, anti-mitochondrial M2 antibodies (AMA), anti-sp100 antibodies (anti-sp100), and anti-gp210 antibodies (anti-gp210); findings included that "37 (16.4%) had AMA, 13 (5.8%) had anti-sp100, and 3 (1.3%) had anti-gp210. Three patients were positive for both AMA and anti-sp100, and 2 were positive for both AMA and anti-gp210. PBC was found in 22 (9.8%) patients positive for AMA with or without anti-sp100 or anti-gp210, but not in those with anti-sp100 or anti-gp210 without AMA. Furthermore, 13 patients lacking these three antibodies were diagnosed with or suspected of PBC by liver biopsy and/or their clinical manifestation. Multivariable analysis revealed that AMA and anti-centromere antibodies were independently associated with PBC in SSc patients, while anti-sp100 and anti-gp210 were not. CONCLUSIONS: This study has demonstrated even higher prevalence of both PBC-associated autoantibodies and PBC in the Japanese SSc population than in the Caucasian SSc population. AMA and anti-centromere antibodies are likely to indicate increasing risk of PBC in SSc patients."[747]

- **Imaging**:
  - ECG abnormalities are common and can include ventricular ectopy, which is correlated with sudden cardiac death
  - Radiography, pulmonary function tests, and CT imaging may be used to detect fibrosing alveolitis and scleroderma-associated pulmonary decline
- **Establishing the diagnosis**:
  - Clinical assessment is sufficient in patients with classic full-blown disease
  - Combination of serologic evidence of autoimmunity and dermal induration

Complications:

- **General: Generalized fibrosis leads to thickening of skin (most obvious), obliteration of the lumen of small arteries (most pathologic), and reduced intestinal motility.**
- Cardiopulmonary and renal: Sudden cardiac death, pulmonary fibrosis/hypertension/failure, hypertension secondary to scleroderma-induced renal damage, renal insufficiency/failure.
- Gastrointestinal: 33% of patients will develop Barrett's esophagus and are at increased risk for cancer; periodic endoscopic surveillance is warranted; referral to gastroenterologist is recommended. To the extent possible, acid-blocking (proton pump-inhibiting) drugs should be avoided because the iatrogenic hypochlorhydria will exacerbate the small bowel bacterial overgrowth and thereby perpetuate the systemic inflammatory state. Malabsorption and resultant malnutrition are due to intestinal hypomotility and SIBO/dysbiosis; from the medical perspective—which in this case is largely correct except for failure to include dietary modification, "Antibiotics, including rifaximin (Xifaxan), and correction of nutritional deficiencies are the mainstays of therapy for intestinal overgrowth."[748] Nonpharmacologic treatments for SIBO include dietary modification especially exclusion of high-fermentation foods such as wheat and potatoes, berberine 1,000-1,500 mg/d, oregano oil (time-released emulsified) 300-600 mg/d, and ascorbate and magnesium to promote bowel clearance.
- Cancer: Increased incidence of breast and lung cancer

---

[746] "AFA identifies young SSc patients with frequent internal organ involvement, especially pulmonary hypertension, myositis and renal disease." Tormey VJ, Bunn CC, Denton CP, Black CM. Anti-fibrillarin antibodies in systemic sclerosis. *Rheumatology* (Oxford). 2001 Oct;40(10):1157-62 rheumatology.oxfordjournals.org/cgi/content/full/40/10/1157
[747] Imura-Kumada et al. High prevalence of primary biliary cirrhosis and disease-associated autoantibodies in Japanese patients with systemic sclerosis. *Mod Rheumatol*. 2012 Nov;22(6):892-8
[748] Hinchcliff M, Varga J. Systemic sclerosis/scleroderma: a treatable multisystem disease. *Am Fam Physician*. 2008 Oct 15;78(8):961-8

Clinical management:
- Address underlying causative contributors; apply Functional Inflammology protocol.
- Monitor for complications such as systemic hypertension, pulmonary hypertension, renal failure.
    - All patients with systemic sclerosis are advised to check their blood pressure at home on a regular basis. Any persistent elevations should prompt medical evaluation and treatment with ACEi.
- Referral if clinical outcome is unsatisfactory or if serious complications are possible/evident.
- Treat complications such as HTN and GERD.

> **Diagnostic evaluation for SSc: Additional rationale for specialist comanagement**
>
> "Clinical evaluation and laboratory testing, along with pulmonary function testing, Doppler echocardiography, and high-resolution computed tomography of the chest [single-photon emission CT for detection of cardiocirculatory abnormalities], establish the diagnosis and detect visceral involvement."
>
> Hinchcliff, Varga. *Am Fam Physician*. 2008 Oct

Treatments:
- Drug treatments: "Treatment of progressive systemic sclerosis is symptomatic and supportive. … Prednisone has little or no role in the treatment of scleroderma."[749] Per 2008 review, "No disease-modifying agent has been proven to prevent or reverse fibrosis, although retrospective studies and case series show that d-penicillamine (Cuprimine), mycophenolate mofetil (Cellcept), and cyclophosphamide (Cytoxan) may be effective in some patients"[750]; other allopathic treatments have been reviewed in articles freely available on-line.[751]
    - Prednisone or other corticosteroid is used for myositis, MCTD, and arthritis; known to exacerbate renal disease when administered in high doses, i.e., greater than 15 mg/d.
    - Penicillamine started at 250 mg/d and gradually increased to 0.5-1.0 g/d can reduce dermal and systemic involvement
    - Tetracycline: one gram per day for bacterial overgrowth[752]
    - ACE inhibitors are the drugs of choice for scleroderma renal disease and hypertension
    - Calcium channel blockers and angiotensin-II receptor blockers for Raynaud phenomenon
    - Endothelin-1 receptor blockers and phosphodiesterase-5 inhibitors for pulmonary arterial hypertension
- **FOOD & NUTRITION: 5-part "supplemented Paleo-Mediterranean diet" (SPMD)** The 5-part "supplemented Paleo-Mediterranean diet" (SPMD—reviewed in Chapter 4) consists of ❶ foundational plant-based low-carbohydrate diet of fruits, vegetables, nuts, seeds, berries and lean sources of protein, ❷ multivitamin and multimineral supplementation, ❸ physiologic doses of vitamin D3 (range 2,000-10,000 IU/d), ❹ combination fatty acid therapy (CFAT) with n3-ALA, n6-GLA, n3-EPA, n3-DHA, and phytochemical-rich olive oil which contains n9-oleate, and ❺ probiotics.
    - Supplemented Paleo-Mediterranean diet: The health-promoting diet of choice for the majority of people is a diet based on abundant consumption of fruits, vegetables, seeds, nuts, omega-3 and monounsaturated fatty acids, and lean sources of protein such as lean meats, fatty cold-water fish, soy and whey proteins. Although this diet is the most-nutrient dense diet available, rational supplementation with vitamins, minerals, and health promoting fatty acids (i.e., ALA, GLA, EPA, DHA) makes this the best practical diet that can possibly be conceived and implemented. **For scleroderma patients whose diets have habitually been low in fiber, dietary improvement which increases fiber consumption should be implemented slowly to avoid phytobezoar formation and intestinal obstruction**[753]; **consumption of water/fluids with meals is reasonable, as is periodic or regular use of osmotic laxative and stool-softening agents such as magnesium and ascorbate.** The specifications of the specific carbohydrate diet detailed by Gottschall[754] are met with adherence to the Paleo diet by Cordain.[755] The combination of both approaches will give patients an excellent combination of informational understanding and culinary versatility. In accord with both of these dietary programs, the diet must

---

[749] Tierney ML. McPhee SJ, Papadakis MA (eds). *Current Medical Diagnosis and Treatment. 35th edition*. Stamford: Appleton and Lange, 1996 page 747
[750] Hinchcliff M, Varga J. Systemic sclerosis/scleroderma: a treatable multisystem disease. Am Fam Physician. 2008 Oct 15;78(8):961-8
[751] Sapadin AN, Fleischmajer R. Treatment of scleroderma. *Arch Dermatol*. 2002 Jan;138(1):99-105. archderm.ama-assn.org/cgi/content/full/138/1/99
[752] Beers MH, Berkow R (eds). *The Merck Manual. Seventeenth Edition*. Whitehouse Station; Merck Research Laboratories 1999 Page 433
[753] Gough et al. Dietary advice in systemic sclerosis: the dangers of a high fibre diet. *Ann Rheum Dis*. 1998;57(11):641-2 ard.bmjjournals.com/cgi/content/full/57/11/641
[754] Gotschall E. *Breaking the Vicious Cycle: Intestinal health though diet*. Kirkton Press; Rev edition (August, 1994) scdiet.com
[755] Cordain L: *The Paleo Diet*. John Wiley & Sons Inc., New York 2002 thepaleodiet.com/

remain free of gluten-containing grains such as wheat, since **some patients with scleroderma have celiac disease**[756,757], and since **wheat, like most grains (except rice), promotes bacterial overgrowth of the intestine due to its high quantity of indigestible oligosaccharides**.[758] Patients with facial involvement and resulting restricted oral aperture will need to use smaller bites of food; consider using a food processor, smoothies—same applies for patients with esophageal dysmotility or restriction.

- Overt malnutrition, micronutrient deficiencies, increased oxidative stress are common in SSc: SSc patients often show overt malnutrition, deficiencies of folate, cobalamin, lipoate, iron, copper, selenium, ascorbic acid, tocopherols, carnitine, and beta-carotene, and enhanced oxidative stress.[759] Very importantly, deficiency of antioxidants in general and selenium in particular is expected to result in enhanced viral replication and mutagenicity, an important realization considering the important role that viral infections appear to play in disease pathogenesis. From a practical clinical standpoint, iron status should be tested with ferritin while other nutritional deficiencies are—generally—treated empirically as discussed in chapters 1 and 4; individual testing of each nutrient is impractical, unnecessarily expensive, and an inappropriate use of time/effort/focus/money. Testing for vitamin B-12 status is notoriously inaccurate, and empiric treatment with 2,000 mcg/d PO is generally warranted for patients with suspected deficiency; however, given the high prevalence of malabsorption in patients with scleroderma/SSc, consideration should be given to laboratory assessments and parenteral administration.

- Daily use of a broad-spectrum high-potency multivitamin and multimineral supplement: **Vitamin and mineral supplementation is important for patients with scleroderma.** Vitamin supplementation (particularly with pyridoxine and riboflavin) appears warranted in patients with **systemic sclerosis** based on a small (n=5) study that documented the normalization of aberrant tryptophan metabolism in most patients following the administration of pyridoxine with riboflavin; the authors concluded that this was evidence of combined vitamin deficiency in patients with scleroderma.[760] This combined deficiency is not surprising given the high incidence of bacterial overgrowth and malabsorption in scleroderma patients. Deficiencies of ascorbate and selenium have also been documented in patients with scleroderma.[761] Reduced folate and cobalamin and elevated homocysteine have also been noted in patients with scleroderma.[762]

- Avoidance of allergenic foods: Any patient may be allergic to any food, even if the food is generally considered a health-promoting food. Generally speaking, the most notorious allergens are wheat, citrus (especially juice due to the industrial use of fungal hemicellulases), cow's milk, eggs, peanuts, chocolate, and yeast-containing foods; according to a study in patients with migraine, some patients will have to avoid as many as 10 specific foods in order to become symptom-free.[763] **Celiac disease is not uncommon in patients with scleroderma, and their scleroderma diagnosis may precede the recognition of celiac disease by many years.**[764,765] Clinicians must explain to their patients that celiac disease and wheat allergy

---

[756] "Coeliac disease may account for malabsorption in scleroderma patients even when test suggest bacterial overgrowth." Marguerie C, Kaye S, Vyse T, Mackworth-Young C, Walport MJ, Black C. Malabsorption caused by coeliac disease in patients who have scleroderma. *Br J Rheumatol*. 1995 Sep;34(9):858-61

[757] Gomez-Puerta et al. Coeliac disease associated with systemic sclerosis. *Ann Rheum Dis*. 2004 Jan;63(1):104-5 ard.bmjjournals.com/cgi/content/full/63/1/104

[758] "Short-chain fructooligosaccharides occur in a number of edible plants, such as chicory, onions, asparagus, wheat... Short-chain fructooligosaccharides, to a large extent, escape digestion in the human upper intestine and reach the colon where they are totally fermented mostly to lactate, short chain fatty acids (acetate, propionate and butyrate), and gas, like dietary fibres." Bornet FR, Brouns F, Tashiro Y, Duvillier V. Nutritional aspects of short-chain fructooligosaccharides: natural occurrence, chemistry, physiology and health implications. *Dig Liver Dis*. 2002 Sep;34 Suppl 2:S111-20

[759] "Half of the patients had a subnormal arm muscle circumference, and two patients also had a subnormal triceps skinfold thickness, indicating severe malnutrition. The concentration of ascorbic acid, alpha-tocopherol, carotene, selenium, and also the proportion of linoleic acid (18:2) in serum phosphatidylcholine was lower in patients than in control subjects." Lundberg et al. Dietary intake and nutritional status in patients with systemic sclerosis. *Ann Rheum Dis*. 1992 Oct;51(10):1143-8 "Selenium levels were lower in patients than in controls (p=0.012). Within the patient cohort, copper correlated inversely with the total skin score (r=-0.52, p=0.03). Our findings provide further evidence that lipid peroxidation is increased and antioxidant capacity is reduced in SSc." Tikly et al. Lipid peroxidation and trace elements in systemic sclerosis. *Clin Rheumatol*. 2006 May;25(3):320-4. "In Raynaud's phenomenon (RP) and Systemic Sclerosis (SSc), a reduced concentration of ascorbic acid, alpha-tocopherol and beta-carotene as well as low values of Selenium have been reported." Simonini et al. Emerging potentials for an antioxidant therapy as a new approach to the treatment of systemic sclerosis. *Toxicology*. 2000 Nov 30;155(1-3):1-15. Famularo et al. Carnitine deficiency in scleroderma—letter. *Immunology Today* 1999 May; 246

[760] "But the simultaneous administration of pyridoxine and nicotinamide to three of these patients normalized the excretory picture after tryptophan loading." De Antoni A, Muggeo M, Costa C, Allegri G, Crepaldi G. Tryptophan metabolism "via" nicotinic acid in patients with scleroderma. *Acta Vitaminol Enzymol*. 1976;30(4-6):134-9

[761] "Plasma ascorbic acid was reduced in all 3 groups of patients: median level 10.6 mg/l in controls, 4.8 mg/l in PRP (p < 0.01), 2.5 mg/l in ISSc (p < 0.01) and 6.8 mg/l in dSSc (p < 0.05). A reduction in serum selenium was especially found in dSSc (median 75 micrograms/l compared to 100 micrograms/l in controls, p < 0.05)." Herrick et al. Micronutrient antioxidant status in patients with primary Raynaud's phenomenon and systemic sclerosis. *J Rheumatol*. 1994 Aug;21(8):1477-83

[762] "Patients with SSc had higher Hcy and vWF concentrations than those with RP or controls. Folic acid and vitamin B12 were lower in SSc than in RP or controls." Marasini et al. Homocysteine concentration in primary and systemic sclerosis associated Raynaud's phenomenon. *J Rheumatol*. 2000 Nov;27(11):2621-3

[763] Grant EC. Food allergies and migraine. *Lancet*. 1979 May 5;1(8123):966-9

[764] Gomez-Puerta et al. Coeliac disease associated with systemic sclerosis. *Ann Rheum Dis*. 2004 Jan;63(1):104-5 ard.bmjjournals.com/cgi/content/full/63/1/104

[765] "Coeliac disease may account for malabsorption in scleroderma patients even when test suggest bacterial overgrowth." Marguerie et al. Malabsorption caused by coeliac disease in patients who have scleroderma. *Br J Rheumatol*. 1995 Sep;34(9):858-61

are two different clinical entities and that exclusion of one does not exclude the other, and in neither case does mutual exclusion obviate the **promotion of intestinal bacterial overgrowth (i.e., proinflammatory dysbiosis) by indigestible wheat oligosaccharides**. Rapid implementation of high fiber diets may precipitate bowel obstruction.[766]

- Vitamin D3 supplementation with physiologic doses and/or tailored to serum 25(OH)D and serum calcium levels : Vitamin D deficiency is common in the general population and is even more common in patients with chronic illness and chronic musculoskeletal pain.[767] Correction of vitamin D deficiency provides a clinically significant anti-inflammatory and immunomodulatory benefit.[768] **Oral administration of active vitamin D3 (1,25-dihydroxyvitamin D) has led to clinical improvement in patients with scleroderma**.[769] Reasonable daily doses for children and adults are 2,000 and 4,000 IU, respectively, as defined by Vasquez, et al.[770] Deficiency and response to treatment are monitored with serum 25(OH)vitamin D while safety is monitored with serum calcium; inflammatory granulomatous diseases and certain drugs such as hydrochlorothiazide greatly increase the propensity for hypercalcemia and warrant increment dosing and frequent monitoring of serum calcium.

- Broad-spectrum fatty acid therapy with ALA, EPA, DHA, GLA and oleic acid: "Sophisticated manipulation of EFA metabolism" may prove clinically beneficial for **scleroderma** patients according to a review by the late David Horrobin[771]; however, a six-month clinical trial of fatty acid supplementation showed no benefit[772], thus proving the ineffectiveness of one-dimensional intervention and of fatty acid supplementation in a condition known to have a high prevalence of untreated malabsorption. Nonetheless, as part of a *comprehensive program*, fatty acid supplementation should be delivered in the form of combination therapy with ALA, GLA, DHA, and EPA. Fish oil provides EPA and DHA which have well-proven anti-inflammatory benefits in rheumatoid arthritis[773,774,775] and lupus.[776,777] ALA, EPA, DHA, and GLA need to be provided in the form of supplements; when using high doses of therapeutic oils, liquid supplements that can be mixed in juice or a smoothie are generally more convenient and palatable than capsules. Therapeutic amounts of oleic acid can be obtained from generous use of olive oil, preferably on fresh vegetables. Supplementation with polyunsaturated fatty acids warrants increased intake of antioxidants from diet, fruit and vegetable juices, and properly formulated supplements; since patients with systemic inflammation are generally in a pro-oxidative state, consideration must be given to the timing and starting dose of fatty acid supplementation and the need for antioxidant protection.

- Probiotics for the treatment of systemic sclerosis-associated gastrointestinal bloating/ distention (*Clin Exp Rheumatol.* 2011 Mar[778]): "We compared the GIT 2.0 scores at baseline and after 2 months of use of Align (Bifidobacterium infantis; 10⁹ CFU per capsule) or Culturelle (Lactobacillus GG; 10⁹ CFU per capsule) using paired t-test and calculated effect size (ES). Significant improvement in total GIT 2.0 score (ES = 0.82), reflux (ES = 0.33), bloating/distention (ES = 1.76), and emotional scales (ES = 0.18) were reported after two months of daily probiotic use. This pilot study suggests probiotics significantly improve the reflux, distention/ bloating, and total GIT scales in SSc patients. As hypothesized, the largest effect was seen in distention/bloating scale. Probiotics may be useful for treatment of SSc-associated distention/ bloating."

---

[766] Gough et al. Dietary advice in systemic sclerosis: the dangers of a high fibre diet. *Ann Rheum Dis.* 1998 Nov;57(11):641-2 ard.bmjjournals.com/cgi/content/full/57/11/641
[767] Plotnikoff GA, Quigley JM. Prevalence of severe hypovitaminosis D in patients with persistent, nonspecific musculoskeletal pain. *Mayo Clin Proc.* 2003 Dec;78(12):1463-70
[768] Timms PM, Mannan N, Hitman GA, Noonan K, Mills PG, Syndercombe-Court D, Aganna E, Price CP, Boucher BJ. Circulating MMP9, vitamin D and variation in the TIMP-1 response with VDR genotype: mechanisms for inflammatory damage in chronic disorders? *QJM.* 2002 Dec;95(12):787-96 qjmed.oxfordjournals.org/cgi/content/full/95/12/787
[769] "After the treatment period (6 months to 3 years), a significant improvement, as compared with baseline values, was observed. No serious side-effects were observed." Humbert et al. Treatment of scleroderma with oral 1,25-dihydroxyvitamin D3: evaluation of skin involvement using non-invasive techniques. *Acta Derm Venereol.* 1993 Dec;73(6):449-51
[770] Vasquez et al. Clinical importance of vitamin D: a paradigm shift with implications for all healthcare providers. *Altern Ther Health Med.* 2004 Sep-Oct;10(5):28-36
[771] "Controlled clinical trials of supplementation with gamma-linolenic acid (GLA) as evening primrose oil (Efamol) in both primary Sjogren's syndrome and systemic sclerosis have given positive results." Horrobin DF. Essential fatty acid and prostaglandin metabolism in Sjogren's syndrome, systemic sclerosis and rheumatoid arthritis. *Scand J Rheumatol* Suppl 1986;61:242-5
[772] "Dietary essential fatty acids have no role in the treatment of vascular symptoms in established systemic sclerosis." Stainforth JM, Layton AM, Goodfield MJ. Clinical aspects of the use of gamma linolenic acid in systemic sclerosis. *Acta Derm Venereol* 1996 Mar;76(2):144-6
[773] Adam et al. Anti-inflammatory effects of a low arachidonic acid diet and fish oil in patients with rheumatoid arthritis. *Rheumatol Int*. 2003 Jan;23(1):27-36
[774] Lau et al. Effects of fish oil supplementation on non-steroidal anti-inflammatory drug requirement in patients with mild rheumatoid arthritis. *Br J Rheumatol.* 1993 Nov:982-9
[775] Kremer et al. Fish-oil fatty acid supplementation in active rheumatoid arthritis. A double-blinded, controlled, crossover study. *Ann Intern Med.* 1987 Apr;106(4):497-503
[776] Walton et al. Dietary fish oil and the severity of symptoms in patients with systemic lupus erythematosus. *Ann Rheum Dis.* 1991 Jul;50(7):463-6
[777] Duffy et al. The clinical effect of dietary supplementation with omega-3 fish oils and/or copper in systemic lupus erythematosus. *J Rheumatol.* 2004 Aug;31(8):1551-6
[778] Frech et al. Probiotics for the treatment of systemic sclerosis-associated gastrointestinal bloating/ distention. *Clin Exp Rheumatol.* 2011 Mar-Apr;29(2 Suppl 65):S22-5

- **INFECTIONS & DYSBIOSIS:** ❶ antimicrobial treatments, ❷ immunorestoration, ❸ immunotolerance via Treg induction   Essentially all autoimmune/rheumatic disorders are associated with microbial colonization and intolerance to same; the presence of persistent microbial colonization is *prima facie* evidence of immunosuppression. The eight areas of dysbiosis (multifocal) are: ❶ sinorespiratory, ❷ orodental, ❸ gastrointestinal, ❹ urogenital/genitourinary, ❺ parenchymal/tissue, ❻ microbial, ❼ dermal/cutaneous, and ❽ environmental. What emerges from the research on SSc and microbes is a complex model of microbial interplay where in some microbes infect vascular cells (e.g., parvovirus B19, EBV, CMV) where as other microbes promote the necessary cytokine response to promote fibrosis (e.g., EBV, *H pylori*, parvovirus B19); readers will find in the following table sufficient evidence to justify testing for viral and bacterial infections and treating, either specifically or empirically. Recall that most components of my antiviral protocol are outlined in Chapter 4 in the section on Microbial Mitochondriopathy.
    - Microbial contributions to scleroderma/SSC:
        - **Gastrointestinal dysbiosis and SIBO** (small intestinal bacterial overgrowth): "The prevalence of SIBO was 43.1% in our SSc patients. ... Our study underscores that SIBO often occurs in SSc patients."[779] A growing body of literature implicates infectious agents in the etiology of **scleroderma**.[780] Regarding dermal dysbiosis, several articles by Cantwell et al[781,782] suggest epidermal and/or intradermal dysbiosis with pleomorphic bacteria, specifically acid-fast cell-wall-deficient mycobacteria. Regarding gastrointestinal dysbiosis, at the very least, we must acknowledge that 1) **bacterial overgrowth of the small bowel is common (33%) in patients with scleroderma**[783] due to impaired gastrointestinal motility, 2) **scleroderma patients show increased levels of deconjugating bacteria**[784], which inactivate bile acids and promote enterohepatic recirculation of endogenous and exogenous toxins, 3) **these patients have a high incidence of *Helicobacter pylori* infection (66% of patients with scleroderma, 78% of patients with scleroderma and Sicca syndrome**[785]), and 4) approximately **44% of scleroderma patients have esophageal overgrowth of *Candida albicans*.**[786] For these and other reasons (detailed in Chapter 4), **patients with scleroderma are presumed to have gastrointestinal dysbiosis until proven otherwise by the combination of 1) three-sample comprehensive parasitology examinations performed by a specialty laboratory and 2) clinical response to at least two 2-4 week courses of broad-spectrum antimicrobial treatment.** Yeast, bacteria, and parasites are treated as indicated based on identification and sensitivity results from comprehensive parasitology assessments. Breath hydrogen/methane testing is inferior to stool testing because it does not allow for identification and sensitivity testing of microbes. Other dysbiotic loci should be investigated as discussed in Chapter 4 in the section on multifocal dysbiosis. Attentive readers may have already surmised that treatment of gastrointestinal dysbiosis in patients with long-standing scleroderma is likely to be particularly

---

[779] Marie et al. Small intestinal bacterial overgrowth in systemic sclerosis. *Rheumatology* (Oxford). 2009 Oct;48(10):1314-9

[780] "...increasing evidence has accumulated to implicate infectious agents in the etiology of systemic sclerosis (SSc)... ...increased antibody titers, a preponderance of specific strains in patients with SSc, and evidence of molecular mimicry inducing autoimmune responses suggest mechanisms by which infectious agents may contribute to the development and progression of SSc." Hamamdzic et al. The role of infectious agents in the pathogenesis of systemic sclerosis. *Curr Opin Rheumatol*. 2002 Nov;14(6):694-8

[781] Disabling pansclerotic morphea (DPM): "The organism could be identified as Staphylococcus epidermidis, but it also had stages of growth with morphologic forms more characteristic of a Corynebacterium-like or actinomycetelike microbe." Cantwell AR Jr, Jones JE, Kelso DW. Pleomorphic, variably acid-fast bacteria in an adult patient with disabling pansclerotic morphea. *Arch Dermatol*. 1984 May;120(5):656-61

[782] "Variably acid-fast coccoid forms, suggestive of cell wall deficient forms of mycobacteria, were observed in the dermis in microscopic sections of skin from six patients with generalized scleroderma, 10 patients with localized scleroderma (morphea), and four patients with lichen sclerosus et atrophicus (LSA)." Cantwell AR Jr. Histologic observations of pleomorphic, variably acid-fast bacteria in scleroderma, morphea, and lichen sclerosus et atrophicus. *Int J Dermatol*. 1984 Jan-Feb;23(1):45-52

[783] "Eight patients (33%) had significant bacterial counts: > 10(5) colony forming units per ml (cfu/ml) of jejunal fluid." Kaye SA, Lim SG, Taylor M, Patel S, Gillespie S, Black CM. Small bowel bacterial overgrowth in systemic sclerosis: detection using direct and indirect methods and treatment outcome. *Br J Rheumatol*. 1995 Mar;34(3):265-9

[784] "Our results demonstrated that some of the bacterial species that overgrow in the upper small intestine of patients with progressive systemic sclerosis can deconjugate bile acids, and that a shift to neutral pH in gastric juice, may promote the bacterial overgrowth related to their impaired peristaltic activity." Shindo et al. Deconjugation ability of bacteria isolated from the jejunal fluid of patients with progressive systemic sclerosis and its gastric pH. *Hepatogastroenterology*. 1998 Sep-Oct;45(23):1643-50

[785] "Urease test demonstrated the presence of HP in 23 patients out of 35 (66%); 12 of them were negative to colonization. A Sicca syndrome, with abnormal Schirmers test and dry mouth was detected in 66% of the patients. 78% of the patients with Sicca syndrome had a concomitant HP infection..." Farina et al. High incidence of Helicobacter pylori infection in patients with systemic sclerosis: association with Sicca Syndrome. *Int J Immunopathol Pharmacol*. 2001 May;14(2):81-85

[786] "Esophageal mucosal brushings from 51 consecutive patients with progressive systemic sclerosis (PSS) (group I), 18 PSS patients continuously treated with high-dose ranitidine or omeprazole (group II), 34 controls referred to the outpatient clinic for endoscopy (group III), and 10 patients receiving long-term potent antireflux therapy for idiopathic gastroesophageal reflux (group IV) were cultured for Candida albicans. There were 44%, 89%, 9%, and 0% Candida albicans culture-positive patients in groups I through IV, respectively." Hendel et al. Esophageal candidosis in progressive systemic sclerosis: occurrence, significance, and treatment with fluconazole. *Scand J Gastroenterol*. 1988 Dec;23(10):1182-6

difficult due to the neuropathic and myopathic **intestinal dysmotility[787] that will serve to perpetuate bacterial overgrowth and dysbiosis, thus necessitating vigilant and long-term treatment**; understanding and due persistence on the part of physician and patient are necessary to see this treatment through to completion—a combination of pharmaceutical/botanical antimicrobials and promotility agents, including the universally safe and effective osmotic laxative magnesium, is reasonable. By this time, readers should appreciate the clinical implications of SIBO (as discussed in Chapter 4), including but not limited to malabsorption due to damage to the intestinal mucosa and mucosal enzymes, increased intestinal permeability, increased bacterial translocation, microbial mitochondriopathy, systemic inflammation, activation of DAMP, PAMP, and TLR receptors—all of these pro-inflammatory effects should be expected to promote the oxidative stress, autoimmunity, and fibrosis that characterize SSc.

- Octreotide (prescription drug): Descamps et al[788] describe the case of a 53-year-old black woman with progressive and severe systemic scleroderma, with diffuse skin sclerosis, myositis with intestinal pseudo-obstruction and bacterial overgrowth who experienced a "spectacular" normalization of clinical status and skin induration following several months of octreotide (75 mug/d). This drug is a somatostatin analog used in the treatment of acromegaly[789] and it also promotes intestinal motility and thus reduces dysbiotic intestinal bacterial overgrowth in patients with scleroderma.[790] Efficacy of octreotide in improving clinical manifestations of scleroderma is probably mediated *at least in part* by reducing the pro-inflammatory effects of dysbiotic intestinal bacterial overgrowth, which can be addressed by other means as well.

- Ciprofloxacin: Over and Bucknall[791] published a case report of a progressive scleroderma patient who experienced marked clinical improvement and biopsy-proven regression of skin changes following administration of ciprofloxacin 500 mg bid which was eventually reduced to 250 mg/d. This case report strongly supports the theory that intestinal dysbiosis is a major contributor to scleroderma. As with all antibacterial treatments, use empiric antifungal treatment with Nystatin 500,000 units bid and/or emulsified oregano 150 mg tid-qid.[792,793]

- *Artemisia annua*: Artemisinin has been safely used for centuries in Asia for the treatment of malaria, and it also has effectiveness against anaerobic bacteria due to the pro-oxidative sesquiterpene endoperoxide.[794,795] I commonly use artemisinin at 200 mg per day in divided doses for adults with dysbiosis. Evidence of past/current *H. pylori* infection is common (~40-60%) in patients with scleroderma[796], and some doctors—such as Jonathan V Wright MD—have reported anecdotally that *Artemisia annua* helps eradicate *H. pylori*. Conversely, we might reasonably look for a non-pro-oxidative treatment alternative to Artemisia, such as mastic.

- Erythromycin: 250-500 mg TID-QID; this drug is a widely used antibiotic that also has intestinal promotility benefits (thus making it an ideal treatment for intestinal bacterial overgrowth associated with or caused by intestinal dysmotility/hypomotility such as seen in

---

[787] "We found ultrastructural signs of axonal degeneration and cytoskeletal abnormalities in the bundles of unmyelinated fibers. There was also focal degeneration of smooth muscle cells, often in association with the presence of partially degranulated mast cells." Malandrini et al. Autonomic nervous system and smooth muscle cell involvement in systemic sclerosis: ultrastructural study of 3 cases. *J Rheumatol*. 2000 May;27(5):1203-6

[788] "After 8 months of treatment, normal weight was obtained and skin induration was spectacularly reduced and pigmentation returned to a normal state." Descamps V, Duval X, Crickx B, Bouscarat F, Coffin B, Belaich S. Global improvement of systemic scleroderma under long-term administration of octreotide. *Eur J Dermatol* 1999 Sep;9(6):446-8

[789] us.sandostatin.com/info/about/home.jsp Accessed December 16, 2005

[790] "Octreotide stimulates intestinal motility in normal subjects and in patients with scleroderma. In such patients, the short-term administration of octreotide reduces bacterial overgrowth and improves abdominal symptoms." Soudah et al. Effect of octreotide on intestinal motility and bacterial overgrowth in scleroderma. *N Engl J Med* 1991 Nov:1461-7

[791] Over et al. Regression of skin changes in a patient with systemic sclerosis following treatment for bacterial overgrowth with ciprofloxacin. *Br J Rheumatol*. 1998 Jun;37(6):696

[792] Stiles JC, Sparks W, Ronzio RA. The inhibition of Candida albicans by oregano. *J Applied Nutr* 1995;47:96–102

[793] Force M, Sparks WS, Ronzio RA. Inhibition of enteric parasites by emulsified oil of oregano in vivo. *Phytother Res*. 2000 May;14(3):213-4

[794] Dien et al. Effect of food intake on pharmacokinetics of oral artemisinin in healthy Vietnamese subjects. *Antimicrob Agents Chemother*. 1997 May;41(5):1069-72

[795] Giao et al. Artemisinin for treatment of uncomplicated falciparum malaria: is there a place for monotherapy? *Am J Trop Med Hyg*. 2001 Dec;65(6):690-5

[796] "Patients with SSc have H. pylori infection at a higher prevalence than the general population." Yazawa et al. High seroprevalence of Helicobacter pylori infection in patients with systemic sclerosis: association with esophageal involvement. *J Rheumatol*. 1998 Apr;25(4):650-3

scleroderma[797,798]). Do not combine erythromycin with the promotility drug cisapride due to risk for serious cardiac arrhythmia.
- Nystatin: Nystatin 500,000 units bid with food; duration of treatment begins with a minimum duration of 2-4 weeks and may continue as long as the patient is deriving benefit.

Aspects of scleroderma: diagram by Vasquez; quotes from Radić et al and Svegliati et al: "Systemic sclerosis is an autoimmune disease characterized by vascular obliteration, excessive extracellular matrix deposition and fibrosis of the connective tissues of the skin, lungs, gastrointestinal tract, heart, and kidneys. The pathogenesis of systemic sclerosis is extremely complex; at present, no single unifying hypothesis explains all aspects. Over the last 20 years increasing evidence has accumulated to implicate infectious agents in the etiology of systemic sclerosis. Increased antibody titers, a preponderance of specific strains in patients with systemic sclerosis, and evidence of molecular mimicry inducing autoimmune responses suggest mechanisms by which infectious agents may contribute to the development and progression of systemic sclerosis."[799] "Trichostatin A, an HDAC inhibitor, prevented WIF-1 loss, β-catenin induction, and collagen accumulation in an experimental fibrosis model. Our findings suggest that oxidative DNA damage induced by SSc autoreactive antibodies enables Wnt activation that contributes to fibrosis."[800]

- **Cytomegalovirus**—Induction of vasculopathy via direction infection and induction of pro-inflammatory cytokines, molecular mimicry: CMV causes experimental vasculopathy resembling SSc; interestingly and consistent with my (DrV) model of dysbiosis which appreciates immunosuppression as (pre)requisite, experimental CMV-induced vasculopathy requires immunosuppression: "A viral agent known for its ability to damage vessel walls is cytomegalovirus (CMV). ... Infected immunocompetent animals exhibited only perivascular inflammation, suggesting that infection and immunosuppression were co-requisites of [vasculopathy] neointima formation. ... Induction of TGF-β1, the canonical pro-fibrotic cytokine, by human CMV (HCMV) was reported by other authors (16), implicating that a primary endothelial cell infection by HCMV

---

[797] "Prokinetic agents effective in pseudoobstruction include metoclopramide, domperidone, cisapride, octreotide, and erythromycin. ... The combination of octreotide and erythromycin may be particularly effective in systemic sclerosis." Sjogren RW. Gastrointestinal features of scleroderma. *Curr Opin Rheumatol*. 1996 Nov;8(6):569-75
[798] "Erythromycin accelerates gastric and gallbladder emptying in scleroderma patients and might be helpful in the treatment of gastrointestinal motor abnormalities in these patients." Fiorucci et al. Effect of erythromycin administration on upper gastrointestinal motility in scleroderma patients. *Scand J Gastroenterol*. 1994 Sep;29(9):807-13
[799] Radić M, Martinović Kaliterna D, Radić J. Infectious disease as aetiological factor in the pathogenesis of systemic sclerosis. *Neth J Med*. 2010 Nov;68(11):348-53
[800] Svegliati et al. Oxidative DNA damage induces ATM-mediated transcriptional suppression of Wnt inhibitor WIF-1 in systemic sclerosis and fibrosis. *Sci Signal* 2014 Sept;ra84

may induce myofibroblast activation in the vessel wall under the effect of this cytokine."[801] "...higher prevalence of IgA antihuman cytomegalovirus antibodies in patients with SSc. ... CMV infection may play a part in SSc pathogenesis due to its ability to infect both endothelial and monocyte/macrophage cells and through the upregulation of fibrogenic cytokines and induction of immune dysregulation. ... association between increased serum levels of CMV-specific antibodies and the prevalence of SSc-related autoantibodies in patients with SSc. ... Molecular mimicry is a mechanism that may explain the pathogenicity of antibodies against viral proteins in SSc. Infection with HCMV may generate a host-antiviral response that is self-reactive toward autoantigens and endothelial cells."[802] Vulnerably to CMV-induced SSc may include genetic factors and fetomaternal/transfusional microchimerism, noted to be more common in women with SSc.

> **CMV meets pathogenic criteria for SSc**
> - Direct infection of endothelial cells and immune cells
> - Induction of pro-fibrotic cytokines
> - Higher levels of CMV antibodies in SSc patients
> - Exact molecular mimicry between HCMV late protein UL94 and human endothelial cell surface integrin–NAG-2 protein complex
> - Cross-reacting CMV-endothelial antibodies kill endothelial cells and cause fibrosis
> - Anti-UL94 antibodies bind to dermal fibroblasts and convert them to a scleroderma phenotype
>
> Moroncini et al. *Clin Exp Rheumatol.* 2013 Mar

- **Epstein-Barr virus**—Localized infection in skin fibroblasts and endothelial cells, upregulation of cytokine production: "Here we show that EBV establishes infection in the majority of fibroblasts and endothelial cells in the skin of SSc patients, characterized by the expression of the EBV noncoding small RNAs (EBERs) and the increased expression of immediate-early lytic and latency mRNAs and proteins. We report that EBV is able to persistently infect human SSc fibroblasts in vitro, inducing an aberrant innate immune response in infected cells. EBV-Toll-like receptor (TLR) aberrant activation induces the expression of selected IFN-regulatory factors (IRFs), IFN-stimulated genes (ISGs), transforming growth factor-β1 (TGFβ1), and several markers of fibroblast activation, such as smooth muscle actin and Endothelin-1, and all of these genes play a key role in determining the profibrotic phenotype in SSc fibroblasts. These findings imply that EBV infection occurring in mesenchymal, endothelial, and immune cells of SSc patients may underlie the main pathological features of SSc including autoimmunity, vasculopathy, and fibrosis, and provide a unified disease mechanism represented by EBV reactivation."[803]

> **EBV meets pathogenic criteria for SSc**
> - Majority of SSc patients show active infection in vascular and dermal cells
> - Virus-induced gene induction promotes the profibrotic scleroderma phenotype
>
> Farina et al. *J Invest Dermatol.* 2014 Apr

- **Parvovirus B19**—Induction of fibrosis: "The presence of parvovirus B19 DNA was demonstrated in a significant percentage of bone marrow biopsies from SSc patients and was never detected in the control group. ... These patients showed the most severe active endothelial injury and perivascular inflammation. ...incubation with parvovirus B19-containing serum induced an invasive phenotype in normal human synovial fibroblasts."[804] Note that bone marrow-derived fibrocytes are involved in the pathogenesis of SSC; therefore, the strong positive correlation

> **PvB19 meets pathogenic criteria for SSc**
> - Direct infection of endothelial cells, immune cells, and dermal epithelial cells
> - Induction of pro-fibrotic cytokines
> - Bone marrow infection is seen in many SSc patients, correlates directly with disease severity, and is never noted in health patients; bone marrow fibrocytes contribute to SSc.
> - PvB19 infection triggers formation of multiple autoantibodies: nuclear antigens (ANA), rheumatoid factor (RF), neutrophils cytoplasmic antigens, mitochondrial antigens (AMA), smooth muscle, gastric parietal antigens and phospholipids.
>
> Moroncini et al. *Clin Exp Rheumatol.* 2013 Mar

---

[801] Moroncini et al. Role of viral infections in the etiopathogenesis of systemic sclerosis. *Clin Exp Rheumatol.* 2013 Mar-Apr;31(2 Suppl 76):3-7
[802] Radić et al. Infectious disease as aetiological factor in the pathogenesis of systemic sclerosis. *Neth J Med.* 2010 Nov;68(11):348-53
[803] Farina et al. Epstein-Barr virus infection induces aberrant TLR activation pathway and fibroblast-myofibroblast conversion in scleroderma. *J Invest Dermatol.* 2014 Apr:954-64
[804] Radić et al. Infectious disease as aetiological factor in the pathogenesis of systemic sclerosis. *Neth J Med.* 2010 Nov;68(11):348-53

between B19 positivity and SSc and the negative correlation seen with B19 negativity and health suggests a likelihood of direct cause and effect.

- ***Helicobacter pylori*, especially the virulent CagA strain**—Induction of systemic inflammation and cytokine response: "...despite the absence of a difference in *H. pylori* infection rates between SSc patients and control subjects, 90% of patients with SSc were infected with the virulent CagA strain compared with only 37% of the infected control subjects..." "Our data suggest that *H. pylori* infection correlates with severity of skin, gastrointestinal, and joint/tendon involvement in SSc patients. *H. pylori*-positive SSc patients showed higher severity score compared to *H. pylori*-negative. Therefore, *H. pylori* infection may play a role in the pathogenesis of SSc and also can provide some prognostic information."[805] "There are two general lines of evidence implicating bacterial infections in the pathogenesis of SSc. One is anecdotal evidence that treatment with antibiotics relieves SSc symptoms in some patients. The other is that graft-versus-host disease, which is recognized as having many similarities to SSc, cannot be induced in germ-free animals and is significantly reduced in children pre-treated with antibiotics to eradicate their normal bacterial flora."[806]

- ***Toxoplasma gondii* and hepatitis B virus**: "Patients with SSc had elevated IgM and IgG against *Toxoplasma gondii* and against CMV. Higher titers were also detected against the hepatitis B virus core protein (recombinant HBc antigen) using MONOLISA anti-HBc Plus commercial kit (Bio-Rad). A significantly higher rate of IgM antibodies against the capsid antigen of the EBV was detected in SSc patients compared with healthy controls, as well."[807]

- **Clinical implications of polymicrobial dysbiosis in scleroderma**: At the risk of redundancy and stating what should be obvious by now to readers who have studied the material in this book—especially chapter 4—here I will outline the implications of the information presented up to this point in this section on scleroderma/SSc. Quite obviously, the typical patient with scleroderma has multiple active microbial infections/colonizations and is therefore—by definition—demonstrating immunosuppression. Thus, two of the three components of my three-part dysbiosis model are established in SSC, and the third component—nutritional immunomodulation—is discussed in the following section. Given the solid data demonstrating polyviral activity for what I will describe as "popular viruses"—EBV, CMV, PvB19—we should reasonably assume that increased transcription of other viruses such as HSV (type-1 in 50% of the adult population; type-2 in 20% of the adult population) and the HERVs—human indigenous retroviruses—is also occurring. Serologic, newer generation PCR testing, and specialty tests—such as western blot for HSV infections—should ideally be performed to assess for the presence and severity/level of viral replication. Per previous discussions, clinicians must appreciate the total microbial load (TML) and not simply the presence/absence of these infections; bacterial quantifications—especially *H pylori*—must also be made if the initial laboratory evaluation is to be considered partly complete. Thereafter, the antimicrobial mission becomes on of search and destroy, using a combination of direct antiviral/antimicrobial agents as well as immunorestoration. My opinion and perspective is that antiviral pharmaceutic drugs—which by definition target single pathways in single viruses and are therefore easily bypassed by viral mutations and which have limited efficacy on the total viral load (TVL), respectively—are of limited clinical value but may still be used if found efficacious in individual patients; any failure of pharmacologic antiviral intervention in autoimmunity does not refute the viral etiology of autoimmunity but is rather to be expected from the failure to effectively address the larger viral load and to restore various aspects of disturbed homeodynamics. Attention should be directed toward a global or generalized antiviral approach to reduce TVL for various categories of viruses *concretely* and TVL *conceptually*, reasonably described here as ❶ common/popular viruses—these are the common viruses most commonly considered by clinicians and patients and for which we have readily available diagnostic tests, namely HIV, HBV, HCV, HSV

---

[805] Radić et al. Is Helicobacter pylori infection a risk factor for disease severity in systemic sclerosis? *Rheumatol Int.* 2013 Nov;33(11):2943-8
[806] Radić et al. Infectious disease as aetiological factor in the pathogenesis of systemic sclerosis. *Neth J Med.* 2010 Nov;68(11):348-53
[807] Arnson et al. The role of infections in the immunopathogensis of systemic sclerosis--evidence from serological studies. *Ann N Y Acad Sci.* 2009 Sep;1173:627-32

1 and 2, CMV, EBV, PvB19; readers should note from the above that SSC patients show viral infections that are not simply *more active* but are *active in different locations* compared to nonSSC persons, ❷ human endogenous retroviruses—viruses permanently embedded in the human genome, for which laboratory assessments are generally not clinically available; clinicians should consider this category to be an occult contributor to the TVL and thus TML and thus **TIL—total inflammatory/immunogenic load**, ❸ bacteriophage load—the **total bacterial load (TBL)** of the body and in particular the biomass in the intestines houses the bacteria-specific viruses known as bacteriophages, and these viruses-specific-for-bacteria contribute significantly to the TML of the gut in particular; thus, consideration to reducing/improving TBL in the gut would be expected to reduce the TVL as well, benignly promoting a reduction in the TIL, ❹ other means of reducing TVL— reducing inflammation and bacterial load: Bacterial debris such as LPS/endotoxin, other viral infections (via "transactivation"), and any other inflammatory stimuli that activate NFkB would be expected to promote viral replication via the NFkB pathway and other pathways that are "hijacked" or reappropriated[808] by viruses to promote their replication. In this manner, reducing the TBL lowers the TVL and thus the TIL. Extending the understanding and implications: Understanding this helps clinicians and researchers make sense of the confusion seen particularly in the research on CFS [caused by SIBO and GI dysbiosis] which is commonly complicated by evidence of increased viral replication; what I think is occurring here is that bacterial debris/LPS from SIBO is promoting viral replication via pathways including NFkB. Problematically, the LPS from SIBO also contributes to other problems such as impairment of cytochrome p450 which leads to xenobiotic accumulation and the resulting multiple chemical sensitivity [MCS], the persistent low-grade inflammatory and oxidative state which impairs the HPA axis and mitochondrial function; SIBO can cause deficiency of tryptophan and thus serotonin and perhaps melatonin via bacterial tryptophanase and deficiency of vitamin B-12 due to increased binding/chelation of B-12 with bacterial H2S.

- **NUTRITIONAL IMMUNOMODULATION: Treg induction for modulation of Th-1/2/17 inflammation**
Nutrients and therapeutic approaches that promote Treg or IL-10 induction and/or Th-17, IL-17 suppression include 1) mitochondrial optimization and mTOR suppression, 2) biotin, 3) vitamin E, 4) sodium avoidance, 5) transgenic/GMO food avoidance, 6) probiotics, 7) lipoic acid, 8) vitamin A, 9) inflammation reduction, 10) vitamin D, 11) fatty acid supplementation with GLA and n3, 12) infection and dysbiosis remediation, 13) green tea EGCG. Acronym: MiBESTPLAIDFIG.
    - Vitamin E: Morelli et al[809] describe a 60-year-old woman with **systemic sclerosis** complicated by hypertension, renal failure, and heart failure; although allopathic drug treatments were of no benefit, **the addition of "vitamin E (600 mg daily)" lead to rapid and significant clinical improvement.** Ayres and Mihan[810] wrote that vitamin E was effective in the clinical management of scleroderma, discoid lupus erythematosus[811], porphyria cutanea tarda, several types of vasculitis, and polymyositis.[812] Given that vitamin E is not a single compound but rather a family of closely related tocopherols, most clinicians prefer to use a source of "mixed tocopherols" inclusive of alpha, beta, delta, and—perhaps most importantly—gamma tocopherol.[813] Vitamin E has a wide margin of safety and although daily doses are kept in the range of 400-1200 IU, doses up to 3,200 IU are generally considered non-toxic. Tocopherols are now known to provide an anti-inflammatory immunomodulatory effect by elevating cAMP and thereby reducing TNF-alpha and increasing IL-10 as reviewed in Chapter 4 in the section on Nutritional Immunomodulation.

---

[808] "As viruses evolve under the highly selective pressures of the immune system, they acquire the capacity to target critical steps in the host cell life, hijacking vital cellular functions to promote viral pathogenesis. Many viruses have evolved mechanisms to target the NF-kB pathway to facilitate their replication, cell survival, and evasion of immune responses." Hiscott et al. Hostile takeovers: viral appropriation of the NF-kappaB pathway. *J Clin Invest*. 2001 Jan;107(2):143-51

[809] "Casually, vitamin E (600 mg daily) was added. After 6 months, clinical manifestations of heart failure were disappeared and the echocardiogram showed a normally-sized left ventricle with normal wall motion." Morelli S, Sgreccia A, Bernardo ML, Gurgo Di Castelmenardo A, Petrilli AC, De Leva R, Nuccio F, Calvieri S. Systemic sclerosis (scleroderma). A case of recovery of cardiomyopathy after vitamin E treatment. *Minerva Cardioangiol*. 2001 Apr;49(2):127-30

[810] "Among the diseases that were successfully controlled were a number in the autoimmune category, including scleroderma, discoid lupus erythematosus, porphyria cutanea tarda, several types of vasculitis, and polymyositis." Ayres S Jr, Mihan R. Is vitamin E involved in the autoimmune mechanism? *Cutis*. 1978 Mar;21(3):321-5

[811] "Despite conflicting opinions, our personal experience and a number of reviewed clinical reports indicate that vitamin E, properly administered in adequate doses, is a safe and effective treatment for chronic discoid lupus erythematosus, and may be of value in treating other types of the disease." Ayres S Jr, Mihan R. Lupus erythematosus and vitamin E: an effective and nontoxic therapy. *Cutis*. 1979;23(1):49-52, 54

[812] "She then made a dramatic improvement when large doses of vitamin E (d, alpha-tocopheryl acetate) were administered." Killeen RN, Ayres S Jr, Mihan R. Polymyositis: response to vitamin E. *South Med J*. 1976 Oct;69(10):1372-4

[813] Jiang et al. gamma-tocopherol, the major form of vitamin E in the US diet, deserves more attention. *Am J Clin Nutr*. 2001 Dec;74(6):714-22 ajcn.org/cgi/content/full/74/6/714

- **DYSMETABOLISM & DYSFUNCTIONAL MITOCHONDRIA: MitoDys, ERS-UPR, AGE/RAGE, hyperglycemia and ceramide** The major clinical considerations in this section are mitochondrial dysfunction, endoplasmic reticulum stress, unfolded protein response, TLR activation, and the dysmetabolic effects of sustained hyperglycemia and hyperinsulinemia and resultant oxidative stress, inflammation, RAGE activation, and accumulation of AGE, palmitate and ceramide. The review of this information in Chapter 4 covered approximately 30 interventions relevant to dysmetabolism, mitochondrial dysfunction, ERS-UPR, etc; these will not be reviewed here except to mention those most commonly, easily, empirically, synergistically, and effectively used: 1) low-carbohydrate diet with 2) moderate exercise, 3) CoQ-10, 4) acetyl-carnitine with 5) lipoic acid, 6) NAC, 7) resveratrol, and 8) melatonin.
    - Mitochondrial dysfunction in scleroderma—a cause of a fibrotic phenotype: My (DrV) intuitive sense is that mitochondrial dysfunction—likely induced by bacteria, viruses and/or xenobiotic exposure—induces a fibrotic phenotype in scleroderma patients; research data supporting this concept is indirect. However, noted is the observation that worsening systemic inflammation (measured by hsCRP) correlates with antimitochondrial antibodies in patients with scleroderma.[814]
    - Liver giant mitochondria: an almost constant lesion in systemic scleroderma (*Virchows Arch A Pathol Anat Histol 1977 Jun*[815]): "Liver electron microscopic studies were performed in 14 patients with systemic scleroderma. In 13 of these patients, giant mitochondria were demonstrated in the hepatocytes. This ultrastructural abnormality was present whatever the type and duration of the disease and was also present even when the liver was histologically normal. The mechanism of formation of giant mitochondria in systemic scleroderma is unknown."
    - Carnitine: According to the final sentence in a short report by Famularo et al[816], "Interestingly, early uncontrolled studies reported that the administration of L-carnitine had a favorable impact on the course of the disease in and this improvement was paralleled by a reduction in serum immunoglobulin levels." The use of carnitine is reviewed in Chapter 4 in the section on mitochondrial dysfunction.

- **STYLE OF LIVING (LIFESTYLE) & SPECIAL CONSIDERATIONS: Sleep optimization, SocioPsychology, Stress management/avoidance, Somatic treatments, Special Supplementation, Sweat/exercise, Sauna/detoxification, Surgery, Stamp your passport and vacate current reality, Sensory deprivation therapy** This is a buffet of mostly lifestyle-based interventions yet also including considerations such as somatic treatments, additional supplementation, and surgery.
    - PABA—para-amino benzoic acid: **Ninety percent of patients treated with PABA experience clinical benefit, especially skin softening.**[817] **PABA therapy prolongs survival in patients with scleroderma.**[818] "Potaba" is a well-tolerated prescription form of PABA.[819] Wright and Gaby[820] recommend "PABA, 2-3 g, 4 times a day." A 2006 review by Gaby[821] noted that PABA administered as potassium para-aminobenzoate (KPAB) was able to preserve pulmonary function and improve survival at five years (88.5% versus 69.8%) and 10 years (76.6% versus 56.6%) among patients treated with 12-12.5 g per day for three months to 20.6 years (average, 4.2 years). Adverse effects attributable to PABA are dose-dependent and include low blood sugar, rash, fever, and liver damage; one case of fatal toxic hepatitis has been reported. Adverse effects may be seen with doses approximating or exceeding eight grams per day; thus serial serum chemistries (e.g., monthly at first, then bimonthly, then quarterly) are warranted, especially when using high doses.

---

[814] "Occurrence rate of anti-mitochondria antibody in high-sensitivity CRP elevated SSc patients (8/14, 57.1%) was significantly elevated compared with that of high-sensitivity CRP low SSc patients (3/26, 11.5%) (P < 0.01). These results led us to conclusion that elevated high-sensitivity CRP shows relation to the occurrence of anti-mitochondria antibody." Ohtsuka T. Relation between elevated high-sensitivity C-reactive protein and anti-mitochondria antibody in patients with systemic sclerosis. *J Dermatol*. 2008 Feb;70-5
[815] Feldmann et al. Hepatocyte giant mitochondria: an almost constant lesion in systemic scleroderma. *Virchows Arch A Pathol Anat Histol*. 1977 Jun 23;374(3):215-27
[816] Famularo et al. Carnitine deficiency in scleroderma—letter. *Immunology Today* 1999 May; 246
[817] "Ninety percent of 224 patients treated with KPAB experienced mild, moderate, or marked skin softening." Zarafonetis CJ, Dabich L, Skovronski JJ, DeVol EB, Negri D, Yuan W, Wolfe R. Retrospective studies in scleroderma: skin response to potassium para-aminobenzoate therapy. *Clin Exp Rheumatol*. 1988 Jul-Sep;6(3):261-8
[818] "For the entire group an estimated 81.4% survived 5 years from diagnosis and 69.4% survived 10 years. …adequate treatment with potassium para-aminobenzoate (Potaba KPAB) was associated with improved survival (p less than 0.01); 88.5% 5 year survival rate and 76.6% 10 year survival rate for adequately treated patients." Zarafonetis CJ, et al. Retrospective studies in scleroderma: effect of potassium para-aminobenzoate on survival. *J Clin Epidemiol*. 1988;41(2):193-205
[819] glenwood-llc.com/potaba.html
[820] Gaby A, Wright JV. Nutritional Protocols. © 1998 by Nutrition Seminars.
[821] Gaby AR. Natural remedies for scleroderma. *Altern Med Rev*. 2006 Sep;11(3):188-95

- *Centella asiatica* (Gotu cola): This botanical has been reported to favorably influence scleroderma.[822] Available forms include teas, tinctures, standardized capsules/tablets, topical ointments, and injectable preparations. The **proprietary product "Madecassol" containing madecassic acid, asiatic acid and asiaticoside has been used in several studies and has demonstrated clinical benefit in scleroderma**[823]; some preparations of this product apparently contain nitrofural, a topically and orally active antibiotic. Contact dermatitis has been reported.
- CoQ10: CoQ10 is a powerful antioxidant with a wide margin of safety and excellent clinical tolerability. **At least four studies have documented its powerful blood-pressure-lowering ability, which often surpasses the clinical effectiveness of antihypertensive drugs.**[824,825,826,827] **Furthermore, at least two published papers**[828,829] **and one case report**[830] **advocate that CoQ10 has powerful renoprotective and renorestorative benefits.** CoQ10 levels are low in patients with allergies[831], and the symptomatic relief that many allergic patients experience following supplementation with CoQ10 suggests that CoQ10 has an immunomodulatory effect. Common doses start at > 100 mg per day with food; doses of 200 mg per day are not uncommon, and doses up to 1,000 mg per day are clinically well tolerated though the high financial toll approximates that of many pharmaceutical drugs.
    - Coenzyme Q supplementation in pulmonary arterial hypertension (*Redox Biol* 2014 Jul[832]): In this controlled clinical trial, 300 mg daily of the reduced form of CoQ-10 were given to eight PAH patients. "Cardiac parameters improved with CoQ supplementation, although 6-minute walk distances and BNP levels did not significantly change. Consistent with improved mitochondrial synthetic function, hemoglobin increased and red cell distribution width (RDW) decreased in PAH patients with CoQ, while hemoglobin declined slightly and RDW did not change in healthy controls. In contrast, metabolic and redox parameters, including lactate, pyruvate and reduced or oxidized glutathione, did not change in PAH patients with CoQ. In summary, CoQ improved hemoglobin and red cell maturation in PAH, but longer studies and/or higher doses with a randomized placebo-controlled controlled design are necessary to evaluate the clinical benefit of this simple nutritional supplement."
- N-acetyl-cysteine (NAC): **Oxidative stress promotes a fibrotic phenotype in scleroderma fibroblasts, which was normalized by administration of NAC *in vitro*.**[833] NAC is well-tolerated, inhibits NF-kappaB, functions as an antioxidant, is a powerful and clinically important antiviral agent, and promotes detoxification via hepatoprotection and glutathione conjugation. In patients with scleroderma/SSC, studies using oral and IV NAC have been performed; benefits include improved hepatic (one-day study[834]), renal (one-day study[835]), and brachial/digital (three-year study[836]) perfusion following IV NAC.
    - Measurement of clinical change in progressive systemic sclerosis: a 1 year double-blind placebo-controlled trial of N-acetylcysteine (*Ann Rheum Dis.* 1979 Aug[837]): "Identically appearing 500 mg

---

[822] "Titrated extract of Centella asiatica (TECA) contains three principal ingredients, asiaticoside (AS), asiatic acid (AA), and madecassic acid (MA). These components are known to be clinically effective on systemic scleroderma, abnormal scar formation, and keloids." Hong SS, Kim JH, Li H, Shim CK. Advanced formulation and pharmacological activity of hydrogel of the titrated extract of C. asiatica. *Arch Pharm Res*. 2005 Apr;28(4):502-8
[823] "Madecassol is effective and well tolerated and therefore recommended for oral and local use in combined treatment of SS adn FS." Guseva NG, Starovoitova MN, Mach ES. [Madecassol treatment of systemic and localized scleroderma]. *Ter Arkh*. 1998;70(5):58-61. Article in Russian; information from abstract.
[824] Burke et al. Randomized, double-blind, placebo-controlled trial of coenzyme Q10 in isolated systolic hypertension. *South Med J*. 2001 Nov;94(11):1112-7
[825] Singh et al. Effect of hydrosoluble coenzyme Q10 on blood pressures and insulin resistance in hypertensive patients with CAD. *J Hum Hypertens*. 1999 Mar;13(3):203-8
[826] Digiesi et al. Coenzyme Q10 in essential hypertension. *Mol Aspects Med*. 1994;15 Suppl:s257-63
[827] Langsjoen P, Langsjoen P, Willis R, Folkers K. Treatment of essential hypertension with coenzyme Q10. *Mol Aspects Med*. 1994;15 Suppl:S265-72
[828] Singh et al. Randomized, double-blind placebo-controlled trial of coenzyme Q10 in chronic renal failure: discovery of a new role. *J Nutr Environ Med* 2000;10:281-8
[829] Singh et al. Randomized, Double-blind, Placebo-controlled Trial of Coenzyme Q10 in Patients with End-stage Renal Failure. *J Nutr Environ Med* 2003:13;13–22
[830] Singh RB, Singh MM. Effects of CoQ10 in new indications with antioxidant vitamin deficiency. *J Nutr Environ Med* 1999; 9:223-228
[831] Ye CQ, Folkers K, et al. A modified determination of coenzyme Q10 in human blood and CoQ10 blood levels in diverse patients with allergies. *Biofactors*. 1988 Dec;1:303-6
[832] Sharp et al. Coenzyme Q supplementation in pulmonary arterial hypertension. *Redox Biol*. 2014 Jul 31;2:884-91
[833] "Treatment of SSc fibroblasts with the membrane-permeant antioxidant N-acetyl-L-cysteine inhibited ROS production, and this was accompanied by decreased proliferation of these cells and down-regulation of alpha1(I) and alpha2(I) collagen messenger RNA." Sambo et al. Oxidative stress in scleroderma: maintenance of scleroderma fibroblast phenotype by the constitutive up-regulation of reactive oxygen species generation through the NADPH oxidase complex pathway. *Arthritis Rheum* 2001 Nov;44(11):2653-64
[834] "In an open-label study 40 patients with systemic sclerosis (SSc) were treated with 15 mg/kg/hour intravenous N-acetylcysteine for 5 consecutive hours in a single day. ... The results of our study demonstrate that NAC is able to increase HFV and total liver perfusion after a single infusion in SSc patients with low disease activity and severity scores." Rosato et al. N-acetylcysteine infusion improves hepatic perfusion in the early stages of systemic sclerosis. *Int J Immunopathol Pharmacol*. 2009 Jul-Sep;22(3):763-72
[835] "In an open-label study 40 patients with systemic sclerosis (SSc) were treated with N-acetylcysteine (NAC) iv infusion over 5 consecutive hours, at a dose of 0.015 g x kg(-1) x h(-1). ... In patients with low disease severity NAC ameliorates vascular renal function." Rosato et al. N-acetylcysteine infusion reduces the resistance index of renal artery in the early stage of systemic sclerosis. *Acta Pharmacol Sin*. 2009 Sep;30(9):1283-8
[836] "The aim of this study was to report long-term outcome (median follow-up 3 years) in a prospective study of a cohort of 50 consecutive patients with SSc who received N-acetylcysteine (NAC) infusional therapy every 2 weeks. ... In conclusion, long-term therapy with NAC, in patients with SSc, has a durable effectiveness on ischemic ulcers and Raynaud's phenomenon." Rosato et al. The treatment with N-acetylcysteine of Raynaud's phenomenon and ischemic ulcers therapy in sclerodermic patients: a prospective observational study of 50 patients. *Clin Rheumatol*. 2009 Dec;28(12):1379-84
[837] Furst et al. Measurement of clinical change in progressive systemic sclerosis. *Ann Rheum Dis*. 1979 Aug;38(4):356-61

capsules of NAC or placebo were dispensed. ... Therapy was begun with 2-4 capsules daily and increased to a maximum of 20 capsules daily given in equally divided doses over a 2-month period. If the full dose was not tolerated, the highest tolerated dose was used. ... In the NAC-treated group, [pulmonary] residual volume increased significantly. Oral aperture increased significantly in the NAC-treated group and latex titers decreased statistically significantly."

- Long-term N-acetylcysteine therapy in systemic sclerosis interstitial lung disease (*Int J Immunopathol Pharmacol* 2011 Jul[838]): "The primary endpoints of this study were changes between baseline and month 24 in single-breath carbon monoxide diffusing capacity (DLco). The secondary endpoints were: vital capacity (VC), forced expired volume in 1 sec (FEV1), total lung capacity (TLC), scores of high resolution computed tomography (HRCT) of the chest, number of adverse effects. In this study, we retrospectively investigated data from SSc patients who had undergone therapy with high-dose *intravenous* N-acetylcysteine (NAC) at a dosage of 15 mg/Kg/h for 5 consecutive hours every 14 days. After NAC therapy median values of DLco (69.5 vs 77.7%), VC (99 vs 101.3%) and TLC (93 vs 98.3%) significantly increased. We did not observe any significant changes from baseline in FEV1 value and HRTC score. The improvement in lung function was more evident in SSc patients without radiological signs of pulmonary fibrosis than in patients with pulmonary fibrosis. In SSc patients with mild-moderate pulmonary fibrosis intravenous NAC administration slows the rate of deterioration of DLco, VC and TLC. In conclusion, this retrospective study demonstrates that long-term therapy with intravenous NAC ameliorates pulmonary function tests in SSc patients."

o Comprehensive antioxidation: **As previously mentioned, patients with scleroderma have evidence of increased oxidative stress demonstrated by a doubling of urinary isoprostane excretion.**[839] Oxidative stress results from and contributes to systemic inflammation because 1) increased immune activity results in elaboration of oxidants, and 2) oxidative stress upregulates NF-kappaB (and other pathways) for additive immune activation. *Antioxidant supplementation* alone is clinically and biochemically inferior to a *comprehensive program* that includes both antioxidant supplementation and dietary modification (i.e., the supplemented Paleo-Mediterranean diet, as described previously) that includes heavy reliance upon fruits, vegetables, low-glycemic juices, nuts, seeds, and berries for their additive and synergistic antioxidant benefits.[840]

- In vitro modulation of collagen type I, fibronectin and dermal fibroblast function and activity, in systemic sclerosis by the antioxidant epigallocatechin-3-gallate (*Rheumatology* 2010 Nov[841]): Dermal fibroblasts from a cell line (AG), healthy individuals (CON) and SSc patients were treated with EGCG, one of the main constituents of green tea. "The results suggest that the antioxidant, EGCG, can reduce ECM production, the fibrotic marker CTGF and inhibit contraction of dermal fibroblasts from SSc patients. Furthermore, EGCG was able to suppress intracellular ROS, ERK1/2 kinase signaling and NFkB activity. Taken together, EGCG may be a possible candidate for therapeutic treatment aimed at reducing both oxidant stress and the fibrotic effects associated with SSc."

o Oral enzyme therapy with proteolytic/pancreatic enzymes: Polyenzyme supplementation is used to ameliorate the pathophysiology induced by immune complexes.[842] Immune complexes are detected in the majority of patients with scleroderma[843] and correlate with disease severity and visceral involvement.[844] Orally administered polyenzyme preparations have an "immune stimulating" action[845]

---

[838] Rosato et al. Long-term N-acetylcysteine therapy in systemic sclerosis interstitial lung disease: a retrospective study. *Int J Immunopathol Pharmacol*. 2011 Jul-Sep;24:727-33
[839] "CONCLUSION: This study provides evidence of enhanced lipid peroxidation in both SSc and UCTD, and suggests a rationale for antioxidant treatment of SSc." Cracowski JL, et al. Enhanced in vivo lipid peroxidation in scleroderma spectrum disorders. *Arthritis Rheum* 2001 May;44(5):1143-8
[840] Liu RH. Health benefits of fruit and vegetables are from additive and synergistic combinations of phytochemicals. *Am J Clin Nutr*. 2003 Sep;78(3 Suppl):517S-520S
[841] Dooley et al. Modulation of collagen type I, fibronectin and dermal fibroblast function and activity, in systemic sclerosis by the antioxidant epigallocatechin-3-gallate. *Rheumatology* 2010 Nov;49(11):2024-36
[842] Galebskaya et al. Human complement system state after wobenzyme intake. *Vestnik Moskovskogo Universiteta Khimiya*. 2000:41; Supplement 148-149
[843] "Serum immune complexes were measured in 92 patients with progressive systemic sclerosis, and elevated levels were found as follows: Raji cell assay 72% (59% after pronase treatment of Raji cell), agarose gel electrophoresis 52%, and C1q binding 24%." Seibold JR, Medsger TA Jr, Winkelstein A, Kelly RH, Rodnan GP. Immune complexes in progressive systemic sclerosis (scleroderma). *Arthritis Rheum*. 1982 Oct;25(10):1167-73
[844] "Patients with SS showed an incidence of circulating immune complexes comparable to that found in SLE, with 20 patients (58.5%),...associated with both elevation of serum IgG and IgA levels and extensive visceral involvement by the disease." Hughes P, Cunningham J, Day M, Fitzgerald JC, French MA, Wright JK, Rowell NR. Immune complexes in systemic sclerosis; detection by C1q binding, K-cell inhibition and Raji cell radioimmunoassays. *J Clin Lab Immunol*. 1983 Mar;10(3):133-8
[845] Zavadova E, Desser L, Mohr T. Stimulation of reactive oxygen species production and cytotoxicity in human neutrophils in vitro and after oral administration of a polyenzyme preparation. *Cancer Biother*. 1995 Summer;10(2):147-52

and promote degradation of microbial biofilms and increased immune and antimicrobial penetration into infectious foci.[846] Given that maldigestion, malabsorption, and pancreatic insufficiency are not uncommon in patients with scleroderma[847], enzymes may be given with food for optimal benefit.

- **ENDOCRINE IMBALANCE & OPTIMIZATION: Prolactin, Insulin, Estrogen, DHEA, Cortisol, Testosterone, Thyroid** Common hormonal imbalances seen among autoimmune/inflammatory patients are: ❶ *elevated* prolactin, ❷ *elevated* estrogen, ❸ *elevated* insulin, and ❹ *reduced* DHEA, ❺ *reduced* cortisol, and ❻ *reduced* testosterone; see Chapter 4 for discussion of these hormones and respective interventions. Thyroid evaluation (patient + labs) should be comprehensive, as discussed in Chapter 1, with a low threshold for empiric treatment.
    - High incidence of thyroid disorders in systemic sclerosis (*J Clin Endocrinol Metab* 2013 Jul[848]): "Our study shows a high incidence of new cases of hypothyroidism and thyroid dysfunction in female sclerodermic patients. Female sclerodermic patients, who are at high risk (a borderline high [even if in the normal range] TSH value, anti-thyroperoxidase antibody positivity, and a hypoechoic and small thyroid) should have periodic thyroid function follow-up."
    - Low DHEA sulphate serum levels in premenopausal systemic sclerosis (*Clin Exp Rheumatol* 2001 Jan[849]): "Mean serum levels of DHEAS in SSc women of childbearing age were significantly lower than in controls (0.87 +/- 0.85 microgram/ml versus 2.75 +/- 0.42 micrograms/ml; $p < 0.001$). On the contrary, no difference was found between postmenopausal women and controls. A reduction below the 95% confidence limits was found in 10 out of 11 patients of childbearing age and in 8 out of 29 postmenopausal women, respectively. In 5 out of 11 patients of childbearing age taking steroids for their SSc (< 10 mg/daily) DHEAS levels were significantly lower than in patients not taking steroids ($p = 0.01$). ... Our data show that, as in other autoimmune diseases, low serum DHEAS is a feature of premenopausal SSc patients. More extensive prospective studies are needed to define the exact role of DHEAS dysregulation in SSc."
    - High prolactin and low dehydroepiandrosterone sulphate serum levels correlate with disease activity in patients with severe systemic sclerosis (*Br J Rheumatol.* 1997 Apr[850]): "Compared to SSc with <9 disease manifestations, patients with > or =9 disease manifestations had higher PRL ($P = 0.044$), higher soluble interleukin 2 receptor (sIL-2R, $P = 0.004$) and vascular cell adhesion molecule (sVCAM, $P = 0.044$), and lower DHEAS ($P = 0.029$). PRL (R(Rank) = 0.490, $P = 0.003$) and DHEAS (R(Rank) = -0.399, $P = 0.013$) were significantly correlated with the number of disease manifestations. The inverse correlation between PRL and DHEAS showed a trend ($P = 0.059$). PRL correlated with sIL-2R (R(Rank) = 0.553, $P = 0.001$) and sVCAM (R(Rank) = 0.520, $P = 0.002$). The number of disease manifestations and sIL-2R correlated significantly (R(Rank) = 0.463, $P = 0.006$)."
    - Melatonin: **In an *in vitro* study with fibroblasts from normal and scleroderma patients, melatonin was shown to inhibit fibroblast proliferation**[851]; future trials may demonstrate that melatonin has an antifibrotic/antisclerodermatous benefit. Melatonin is a pineal hormone with well-known sleep-inducing and immunomodulatory properties, and it is commonly administered in doses of 1-40 mg in the evening, before bedtime. Its exceptional safety is well documented. In contrast to implementing treatment with high doses of 20-40 mg, starting with a relatively low dose (e.g., 1-5 mg) and increasing as tolerated is recommended. Melatonin (20 mg hs) appears to have cured two patients with drug-resistant sarcoidosis[852] and 3 mg provided immediate short-term benefit to a patient with multiple sclerosis.[853] Immunostimulatory anti-infective action of melatonin was demonstrated in a clinical trial wherein septic newborns administered 20 mg melatonin showed significantly increased survival over nontreated

---

[846] "The enzymes were shown to inhibit the biofilm formation. When apliplied to the formed associations, the enzymes potentiated the effect of antibiotics on the bacteria located in them." Tets VV, et al. [Impact of exogenic proteolytic enzymes on bacteria][Article in Russian] *Antibiot Khimioter*. 2004;49(12):9-13
[847] Of 20 patients: "Three patients had very low levels of tryptic activity in their intestinal juice and only nine had results which were unequivocally normal." Cobden I, Axon AT, Rowell NR. Pancreatic exocrine function in systemic sclerosis. *Br J Dermatol* 1981 Aug;105(2):189-93
[848] Antonelli et al. Incidence of thyroid disorders in systemic sclerosis: results from a longitudinal follow-up. *J Clin Endocrinol Metab*. 2013 Jul;98(7):E1198-202
[849] La Montagna, et al. Dehydroepiandrosterone sulphate serum levels in systemic sclerosis. *Clin Exp Rheumatol*. 2001 Jan-Feb;19(1):21-6
[850] Straub et al. High prolactin and low dehydroepiandrosterone sulphate serum levels in patients with severe systemic sclerosis. *Br J Rheumatol*. 1997 Apr;36(4):426-32
[851] "These results suggest that MLT, at higher dosages, is a potent inhibitor of the proliferation of fibroblasts derived from the skin of healthy and SSc patients." Carossino AM, et al. Effect of melatonin on normal and sclerodermic skin fibroblast proliferation. *Clin Exp Rheumatol*. 1996 Sep-Oct;14(5):493-8.
[852] Cagnoni et al. Melatonin for treatment of chronic refractory sarcoidosis. *Lancet*. 1995 Nov 4;346(8984):1229-30
[853] "...administration of melatonin (3 mg, orally) at 2:00 p.m., when the patient experienced severe blurring of vision, resulted within 15 minutes in a dramatic improvement in visual acuity and in normalization of the visual evoked potential latency after stimulation of the left eye." Sandyk R. Diurnal variations in vision and relations to circadian melatonin secretion in multiple sclerosis. *Int J Neurosci*. 1995 Nov;83(1-2):1-6

controls[854]; given that scleroderma is associated with subclinical "infections", melatonin may provide therapeutic benefit by virtue of its anti-infective properties.
- o Estrogen (excess): **Research suggests that estrogen is immunodysregulatory and an important contributor to autoimmune disease**, perhaps explaining the greatly higher incidence of autoimmune diseases in women compared to men. So-called **"estrogen-replacement therapy" used in postmenopausal women increases the risk for lupus and scleroderma.**[855] Men with rheumatoid arthritis show an excess of estradiol and a decrease in DHEA, and the excess estrogen is proportional to the degree of inflammation.[856] Serum estradiol is commonly used to assess estrogen status; estrogens can also be measured in 24-hour urine samples. Interventions to combat high estrogen levels may include any effective combination of the following:
    - Weight loss and weight optimization: In overweight patients, weight loss is the means to attaining the goal of weight optimization; the task is not complete until the body mass index is normalized/optimized. Excess adiposity and obesity raise estrogen levels due to high levels of aromatase (the hormone that makes estrogen) in adipose tissue; weight optimization and loss of excess fat helps normalize hormone levels and reduce inflammation.
    - Avoidance of ethanol: Estrogen production is stimulated by ethanol intake.
    - Consider surgical correction of varicocele in affected men: Men with varicocele have higher estrogen levels due to temperature-induced alterations in enzyme function in the testes; surgical correction of the varicocele lowers estrogen levels.
    - "Anti-estrogen diet": Foods and supplements such as green tea, DIM, I3C, licorice, and a high-fiber "anti-estrogenic diet" can also be used; monitoring clinical status and serum estradiol will prove or disprove efficacy.
    - Anastrozole/Arimidex: In our office, we commonly measure serum estradiol in men and administer the aromatase inhibitor anastrozole/Arimidex 1 mg (2-3 doses per week) to men whose estradiol level is greater than ~20 picogram/mL; we consider estradiol 10-24 picogram/mL to be optimal for a man.[857] Clinical studies using anastrozole/Arimidex in men have shown that aromatase blockade lowers estradiol and raises testosterone[858]; generally speaking, this is exactly the result that we want in patients with severe systemic autoimmunity. Frequency of dosing is based on serum and clinical response. Letrozole/Femara is another aromatase inhibitor, one that should generally be avoided due to its ability to block androgen receptors.

- **XENOBIOTIC ACCUMULATION & DETOXIFICATION: Chemical avoidance, nutritional support for detoxification pathways, urine alkalinization** The clinical relevance and pathogenic mechanisms of xenobiotic accumulation are irrefutably well documented and described. Clinical assessments include history, physical examination, and laboratory assessment (using serum, whole blood, urine or—rarely yet accurately—fat biopsy), and response to treatment. Treatments include nutritional support for Phases 1 and 2 of detoxification (e.g., oxidation and conjugation) and excretion via bile and urine; for the latter, urinary alkalinization is generally recommended. Chemical toxins can be bound in the gut using activated charcoal, cholestyramine, or *Chlorella*—all of these three treatments have documented safety and effectiveness; clinically and empirically, phytochelatin (plant-derived peptides that bind toxic metals) concentrates appear safe and effective despite lack of conclusive published data supporting clinical use.

---

[854] Gitto et al. Effects of melatonin treatment in septic newborns. *Pediatr Res*. 2001 Dec;50(6):756-60 pedresearch.org/cgi/content/full/50/6/756
[855] "These studies indicate that estrogen replacement therapy in postmenopausal women increases the risk of developing lupus, scleroderma, and Raynaud disease..." Mayes MD. Epidemiologic studies of environmental agents and systemic autoimmune diseases. *Environ Health Perspect*. 1999 Oct;107 Suppl 5:743-8
[856] "DHEAS and estrone concentrations were lower and estradiol was higher in patients compared with healthy controls. DHEAS differed between RF positive and RF negative patients. Estrone did not correlate with any disease variable, whereas estradiol correlated strongly and positively with all measured indices of inflammation." Tengstrand et al. Abnormal levels of serum dehydroepiandrosterone, estrone, and estradiol in men with rheumatoid arthritis: high correlation between serum estradiol and current degree of inflammation. *J Rheumatol*. 2003 Nov;30(11):2338-43
[857] Male Hormone Modulation Therapy, Page 4 Of 7: lef.org/protocols/prtcl-130c.shtml Accessed October 30, 2005
[858] "These data demonstrate that aromatase inhibition increases serum bioavailable and total testosterone levels to the youthful normal range in older men with mild hypogonadism." Leder et al. Effects of aromatase inhibition in elderly men with low or borderline-low serum testosterone levels. *J Clin Endocrinol Metab*. 2004 Mar;89:1174-80

- o Xenobiotic immunotoxicity: Given that **antifibrillarin antibodies are specifically seen in patients with scleroderma**[859] and that **mercury exposure induces antifibrillarin autoimmunity in susceptible mice**[860], clinicians may be justified in searching for and treating evidence of mercury exposure in patients with autoimmunity in general and scleroderma in particular. Detailed history, dental examination for mercury-containing amalgams, and post-DMSA urine metal analysis are suggested.
- **ADDITIONAL CONSIDERATIONS FOR COMMON COMPLICATIONS: Raynaud's & GERD**
  - Esophageal dysfunction and GERD in scleroderma—specific treatments:
    - Low carbohydrate diet, specific carbohydrate diet: The gastroesophageal dysfunction that contributes to the high incidence of Barrett's esophagus is likely the result of a confluence of different factors: neurogenic, myogenic, and dysbiotic. With regard to the latter, clinicians must be diligent in the eradication of small intestine bacterial overgrowth, since microbial products of fermentation lead to relaxation of the so-called lower esophageal sphincter.[861,862] This is why diets low in carbohydrate and fermentable fibers (such as those found in grains)—in other words: "**low fermentation diets**"—are effective in the treatment of esophageal reflux; low-carbohydrate diets deprive gut microbes of substrate for fermentation into metabolites that relax the lower esophageal sphincter and thereby contribute to symptomatic improvement in patients with gastroesophageal reflux.[863] This is part of the reason why the diet for these patients must be as low as possible in the difficult-to-digest and easy-to-ferment carbohydrates that are common in the Standard American Diet (SAD) from corn, potatoes, wheat, oats, and disaccharides such as lactose and sucrose; see *Breaking the Vicious Cycle*[864] by the late Elaine Gottschall for more details and recipes for the specific carbohydrate diet. Similarly, a low-carbohydrate Atkins-type diet[865] might also be considered, particularly for short-term use and particularly if modified away from proinflammatory saturated fats and arachidonic acid. As emphasized previously, high-fiber diets increase the risk for bowel obstruction in scleroderma patients, especially if implemented rapidly; slow implementation of dietary fiber increase along with an osmotic stool softener such as magnesium and/or ascorbate is advised.
    - Alginate: Alginate is a processed extract from seaweed that is the active ingredient in the FDA-approved OTC anti-heartburn drug Gaviscon.[866] When mixed with stomach acid, alginate forms a foam "raft" that creates a barrier of protection for the esophagus, and it significantly reduces the number of acidic reflux events. Clinical studies have proven the effectiveness of alginate for treating GERD; however pure supplements of sodium alginate may be preferred over Gaviscon due to the latter's inclusion of aluminum (hydroxide)[867], a metal correlated with adverse effects and increased risk for neurologic disease. Alginate is also said to bind toxic metals and may therefore reduce enterohepatic recirculation of these proinflammatory immunotoxins.
    - Betaine hydrochloric acid (betaine HCL): Many patients with gastroesophageal reflux are cured with the administration of supplemental HCL. Although the addition of acid rather than the suppression of acid goes against the well-funded acid-blocking drug paradigm, the truth remains that—*physiologically*—gastric emptying is promoted by acidification and—*clinically*—the treatment works for a significant number of patients with GERD. Furthermore, correction of hypochlorhydria by supplementation with betaine HCL helps to reduce bacterial/yeast counts in the stomach and upper small intestine, thereby alleviating GERD by reducing the bacteria/yeast available for

---

[859] "Since anti-fibrillarin antibodies are specific markers of scleroderma, the present animal model may be valuable for studies of the immunological aberrations which are likely to induce this autoimmune response." Hultman et al. Anti-fibrillarin autoantibodies in mercury-treated mice. *Clin Exp Immunol*. 1989 Dec;78(3):470-7
[860] Nielsen et al. Mercury-induced autoimmunity in mice. *Environ Health Perspect*. 2002 Oct;110 Sup 5:877-81 ehp.niehs.nih.gov/docs/2002/suppl-5/877-881nielsen/abstract.html
[861] "Colonic fermentation of indigestible carbohydrates increases the rate of TLESRs [transient lower esophageal sphincter relaxations], the number of acid reflux episodes, and the symptoms of GERD." Piche et al. Colonic fermentation influences lower esophageal sphincter function in gastroesophageal reflux disease. *Gastroenterology*. 2003 Apr;124(4):894-902
[862] Piche et al. Modulation by colonic fermentation of LES function in humans. *Am J Physiol Gastrointest Liver Physiol*. 2000 Apr;278(4):G578-84
[863] "The 5 individuals described in these case reports experienced resolution of GERD symptoms after self-initiation of a low-carbohydrate diet." Yancy et al. Improvement of gastroesophageal reflux disease after initiation of a low-carbohydrate diet: five brief case reports. *Altern Ther Health Med*. 2001 Nov-Dec;7(6):120, 116-9
[864] Gotschall E. *Breaking the Vicious Cycle: Intestinal health though diet*. Kirkton Press; Rev edition (August, 1994) scdiet.com/
[865] Atkins, RC. *Dr. Atkins' New Diet Revolution (revised and updated)*. New York: Avon Books, 1999
[866] "For this population, sodium alginate was assessed as significantly superior by both investigators and patients at week two (p < 0.001 and p = 0.004, respectively) and at week four (p = 0.001 and p < 0.001, respectively)." Chatfield S. A comparison of the efficacy of the alginate preparation, Gaviscon Advance, with placebo in the treatment of gastro-oesophageal reflux disease. *Curr Med Res Opin*. 1999;15(3):152-9
[867] gaviscon.com/info.htm

fermentation; recall that microbial fermentation is one of the primary driving influences for gastroesophageal reflux.[868]
- **GLA**: Numerous studies have documented the anti-cancer effects of GLA, and these have specifically been documented in esophageal cancer cell lines.[869] Thus, GLA consumption may help protect against the development of esophageal cancer, in addition to its important anti-inflammatory and vasodilating actions.
- <u>Vitamin B12</u>: Vitamin B-12 levels are low in patients with malabsorption, and vitamin B-12 administration (4,000 mcg/d orally, or 1,000-2,000 mcg intramuscularly/ 2-3 times weekly) promotes intestinal motility.

o <u>Raynaud's phenomenon—specific treatments</u>: See section/minimonograph at the end of this chapter.

---

[868] "Colonic fermentation of indigestible carbohydrates increases the rate of TLESRs [transient lower esophageal sphincter relaxations], the number of acid reflux episodes, and the symptoms of GERD." Piche et al. Colonic fermentation influences lower esophageal sphincter function in gastroesophageal reflux disease. *Gastroenterology*. 2003 Apr;124(4):894-902

[869] "A statistically highly significant growth-suppressive effect of the prostaglandin precursor gamma-linolenic acid (GLA) on MG63 human osteogenic sarcoma and oesophageal carcinoma cells in culture was found." Booyens et al. The effect of gamma-linolenic acid on the growth of human osteogenic sarcoma and oesophageal carcinoma cells in culture. *S Afr Med J*. 1984 Feb 18;65(7):240-2

Vasculitic Diseases & Wegener's Granulomatosis

Introduction:

Vasculitic diseases are largely considered to be mediated by deposition of circulating immune complexes (CIC) into/on the vascular endothelium, resulting in a localized activation of cell-mediated inflammation and activation of the complement cascade. From an allopathic perspective, these conditions are generally considered idiopathic and thus necessarily requiring long-term immunosuppression, in various forms.

From the perspective of logic and with a desire to deconstruct complex clinical phenomena, one can approach diseases that are mediated by immune complex deposition by deciphering the components into their elemental parts. *Por ejemplo*/For example, given that vasculitic disease are mediated by endothelial deposition of immune complexes, and that immune complexes are chains of antigens and antibodies, one can then ask "*What are the major sources of antigens to which the immune system is exposed?*" and the correct answers are: "*Self, diet, microbes.*" One can then ponder the source of the antibodies, and ask if the presumed overproduction of antibodies is a *qualitative* problem or a *quantitative* problem, i.e., "Is the immune system 'wrong' in making antibodies to an antigen to which it is exposed [qualitative problem, error in action], *or* is the immune system 'correct' in its action but simply over-producing antibodies to perhaps otherwise benign antigens, whether these are self, diet, and/or microbes [quantitative problem, error in regulation]? From these questions, we arrive at answers other than crisis management and perpetual medicalization and pharmacologic immunosuppression; we arrive at the opportunity to reduce exposure to antigens from self (via antioxidant therapy to prevent molecular alteration of "self" structures), food (via food allergy avoidance and healing of intestinal hyperpermeability, and microbes (reducing dysbiosis and total microbial load [TML]) while also reducing the likely overzealous production of corresponding immunoglobulins via nutritional immunomodulation: induction of Treg for the reciprocal inhibition Th1, Th2, and Th17.

Description/pathophysiology, and clinical presentations:

- "Vasculitis" refers to a heterogeneous group of inflammatory disorders primarily affecting blood vessels, particularly the arteries and arterioles. Although the underlying pathomechanisms are similar among different disorders, these diseases differ in the location/size and number of affected vessels, and thus the clinical presentations and complications differ accordingly. Polymyalgia rheumatica / giant cell arteritis, Wegener's granulomatosis, and Behcet's disease are subtypes of vasculitis that are discussed in their respective chapters. As shown in the table at the right, several subtypes of vasculitis can be categorized based on the size/location of the vessel affected, and whether or not the cause of the vasculitis has been determined.
- Systemic manifestations are comparable to many other autoimmune disorders: insidious onset of fever, malaise, weight loss, generalized aches/pains.
- The autoimmune and immune-mediated pathogenesis of the vasculitides includes the following:
  - <u>Antibody-antigen binding</u>: *Example*: Goodpasture syndrome.
  - <u>Delayed hypersensitivity reactions</u>: Especially in lesions characterized with granulomas formation. *Example*: temporal arteritis.
  - <u>Deposition of circulating immune complexes</u>: The majority of the vasculitides are characterized by intra-arterial deposition of circulating immune complexes, which provoke activation of the complement cascade and leukocyte migration and

Overview of common vasculopathic disorders

Primary vasculitides

Large vessel diseases
- Takayasu's arteritis
- Behcet's disease

Medium vessel diseases
- Polyarteritis nodosa
- Buerger's disease
- Giant cell arteritis

Small vessel diseases
Immune-complex mediated
- Cutaneous leukocystoclastic vasculitis
- Henoch-Schonlein purpura
- Cryoglobulinemia

ANCA-associated disorders
- Wegener's granulomatosis
- Microscopic polyangiitis: microscopic polyarteritis, leukocytoclastic vasculitis ; variants include allergic granulomatosis and angiitis also known as Churg-Strauss syndrome

Secondary vasculitides
- Infections, dysbiosis
- Other autoimmune disease
- Crohn's disease or ulcerative colitis
- Cancer
- Drug reactions
- Food allergies

activation for the resultant vascular damage, which often includes necrosis, fibrinous occlusion, and thrombosis. *Example*: acute arteritis in SLE.

Schematized illustration of an immune complex: Immunoglobulins/antibodies—represented by the Y-shaped molecule—and antigens such as molecular fragments and peptides—represented by the ovoid molecule—form "chains" of alternating antigens-and-antibodies which in the circulation become lodged in the skin (dermatitis), vascular endothelium (vasculitis), kidney (nephritis), serosal surfaces (serositis), and synovial joints (arthritis). Readers must note that the location of the immune complex deposition is "innocent"; in immune complex disease, the location of the inflammation and complement activation (i.e., skin, vascular endothelium, kidney, synovial joints, serosa, and synovial joints) is simply a convenient molecular depot for the circulating immune complexes (CIC). Once deposited and following sufficient accumulation, immune complexes incite activation of the complement cascade and a local cell-mediated immune response, which causes local tissue inflammation and progressive destruction. Thus, for example, the joint or the skin or the kidney will be inflamed, but the actual problem of excess antigen exposure originated elsewhere, and the corresponding excess antibody production may have simply been a normal physiologic response to antigen exposure or may have been facilitated by a pro-inflammatory state and—synergistically yet distinctly—immunophenotypic imbalance.

Major differential diagnoses:
- Infection
- Cancer, especially leukemia, lymphoma, and multiple myeloma
- Autoimmunity: Concomitant or independent
- Trauma or abuse: Numerous unexplainable bruises/purpura may indicate abuse
- Adverse drug reaction
- Atherosclerosis, peripheral vascular disease, aneurysm

Clinical assessments:
- **History/subjective**:
  - See clinical presentations
- **Physical examination/objective**:
  - General physical examination with emphasis placed on symptomatic regions, circulatory examination, and dermal lesions
- **Laboratory assessments**:
  - Chemistry/metabolic panel: Assess for complications, especially renal insufficiency
  - Urinalysis: Assess for renal involvement
  - CRP/ESR: Generally elevated
  - Serum immune complexes: Most vasculopathies are due to immune complex deposition: Immune Complexes Reference Range (Raji cell technique, quantitative analysis):
    - Normal: ≤ 15.0 μg Eq/mL
    - Equivocal: 15.1-19.9 μg Eq/mL
    - Positive: ≥20.0 μg Eq/mL
  - Testing for multifocal dysbiosis: As discussed in Chapter 4
  - ANA
  - CH50: Complement levels may be low during exacerbations of immune complex mediated disease as the complement cascade is activated and complement proteins are consumed in the process, thus leading to a reduction in serum levels.

- ANCA: Many of the vasculopathies, particularly those affecting the small vessels, are characterized by the presence of anti-neutrophilic cytoplasmic autoantibodies (ANCA), which can be segregated into two distinct subtypes: ❶ **cytoplasmic-ANCA** (C-ANCA, major antigen: proteinase 3) associated with Wegener granulomatosis, and ❷ **perinuclear-ANCA** (P-ANCA, major antigen: myeloperoxidase) associated with microscopic polyangiitis, or Churg-Strauss syndrome. Clinicians should note that neither P-ANCA nor C-ANCA is specific for a particular diagnosis, and that 10% of patients with biopsy-proved small vessel vasculitis do not show either ANCA subtype. In patients with small vessel vasculitis, levels of ANCA correlate with disease severity, especially C-ANCA in patients with Wegener granulomatosis.

- **Imaging and biopsy**:
  - Angiography is commonly used in the evaluation of vasculitic syndromes affecting larger vessels; Doppler ultrasound imaging can also be used.
  - Biopsy of dermal lesions, superficial arteries, and other tissues can support the diagnosis
- **Establishing the diagnosis**:
  - Based on clinical, laboratory, and biopsy/imaging findings

Major complications:
- Tissue necrosis: Complications depend on location of hypoxia and can include dermal necrosis, myocardial infarction, stroke, and intestinal infarction
- Infection secondary to immunosuppression
- Renal damage

Clinical management:
- Exacerbations are best managed pharmaceutically with appropriate immunosuppression. Patients may require hospital admission.
- An overview/survey of various inflammatory vascular disorders is presented on the following two pages.

> **Timely referral and comanagement**
> Generally speaking, patients with these conditions should be co-managed with a specialist (e.g., Internal Medicine, Rheumatology) because complications such as transverse myelitis and vascular occlusion leading to distal tissue ischemia—blindness, digital necrosis, mesenteric ischemia—can present quickly and require immediate immunosuppression in a hospital setting.

Overview of Vasculitic Diseases

Vasculitis subtype	Unique characteristics	Assessment and treatment considerations
Giant Cell (Temporal) Arteritis (outlined here and detailed in following subsection before the therapeutics section): Three subtypes exist along a continuum: • Granulomatous vasculitis (2/3 of cases) • Leukocytic infiltration of vessel wall • Intimal fibrosis with lumenal narrowing	• GCA is the most common form of vasculitis; elevated ESR is classic • Granulomatous inflammation of medium and small arteries, particularly of the head; involvement of the aorta (giant cell aortitis) is a rare variant • Jaw claudication is highly suggestive • Classic presentation includes headache and facial pain; 50% of patients have PMR: polymyalgia rheumatica	• Biopsy is the gold standard for diagnosis, although it may be normal in one-third of patients due to lesion focality/locality. • **Patients can transition from asymptomatic to blind—vision loss due to occlusion of ophthalmic artery—within days; therefore, this condition is generally considered a medical emergency/urgency mandating immediate implementation of prednisone, typically starting at 60 mg/d or 1 mg/kg/d.**
Wegener granulomatosis (outlined here and detailed in following subsection before the therapeutics section): • Affects small arteries all the way through to veins	• Granulomatous vasculitis affecting the upper respiratory tract	• Most patients have C-ANCA (cytoplasmic anti-proteinase 3 antibodies); small percentage of patients have P-ANCA (perinuclear anti-myeloperoxidase antibodies)

Overview of Vasculitic Diseases—*continued*

Vasculitis subtype	Unique characteristics	Assessment and treatment considerations
Takayasu arteritis: "pulseless disease" • Leukocytic infiltration of the vasa vasorum followed by medial fibrosis and granulomatosis	• Granulomatous vasculitis of large and medium arteries • Fibrous thickening of the aortic arch and occlusion of large arteries • Presentation typically includes neuro-ocular disturbances, reduced arm pulses; may include aortic valve insufficiency, and hypertension due to renal artery stenosis	• Clinical assessment with aortogram
Polyarteritis nodosa (PAN): • Immune-complex vasculitis • 10-30% of patients have Hepatitis B—testing for hepatitis B is mandatory[870] • Generally fatal if untreated; estimated 5-year survival 13% • Without treatment, only 20% of patients survive 5 years; with treatment, survival improves to 60-90% at 5 years	• Necrotizing vasculitic ischemia of numerous systems, thrombosis and ischemia at sites distal to lesion • <u>Gut</u>: abdominal pain, nausea, vomiting exacerbated by eating (due to ischemia) • <u>Nerves</u>: mononeuritis multiplex, vasculitic neuropathy; foot drop is most common manifestation • <u>Skin</u>: dermal lesions include sharply-demarcated nodules, erythema, and ulceration; lesions are **non-palpable** and are in **different stages** of development • <u>Kidneys</u>: hypertension due to renal involvement • *Pulmonary involvement is rare* • Can be categorized as *infectious and ANCA-negative* or *noninfectious and P-ANCA-positive*	• Clinical presentation is varied depending on location of arterial lesion(s) and severity of systemic inflammation; typical population is young adults • Anemia, elevated ESR, leukocytosis • Autoantibodies commonly normal or low-positive • Diagnosis is established with biopsy or angiogram • <u>Pharmacotherapy</u>: prednisone: 60 mg/d; pulsed methylprednisolone: 1 gram IV daily for 3 days; cyclophosphamide or other immunosuppressant drug • Plasmapheresis • Treatment of underlying hepatitis: must balance immunosuppression with anti-infective treatments
Mixed cryoglobulinemia: • Many patients have underlying hepatitis C • Many patient respond to avoidance of foods to which they are allergic	• Purpura • Peripheral neuropathy • Glomerulonephritis • Abdominal pain • Hepatitis • May have pulmonary involvement	• Diagnosis is based on clinical picture and serology for cryoglobulins • Testing for and treatment of underlying hepatitis is essential • Immunosuppression may exacerbate viral replication • **Avoidance of food allergens is highly beneficial**[871,872]

---

[870] Tierney ML. McPhee SJ, Papadakis MA (eds). *Current Medical Diagnosis and Treatment 2006. 45th edition*. New York; Lange Medical Books: 2006, pages 844-850
[871] "CONCLUSION: These data show that an LAC diet decreases the amount of circulating immune complexes in MC and can modify certain signs and symptoms of the disease." Ferri C, Pietrogrande M, Cecchetti R, et al. Low-antigen-content diet in the treatment of patients with mixed cryoglobulinemia. *Am J Med*. 1989 Nov;87:519-24
[872] Pietrogrande M, Cefalo A, Nicora F, Marchesini D. Dietetic treatment of essential mixed cryoglobulinemia. *Ric Clin Lab*. 1986 Apr-Jun;16(2):413-6

Overview of Vasculitic Diseases—*continued*

Vasculitis subtype	Unique characteristics	Assessment and treatment considerations
Henoch-Schonlein purpura: IgA vasculitis Note: These terms are easy to intermix and confuse: • Buerger's disease: thromboangiitis obliterans • Berger's disease: IgA nephropathy	• Dermal purpura • Abdominal pain • Arthritis • Hematuria associated with renal involvement; IgA nephropathy (Berger's disease) is generally considered a glomerular variant of Henoch-Schonlein purpura	• The disease is generally self-limiting to 1-6 weeks, subsiding without complications if renal involvement is mild • Monitor renal function • No generally effective allopathic treatment is known
Microscopic polyangiitis, microscopic polyarteritis, leukocytoclastic vasculitis: • Affects small arterioles, capillaries, and venules; affected organs may include skin, lung, brain, heart, and kidneys (necrotizing glomerulonephritis) • Associated with relatively acute events, such as infection (including dysbiosis), drug administration, cancer, or administration of foreign protein	• Necrotizing vasculitis • Dermal lesions are differentiated from those of PAN because lesions of leukocytoclastic vasculitis are all at the **same stage of development** (due to acute event) and these lesions are **palpable due to acute inflammation** • P-ANCA is generally positive • Immune complexes are *not* characteristic of the vascular lesions	• P-ANCA is generally positive • "In general, the disease responds well to removal of the offending agent."[873]
Churg-Strauss syndrome, allergic granulomatous angiitis: affects small arteries all the way through to veins; variant of leukocytoclastic vasculitis	• Eosinophilia with bronchial asthma and sinusitis; mimics allergic sinusitis and allergic asthma • Pulmonary and splenic vessel involvement; granulomas • Associated with Henoch-Schonlein purpura, essential mixed cryoglobulinemia, and vasculitis of malignancy	• ANCA, particularly P-ANCA • Eosinophilia
Kawasaki disease; mucocutaneous lymph node syndrome: affects small-large arteries, classically the coronary arteries of children	• Arteritis of the coronary arteries in children • Mucocutaneous lymph node syndrome	• Coronary angiography • High-dose aspirin therapy

---

[873] Mitchell RN, et al. *Pocket Companion to Robbins and Cotran Pathologic Basis of Disease, Seventh Edition*. Philadelphia; Saunders Elsevier: 2006, page 279

Clinical Applications: Rheumatology

Brief Mention / Additional Emphasis
Polymyalgia Rheumatica (PMR), Giant Cell Arteritis (GCA, previously Temporal Arteritis)

> **Introduction:**
> Giant cell arteritis (previously called temporal arteritis) and polymyalgia rheumatica are related conditions characterized histopathologically by inflammatory occlusion of small arteries and arterioles in the upper body: head, neck, shoulders. The possibility of arterial occlusion leading to blindness due to occlusion of the ophthalmic artery mandates early implementation of immunosuppressive prednisone (generally at 60mg/d or 1mg/kg/d). These patients must be co-managed with an Internal Medicine or Rheumatology specialist, while components of the Functional Inflammology protocol are appropriately applied.

<u>Description/pathophysiology</u>:
- This group of tightly related and largely synonymous disorders is described as "idiopathic" by medical textbooks.
- **Polymyalgia rheumatica (PMR)**: This disorder typically presents with painful inflammation of the shoulder/neck and hip muscles along with systemic manifestations of fever, malaise, and weight loss. When present in isolation (i.e., not with giant cell arteritis), it does not lead to blindness, and the condition responds to low-dose (10-20 mg) prednisone.
- **Giant Cell Arteritis (GCA):** When treated allopathically, GCA requires higher daily doses (40-60 mg) of prednisone than PMR. **GCA can result in rapid-onset blindness and therefore any evidence of ocular involvement in a patient with GCA must be treated as a medical emergency.** Indeed, the diagnosis of GCA itself is considered urgent due to ability of blindness to occur rapidly and without warning. GCA was previously called temporal arteritis. Approximately 50% of patients with GCA have PMR.

<u>Clinical presentations</u>:
- Pain and stiffness in proximal muscle groups: shoulders, neck, and hips; weakness—if any—is secondary to pain, disuse atrophy, drug side-effect (e.g., "steroid myopathy"), or other concomitant disorder. Presentations are consistent with muscle/tissue ischemia due to the underlying panarteritis which results in vessel occlusion: head pain, jaw claudication, blindness.
- Generally presents after age 50 years. The later age of onset helps distinguish PMR from fibromyalgia, which generally affects young adult patients between the ages of 20-40 years.
- 2x more common in women than in men.
- Typical autoimmune systemic manifestations: fatigue, malaise, fever, anorexia, and weight loss.
- Patients may have high fever and chills with disease initiation and/or exacerbation.

<u>Major differential diagnoses</u>:
- <u>Fibromyalgia</u>: ESR is normal, age of onset is nearly always before 50 years.
- <u>Dermatomyositis, polymyositis</u>: These conditions cause muscle weakness, which is characteristically absent in patients with PMR. Muscle enzymes are elevated in patients with dermatomyositis/polymyositis but are normal in patients with PMR.
- <u>Cancer, particularly multiple myeloma</u>
- <u>Hypothyroidism</u>: Hypothyroidism can easily mimic PMR by producing an inflammatory myopathy that affects the shoulder muscles and which remits following normalization of thyroid status.
- <u>Rheumatoid arthritis, SLE, vasculitis, or other autoimmune disorder</u>
- <u>Infection</u>: WBC count is normal in GCA/PMR and is generally elevated in patients with severe infection.
- <u>Cervical spondylosis</u>: Normal ESR and no anemia

Clinical assessments:
- **History/subjective**:
  - See clinical presentations
- **Physical examination/objective**:
  - Palpate pulses for strength and symmetry:
    - Carotid artery in the anterior neck
    - Axillary/brachial in the axilla and inner arm, respectively
    - Radial pulse at the distal radius
    - Aorta in the abdomen
    - Femoral pulses in the groin
    - Dorsalis pedis and posterior tibial arteries at the ankle/foot
- **Laboratory assessments**:
  - ESR: Most patients will have a very high ESR > 50 mm/h.
  - CBC: Anemia is common.
  - Chemistry/metabolic panel: Hepatic alkaline phosphatase is elevated in 20% of patients.
  - RF: generally negative
  - Muscle enzymes: are almost always normal.
  - Protein in urine, serum protein electrophoresis: No evidence of proteinuria or monoclonal gammopathy, as seen in MM.
- **Imaging**:
  - Not generally indicated except when looking for complications or concomitant disease
- **Establishing the diagnosis**:
  - PMR is a clinical diagnosis based on 1) painful inflammation of the shoulder/neck and hip muscles along with 2) systemic manifestations of fever, malaise, and weight loss and 3) the absence of evidence supporting an alternate diagnosis.[874]
  - GCA is classically diagnosed following biopsy of the temporal artery.
  - Pattern recognition (proximal muscle pain with no other explanation) and evidence of inflammation in an elderly patient when other diseases have been ruled out.

Complications:
- GCA can lead to blindness.
- Dry cough is seen in some patients and may be the presenting complaint.
- Mononeuritis multiplex may cause (shoulder) paralysis.
- Aneurysms of the thoracic aorta are 17x more common in patients with GCA than the general population

Clinical management:
- Assess for temporal arteritis—educate patient about the significance of the onset of eye symptoms, headache, and jaw claudication.
- A few patients treated with prednisone will have permanent remission within 2 years.

Treatments: Use this section in association with previously mentioned assessments and interventions.
  Drug treatments: This condition requires early implementation of prednisone immunosuppression; comanagement with a specialist—Internal Medicine or Rheumatology—is mandatory.
- Prednisone: 10-20 mg per day for PMR should result in "dramatic improvement" within 72 hours.[875] Prednisone dose for GCA is typically 60 mg per day at the start of treatment in order to prevent one of the most feared complications—blindness. Dose is tapered after clinical remission. Low-dose aspirin appears to reduce the risk of blindness and stroke in GCA patients.

---

[874] Tierney ML. McPhee SJ, Papadakis MA. *Current Medical Diagnosis and Treatment. 35th edition*. Stamford: Appleton and Lange, 1996 page 751. Tierney ML. McPhee SJ, Papadakis MA (eds). *Current Medical Diagnosis and Treatment 2006. 45th edition*. New York; Lange Medical Books: 2006, pages 486
[875] Tierney ML. McPhee SJ, Papadakis MA (eds). *Current Medical Diagnosis and Treatment 2006. 45th edition*. New York; Lange Medical Books: 2006, pages 487

Brief Mention / Additional Emphasis
Wegener's Granulomatosis

> **Introduction:**
> Wegener's is a granulomatous and vasculitic disease with a high mortality. Insight into the molecular basis of the condition—electrostatic haptenization of the *Staphylococcus aureus* enzyme acid phosphatase with endothelial cells—provides brilliant insight into the disease and its treatment. The possible role of other microbes, along with other factors such as immunophenotype imbalance should be intuitive by this time to readers who have read the other chapters.

Description/pathophysiology:
- This inflammatory condition generally begins with granulomatous involvement of the upper or lower respiratory tract and then progresses to systemic vasculitis and glomerulonephritis.
- Biopsy of nasopharyngeal/pulmonary/renal lesions reveals granulomatous/inflammatory tissue.
- Allopathic textbooks generally describe this condition as *idiopathic*, although the condition is increasingly associated with occult sinorespiratory dysbiosis with *Staphylococcus aureus*.[876,877] Additionally, *Klebsiella aerogenes, Haemophilus influenzae,* and *Bacillus subtilis* have been implicated.[878]
- Immune complexes contribute to pathophysiology

Clinical presentations:
- Twice as common in males as in females
- Sinorespiratory symptoms:
    - Mucosal ulcerations/friability, hemorrhagic rhinorrhea
    - Persistent sinusitis; increased incidence of otitis media
    - Cough, hemoptosis due to intraalveolar hemorrhage, pleuritis
- Renal complications are inevitable without effective/immunosuppressive treatment
- Typical autoimmune systemic manifestations: fatigue, malaise, low-grade fever, anorexia, and weight loss, polyarthritis.

Major differential diagnoses:
- Extramedullary plasmacytoma of multiple myeloma (typically occurs in the nasopharyngeal region)
- Sinus infection
- Lung cancer
- Tuberculosis
- Septicemia or septic arthritis
- Lymphoma
- Other systemic/inflammatory disorder such as lupus (ANA and low complement)
- Bacterial endocarditis

Clinical assessments:
- **History/subjective**: See clinical presentations.
- **Physical examination/objective**:
    - Examination of oral and nasal mucosa
    - Pulmonary auscultation
    - Dermatologic screen for cutaneous vasculitis

---
[876] Brons RH, Bakker HI, Van Wijk RT, et al. Staphylococcal acid phosphatase binds to endothelial cells via charge interaction; a pathogenic role in Wegener's granulomatosis? *Clin Exp Immunol*. 2000 Mar;119(3):566-73 blackwell-synergy.com/doi/abs/10.1046/j.1365-2249.2000.01172.x
[877] Popa ER, et al. Staphylococcus aureus and Wegener's granulomatosis. *Arthritis Res*. 2002;4(2):77-9 arthritis-research.com/content/4/2/77
[878] George J, et al. Infections and Wegener's granulomatosis—a cause and effect relationship? *QJM*. 1997 May;90(5):367-73 qjmed.oxfordjournals.org/cgi/reprint/90/5/367

- **Laboratory assessments**:
    - Urinalysis for assessment of renal status
    - Chemistry/metabolic panel for BUN and creatinine, etc.
    - Microbial assessments—reviewed in Chapters 1 and 4.
    - Nasal culture for *Staphylococcus aureus*[879] and other bacterial or fungal contaminants
    - Complement levels are normal or elevated
    - ESR/CRP is elevated
    - CBC may reveal leukocytosis and anemia
    - **ANA (antinuclear antibodies) are generally absent**
    - **ANCA are almost always present and strongly support the diagnosis of this condition.** The finding of the more specific C-ANCA is 97% specific for the diagnosis of Wegener's granulomatosis.[880] Interestingly, ANCA can also be induced by gastrointestinal parasitic infections.
- **Imaging**: Generally not required; only indicated as needed
- **Establishing the diagnosis**: Based on clinical, serologic, and biopsy findings.
    - Respiratory tract symptoms and mucosal lesions; biopsy of granulomas.
    - C-ANCA: positive C-ANCA result can replace biopsy in a patient with a clinical picture of Wegener's granulomatosis.[881]

Complications:
- Severe anemia requiring blood transfusion
- Secondary bacterial infections on ulcerated mucosa
- Respiratory and renal failure
- Hypoxic complications due to vasculitis

Clinical management:
- Referral to internist/rheumatologist for additional treatment and defensive management as indicated. Unless you are a specialist, you need to have a specialist as part of the care team who can help you manage acute exacerbations which can occur with any autoimmune/inflammatory disease.

Therapeutic considerations: Medical treatment routinely includes the following:[882]
- Cyclophosphamide: 1-2 mg/kg/d PO or IV: associated with increased risk for cancer, particularly bladder cancer
- Prednisone: 1 mg/kg/d po; use the lowest dose possible
- Methotrexate: pulse treatment < 20-30 mg per week po
- **Antibiotic treatment: Bactrim / trimeth-sulfa 160/800 up to 480/2400 mg/d po**
- Blood transfusions for anemia
- **Assessment for multifocal dysbiosis: emphasis on gastrointestinal and sinorespiratory dysbiosis**
    - ***Staphylococcus aureus*: Produces an antigenic acid phosphatase which haptenizes with endothelial cells for the induction of autoimmune vasculitis in Wegener's granulomatosis.**[883]
        - Drugs: Antimicrobial treatment—typically with Bactrim—to eradicate *Staphylococcus aureus* results in clinical remission of the "autoimmune" disease, thus proving the microbe-rheumatic link.[884]
        - Herbs: Hyperforin from *Hypericum perforatum* shows in vitro effectiveness against *Staphylococcus aureus*.[885]
        - Topical antiseptic: Intranasal 5% povidone iodine is highly effective against *Staphylococcus aureus*; Among 1,697 patients undergoing arthroplasty or spine fusion surgery, 5% povidone iodine proved

---

[879] Brons RH, Bakker HI, Van Wijk RT, et al. Staphylococcal acid phosphatase binds to endothelial cells via charge interaction; a pathogenic role in Wegener's granulomatosis? *Clin Exp Immunol*. 2000 Mar;119(3):566-73 blackwell-synergy.com/doi/abs/10.1046/j.1365-2249.2000.01172.x P
[880] Beers MH, Berkow R (eds). *The Merck Manual. Seventeenth Edition*. Whitehouse Station; Merck Research Laboratories 1999 Page 443
[881] Shojania K. Rheumatology: 2. What laboratory tests are needed? *CMAJ*. 2000 Apr 18;162(8):1157-63 cmaj.ca/cgi/content/full/162/8/1157
[882] Beers MH, Berkow R (eds). *The Merck Manual. Seventeenth Edition*. Whitehouse Station; Merck Research Laboratories 1999 Page 443
[883] Brons et al. Staphylococcal acid phosphatase binds to endothelial cells via charge interaction in Wegener's granulomatosis? *Clin Exp Immunol*. 2000 Mar;119(3):566-73
[884] Popa ER, et al. Staphylococcus aureus and Wegener's granulomatosis. *Arthritis Res*. 2002;4(2):77-9 arthritis-research.com/content/4/2/077
[885] Schempp et al. Antibacterial activity of hyperforin from St John's wort, against multiresistant Staphylococcus aureus and gram-positive bacteria. *Lancet*. 1999 Jun;353:2129

better tolerated, safer, less expensive and more effective with greater compliance compared with intranasal mupirocin.[886]
- *Entamoeba histolytica*: *Entamoeba histolytica* induces formation of antineutrophil cytoplasmic antibodies (ANCA).[887] Stool testing with a specialty laboratory is recommended.
- Other microbes such as *Klebsiella aerogenes, Haemophilus influenzae* and *Bacillus subtilis*: These have also been implicated in Wegener's granulomatosis.[888]

- Vitamin D3 supplementation with physiologic doses and/or tailored to serum 25(OH)D levels: Since Wegener's *granulomatosis* is a *granulomatous* disease, caution and frequent monitoring must be employed when optimizing vitamin D status to avoid hypercalcemia; Wegener's granulomatosis can result in hypercalcemia mediated by elevated 1,25-dihydroxyvitamin D [1,25(OH)2D].[889] A reasonable clinical approach would be to start with testing of serum 25(OD)D, serum 1,25(OH)2D, and serum calcium (See Chapter 1 for review of Laboratory Association); thereafter, if necessary, start with a relatively low dose cholecalciferol 1,000-2,000 IU/d following the exclusion of hypercalcemia. Thereafter, serum calcium can be measured at 2 weeks, 4 weeks, 6 weeks, 8 weeks, and monthly/periodically thereafter.
- Orthoendocrinology: Assess prolactin, cortisol, DHEA, free and total testosterone, serum estradiol, and thyroid status (e.g., TSH, T4, *and* anti-thyroid peroxidase antibodies). Correct effectively.
- Assess for heavy metals, especially mercury: Exposure to mercury and lead is associated with increased risk of developing Wegener's granulomatosis.[890] Consider urine toxic metal assessment following 10-30 mg/kg DMSA as described in Chapter 4 and as described elsewhere for the assessment of heavy metals in patients with autism.[891]
- Proteolytic enzymes: Wegener's granulomatosis is mediated in large part by IgG and IgA immune complexes, which directly contribute to vasculitis and nephritis.[892] Polyenzyme supplementation has been used to ameliorate the pathophysiology induced by immune complexes in other conditions.[893]

> **Review of treatments**
> General and specific treatment considerations for the aforementioned conditions are reviewed starting on the next page; see Chapter 4 for the complete details of these protocols—their rationale, application, and exceptions.

---

[886] London S. Nasal povidone-iodine cuts postop infections. *Internal Medicine News Digital Network* 2012 Nov. internalmedicinenews.com/news/conference-news/idweek-2012/single-article/nasal-povidone-iodine-cuts-postop-infections/fabb79e1a44f38b7318f060284a6018f.html
[887] George J, Levy Y, Kallenberg CG, Shoenfeld Y. Infections and Wegener's granulomatosis—a cause and effect relationship? *QJM*. 1997 May;90(5):367-73
[888] George J, Levy Y, Kallenberg CG, Shoenfeld Y. Infections and Wegener's granulomatosis—a cause and effect relationship? *QJM*. 1997 May;90(5):367-73
[889] "Furthermore, in view of this case and two other recently reported cases, we believe that Wegener's granulomatosis must be definitively added to the list of granulomatous diseases that are responsible for 1,25(OH)2D-mediated hypercalcemia." Bosch et al. Vitamin D metabolite-mediated hypercalcemia in Wegener's granulomatosis. *Mayo Clin Proc*. 1997 May;72(5):440-4
[890] "Results suggest that mercury and perhaps lead exposure were positively associated with WG as compared with either control group, although the number of patients exposed was small... CONCLUSION: We conclude that heavy metal exposure and a prior history of allergy may play a role in the etiopathogenesis of Wegener's granulomatosis." Albert D, et al. Wegener's granulomatosis: Possible role of environmental agents in its pathogenesis. *Arthritis Rheum*. 2004 Aug 15;51(4):656-64
[891] Bradstreet et al. A case-control study of mercury burden in children with autistic spectrum disorders. *J Am Physicians Surgeons* 2003; 8: 76-79 jpands.org/vol8no3/geier.pdf
[892] "RESULTS: Four of 11 biopsies taken at initial presentation and four of 21 biopsies taken at the onset of a relapse of WG showed IgG and/or IgA containing immune deposits in the subepidermal blood vessels. ...CONCLUSION: A substantial number of skin biopsies showed immune deposits during active disease. These results could support the hypothesis that immune complexes may trigger vasculitic lesions in WG." Brons RH, et al. Detection of immune deposits in skin lesions of patients with Wegener's granulomatosis. *Ann Rheum Dis*. 2001 Dec;60(12):1097-102 ard.bmjjournals.com/cgi/content/full/60/12/1097
[893] Galebskaya et al. Human complement system state after wobenzyme intake. *Vestnik Moskovskogo Universiteta (Seriya 2: Khimiya)*. 2000:41(6 Suppl): 148-149

Integrative and Nonpharmacologic Considerations for the Vasculopathic Diseases discussed previously:
- **FOOD & NUTRITION: 5-part "supplemented Paleo-Mediterranean diet" (SPMD)** The 5-part "supplemented Paleo-Mediterranean diet" (SPMD—reviewed in Chapter 4) consists of ❶ foundational plant-based low-carbohydrate diet of fruits, vegetables, nuts, seeds, berries and lean sources of protein, ❷ multivitamin and multimineral supplementation, ❸ physiologic doses of vitamin D3 (range 2,000-10,000 IU/d), ❹ combination fatty acid therapy (CFAT) with n3-ALA, n6-GLA, n3-EPA, n3-DHA, and phytochemical-rich olive oil which contains n9-oleate, and ❺ probiotics.
    - Avoidance of allergenic, inflammatory, and SIBO-promoting foods: Hypoallergenic diets can benefit patients with immune-complex-mediated diseases such as mixed cryoglobulinemia[894,895], hypersensitivity vasculitis[896], and leukocystoclastic vasculitis with arthritis.[897] Any patient may be allergic to any food, even if the food is generally considered a health-promoting food. Generally speaking, the most notorious allergens are wheat, citrus (especially juice due to the industrial use of fungal hemicellulases), cow's milk, eggs, peanuts, chocolate, and yeast-containing foods. According to a study in patients with migraine, some patients will have to avoid as many as 10 specific foods in order to become symptom-free.[898] The severe wheat allergy *celiac disease* can present with inflammatory oligoarthritis[899,900], and celiac disease can also present as cryoglobulinemia and vasculitis[901], cutaneous leukocystoclastic vasculitis[902], including cerebral vasculitis[903] and pediatric stroke.[904] High glycemic foods suppress immune function[905,906] and thus promote the perpetuation of infection/dysbiosis. Delivery of a high carbohydrate load to the gastrointestinal lumen promotes bacterial overgrowth[907,908], which is inherently pro-inflammatory[909,910] and which promotes immune complex formation. Wheat consumption induces formation for immune complexes in virtually everyone (i.e., people who are "apparently healthy")[911], including as expected (but certainly not limited to) patients with dermatitis herpetiformis.[912] Vegetarian/vegan diets have a place in the treatment plan of all patients with autoimmune/inflammatory disorders[913,914]; this is also true for patients for whom long-term exclusive reliance on a meat-free vegetarian diet is either not appropriate or not appealing. No legitimate scientist or literate clinician doubts the antirheumatic power and anti-inflammatory advantages of vegetarian diets, whether used

---

[894] "CONCLUSION: These data show that an LAC diet decreases the amount of circulating immune complexes in MC and can modify certain signs and symptoms of the disease." Ferri C, Pietrogrande M, Cecchetti R, et al. Low-antigen-content diet in the treatment of patients with mixed cryoglobulinemia. *Am J Med.* 1989 Nov;87:519-24

[895] Pietrogrande M, Cefalo A, Nicora F, Marchesini D. Dietetic treatment of essential mixed cryoglobulinemia. *Ric Clin Lab.* 1986 Apr-Jun;16(2):413-6

[896] "In three cases the vasculitis relapsed following the introduction of food additives; in one case with the addition of potatoes and green vegetables (i.e., beans and green peas) and in the last case with the addition of eggs to the diet." Lunardi et al. Elimination diet in the treatment of selected patients with hypersensitivity vasculitis. *Clin Exp Rheumatol.* 1992 Mar-Apr;10(2):131-5

[897] "Described in this report are two children with severe vasculitis caused by specific foods." Businco et al. Severe food-induced vasculitis in two children. *Pediatr Allergy Immunol.* 2002 Feb;13(1):68-71

[898] Grant EC. Food allergies and migraine. *Lancet.* 1979 May 5;1(8123):966-9

[899] "We report six patients with coeliac disease in whom arthritis was prominent at diagnosis and who improved with dietary therapy. Joint pain preceded diagnosis by up to three years in five patients and 15 years in one patient." Bourne et al. Arthritis and coeliac disease. *Ann Rheum Dis.* 1985 Sep;44(9):592-8

[900] "A 15-year-old girl, with synovitis of the knees and ankles for 3 years before a diagnosis of gluten-sensitive enteropathy, is described." Pinals RS. Arthritis associated with gluten-sensitive enteropathy. *J Rheumatol.* 1986 Feb;13(1):201-4

[901] "Immunosuppressive treatment led to a normalization of transaminase levels and resolved the cryoglobulinaemic vasculitis. In addition, the patient exhibited low ferritin and iron levels, which led to the diagnosis of coeliac disease." Biecker E, Stieger M, Zimmermann A, Reichen J. Autoimmune hepatitis, cryoglobulinaemia and untreated coeliac disease: a case report. *Eur J Gastroenterol Hepatol.* 2003 Apr;15(4):423-7

[902] "A 38 year old female, with chronic uncontrolled coeliac disease, presented with the rare complication of cutaneous leucocystoclastic vasculitis." Meyers S, Dikman S, Spiera H, Schultz N, Janowitz HD. Cutaneous vasculitis complicating coeliac disease. *Gut.* 1981 Jan;22(1):61-4

[903] "A 51-year-old white man with celiac disease presented with seizures unresponsive to medical therapy." Rush PJ, Inman R, Bernstein M, Carlen P, Resch L. Isolated vasculitis of the central nervous system in a patient with celiac disease. *Am J Med.* 1986 Dec;81(6):1092-4

[904] "Because celiac disease is a potentially treatable cause of cerebral vasculopathy, serology-specifically antitissue transglutaminase antibodies-should be included in the evaluation for cryptogenic stroke in childhood, even in absence of typical gut symptoms." Goodwin et al. Celiac disease and childhood stroke. *Pediatr Neurol* 2004 Aug;31:139-42

[905] Sanchez A, Reeser JL, Lau HS, et al. Role of sugars in human neutrophilic phagocytosis. *Am J Clin Nutr.* 1973 Nov;26(11):1180-4

[906] "Postoperative infusion of carbohydrate solution leads to moderate fall in the serum concentration of inorganic phosphate. ... The hypophosphatemia was associated with significant reduction of neutrophil phagocytosis, intracellular killing, consumption of oxygen and generation of superoxide during phagocytosis." Rasmussen A, Segel E, Hessov I, Borregaard N. Reduced function of neutrophils during routine postoperative glucose infusion. *Acta Chir Scand.* 1988 Jul-Aug;154(7-8):429-33

[907] Ramakrishnan T, Stokes P. Beneficial effects of fasting and low carbohydrate diet in D-lactic acidosis associated with short-bowel syndrome. *JPEN J Parenter Enteral Nutr.* 1985 May-Jun;9(3):361-3

[908] Gottschall E. *Breaking the Vicious Cycle: Intestinal Health through Diet.* Kirkton Press; Rev edition (August 1, 1994)

[909] Lin HC. Small intestinal bacterial overgrowth: a framework for understanding irritable bowel syndrome. *JAMA.* 2004 Aug 18;292(7):852-8

[910] Lichtman et al. Reactivation of arthritis induced by small bowel bacterial overgrowth in rats: role of cytokines, bacteria, and bacterial polymers. *Infect Immun.* 1995 Jun;63(6):2295-301

[911] Eisenmann A, Murr C, Fuchs D, Ledochowski M. Gliadin IgG antibodies and circulating immune complexes. *Scand J Gastroenterol.* 2009;44(2):168-71

[912] Zone JJ, et al. Induction of IgA circulating immune complexes after wheat feeding in dermatitis herpetiformis patients. *J Invest Dermatol.* 1982 May;78(5):375-80

[913] "After four weeks at the health farm the diet group showed a significant improvement in number of tender joints, Ritchie's articular index, number of swollen joints, pain score, duration of morning stiffness, grip strength, erythrocyte sedimentation rate, C-reactive protein, white blood cell count, and a health assessment questionnaire score." Kjeldsen-Kragh J, et al. Controlled trial of fasting and one-year vegetarian diet in rheumatoid arthritis. *Lancet.* 1991 Oct 12;338(8772):899-902

[914] "During the vegan diet, both signs and symptoms returned in most patients, with the exception of some patients with psoriasis who experienced an improvement." Lithell H, et al. A fasting and vegetarian diet treatment trial on chronic inflammatory disorders. *Acta Derm Venereol.* 1983;63(5):397-403

short-term or long term.[915] Patients who rely on the Paleo-Mediterranean Diet can use vegetarian meals, on a daily basis or for days at a time, for example, by having a daily vegetarian meal, or one week per month of vegetarianism. Of course, some (not all) patients can use a purely vegetarian diet long-term provided that nutritional needs (especially protein and cobalamin) are consistently met.

- **INFECTIONS & DYSBIOSIS:** ❶ antimicrobial treatments, ❷ immunorestoration, ❸ immunotolerance via Treg induction Essentially all autoimmune/rheumatic disorders are associated with microbial colonization and intolerance to same; the presence of persistent microbial colonization is *prima facie* evidence of immunosuppression. The eight areas of dysbiosis (multifocal) are: ❶ sinorespiratory, ❷ orodental, ❸ gastrointestinal, ❹ urogenital/genitourinary, ❺ parenchymal/tissue, ❻ microbial, ❼ dermal/cutaneous, and ❽ environmental. The following survey of the literature serves to remind clinicians of possible underlying infectious contributions to vasculitic diseases:

  o Viral infections associated with Kawasaki disease (*J Formos Med Assoc.* 2014 Mar[916]): "We enrolled 226 children with KD and 226 age- and sex-matched healthy children from February 2004 to March 2010. Throat and nasopharyngeal swabs were taken for both viral isolation and polymerase chain reaction (PCR) for various viruses. ...Cases of KD had a significantly higher positive rate of viral isolation in comparison with the control group (7.5% vs. 2.2%, p = 0.02). Compared with the control group, cases of KD were more likely to have overall positive rates of viral PCR (50.4% vs. 16.4%, p < 0.001) and for various viruses including enterovirus (16.8% vs. 4.4%, p < 0.001), adenovirus (8.0% vs. 1.8%, p = 0.007), human rhinovirus (26.5% vs. 9.7%, p < 0.001), and coronavirus (7.1% vs. 0.9%, p = 0.003)."

  o Ischemic retinal vasculitis in an 18-year-old man with chickenpox infection (*Clin Ophthalmol.* 2014 Feb[917]): "We report a case of a healthy 18-year-old man who presented with unilateral ischemic retinal vasculitis 10 days after the onset of chickenpox. ... Fundus imaging, optical coherence tomography, fundus fluorescence angiography, and electrophysiologic studies confirmed the diagnosis of retinal vasculitis, which led to generalized retinal ischemia."

  o Antineutrophil cytoplasmic antibody-associated vasculitis associated with Epstein-Barr virus infection (*Infection* 2014 Jun[918]): "Although a previous study indicated that there was a high positive rate of ANCA in the sera positive for IgM antibodies to EBV and EBV infection might trigger the relapse of AAV, this is the first case of incipient AAV associated with acute EBV infection. One possible explanation might be that EBV infection stimulated the production of ANCA."

Wheat and circulating immune complexes in "healthy" disease-free persons

- Circulating immune complexes (CICs) in blood are associated with autoimmune-diseases such as systemic lupus erythematosus, immune complex glomerulonephritis, rheumatoid arthritis and vasculitis. However, slightly increased serum concentrations of such CICs are sometimes also found in healthy individuals. The objective of the current study was to assess whether food antigens could play a role in the formation of CICs.
- MATERIAL AND METHODS: A total of **352 (265 F, 87 M), so far, healthy individuals** were tested for CICs containing C1q and immunoglobulin G (IgG) as well as for gliadin IgG antibodies using the ELISA technique. Additionally, fructose and lactose malabsorption was assessed using hydrogen breath tests.
- RESULTS: In our study, 15.3% (54/352) of the patients presented with elevated CIC concentrations (above 50 microg/ml) and 6.5% (23/352) of the study population were positive for gliadin IgG antibodies (above 20 U/ml). **CIC concentration levels were significantly higher in the group with elevated gliadin IgG antibodies** (CIC median: 49.0 microg/ml **compared with the group with normal levels of gliadin IgG antibodies** (CIC median: 30.0 microg/ml; Mann-Whitney U-test, U=1992; p <0.001). ...
- CONCLUSIONS: **The results of this study indicate that certain food antigens (e.g. gluten) could play a role in the formation of CICs.** ...

Eisenmann et al. *Scand J Gastroenterol.* 2009

---

[915] "For the patients who were randomised to the vegetarian diet there was a significant decrease in platelet count, leukocyte count, calprotectin, total IgG, IgM rheumatoid factor (RF), C3-activation products, and the complement components C3 and C4 after one month of treatment." Kjeldsen-Kragh J, Mellbye OJ, Haugen M, et al. Changes in laboratory variables in rheumatoid arthritis patients during a trial of fasting and one-year vegetarian diet. *Scand J Rheumatol.* 1995;24(2):85-93
[916] Chang et al. Viral infections associated with Kawasaki disease. *J Formos Med Assoc.* 2014 Mar;113(3):148-54
[917] Poonyathalang et al. Ischemic retinal vasculitis in an 18-year-old man with chickenpox infection. *Clin Ophthalmol.* 2014 Feb 24;8:441-3
[918] Xu et al. Antineutrophil cytoplasmic antibody-associated vasculitis associated with Epstein-Barr virus infection: a case report and review of the literature. *Infection.* 2014 Jun;42(3):591-4

- o Cytomegalovirus-related necrotizing vasculitis mimicking Henoch-Schönlein syndrome (*Clin Exp Rheumatol*. 2014 May[919]): "The causative role of viral infection was revealed by the presence of CMV DNA in patient's blood and positive IgG titer against the virus. … Our report suggests that CMV vasculitis is probably more frequent than previously thought, even in immunocompetent patients, with a protean clinical presentation, mimicking other types of vasculitides."
  - o Hepatitis C virus infection and its rheumatologic implications. *Gastroenterol Hepatol* 2014 May[920]): "Symptoms of HCV infection and rheumatic diseases may be similar and include arthralgia, myalgia, arthritis, and vasculitis. …It is imperative to distinguish whether symptoms such as arthralgia, myalgia, and arthritis occur in patients with HCV infection due to primary chronic HCV infection or to a newly developed rheumatologic disease process."
  - o Vasculitis and anaphylactoid shock induced in mice by cell wall extract of the fungus Candida metapsilosis (*Pol J Microbiol*. 2014[921]): "Our results show that intraperitoneal injection of cell wall extracts induced severe coronary arteritis, and intravenous injection induced acute anaphylactoid shock similar to extracts from Candida albicans (C. albicans)."
  - o Varicella zoster virus in the temporal artery of a patient with giant cell arteritis (*J Neurol Sci*. 2013 Dec[922]): "We recently detected varicella zoster virus (VZV) in the temporal arteries (TA) of 5/24 patients with clinically suspect giant cell arteritis (GCA) whose TAs were GCA-negative pathologically; in those GCA-negative, VZV+TAs, virus antigen predominated in the arterial adventitia, but without medial necrosis and multinucleated giant cells. During our continuing search for VZV antigen in GCA-negative TAs, in the TA of one subject, we found abundant VZV antigen, as well as VZV DNA, in multiple regions (skip areas) of the TA spanning 350 [micrometers], as well as in skeletal muscle adjacent to the infected TA."
  - o Is giant cell arteritis an infectious disease? (*Presse Med*. 2004 Nov[923]): "Simultaneous occurrence of peaks of GCA/PMR and respiratory infections have been observed in Denmark. Several viruses have been suspected as triggers and assessed by serological testing, PCR or immunostaining on temporal artery biopsies, or both techniques: the hepatitis B virus can be ruled out, as well as Herpes simplex 1 and 2, Herpes varicellae, Epstein-Barr virus and cytomegalovirus. Recent studies focused on parainfluenza virus, Parvovirus B19 and Chlamydia pneumoniae. Immunological studies suggest, at the origin of the inflammatory reaction leading to the typical pathological features of giant cell arteritis, the existence of a triggering antigen of unknown nature activating T-cells in the artery wall."

- **NUTRITIONAL IMMUNOMODULATION: Treg induction for modulation of Th-1/2/17 inflammation** Nutrients and therapeutic approaches that promote Treg or IL-10 induction and/or Th-17, IL-17 suppression include 1) mitochondrial optimization and mTOR suppression, 2) biotin, 3) vitamin E, 4) sodium avoidance, 5) transgenic/GMO food avoidance, 6) probiotics, 7) lipoic acid, 8) vitamin A, 9) inflammation reduction, 10) vitamin D, 11) fatty acid supplementation with GLA and n3, 12) infection and dysbiosis remediation, 13) green tea EGCG. Acronym: MiBESTPLAIDFIG.

- **DYSMETABOLISM & DYSFUNCTIONAL MITOCHONDRIA: MitoDys, ERS-UPR, AGE/RAGE, hyperglycemia and ceramide** The major clinical considerations in this section are mitochondrial dysfunction, endoplasmic reticulum stress, unfolded protein response, TLR activation, and the dysmetabolic effects of sustained hyperglycemia and hyperinsulinemia and resultant oxidative stress, inflammation, RAGE activation, and accumulation of AGE, palmitate and ceramide. The review of this information in Chapter 4 covered approximately 30 interventions relevant to dysmetabolism, mitochondrial dysfunction, ERS-UPR, etc; these will not be reviewed here except to mention those most commonly, easily, empirically, synergistically, and effectively used: 1) low-carbohydrate diet with 2) moderate exercise, 3) CoQ-10, 4) acetyl-carnitine with 5) lipoic acid, 6) NAC, 7) resveratrol, and 8) melatonin.

- **STYLE OF LIVING (LIFESTYLE) & SPECIAL CONSIDERATIONS: Sleep optimization, SocioPsychology, Stress management/avoidance, Somatic treatments, Special Supplementation, Sweat/exercise, Sauna/detoxification, Surgery, Stamp your passport and vacate current reality, Sensory deprivation therapy**

---

[919] D'Alessandro et al. Cytomegalovirus-related necrotising vasculitis mimicking Henoch-Schönlein syndrome. *Clin Exp Rheumatol*. 2014 May-Jun;32(3 Suppl 82):S73-5
[920] Sayiner et al. Hepatitis C virus infection and its rheumatologic implications. *Gastroenterol Hepatol* 2014 May;10(5):287-93
[921] Tada et al. Vasculitis and anaphylactoid shock induced in mice by cell wall extract of the fungus Candida metapsilosis. *Pol J Microbiol*. 2014;63(2):223-30
[922] Nagel et al. Varicella zoster virus in the temporal artery of a patient with giant cell arteritis. *J Neurol Sci*. 2013 Dec 15;335(1-2):228-30
[923] Duhaut P, Bosshard S, Ducroix JP. Is giant cell arteritis an infectious disease? *Presse Med*. 2004 Nov 6;33(19 Pt 2):1403-8

This is a buffet of mostly lifestyle-based interventions yet also including considerations such as somatic treatments, additional supplementation, and surgery.

- **ENDOCRINE IMBALANCE & OPTIMIZATION: Prolactin, Insulin, Estrogen, DHEA, Cortisol, Testosterone, Thyroid** Common hormonal imbalances seen among autoimmune/inflammatory patients are: ❶ *elevated* prolactin, ❷ *elevated* estrogen, ❸ *elevated* insulin, and ❹ *reduced* DHEA, ❺ *reduced* cortisol, and ❻ *reduced* testosterone; see Chapter 4 for discussion of these hormones and respective interventions. Thyroid evaluation (patient + labs) should be comprehensive, as discussed in Chapter 1, with a low threshold for empiric treatment.
    - Orthoendocrinology and Dysendocrinism: Assess prolactin, cortisol, DHEA, free and total testosterone, serum estradiol, and thyroid status (e.g., TSH, T4, *and* anti-thyroid peroxidase antibodies). Correct as indicated (see Chapter 4). **Prolactin levels are typically elevated in patients with PMR and correlate with clinical symptomatology.**[924] Adrenal hypofunction in patients with PR/GCA is suggested by the relative insufficiencies of cortisol and DHEA.[925] **DHEA (insufficiency and supraphysiologic supplementation):** Patients with autoimmunity should be tested for DHEA insufficiency by measurement of serum DHEA-sulfate; insufficiencies should generally be corrected except in cases of concomitant hormone-responsive cancer such as breast cancer or prostate cancer. The rationale for using high-dose DHEA in patients with autoimmune diseases is reviewed in Chapter 4.

> **Endocrine imbalance in PMR/GCA**
> "Patients with PMR/GCA with new-onset active disease before steroid treatment have inappropriately normal cortisol levels regarding the ongoing inflammation, and significantly lower levels of DHEAS compared to the age- and sex-matched healthy control subjects. These data support the existence of a relative adrenal hypofunction in PMR and GCA."
>
> Narvaez et al. *J Rheumatol* 2006;33:1293-8

- **XENOBIOTIC ACCUMULATION & DETOXIFICATION: Chemical avoidance, nutritional support for detoxification pathways, urine alkalinization** The clinical relevance and pathogenic mechanisms of xenobiotic accumulation are irrefutably well documented and described. Clinical assessments include history, physical examination, and laboratory assessment (using serum, whole blood, urine or—rarely yet accurately—fat biopsy), and response to treatment. Treatments include nutritional support for Phases 1 and 2 of detoxification (e.g., oxidation and conjugation) and excretion via bile and urine; for the latter, urinary alkalinization is generally recommended. Chemical toxins can be bound in the gut using activated charcoal, cholestyramine, or *Chlorella*—all of these three treatments have documented safety and effectiveness; clinically and empirically, phytochelatin (plant-derived peptides that bind toxic metals) concentrates appear safe and effective despite lack of conclusive published data supporting clinical use.

---

[924] Straub RH, Georgi J, Helmke K, Vaith P, Lang B. In polymyalgia rheumatica serum prolactin is positively correlated with the number of typical symptoms but not with typical inflammatory markers. *Rheumatology* (Oxford). 2002 Apr;41(4):423-9 rheumatology.oxfordjournals.org/cgi/content/full/41/4/423

[925] "Patients with PMR/GCA with new-onset active disease before steroid treatment have inappropriately normal cortisol levels regarding the ongoing inflammation, and significantly lower levels of DHEAS compared to the age- and sex-matched healthy control subjects. These data support the existence of a relative adrenal hypofunction in PMR and GCA." Narvaez et al. Low serum levels of DHEAS in untreated polymyalgia rheumatica/giant cell arteritis. *J Rheumatol*. 2006 Jul;33(7):1293-8. Epub 2006 Jun 15

Spondyloarthropathies: Axial Inflammatory Conditions
Ankylosing spondylitis
Reactive arthritis (previously Reiter's syndrome)
Enteropathic spondyloarthropathy, enteropathic arthritis

> **Axial inflammation as yet another *pattern of inflammation***
> Spinal/axial inflammatory conditions are patterns of inflammation with etiologic factors consistent with the pattern reviewed throughout this textbook and surveyed in Chapter 4; likewise therefore, similar therapeutic concepts are applicable. As always, pharmacologic immunosuppression may be urgently needed if a patient experiences exacerbation or inflammatory complication; however, routine "chronic" pharmacologic immunosuppression offers no hope of authentically curing the disease and correcting the underlying imbalances: it only suppresses manifestations of underlying physiologic imbalances.

Description/pathophysiology:
- Inflammatory arthropathies affecting the spine and sacroiliac joints are termed "spondyloarthropathies" and like other arthritic conditions are termed *seronegative* if not related to rheumatoid arthritis in general and RF positivity in particular. **The spondyloarthropathies differ in some aspects of their etiologies, affected populations, clinical presentations, and treatment; however—regarding etiology and treatment—the similarities far outnumber the differences.** Regarding clinical management, from both allopathic and integrative/naturopathic perspectives, the treatment and management of these different conditions is virtually identical, save for a few important nuances.
- Spondyloarthropathies and reactive arthritis differ from the classic pattern of other autoimmune conditions in that 1) most patients affected are male, 2) they are highly correlated with HLA-B27, 3) serologic evidence of autoimmunity is generally absent, 4) they are strongly associated with dysbiosis, infections, and/or occult or overt enteropathy.[926,927]
- Some variation exists in the conditions that are included under the heading of *Spondyloarthropathies*. Most medical textbooks include four disorders under the heading of spondyloarthropathies: 1) ankylosing spondylitis, 2) psoriatic arthritis, 3) reactive arthritis, and 4) enteropathic spondyloarthropathy (ES), while a few others go on to include 5) juvenile spondyloarthropathy, and 6) rheumatoid arthritis. Psoriatic arthritis (PsA) and rheumatoid arthritis (RA) are detailed in their own chapters in this book and therefore will not be discussed in great detail here.
- Although ankylosing spondylitis (AS) is the prototype of the spondyloarthropathies, reactive arthritis (ReA) is the best-known and most well accepted model for microbe-induced musculoskeletal autoimmunity. Despite nearly overwhelming research demonstrating that all of these conditions are triggered by exposure to microbes, major medical textbooks[928] still describe these conditions as *idiopathic*. Enteropathic arthritis and enteropathic spondyloarthropathy (EAES) demonstrate how gastrointestinal dysbiosis, hormonal imbalances, increased intestinal permeability ("leaky gut"), and non-musculoskeletal systemic inflammation can spill-over into peripheral and axial arthritis. As detailed in the separate chapter on psoriasis and psoriatic arthritis (PsA), PsA is clearly a microbe-triggered disease, and its similarity to AS suggests a common physiologic etiology. The common themes that weave these disorders together are 1) dysbiosis-induced musculoskeletal inflammation, 2) hormonal imbalances, and 3) increased intestinal/mucosal permeability—the latter is the most voluminous route of absorption of arthritogenic antigens, immunogens, and antimetabolites—see Chapter 4 for overview and details.
- All of these conditions are *systemic* inflammatory disorders that show clear evidence of immune-mediated tissue damage and are therefore worthy of being dubbed *autoimmune*. The systemic nature of these disorders carries important clinical implications because both doctor and patient need to be aware of *non-musculoskeletal*

---

[926] Colmegna I, Cuchacovich R, Espinoza LR. HLA-B27-associated reactive arthritis: pathogenetic and clinical considerations. *Clin Microbiol Rev*. 2004 Apr;17(2):348-69
[927] Ringrose JH. HLA-B27 associated spondyloarthropathy, an autoimmune disease based on crossreactivity between bacteria and HLA-B27? *Ann Rheum Dis*. 1999 Oct;:598-610
[928] Klippel JH (ed). *Primer on the rheumatic diseases. 11th edition*. Atlanta: Arthritis Foundation; 1997, page 181

complications. Non-musculoskeletal complications of these disorders include renal failure secondary to amyloidosis[929,930], cardiovascular and pulmonary complications, and increased risk of trauma, violent death, poisonings, and alcohol misuse.[931,932,933] Not surprisingly, the risk of pulmonary, renal, neurologic, ocular and cardiac complications is increased in patients with long-standing and severe disease.

Differentiating Characteristics of the Spondyloarthropathies

Condition	Etiopathogenesis	Unique presentation	Specific emphasis
Ankylosing spondylitis	• *Allopathic*: idiopathic • *Integrative*: dysbiosis is paramount	• Insidious onset of low-back pain in young patient • Ankylosis begins in lumbopelvis and can progress to thorax, neck, hips and knees. • 90% positive HLA-B27	• *Allopathic*: anti-inflammatory drugs • *Integrative*: Antidysbiosis and orthoendocrinology are treatment cornerstones
Reactive arthritis (previously Reiter's syndrome[934])	• *Allopathic*: infection-triggered arthritis • *Integrative*: infection-triggered arthritis in a patient with dietary and endocrinologic predispositions.	• Classically associated with a recent infection, particularly a genitourinary infection or gastrointestinal infection. • Inflammation is characteristically located at the low-back, iris, and heels. • 75% positive HLA-B27	• Antimicrobial treatment for acute and chronic infections is the mainstay of treatment although in a large percentage of patients the arthropathy continues despite apparent clearance of the primary infection.
Enteropathic spondylo-arthropathy, enteropathic arthritis	• *Allopathic*: idiopathic • *Integrative*: dysbiosis-triggered arthritis in a patient with dietary and endocrinologic predispositions	• Arthropathy of the peripheral joints and/or spine in a patient with inflammatory bowel disease—Crohn's disease or ulcerative colitis • 50% positive HLA-B27	• *Allopathic*: anti-inflammatory drugs • *Integrative*: Antidysbiosis and orthoendocrinology are treatment cornerstones • Treatment is similar to other treatments except with a greater focus on addressing the intestinal lesions

---

[929] "The mechanism of death in these patients was secondary amyloidosis in 19, cardiovascular complications in six, fracture of the spine in one, and it was not known in one patient. Excess deaths due to circulatory, gastrointestinal and renal diseases, and violence were also observed." Lehtinen K. Mortality and causes of death in 398 patients admitted to hospital with ankylosing spondylitis. *Ann Rheum Dis*. 1993 Mar;52(3):174-6

[930] "During an outbreak of Yersinia pseudotuberculosis III, one of two HLA-B27 positive brothers developed reactive arthritis (ReA), mild at first, but later severely destructive and ultimately fatal. The reactivation of ReA was possibly triggered by an oral polio vaccine. The cause of death was severe secondary amyloidosis." Yli-Kerttula T, Mottonen T, Toivanen A. Different course of reactive arthritis in two HLA-B27 positive brothers with fatal outcome in one. *J Rheumatol*. 1997 Oct;24(10):2047-50

[931] "A marked sex-associated effect was noted among deaths caused by injuries/poisoning, since 6 of the deaths occurred in men and only 1 was in a woman. CONCLUSION: Patients with PsA are at an increased risk of death compared with the general population." Gladman DD, Farewell VT, Wong K, Husted J.Mortality studies in psoriatic arthritis: results from a single outpatient center. II. Prognostic indicators for death. *Arthritis Rheum*. 1998 Jun;41(6):1103-10

[932] "The 4 leading causes of death were diseases of the circulatory (36.2%) or respiratory (21.3%) system, malignant neoplasms (17.0%), and injuries/poisoning (14.9%). The SMR for the female cohort was 1.59, and for the men, it was 1.65, indicating a 59% and 65% increase in the death rate, respectively. Deaths due to respiratory causes were particularly increased in these patients." Wong K, Gladman DD, Husted J, Long JA, Farewell VT. Mortality studies in psoriatic arthritis: results from a single outpatient clinic. I. Causes and risk of death. *Arthritis Rheum*. 1997 Oct;40(10):1868-72

[933] "Subjects with ankylosing spondylitis (AS) have an increased incidence of deaths from accidents and violence, which is due in part, but perhaps not entirely, to the vulnerability of the affected spine to fractures... Uncontrolled use of alcohol is an important determinant in the surplus of deaths from accidents and violence in Finnish patients with AS." Myllykangas-Luosujarvi et al. Increased incidence of alcohol-related deaths from accidents and violence in subjects with ankylosing spondylitis. *Br J Rheumatol*. 1998 Jun;37(6):688-90

[934] The term "Reiter's syndrome" has fallen out of favor due to the increasing acknowledgement that Dr Hans Reiter was affiliated with Nazi atrocities during World War II. See the following for additional information: "During World War II, Reiter, a physician leader of the Nazi party, authorized medical experiments on concentration camp prisoners." Lu DW, Katz KA. Declining use of the eponym "Reiter's syndrome" in the medical literature, 1998-2003. *J Am Acad Dermatol*. 2005 Oct;53(4):720-3 and "There is more than ample evidence that Hans Reiter, whose name has been eponymously linked to a rheumatologic syndrome, was a Nazi war criminal. He was responsible for heinous atrocities that violated the precepts of humanity, ethics, and professionalism." Panush et al. The tainted legacy of Hans Reiter. *Semin Arthritis Rheum*. 2003 Feb;32(4):231-6

Differentiating Characteristics of the Spondyloarthropathies — *continued*

Condition	Etiopathogenesis	Unique presentation	Specific emphasis
Juvenile spondyloarthropathy	• *Allopathic*: idiopathic • *Integrative*: dysbiosis[935]	• Generally occurs in boys aged 8-18 years • Peripheral arthritis (90%) is more common than spondylitis (50%)	• *Allopathic*: anti-inflammatory drugs • *Integrative*: Antidysbiosis
Psoriatic arthritis	• *Allopathic*: idiopathic • *Integrative*: Food allergies and dysbiosis are paramount	• Arthropathy of the peripheral joints and/or spine in a patient with psoriasis • 50% positive HLA-B27	• *Allopathic*: anti-inflammatory drugs • *Integrative*: Antidysbiosis and orthoendocrinology are treatment cornerstones
Rheumatoid arthritis	• *Allopathic*: idiopathic • *Integrative*: dysbiosis-triggered arthritis in a patient with dietary and endocrinologic predisposition	• Inflammatory peripheral arthropathy generally precedes axial joints • Sacroiliac joints are generally spared • RF is frequently positive	• *Allopathic*: anti-inflammatory drugs • *Integrative*: Antidysbiosis and orthoendocrinology are treatment cornerstones

Clinical presentations:
- Musculoskeletal:
  - <u>Pain and limited motion in the low-back sacroiliac joints</u>: This is an aspect of all of the spondyloarthropathies, especially AS and ReA. Back pain is generally worse in the morning and alleviated by motion, including passive motion such as spinal manipulation.
  - <u>Thoracic spine pain and decreased rib expansion/excursion</u>: Although it typically begins in the lumbar spine and sacroiliac joints, AS commonly progresses to involve the thoracic spine and rib cage. Decreased mobility of the ribs limit respiration, and thus respirometry is used in the clinical assessment of patients with AS.
  - <u>Neck pain</u>: particularly common in RA and AS, two conditions associated with spontaneous atlantoaxial instability
  - <u>Atlantoaxial instability</u>: May be the presenting manifestation of AS[936] and is a common long-term complication of RA. Particularly in patients with neck pain and/or long-standing inflammation, cervical radiographs including APOM and measurement of the atlantodental interval should be performed before the clinical use of forceful cervical spine manipulation as well as esophageal/tracheal endoscopy.
  - <u>Enthesopathies</u>: Inflammation at the site of ligament insertion into bone—classically seen at the insertion of the Achilles' tendon at the calcaneus—is a characteristic finding and complaint in patients with ReA.
  - <u>Non-erosive asymmetrical peripheral arthritis</u>: 50% of patients with AS experience a temporary peripheral arthritis, while in 25% of patients the peripheral arthritis is permanent.
- Pulmonary: Pleurisy (painful inflammation of the pleural lining of the internal thoracic cavity) may be a complication of nearly all rheumatic/inflammatory disorders. Patients with AS may develop pulmonary fibrosis.
- Cardiac: "Spondylitic heart disease" is seen in patients with AS and commonly includes atrioventricular conduction defects and aortic regurgitation.[937]

---

[935] "Our findings provide clear evidence of ReA diagnosis following an acute M. pneumoniae infection that in four patients progressed to chronic jSpA. Our results suggest that detecting M. pneumoniae-specific antibodies in serological screening of jSpA patients might be useful." Harjacek M, Ostojic J, Djakovic Rode O. Juvenile spondyloarthropathies associated with Mycoplasma pneumoniae infection. *Clin Rheumatol*. 2006 Jan 4;:1-6

[936] Thompson et al. Spontaneous atlantoaxial subluxation as a presenting manifestation of juvenile ankylosing spondylitis. A case report. *Spine* 1982 Jan-Feb;7(1):78-9

[937] Tierney ML. McPhee SJ, Papadakis MA (eds). Current Medical Diagnosis and Treatment 2006. 45th edition. New York; Lange Medical Books: 2006, pages 851-855

- GI tract: Oral ulcers, intestinal inflammation, increased intestinal permeability
- Skin/mucosal lesions: Dermal lesions are particularly common in patients with ReA and PsA. Psoriatic lesions are typically well-demarcated erythematous patches with white/silvery scales. Dermal lesions of ReA can include pustular lesions on the feet and hands (palmoplantar pustulosis) in addition to genital lesions in patients with sexually transmitted diseases.
- Renal complications: These can be seen in nearly all rheumatic disorders, either as a result of the systemic inflammation (particularly immune complexes), amyloidosis, or as a result of NSAIDs or other pharmaceutical drugs.
- Neurological complications: Cerebral necrosis, corticosteroid psychosis, and transverse myelitis may occur. Atlantoaxial subluxation can present with myelopathic signs.
- Ocular complications: Anterior uveitis is seen in ~25% of patients with AS and is a characteristic finding in patients with ReA.

Major differential diagnoses:
- Initial evaluation of patients with spondyloarthropathy must include consideration of numerous differential diagnoses which may mimic or co-exist with inflammatory spondyloarthropathy. See table of *Differential Diagnoses* at the end of this chapter, as well as *algorithm for patient assessment and management*. Useful categories during the evaluation of low-back pain include the following:
    - Serious organic diseases requiring immediate attention: Metastatic disease, viscerosomatic referral, osteomyelitis/discitis, aortic aneurysm.
    - Serious musculoskeletal disorders requiring immediate attention: Recent fracture (pathologic fracture, osteoporosis, compression fracture, fall from a height, major motor vehicle accident), cauda equina syndrome, and severe radiculopathy (i.e., severe pain or progressive muscular deficits).
    - Rheumatologic disorders affecting the low back and pelvis: Ankylosing spondylitis, reactive arthritis, enteropathic spondyloarthropathy, psoriatic arthritis, rheumatoid arthritis, and fibromyalgia.
    - Psychogenic: Emotional overlay, symptom amplification, secondary gain, depression.
    - Benign musculoskeletal disorders requiring conservative treatment and monitoring: Muscle spasm, facet irritation, disc injuries causing radiculitis or radiculopathy, self-limiting inflammation due to injury.
    - Functional, metabolic, allergic or nutritional causes of low-back pain: Food allergies, obesity leading to a systemic inflammatory state as well as biomechanical stress on the lumbar spine, vitamin D deficiency[938], acidifying diet[939] (i.e., the Standard American Diet[940,941]).

---

[938] Al Faraj S, Al Mutairi K. Vitamin D deficiency and chronic low back pain in Saudi Arabia. *Spine*. 2003 Jan 15;28(2):177-9
[939] "The results show that a disturbed acid-base balance may contribute to the symptoms of low back pain. The simple and safe addition of an alkaline multimineral preparate was able to reduce the pain symptoms in these patients with chronic low back pain." Vormann J,Worlitschek M,Goedecke T,Silver B. Supplementation with alkaline minerals reduces symptoms in patients with chronic low back pain. *J Trace Elem Med Biol*. 2001;15(2-3):179-83
[940] Seaman DR. The diet-induced proinflammatory state: a cause of chronic pain and other degenerative diseases? *J Manipulative Physiol Ther*. 2002 Mar-Apr;25(3):168-79
[941] Cordain L. *The Paleo Diet*. John Wiley & Sons Inc., New York 2002

Low Back Pain: Differential Diagnostic Considerations

	DDX Category	Examples:
V	Vascular Visceral referral	Aortic aneurysm Pancreatic disease/cancer
I	Infectious Inflammatory Immunologic	Ankylosing spondylitis, Reiter's syndrome Rheumatoid arthritis Psoriatic arthritis Enteropathic spondyloarthropathy Lymphoma, leukemia Bone/ tissue infections Gastrointestinal disease Kidney infection Psoriatic arthritis Herpes zoster
N	Neurologic Nutritional New growth: neoplasia, pregnancy	Metastatic disease, primary bone tumors, multiple myeloma Herpes zoster Cauda equina syndrome
D	Deficiency Degenerative Developmental	Degenerative joint/spine disease Congenital malformations of bones/ viscera Scoliosis Postural syndromes Disc herniation Varicose veins in the leg mimicking sciatica
I	Iatrogenic (drug related) Intoxication Idiosyncratic	Anticoagulants predispose to epidural or spinal cord bleeding[942] Prednisone use promotes osteoporosis and spinal fractures Excess alcohol consumption[943]
C	Congenital	Congenital malformations of bones: hemivertebrae, leg length inequality, etc.
A	Allergy Autoimmune Abuse	Ankylosing spondylitis Fractures, injuries
T	Trauma	Fractures: injuries to vertebrae, ribs, muscles
E	Endocrine Exposure	Diabetes mellitus
S	"Subluxation", somatic dysfunction Structural Stress Secondary gain	Segmental dysfunction of lumbar spine and pelvis Muscle tension
M	Mental Malpractice Mental disorder Malignancy Metabolic disease Menstrual Myofascial	Anxiety Depression Endometriosis, hematocolpos[944] Ovarian tumor Nephrolithiasis Metastasis to spine Myofascial trigger points in quadratus lumborum, piriformis, iliacus, psoas

---

[942] Souza TA. Differential Diagnosis for the Chiropractor: Protocols and Algorithms. Gaithersburg: Aspen Publications. 1997 page 110
[943] "Alcohol abuse was significantly more frequent among the male low back patients." Sandstrom J, Andersson GB, Wallerstedt S. The role of alcohol abuse in working disability in patients with low back pain. *Scand J Rehabil Med*. 1984;16(4):147-9
[944] London NJ, Sefton GK. Hematocolpos. An unusual cause of sciatica in an adolescent girl. *Spine*. 1996 Jun 1;21(11):1381-2

Specific differential diagnoses
- Mechanical low back pain, traumatic low back pain, spinal strain/sprain
- Cauda equina syndrome
- Vitamin D deficiency: Vitamin D deficiency causes inflammation and low-back pain. Measure 25(OH)vitamin D in serum or supplement with 4,000-10,000 IU daily for at least three months[945] unless contraindicated by drugs (e.g., hydrochlorothiazide) or hypercalcemic condition (e.g., sarcoidosis, cancer, or hyperparathyroidism, etc.).[946]
- Spinal degeneration, degenerative arthritis of the spine
- Spinal fracture: Patients with AS may experience fracture following trivial "injury" such as rolling over in bed: "Fracture should be suspected whenever a [AS] patient complains of new back pain."[947]
- Osteitis condensans ilii
- Cancer, malignant disease
- Vertebral osteomyelitis, infectious discitis
- Developmental/congenital sacralization of the lumbar vertebrae
- Other autoimmune disease
- Lung disease: Asthma, COPD, bronchitis, tuberculosis
- Iron overload: Hemochromatosis may resemble ankylosing spondylitis clinically and radiographically.[948]
- Fibromyalgia: ESR, CRP, thyroid tests, ANA and most other 'basic' tests are normal; assess and treat for bacterial overgrowth of the small bowel.[949]
- Diffuse idiopathic skeletal hyperostosis (DISH): DISH generally affects the longitudinal ligaments of the spine rather than the intervertebral discs. Cervical involvement generally precedes that of the lumbar spine, and the condition is strongly associated with diabetes mellitus.

Clinical assessments:
- History/subjective: See clinical presentations
  - **Typical presentation is that of dull achy pain in the low-back—worse in the morning and improving as the day progresses and/or with activity.**
  - **Systemic manifestations may or may not be present in the early stages of disease.**
- Physical examination/objective:
  - ROM, neurologic assessments; orthopedic assessments
  - Specialty examinations may be indicated:
    - Eye exam: For retinal and anterior chamber abnormalities; external exam for scleritis
    - Genital examination and/or assessment for UTI and STDs: Indicated in patients with ReA due to high association with sexually transmitted diseases. Urethral swab for culture and DNA probes are commonly indicated.
    - Cardiopulmonary assessment: Common considerations include auscultation, measurement of thoracic excursion, and spirometry. Chest radiographs may be indicated.
    - Neurologic examination: A screening neurologic examination should be performed as part of the initial assessment of all patients and more detailed examinations are carried out when indicated.
    - Schober test: Draw a line over the spinous process of L5, then mark a line 10 cm above and 5 cm below; with lumbar flexion, the total distance should increase from 15 cm to 20 cm—less than 5 cm excursion indicates spinal rigidity, consistent with AS.
    - Occiput-to-wall distance: This assessment can be used to quantify progression/regression of cervical flexion in patients with AS.
    - Chest expansion: Use tape measure around lower thorax; measure chest circumference before and after inhalation; use along with spirometry to monitor thoracic stiffness in patients with AS.

---

[945] Al Faraj S, Al Mutairi K. Vitamin D deficiency and chronic low back pain in Saudi Arabia. *Spine*. 2003 Jan 15;28(2):177-9
[946] Vasquez et al. The clinical importance of vitamin D: a paradigm shift with implications for all healthcare providers. *Altern Ther Health Med*. 2004 Sep-Oct;10(5):28-36
[947] Harley JB, Scofield RH. The spectrum of ankylosing spondylitis. *Hosp Pract (Off Ed)* 1995 Jul 15;30(7):37-43, 46
[948] Bywaters EGL, Hamilton EBD, Williams R. The spine in idiopathic hemochromatosis. *Ann Rheum Dis* 1971; 30: 453-65
[949] Pimentel M, et al. A link between irritable bowel syndrome and fibromyalgia may be related to findings on lactulose breath testing. *Ann Rheum Dis*. 2004 Apr;63:450-2

- **Laboratory assessments**:
  - ESR or CRP: These are generally elevated, and neither test is superior to the other in the assessment of patients with AS. One study[950] used a unique approach to differentiate active disease from inactive disease in patients with AS; they added ESR value (mm/h) and CRP value (mg/L) and classified patients as having active inflammatory disease if the total was greater than thirty (30).
  - Rheumatoid factor (RF): Characteristically **negative** *by definition* in patients with sero**negative** spondyloarthropathies. Positivity suggests rheumatoid spondylitis or concomitant RA with another spondyloarthropathy.
  - CBC: Look for evidence of true *infection* (in contrast to *dysbiosis*); also assess for anemia, which may be secondary to renal failure, NSAID gastropathy, chronic inflammation, or nutritional inadequacy.
  - Comprehensive metabolic panel: Assess as indicated for complications and concomitant disease.
  - Comprehensive stool analysis with comprehensive parasitology: **All patients with AS, RA, and PsA have gastrointestinal dysbiosis until proven otherwise.** Use of comprehensive stool tests should be the standard of care for all patients with AS, RA, PsA, and of course those with enteropathic spondyloarthropathy. Patients with ReA due to gastroenteritis or those whose primary infection has not been identified/eliminated are also obvious candidates for stool testing; the most commonly implicated microbes are *Salmonella*, *Shigella*, and *Yersinia*. Regarding the etiopathogenesis of AS, the most commonly implicated microbes are *Klebsiella* and *E. coli*. However, it is more accurate to see that microbes incite autoimmunity/inflammation by numerous mechanisms and that exposure to numerous microbes—each one of which *in isolation* may be innocuous—in combination leads to additive and synergistic proinflammatory effects, as reviewed in Chapter 4 in the section on multifocal dysbiosis and elsewhere in a recent publication by the current author.[951]

Microorganisms clinically or molecularly associated with induction of seronegative spondyloarthropathy, ankylosing spondylitis, and reactive arthritis
• *Campylobacter* spp
• *Chlamydia trachomatis*
• *Citrobacter freundii*
• *E. coli*
• *Giardia lamblia*
• *Helicobacter pylori*
• *Klebsiella pneumoniae*
• *Mycoplasma* spp
• *Proteus mirabilis*
• *Salmonella typhimurium*
• *Shigella flexneri*
• *Shigella sonnei*
• *Staphylococcus aureus*
• *Streptococcus pyogenes*
• *Ureaplasma* spp
• *Yersinia enterocolitica*

  - Serologic and genital tests for sexually transmitted diseases: These tests are particularly indicated in patients with ReA due to the frequent association of this disorder with genitourinary infections, particularly those caused by *Chlamydia*. Numerous articles have shown that patients with long-term idiopathic oligoarthritis harbor "silent infections"—otherwise known as dysbiosis—in the genitourinary and gastrointestinal tracts; the most commonly identified organisms are *Chlamydia trachomatis*, *Yersinia*, *Salmonella*, *Mycoplasma*, and *Ureaplasma*.[952,953]
  - Serum vitamin D: Measure 25(OH)vitamin D in all patients and/or begin empiric treatment with physiologic doses of vitamin D3. Emulsified cholecalciferol is particularly efficacious in older patients and those with malabsorption due to enteropathy.[954] According to research by Falkenbach et al[955], **"Patients with ankylosing spondylitis may have extremely low levels of 25(OH)D."** Vitamin D deficiency appears common in patients with low-back pain[956], limb pain[957], chronic persistent

---

[950] Maki-Ikola O, Lehtinen K, Nissila M, Granfors K. IgM, IgA and IgG class serum antibodies against Klebsiella pneumoniae and Escherichia coli lipopolysaccharides in patients with ankylosing spondylitis. *Br J Rheumatol* 1994 Nov;33(11):1025-9

[951] Vasquez A. Nutritional and Botanical Treatments against "Silent Infections" and Gastrointestinal Dysbiosis. *Nutritional Perspectives* 2006; January

[952] "Urogenital swab cultures showed a microbial infection in 44% of the patients with oligoarthritis (15% Chlamydia, 14% Mycoplasma, 28% Ureaplasma), whereas in the control group only 26% had a positive result (4% Chlamydia, 7% Mycoplasma, 21% Ureaplasma)." Erlacher et al. Reactive arthritis: urogenital swab culture is the only useful diagnostic method for the detection of the arthritogenic infection in extra-articularly asymptomatic patients with undifferentiated oligoarthritis. *Br J Rheumatol*. 1995 Sep;34(9):838-42

[953] Fendler C, et al. Frequency of triggering bacteria in patients with reactive arthritis and undifferentiated oligoarthritis and the relative importance of the tests used for diagnosis. *Ann Rheum Dis*. 2001 Apr;60(4):337-43 ard.bmjjournals.com/cgi/content/full/60/4/337

[954] Vasquez A. Subphysiologic Doses of Vitamin D are Subtherapeutic: Comment on the Study by The Record Trial Group. *The Lancet* Published on-line May 6, 2005

[955] "Patients with ankylosing spondylitis may have extremely low levels of 25(OH)D." Falkenbach et al. Serum 25-hydroxyvitamin D and parathyroid hormone in patients with ankylosing spondylitis before and after a three-week rehabilitation treatment at high altitude during winter and spring. *Wien Klin Wochenschr*. 2001 Apr 30;113(9):328-32

[956] Al Faraj S, Al Mutairi K. Vitamin D deficiency and chronic low back pain in Saudi Arabia. *Spine*. 2003 Jan 15;28(2):177-9

[957] Masood H, Narang AP, Bhat IA, Shah GN. Persistent limb pain and raised serum alkaline phosphatase the earliest markers of subclinical hypovitaminosis D in Kashmir. *Indian J Physiol Pharmacol*. 1989 Oct-Dec;33(4):259-61

musculoskeletal pain[958], and in general medical patients.[959] [960] In our review of the literature[961], we concluded that **optimal serum 25(OH)-vitamin D levels should be defined as 40 – 65 ng/mL (100 - 160 nmol/L)** and that, "Until proven otherwise, the balance of the research clearly indicates that oral supplementation in the range of 1,000 IU per day for infants, 2,000 IU per day for children and **4,000 IU per day for adults** is safe and reasonable to meet physiologic requirements, to promote optimal health, and to reduce the risk of several serious diseases. Safety and effectiveness of supplementation are assured by periodic monitoring of serum 25(OH)D and serum calcium." Vitamin D supplementation 5,000 – 10,000 IU per day for adults was shown to alleviate low-back pain after 3 months in nearly all patients with low initial serum levels of vitamin D.[962]
   - Testing for multifocal dysbiosis: If the intestinal and genitourinary tracts appear clear of infection following direct testing, then empiric antimicrobial treatment should be considered. Following this, searching for other loci of infection—namely the mouth, throat, nose, sinuses, lungs, and skin—should be pursued as discussed in Chapter 4.
   - HLA-B27: This marker is seen with increased prevalence in patients with AS and ReA. The test can be used to support the diagnosis, particularly early in the course of the illness when radiographs are *negative*.
   - Hormone assessments: These should be performed as detailed in Chapter 4 and/or as indicated per patient.
- **Imaging**:
   - Plain radiographs: In contrast to most of the other rheumatic disorders wherein radiographs are generally unnecessary in early stages of the disease, plain radiographs are of tremendous value in the assessment of spondylitis and sacroiliitis and are generally diagnostic once the diagnostic threshold has been crossed; i.e., they may be negative in early disease, but become positive after a given amount of time, which varies per patient and per disease. Characteristic initial findings in AS are lumbar syndesmophytes and sacroiliitis.
   - MRI and CT imaging: Generally reserved for the evaluation of spinal stenosis and inflammatory myelopathy. **CT imaging is more sensitive than plain radiography for the initial evaluation of sacroiliitis**.[963] Also used for assessment of other complications as indicated.
- **Establishing the diagnosis**:
   - Inflammatory spondyloarthropathy as a general term can be diagnosed with a combination of serologic, clinical, and radiographic findings. The subtype of spondyloarthropathy—AS, ReA, PsA, RA, ES, etc—is then distinguished based on the details of the clinical history (e.g., inflammatory bowel disease or recent infection), presentation, clinical findings, serologic tests, and radiographic characteristics.

Complications:
- Chronic pain, significant physical limitations and significant morbidity
- Renal failure, secondary to amyloidosis or medications such as sulfasalazine or NSAID's
- Spinal fracture (in patients with spinal ankylosis following minor trauma)
- Respiratory insufficiency
- Permanent disability due to rigid spinal flexion secondary to bony ankylosis resulting in loss of spinal motion
- Neurologic compromise: due to spinal stenosis, transverse myelopathy, atlantoaxial subluxation, cauda equina fibrosis, or cauda equina syndrome

Clinical management:
- Referral if clinical outcome is unsatisfactory or as otherwise indicated.

---

[958] Plotnikoff GA, Quigley JM. Prevalence of severe hypovitaminosis D in patients with persistent, nonspecific musculoskeletal pain. *Mayo Clin Proc*. 2003 Dec;78(12):1463-70
[959] Thomas et al. Hypovitaminosis D in medical inpatients. *N Engl J Med*. 1998 Mar 19;338(12):777-83
[960] Kauppinen-Makelin et al. A high prevalence of hypovitaminosis D in Finnish medical in- and outpatients. *J Intern Med*. 2001 Jun;249(6):559-63
[961] Vasquez A, Manso G, Cannell J. The Clinical Importance of Vitamin D (Cholecalciferol). *Alternative Therapies in Health and Medicine* InflammationMastery.com/reprints
[962] Al Faraj S, Al Mutairi K. Vitamin D deficiency and chronic low back pain in Saudi Arabia. *Spine*. 2003 Jan 15;28(2):177-9
[963] Tierney ML. McPhee SJ, Papadakis MA. *Current Medical Diagnosis and Treatment 2006. 45th edition*. New York; Lange Medical Books: 2006, pages 851-855

Treatments[964]
- NSAIDs, especially indomethacin 25-50 mg thrice daily—"side effects" of indomethacin include headache, giddiness, psychosis, depression, nausea, vomiting, gastric ulcer, and renal impairment. Sulfasalazine: 1,000 mg twice daily.
- Corticosteroids are notably ineffective in the treatment of spondyloarthropathy, though they are commonly used against complications such as uveitis.
- TNF inhibitors: Etanercept 25 mg subcutaneously twice weekly, or infliximab 5 mg/kg every other month. These drugs are clinically effective from the perspective of anti-inflammation, but they are associated with increased risks for lymphoma, serious infections including pulmonary tuberculosis, congestive heart failure, demyelinating diseases, and systemic lupus erythematosus.
- Methotrexate: Used for recalcitrant psoriatic arthritis.[965]
- **FOOD & NUTRITION: 5-part "supplemented Paleo-Mediterranean diet" (SPMD)** The 5-part "supplemented Paleo-Mediterranean diet" (SPMD—reviewed in Chapter 4) consists of ❶ foundational plant-based low-carbohydrate diet of fruits, vegetables, nuts, seeds, berries and lean sources of protein, ❷ multivitamin and multimineral supplementation, ❸ physiologic doses of vitamin D3 (range 2,000-10,000 IU/d), ❹ combination fatty acid therapy (CFAT) with n3-ALA, n6-GLA, n3-EPA, n3-DHA, and phytochemical-rich olive oil which contains n9-oleate, and ❺ probiotics.
  - The use of a low starch diet in the treatment of patients suffering from ankylosing spondylitis: alleviation of dysbiosis and immune complex formation via nutritional intervention (*Clin Rheumatol* 1996 Jan[966]): "The majority of ankylosing spondylitis (AS) patients not only possess HLA-B27, but during active phases of the disease have elevated levels of total serum IgA, suggesting that a microbe from the bowel flora is acting across the gut mucosa. .... Furthermore AS patients from 10 different countries have been found to have elevated levels of specific antibodies against Klebsiella bacteria. It has been suggested that these Klebsiella microbes, found in the bowel flora, might be the trigger factors in this disease and therefore reduction in the size of the bowel flora could be of benefit in the treatment of AS patients. Microbes from the bowel flora depend on dietary starch for their growth and therefore a reduction in starch intake might be beneficial in AS patients. A "low starch diet" involving a reduced intake of "bread, potatoes, cakes and pasta" has been devised and tested in healthy control subjects and AS patients. The "low starch diet" leads to a reduction of total serum IgA in both healthy controls as well as patients, and furthermore to a decrease in inflammation and symptoms in the AS patients."
- **INFECTIONS & DYSBIOSIS: ❶ antimicrobial treatments, ❷ immunorestoration, ❸ immunotolerance via Treg induction** Essentially all autoimmune/rheumatic disorders are associated with microbial colonization and intolerance to same; the presence of persistent microbial colonization is *prima facie* evidence of immunosuppression. The eight areas of dysbiosis (multifocal) are: ❶ sinorespiratory, ❷ orodental, ❸ gastrointestinal, ❹ urogenital/genitourinary, ❺ parenchymal/tissue, ❻ microbial, ❼ dermal/cutaneous, and ❽ environmental.
  - Rational assumption of polymicrobial dysbiosis: The association of spondyloarthropathies and reactive arthritis with microbial infection/colonization is so strong and consistent throughout decades of research that a review or substantiation here, notwithstanding a few relevant samples, would be superfluous; rather, the 3-part anti-dysbiosis protocols and concepts reviewed in Chapter 4 should be implemented. See also the laboratory (microbial) assessments and concepts in Chapter 1. The examples that follow should be viewed concretely for the data provided, but also as metaphorical and representative of the microbe-autoimmunity connection.
  - Helicobacter pylori eradication therapy on gastrointestinal permeability in seronegative spondyloarthritis (*J Rheumatol.* 2005 Feb[967]): "Disruption of intestinal barrier function, followed by increased antigen load, may possibly trigger joint inflammation. In seronegative spondyloarthritis (SpA) both gut inflammation and altered intestinal permeability have been reported. We evaluated ...20 SpA

---

[964] Tierney ML. McPhee SJ, Papadakis MA. *Current Medical Diagnosis and Treatment 2006. 45th edition.* New York; Lange Medical Books: 2006, pages 851-855
[965] Tierney ML. McPhee SJ, Papadakis MA. *Current Medical Diagnosis and Treatment 2006. 45th edition.* New York; Lange Medical Books: 2006, pages 851-855
[966] Ebringer A, Wilson C. The use of a low starch diet in the treatment of patients suffering from ankylosing spondylitis. *Clin Rheumatol.* 1996 Jan;15 Suppl 1:62-66
[967] Di Leo et al. Effect of Helicobacter pylori and eradication therapy on gastrointestinal permeability. Implications for patients with seronegative spondyloarthritis. *J Rheumatol.* 2005 Feb;32(2):295-300

patients, 30 patients with endoscopic gastritis (EndG), and 35 healthy controls... H. pylori affected GI permeability in both SpA and EndG patients. After eradication therapy, sucrose excretion remained increased in SpA and reverted to normal in EndG patients, whereas lactulose/mannitol test became comparable to controls in both groups. SpA patients taking chronic NSAID had increased gastroduodenal permeability only when H. pylori-positive. In SpA patients, GI permeability did not correlate with clinical activity or biochemical inflammation. CONCLUSION: In SpA, H. pylori and NSAID contribute to impaired GI permeability. Eradication therapy may help to maintain epithelial barrier function and possibly influence clinical improvement in patients with SpA."

- Reactive arthritis responding to antiretroviral therapy in an HIV-1-infected individual (*Int J STD AIDS. 2012 May*[968]): "Reactive arthritis (ReA) is an autoimmune seronegative spondyloarthropathy that occurs in response to a urogenital or enteric infection. Several studies have reported a link between ReA and HIV infection. We report a case of an HIV-1-infected patient diagnosed with a disabling ReA who failed to respond to conventional therapy but whose symptoms resolved rapidly after starting antiretroviral therapy (ART)."

- Human immunodeficiency virus associated spondyloarthropathy (*Ann Rheum Dis.* 2001 Jul[969]): "In this case report a patient is described with severe HIV associated reactive arthritis, who on magnetic resonance imaging and sonographic imaging of inflamed knees had extensive polyenthesitis and adjacent osteitis. The arthritis deteriorated despite conventional antirheumatic treatment, but improved dramatically after highly active antiretroviral treatment, which was accompanied by a significant rise in CD4 T lymphocyte counts."

- Reactive arthritis: urogenital swab culture is the only useful diagnostic method for the detection of the arthritogenic infection in extra-articularly asymptomatic patients with undifferentiated oligoarthritis (*Br J Rheumatol.* 1995 Sep[970]): "Reactive arthritis (ReA) is a seronegative oligoarthritis triggered by a preceding extra-articular infection. ... In a retrospective study, we evaluated the usefulness of urogenital swab cultures, serology and stool culture to identify infections in 234 patients with undifferentiated oligoarthritis. One hundred and forty-four patients complaining about joint pain who had no sign or history of inflammatory arthritis served as controls. Urogenital swab cultures showed a microbial infection in 44% of the patients with oligoarthritis (15% Chlamydia, 14% Mycoplasma, 28% Ureaplasma), whereas in the control group only 26% had a positive result (4% Chlamydia, 7% Mycoplasma, 21% Ureaplasma). A Chlamydia IgG-antibody titer > or = 1:256 was found in 22% of the patients in the oligoarthritis group and in 9% of the controls (P < 0.01). However, for only half of Chlamydia IgG-positive patients could a Chlamydia infection be confirmed by urogenital swab culture. Twenty-one per cent of patients with oligoarthritis vs 23% of the controls had positive antibody titers for Salmonella (not significant), 15% vs 5% for Yersinia (P < 0.05) and 17% vs 3% for Borrelia IgG (P < 0.01). In two patients, stool cultures were positive for Campylobacter. Urogenital swab culture is a sensitive diagnostic method to identify the triggering infection in ReA."

- **NUTRITIONAL IMMUNOMODULATION: Treg induction for modulation of Th-1/2/17 inflammation** Nutrients and therapeutic approaches that promote Treg or IL-10 induction and/or Th-17, IL-17 suppression include 1) mitochondrial optimization and mTOR suppression, 2) biotin, 3) vitamin E, 4) sodium avoidance, 5) transgenic/GMO food avoidance, 6) probiotics, 7) lipoic acid, 8) vitamin A, 9) inflammation reduction, 10) vitamin D, 11) fatty acid supplementation with GLA and n3, 12) infection and dysbiosis remediation, 13) green tea EGCG. Acronym: MiBESTPLAIDFIG.

- **DYSMETABOLISM & DYSFUNCTIONAL MITOCHONDRIA: MitoDys, ERS-UPR, AGE/RAGE, hyperglycemia and ceramide** The major clinical considerations in this section are mitochondrial dysfunction, endoplasmic reticulum stress, unfolded protein response, TLR activation, and the dysmetabolic effects of sustained hyperglycemia and hyperinsulinemia and resultant oxidative stress, inflammation, RAGE activation, and accumulation of AGE, palmitate and ceramide. The review of this information in Chapter 4 covered

---

[968] Scott et al. Reactive arthritis responding to antiretroviral therapy in an HIV-1-infected individual. *Int J STD AIDS.* 2012 May;23(5):373-4
[969] McGonagle et al. Human immunodeficiency virus associated spondyloarthropathy. *Ann Rheum Dis.* 2001 Jul;60(7):696-8
[970] Erlacher et al. Reactive arthritis: urogenital swab culture is the only useful diagnostic method for the detection of the arthritogenic infection in extra-articularly asymptomatic patients with undifferentiated oligoarthritis. *Br J Rheumatol.* 1995 Sep;34(9):838-42

approximately 30 interventions relevant to dysmetabolism, mitochondrial dysfunction, ERS-UPR, etc; these will not be reviewed here except to mention those most commonly, easily, empirically, synergistically, and effectively used: 1) low-carbohydrate diet with 2) moderate exercise, 3) CoQ-10, 4) acetyl-carnitine with 5) lipoic acid, 6) NAC, 7) resveratrol, and 8) melatonin.

- **STYLE OF LIVING (LIFESTYLE) & SPECIAL CONSIDERATIONS: S**leep optimization, **S**ocioPsychology, **S**tress management/avoidance, **S**omatic treatments, **S**pecial **S**upplementation, **S**weat/exercise, **S**auna/detoxification, **S**urgery, **S**tamp your passport and vacate current reality, **S**ensory deprivation therapy
This is a buffet of mostly lifestyle-based interventions yet also including considerations such as somatic treatments, additional supplementation, and surgery.

- **ENDOCRINE IMBALANCE & OPTIMIZATION: Prolactin, Insulin, Estrogen, DHEA, Cortisol, Testosterone, Thyroid** Common hormonal imbalances seen among autoimmune/inflammatory patients are: ❶ *elevated* prolactin, ❷ *elevated* estrogen, ❸ *elevated* insulin, and ❹ *reduced* DHEA, ❺ *reduced* cortisol, and ❻ *reduced* testosterone; see Chapter 4 for discussion of these hormones and respective interventions. Thyroid evaluation (patient + labs) should be comprehensive, as discussed in Chapter 1, with a low threshold for empiric treatment.

- **XENOBIOTIC ACCUMULATION & DETOXIFICATION: Chemical avoidance, nutritional support for detoxification pathways, urine alkalinization** The clinical relevance and pathogenic mechanisms of xenobiotic accumulation are irrefutably well documented and described. Clinical assessments include history, physical examination, and laboratory assessment (using serum, whole blood, urine or—rarely yet accurately—fat biopsy), and response to treatment. Treatments include nutritional support for Phases 1 and 2 of detoxification (e.g., oxidation and conjugation) and excretion via bile and urine; for the latter, urinary alkalinization is generally recommended. Chemical toxins can be bound in the gut using activated charcoal, cholestyramine, or *Chlorella*—all of these three treatments have documented safety and effectiveness; clinically and empirically, phytochelatin (plant-derived peptides that bind toxic metals) concentrates appear safe and effective despite lack of conclusive published data supporting clinical use.

Sjögren Syndrome/Disease

Introduction:
Sjögren Syndrome/Disease is a sustained inflammatory disorder characterized by inflammatory and destructive lymphocytic infiltrates in exocrine organs, leading to failure of these glands and the resultant complications reviewed in the section that follows. Common to other inflammatory and autoimmune disorders, the condition is multifactorial in accord with most of the categories addressed by the Functional Inflammology protocol and recalled by the FINDSEX acronym detailed in Chapter 4 and the accompanying videos. Readers are expected to have read Chapters 1 and 4 so that this chapter can focus on the more salient points specific for Sjögren Syndrome/Disease. The condition is inaccurately named a "syndrome"—implying that it is a "group of symptoms that collectively indicate or characterize a disease or disorder"; however, this condition—like fibromyalgia—has distinct clinical and histopathological findings and is therefore more accurately described and legitimized as a "disease", which it properly is.

Description/pathophysiology:
- **Autoimmune condition affecting the exocrine glands; mucosal surfaces become dry, irritated and prone to microbial colonization.** Clinically manifested as "*sicca* syndrome" which implies a group of symptoms caused by *dryness* of mucosal surfaces.
- Like most conditions, it is generally described as "idiopathic" by medical textbooks and journal articles.[971] More common than SLE, less common than RA; Sjogren's syndrome is considered by some references to be as common as RA.
- Occurs in two general forms:
    - Primary—only Sjogren's/Sicca syndrome *without evidence of systemic autoimmunity*
    - Secondary—the occurrence of Sjogren's syndrome *along with another autoimmune disease*, especially rheumatoid arthritis, but also SLE, systemic sclerosis, primary biliary cirrhosis, polymyositis, Hashimoto's thyroiditis, polyarteritis, interstitial pulmonary fibrosis

Clinical presentations:
- Much more common in women—90% of patients with Sjogren's disease are female[972]
- Average age of onset is 50 years (typical range 40-60 years)
- **"Sicca syndrome"** denotes dryness of mucus membranes:
    - Dry eyes, keratoconjunctivitis sicca: Lymphocyte and plasma cells cause destruction of lacrimal glands; subjective complaints are more prominent than objective evidence: dry eyes, burning, itching, inability to wear contact lenses, thick mucus, photophobia, corneal ulceration—the latter can lead to infection, vision loss.
    - Dry mouth, xerostomia: this is generally more problematic than keratoconjunctivitis sicca; dental carries ("cavities") are greatly increased; 33% of patients will have parotid gland tenderness (can be treated with analgesics) and fluctuations in gland size.
    - Nose, throat, bronchi, and vagina may also be affected.
- Joint pain: Similar distribution to RA but less severe and nondestructive; minimal swelling: PIP and knees most common
- Classic presentation: Woman (90%) aged 40-60 years with dry mouth, dry eyes, and arthritis that mimics RA; other common presentations include:
    - Photosensitivity, skin rash, hair loss
    - Mouth lesions, carries
    - Chest pain (caused by pleurisy) or breathlessness
    - Raynaud's phenomenon

---
[971] "In spite of [the fact that we have no evidence-based solutions to the etiology and pathogenesis of autoimmune diseases], consensus is often taken as a truth, which may hamper the production, funding and/or publication of new and original ideas and views." Konttinen YT, Kasna-Ronkainen L. Sjogren's syndrome: viewpoint on pathogenesis. One of the reasons I was never asked to write a textbook chapter on it. *Scand J Rheumatol Suppl* 2002;(116):15-22
[972] Tierney ML. McPhee SJ, Papadakis MA. *Current Medical Diagnosis and Treatment 2006. 45th edition*. New York; Lange Medical Books: 2006, pages 842-843

Major differential diagnoses:
- Dehydration, exposure to excessively dry air (furnaces, dehumidifiers, etc.)
- Another autoimmune disease may mimic or occur concomitantly: RA, SLE, scleroderma, polymyositis, autoimmune thyroid disease, arteritis—none of these conditions by itself will cause sicca/dryness.
- Medication side effects (dry eyes and dry mouth are common side effects of many drugs)
- Systemic illness: HIV, lymphoma, sarcoidosis
- Hepatitis C—may possibly induce Sjogren's syndrome[973]
- Mumps (swollen parotid glands)
- Menopause
- Normal aging
- Salivary gland atrophy/fibrosis due to previous radiation to head and neck

Clinical assessments:
- **History/subjective**:
  - See clinical presentations
- **Physical examination/objective**:
  - Schirmer test: Use filter paper to assess adequacy of lacrimation for 5 minutes; less than 5 mm of wetness is abnormal
  - Rose Bengal staining: Used to assess the health of the cornea and to thus search for objective evidence of keratoconjunctivitis sicca
- **Laboratory assessments**:
  - ANA: positive in >95%
    - If ANA is negative, consider HIV, lymphoma, sarcoidosis, hepatitis C.
    - Supportive evidence with **anti-SS-A (anti-Ro)** and **anti-SS-B (anti-La)**, neither of which are specific
    - Autoimmunity directed toward glands/tissues such as stomach, adrenal, and neurons may also be noted[974]
  - RF: Positive in 70%
  - ESR: Elevated in 70%
  - CBC: Shows anemia (33%), leukopenia and eosinophilia (25%)
  - Thyroid disorders: Thyroid autoimmunity is common in patients with Sjogren's syndrome; test anti-thyroid peroxidase antibodies and anti-thyroglobulin antibodies along with TSH, T4, and perhaps T3—see Chapter 1 for discussions on thyroid assessments and interventions.
  - HLA markers: DR2 and DR3 are more common in patients who have Sjogren's syndrome *without rheumatoid arthritis.*
  - Schirmer test: Measures quantity of tears and thus objectively quantifies keratoconjunctivitis sicca.
  - Salivary gland biopsy: Not commonly performed except for atypical presentations such as unilateral involvement and to exclude malignancy.
  - Anti-parietal cell antibodies: Noted in various autoimmune conditions (e.g., approximately 33% of patients with Hashimoto thyroiditis); leads to gastric atrophy and associated hypochlorhydria, cobalamin malabsorption, and microbial overgrowth.
  - Assess patient as indicated for other conditions and complications.
- **Imaging**: Used as indicated per patient; generally not part of assessment
- **Establishing the diagnosis**: Both of the following must be present:
  1. Autoantibodies—ANA or variant: Preferably in combination with the gold standard in allopathic medicine: salivary gland biopsy—this is necessary for "definite diagnosis" but is not necessary for clinical purposes based on "probable diagnosis."
  2. Evidence of exocrine damage: keratoconjunctivitis sicca and/or xerostomia.

---

[973] Siegel LB, Gall EP. Viral infection as a cause of arthritis. *Am Fam Physician* 1996 Nov 1;54(6):2009-15
[974] Rehman HU. Sjogren's syndrome. *Yonsei Med J*. 2003 Dec 30;44(6):947-54 eymj.org/2003/pdf/12947.pdf

Clinical Applications: Rheumatology

Complications:
- Vision impairment, vision loss due to corneal lesion, ulceration and secondary infection
- Dental carries
- Malnutrition, especially vitamin B-12 deficiency
- Inflammatory polyarthropathy
- Salivary stones
- Pneumonia: can be fatal
- Pancreatitis
- Raynaud's phenomenon is seen in ~20%
- Sensory neuropathy, peripheral neuropathy: immune complex neuropathy, nutrient/B12 deficiencies
- Renal tubular acidosis
- Renal insufficiency and failure: can be fatal
- Nephritis (immune complex disorder)
- Vasculitis (immune complex disorder)
- Cryoglobulinemia (immune complex disorder)
- **Lymphoma: Up to 3-10% of patients with Sjogren's syndrome develop lymphoma**; risk is increased in patients with severe dryness and systemic complications such as vasculitis, splenomegaly, and cryoglobulinemia.
- Waldenstrom's macroglobulinemia

Clinical management:
- Medical treatment: "Treatment is symptomatic and supportive."[975] "There is no specific [allopathic] treatment for the basic process. Local manifestations can be treated symptomatically."[976]
- Referral if clinical outcome is unsatisfactory or if serious complications are possible.

Treatments:
- Drug treatments include pilocarpine (5 mg 4 times daily) and/or cevimeline (30 mg three times daily) to promote salivation. Associated rheumatic diseases are treated as indicated; prednisone is commonly used.
- Eye drops: Consider vitamin-A-containing eye drops, available OTC or by a compounding pharmacist
- For dry mouth:
    - Sip fluids throughout the day.
    - Chew sugarless gum to promote saliva flow; xylitol chewing gum can stimulate saliva flow and inhibit the growth of cariogenic bacteria.
    - Saliva substitute with carboxymethylcellulose.
    - Fastidious oral hygiene (brushing, flossing, oral antiseptics) and regular dental care are important.
    - Liquid folic acid supplementation swished in the mouth may help alleviate mouth sores; likewise, topical vitamin E and glutamine may help (as they do with chemotherapy-induced mucositis); chewable deglycyrrhizinated licorice benefits some patients.
    - Acupuncture improves salivary flow rates in patients with Sjogren's syndrome.[977,978]
- **FOOD & NUTRITION: 5-part "supplemented Paleo-Mediterranean diet" (SPMD)** The 5-part "supplemented Paleo-Mediterranean diet" (SPMD—reviewed in Chapter 4) consists of ❶ foundational plant-based low-carbohydrate diet of fruits, vegetables, nuts, seeds, berries and lean sources of protein, ❷ multivitamin and multimineral supplementation, ❸ physiologic doses of vitamin D3 (range 2,000-10,000 IU/d),

---

[975] Tierney ML. McPhee SJ, Papadakis MA. *Current Medical Diagnosis and Treatment. 35th edition*. Stamford: Appleton and Lange, 1996 page 749 and Tierney ML. McPhee SJ, Papadakis MA. *Current Medical Diagnosis and Treatment 2006. 45th edition*. New York; Lange Medical Books: 2006, pages 842-843
[976] Beers MH, Berkow R (eds). *The Merck Manual. Seventeenth Edition*. Whitehouse Station; Merck Research Laboratories 1999 Page 424
[977] "CONCLUSIONS: This study shows that acupuncture treatment results in statistically significant improvements in SFR in patients with xerostomia up to 6 months. It suggests that additional acupuncture therapy can maintain this improvement in SFR for up to 3 years." Blom M, Lundeberg T. Long-term follow-up of patients treated with acupuncture for xerostomia and the influence of additional treatment. *Oral Dis* 2000 Jan;6(1):15-24
[978] "A majority of the patients subjectively reported some improvement after treatment, and a significant increase in paraffin-stimulated saliva secretion was found after treatment." List et al. The effect of acupuncture in the treatment of patients with primary Sjogren's syndrome. A controlled study. *Acta Odontol Scand* 1998 Apr;56(2):95-9

❹ combination fatty acid therapy (CFAT) with n3-ALA, n6-GLA, n3-EPA, n3-DHA, and phytochemical-rich olive oil which contains n9-oleate, and ❺ probiotics.

- Avoidance of allergenic foods: Any patient may be allergic to any food, even if the food is generally considered a health-promoting food. Generally speaking, the most notorious allergens are wheat, citrus (especially juice due to the industrial use of fungal hemicellulases), cow's milk, eggs, peanuts, chocolate, and yeast-containing foods. **Patients with celiac disease have an increased prevalence of Sjogren's syndrome[979], and patients with Sjogren's syndrome have an increased prevalence of celiac disease.[980] In one study, the estimated prevalence of celiac disease in Sjogren's patients was nearly 1 in 20.[981]** Celiac disease can present with inflammatory oligoarthritis that resembles rheumatoid arthritis and which remits with avoidance of wheat/gluten; the inflammatory arthropathy of celiac disease has preceded bowel symptoms and/or an accurate diagnosis by as many as 3-15 years.[982,983] Clinicians must explain to their patients that celiac disease and wheat allergy are two different clinical entities and that exclusion of one does not exclude the other, and in neither case does mutual exclusion obviate the promotion of intestinal bacterial overgrowth (i.e., proinflammatory dysbiosis) by indigestible wheat oligosaccharides.

- Broad-spectrum fatty acid therapy with ALA, EPA, DHA, GLA and oleic acid: Fatty acid supplementation should be delivered in the form of combination therapy with ALA, GLA, DHA, and EPA. Given at doses of 3,000 – 9,000 mg per day, ALA from flax oil has impressive anti-inflammatory benefits demonstrated by its ability to halve prostaglandin production in humans.[984] **Patients with Sjogren's syndrome have lower levels of GLA/DGLA[985] and fatty acid supplementation—particularly with GLA (along with vitamin C)—is safe and may be beneficial (positive reports[986,987], neutral report[988], negative report[989]).**

- Vitamin D3 supplementation with physiologic doses and/or tailored to serum 25(OH)D levels: **Vitamin D insufficiency has been reported in patients with Sjogren's syndrome, presumably due to reduced intake and/or malabsorption.** Vitamin D deficiency is common in the general population and is even more common in patients with chronic illness and chronic musculoskeletal pain.[990] Correction of vitamin D deficiency supports normal immune function against infection and provides a clinically significant anti-inflammatory[991] and analgesic benefit in patients with back pain[992] and limb pain.[993] **Vitamin D status is inversely associated with inflammation in patients with Sjogren's syndrome.[994,995]** Reasonable daily doses for children and adults are 2,000 and 4,000 IU, respectively, as defined by Vasquez, et al.[996] Deficiency

---

[979] "Sjogren's syndrome occurred in 3.3% of coeliac patients and in 0.3% of controls." Collin et al. Coeliac disease—associated disorders and survival. *Gut.* 1994 Sep;35:1215-8.
[980] "Further, our study shows that anti-tTG is more prevalent in SS than in other systemic rheumatic diseases." Luft LM, Barr SG, Martin LO, Chan EK, Fritzler MJ. Autoantibodies to tissue transglutaminase in Sjogren's syndrome and related rheumatic diseases. *J Rheumatol.* 2003 Dec;30(12):2613-9
[981] "The frequency of CD in the SS population was significantly higher than in the non-SS European population (4.5:100 vs 4.5-5.5:1,000)." Szodoray et al. Coeliac disease in Sjogren's syndrome--a study of 111 Hungarian patients. *Rheumatol Int.* 2004 Sep;24(5):278-82
[982] "We report six patients with coeliac disease in whom arthritis was prominent at diagnosis and who improved with dietary therapy. Joint pain preceded diagnosis by up to three years in five patients and 15 years in one patient." Bourne et al. Arthritis and coeliac disease. *Ann Rheum Dis.* 1985 Sep;44(9):592-8
[983] "A 15-year-old girl, with synovitis of the knees and ankles for 3 years before a diagnosis of gluten-sensitive enteropathy, is described." Pinals RS. Arthritis associated with gluten-sensitive enteropathy. *J Rheumatol.* 1986 Feb;13(1):201-4
[984] Adam et al. Effect of alpha-linolenic acid in the human diet on linoleic acid metabolism and prostaglandin biosynthesis. *J Lipid Res.* 1986 Apr;27(4):421-6
[985] "We found MD levels of 20:3n6 (dihommo-gamma-linolenic acid), and basal and indomethacin-enhanced NK cell activity significantly reduced, in 10 primary Sjogren's syndrome patients as compared with 10 healthy controls." Oxholm P, Pedersen BK, Horrobin DF. Natural killer cell functions are related to the cell membrane composition of essential fatty acids: differences in healthy persons and patients with primary Sjogren's syndrome. *Clin Exp Rheumatol.* 1992 May-Jun;10(3):229-34
[986] "An attempt to treat humans with Sjogren's syndrome by raising endogenous PGE1 production by administration of essential fatty acid PGE1 precursors, of pyridoxine and of vitamin C was successful in raising the rates of tear and saliva production." Horrobin DF, Campbell A. Sjogren's syndrome and the sicca syndrome: the role of prostaglandin E1 deficiency. Treatment with essential fatty acids and vitamin C. *Med Hypotheses.* 1980 Mar;6(3):225-32
[987] "Efamol treatment improved the Schirmer-I-test..." Manthorpe R, Hagen Petersen S, Prause JU. Primary Sjogren's syndrome treated with Efamol/Efavit. A double-blind cross-over investigation. *Rheumatol Int.* 1984;4(4):165-7. The duration of this study was ridiculously short—only 3 weeks.
[988] "The objective ocular status, evaluated by a combined ocular score, including the results from Schirmer-I test, break-up time and van Bijsterveld score, improved significantly during Efamol treatment when compared with Efamol start-values (p less than 0.05), but not when compared with placebo values (p less than 0.2)." Oxholm P, Manthorpe R, Prause JU, Horrobin D. Patients with primary Sjogren's syndrome treated for two months with evening primrose oil. *Scand J Rheumatol.* 1986;15:103-8
[989] "There was no significant improvement in any of the patients during the treatment period compared to assessments done pre and post treatment." McKendry RJ. Treatment of Sjogren's syndrome with essential fatty acids, pyridoxine and vitamin C. *Prostaglandins Leukot Med.* 1982 Apr;8(4):403-8
[990] Plotnikoff GA, Quigley JM. Prevalence of severe hypovitaminosis D in patients with persistent, nonspecific musculoskeletal pain. *Mayo Clin Proc.* 2003 Dec;78(12):1463-70
[991] Timms PM, et al. Circulating MMP9, vitamin D and variation in the TIMP-1 response with VDR genotype. *QJM.* 2002 Dec;95(12):787-96
[992] Al Faraj S, Al Mutairi K. Vitamin D deficiency and chronic low back pain in Saudi Arabia. *Spine.* 2003 Jan 15;28(2):177-9
[993] Masood H, Narang AP, Bhat IA, Shah GN. Persistent limb pain and raised serum alkaline phosphatase the earliest markers of subclinical hypovitaminosis D in Kashmir. *Indian J Physiol Pharmacol.* 1989 Oct-Dec;33(4):259-61
[994] "In conclusion the inverse correlations found between levels of 25 OH D and measures of clinical and immunoinflammatory status support the notion that vitamin D metabolism may be involved in the pathogenesis of primary SS." Bang B, Asmussen K, Sorensen OH, Oxholm P. Reduced 25-hydroxyvitamin D levels in primary Sjogren's syndrome. Correlations to disease manifestations. *Scand J Rheumatol.* 1999;28(3):180-3
[995] "Among patients with increased concentrations of IgM rheumatoid factor there was a significant negative correlation between the serum titres of IgM rheumatoid factor and 25-OHD3 concentrations." Muller K, et al. Abnormal vitamin D3 metabolism in patients with primary Sjogren's syndrome. *Ann Rheum Dis.* 1990 Sep;49(9):682-4
[996] Vasquez et al. The clinical importance of vitamin D: a paradigm shift with implications for all healthcare providers. *Altern Ther Health Med.* 2004 Sep-Oct;10(5):28-36

and response to treatment are monitored with serum 25(OH)vitamin D while safety is monitored with serum calcium; inflammatory granulomatous diseases and certain drugs such as hydrochlorothiazide greatly increase the propensity for hypercalcemia and warrant increment dosing and frequent monitoring of serum calcium.

- o Green tea, green tea extract (EGCG), and other phytonutritional antioxidants and anti-inflammatories: Very interestingly, an *in vitro* study[997] showed that epigallocatechin gallate inhibited the expression of major autoantigens, including those which are characteristic of Sjogren's syndrome: SS-B/La, SS-A/Ro. Given its antioxidant properties and anti-inflammatory actions (specifically via inhibition of NF-kappaB[998]), green tea and related supplements may prove beneficial for patients with Sjogren's syndrome.
- o High-dose short-term oral vitamin A: Szocsik et al[999] administered vitamin A 100,000 IU per day for two weeks and obtained improved immune function, such as improved natural killer cell function, in patients with Sjogren's syndrome.

- **INFECTIONS & DYSBIOSIS: ❶ antimicrobial treatments, ❷ immunorestoration, ❸ immunotolerance via Treg induction** Essentially all autoimmune/rheumatic disorders are associated with microbial colonization and intolerance to same; the presence of persistent microbial colonization is *prima facie* evidence of immunosuppression. The eight areas of dysbiosis (multifocal) are: ❶ sinorespiratory, ❷ orodental, ❸ gastrointestinal, ❹ urogenital/genitourinary, ❺ parenchymal/tissue, ❻ microbial, ❼ dermal/cutaneous, and ❽ environmental.

    - o T-cell epitope mimicry between Sjögren's syndrome Antigen A (SSA)/Ro60 and oral, gut, skin and vaginal bacteria (*Clin Immunol.* 2014 May[1000]): "Amongst these, a peptide from the von Willebrand factor type A domain protein (vWFA) from the oral microbe *Capnocytophaga ochracea* was the most potent activator. Further, Ro60-reactive T cells were activated by recombinant vWFA protein and whole *Escherichia coli* expressing this protein. These results demonstrate that peptides derived from normal human microbiota can activate Ro60-reactive T cells."
    - o Epstein-Barr virus in Sjögren's syndrome salivary glands drives local autoimmunity (*Nat Rev Rheumatol.* 2014 Jul[1001]): Paraphrasing from the original article: "Ectopic lymphoid structures (ELS) within the salivary glands of patients with Sjögren's syndrome serve as niches for latency and reactivation of EBV and contribute to the activation and differentiation of plasma cells. ... EBV is aberrantly expressed in the salivary glands of patients with Sjögren's syndrome, specifically in those glands that displayed ELS, as revealed by the presence of EBV-encoded small RNA (EBER) transcripts and EBER+ cells within infiltrating cells. ... EBV reactivation occurs in a substantial proportion of perifollicular plasma cells that produce anti-Ro52 antibodies."
    - o Epstein-Barr Virus Infection in Disease-Specific Autoreactive B Cell Activation in Ectopic Lymphoid Structures of Sjögren's Syndrome (*Arthritis Rheumatol.* 2014 Sep[1002]): "Active EBV infection is selectively associated with ELS in the salivary glands of patients with SS and appears to contribute to local growth and differentiation of disease-specific autoreactive B cells."
    - o Epstein-Barr Virus Infection, Vitamin D Deficiency, and Steps to Autoimmunity: A Unifying Hypothesis (*Autoimmune Dis.* 2012[1003]): Per this model, "Autoimmunity is postulated to evolve in the following steps: (1) CD8+ T-cell deficiency, (2) primary EBV infection, (3) decreased CD8+ T-cell control of EBV, (4) increased EBV load and increased anti-EBV antibodies, (5) EBV infection in the target organ, (6) clonal

---

[997] "EGCG inhibited the transcription and translation of major autoantigens, including SS-B/La, SS-A/Ro, coilin, DNA topoisomerase I, and alpha-fodrin. These findings, taken together with green tea's anti-inflammatory and antiapoptotic effects, suggest that green tea polyphenols could serve as an important component in novel approaches to combat autoimmune disorders in humans." Hsu et al. Inhibition of autoantigen expression by (-)-epigallocatechin-3-gallate (the major constituent of green tea) in normal human cells. *J Pharmacol Exp Ther.* 2005 Nov;315(2):805-11

[998] "In conclusion, EGCG is an effective inhibitor of IKK activity. This may explain, at least in part, some of the reported anti-inflammatory and anti-cancer effects of green tea." Yang et al. The green tea polyphenol (-)-epigallocatechin-3-gallate blocks nuclear factor-kappa B activation by inhibiting I kappa B kinase activity in the intestinal epithelial cell line IEC-6. *Mol Pharmacol.* 2001 Sep;60(3):528-33

[999] "Patients with Sjogren's syndrome were treated with vitamin A (100,000 U) daily during a two-week period. The vitamin treatment significantly elevated their ADCC and NK activity." Szocsik et al. Effect of vitamin A treatment on immune reactivity and lipid peroxidation in patients with Sjogren's syndrome. *Clin Rheumatol.* 1988 Dec;7(4):514-9

[1000] Szymula et al. T cell epitope mimicry between Sjögren's syndrome Antigen A (SSA)/Ro60 and oral, gut, skin and vaginal bacteria. *Clin Immunol.* 2014 May-Jun;152(1-2):1-9

[1001] Onuora S. Connective tissue diseases: Epstein-Barr virus in Sjögren's syndrome salivary glands drives local autoimmunity. *Nat Rev Rheumatol.* 2014 Jul;10(7):384

[1002] Croia et al. Implication of Epstein-Barr Virus Infection in Disease-Specific Autoreactive B Cell Activation in Ectopic Lymphoid Structures of Sjögren's Syndrome. *Arthritis Rheumatol.* 2014 Sep;66(9):2545-57

[1003] Pender MP. CD8+ T-Cell Deficiency, Epstein-Barr Virus Infection, Vitamin D Deficiency, and Steps to Autoimmunity. *Autoimmune Dis.* 2012;2012:189096 expansion of EBV-infected autoreactive B cells in the target organ, (7) infiltration of autoreactive T cells into the target organ, and (8) development of ectopic lymphoid follicles in the target organ [which drive the tissue damage and autoantibody production as recently demonstrated per *Nat Rev Rheumatol* 2014 Jul[1004] and *Arthritis Rheumatol* 2014 Sep[1005]]. It is also proposed that deprivation of sunlight and vitamin D at higher latitudes facilitates the development of autoimmune diseases by aggravating the CD8+ T-cell deficiency and thereby further impairing control of EBV." Congratulations to this author—Pender—for predicting two years in advance the research that would later support this model.

- o Aryl hydrocarbon receptor-mediated induction of EBV reactivation as a risk factor for Sjögren's syndrome (*J Immunol* 2012 May[1006]): This is very impressive research, connecting xenobiotic exposure with viral reactivation. "The aryl hydrocarbon receptor (AhR) is a ligand-activated transcription factor that mediates a variety of biological effects by binding to environmental pollutants, including 2,3,7,8-tetrachlorodibenzo-p-dioxin (TCDD or dioxin). … This study evaluated the possibility that ligand-activated AhR reactivates EBV. … TCDD enhanced BZLF1 transcription, which mediates the switch from the latent to the lytic form of EBV infection in EBV-positive B cell lines and in a salivary gland epithelial cell line. Moreover, TCDD-induced increases in BZLF1 mRNA and EBV genomic DNA levels were confirmed in the B cell lines. Saliva from SS patients activated the transcription of both CYP1A1 and BZLF1. Additionally, there was a positive correlation between CYP1A1 and BZLF1 promoter activities. AhR ligands elicited the reactivation of EBV in activated B cells and salivary epithelial cells, and these ligands are involved in SS." This is stunning research: it provides direct links between infections, xenobiotic exposure, and autoimmunity; further, by extension, this research also suggests that xenobiotic exposure could also enhance transcription of HERVs (directly, or indirectly via viral transactivation) which also contributes to autoimmunity.

- o Assess for and treat dysbiosis: Insufficient flow of saliva and other fluids promotes microbial colonization of mucosal surfaces, particularly the digestive and respiratory tracts. Gastrointestinal infection/dysbiosis can cause nutrient malabsorption, and the resultant nutritional insufficiencies can exacerbate the sicca symptoms.[1007] Patients with Sjögren's syndrome may have an increased prevalence of infection/colonization with *H. pylori*[1008], an organism known to incite systemic inflammation and to produce pro-inflammatory endotoxin and antigens; eradication of this microbe—or others per patient—may alleviate clinical manifestations by addressing one of the inciting causes. Of particular note is that *H. pylori* promotes gastric autoimmunity, sicca syndrome, as well as intestinal lymphoma—all of which are noted in Sjögren's syndrome.

    - *H pylori* and gastrointestinal cancer: "*H. pylori* infection is a major cause of gastric (stomach) cancer, specifically non-cardia gastric cancer (cancer in all areas of the stomach, except for the top portion near where it joins the esophagus). *H. pylori* infection also causes gastric mucosa-associated lymphoid tissue (MALT) lymphoma. *H. pylori* infection is associated with a decreased risk of some other cancers, including gastric cardia cancer (cancer in the top portion of the stomach) and esophageal adenocarcinoma."[1009]

- **NUTRITIONAL IMMUNOMODULATION: Treg induction for modulation of Th-1/2/17 inflammation**
Nutrients and therapeutic approaches that promote Treg or IL-10 induction and/or Th-17, IL-17 suppression include 1) mitochondrial optimization and mTOR suppression, 2) biotin, 3) vitamin E, 4) sodium avoidance, 5) transgenic/GMO food avoidance, 6) probiotics, 7) lipoic acid, 8) vitamin A, 9) inflammation reduction, 10) vitamin D, 11) fatty acid supplementation with GLA and n3, 12) infection and dysbiosis remediation, 13) green tea EGCG. Acronym: MiBESTPLAIDFIG.

[1004] Onuora S. Connective tissue diseases: Epstein-Barr virus in Sjögren's syndrome salivary glands drives local autoimmunity. *Nat Rev Rheumatol*. 2014 Jul;10(7):384
[1005] Croia et al. Implication of Epstein-Barr Virus Infection in Disease-Specific Autoreactive B Cell Activation in Ectopic Lymphoid Structures of Sjögren's Syndrome. *Arthritis Rheumatol*. 2014 Sep;66(9):2545-57
[1006] Inoue et al. Aryl hydrocarbon receptor-mediated induction of EBV reactivation as a risk factor for Sjögren's syndrome. *J Immunol*. 2012 May 1;188(9):4654-62
[1007] Bosman et al. Sicca syndrome associated with Tropheryma whipplei intestinal infection. *J Clin Microbiol*. 2002 Aug;40(8):3104-6
[1008] "Patients with SS are more prone to have H. pylori infection in comparison to other connective tissue diseases. Serum antibody titer to H. pylori correlated with index for clinical disease manifestations, age, disease duration and CRP." El Miedany et al. Sjogren's syndrome: concomitant H. pylori infection and possible correlation with clinical parameters. *Joint Bone Spine*. 2005 Mar;72(2):135-41
[1009] cancer.gov/cancertopics/factsheet/Risk/h-pylori-cancer

- IL-17-producing T cells are expanded in the peripheral blood, infiltrate salivary glands and are resistant to corticosteroids in patients with primary Sjogren's syndrome (*Ann Rheum Dis*. 2013 Feb[1010]): "It has been recently observed that a T-cell subset, lacking of both CD4 and CD8 molecules and defined as double negative (DN), is expanded in the blood of patients with systemic lupus erythematosus, produces IL-17 and accumulates in the kidney during nephritis. Since IL-17 production is enhanced in salivary gland infiltrates of primary Sjögren's syndrome (SS) patients, we investigated whether DN T cells may be involved in the pathogenesis of salivary gland damage. ... CD3(+)CD4(-)CD8(-) DN T cells were major producers of IL-17 in SS and expressed ROR-γt. They were expanded in the peripheral blood, spontaneously produced IL-17 and infiltrated salivary glands. In addition, the expansion of αβ-TCR(+) DN T cells was associated with disease activity. Notably, IL-17-producing DN T cells from SS patients, but not from healthy controls, were strongly resistant to the in vitro effect of dexamethasone." Readers should by now (following discussion in Chapter 4) appreciate that IL-17 production and tissue infiltration are synonymous with autoimmune-type tissue damage and inflammation.

- **DYSMETABOLISM & DYSFUNCTIONAL MITOCHONDRIA: MitoDys, ERS-UPR, AGE/RAGE, hyperglycemia and ceramide** The major clinical considerations in this section are mitochondrial dysfunction, endoplasmic reticulum stress, unfolded protein response, TLR activation, and the dysmetabolic effects of sustained hyperglycemia and hyperinsulinemia and resultant oxidative stress, inflammation, RAGE activation, and accumulation of AGE, palmitate and ceramide. The review of this information in Chapter 4 covered approximately 30 interventions relevant to dysmetabolism, mitochondrial dysfunction, ERS-UPR, etc; these will not be reviewed here except to mention those most commonly, easily, empirically, synergistically, and effectively used: 1) low-carbohydrate diet with 2) moderate exercise, 3) CoQ-10, 4) acetyl-carnitine with 5) lipoic acid, 6) NAC, 7) resveratrol, and 8) melatonin.

- **STYLE OF LIVING (LIFESTYLE) & SPECIAL CONSIDERATIONS** This is a buffet of mostly lifestyle-based interventions yet also including considerations such as additional supplementation and surgery.
    - Individualized homeopathy: A small randomized placebo-controlled trial found homeopathy beneficial for xerostomia.[1011]
    - Replacement of gastric HCL: Tablets/capsules of betaine HCL may improve digestion, nutrient assimilation, and also alleviate intestinal microbial overgrowth; antiparietal cell antibodies may be noted.

- **ENDOCRINE IMBALANCE & OPTIMIZATION: Prolactin, Insulin, Estrogen, DHEA, Cortisol, Testosterone, Thyroid** Common hormonal imbalances seen among autoimmune/inflammatory patients are: ❶ *elevated* prolactin, ❷ *elevated* estrogen, ❸ *elevated* insulin, and ❹ *reduced* DHEA, ❺ *reduced* cortisol, and ❻ *reduced* testosterone; see Chapter 4 for discussion of these hormones and respective interventions. Thyroid evaluation should be comprehensive, as discussed in Chapter 1, with a low threshold for empiric treatment.
    - Endocrine alterations in primary Sjogren's syndrome (*J Autoimmun*. 2012 Dec[1012]): "Heightened serum and salivary gland tissue prolactin levels in primary SS patients have been also suggested as contributors in disease pathogenesis. Finally, autoimmune thyroid disease (ATD) occurs quiet commonly in the setting of primary SS and subclinical hypothyroidism is the main functional abnormality observed in these patients."
    - DHEA in Sjogren's syndrome—a hormonal deficiency and potential treatment in search of clinical significance: Generally, the finding of low DHEA and the correction/normalization of low DHEA in patients with autoimmunity/inflammation/autoinflammation correlates with clinical improvement; such has not been the situation with Sjogren's syndrome, which has been consistently resistant to improvement following DHEA administration, a fact which I have noted since the first publication of *Integrative Rheumatology* in 2006. I think what is likely here is that the DHEA deficiency is important, but that isolated DHEA supplementation is insufficient to elicit a significant clinical improvement as monotherapy.

[1010] Alunno et al. IL-17-producing CD4-CD8- T cells are expanded in the peripheral blood, infiltrate salivary glands and are resistant to corticosteroids in patients with primary Sjogren's syndrome. *Ann Rheum Dis*. 2013 Feb;72(2):286-92
[1011] "Our results suggest that individually prescribed homeopathic medicine could be a valuable adjunct to the treatment of oral discomfort and xerostomic symptoms." Haila et al. Effects of homeopathic treatment on salivary flow rate and subjective symptoms in patients with oral dryness: a randomized trial. *Homeopathy*. 2005 Jul;94(3):175-81
[1012] Mavragani et al. Endocrine alterations in primary Sjogren's syndrome: an overview. *J Autoimmun*. 2012 Dec;39(4):354-8

- Low serum dehydroepiandrosterone sulfate in women with primary Sjögren's syndrome as an isolated sign of impaired HPA axis function (*J Rheumatol*. 2001 Jun[1013]): "The results show that women with pSS have intact cortisol synthesis but decreased serum concentrations of DHEA-S and increased cortisol/DHEA-S ratio compared with healthy controls. The findings may reflect a constitutional or disease mediated influence on adrenal steroid synthesis. The thyroid axis and gonadotropin secretion were similar in patients and controls."
  - DHEA versus placebo for Sjögren's syndrome (*Arthritis Rheum*. 2004 Aug[1014]): "A 24-week randomized, double-blinded, pilot trial of oral DHEA (200 mg/day) versus placebo was conducted. ... Apart from changes over the trial in dry mouth symptoms, no significant differences were noted between the DHEA and placebo groups for dry eye symptoms, objective measures of ocular dryness, stimulated salivary flow; IgG, or ESR. ... DHEA showed no evidence of efficacy in SS. Without evidence for efficacy, patients with SS should avoid using unregulated DHEA supplements, since long-term adverse consequences of exposure to this hormone are unknown."
  - Dehydroepiandrosterone (DHEA) treatment for severe fatigue in DHEA-deficient patients with primary Sjögren's syndrome (*Arthritis Care Res* 2010 Jan[1015]): "A multicenter, investigator-based, powered, randomized controlled clinical trial (crossover, washout design) using fatigue as the primary outcome measure was performed on patients with primary SS (n = 107) who had a general fatigue score > or =14 on the 20-item Multiple Fatigue Inventory (MFI-20), combined with age- and sex-adjusted serum DHEAS values below the mean. ... Similar to earlier results using pharmacologic doses, substitution treatment with 50 mg of DHEA in DHEA-deficient and severely tired primary SS patients does not help against fatigue better than placebo."

- **XENOBIOTIC ACCUMULATION & DETOXIFICATION: Chemical avoidance, nutritional support for detoxification pathways, urine alkalinization** The clinical relevance and pathogenic mechanisms of xenobiotic accumulation are irrefutably well documented and described. Clinical assessments include history, physical examination, and laboratory assessment (using serum, whole blood, urine or—rarely yet accurately—fat biopsy), and response to treatment. Treatments include nutritional support for Phases 1 and 2 of detoxification (e.g., oxidation and conjugation) and excretion via bile and urine; for the latter, urinary alkalinization is generally recommended. Chemical toxins can be bound in the gut using activated charcoal, cholestyramine, or *Chlorella*—all of these three treatments have documented safety and effectiveness; clinically and empirically, phytochelatin (plant-derived peptides that bind toxic metals) concentrates appear safe and effective despite lack of conclusive published data supporting clinical use.
  - Aryl hydrocarbon receptor-mediated induction of EBV reactivation as a risk factor for Sjögren's syndrome (*J Immunol* 2012 May[1016]): This is very impressive research, connecting xenobiotic exposure with viral reactivation. "The aryl hydrocarbon receptor (AhR) is a ligand-activated transcription factor that mediates a variety of biological effects by binding to environmental pollutants, including 2,3,7,8-tetrachlorodibenzo-p-dioxin (TCDD or dioxin). ... This study evaluated the possibility that ligand-activated AhR reactivates EBV. ... TCDD enhanced BZLF1 transcription, which mediates the switch from the latent to the lytic form of EBV infection in EBV-positive B cell lines and in a salivary gland epithelial cell line. Moreover, TCDD-induced increases in BZLF1 mRNA and EBV genomic DNA levels were confirmed in the B cell lines. Saliva from SS patients activated the transcription of both CYP1A1 and BZLF1. Additionally, there was a positive correlation between CYP1A1 and BZLF1 promoter activities. AhR ligands elicited the reactivation of EBV in activated B cells and salivary epithelial cells, and these ligands are involved in SS." This is stunning research: it provides direct links between infections, xenobiotic exposure, and autoimmunity; further, by extension, this research also suggests that xenobiotic exposure could also enhance transcription of HERVs (directly, or indirectly via viral transactivation) which also contributes to autoimmunity.

[1013] Valtysdóttir et al. Low serum dehydroepiandrosterone sulfate in women with primary Sjögren's syndrome as an isolated sign of impaired HPA axis function. *J Rheumatol.* 2001 Jun;28(6):1259-65
[1014] Pillemer et al. Pilot clinical trial of dehydroepiandrosterone (DHEA) versus placebo for Sjögren's syndrome. *Arthritis Rheum.* 2004 Aug 15;51(4):601-4
[1015] Virkki et al. Dehydroepiandrosterone (DHEA) substitution treatment for severe fatigue in DHEA-deficient patients with primary Sjögren's syndrome. *Arthritis Care Res* (Hoboken). 2010 Jan 15;62(1):118-24
[1016] Inoue et al. Aryl hydrocarbon receptor-mediated induction of EBV reactivation as a risk factor for Sjögren's syndrome. *J Immunol.* 2012 May 1;188(9):4654-62

Raynaud's Phenomenon

> **Introduction:**
> Raynaud's Phenomenon is a disorder of periodic vasoconstriction mainly affecting the hands/fingers; it is a manifestation of autonomic dysfunction associated with and often preceding autoimmune diseases, especially scleroderma. Per the 2010 criteria for fibromyalgia (FM), Raynaud's is now associated with that condition as well; this is utterly absurd except that both Raynaud's and FM are causatively associated with microbial dysbiosis, especially in the intestines, i.e., *Helicobacter pylori* with Raynaud's and SIBO with FM. The condition responds poorly to medical/pharmacologic treatment that focuses on vasodilation; the condition responds very well to integrative treatment, especially that which focuses on dysbiosis eradication, antioxidant supplementation, hormonal correction/supplementation, and other components of the Functional Inflammology protocol.

Introduction and Diagnosis
- Introduction and terminology: Raynaud's phenomenon is periodic recurrent severe vasoconstriction-induced hypoperfusion accompanied by discomfort most commonly affecting the fingers.
  - Primary Raynaud's phenomenon—formerly "Raynaud's disease": Not associated with a concomitant disease; therefore, in this case the vasospasm is considered its own problem, hence the previously used term "disease" when describing primary Raynaud's phenomenon.
  - Secondary Raynaud's phenomenon—formerly "Raynaud's syndrome": Associated with a concomitant disease, especially autoimmunity, especially scleroderma.
- Diagnosis and Evaluation: Assessment for the presence/absence of systemic disease is important; Raynaud's can precede systemic autoimmunity by several years, for example in scleroderma.
  - Digital artery blood pressure: A decrease of > 15 mmHg is consistent with vasoconstriction.
  - Doppler ultrasound: Can be used to measure blood flow.
  - Routine labs: CBC, chemistry/metabolic panel, ANA, CRP, and the full thyroid evaluation in Chapter 1..
  - Nailfold capillaroscopy: Reveals microvascular changes consistent with autoimmunity and autoimmune-expedited cardiovascular disease. Per Cutolo et al[1017], "Raynaud's phenomenon (RP) represents the most frequent clinical aspect of cardio/microvascular involvement and is a key feature of several autoimmune rheumatic diseases. Moreover, RP is associated in a statistically significant manner with many coronary diseases. In normal conditions or in primary RP (excluding during the cold-exposure test), the normal nailfold capillaroscopic pattern shows a regular disposition of the capillary loops along with the nailbed. On the contrary, in subjects suffering from secondary RP, one or more alterations of the capillaroscopic findings should alert the physician of the possibility of a connective tissue disease not yet detected. Nailfold capillaroscopy (NV) represents the best method to analyze microvascular abnormalities in autoimmune rheumatic diseases. Architectural disorganization, giant capillaries, hemorrhages, loss of capillaries, angiogenesis and avascular areas characterize >95% of patients with overt scleroderma (SSc)."
- Complications: Long-term recurrent vasoconstriction can result in atrophy of the skin and subcutaneous tissues including muscle; digital ulceration and ischemic gangrene can result. Recurrent vasospasm-induced tissue hypoxia appears to increase inflammation via oxidative stress and possibly via elaboration of damage-associated molecular patterns.

Clinical Applications and Interventions
- Raynaud's phenomenon—specific treatments: Treatment of Raynaud's phenomenon should not be trivialized as merely symptomatic; the pain experienced by some patients with Raynaud's phenomenon is truly excruciating. Additionally, a wonderfully insightful comment by Simonini et al[1018] in 2000 stated that the tissue ischemia induced by Raynaud's phenomenon is *pathogenic* because it promotes oxidative stress

---

[1017] Cutolo M, Sulli A, Secchi ME, Paolino S, Pizzorni C. Nailfold capillaroscopy is useful for the diagnosis and follow-up of autoimmune rheumatic diseases. A future tool for the analysis of microvascular heart involvement? *Rheumatology* (Oxford). 2006 Oct;45 Suppl 4:iv43-6 rheumatology.oxfordjournals.org/content/45/suppl_4/iv43.full.pdf

[1018] "…daily episodes of hypoxia-reperfusion injury, produces several episodes of free radicals-mediated endothelial derangement. These events results in a positive feedback effect of luminal narrowing and ischemia and therefore to the birth of a vicious cycle of oxygen free radicals (OFR) generation, leading to endothelial damage, intimal thickening and fibrosis." Simonini et al. Emerging potentials for an antioxidant therapy as a new approach to the treatment of systemic sclerosis. *Toxicology*. 2000 Nov 30;155(1-3):1-15 and the vicious cycle of inflammation; the recurrent ischemia and reperfusion of hypoxic Raynaud's phenomenon could be thought of somewhat as a "recurrent, mild heart attack [or stroke] of the hands" causing tissue damage and cell apoptosis/necrosis leading to release of damage-associated molecular patterns (DAMP) and the resultant immune activation, systemic inflammation, mitochondrial dysfunction, proinflammatory immunophenotype switch toward Th1/Th2/Th17 and resultant fibrosis and autoimmunity. Remarkably, Mahoney et al[1019] proposed a similar model in 2011 when they wrote, "We propose that a recent change in the conception of the role of type 1 interferon and the identification of adventitial stem cells suggests a unifying hypothesis for scleroderma. This hypothesis begins with vasospasm. Vasospasm is fully reversible unless, as proposed here, the resulting ischemia leads to apoptosis and activation of type 1 interferon. The interferon, we propose, initiates immune amplification, including characteristic scleroderma-specific antibodies." Thus, treatments to maintain vasodilation and quench the free radicals resultant from recurrent hypoxic events are necessary. Antioxidants have been discussed previously and should be common knowledge to readers of this text. Vasodilation in Raynaud's phenomenon can be supported with any/all of the following:

- Eradication of *Helicobacter pylori*: Eradication of *Helicobacter pylori* is one of the most effective treatments of Raynaud's disease/syndrome/phenomenon and should therefore be pursued in all affected patients.
    - Helicobacter pylori eradication ameliorates primary Raynaud's phenomenon (*Dig Dis Sci* 1998 Aug[1020]): "Forty-six patients affected by primary Raynaud's phenomenon were evaluated. *H. pylori* infection was assessed by [13C]urea breath test. Eradication therapy was given to infected patients for seven days. … **Attacks of Raynaud's phenomenon completely disappeared in 17% of the patients with *H. pylori* eradication. Discomfort and the duration and frequency of attacks of Raynaud's phenomenon were significantly reduced in 72% of the remaining patients.** … The study shows that *H. pylori* eradication causes a significant decrease in clinical attacks of Raynaud's disease. The reduction of vasoactive substances determined by the eradication of the bacterium may be the pathogenetic mechanism underlying the phenomenon."
- Inositol hexaniacinate: 3,000-4,000 mg/d *po* in divided doses[1021,1022,1023]
- *Ginkgo biloba*: Ginkgo reduces the number of daily Raynaud's attacks in patients with primary Raynaud's disease[1024], and it is also an excellent antioxidant with potent anti-inflammatory benefits.
- Magnesium: 300-500 mg/d or bowel tolerance; systemic alkalinization to achieve urine alkalinity of 7.5 promotes renal retention of magnesium and systemic cellular uptake.
- Combination fatty acid therapy: must include GLA (minimum 500 mg) and EPA (minimum 2,000 mg)
- L-arginine: L-arginine is the biochemical precursor to nitric oxide, which has vasodilating actions. L-arginine supplementation in patients with Raynaud's phenomenon showed benefit in one study[1025] and no benefit in another.[1026] However, arginine supplementation was tremendously beneficial in 4 case reports of scleroderma patients with Raynaud's-induced digital necrosis.[1027] Excess arginine supplementation may lead to an overproduction of nitric oxide, which can be harmful in excess due to its free radical behavior and its contribution to peroxynitrite. Additionally, metabolism of arginine requires methyl groups, and therefore supplementation with methyl donors such as

---

[1019] Mahoney et al. A unifying hypothesis for scleroderma: identifying a target cell for scleroderma. *Curr Rheumatol Rep*. 2011 Feb;13:28-36
[1020] Gasbarrini A et al. Helicobacter pylori eradication ameliorates primary Raynaud's phenomenon. *Dig Dis Sci*. 1998 Aug;43(8):1641-5
[1021] "It appears to be a safe and well tolerated drug, which, together with other symptomatic measures, merits to be used in the management of vasospastic disease of the extremities even in the presence of partial obliteration of the microcirculation." Holti G. An experimentally controlled evaluation of the effect of inositol nicotinate upon the digital blood flow in patients with Raynaud's phenomenon. *J Int Med Res*. 1979;7(6):473-83
[1022] "Although the mechanism of action remains unclear Hexopal is safe and is effective in reducing the vasospasm of primary Raynaud's disease during the winter months." Sunderland et al. A double blind randomised placebo controlled trial of hexopal in primary Raynaud's disease. *Clin Rheumatol*. 1988 Mar;7(1):46-9
[1023] "It is suggested that long-term treatment with nicotinate acid derivatives may produce improvement in the peripheral circulation by a different mechanism than the transient effect detected by short-term studies." Ring et al. Quantitative thermographic assessment of inositol nicotinate therapy in Raynaud's phenomena. J Int Med Res. 1977;5(4):217-22
[1024] "Ginkgo biloba phytosome may be effective in reducing the number of Raynaud's attacks per week in patients suffering from Raynaud's disease." Muir et al. The use of Ginkgo biloba in Raynaud's disease: a double-blind placebo-controlled trial. *Vasc Med*. 2002;7(4):265-7
[1025] "After therapy, patients with Raynaud's phenomenon secondary to systemic sclerosis showed: (1) higher digital vasodilation after local warming, (2) cold-induced digital vasodilation, and (3) increase of plasma levels of tissue-type plasminogen activator." Agostoni A, Marasini B, Biondi ML, Bassani C, Cazzaniga A, Bottasso B, Cugno M. L-arginine therapy in Raynaud's phenomenon? *Int J Clin Lab Res*. 1991;21(2):202-3
[1026] "L-arginine supplementation, however, had no significant effect on vascular responses to acetylcholine and sodium nitroprusside." Khan F, Belch JJ. Skin blood flow in patients with systemic sclerosis and Raynaud's phenomenon: effects of oral L-arginine supplementation. *J Rheumatol*. 1999 Nov;26(11):2389-94
[1027] "We report two cases in which oral L-arginine reversed digital necrosis in Raynaud's phenomenon and two additional cases in which the symptoms of severe Raynaud's phenomenon were improved with oral L-arginine." Rembold et al. Oral L-arginine can reverse digital necrosis in Raynaud's phenomenon. *Mol Cell Biochem*. 2003 Feb;244:139-41

methylfolate/folinate, cobalamin, betaine, et al should be used anytime supplemental arginine is used for long periods of time; homocysteine levels should occasionally be measured.
- NAC 500-1,500mg *po tid ic*: NAC is pleiotropically beneficial, via antiviral, antioxidant, GSH-supporting, and mTOR inhibiting actions.
  - Intravenous N-acetylcysteine for treatment of Raynaud's phenomenon secondary to systemic sclerosis (*J Rheumatol* 2001 Oct[1028])—paraphrased/quoted as follows: "Twenty-two patients with RP secondary to SSc were enrolled in a multicenter, open clinical trial lasting 11 weeks and conducted in winter. Primary outcome measures were frequency and severity of RP attacks, and number of digital ulcers. Secondary outcome measure was improvement in digital cold challenge test assessed by photoelectric plethysmography. Patients received a continuous 5 day intravenous infusion of NAC starting with a 2 h loading dose of 150 mg/kg subsequently adjusted to 15 mg/kg/h. RESULTS: … Both frequency and severity of RP attacks decreased significantly compared to pretreatment values. Active ulcers were significantly less numerous at all follow-up visits (25% of baseline count on Day 33 from the beginning of infusion). In the cold challenge test, mean recovery time fell by 69%, 67%, 71%, and 71% on Days 12, 19, 33, and 61 from the beginning of treatment. Side effects were minor, easily controlled, and reversible. CONCLUSION: N-acetylcysteine appears to be safe for the treatment of RP secondary to SSc. These preliminary data warrant further controlled studies."
- Acupuncture, biofeedback, counseling, stress reduction, cold avoidance, smoking cessation: Since stressful events, cold exposure, and cigarette smoking are all vasoconstrictive, these should be avoided/modified to the highest extent possible. Stress reduction and modification of inter- and intra-personal socioemotional exchange would be beneficial for anyone.
  - Freedman et al. Biofeedback treatment of Raynaud's disease and phenomenon (*Biofeedback Self Regul.* 1981 Sep[1029]): "Six Raynaud's disease [primary] and four Raynaud's phenomenon [secondary] patients were treated with 12 sessions of finger temperature biofeedback. The mean frequency of vasospastic attacks was reduced to 7.5% of that reported during the pretreatment baseline and was maintained for a 1 year follow-up period. … Raynaud's phenomenon [secondary] patients showed significantly greater temperature increases during feedback periods than Raynaud's disease [primary] patients."
- Hormonal interventions: Annotated below:
  - Treatment of Raynaud's phenomenon with large doses of triiodothyronine [T3] (*Ann Rheum Dis.* 1987 Dec[1030]): Triiodothyronine was prescribed at a dosage of 80 mcg/d to 9 female patients with autoimmunity (SLE, SSc, RA, overlap syndrome [OS]); they all experienced safe and significant remission of their Raynaud's symptoms. Patients who could not tolerate 80 mcg/d due to anticipated heat intolerance and palpitations were treated with lower doses of 40-60 mcg/d. "In all patients, blood pressure, pulse pressure, and pulse rate remained essentially unchanged and thyroid function tests were confirmatory of drug compliance. … In the first place, every one of them described a substantial, if not dramatic, improvement in their condition. … Large dosages of T3 were found in this study to be a highly effective treatment for Raynaud's phenomenon and one principally free from side effects."
  - Treatment of Raynaud's phenomenon with triiodothyronine [T3] corrects co-existent autonomic dysfunction (*Postgrad Med J* 1992 Apr[1031]): Nine female patients with autoimmunity and Raynaud's phenomenon showed a high prevalence of cardiovascular autonomic dysfunction as assessed by five standard non-invasive tests (3 of heart rate and 2 of blood pressure). "The subjects were given triiodothyronine, 60 to 80 micrograms per day, for vasospastic attacks. … Test results [of autonomic function] showed a considerable improvement. … Adverse side effects to triiodothyronine occurred in a single subject and were readily controlled. … Triiodothyronine may have corrected autonomic

---

[1028] Sambo et al. Intravenous N-acetylcysteine for treatment of Raynaud's phenomenon secondary to systemic sclerosis: a pilot study. *J Rheumatol*. 2001 Oct;28(10):2257-62
[1029] Freedman et al. Biofeedback treatment of Raynaud's disease and phenomenon. *Biofeedback Self Regul*. 1981 Sep;6(3):355-65
[1030] Dessein PH, Gledhill RF. Treatment of Raynaud's phenomenon with large doses of triiodothyronine: a pilot study. *Ann Rheum Dis*. 1987 Dec;46(12):944-5
[1031] Gledhill et al. Treatment of Raynaud's phenomenon with triiodothyronine corrects co-existent autonomic dysfunction. *Postgrad Med J*. 1992 Apr;68(798):263-7

dysfunction by increasing blood flow to ischemic peripheral nerves or by acting on the autonomic system more directly."

- Successful treatment of Raynaud's phenomenon with L-thyroxine [T4] (*Med Hypotheses* 2003 Mar[1032]): "A 50-year old patient a 15-year history of Raynaud's phenomenon developed thyroid deficiency with exacerbation of the symptoms of Raynaud's. After substitution therapy with L-thyroxine, the patient became euthyroid and the symptoms of Raynaud's phenomenon disappeared. Similarly, several patients with Raynaud's phenomenon were found to be hypothyroid and replacement therapy again eliminated the symptoms."
- 7-oxo-DHEA contra Raynaud's phenomenon (*Med Hypotheses* 2003 Mar[1033]): The authors of this report basically provide a review of the literature on Raynaud's phenomenon—its assessments and treatments—and then provide a single case report of improvement; the dose and duration of treatment are not provided. "An initial result is encouraging. A 46-year old patient had increasingly frequent vasospastic attacks accompanied by pain and pallor in her left fingers except the thumb. Precipitating factors included being in an excessively air-conditioned environment, touching cold objects, and digging in cold, wet earth. The episodes were less than 10 min duration. The patient had no other complaints, denied other illnesses, and does not take any prescription medications. The patient does not smoke, and consumes minimal amounts of alcohol occasionally. On examination, her hands were without any abnormalities with normal skin and color appearance. These vasospastic attacks did not occur after taking 7-oxo-DHEA but returned within one week of discontinuing the medication, and disappeared again on resuming the medication." Obviously that is a pretty weak case report, but nonetheless, clinicians might consider using this generally considered as safe nonprescription agent in conjunction with the treatments aforementioned.

Lago Azul (Blue Lake) near Villa de Leyva, Colombia: 2014, photo by DrV

[1032] Ihler et al. 7-oxo-DHEA and Raynaud's phenomenon. *Med Hypotheses.* 2003 Mar;60(3):391-7
[1033] Ihler et al. 7-oxo-DHEA and Raynaud's phenomenon. *Med Hypotheses.* 2003 Mar;60(3):391-7

Do the Benefits of Botanical and Physiotherapeutic Hepatobiliary Stimulation Result From Enhanced Excretion of IgA Immune Complexes?

This article was originally published in *Naturopathy Digest* 2006
InflammationMastery.com/reprints/2006IgAhepatobiliary.html

Antigen-IgA complexes are phagocytized by hepatocytes and delivered largely intact directly into the bile. This is the most efficient means of disposing of antigens resistant to hydrolytic degradation due either to their size or physiochemical configuration. IgA immune complexes are taken up by hepatocytes and then secreted into the bile for elimination. The fact that bile duct obstruction retards systemic clearance of IgA immune complexes and that restoration of bile flow reduces serum IgA levels by enhancing biliary IgA excretion in animals and humans proves the importance of ensuring optimal hepatobiliary function and supports the use of botanical and physiological therapeutics that facilitate bile flow. Evidence from journals such as the *Archives of Internal Medicine* suggests the primary physiotherapeutic intervention for the stimulation of bile flow is the enema. Enemas are differentiated from colonics in that enemas generally are delivered as a single insertion of water with a modest volume (generally 1-2 quarts [1-2 liters]), whereas colonics generally employ numerous insertions and removals of water, the total volume of which might exceed several gallons (>4-8 liters). Relatedly, the purpose of an enema is to stimulate normal function, while colonics are used to mechanically cleanse the bowel of debris in a manner analogous to the removal of dirt by hand-washing under running water. Colon irrigations were endorsed by the American Medical Association for the adjunctive treatment of numerous health problems as late as 1932, when Bastedo published a review in *Journal of the American Medical Association* endorsing and encouraging their use. In that same year, the *New England Journal of Medicine* documented the value of colon irrigation in the treatment of mental disease. In 1939, Snyder wrote a review article published in the prestigious *Medical Clinics of North America* in which he extolled the clinical benefits of colonics and enemas and lamented the decline in their use, which he attributed to doctors and nurses not having the time or inclination to administer the procedure.

Treatments to reduce the adverse effects of autoantibodies and immune complexes: a conceptual overview with interventional considerations

Goal	Strategic means	Technical means
Reduce *de novo* formation of autoantibodies	→ Biological immunomodulation	→ Orthoendocrinology, particularly supraphysiologic DHEA supplementation → Anti-inflammatory hypoallergenic diet → Anti-inflammatory nutrition: ALA, GLA, EPA, DHA, cholecalciferol, antioxidants, NF-kappaB inhibitors, and anti-inflammatory botanicals → Xenobiotic detoxification
	→ Pharmacologic immunosuppression	→ Prednisone and other corticosteroids → Antibiologics such as hydroxychloroquine which exert their clinical benefits via interfering with normal immunologic function, not by improving overall health or addressing underlying etiologic factors
	→ Removal/correction of primary stimuli for antibody formation *per patient*	→ Orthoendocrinology → Xenobiotic detoxification → Mitochondrial resuscitation → Antidysbiotic interventions: assessment and correction of multifocal dysbiosis
Reduce effects of autoantibodies	→ Anti-inflammatory treatments	→ Anti-inflammatory nutrition: ALA, GLA, EPA, DHA, cholecalciferol, antioxidants, NF-kappaB inhibitors, and anti-inflammatory botanicals

Treatments to reduce the adverse effects of autoantibodies and immune complexes: a conceptual overview with interventional considerations—*continued*

Goal	Strategic means	Technical means
Reduce effects of autoantibodies —*continued*	→ Proteolytic enzymes	→ Proteolytic/pancreatic enzymes appear to reduce *de novo* formation of immune complexes
Enhance clearance of autoantibodies	→ Allopathic interventions	→ Immunoadsorption[1034] → Plasmapheresis[1035,1036]
	→ Naturopathic interventions (theoretical[1037])	→ Choleretic and cholagogic botanicals: beets, ginger[1038], curcumin[1039], *Picrorhiza*[1040], milk thistle[1041], *Andrographis paniculata*[1042] and *Boerhaavia diffusa*.[1043] → Low-volume enemas[1044]

Multifocal Dysbiosis: Pathophysiology, Relevance for Inflammatory and Autoimmune Diseases, and Treatment With Nutritional and Botanical Interventions

This article was originally published in Naturopathy Digest *2006*
InflammationMastery.com/reprints/2006dysbiosis.html

At least 70 percent of patients with chronic arthritis are carriers of "silent infections," according to a 1992 article published in the peer-reviewed medical journal *Annals of the Rheumatic Diseases*. A 2001 article in that same journal which focused exclusively on five bacteria showed that 56 percent of patients with idiopathic inflammatory arthritis had gastrointestinal or genitourinary dysbiosis. Indeed, published research strongly and consistently indicates that bacteria, yeast/fungi, amoebas, protozoa, and other "parasites" (rarely including helminths/worms) are underappreciated causes of neuromusculoskeletal inflammation. In my own clinical practice, gastrointestinal dysbiosis is so common in patients with autoimmune/inflammatory disorders that I consider all of these patients to have dysbiosis until proven otherwise. We perform stool testing with a specialty laboratory, and I am rarely "disappointed" with the finding of normal stool analysis and parasitology. Overall, including patients without autoimmune/inflammatory disorders, I estimate that in my practice, approximately 80 percent of stool and parasitology examinations return with at least one clinically relevant abnormality that, when corrected, provides either subjective or objective improvement in the patient's primary complaint. My experience is consistent with that of other authors and researchers, who note a prevalence of dysbiosis in the range of 70 percent to 100 percent in patients with inflammatory disorders. Recognizing the need to appreciate and transcend the contributions by Koch and Pasture, I've defined dysbiosis as "a relationship of non-acute non-infectious host-microorganism interaction that adversely affects the human host." When used without additional specification, the term "dysbiosis" generally is meant to imply "gastrointestinal dysbiosis." However, as research has continued to progress in this arena, clinicians are now obligated to appreciate the concept of "multifocal dysbiosis" because patients might have dysbiosis in extra-intestinal sites, namely their skin, mouth, sinuses, respiratory tract, genitourinary tract, surrounding environment, and parenchymal tissues. We might reasonably describe multifocal dysbiosis as "a clinical condition characterized by a patient's simultaneously having more than one foci/location of dysbiosis;

[1034] Braun et al. Immunoadsorption onto protein A induces remission in severe systemic lupus erythematosus. *Nephrol Dial Transplant*. 2000 Sep;15(9):1367-72
[1035] Santos-Ocampo AS, Mandell BF, Fessler BJ. Alveolar hemorrhage in systemic lupus erythematosus: presentation and management. *Chest*. 2000 Oct;118(4):1083-90
[1036] Choi BG, Yoo WH. Successful treatment of pure red cell aplasia with plasmapheresis in a patient with systemic lupus erythematosus. *Yonsei Med J*. 2002 Apr;4):274-8
[1037] Vasquez A. Do Benefits of Botanical and Physiotherapeutic Hepatobiliary Stimulation Result From Enhanced Excretion of IgA Immune Complexes? *Naturo Digest* 2006 Jan
[1038] "Further analyses for the active constituents of the acetone extracts through column chromatography indicated that [6]-gingerol and [10]-gingerol, which are the pungent principles, are mainly responsible for the cholagogic effect of ginger." Yamahara et al. Cholagogic effect of ginger and its active constituents. *J Ethnopharmacol*. 1985;13:217-25
[1039] "On the basis of the present findings, it appears that curcumin induces contraction of the human gall-bladder." Rasyid A, Lelo A. The effect of curcumin and placebo on human gall-bladder function: an ultrasound study. *Aliment Pharmacol Ther*. 1999 Feb;13(2):245-9
[1040] "Significant anticholestatic activity was also observed against carbon tetrachloride induced cholestasis in conscious rat, anaesthetized guinea pig and cat. Picroliv was more active than the known hepatoprotective drug silymarin." Saraswat B, Visen PK, Patnaik GK, Dhawan BN. Anticholestatic effect of picroliv, active hepatoprotective principle of Picrorhiza kurrooa, against carbon tetrachloride induced cholestasis. *Indian J Exp Biol*. 1993 Apr;31(4):316-8
[1041] Crocenzi et al. Preventive effect of silymarin against taurolithocholate-induced cholestasis in the rat. *Biochem Pharmacol*. 2003 Jul 15;66(2):355-64
[1042] Shukla B, Visen PK, Patnaik GK, Dhawan BN. Choleretic effect of andrographolide in rats and guinea pigs. *Planta Med*. 1992 Apr;58(2):146-9
[1043] Chandan BK, Sharma AK, Anand KK. Boerhaavia diffusa: a study of its hepatoprotective activity. *J Ethnopharmacol*. 1991 Mar;31(3):299-307
[1044] Garbat AL, Jacobi HG. Secretion of Bile in Response to Rectal Installations. *Arch Intern Med* 1929; 44: 455-462

generally the adverse physiologic and clinical consequences are additive and synergistic." Although different foci of dysbiosis generally require different types of treatment (e.g., oral versus topical versus environmental), the pathophysiologic mechanisms and clinical consequences are largely identical. Thus, sinorespiratory dysbiosis or genitourinary dysbiosis can be just as devastating as gastrointestinal dysbiosis, and therefore requires appropriate clinical consideration, particularly in patients with autoimmune/inflammatory disorders such as lupus, rheumatoid arthritis, psoriasis, polymyositis, ankylosing spondylitis, and various types of vasculitis.

Dysbiotic Emphases and Therapeutic Prioritization and Contextualization

With the concepts and data that I have presented in Chapters 1, 4, and here in 5, readers are hopefully gaining an appreciation of 1) the great importance of dysbiosis in inflammatory and autoimmune disorders, and 2) the relative importance of the various types and combinations of dysbiosis that are more compellingly implicated in various conditions. Hopefully, clinicians will also not lose sight of the fact that patient-specific variations on these themes clearly exist; yet despite the importance of patient specificity and biochemical individuality, clear patterns do exist, and I have roughly represented these emphases and relationships in the image that follows. Again, clear delineations are impossible in complex living systems affected simultaneously by all of these (and other) variables.

Dysbiotic emphases in various disease states: A rough estimates based on overview of research literature and clinical experience; my hope is that readers will appreciate the disease-specific information presented in this book within its disease-specific context and then break free from that context to see how the information applies to other diseases generally and individual patients specifically.

Excerpt from _Chiropractic and Naturopathic Mastery of Common Clinical Disorders_ (2009):
Research and Biologic Support for a Dietary and (Phyto)Nutritional Antiviral Protocol—Excerpt added *In Press*

To access the information in this section, readers will have to indulge the time lapse and evolution of style

Therapeutic and Interventional Considerations for Use in Patients *with* and *Who Wish to Avoid* Viral Infections: Clinicians can use any combination of safe noncontraindicated nutrients, botanicals, and dietary modifications to support immune function and the clearance or amelioration of acute or chronic viral infections. These treatments are listed by the current author's preference, with appreciation for naturopathy's hierarchy of therapeutics, and/or by the level of available evidence (i.e., clinical trials over in vitro studies), given the current healthcare trend in favor of evidence-based medicine. General benefits derived from the use of immunonutrition are reductions in severity/frequency/duration of major infections, abbreviated hospitalization (i.e., early discharge due to expedited healing and recovery), reductions in the need for medications, significant improvements in survival, and hospital savings.[1045,1046,1047,1048,1049,1050,1051] Doses listed here and throughout this book are for adults unless otherwise specified. Doctors are expected to use these interventions in combination, with individual nutrients and doses customized for each patient.

> **Perspective & Context**
> Although these interventional considerations are presented in the context of the treatment and prevention of acute and chronic viral infections, several of these treatments are also applicable to bacterial and fungal infections as well. Viral infections are chosen as the emphasis of this chapter because of their enigmatic nature, their high frequency, and the documented inefficacy and high costs of "medical" treatments. This review is also intended to be practical (rather than exhaustive, and exhausting) so that clinicians can focus on the most established and accessible treatments.

- **Paleo-Mediterranean Diet**: The health-promoting diet of choice for the majority of people is a diet based on abundant consumption of fruits, vegetables, seeds, nuts, omega-3 and monounsaturated fatty acids, and lean sources of protein such as lean meats, fatty cold-water fish, soy and whey proteins. This diet prohibits and obviates overconsumption of chemical preservatives, artificial sweeteners, and carbohydrate-dominant foods such as candies, pastries, breads, potatoes, grains, and other foods with a high glycemic load and high glycemic index. This "Paleo-Mediterranean Diet" is a combination of the "Paleolithic" or "Paleo diet" and the well-known "Mediterranean diet", both of which are well described in peer-reviewed journals and the lay press. The Mediterranean diet is characterized by increased proportions of legumes, nuts, seeds, whole grain products, fruits, vegetables (including potatoes), fish and lean meats, and monounsaturated and n-3 fatty acids.[1052] Consumption of this diet is consistently associated with improvements in insulin sensitivity and

> **Importance of Whole-Foods Nutrition**
> "Given the increased micronutrient requirements, **nutrition counseling with HIV-infected youths should focus on early increase of intake of foods rich in micronutrients** to improve growth, slow disease progression, and increase survival. ... Young patients with HIV are at highest risk of being deficient in vitamins A and E and zinc."
>
> Kruzich et al. US youths in the early stages of HIV disease have low intakes of some micronutrients important for optimal immune function. *J Am Diet Assoc.* 2004 Jul

---

[1045] "To evaluate the metabolic and immune effects of dietary arginine, glutamine and omega-3 fatty acids (fish oil) supplementation, we performed a prospective study... CONCLUSIONS: The feeding of Neomune in critically injured patients was well tolerated as Traumacal and significant improvement was observed in serum protein. Shorten ICU stay and wean-off respirator day may benefit from using the immunonutrition formula." Chuntrasakul et al. Comparison of a immunonutrition formula enriched arginine, glutamine and omega-3 fatty acid, with a currently high-enriched enteral nutrition for trauma patients. *J Med Assoc Thai.* 2003 Jun;86(6):552-6

[1046] "CONCLUSIONS: In conclusion, arginine-enhanced formula improves fistula rates in postoperative head and neck cancer patients and decreases length of stay." de Luis et al. Randomized clinical trial with an enteral arginine-enhanced formula in early postsurgical head and neck cancer patients. *Eur J Clin Nutr.* 2004;58(11):1505-8

[1047] "In this prospective, randomised, double-blind, placebo-controlled study, we randomly assigned 50 patients who were scheduled to undergo coronary artery bypass to receive either an oral immune-enhancing nutritional supplement containing L-arginine, omega3 polyunsaturated fatty acids, and yeast RNA (n=25), or a control (n=25) for a minimum of 5 days... Intake of an oral immune-enhancing nutritional supplement for a minimum of 5 days before surgery can improve outlook in high-risk patients who are undergoing elective cardiac surgery." Tepaske et al. Effect of preoperative oral immune-enhancing nutritional supplement on patients at high risk of infection after cardiac surgery: a randomised placebo-controlled trial. *Lancet.* 2001 Sep 1;358(9283):696-701

[1048] "The feeding of IMMUNE FORMULA was well tolerated and significant improvement was observed in nutritional and immunologic parameters as in other immunoenhancing diets. Further clinical trials of prospective double-blind randomized design are necessary to address the so that the necessity of using immunonutrition in critically ill patients will be clarified." Chuntrasakul et al. Metabolic and immune effects of dietary arginine, glutamine and omega-3 fatty acids supplementation in immunocompromised patients. *J Med Assoc Thai.* 1998 May;81(5):334-43

[1049] "enteral diet supplemented with arginine, dietary nucleotides, and omega-3 fatty acids (IMPACT, Sandoz Nutrition, Bern, Switzerland)" Senkal et al. Early postoperative enteral immunonutrition: clinical outcome and cost-comparison analysis in surgical patients. *Crit Care Med* 1997;25(9):1489-96

[1050] "...supplemented diet with glutamine, arginine and omega-3-fatty acids... It was clearly established in this trial that early postoperative enteral feeding is safe in patients who have undergone major operations for gastrointestinal cancer. Supplementation of enteral nutrition with glutamine, arginine, and omega-3-fatty acids positively modulated postsurgical immunosuppressive and inflammatory responses." Wu et al. Modulation of postoperative immune and inflammatory response by immune-enhancing enteral diet in gastrointestinal cancer patients. *World J Gastroenterol.* 2001 Jun;7(3):357-62 wjgnet.com/1007-9327/7/357.pdf

[1051] "using a formula supplemented with arginine, mRNA, and omega-3 fatty acids from fish oil (Impact)... CONCLUSIONS: Immune-enhancing enteral nutrition resulted in a significant reduction in the mortality rate and infection rate in septic patients admitted to the ICU. These reductions were greater for patients with less severe illness." Galban et al. An immune-enhancing enteral diet reduces mortality rate and episodes of bacteremia in septic intensive care unit patients. *Crit Care Med.* 2000 Mar;28(3):643-8

[1052] Curtis et al. Understanding the Mediterranean diet. Could this be the new "gold standard" for heart disease prevention? *Postgrad Med.* 2002 Aug;112(2):35-8, 41-5 reductions in cardiovascular disease, diabetes, cancer, and all-cause mortality.[1053] The Paleolithic diet detailed by collaborators Eaton, O'Keefe, and Cordain[1054] is similar to the Mediterranean diet except for stronger emphasis on fruits and vegetables (preferably raw or minimally cooked), omega-3-rich lean meats, and reduced consumption of starchy foods such as potatoes and grains, the latter of which were not staples in the human diet until the last few thousand years. The current author expects that habitual consumption of this Paleo-Mediterranean Diet is immunosupportive/immunoempowering due to both ❶ increased intake of micronutrients, phytonutrients, and the alkalinizing pro-homeostatic benefits in addition to ❷ avoidance of nutrient-poor high-carbohydrate high-fat foods which are immunosuppressive and pro-inflammatory. Given that the pro-inflammatory effect of high-carbohydrate and/or high-fat foods is mediated at least in part via NFkB, and that NFkB stimulation is important for viral replication, we can easily see how a high-carbohydrate high-fat diet can promote viral replication by enhancing activity of NFkB. High-carbohydrate diets deal a double-punch to the human host; first, consumption of a high-carbohydrate load causes immunosuppression, and then secondly the high-carbohydrate load promotes activation of NFkB which then promotes viral replication. Although raw fruits and vegetables have—by definition and virtue of their "rawness"—not been exposed to the potentially near-sterilizing heat of cooking, the bacterial loads of raw fruit and vegetable consumption do not appear to present a risk to immunosuppressed patients[1055,1056], even though such patients should not take undue culinary risks. The Mediterranean diet has shown unparalleled safety and efficacy in the prevention of cardiovascular disease, cancer, and all-cause mortality; its specific application in reducing the burden of infectious diseases has not been adequately studied in clinical trials, other than by the indirect inference that a reduction in all-cause mortality by the Mediterranean diet implies a reduction in infection-related mortality. Absence of *direct* evidence is not *direct* evidence of absence. We must also appreciate that diet-and-lifestyle studies are much more complicated to implement than are "pill-based" studies; diet and lifestyle interventions reflect the complexity of human physiology and are thus at odds with the medical model of single-intervention double-blind clinical trials.

- o <u>Negative effects of the standard American diet (SAD): Increase in intranuclear nuclear factor kappaB and decrease in inhibitor kappaB in mononuclear cells after a mixed meal</u>: Consumption of the standard American diet (SAD) causes oxidative stress, systemic inflammation, and activation of NFkB; clinicians must appreciate that each of these three adverse effects leads to a biochemical milieu that supports the development and perpetuation of infections, particularly viral infections. Subjects in this study consumed an egg-muffin and sausage-muffin sandwiches and 2 hash browns, which contained 81 g carbohydrate, 51 g fat, and 32 g protein "RESULTS: ROS generation by mononuclear cells and polymorphonuclear leukocytes and p47(phox) expression increased significantly. The expression of IKKalpha and IKKbeta and DNA-binding activity of NF-kappaB increased significantly, whereas IkappaBalpha expression decreased. Plasma CRP concentrations increased. The intake of 300 mL water did not induce a change in any of the above indexes. CONCLUSIONS: These data show that the intake of a mixed meal results in significant inflammatory changes characterized by a decrease in IkappaBalpha and an increase in NF-kappaB binding, plasma CRP, and the expression of IKKalpha, IKKbeta, and p47(phox) subunit. These proinflammatory changes are probably relevant to the state of chronic hypertension and obesity and to its association with atherosclerosis."[1057] Thus, some of the benefit of the Paleo-Mediterranean diet comes not only from the inherent benefits of the diet itself, but also from the avoidance of the negative effects of the SAD eating pattern that is typical in industrialized nations.
- o <u>Negative effects of glucose ingestion: Glucose ingestion induces an increase in intranuclear nuclear factor kappaB, a fall in cellular inhibitor kappaB, and an increase in tumor necrosis factor alpha messenger RNA by mononuclear cells in healthy human subjects</u>: Subjects in this study received glucose ingestion

---

[1053] Knoops et al. Mediterranean diet, lifestyle factors, and 10-year mortality in elderly European men and women: the HALE project. *JAMA*. 2004 Sep 22;292(12):1433-9
[1054] Cordain L, Eaton SB, Sebastian A, Mann N, Lindeberg S, Watkins BA, O'Keefe JH, Brand-Miller J. Origins and evolution of the Western diet: health implications for the 21st century. *Am J Clin Nutr*. 2005 Feb;81(2):341-54
[1055] "No clear evidence exists that the neutropenic diet makes a difference in overall rates of infection." DeMille et al. The effect of the neutropenic diet in the outpatient setting: a pilot study. *Oncol Nurs Forum*. 2006 Nov 3;33(2):337-43
[1056] "CONCLUSION: In patients treated in a [protected environment], a neutropenic diet did not prevent major infection or death." Gardner et al. Randomized comparison of cooked and noncooked diets in patients undergoing remission induction therapy for acute myeloid leukemia. *J Clin Oncol*. 2008 Dec 10;26(35):5684-8
[1057] Aljada et al. Increase in intranuclear nuclear factor kappaB and decrease in inhibitor kappaB in mononuclear cells after a mixed meal. *Am J Clin Nutr*. 2004 Apr;79(4):682-90

consistent with normal dietary habits: 300 kcal (75 g) glucose in water (300 mL). Results showed that 300 kcal of glucose causes NFkB activation, systemic inflammation, and increased expression of pro-inflammatory TNF-alpha. Clinicians should appreciate that many of the new drugs for rheumatic diseases specifically target TNF-alpha. "We conclude that glucose intake induces an immediate increase in intranuclear NF-kappaB binding, a fall in IkappaBalpha, an increase in IKKalpha, IKKbeta, IKK activity, and messenger RNA expression of TNF-alpha in MNCs (mononuclear cells) in healthy subjects. These data are consistent with profound acute pro-inflammatory changes in MNCs after glucose intake."[1058] When patients overconsume simple carbohydrates several times per day, they are inducing a clinically significant oxidative stress and pro-inflammatory state several times per day that lasts for several hours. Thus, by following the SAD eating pattern and lifestyle, patients unwittingly cause in themselves the oxidative stress and pro-inflammatory milieu that predisposes them toward diseases in general and acute and chronic viral infections in particular; additional details to follow.

- Review: Acute hyperglycemia adversely impacts the innate immune system: "The most obvious findings related to hyperglycemia included reduced neutrophil activity (e.g., chemotaxis, formation of reactive oxygen species, phagocytosis of bacteria), despite accelerated diapedesis of leukocytes into peripheral tissue, as well as specific alterations of cytokine patterns with increased concentrations of the early proinflammatory cytokines tumor necrosis factor-alpha and interleukin-6. Furthermore, a reduction of endothelial nitric oxide formation takes place, thus decreasing microvascular reactivity to dilating agents such as bradykinin, and complement function (e.g., opsonization, chemotaxis) is impaired, despite elevations of certain complement factors. CONCLUSIONS: Acute, short-term hyperglycemia affects all major components of innate immunity and impairs the ability of the host to combat infection."[1059]

- Cohort study of the Mediterranean diet in elderly humans: "Among individuals aged 70 to 90 years, adherence to a Mediterranean diet and healthful lifestyle is associated with a more than 50% lower rate of all-causes and cause-specific mortality."[1060] The Mediterranean diet has shown unparalleled safety and efficacy in the prevention of cardiovascular disease, cancer, and all-cause mortality; its specific application in reducing the burden of infectious diseases has not been adequately studied in clinical trials, other than by the indirect inference that a reduction in all-cause mortality by the Mediterranean diet implies a reduction in infection-related mortality.

- Cross-sectional study: "HIV-infected youths may have increased micronutrient needs related to impaired immune function and metabolic complications of the disease. Dietitians and health care professionals should focus on setting individualized behavioral goals with HIV-infected youths, emphasizing foods rich in micronutrients early in the infection."[1061]

- Cross-sectional study in 285 adolescent boys and girls aged 13 to 17 years: In this study, serologic markers of inflammation and oxidative stress were correlated with dietary intake. Urinary F(2)-isoprostane (a combined marker for inflammation, oxidative stress, and arachidonate intake), interleukin-6 (IL-6), tumor necrosis factor-alpha (TNF), and C-reactive protein (CRP) were inversely correlated with intakes of total fruit and vegetables, legumes, vitamin C, beta carotene, luteolin, folate, and flavonoids; in other words, the lower the intake of fruits and phytonutrients, the higher the level of isoprostane, CRP, TNF, and IL-6.[1062]

- Retrospective cohort of 1034 North American women: Fruit and vegetable intake and risk of upper respiratory tract infection (URTI) in pregnant women: Subjects were asked retrospectively about their fruit/vegetable intake during the six months before the pregnancy and their occurrences of URTI during the first half of pregnancy "CONCLUSIONS: Women who consume more fruits and vegetables have a moderate reduction in risk of URTI during pregnancy, and this benefit appears to be derived from both fruits and vegetables instead of either alone."[1063]

[1058] Aljada et al. Glucose ingestion induces an increase in intranuclear nuclear factor kappaB, a fall in cellular inhibitor kappaB, and an increase in tumor necrosis factor alpha messenger RNA by mononuclear cells in healthy human subjects. *Metabolism*. 2006 Sep;55(9):1177-85
[1059] Turina et al. Acute hyperglycemia and the innate immune system: clinical, cellular, and molecular aspects. *Crit Care Med*. 2005;33(7):1624-33
[1060] Knoops et al. Mediterranean diet, lifestyle factors, and 10-year mortality in elderly European men and women: the HALE project. *JAMA*. 2004 Sep 22;292(12):1433-9
[1061] Kruzich et al. US youths in the early stages of HIV disease have low intakes of some micronutrients important for optimal immune function. *J Am Diet Assoc*. 2004 Jul;104(7):1095-101
[1062] Holt et al. Fruit and vegetable consumption and its relation to markers of inflammation and oxidative stress in adolescents. *J Am Diet Assoc*. 2009 Mar;109(3):414-21
[1063] Li L, Werler MM. Fruit and vegetable intake and risk of upper respiratory tract infection in pregnant women. *Public Health Nutr*. 2009 Jun 25:1-7

o Double-blinded placebo-controlled clinical trial: Regulatory effects of a fermented food concentrate on immune function parameters in healthy volunteers: This study sought to assess the influence of a "cascade-fermented food consisting of fruits, nuts, and vegetables rich in polyphenols (Regulat)" twice daily for 4 weeks on the immune system in healthy volunteers: 48 healthy men 20-48 y of age with regular low to moderate intake of fruit and vegetables. "The intake of Regulat significantly enhanced intracellular glutathione content in lymphocytes, monocytes, and natural killer cells. Furthermore, activation of natural killer cell cytotoxicity in response to interleukin-2 stimulation...were found in the Regulat but not in the placebo group." Other biochemical benefits included reductions of the following: total lipid peroxidation, soluble vascular cell adhesion molecule-1, soluble intercellular adhesion molecule-1—each of these serve as blood markers for inflammation.[1064] Regulat is produced under patent by a "cascade fermentation process" and is made mainly from fruits, vegetables, and nuts (lemons, dates, figs, walnuts, soy beans, coconuts, onions, sprouts, celery, artichokes, millet, peas, spices, saffron). This mixture is fermented over several weeks in various steps with the aid of five different strains of *Lactobacilli* probiotics. In the final product, no viable *Lactobacilli* are present.

- **Multivitamin/multimineral supplementation**: As would be expected, clinical trials of multivitamin supplementation are impressively heterogeneous. In some studies, "multivitamin" is used to describe supplementation with only a handful of vitamins (this should be called ***oligo***vitamin supplementation rather than ***multi***vitamin supplementation), often in doses so low that they hardly would seem worthwhile to any practitioner of integrative/functional nutrition. In other studies, "multivitamin" does indeed include a broader spectrum of nutrients, but often these are in poor form, for example, cyanocobalamin rather than hydroxy-/methyl-/adenosyl-cobalamin, ergocalciferol rather than cholecalciferol, and pyridoxine HCl rather than pyridoxal-5-phosphate. In essentially 100% of these studies, no consideration is given to nutrients such as magnesium, nor to phytonutrients, nor to the critically important effects of whole-foods nutrition such as urinary/systemic alkalinization to overcome the acidogenic effect of the Western diet which causes mild diet-induced chronic metabolic acidosis.[1065]
    o Review: Vitamins for chronic disease prevention in adults: clinical applications: "Most people do not consume an optimal amount of all vitamins by diet alone. ...it appears prudent for all adults to take vitamin supplements. ... Physicians should...ensure that [patients] are taking vitamins they should..."[1066]
    o Review: Selected vitamins and trace elements support immune function by strengthening epithelial barriers and cellular and humoral immune responses: The abstract from the review published in 2007 by Maggini, Wintergerst, Beveridge, and Hornig[1067] is so succinct and clear that I feel compelled to quote it here in its entirety for the benefit of clinicians and our worldwide audience of patients in order to give appropriate credit to those authors for their skill in distilling massive amounts of information into a comprehensible summary of the effect of nutrients in immune function. Readers are encouraged to obtain the full text of the article from the publisher's website at journals.cambridge.org:

        "Adequate intakes of micronutrients are required for the immune system to function efficiently. Micronutrient deficiency suppresses immunity by affecting innate, T cell mediated and adaptive antibody responses, leading to dysregulation of the balanced host response. This situation increases susceptibility to infections, with increased morbidity and mortality. In turn, infections aggravate micronutrient deficiencies by reducing nutrient intake, increasing losses, and interfering with utilization by altering metabolic pathways. Insufficient intake of micronutrients occurs in people with eating disorders, in smokers (active and passive), in individuals with chronic alcohol abuse, in certain diseases, during pregnancy and lactation, and in the elderly. This paper summarizes the roles of selected vitamins and trace elements in immune function. Micronutrients contribute to the body's natural defenses on three levels by supporting physical barriers (skin/mucosa), cellular immunity and antibody production. Vitamins A, C, E and the trace element

---

[1064] Schoen C, Schulz A, Schweikart J, Schütt S, von Baehr V. Regulatory effects of a fermented food concentrate on immune function parameters in healthy volunteers. *Nutrition*. 2009 May;25(5):499-505
[1065] Cordain et al. Origins and evolution of the Western diet: health implications for the 21st century. *Am J Clin Nutr*. 2005 Feb;81(2):341-54
[1066] Fletcher RH, Fairfield KM. Vitamins for chronic disease prevention in adults: clinical applications. *JAMA*. 2002 Jun 19;287(23):3127-9
[1067] Maggini et al. Selected vitamins and trace elements support immune function by strengthening epithelial barriers and cellular and humoral immune responses. *Br J Nutr*. 2007 Oct;98 Suppl 1:S29-35

zinc assist in enhancing the skin barrier function. The vitamins A, B6, B12, C, D, E and folic acid and the trace elements iron, zinc, copper and selenium **work in synergy to support the protective activities of the immune cells**. Finally, all these micronutrients, with the exception of vitamin C and iron, are essential for antibody production. Overall, inadequate intake and status of these vitamins and trace elements may lead to suppressed immunity, which predisposes to infections and aggravates malnutrition. Therefore, supplementation with these selected micronutrients can support the body's natural defense system by enhancing all three levels of immunity."[1068]

- Clinical trial: Effect of a multivitamin and mineral supplement on infection and quality of life. A randomized, double-blind, placebo-controlled trial.: "A multivitamin and mineral supplement reduced the incidence of participant-reported infection and related absenteeism in a sample of participants with type 2 diabetes mellitus and a high prevalence of subclinical micronutrient deficiency."[1069]

- Review: Contribution of selected vitamins and trace elements to immune function: "Adequate intake of vitamins B(6), folate, B(12), C, E, and of selenium, zinc, copper, and iron supports a Th-1 cytokine-mediated immune response with sufficient production of proinflammatory cytokines, which maintains an effective immune response and avoids a shift to an anti-inflammatory Th2 cell-mediated immune response and an increased risk of extracellular infections."[1070]

- Review: Nutritional strategies to boost immunity and prevent infection in elderly individuals: "Nutritional supplementation strategies can reduce this risk and reverse some of the immune dysfunction associated with advanced age. ... The data support use of a daily multivitamin or trace-mineral supplement that includes zinc (elemental zinc, >20 mg/day) and selenium (100 microg/day), with additional vitamin E, to achieve a daily dosage of 200 mg/day."[1071]

- Clinical trial: Nutritional supplements [cod liver oil and a children's multivitamin-mineral with selenium] as adjunctive therapy for children with chronic/recurrent sinusitis: pilot research: "Four, six, and eight weeks after beginning study supplements, the responders had decreased sinus symptoms, fewer episodes of acute sinusitis, and fewer doctor visits for acute illnesses. Their parents reported that they had begun to recover from upper respiratory illnesses without complications, which was unusual for these children..."[1072]

- Clinical trial: Lemon-flavored cod liver oil and a multivitamin-mineral supplement for the secondary prevention of otitis media in young children: "...8 children received 1 teaspoon of lemon-flavored cod liver oil (containing both EPA and vitamin A) and 1 half-tablet of a selenium-containing children's chewable multivitamin-mineral tablet per day. During this OM season, study subjects received antibiotics for OM for 12.3% fewer days during supplementation than before supplementation."[1073]

- Clinical trial: Effect of daily cod liver oil and a multivitamin-mineral supplement with selenium on upper respiratory tract pediatric visits by young, inner-city, Latino children: "The supplementation group had a statistically significant decrease in the mean number of upper respiratory tract [infection] visits over time... Use of these nutritional supplements was acceptable to the inner-city Latino families and their young children, and was associated with a decrease in upper respiratory tract [infection] pediatric visits over time...."[1074]

- Clinical trial: A randomized trial of multivitamin supplements and HIV disease progression and mortality: "Multivitamins also resulted in significantly higher CD4+ and CD8+ cell counts and significantly lower viral loads. ... Multivitamin supplements delay the progression of HIV disease and provide an effective, low-cost means of delaying the initiation of antiretroviral therapy in HIV-infected women."[1075]

[1068] The exact location for accessing this article from the publisher is: journals.cambridge.org/action/displayAbstract?fromPage=online&aid=1364128 2009
[1069] Barringer et al. Effect of a multivitamin and mineral supplement on infection and quality of life. A randomized, double-blind, placebo-controlled trial. *Ann Intern Med*. 2003 Mar 4;138(5):365-71
[1070] Wintergerst et al. Contribution of selected vitamins and trace elements to immune function. *Ann Nutr Metab*. 2007;51(4):301-23
[1071] High KP. Nutritional strategies to boost immunity and prevent infection in elderly individuals. *Clin Infect Dis*. 2001 Dec 1;33(11):1892-900
[1072] Linday et al. Nutritional supplements as adjunctive therapy for children with chronic/recurrent sinusitis: pilot research. *Int J Pediatr Otorhinolaryngol*. 2004 Jun;68(6):785-93
[1073] Linday et al. Lemon-flavored cod liver oil and a multivitamin-mineral supplement for secondary prevention of otitis media in young children. *Ann Otol Rhinol Laryngol*. 2002 Jul;111(7 Pt 1):642-52
[1074] Linday et al. Effect of daily cod liver oil and a multivitamin-mineral supplement with selenium on upper respiratory tract pediatric visits by young, inner-city, Latino children: randomized pediatric sites. *Ann Otol Rhinol Laryngol*. 2004 Nov;113(11):891-901
[1075] Fawzi et al. A randomized trial of multivitamin supplements and HIV disease progression and mortality. *N Engl J Med*. 2004 Jul 1;351(1):23-32

- Review: Effects of antioxidant and non-antioxidant vitamin supplementation on immune function: "There is evidence to support causal effects of supplementation with vitamins E and C and the carotenoids singly and in combination on selected aspects of immunity, including the functional capacity of innate immune cells, lymphocyte proliferation, and the delayed-type hypersensitivity (DTH) response. Controlled intervention trials of B vitamin-containing multivitamin supplements suggest beneficial effects on immune parameters and clinical outcomes in HIV-positive individuals."[1076]
- Clinical trial: Effects of maternal vitamin supplements on malaria in children born to HIV-infected women: "Compared with placebo, multivitamins excluding VA/BC [vitamin A / beta-carotene] reduced the incidence of clinical malaria by 71% (95% CI = 11-91%; P = 0.02), whereas VA/BC alone resulted in a nonsignificant 63% reduction (95% CI = -4% to 87%; P = 0.06). Multivitamins including VA/BC significantly reduced the incidence of high parasitemia by 43% (95% CI = 2-67%; P = 0.04)."[1077]
- Clinical trial: Multivitamin supplementation improves hematologic status in HIV-infected women and their children in Tanzania: "Multivitamin supplementation provided during pregnancy and in the postpartum period resulted in significant improvements in hematologic status among HIV-infected women and their children, which provides further support for the value of multivitamin supplementation in HIV-infected adults."[1078]
- Randomized controlled trial: Multivitamin supplementation (vitamins B, C, and E) in HIV-positive pregnant women: impact on depression and quality of life in a resource-poor setting: "Multivitamin supplementation (B-complex, C and E) resulted in a reduction in risk of elevated depressive symptoms comparable to MDD [major depressive disorder] and improvement in quality of life in HIV-positive pregnant women in Tanzania."[1079] This article reminds us of two important clinical considerations: 1) that the negative effects of any illness extend beyond the illness/infection itself—in this case to include depression, and 2) that nutritional supplementation can help correct the biochemical imbalances that contribute to the psychosocial experience and clinical manifestations of depression. Clinicians would be wise to consider nutritional deficiencies in their depressed patients before jumping to the conclusion that the patient has a Prozac deficiency or insufficiency of electroconvulsive shocks, now again increasingly used in the "medical" management of mental depression, especially among older patients[1080]—that is, among patients most likely to have the nutritional deficiencies known to cause depression.[1081]
- Review: Effects of vitamins, including vitamin A, on HIV/AIDS patients: "Further, multivitamin supplementation reduces the rate of HIV disease progression among patients in early stage of disease, thus delaying the need for ART [antiretroviral treatment] by prolonging the pre-ART stage. In brief, there is no evidence to recommend vitamin A supplementation of HIV-infected pregnant women; however, periodic vitamin A supplementation of HIV-infected infants and children is beneficial in reducing all-cause mortality and morbidity and is recommended. Similarly, multivitamin supplementation of people infected with HIV, particularly pregnant women, is strongly suggested."[1082]
- Prospective randomized, placebo-controlled trial of intravenous copper, selenium, and zinc in burn patients: Trace element supplementation after major burns modulates antioxidant status and clinical course by way of increased tissue trace element concentrations: Due to increased metabolic needs compounded by fluid losses through skin and secondary to hyperhydration, trace element (TE) deficiencies are common in multi-trauma and burn patients. This study used "large, intravenous doses of TE supplements" containing copper, selenium, and zinc. "The number of infections in the first 30 d

---

[1076] Webb AL, Villamor E. Update: effects of antioxidant and non-antioxidant vitamin supplementation on immune function. *Nutr Rev.* 2007 May;65(5):181-217
[1077] Villamor et al. Effects of maternal vitamin supplements on malaria in children born to HIV-infected women. *Am J Trop Med Hyg.* 2007 Jun;76(6):1066-71
[1078] Fawzi et al. Multivitamin supplementation improves hematologic status in HIV-infected women and their children in Tanzania. *Am J Clin Nutr.* 2007 May;85(5):1335-43
[1079] Smith Fawzi et al. Multivitamin supplementation in HIV-positive pregnant women: impact on depression and quality of life in a resource-poor setting. *HIV Med.* 2007 May;8(4):203-12
[1080] "Electroconvulsive therapy (ECT) is used increasingly in the older adult population for major depression, particularly when depression is not responsive to medications, when antidepressants are not tolerated due to side effects, ..." Kelly KG, Zisselman M. Update on electroconvulsive therapy (ECT) in older adults. *J Am Geriatr Soc.* 2000 May;48(5):560-6
[1081] "A low serum vitamin B-12 concentration was found in 6% and 5%, low folate in 5% and 19%, and low vitamin B-6 in 9% and 51%, and one or more metabolites were elevated in 63% and 83% of healthy elderly subjects and elderly hospitalized patients, respectively. These results strongly suggest that the prevalence of tissue deficiencies of vitamin B-12, folate, and vitamin B-6 as demonstrated by the elevated metabolite concentrations is substantially higher than that estimated by measuring concentrations of the vitamins." Joosten et al. Metabolic evidence that deficiencies of vitamin B-12 (cobalamin), folate, and vitamin B-6 occur commonly in elderly people. *Am J Clin Nutr.* 1993 Oct;58(4):468-76
[1082] Mehta S, Fawzi W. Effects of vitamins, including vitamin A, on HIV/AIDS patients. *Vitam Horm.* 2007;75:355-83

was significantly lower in the TE group (P=0.015), with a median number of 2 versus 4 infections per patient in the TE and V groups, respectively, as a result of a reduction in pulmonary infections (P=0.03)."[1083]

- o Review: Antioxidants and viral infections: host immune response and viral pathogenicity: "Work in our laboratory has demonstrated that not only is the host affected by the nutritional deficiency, but the invading pathogen is as well. … The immune system was altered in the Se-deficient animals, as was the viral pathogen itself." Dr Beck goes on to note that viral isolates recovered from Se-deficient mice demonstrated mutations in the viral genome of both coxsackievirus and influenza virus, and that these changes in the viral genome are associated with increased pathogenicity of the virus. Many of the antiviral/immunosupportive benefits of selenium appear to be mediated though the antioxidant selenoenzyme, glutathione peroxidase-1, given that glutathione peroxidase knockout mice developed myocarditis, similar to the Se-deficient mice, when infected with the benign strain of myocarditis.[1084]
- o Review: Nutritionally induced oxidative stress: effect on viral disease: "The nutritional status of the host can have a profound influence on a virus, so that a normally avirulent virus becomes virulent because of changes in the viral genome."[1085]

- **Selenium: 600-1,000 mcg per day, limit duration of highest doses**:
  - o Review: Selenium and vitamin E status: impact on viral pathogenicity: "Recent work has demonstrated that deficiencies in either Se or vitamin E result in increased viral pathogenicity and altered immune responses. Furthermore, deficiencies in either Se or vitamin E results in specific viral mutations, changing relatively benign viruses into virulent ones."[1086]

> **Nutritional deficiencies impair host immune responses and mucosal defenses, and promote viral mutations that lead to more severe and recalcitrant infections**
>
> "Many viral infections, for example infections with rotavirus, measles, and parainfluenza virus, are much more severe in malnourished hosts as compared with well-nourished hosts. … With the current interest in emerging infectious diseases, it would be important to consider the **host nutritional status as a driving force for viral mutations**."
>
> Beck MA. Antioxidants and viral infections: host immune response and viral pathogenicity. *J Am Coll Nutr.* 2001

  - o Review: Selenium and host defense towards viruses: Nutritional deficiencies cause immunosuppression—this point has been made very clear and is medically irrefutable, despite the fact that it is commonly medically ignored. In this review, Dr Beck again reminds us that the adverse alterations due to nutritional deficiency are not limited to the effect on the human host; when the human host is nutritionally deficient, the changes in the biochemical milieu also affect the replication and level of mutagenicity within the viral invader. Nutritional deficiency leads to increased oxidative stress; increased oxidative stress promotes additional mutations within the virus, and these additional mutations cause the virus to behave more aggressively, thereby increasing the severity of the viral infection while also increasing the infectivity of the virus to include nutritionally-replete hosts. "Six nucleotide changes were found in the virus that replicated in the deficient mice, and once these mutations occurred, even mice with normal nutrition became susceptible to disease. Thus, the nutritional status of the host was able to transform an avirulent virus into a virulent one due to genomic changes in the virus."[1087]
  - o Double-blind, randomized, placebo-controlled trial clinical trial: Suppression of human immunodeficiency virus type 1 viral load with selenium supplementation: a randomized controlled trial: This study used "High selenium yeast supplementation (200 mcg/d)" to evaluate effect on HIV-1 viral load and CD4 count after 9 months of treatment among 262 HIV-positive men and women. Evidence of dose-response was noted, with higher selenium levels correlating with lower HIV viral load and higher CD4 count. The authors conclude that, "Daily selenium supplementation can suppress the progression of HIV-1 viral burden and provide indirect improvement of CD4 count. The results support the use of selenium as a simple, inexpensive, and safe adjunct therapy in HIV spectrum disease."[1088]

[1083] Berger et al. Trace element supplementation after major burns modulates antioxidant status and clinical course by way of increased tissue trace element concentrations. *Am J Clin Nutr.* 2007 May;85(5):1293-300
[1084] Beck MA. Antioxidants and viral infections: host immune response and viral pathogenicity. *J Am Coll Nutr.* 2001 Oct;20(5 Suppl):384S-388S
[1085] Beck MA. Nutritionally induced oxidative stress: effect on viral disease. *Am J Clin Nutr.* 2000 Jun;71(6 Suppl):1676S-81S
[1086] Beck MA. Selenium and vitamin E status: impact on viral pathogenicity. *J Nutr.* 2007 May;137(5):1338-40
[1087] Beck MA. Selenium and host defence towards viruses. *Proc Nutr Soc.* 1999 Aug;58(3):707-11
[1088] Hurwitz et al. Suppression of human immunodeficiency virus type 1 viral load with selenium supplementation. *Arch Intern Med.* 2007 Jan 22;167(2):148-54

- o Clinical trial: Selenium in Intensive Care (SIC): results of a prospective randomized, placebo-controlled, multiple-center study in patients with severe systemic inflammatory response syndrome, sepsis, and septic shock: This trial took place among eleven intensive care units in Germany among 249 patients with severe systemic inflammatory response syndrome, sepsis, and septic shock. Acute Physiology and Chronic Health Evaluation (APACHE) III score was >70. Patients received 1000 microg of sodium-selenite as a 30-min bolus injection, followed by 14 daily continuous infusions of 1000 microg intravenously, or placebo. "The intention-to-treat analysis of the remaining 238 patients revealed a mortality rate of 50.0% in the placebo group and 39.7% in the selenium-treated group. ... the 28-day mortality rate was significantly reduced to 42.4% compared with 56.7% in 97 patients of the placebo group." No side effects were observed due to high-dose sodium-selenite treatment.[1089] Orally administered 1000 mcg of selenium is a reasonable dose for in-office use; duration can optionally be limited to a few days or a few weeks but should not extend for more than about two months unless professionally supervised and clinically indicated.
- o Clinical trial: Effects of high doses of selenium, as sodium selenite, in septic shock: a placebo-controlled, randomized, double-blind, phase II study: "CONCLUSION: Continuous infusion of selenium as sodium selenite (4,000 microg on the first day, 1,000 microg/day on the nine following days) had no obvious toxicity but did not improve the clinical outcome in septic shock patients."[1090] The importance of this study—beyond confirming the lack of toxicity of 4,000 mcg followed by 1,000 mcg of selenium—is that it suggests that 4,000 mcg is too much selenium to give as a loading dose; this appears to be the only protocol variable in the study that differentiates it from the more successful study listed previously that showed significant benefit when 1,000 mcg was used as the loading dose.
- **Vitamin D3 (cholecalciferol, not ergocalciferol): 4,000-10,000 IU per day; for acute infections in deficient patients consider a one-time loading dose of 100,000-300,000 IU followed by a more conservative maintenance dose**: In our 2004 monograph by Vasquez, Manso, and Cannell, we fulfilled our promise of creating a "paradigm shift" that summarized new applications for the clinical use of vitamin D beyond its application in patients with osteoporosis or malabsorption to include the mandate of empiric treatment or laboratory assessment of all patients seen in clinical practice.[1091] Vitamin D3 has a particularly relevant role in the prevention of viral infections, especially viral infections of the respiratory tract, including influenza. Daily doses generally average between 4,000-10,000 IU/d for adults, with an acceptable one-time loading dose of 100,000-300,000 IU in patients for whom it is advantageous and safe to raise serum 25-hydroxy-vitamin D levels quickly and without concern for compliance failure; the logistical goal with vitamin D supplementation is to get serum 25-hydroxy-vitamin D levels into the optimal range, as defined in the illustration.
    - o Review: Acute lower respiratory infections in childhood: opportunities for reducing the global burden through nutritional interventions: "The active form of vitamin D affects a variety of immune functions, including the synthesis of endogenous antimicrobial peptides."[1092]
    - o Review: Vitamin D for Treatment and Prevention of Infectious Diseases: A Systematic Review of Randomized Controlled Trials: "Based on studies reviewed to date, the strongest evidence supports further research into adjunctive vitamin D therapy for tuberculosis, influenza, and viral upper respiratory illnesses."[1093]
    - o Review: Vitamin D signaling, infectious diseases, and regulation of innate immunity: Evidence is accumulating that vitamin D sufficiency confers protection against tuberculosis and a wide range of other bacterial as well as viral infections. Studies support a role for vitamin D in protection against upper and lower respiratory tract infections, most of which are typically caused by viruses, and some of which are then later complicated by secondary bacterial infection (after the viral infection has exacerbated nutritional depletion and lead to damage of respiratory epithelium). Subclinical vitamin D deficiency increases the risk for severe pneumonia and was associated with a 13-fold-increased risk of pneumonia

---

[1089] Angstwurm et al. Selenium in Intensive Care (SIC): results of a prospective randomized, placebo-controlled, multiple-center study in patients with severe systemic inflammatory response syndrome, sepsis, and septic shock. *Crit Care Med*. 2007 Jan;35(1):118-26
[1090] Forceville et al. Effects of high doses of selenium, as sodium selenite, in septic shock: a placebo-controlled, randomized, double-blind, phase II study. *Crit Care*. 2007;11:R73
[1091] Vasquez A, Manso G, Cannell J. The clinical importance of vitamin D (cholecalciferol). *Altern Ther Health Med*. 2004 Sep-Oct;10(5):28-36
[1092] Roth et al. Acute lower respiratory infections in childhood: reducing the global burden through nutritional interventions. *Bull World Health Organ*. 2008 May;86(5):356-64
[1093] Yamshchikov et al. Vitamin D for Treatment and Prevention of Infectious Diseases: A Systematic Review of Randomized Controlled Trials. *Endocr Pract*. 2009 Jun 2:1-29

in Ethiopian children. Readers should revisit the illustrated optimal range in this section in light of the quote, "A Finnish study found that there was an association between serum 25D concentrations of less than 40 nM (16 ng/ml) and a range of acute respiratory infections (sinusitis, tonsillitis, otitis, bronchitis, pneumonia, pharyngitis, and laryngitis) in young army recruits."[1094]

- o Expert literature review: Epidemic influenza and vitamin D: Vitamin D3 stimulates the expression of potent anti-microbial peptides from neutrophils, monocytes, natural killer cells, and in epithelial cells lining the respiratory tract. "An interventional study showed that vitamin D reduces the incidence of respiratory infections in children."[1095]
- o Meta-analysis of randomized controlled trials: Vitamin D supplementation and total mortality: "Intake of ordinary doses of vitamin D supplements seems to be associated with decreases in total mortality rates."[1096] Most of the studies reviewed in this meta-analysis used subphysiologic doses of vitamin D; yet they still produced benefit in terms of reduced total mortality, some of which is likely attributable to reductions in the incidence and severity of infections, including viral infections.
- o Hypothesis—Ultraviolet-B irradiance and vitamin D reduce the risk of viral infections and thus their sequelae, including autoimmune diseases and some cancers: "Vitamin D, through induction of cathelicidin, which effectively combats both bacterial and viral infections, may reduce the risk of several autoimmune diseases and cancers by reducing the development of viral infections."[1097]

- **Zinc: up to 150 mg per day of elemental zinc for adults; limit duration and/or co-administer copper to avoid zinc-induced copper deficiency**: Zinc ions are directly antiviral, and this is the rationale behind the use of zinc throat lozenges, which generally show significant benefit in the prevention and treatment of respiratory tract infections, including influenza.[1098] Zinc is also required for the proper production of thymulin, which is an immune-supporting peptide hormone made by the thymus gland required for maturation of T-helper cells; in zinc-depleted chronically infected patients, their undetectable levels of thymulin can be raised to the normal level following zinc supplementation with a corresponding restoration of immune function. Zinc has an important role in cell-mediated immune functions and also functions as anti-inflammatory and antioxidant agent[1099]; thus, the state of zinc deficiency (which can be assessed by measuring serum zinc, among other methods) is a state of immunodysfunction/immunosuppression, and superfluous pro-inflammation and oxidative stress. Per the review by Hadden[1100], the adverse effects on the immune system caused by zinc deficiency include but are not limited to thymic involution, thymocyte depletion in thymus, depression of serum thymopoietin and thymulin, depression of delayed type hypersensitivity, depressed peripheral T-lymphocyte and/or T-cell numbers, depressed T-cell mitogen responses, depressed primary and secondary responses to sheep red blood cells, depressed T-helper function, depressed natural killer function. Furthermore, per the review by Prasad[1101], in zinc deficiency, the CD4+ to CD8+ ratio is decreased and Th-1 cytokines IL-2 and IFN-gamma are both decreased; this would obviously favor the acquisition and persistence of viral infections.
  - o Clinical trial contrasting oral zinc (20 mg/d) plus multivitamin syrup or multivitamin syrup alone: Impact of zinc supplementation on subsequent growth and morbidity in Bangladeshi children with acute diarrhea: "These results suggest that a short course of zinc supplementation (20 mg/d) to malnourished children during acute diarrhea reduces growth-faltering and diarrhea and respiratory [infection] morbidity during subsequent two months."[1102]
  - o Double-blind, controlled trial: Zinc supplementation (10 mg/d) reduces the incidence of acute lower respiratory infections in infants and preschool children (n=298 vs 311 controls): "Zinc-supplemented children had 0.19 acute lower respiratory infection episodes/child/year compared with 0.35 episodes/child/year in the control children. After correction for correlation of data using generalized

---

[1094] White JH. Vitamin D signaling, infectious diseases, and regulation of innate immunity. *Infect Immun*. 2008 Sep;76(9):3837-43
[1095] Cannell et al. Epidemic influenza and vitamin D. *Epidemiol Infect*. 2006;134(6):1129-40
[1096] Autier P, Gandini S. Vitamin D supplementation and total mortality: a meta-analysis of randomized controlled trials. *Arch Intern Med*. 2007 Sep 10;167(16):1730-7
[1097] Grant WB. Hypothesis—ultraviolet-B irradiance and vitamin D reduce the risk of viral infections and thus their sequelae, including autoimmune diseases and some cancers. *Photochem Photobiol*. 2008 Mar-Apr;84(2):356-65
[1098] Roxas M, Jurenka J. Colds and influenza: a review of diagnosis and conventional, botanical, and nutritional considerations. *Altern Med Rev*. 2007 Mar;12(1):25-4
[1099] Prasad AS. Zinc: mechanisms of host defense. *J Nutr*. 2007 May;137(5):1345-9
[1100] Hadden JW. The treatment of zinc deficiency is an immunotherapy. *Int J Immunopharmacol*. 1995 Sep;17(9):697-701
[1101] Prasad AS. Zinc: mechanisms of host defense. *J Nutr*. 2007 May;137(5):1345-9
[1102] Roy et al. Impact of zinc supplementation on subsequent growth and morbidity in Bangladeshi children with acute diarrhoea. *Eur J Clin Nutr*. 1999 Jul;53(7):529-34

estimating equation regression methods, there was a reduction of 45% in the incidence of acute lower respiratory infections in zinc-supplemented children."[1103] These results are impressive for low-dose zinc monotherapy.
   - o Clinical trial of zinc (10-20 mg/d) with or without a single large dose of vitamin A (100,000-200,00 IU): Effect of routine zinc supplementation on acute lower respiratory tract infections and pneumonia in children aged 6 months to 3 years: randomized controlled trial in an urban slum: "Zinc supplementation resulted in a lower incidence of pneumonia than placebo... CONCLUSIONS: Zinc supplementation substantially reduced the incidence of pneumonia in children who had received vitamin A."[1104]
- **Vitamin C (ascorbic acid)**: Ascorbate as treatment for the common cold and other respiratory viral infections may not have lived up to Dr Pauling's high expectations, but the overall evidence suggests some efficacy when used in isolation.[1105] We would tend to expect better results if this agent is used in an appropriate combination approach since this more accurately reflects the interconnected nature of nutritional biochemistry and immune physiology. The combination of modest efficacy and a near absence of adverse effects produces a sufficiently high benefit:risk ratio at low cost to make vitamin C worthy of clinical utilization.
- **Vitamin A: load with 300,000 IU per day for about 3-5 days, then 25-000-50,000 IU per day until well; limit 2-4 weeks; monitor for toxicity (headaches, dry skin, cracked lips, bone pain)**: Vitamin A clearly shows immunosupportive benefits. Vitamin A stores are depleted by the stress of infection and injury because reduced hepatic production of retinol-binding protein paradoxically results in increased renal loss of retinol exactly at the time it is critically needed in order to support

> **Historical and Clinical Perspective**
> The most frequently studied nutritional interventions to reduce the clinical impact of respiratory infections in children *of developing nations* are ❶ breast-feeding (preferably from a well-nourished mother), ❷ vitamin A, ❸ zinc, ❹ folic acid, and ❺ iron.

function of the immune system and maintenance/repair of epithelial tissue. In a patient with vitamin A sufficiency, whose tissue stores of this fat-soluble vitamin are well stocked, the reduced production of retinol binding protein serves to liberate retinol for uptake by cells; in patients with marginal or depleted vitamin A status, they do not have the *tissue nutrient reserve* to supply immune and epithelial cells at the same time that retinol is increasingly lost in the urine. Further, not all of the benefits of vitamin A for immune function are available on an acute basis; the maintenance of proper respiratory epithelial structure/function requires vitamin A, but in a vitamin A-deficient patient, acute administration of vitamin A does not immediately restore the respiratory epithelium to promote clearance of the infection, even though other aspects of immune function will recover more quickly. From a practical clinical perspective, consider giving 200,000-300,000 IU per day of retinol palmitate (the least toxic form) for 1-2 weeks, then taper; reduce dose or discontinue with onset of toxicity symptoms such as skin problems (dry skin, flaking skin, chapped or split lips, red skin rash, hair loss), joint pain, bone pain, headaches, anorexia (loss of appetite), edema (water retention, weight gain, swollen ankles, difficulty breathing), fatigue, and/or liver damage. Patients should be given written instructions that clearly delineate the time limit for high-dose vitamin A supplementation and advise them of the potential adverse effects. Women who are pregnant or might become pregnant and who are planning to carry the baby to full term delivery should not ingest more than 10,000 IU of vitamin A per day. Several studies are listed below documenting the precedent use of high-dose vitamin A; clinicians must be aware of the potential adverse effects, must monitor and select patients appropriately, and should generally not use these high doses for the durations listed in these clinical trials.
   - o Documentation of the use and safety of high-dose vitamin A: Adjuvant treatment of stage I lung cancer with high-dose vitamin A: "...retinol palmitate administration (orally 300,000 IU daily for 12 months) ... CONCLUSION: Daily oral administration of high-dose vitamin A is effective in reducing the number of new primary tumors related to tobacco consumption and may improve the disease-free interval in patients curatively resected for stage I lung cancer."[1106]
   - o Documentation of the use and safety of high-dose vitamin A: Safety of high-dose vitamin A. Randomized trial on lung cancer chemoprevention: After administering retinol palmitate (300,000 IU daily for at least

---

[1103] Sazawal et al. Zinc supplementation reduces the incidence of acute lower respiratory infections in infants and preschool children. *Pediatrics*. 1998 Jul;102(1 Pt 1):1-5
[1104] Bhandari et al. Effect of routine zinc supplementation on pneumonia in children aged 6 months to 3 years. *BMJ*. 2002 Jun 8;324(7350):1358
[1105] Roxas M, Jurenka J. Colds and influenza: a review of diagnosis and conventional, botanical, and nutritional considerations. *Altern Med Rev*. 2007 Mar;12(1):25-4
[1106] Pastorino et al. Adjuvant treatment of stage I lung cancer with high-dose vitamin A. *J Clin Oncol*. 1993 Jul;11(7):1216-22

12 months), the authors report their experience with the safety of such doses. "Skin dryness and desquamation were the most frequent symptoms, affecting 60% of all treated patients. Other symptoms such as dyspepsia, headache, nosebleeds and mild hair loss occurred in less than 10% of patients, and were self-terminating. Only in 4 patients (3%) was the treatment interrupted because of symptoms potentially related to vitamin A administration."[1107]

- o Documentation of the use and safety of high-dose vitamin A: Laboratory evaluation during high-dose vitamin A administration: a randomized study on lung cancer patients after surgical resection: Adverse effects of high-dose vitamin A in this report included elevations of serum gamma-glutamyltransferase (abnormally elevated in 69% of the treated patients compared to 39% of controls (mean values 149 vs 57 IU/l at 24 months)) and elevations of serum triglyceride concentrations (over 150 mg/dl seen in 74% of treated patients compared to 43% of controls at 12 months; the average concentration was 283 mg/dl compared to 179 mg/dl). "…there was no other laboratory evidence of toxicity attributable to vitamin A. … In our experience **300,000 IU/day of retinyl palmitate can be administered as a possible chemopreventive agent with reasonable safety for up to 2 years**."[1108]

- **Immunonutrition—common components and beneficial effects**: While the nonspecific term "immunonutrition" could probably be accurately applied to any nutrient (and therefore essentially all nutrients) that affect or benefit immune function, immunonutrition generally is relatively specific to the provision of glutamine, arginine, n-3 fatty acids such as EPA and DHA, and dietary nucleotides. These can be used alone, but their benefit, as expected by the interactive and synergistic activity of nutrients and physiological processes, is generally enhanced when used in combination. Numerous multi-site and international studies have consistently demonstrated significant benefit in terms of reduced infection rates, morbidity, mortality, duration of hospitalization, and hospital costs when immunonutrition intervention is utilized in patients with major trauma, burns, and sepsis.
    - o Clinical trial and review: Immunonutrition in patients after multiple trauma: "In the recovery period after trauma (1-72 h after injury) a limitation of the inflammatory response of immunocompetent cells must be achieved as quickly as possible (<72 h). The only strategy available to clinicians caring for trauma patients is immunonutrition, and this should be strongly considered as a rational approach improving immune function and reducing septic complications in critically ill or injured patients."[1109]
    - o Clinical trial: Influence of arginine, omega-3 fatty acids and nucleotide-supplemented enteral support on systemic inflammatory response syndrome and multiple organ failure in patients after severe trauma: This study used an enteral diet supplemented with arginine, omega-3 fatty acids, and nucleotides (Impact, Sandoz Nutrition, Berne, Switzerland) in patients at high risk for systemic inflammatory response syndrome (SIRS) and multiple organ failure (MOF) after severe trauma. Thirty-two patients were enrolled in this prospective, randomized, double-blind, controlled study. "In the test group, significantly fewer SIRS days per patient were found… MOF score was significantly lower in the test group on d 3 and d 8-11. … The results of the study provide further support for beneficial effects of arginine, omega-3-fatty acids and nucleotide-supplemented enteral diet in critically ill patients." These benefits are counterbalanced by neutral findings of no significant differences in T-lymphocyte CD4/CD8 ratio, interleukin-2 receptor expression, infection rate, mortality (2/16 vs. 4/13), and hospital stay between supplemented and unsupplemented patients.[1110]
    - o Randomized, controlled, double-blind trial: Early enteral supplementation with key pharmaconutrients improves Sequential Organ Failure Assessment score in critically ill patients with sepsis: outcome of a randomized, controlled, double-blind trial: This study tested an "enteral pharmaconutrition supplement containing glutamine dipeptides, antioxidative vitamins and trace elements, and butyrate" [Intestamin, Fresenius Kabi] among fifty critically ill, septic patients. Patients receiving the experimental supplement showed significantly faster improvement in daily SOFA [Sequential Organ Failure Assessment] score over time compared with control group, leading the authors to conclude, "In medical patients with

---

[1107] Pastorino et al. Safety of high-dose vitamin A. Randomized trial on lung cancer chemoprevention. *Oncology*. 1991;48(2):131-7
[1108] Infante et al. Laboratory evaluation during high-dose vitamin A administration: a randomized study on lung cancer patients after surgical resection. *J Cancer Res Clin Oncol*. 1991;117(2):156-62
[1109] Bastian L, Weimann A. Immunonutrition in patients after multiple trauma. *Br J Nutr*. 2002 Jan;87 Suppl 1:S133-4
[1110] Weimann et al. Influence of arginine, omega-3 fatty acids and nucleotide-supplemented enteral support on systemic inflammatory response syndrome and multiple organ failure in patients after severe trauma. *Nutrition*. 1998 Feb;14(2):165-72

sepsis, early enteral pharmaconutrition with glutamine dipeptides, vitamin C and E, beta-carotene, selenium, zinc, and butyrate in combination with an immunonutrition formula results in significantly faster recovery of organ function compared with control."[1111]

> **Research Quote**
>
> "Although under most circumstances the systemic inflammatory response is beneficial to the host, improving the eventual outcome of injury, infection, or inflammation, excessive proinflammation (leading to cardiac, hepatic, and mitochondrial dysfunction) or excessive counterinflammation (leading to immune depression) can worsen outcome."
>
> Bistrian BR. Practical recommendations for immune-enhancing diets. *J Nutr.* 2004 Oct

- o Review: Antioxidant supplementation in sepsis and systemic inflammatory response syndrome: "Three antioxidant nutrients have demonstrated clinical benefits and reached level A evidence: a) selenium improves clinical outcome (infections, organ failure); b) glutamine reduces infectious complication in large-sized trials; and c) the association of eicosapentaenoic acid and micronutrients has significant anti-inflammatory effects."[1112]

- **Fatty acids**: Fatty acids (FA) have many interconnected roles in human physiology, and these interactions are at their most critical importance during disorders of inflammation. An excess of pro-inflammatory FA and deficiency of anti-inflammatory FA may have been tolerated by the patient for decades without *obvious* adverse effect. However, during times of illness or injury, these fatty acid imbalances are made more apparent by the biological activation of these generally inert fatty acids into their biologically active—often inflammatory and painful—chemical mediators, including but not limited to prostaglandins, leukotrienes, isoprostanes, and (beneficially) the anti-inflammatory docosatrienes and resolvins. **Part of the benefit of fatty acid supplementation during infection is that it helps modulate inflammatory responses to prevent them from leading to excess tissue damage and vicious cycles of *inflammation-induced inflammation*. Extreme inflammatory responses actually cause immunosuppression (counterinflammation[1113]) that can increase the susceptibility to or severity of infection.** "Fatty acid" supplementation in the context of acute illness, trauma, and sepsis generally means EPA and DHA from fish oil; however, some studies have used EPA without DHA, while others have used EPA with GLA.

  - o Clinical trial: Nutritional supplements [cod liver oil and a children's multivitamin-mineral with selenium] as adjunctive therapy for children with chronic/recurrent sinusitis: pilot research: "Four, six, and eight weeks after beginning study supplements, the responders had decreased sinus symptoms, fewer episodes of acute sinusitis, and fewer doctor visits for acute illnesses. Their parents reported that they had begun to recover from upper respiratory illnesses without complications, which was unusual for these children..."[1114]

  - o Clinical trial: Lemon-flavored cod liver oil and a multivitamin-mineral supplement for the secondary prevention of otitis media in young children: "...8 children received 1 teaspoon of lemon-flavored cod liver oil (containing both EPA and vitamin A) and 1 half-tablet of a selenium-containing children's chewable multivitamin-mineral tablet per day. During this OM season, study subjects received antibiotics for OM for 12.3% fewer days during supplementation than before supplementation."[1115]

  - o Clinical trial: Effect of daily cod liver oil and a multivitamin-mineral supplement with selenium on upper respiratory tract pediatric visits by young, inner-city, Latino children: "The supplementation group had a statistically significant decrease in the mean number of upper respiratory tract [infection] visits over time... Use of these nutritional supplements…was associated with a decrease in upper respiratory tract [infection] pediatric visits over time…."[1116]

  - o Systematic review: Immunonutrition in critically ill patients: a systematic review and analysis of the literature: This systematic review compared studies with various combinations of arginine, glutamine, and/or fish oil and concluded that only fish oil supplementation provided consistent benefit in terms of

---

[1111] Beale et al. Early enteral supplementation with key pharmaconutrients improves Sequential Organ Failure Assessment score in critically ill patients with sepsis: outcome of a randomized, controlled, double-blind trial. *Crit Care Med.* 2008 Jan;36(1):131-44
[1112] Berger MM, Chioléro RL. Antioxidant supplementation in sepsis and systemic inflammatory response syndrome. *Crit Care Med.* 2007 Sep;35(9 Suppl):S584-90
[1113] Bistrian BR. Practical recommendations for immune-enhancing diets. *J Nutr.* 2004;134(10 Sup):2868S-2872S jn.nutrition.org/cgi/content/full/134/10/2868S
[1114] Linday et al. Nutritional supplements as adjunctive therapy for children with chronic/recurrent sinusitis: pilot research. *Int J Pediatr Otorhinolaryngol.* 2004 Jun;68(6):785-93
[1115] Linday et al. Lemon-flavored cod liver oil and a multivitamin-mineral supplement for secondary prevention of otitis media in young children. *Ann Otol Rhinol Laryngol.* 2002 Jul;111(7 Pt 1):642-52
[1116] Linday et al. Effect of daily cod liver oil and a multivitamin-mineral supplement with selenium on upper respiratory tract pediatric visits by young, inner-city, Latino children: randomized pediatric sites. *Ann Otol Rhinol Laryngol.* 2004 Nov;113(11):891-901

mortality and length of stay [LOS]. "Mortality, infections and LOS were significantly lower only in the ICU patients receiving the FO [fish oil] IMD [immuno-modulating diets] (OR 0.42, 95% CI 0.26-0.68; OR 0.45, 95% CI 0.25-0.79 and WMD -6.28 days, 95% CI -9.92 to -2.64, respectively)."[1117] The benefits of fish oil across such a heterogeneous group of patients is due to the following: ❶ deficiency of EPA and DHA is essentially universal among patients consuming an American/Western diet, ❷ the provision of EPA and DHA provides potent anti-inflammatory effects, some of which such as activation of PPAR-alpha is enhanced when the fatty acid ligand (e.g., EPA) is in an oxidized state, and 3) oral consumption of lipid stimulates the vagus nerve, which then provides an anti-inflammatory effect via **neuroimmunomodulation**.

- <u>Glutamine: 3-6 grams x3 between meals</u>: Glutamine (Gln) is a conditionally essential nutrient that is needed by immunocytes and enterocytes in increased amounts during times of trauma and infection. Insufficient glutamine availability is a compound problem resulting in immunosuppression and increased intestinal permeability; clinicians should appreciate that this is the perfect formula for gram-negative sepsis. Further, insufficiency of glutamine would also be expected to result in a deficiency of glutathione and the resultant increase in oxidative stress. All clinicians should know that glutathione (GSH) is a critically important antioxidant that has numerous functions for regulating cell cycle, DNA repair, and inflammatory responses, and that this antioxidant is formed endogenously from three amino acids: cysteine, glycine, and glutamine/glutamate. This explains the benefit of providing cysteine (generally in the form of N-acetyl-cysteine [which has additional benefits independent from its contribution to GSH], supported by many human trials) and glutamine (supported by animal research) to patients with toxic exposures, such as Tylenol/acetaminophen overdose. In clinical practice, 9-18 grams per day between meals (amino acids are generally administered between meals) is reasonable, although higher doses have been used and reported in clinical trials in specific situations. After administering glutamine 26 grams/d to severely burned patients, Garrel et al[1118] concluded that glutamine reduced the risk of infection by 3-fold and that **oral glutamine "may be a life-saving intervention"** in patients with severe burns. A dose of 30 gm/d was used in a clinical trial showing hemodynamic benefit in patients with sickle cell anemia.[1119] The highest glutamine dose that the current author is aware of is the study by Scheltinga et al[1120] who used intravenous glutamine 0.57 gm/kg/day in cancer patients following chemotherapy administration; for a 220-lb-pt, this would be approximately 57 grams/d of glutamine.
    - <u>Ex vivo study: Glutamine-enhanced bacterial killing by neutrophils from postoperative patients</u>: Not all studies have replicated this finding of enhanced antibacterial action of neutrophils following the addition of glutamine; however, these findings provide an excellent *partial* explanation for the anti-infective and immunosupportive effects of glutamine administration to humans, which has been documented in numerous trials. "This finding indicated that as plasma Gln fell, there was an enhancement of neutrophil E. coli-killing activity by neutrophils in *in vitro* tests when the Gln concentration was increased from 500 to 1000 nmol/mL. ... In conclusion, Gln supplementation enhanced the in vitro bactericidal function of neutrophils from postoperative patients."[1121]
    - <u>Clinical trial and documentation of hospital cost savings by the use of glutamine administration in critically ill patients (despite no reduction in mortality): Randomized clinical outcome study of critically ill patients given glutamine-supplemented enteral nutrition</u>: "However, there was a significant reduction in the median postintervention ICU and hospital patient costs in the glutamine recipients $23,000 versus $30,900 in the control patients (P 5 0.036). For patients given glutamine there was a reduced cost per survivor of 30%."[1122] Given the safety and low cost of glutamine, one might wonder why hospitals have

---

[1117] Marik PE, Zaloga GP. Immunonutrition in critically ill patients: a systematic review and analysis of the literature. *Intensive Care Med*. 2008 Nov;34(11):1980-90
[1118] The glutamine dose in this study was "a total of 26 g/day" administered in four divided doses. CONCLUSION: "The results of this prospective randomized clinical trial show that enteral G reduces blood culture positivity, particularly with P. aeruginosa, in adults with severe burns and may be a life-saving intervention." Garrel et al. Decreased mortality and infectious morbidity in adult burn patients given enteral glutamine supplements: a prospective, controlled, randomized clinical trial. *Crit Care Med*. 2003 Oct;31(10):2444-9
[1119] Niihara et al. L-glutamine therapy reduces endothelial adhesion of sickle red blood cells to human umbilical vein endothelial cells. *BMC Blood Disord*. 2005 Jul 25;5:4
[1120] "Subjects with hematologic malignancies in remission underwent a standard treatment of high-dose chemotherapy and total body irradiation before bone marrow transplantation. After completion of this regimen, they were randomized to receive either standard parenteral nutrition (STD, n = 10) or an isocaloric, isonitrogenous nutrient solution enriched with crystalline L-glutamine (0.57 g/kg/day, GLN, n = 10)." Scheltinga et al. Glutamine-enriched intravenous feedings attenuate extracellular fluid expansion after a standard stress. *Ann Surg*. 1991 Oct;214(4):385-93; discussion 393-5 For additional review, see Ziegler TR. Glutamine supplementation in cancer patients receiving bone marrow transplantation and high dose chemotherapy. *J Nutr*. 2001 Sep;131(9 Suppl):2578S-84S
[1121] Furukawa et al. Glutamine-enhanced bacterial killing by neutrophils from postoperative patients. *Nutrition*. 1997 Oct;13(10):863-9
[1122] Jones et al. Randomized clinical outcome study of critically ill patients given glutamine-supplemented enteral nutrition. *Nutrition*. 1999 Feb;15(2):108-15

not already started to implement glutamine therapy on a regular basis, based on this research and other supporting research which also points toward clinical efficacy and lack of adverse effects.
- o Randomized clinical trial: Benefits of early enteral nutrition with glutamine and probiotics in brain injury patients: This clinical trial of brain injury patients showed that an enteral formula containing glutamine and probiotics decreased the infection rate and shortened the stay in the intensive care unit; "The infection rate was higher in controls (100%) when compared with the study group (50%; P=0.03) and the median (range) number of infections per patient was significantly greater (P<0.01) in the control group compared with the study group."[1123]
- o Double-blind, randomized, controlled study of alanyl-glutamine dipeptide-supplemented parenteral nutrition in SICU patients requiring parenteral nutrition: Efficacy of parenteral nutrition supplemented with glutamine dipeptide to decrease hospital infections in critically ill surgical patients: This clinical trial in the surgical intensive care unit (SICU) compared ❶ standard hospital parenteral/intravenous nutrition (STD-PN) against ❷ alanyl-glutamine dipeptide-supplemented parenteral nutrition (GLN-PN) in two different patient populations: 1) SICU patients requiring parenteral nutrition and 2) SICU care after surgery for pancreatic necrosis, cardiac, vascular, or colonic surgery. Nutritional intake was isonitrogenous, either containing no glutamine (standard nutrition) or containing 0.5 g/kg/d glutamine dipeptide. GLN-PN did not alter the incidence of infection after pancreatic necrosis surgery; however, in nonpancreatic surgery patients, GLN-PN was associated with significantly decreased total nosocomial infections (STD-PN 36 vs GLN-PN 13), bloodstream infections (7 vs 0), pneumonias (16 vs 6), and infections attributed to *Staphylococcus aureus*, fungi, and enteric Gram-negative bacteria. The authors concluded, "Glutamine dipeptide-supplemented parenteral nutrition did not alter infection rates following pancreatic necrosis surgery but significantly decreased infections in SICU patients after cardiac, vascular, and colonic surgery."[1124]
- **Dietary nucleotides**: Especially during times of infection/immunoproliferation/immunoactivation and trauma/repair, rapidly proliferating tissues, such as the immune system or the intestine are not able to fulfill the needs of cell nucleotides exclusively by de novo synthesis; in these times, nutritional supplementation with dietary nucleotides can provide therapeutic value by promoting mucosal maintenance/repair and immune responses to infection. Dietary nucleotides have several effects on immune function, including beneficial influence on immunoglobulin response and lymphocyte maturation/activation/proliferation and enhancement of macrophage phagocytosis and (anti)tumor responses.[1125] Similar to glutamine, arginine, EPA, DHA, and GLA, nucleotides appear to be conditionally-essential nutrients for the provision of an adequate supply of purines and pyrimidines for nucleic acid synthesis during times of growth/proliferation such as during infancy and in response to infection/trauma.
  - o Review: The role of nucleotides in adult nutrition: The authors of this study review relevant literature and summarize that dietary RNA is required to maintain immune function, and to restore lost immune function after protein deprivation, following which adequate calories and protein alone do not return immune function to normal. The authors proceed to note that dietary nucleotides can restore lost immune function even during protein starvation and weight loss. "In two separate double blind clinical studies the patients fed the enteral diet containing nucleotides had improved immune function compared with patients receiving a nucleotide free diet. In addition, infectious complications and length of hospital stay were reduced in postoperative cancer patients fed Impact [a commercial nucleotide-containing immunonutrition formula] compared with a control group."[1126]
- **Whey protein isolate**: Whey protein is a mixture of globular proteins isolated from whey, the liquid material created as a by-product of cheese production. The major protein fractions in whey are beta-lactoglobulin, alpha-lactalbumin, bovine serum albumin and immunoglobulins. Whey proteins are rich in cysteine as well as in GSH-precursor peptides. Whey protein isolates are processed to remove fat and lactose and are generally > 90%

[1123] Falcão de Arruda et al. Benefits of early enteral nutrition with glutamine and probiotics in brain injury patients. *Clin Sci* (Lond). 2004 Mar;106(3):287-92
[1124] Estivariz et al. Efficacy of parenteral nutrition supplemented with glutamine dipeptide to decrease hospital infections in critically ill surgical patients. *JPEN J Parenter Enteral Nutr*. 2008 Jul-Aug;32(4):389-402
[1125] Gil A. Modulation of the immune response mediated by dietary nucleotides. *Eur J Clin Nutr*. 2002 Aug;56 Suppl 3:S1-4
[1126] Van Buren et al. The role of nucleotides in adult nutrition. *J Nutr*. 1994 Jan;124(1 Suppl):160S-164S

protein by weight. Although whey proteins are responsible for some "milk allergies", the major allergens in milk are caseins; many "milk allergic" patients can tolerate whey protein isolate even if they are intolerant of other milk/dairy products. Whey protein isolate provides high-quality easily digestible protein to meet body needs, either on an everyday basis or on a special needs basis, such as during infection or recovery from injury. Reviewed in the section below are supporting articles with specific reference to the use of whey protein supplementation in patients with infections. Whey protein isolate can easily be incorporated into even the most noncompliant patient's regimen, either in the form of smoothies or incorporated into raw-foods brownies or other treats; smoothies can be blended with whey protein isolate, fish oil, borage oil, fresh/frozen berries, and fiber sources such as wheat bran or flax seeds.

- o Prospective double-blind clinical trial: Oral supplementation with whey proteins increases plasma glutathione levels of HIV-infected patients: Authors of this study sought to restore glutathione (GSH) levels by providing the semi-essential amino acid cysteine via oral supplementation with two different cysteine-rich whey protein formulas: Protectamin (Fresenius Kabi, Bad Hamburg, Germany) or Immunocal (Immunotec, Vandreuil, Canada). One intervention included the addition of a daily dose of 45 g whey protein to either Protectamin or Immunocal for two weeks. "**Following two weeks of oral supplementation with whey proteins, plasma GSH levels increased in the Protectamin group by 44%** (2.79 microM, P = 0.004) while the difference in the Immunocal group did not reach significance (+ 24.5%, 2.51 microM, P = 0.43)."[1127] This study showed that while both whey protein supplements increased GSH levels, one product (Protectamin) significantly out-performed the other in terms of the difference in plasma GSH levels. This appears to be a significant biochemical difference, although the clinical significance in terms of patient outcomes (which would requires years of study in the same patient group) was not studied here.

- o Clinical trial: Effects of long-term supplementation with whey proteins on plasma glutathione levels of HIV-infected patients: This study reported again that Protectamin outperformed Immunocal insofar as Protectamin lead to higher levels of GSH when given at 45 g whey protein per day. Very interestingly, the biochemical benefits continued to accumulate over at least 6 months of treatment. "After six months, total GSH plasma levels were still significantly elevated compared to baseline (day 1: 1.95 microM vs. month 1: 2.18 microM; month 3: 2.39 microM; month 6: 2.47 microM)."[1128] The authors found that body weight, T-cell counts, and other clinical parameters did not change, and that the most common mild side effect was intestinal disturbance. No severe adverse events occurred. This study supports the importance of long-term adherence to dietary optimization and nutritional supplementation, with the benefits of whey protein supplementation (45 g/d) continuing to accumulate for at least 6 months after the initiation of treatment.

- o Prospective double-blind clinical trial: Features of whey protein concentrate supplementation in children with rapidly progressive HIV infection: This trial lasted 4 months and included 18 vertically HIV-infected children (2-6 years of age), taking antiretroviral therapy, who had received whey protein (treatment), maltodextrin (placebo) or none. "A significant median increase of 16.14 mg/dl (p = 0.018) in erythrocyte glutathione levels was observed in the whey protein-supplemented group; the TCD4/CD8 lymphocyte ratio showed a non-significant increase and **lower occurrence of associated co-infections was also observed.**"[1129]

- o Clinical trial: Beneficial effects of aggressive protein feeding with whey protein in severely burned children: Injured and infected patients are hypermetabolic; nutrient utilization is greatly increased due to physiologic hyperthermia, cell turnover, immune activation, and tissue repair. This hypermetabolic state depletes protein stores (i.e., tissue proteins, such as muscle) and vitamins (either due to metabolic utilization or oxidative destruction). In this study, 18 children with burns averaging 60% total surface area were randomized into two groups and studied for at least six weeks. The first group was given a normal diet with "a balanced nutritional supplement", while the second group was supplemented with milk whey protein. Details of their report were impressive: "The normal protein group received 87.1% of

---

[1127] Micke et al. Oral supplementation with whey proteins increases plasma glutathione levels of HIV-infected patients. *Eur J Clin Invest*. 2001 Feb;31(2):171-8
[1128] Micke et al. Effects of long-term supplementation with whey proteins on plasma glutathione levels of HIV-infected patients. *Eur J Nutr*. 2002 Feb;41(1):12-8
[1129] Moreno et al. Features of whey protein concentrate supplementation in children with rapidly progressive HIV infection. *J Trop Pediatr*. 2006 Feb;52(1):34-8

their desired caloric intake with 16.5% of calories from protein compared to 77.7% of desired caloric intake with 23.0% of calories from protein for the high protein group. Despite a higher caloric intake, the normal protein group had...lower levels of C3 (1371 vs. 1585 micrograms/ml), lower levels of IgG (805 vs. 975 micrograms/ml), lower levels of transferrin (200 vs. 283 mg/dl), lower levels of total serum protein (5.5 vs. 6.3 g/dl), more bacteremic days (11% vs. 8%) and worse survival (5/9--56% vs. 9/9--100%)." As expected, patients receiving the high protein diet had significantly higher plasma levels of amino acids. Plasma asparagine levels positively correlated with better neutrophil function. The authors conclude that, "These studies provide evidence that many immunologic functions are dependent upon optimal availability of specific amino acids, and that routine diets do not provide sufficient protein to satisfy the needs of seriously burned children."[1130]

- **Melatonin: 5-40 mg hs (*hora somni*—Latin: sleep hour)**: Melatonin has proven anti-infectious and immunosupportive properties; it must be taken only at night (within a few hours of sleep) in order to be beneficial.
    - Clinical trial: Effects of melatonin treatment in septic newborns: Immunostimulatory anti-infective action of melatonin was demonstrated in a small clinical trial wherein septic newborns administered 20 mg melatonin showed significantly increased survival over nontreated controls. "Three of 10 septic children who were not treated with melatonin died within 72 h after diagnosis of sepsis; none of the 10 septic newborns treated with melatonin died."[1131]
    - Review: Therapeutic potential of melatonin in immunodeficiency states, viral diseases, and cancer: The clinical benefits of melatonin (MLT) administration have been well documented and consistently documented in patients with various forms of cancer receiving various forms of chemotherapy and/or radiation treatment. In this review, Maestroni[1132] provides a partial review of this research and also adds to clinicians' mechanistic understanding of the immunosupportive and immunostimulatory actions, summarized as, "T-helper cells bear G-protein-coupled MLT cell membrane receptors and, perhaps, MLT nuclear receptors. Activation of MLT receptors enhances the release of T-helper cell cytokines, such as gamma-interferon and interleukin-2 (IL-2), ... MLT has been reported also to enhance the production of interleukin-1, interleukin-6 and interleukin-12 in human monocytes. These mediators may counteract secondary immunodeficiencies, ..."
    - Review: The potential of melatonin in reducing morbidity-mortality after craniocerebral trauma: Actions that make melatonin a reasonable treatment after trauma such as craniocerebral trauma include ❶ neutralization of both oxygen-based and nitrogen-based free radicals, ❷ stimulation of the activities of a variety of antioxidative enzymes (e.g. superoxide dismutase, glutathione peroxidase, glutathione reductase and catalase), ❸ inhibition of pro-inflammatory cytokines and activation-adhesion molecules which consequently reduces lymphocytopenia and **reduces infections by opportunistic organisms**, ❹ reestablishment of the natural circadian rhythm of sleep and wakefulness, ❺ reduction in the toxicity of the drugs used in the treatment of craniocerebral trauma, ❻ enhanced function of drugs used in the treatment of craniocerebral trauma, ❼ reduction in brain contusion volume, and ❽ stabilization of cellular membranes preventing vasospasm and apoptosis of endothelial cells.[1133]

- **Licorice (*Glycyrrhiza glabra*)**: Licorice has been consumed by humans for thousands of years as a food spice, tea, and medicine. Ancient documents from China, India, and Greece all mention its use for symptoms of viral respiratory tract infections and hepatitis. Beyond its sweet taste, licorice is best known medicinally for its use in soothing the gastrointestinal tract as well as for its potent broad-spectrum antiviral effects. The current author has worked with several patients plagued by recurrent, persistent, and pharmacorecalcitrant herpes simplex infections for whom drugs such as acyclovir failed and for whom licorice worked very satisfactorily. The pro-hypertensive sodium-retaining potassium-depleting pseudoaldosterone effect of licorice should be well appreciated by all clinicians with doctorate-level training. Less well known is the ability of licorice to potentiate cortisol and to impair testosterone biosynthesis, with the latter action useful for patients with excess

---

[1130] Alexander et al. Beneficial effects of aggressive protein feeding in severely burned children. *Ann Surg*. 1980;192(4):505-17
[1131] Gitto et al. Effects of melatonin treatment in septic newborns. *Pediatr Res*. 2001 Dec;50(6):756-60 pedresearch.org/cgi/content/full/50/6/756
[1132] Maestroni GJ. Therapeutic potential of melatonin in immunodeficiency states, viral diseases, and cancer. *Adv Exp Med Biol*. 1999;467:217-26
[1133] Maldonado et al. The potential of melatonin in reducing morbidity-mortality after craniocerebral trauma. *J Pineal Res*. 2007 Jan;42(1):1-11

testosterone or estradiol; the effect begins within four days as measured by reductions in serum testosterone (or estradiol).

- o Review: Antiviral effects of *Glycyrrhiza* species: Clinical trials have demonstrated the *Glycyrrhiza glabra* derived compound glycyrrhizin and its derivatives are clinically beneficial in patients with chronic hepatitis B and C, including a reduction in the risk of hepatocellular carcinoma. Animal studies have shown benefit against herpes simplex virus encephalitis and influenza A virus pneumonia. In vitro studies show activity against HIV-1, SARS related coronavirus, respiratory syncytial virus, arboviruses, vaccinia virus and vesicular stomatitis virus. Numerous mechanisms are involved, including direct viral inactivation (anti-viral effect) and enhancement of interferon gamma in T-cells (host-augmenting effect).[1134]

> **Broad-spectrum antiviral activity of licorice**
> "… a component of Glycyrrhiza glabra roots, found to be glycyrrhizie acid, is active against viruses. We report here that this drug inhibits growth and cytopathology of several unrelated DNA and RNA viruses... In addition, glycyrrhizic acid inactivates herpes simplex virus particles irreversibly."
>
> Pompei et al. Glycyrrhizic acid inhibits virus growth and inactivates virus particles. *Nature*. 1979 Oct

- o In vitro research: Glycyrrhizic acid inhibits virus growth and inactivates virus particles: "…a component of Glycyrrhiza glabra roots, found to be glycyrrhizie acid, is active against viruses. We report here that this drug inhibits growth and cytopathology of several unrelated DNA and RNA viruses... In addition, glycyrrhizic acid inactivates herpes simplex virus particles irreversibly."[1135]

- o Ex vivo study: Glycyrrhizin, an active component of licorice roots, and replication of SARS-associated coronavirus: "We assessed the antiviral potential of ribavirin, 6-azauridine, pyrazofurin, mycophenolic acid, and glycyrrhizin against two clinical isolates of coronavirus (FFM-1 and FFM-2) from patients with SARS admitted to the clinical center of Frankfurt University. Of all the compounds, glycyrrhizin was the most active in inhibiting replication of the SARS-associated virus."[1136]

- o Review: The use of alternative medicine in the treatment of hepatitis C: "The active component of licorice root, glycyrrhizin, has been shown to reduce alanine transaminase and aspartate transaminase values in the serum. This protective function has recently been explained as the inhibitory effects of glycyrrhizin on immune-mediated cytotoxicity against hepatocytes and on nuclear factor (NF)-kappa B, …"[1137]

- **Silibinin/silybin from *Silymarin marianum*—special (but not exclusive) application for viral hepatitis**: In the world of botanical medicine, certainly most herbalists and naturopathic physicians would readily but not exclusively associate *Silymarin marianum* with the treatment of liver disorders, ranging from cirrhosis to cholestasis. Herbal preparations are safe, well standardized, and useful "beyond the liver" in support of general detoxification, cancer treatment, and renoprotection.

  - o Triple-blind, randomized, placebo-controlled trial: A randomized controlled trial to assess the safety and efficacy of Silymarin on symptoms, signs and biomarkers of acute hepatitis: This study[1138] enrolled 105 patients with symptoms compatible with acute clinical hepatitis and serum alanine aminotransferase (ALT) levels >2.5 times the upper limit of normal. Per the authors' description, "The intervention consisted of three times daily ingestion of either a standard recommended dose of 140 mg of silymarin (Legalon, MADAUS GmbH, Cologne, Germany), or a vitamin placebo for four weeks with an additional four-week follow-up." No adverse events were noted. Results showed that, "Patients randomized to the silymarin group had quicker resolution of symptoms related to biliary retention: dark urine (p=0.013), jaundice (p=0.02) and scleral icterus (p=0.043). There was a reduction in indirect bilirubin

> **Orally administered antioxidant nutrients and antiviral botanicals used in the study by Melhem et al**
> - Glycyrrhiza: 500 mg bid*
> - Schizandrae: 500 mg tid*
> - Ascorbate: 2,000 mg tid
> - Glutathione: 150 mg bid
> - Silymarin: 250 mg tid*
> - Lipoic acid: 150 mg bid
> - D-alpha-tocopherol: 800 IU/d
>
> *No data was provided about the standardization of the botanicals.
>
> Melhem et al. Treatment of chronic hepatitis C virus infection via antioxidants: results of a phase I clinical trial. *J Clin Gastroenterol*. 2005 Sep;39(8):737-42

[1134] Fiore et al. Antiviral effects of Glycyrrhiza species. *Phytother Res*. 2008 Feb;22(2):141-8
[1135] Pompei et al. Glycyrrhizic acid inhibits virus growth and inactivates virus particles. *Nature*. 1979;281(5733):689-90
[1136] Cinatl et al. Glycyrrhizin, an active component of liquorice roots, and replication of SARS-associated coronavirus. *Lancet*. 2003 Jun 14;361(9374):2045-6
[1137] Bean P. The use of alternative medicine in the treatment of hepatitis C. *Am Clin Lab*. 2002 May;21(4):19-21
[1138] El-Kamary et al. A randomized controlled trial to assess the safety and efficacy of silymarin on symptoms, signs and biomarkers of acute hepatitis. *Phytomedicine*. 2009 May;16(5):391-400

among those assigned to silymarin (p=0.012), but other variables including direct bilirubin, ALT and aspartate aminotransferase (AST) were not significantly reduced."

- o Clinical trial of intravenous silibinin/silybin from *Silymarin marianum*: Silibinin is a potent antiviral agent in patients with chronic hepatitis C not responding to pegylated interferon/ribavirin therapy: Silibinin, also known as silybin, is the major active constituent of silymarin, the mixture of flavonolignans extracted from milk thistle, *Silybum/Silymarin marianum*. Oral dosing of silibinin, like oral dosing of many nutrients, cannot achieve the high serum levels attainable with intravenous treatment. In this study, sixteen patients unresponsive to full-dose pegylated (Peg)-interferon/ribavirin (PegIFN/RBV) received 10 mg/kg/day SIL IV (Legalon Sil; Madaus, Köln, Germany) for 7 days. In a subsequent dose-finding study, 20 patients received 5, 10, 15, or 20 mg/kg/day SIL for 14 days. The authors report that subjects treated with SIL IV showed an "unexpected" temporary reduction in HCV-RNA which was dose dependent and which decreased further after 7 days combined SIL/PegIFN/RBV. In 7 patients on 15 or 20 mg/kg SIL, their viral load became undetectable at week 12 (despite previous nonresponse to PegIFN/RBV. Mild gastrointestinal symptoms were the only adverse effect attributed to IV SIL monotherapy. The authors conclude that, " IV SIL is well tolerated and shows a substantial antiviral effect against HCV in nonresponders."[1139]

- o Review, and a word of caution in the use of silymarin in non-hepatitis viral infections: Immunosuppressive effect of silibinin in experimental autoimmune encephalomyelitis, and Silibinin polarizes Th1/Th2 immune responses through the inhibition of immunostimulatory function of dendritic cells: Silymarin has beneficial effects in models (including human clinical trials) of liver disease; new research is promoting its use in anti-cancer protocols. Silymarin inhibits NFkB and this probably explains a good deal of its anti-inflammatory and anti-fibrotic effects. However, a few articles, such as by Min et al[1140] suggest that silymarin might impair antiviral Th-1 immune responses; they write, "…silibinin Ag-nonspecifically down-regulated the secretion of pro-inflammatory Th1 cytokines and up-regulated the anti-inflammatory Th2 cytokines in vitro. Silibinin also dose-dependently inhibited the production of Th1 cytokines ex vivo. These results indicate that silibinin is both immunosuppressive and immunomodulatory." Identically, Lee et al[1141] found, in an experiment involving dendritic cells (DC) that, "…silibinin-treated DCs evidenced an **impaired induction of Th1 response**, and a normal cell-mediated immune response."

• **NFkB inhibitors**: Many viruses responsible for human disease are dependent upon the NFkB pathway for their replication and thus survival and ability to create disease. Per the review by Hiscott et al[1142], "…certain viruses, including human immunodeficiency virus type I (HIV-I), human T-cell leukemia virus type 1 (HTLV-1), Human herpesvirus 8 (HHV8) and Epstein–Barr virus (EBV), have incorporated aspects of NFkB signaling into their life cycle and pathogenicity, and thus induce NFkB activation." NFkB is also involved in the host defense system; so the paradox of NFkB is that it is necessary for *anti-viral defense* as well as for *viral replication*. Thus, at this time, the goal of intervention in this regard is toward one of NFkB *modulation*, rather than complete suppression or additional activation. Patients following the American/Western lifestyle are adept at activating NFkB through physical inactivity, sarcopenia, excess adiposity, widespread nutritional deficiencies, and overconsumption of dietary fats (especially saturated fats) and simple carbohydrates in large amounts. Phytonutritional modulation of NFkB was reviewed by Vasquez in 2005 (available on-line[1143]) and regularly thereafter, particularly in *Integrative Rheumatology*, especially Chapter 4.[1144]

- o Clinical trial of combination antioxidant nutrients and antiviral botanicals: Treatment of chronic hepatitis C virus infection via [oral and intravenous] antioxidants: results of a phase I clinical trial: The authors of this study correctly begin their introduction with an appreciation of host factors that are important in chronic hepatitis C virus infection when they state, "The pathogenesis of chronic hepatitis C virus (HCV)

[1139] Ferenci et al. Silibinin is a potent antiviral agent in patients with chronic hepatitis C not responding to pegylated interferon/ribavirin therapy. *Gastroenterology*. 2008 Nov;135(5):1561-7
[1140] Min K, Yoon WK, Kim SK, Kim BH. Immunosuppressive effect of silibinin in experimental autoimmune encephalomyelitis. *Arch Pharm Res*. 2007 Oct;30(10):1265-72
[1141] Lee et al. Silibinin polarizes Th1/Th2 immune responses through the inhibition of immunostimulatory function of dendritic cells. *J Cell Physiol*. 2007 Feb;210(2):385-97
[1142] Hiscott et al. Manipulation of the nuclear factor-kappaB pathway and the innate immune response by viruses. *Oncogene*. 2006 Oct 30;25(51):6844-67
[1143] Vasquez A. Nutritional and Botanical Inhibition of NF-kappaB, the Major Intracellular Amplifier of the Inflammatory Cascade. *Nutr Perspect* 2005;Jul: 5-12
[1144] Vasquez A. *Integrative Rheumatology*. IBMRC, 2007 to present. optimalhealthresearch.com/textbooks/rheum

infection is associated with a defective host antiviral immune response and intrahepatic oxidative stress. Oxidative stress and lipid peroxidation play major roles in the fatty liver accumulation (steatosis) that leads to necro-inflammation and necrosis of hepatic cells." In this Phase-1 study, fifty chronic HCV patients were treated for 20 weeks with a combination of seven orally-administered nutritional supplements: glycyrrhizin, schisandra, silymarin, ascorbic acid, lipoic acid, L-glutathione, and alpha-tocopherol); they also received "four different intravenous preparations (glycyrrhizin, ascorbic acid, L-glutathione, B-complex) twice weekly for the first 10 weeks, and followed up for an additional 20 weeks." Assessments included HCV-RNA levels, liver enzymes, and liver histology, while quality of life was assessed using the SF-36 questionnaire. Results showed normalization of liver enzymes in 44% of patients who had elevated pretreatment ALT levels (15 of 34). "A decrease in viral load (one log or more) was observed in 25% of the patients. Histologic improvement (2-point reduction in the HAI score) was noted in 36.1% of the patients. The SF-36 score improved in 26 of 45 patients throughout the course of the trial (58% of the patients). Treatment was well tolerated by all patients. No major adverse reactions were noted."[1145] As may be expected with the use of licorice, hypokalemia was seen in 3 patients (10.7%) and hypertension was seen in 2 patients (3.6%); both problems were mild and were treated symptomatically. Clinicians with any experience in the management of patients with HCV should appreciate the value of these findings, given the debilitating and fatal course of the disease when untreated, and the frequently devastating effects of pharmaceutical drugs that are expensive, toxic, and poorly efficacious.

Nutritional inhibition of NFkB
1. 1,25-dihydroxyvitamin D3
2. Bee propolis (CAPE)
3. Boswellia serratia
4. CoQ-10
5. Curcumin
6. GLA via PPAR-gamma
7. Glycyrrhizin from licorice
8. Grape seed extract
9. Green tea
10. Indole-3-carbinol
11. Isohumulones
12. Lipoic acid
13. N-acetyl-L-cysteine
14. EPA via PPAR-alpha
15. Resveratrol
16. Rosemary
17. Selenium
18. Silibinin, Silymarin
19. Zinc

- **Lipoic acid: 400 mg 3-4 times per day, ensure coverage with multivitamin**: Some clinicians note that because lipoic acid and thiamine work together in certain biochemical pathways (e.g., the pyruvate dehydrogenase complex between glycolysis and the Kreb's cycle) that thiamine should be co-administered when high-dose lipoic acid is used. Integrative clinicians should always cover the nutritional basics with the Paleo-Mediterranean diet and a high-potency broad-spectrum multivitamin/multimineral, so that this concern does not require special attention. Lipoic acid plays important metabolic, antioxidant, and NFkB-inhibiting roles in human physiology.
    - <u>Randomized, double-blinded, placebo-controlled trial conducted at two study sites: Restoration of blood total glutathione status and lymphocyte function following alpha-lipoic acid supplementation (300 mg thrice daily; 900 mg per day total) in patients with HIV infection</u>: This study involved 33 human immunodeficiency virus (HIV)-infected men and women with history of unresponsiveness (viral load >10,000 copies/ml) to highly active antiretroviral treatment (HAART). Results showed that mean blood total glutathione level in ALA-supplemented subjects was increased after 6 months from 0.81 to 1.34 mmol/L in contrast to no change in the placebo control group. Lymphocyte proliferation response was enhanced or stabilized after 6 months of ALA supplementation compared to progressive decline in the placebo group. No significant change was noted in either HIV RNA level or CD4 count. The authors concluded, "Supplementation with alpha-lipoic acid may positively impact patients with HIV and acquired immune deficiency syndrome by restoring blood total glutathione level and improving functional reactivity of lymphocytes to T-cell mitogens." Given that this group of patients had been previously unresponsive to HAART, we could reasonably expect a more severe level of oxidant stress and nutritional depletion; the mono-therapeutic intervention here with lipoate shows short-term safety and some biochemical efficacy; however, more impressive results would have been attained with a more comprehensive intervention.
- **N-acetyl-cysteine (NAC): 500-600 mg tid between meals**: NAC is commonly used in emergency medicine and outpatient integrative care alike. Relevant to the treatment of viral infections in general and respiratory infections in particular, we see that although most clinical trials have used monotherapy and doses that were

---

[1145] Melhem et al. Treatment of chronic hepatitis C virus infection via antioxidants: results of a phase I clinical trial. *J Clin Gastroenterol*. 2005 Sep;39(8):737-42 probably too low to produce optimal efficacy[1146], NAC does show benefit in the treatment and prevention of respiratory infections. Mechanisms of action include serving as a glutathione precursor and thus providing antioxidant protection, inhibiting viral replication—perhaps by potently suppressing NFkB, and thinning mucus to promote expectoration and prevent airway obstruction. In patients with acetaminophen overdose and the resulting hepatotoxicity and oxidative stress, Kelly[1147] reported NAC doses as follows: "...loading dose of 140 mg oral NAC per kg of body weight, followed four hours later by 70 mg per kg given every four hours for an additional 17 doses." These doses are life-saving for a potentially fatal situation. Doses used clinically for routine and preventive purposes are more in the range of 500-600 mg thrice daily between meals; higher doses can be used when indicated.

> **Research Quote**
> "Administration of **N-acetylcysteine during the winter, thus, appears to provide a significant attenuation of influenza and influenza-like episodes**, especially in elderly high-risk individuals. N-acetylcysteine did not prevent A/H1N1 virus influenza infection but **significantly reduced the incidence of clinically apparent disease**."
>
> De Flora et al. Attenuation of influenza-like symptomatology and improvement of cell-mediated immunity with long-term N-acetylcysteine treatment. *Eur Respir J*. 1997 Jul;10(7):1535-41

- Clinical trial: Effect of N-acetylcysteine (NAC) treatment on HIV-1 infection: a double-blind placebo-controlled trial: Authors of this study used low-dose 800 mg/d of NAC in patients with HIV to find that "After treatment the low plasma cysteine level in the NAC group increased to normal, and the decline of the CD4+ lymphocyte count before the study start, was less steep in the NAC group than in the placebo group after treatment."[1148] These are the anticipated findings for an effective antiviral agent.

- Randomized, double-blind trial involving 20 Italian Centers: Attenuation of influenza-like symptomatology and improvement of cell-mediated immunity with long-term N-acetylcysteine treatment (600 mg twice daily): "NAC treatment was well tolerated and resulted in a significant decrease in the frequency of influenza-like episodes, severity, and length of time confined to bed. Both local and systemic symptoms were sharply and significantly reduced in the NAC group."[1149]

- Randomized, 8-week, double-blind, placebo-controlled trial of high-dose NAC (8,000 mg/d) followed by optional open-label trial: N-acetylcysteine replenishes glutathione in HIV infection: Eighty-one HIV-infected, low GSH, CD4 T cells < 500 micro L(-1) with no active opportunistic infections or other debilitation showed serologic increase in GSH following NAC supplementation. The authors concluded, "NAC treatment for 8 weeks safely replenishes whole blood GSH and T cell GSH in HIV-infected individuals. Thus, NAC offers useful adjunct therapy to increase protection against oxidative stress, improve immune system function..."[1150] Many clinicians will be impressed by the high dose of NAC used in this study: 8000 mg of NAC per day in divided doses; the average NAC intake was 7g/d. Such doses are impressively higher than the 500-600 mg thrice daily that is more representative of common clinical practice. NAC should be consumed between meals, and if high doses are used for long periods of time, trace mineral supplementation, especially including copper, is advised. NAC has the ability to chelate minerals from the body; this can be used for life-saving benefit in patients with arsenic poisoning.

- Review: N-acetylcysteine: a new approach to anti-HIV therapy: Paralleling previous themes discussed earlier in this chapter in the topics of selenium and NFkB inhibition, authors of this review note that "NAC is different than many other antiviral drugs in that it inhibits host-mediated stimulation of viral replication arising in normal immune responses..." They go on to note that NAC "inhibits the action of inflammatory cytokines which may mediate cachexia, thereby raising the possibility that it may alleviate the deleterious wasting that accompanies late stage AIDS."[1151] This latter finding is important because the prevention of anorexia supports food intake which resists or reverses the nutrient depletion caused by chronic infection, and which, if left unchecked, causes a progressive decline in immune function and ever increasing susceptibility to progressive and additive infections.

[1146] Roxas M, Jurenka J. Colds and influenza: a review of diagnosis and conventional, botanical, and nutritional considerations. *Altern Med Rev*. 2007 Mar;12(1):25-4
[1147] Kelly GS. Clinical applications of N-acetylcysteine. *Altern Med Rev*. 1998 Apr;3(2):114-27
[1148] Akerlund et al. Effect of N-acetylcysteine(NAC) treatment on HIV-1 infection: a double-blind placebo-controlled trial. *Eur J Clin Pharmacol*. 1996;50(6):457-61
[1149] De Flora et al. Attenuation of influenza-like symptomatology and improvement of cell-mediated immunity with long-term N-acetylcysteine treatment. *Eur Respir J*. 1997 Jul;10(7):1535-41
[1150] De Rosa et al. N-acetylcysteine replenishes glutathione in HIV infection. *Eur J Clin Invest*. 2000 Oct;30(10):915-29
[1151] Roederer M, Ela SW, Staal FJ, Herzenberg LA, Herzenberg LA. N-acetylcysteine: a new approach to anti-HIV therapy. *AIDS Res Hum Retroviruses*. 1992 Feb;8(2):209-17

- Placebo-controlled double-blind multicenter study: Combination therapy with interferon-alpha plus N-acetyl cysteine for chronic hepatitis C: In this study, chronic hepatitis C patients (n=73) were treated with interferon-alpha plus NAC 600 mg thrice daily (IFN+NAC) or IFN alone (n=74) for 6 months with an additional 6-month follow-up. "Amongst patients receiving IFN plus NAC, sustained virological responses were observed in 5.5%, transient responses in 26% and non-response in 68.5%. The figures for patients receiving IFN only were 4.1%, 24.3% and 71.6% respectively."[1152] This study showed biochemical benefit to NAC+IFN therapy over IFN alone, but the benefits are only marginally better than not using NAC. The NAC dose of 600 mg/d is reasonable. Two problems with this study may have contributed to the inefficacy: ❶ In the Materials and Methods section of the full-text of the article, the authors make no mention of advising patients to consume the NAC between meals, on an empty stomach. This subtle yet important oversight may have retarded absorption and thus contributed to the negation of benefit. Clinicians untrained in nutrition would not be attentive to this level of detail, and details like this are clinically important. ❷ Also, the authors failed to test for changes in GSH levels. Such measurement would have provided objective data about the efficacy of the supplement being used, as well as about the compliance of each patient.
- Two randomized trials: Improvement of immune functions in HIV infection by sulfur supplementation: The authors of this study randomized 40 patients on antiretroviral therapy (ART; study 1) and 29 patients without ART (study 2) to treatment for 7 months with NAC or placebo dosed at "an individually adjusted dose according to a defined scheme." The authors report that both studies consistently showed that NAC causes a marked increase in immune functions and plasma albumin concentrations. The effect of NAC on viral load was not consistent. Our findings suggest that the impairment of immunological functions in HIV+ patients results at least partly from cysteine deficiency. The authors conclude by advocating NAC as a means for "**immunoreconstituting**" HIV patients to counter the effect of "HIV-induced cysteine depletion" which is a novel pathogenic mechanism "by which a virus destroys the immune defense of the host and escapes immune elimination."[1153]

- **Polyphenolics and phytonutrients**: Phytonutrients and polyphenolics have immune-modulating and NFkB-suppressing actions that are generally beneficial. Patients should have an optimized foundational whole-foods diet, upon which nutritional supplements, possibly including phytonutrient supplements, are added.
  - Double-blind, randomized, placebo-controlled trial: Immunity and Antioxidant Capacity in Humans Is Enhanced by Consumption of a Dried, Encapsulated Fruit and Vegetable Juice Concentrate: This trial involved oral supplementation with a commercially available encapsulated fruit and vegetable juice powder concentrate (FVJC) to provide phytonutrients; test subjects included 59 healthy law students who consumed either FVJC or placebo capsules for 77 days. "The FVJC group tended to have fewer total symptoms than the placebo group (P < 0.076). ... FVJC consumption during this study period resulted in increased plasma nutrients and antioxidant capacity, reduction in DNA strand breaks, and an increase in circulating gammadelta-T cells."[1154] Plasma levels of vitamin C, beta-carotene, lycopene, and lutein increased significantly from baseline in the FVJC group as did plasma oxygen radical absorptive capacity (50% increase in ORAC).
  - Study: Several indicators of oxidative stress, immunity, and illness improved in trained men consuming an encapsulated juice powder concentrate for 28 weeks: Subjects for this study involving a commercially available encapsulated juice powder concentrate (JPC) included 41 trained men from a homogenous police Special Forces unit, randomly assigned in a double blind manner to either JPC (n = 21) or placebo (n = 20). Subjects consumed 3 capsules twice daily with food; capsules contained dehydrated juice extracts from apple, beet, bilberry, blackberry, black currant, blueberry, broccoli, cabbage, carrot, cherry (acerola), Concord grape, cranberry, elderberry, kale, orange, peach, papaya, parsley, pineapple, raspberry, red currant, spinach, and tomato. Over 28 weeks of treatment, levels of carbonyl groups on protein and TNFalpha were lower in the JPC group. Importantly, "Over the final 20 wk of the study, the

---

[1152] Grant et al. Combination therapy with interferon-alpha plus N-acetyl cysteine for chronic hepatitis C. *J Med Virol*. 2000 Aug;61(4):439-42
[1153] Breitkreutz et al. Improvement of immune functions in HIV infection by sulfur supplementation: two randomized trials. *J Mol Med*. 2000;78(1):55-62
[1154] Nantz et al. Immunity and Antioxidant Capacity in Humans Is Enhanced by Consumption of a Dried, Encapsulated Fruit and Vegetable Juice Concentrate. *J Nutr*. 2006 Oct;136(10):2606-10

placebo group tended to have more days of illness than the JPC group. These data suggest beneficial JPC effects with regard to reduction of duty days lost due to illness..."[1155]

- Clinical trial: Immune Function in Elderly Smokers and Nonsmokers Improves during Supplementation with Fruit and Vegetable Extracts: ""Conclusions: Fruit and vegetable extract supplementation significantly enhanced multiple measures of immune function in elderly subjects, and improved IL-2 levels in smokers. Fruit and vegetable extract supplementation offers a novel way to improve compliance with current nutritional recommendations and may potentially lower disease risk."[1156]

- **Probiotics**: Generally speaking, probiotics are beneficial bacteria which colonize the human gastrointestinal tract; related terms are prebiotics (nutritional substrate such as inulin and fructooligosaccharides [FOS] consumed with the intention of promoting and supporting the intestinal growth of probiotics or endogenous beneficial bacteria) whereas synbiotics are combinations of probiotics and prebiotics.

  > **Research Quote**
  > "These data indicate that the intake of a dietary supplement containing **probiotic bacteria plus vitamins and minerals** during a period of at least three months in winter/spring **may reduce the incidence and the severity of symptoms in common cold infections** in otherwise healthy adults. This may be due to stimulated cellular immunity."
  >
  > Winkler et al. Effect of a dietary supplement containing probiotic bacteria plus vitamins and minerals on common cold infections and cellular immune parameters. *Int J Clin Pharmacol Ther.* 2005 Jul

  - Systematic review: Probiotics for the prevention of respiratory tract infections: In this systematic review, Vouloumanou et al[1157] evaluated the clinical evidence regarding probiotic use for the prevention of respiratory tract infections (RTIs) which ultimately included fourteen randomized controlled trials (RCTs). These studies used various Lactobacillus strains (7 studies), combinations of *Lactobacillus* and *Bifidobacterium* strains (5 studies), and a *Bifidobacterium* strain and a non-pathogenic *Enterococcus faecalis* strain (1 study). While the incidence of RTIs was often not affected (10 studies showed no difference; 4 studies showed reduced frequency of viral RTIs), the severity of the infections was shown to be reduced in 5 of 6 studies. Regarding duration, 3 studies showed a reduction in sick time, while 6 studies reported no difference. The authors wrote, "In conclusion, probiotics may have a beneficial effect on the severity and duration of symptoms of RTIs but do not appear to reduce the incidence of RTIs."

  - Clinical trial: Dietary supplementation of probiotic *Bacillus polyfermenticus*, Bispan strain, modulates natural killer cell and T cell subset populations and immunoglobulin G levels in human subjects: This study used the probiotic *Bacillus polyfermenticus* in twenty-five male subjects, 20-35 years of age, randomly assigned to placebo control or *B. polyfermenticus* tablets at a dose of 3.1 x 10(8) colony-forming units/day for 8 weeks. Results: "The concentration of IgG in the experimental group was 12% higher than in the placebo group after 8 weeks of Bispan supplementation. Also, the percentages of CD4+ helper T cells, CD8+ cytotoxic T cells, and CD56+ NK cells in the Bispan strain-supplemented group were 32%, 28%, and 35% higher, respectively, compared with the control group. Because of a higher increment of the CD4+ T cell subset than CD8+ T cells, the ratio of CD4+/CD8+ T cells was greater in the experimental group. This study suggests that the supplementation of *B. polyfermenticus* has a potentially positive effect on immune function by enhancing IgG production as well as by modulating the number of immune cell population such as CD4+ and CD8+ T cells and NK cells."[1158]

  - Randomized, double-blind, placebo-controlled clinical trial: Effect of a dietary supplement containing probiotic bacteria plus vitamins and minerals on common cold infections and cellular immune parameters: This very large study included 477 healthy men and women (aged 36 +/- 13 years) who had not been vaccinated against influenza; subjects were randomly assigned to daily probiotic/multivitamin/mineral supplement or a placebo, for up to 5.5 months. "RESULTS: The incidence of respiratory tract infections regarded as being virally induced was 13.6% lower in the

---

[1155] Lamprecht et al. Several indicators of oxidative stress, immunity, and illness improved in trained men consuming an encapsulated juice powder concentrate for 28 weeks. *J Nutr.* 2007 Dec;137(12):2737-41
[1156] Inserra et al. Immune Function in Elderly Smokers and Nonsmokers Improves During Supplementation with Fruit and Vegetable Extracts. *Integrative Medicine* 1999: 2; 3-10
[1157] Vouloumanou et al. Probiotics for the prevention of respiratory tract infections: a systematic review. *Int J Antimicrob Agents.* 2009 Jan 27
[1158] Kim et al. Dietary supplementation of probiotic Bacillus polyfermenticus, Bispan strain, modulates natural killer cell and T cell subset populations and immunoglobulin G levels in human subjects. *J Med Food.* 2006 Fall;9(3):321-7

probiotic/multivitamin/mineral supplement group compared to the placebo group."[1159] All symptoms of common cold and influenza-like infection were lower in the probiotic/multivitamin/mineral supplement group. Total symptom score was reduced by 19%, influenza symptoms by 25%, number of days with fever by 54%. Illness duration was not affected. Patients receiving the daily probiotic/multivitamin/mineral supplement showed significantly higher levels of leukocytes, lymphocytes, and in particular T-lymphocytes including CD4+ and CD8+ cells, as well as monocytes during the first 14 days of supplementation compared to placebo.

- o <u>In vitro (cell culture) study: Probiotic *Leuconostoc mesenteroides* ssp. *cremoris* and *Streptococcus thermophilus* induce IL-12 and IFN-γ production</u>: The authors of this study observed responses of human immunocytes in culture following response to probiotic bacteria; their results showed increased production of anti-inflammatory IL-12 and antiviral IFN-γ (gamma-interferon). The authors note that the increased production of IL-12 and IFN-γ is consistent with the TH1 response, which is important for anti-viral immunity. They write, "…novel probiotic *S. thermophilus* and *Leuconostoc* strains were extremely good inducers of these Th1 type cytokines. … A strong Th1 type cytokine response is also an important factor in the fight against viral infections such as that caused by influenza A virus."[1160]

- o <u>Randomized clinical trial: Synbiotics, prebiotics, glutamine, or peptide in early enteral nutrition: a randomized study in trauma patients</u>: One hundred thirteen multiple injured patients were prospectively randomized into 4 groups: group A, glutamine; B, fermentable fiber; C, peptide diet; and D, standard enteral formula with fibers combined with Synbiotic 2000 (Synbiotic 2000 Forte; Medifarm, Sweden), a formula containing live lactobacilli and specific bioactive fibers. Intestinal permeability was evaluated by measuring lactulose-mannitol excretion ratio on days 2, 4, and 7. Results showed no differences in days of mechanical ventilation, duration of intensive care unit stay, or multiple-organ failure scores. Researchers documented a total of 51 infections with 38 pneumonias; of these, only 5 infections and 4 pneumonias occurred in group D, which was significantly less than the infections and pneumonias in groups A, B, and C. Intestinal permeability decreased only in group D, from 0.148 on day 4 to 0.061 on day 7 whereas in group A, the lactulose-mannitol excretion ratio increased significantly from 0.050 on day 2 to 0.159 on day 7. Clearly and appropriately, the authors of this study concluded, "Patients supplemented with synbiotics did better than the others, with lower intestinal permeability and fewer infections."[1161]

- o <u>Clinical trial: Daily ingestion of fermented milk containing *Lactobacillus casei* DN114001 improves innate-defense capacity in healthy middle-aged people</u>: "…the probiotic-treated group increased oxidative burst capacity of monocytes, as well as NK cells tumoricidal activity. Results showed that daily intake of fermented milk containing *Lactobacillus casei* DN114001 could have a positive effect in modulating the innate immune defense in healthy-middle-age people."[1162]

- **Pancreatic and proteolytic enzymes**: Orally administered pancreatic/proteolytic enzyme combinations are remarkably safe and have applicability for a wide range of clinical problems, including resolution of acute and chronic refractory sinusitis (bromelain)[1163], clinical benefit in traumatic contusions, sprains, lacerations, strains (papain-containing preparation)[1164], alleviation of hip[1165] and knee[1166] pain (bromelain), and alleviation of knee pain (bromelain-trypsin-rutosid combination).[1167,1168] For the concentrations and combinations generally available, orally consumed enzymes might be prescribed as 4-8 tablets thrice daily between meals; doctors will have to customize the doses used based on the products chosen and the details of the patient and condition

---

[1159] Winkler et al. Effect of a dietary supplement containing probiotic bacteria plus vitamins and minerals on common cold infections and cellular immune parameters. *Int J Clin Pharmacol Ther*. 2005 Jul;43(7):318-26
[1160] Kekkonen et al. Probiotic Leuconostoc mesenteroides ssp. cremoris and Streptococcus thermophilus induce IL-12 and IFN-gamma production. *World J Gastroenterol*. 2008 Feb 28;14(8):1192-203
[1161] Spindler-Vesel et al. Synbiotics, prebiotics, glutamine, or peptide in early enteral nutrition: a randomized study in trauma patients. *JPEN*. 2007 Mar-Apr;31(2):119-26
[1162] Parra et al. Daily ingestion of fermented milk containing Lactobacillus casei DN114001 improves innate-defense capacity in healthy middle-aged people. *J Physiol Biochem*. 2004 Jun;60(2):85-91
[1163] Taub SJ. The use of bromelains in sinusitis: a double-blind clinical evaluation. Eye Ear Nose Throat Mon. 1967 Mar;46(3):361-5
[1164] Trickett P. Proteolytic enzymes in treatment of athletic injuries. Appl Ther. 1964;30:647-52
[1165] Klein et al. Efficacy and tolerance of an oral enzyme combination in painful osteoarthritis of the hip. *Clin Exp Rheumatol*. 2006 Jan-Feb;24(1):25-30
[1166] Walker et al. Bromelain reduces mild acute knee pain and improves well-being in a dose-dependent fashion in an open study of otherwise healthy adults. *Phytomedicine*. 2002;9:681-6
[1167] Akhtar et al. Oral enzyme combination versus diclofenac in the treatment of osteoarthritis of the knee. *Clin Rheumatol*. 2004 Oct;23(5):410-5
[1168] Tilwe et al. Efficacy and tolerability of oral enzyme therapy as compared to diclofenac in active osteoarthrosis of knee joint. *J Assoc Physicians India*. 2001 Jun;49:617-21

being treated. At the highest end of the dosage spectrum, Gonzalez[1169] reports using as much as "25-40 grams of porcine lyophilized pancreas product daily, taken in capsule form, away from meals, and spread evenly throughout the day. ... The particular formulation for pancreatic enzymes we use tests at 30-80 UPS units of proteolytic activity per milligram and 15-40 units of lipolytic activity per milligram." Relevant to this discussion of infectious diseases, we note that oral consumption of pancreatic/proteolytic enzymes has immunostimulatory actions[1170] as well as anti-edematous and anti-inflammatory actions.[1171]

- o <u>Pilot study in patients with pityriasis lichenoides chronica: Role of bromelain in the treatment of patients with pityriasis lichenoides chronica (PLC)</u>: "RESULTS: All patients showed complete clinical recovery after treatment. ... CONCLUSIONS: In conclusion bromelain **can** be considered an effective therapeutic option for PLC; its efficacy could be related to its anti-inflammatory, immunomodulatory and/or anti-viral properties."[1172]
- o <u>Double-blind, randomized, controlled phase III study at a tertiary care center: Efficacy and safety of phlogenzym—a protease formulation, in sepsis in children</u>: The authors of this study hypothesize that oral administration of proteolytic enzymes may regulate the host's immune system and promote early recovery from sepsis. This study used enteric-coated tablets with bromelain 90 mg, trypsin 48 mg, and rutin 100 mg as adjuvant therapy in treatment of 60 children (aged one month to 12 years) with sepsis; patients were given 1 tablet/10 kg body weight up to maximum six tablets a day in two or three divided doses for 14-21 days along with appropriate antibiotics and supportive treatment. Results are as follows: "Median time taken for fever to subside was three days in the [enzyme] group vs four days in the placebo group; hemodynamic support was needed for two days in the [enzyme] group but three days in the placebo group. The modified Glasgow coma scale score normalized in three days in the [enzyme] group vs 5.5 days in the placebo group. Oral feeds could be started in four days in the [enzyme] group vs five days in the placebo group. Two patients died in the placebo group. CONCLUSION: [Orally administered enzyme therapy] is effective as an adjuvant with antibiotics and supportive treatment for early improvement of pediatric patients with sepsis."[1173]

- **Iodine/iodide: approximately 13 mg per day**: Both iodine and iodide have biological activity in humans. The average daily intake of iodine in Japan is approximately 13 mg per day due to high consumption of seafood (fish, seaweed, etc); this level of nutrient intake is approximately 25x higher than levels consumed in the United States. Beyond thyroid hormone metabolism, iodine/iodide has important roles in estrogen metabolism—both in the modulation of estrogen subfractions as well as in the modulation (downregulation) of cellular estrogen receptors; these "anti-estrogen effects of iodine" contribute to its anticancer benefits. Relevant to this conversation is the antimicrobial effects of iodine/iodide; by their first or second year of professional education, all healthcare students who have had hand-on access to microbiology laboratory work are familiar with Lugol's solution. Lugol's solution is a broad-spectrum antiseptic introduced into medicine/microbiology in 1829 by the French physician Jean Lugol; it is an effective bactericide, fungicide, and virucide made by dissolving 10 parts of potassium iodide and 5 parts of iodine in 85 parts of water. By this time, clinicians should appreciate the potential benefits of routinely employing an essential nutrient with antiestrogen benefits, anticancer benefits, and antimicrobial (antibacterial, antiviral, and antifungal) effects. Human leukocytes preferentially concentrate iodide 1200-fold greater than do erythrocytes; experimental studies have shown that the combination of iodide with hydrogen peroxide and myeloperoxidase greatly increases the bactericidal activity over what is seen with myeloperoxidase alone.[1174] The virucidal effect of 1% Lugol's solution against influenza were shown *in vitro* in 1944 by Dunham and MacNeal.[1175] What is being proposed here is the *potential* for antiviral benefit from the supplemental use of this nutrient; of course, the recognition of this positive potentiality precedes the necessary clinical trials to validate this concept, but the safety and basic science are well established. At the very least, we

---

[1169] Gonzalez et al. Evaluation of pancreatic proteolytic enzyme treatment of adenocarcinoma of the pancreas, with nutrition and detoxification support. *Nutr Cancer*. 1999:117-24
[1170] "Similarly, oral administration of Wobenzym to healthy volunteers (n = 28) resulted in significant increases in ROS production, depending on dose (peak with 20 tablets) and time (peak 4 hours after Wobenzym administration). ... These findings point to an immunomodulatory capacity of WE in adjuvant tumor therapy." Zavadova et al. Stimulation of reactive oxygen species production and cytotoxicity in human neutrophils in vitro and after oral administration of a polyenzyme preparation. *Cancer Biother*. 1995;10(2):147-52
[1171] Taub SJ. The use of bromelains in sinusitis: a double-blind clinical evaluation. *Eye Ear Nose Throat Mon*. 1967 Mar;46(3):361-5
[1172] Massimiliano et al. Role of bromelain in the treatment of patients with pityriasis lichenoides chronica. *J Dermatolog Treat*. 2007;18(4):219-22
[1173] Shahid et al. Efficacy and safety of phlogenzym--a protease formulation, in sepsis in children. *J Assoc Physicians India*. 2002 Apr;50:527-31
[1174] Klebanoff SJ. Iodination of bacteria: a bactericidal mechanism. *J Exp Med*. 1967 Dec 1;126(6):1063-78
[1175] Dunham WB, MacNeal WJ. Inactivation of Influenza Virus by Mild Antiseptics. *Journal of Immunology* 1944; 49: 123-128

could reasonably anticipate that Lugol's solution—whether consumed as liquid drops or in tablet form as is commercially available—would have activity against microbes in the upper gastrointestinal tract, namely *Helicobacter pylori*; again, clinical trials are needed here. Saturated solution of potassium iodide (SSKI) is also used in humans for nutritional and therapeutic purposes. Limited evidence does prove (*not merely suggest*) that orally administered iodine/iodide has systemic antimicrobial benefit in humans.

- o Case report: Rhinofacial zygomycosis (RFZ) successfully treated with oral saturated solution of potassium iodide: a case report: "A diagnosis of RFZ was made and the patient was put on oral SSKI at an initial dose of 0.5 mL three times daily. This was gradually increased by 0.1 mL/dose/day until a dose of 5 mL three times daily was reached."[1176] By the one year of treatment, an 80% reduction in facial swelling.
- o Case reports: Sporotrichosis in childhood: clinical and therapeutic experience in 25 patients: "*Sporothrix schenckii* was isolated in all patients... Nineteen patients were treated and cured clinically and mycologically with potassium iodide... The dose of KI used was 1–3 g/day, starting at 1 g/day and increasing until the dose of 3 g/day was reached."[1177] The authors write that the duration of treatment is generally 3 months, and that side-effects occur in 5% to 10% of patients, mainly consisting of gastrointestinal symptoms, headache, or rhinorrhea; these adverse effects are eliminated when treatment is discontinued or the dose is reduced.

- **Lysine**: Lysine as an amino acid supplement is most famous for its use in the suppression of herpes outbreaks. Herpes simplex virus (HSV) type-1 infects about 50% of the human population, while HSV type-2 infects about 20% of the human population. Many and perhaps most patients are either asymptomatic and/or are unaware that they carry the infection and can transmit it via close contact such as kissing or sexual intercourse. *Lack of a visible outbreak or symptoms in no way indicates lack of transmissibility.* On the other end of the symptomatic spectrum, some unfortunate patients live in perpetual cycles of painful blistering and weeping outbreaks; these patients generally suffer quietly as they receive no time off from work or other compensation during what can be very painful attacks. HSV infects close to 70% of adults worldwide. From a pathologic perspective, HSV-1 is notorious for causing herpes encephalitis, which is a commonly fatal or devastating infection of the brain, generally involving the temporal lobes; this infection is typically fatal when neonates are infected during travel through an *actively herpetic* birth canal. When used for its anti-HSV effects, lysine should be consumed between meals, with avoidance of arginine-containing foods, and in combination with other immunosupportive nutrients such as licorice and lipoic acid and other NFkB inhibitors within a context of improved overall nutrition and lifestyle. There is no "cure" in terms of eradication for herpes—it is a chronic life-long infection, whether symptomatic or asymptomatic, hence the adage, "Love can be fleeting, but herpes is forever."
  - o Double-blind, placebo-controlled, multicenter trial: Success of l-lysine therapy in frequently recurrent herpes simplex infection. Treatment and prophylaxis: Twenty-seven patients were given L-Lysine monohydrochloride tablets (1,000 mg L-lysine per dose) 3 times a day for 6 months and their outcomes were compared to a placebo group. "The L-lysine treatment group had an average of 2.4 less HSV infections [during the 6-month period], symptoms were significantly diminished in severity and healing time was significantly reduced [i.e., faster healing]. L-Lysine appears to be an effective agent for reduction of occurrence, severity and healing time for recurrent HSV infection."[1178] The results of this study are comparable to if not better than the results obtained with several of the new anti-herpes drugs; however this treatment is inexpensive and does not carry the risks of chemical hepatitis and life-threatening drug reactions that are noted with the anti-herpes drugs.
  - o Double-blind, controlled crossover study: Lysine prophylaxis in recurrent herpes simplex labialis: L-lysine has an inhibitory effect on the multiplication of herpes simplex virus in cell cultures. This study used only 1,000 mg L-lysine monohydrochloride daily to find little benefit within 12 weeks; note that the dose used in this study was only 33% of the dose used by Griffith et al[1179] and that the duration was 3 months compared with 6 months. Nonetheless, the authors noted, "...significantly more patients were

---

[1176] Tripathy et al. Rhinofacial zygomycosis successfully treated with oral saturated solution of potassium iodide. *J Eur Acad Dermatol Venereol*. 2007 Jan;21(1):117-9
[1177] Bonifaz et al. Sporotrichosis in childhood: clinical and therapeutic experience in 25 patients. *Pediatr Dermatol*. 2007 Jul-Aug;24(4):369-72
[1178] Griffith et al. Success of l-lysine therapy in frequently recurrent herpes simplex infection. Treatment and prophylaxis. *Dermatologica* 1987;175:183-90
[1179] Griffith et al. Success of l-lysine therapy in frequently recurrent herpes simplex infection. Treatment and prophylaxis. *Dermatologica* 1987;175:183-90

recurrence-free during lysine than during placebo treatment (p = 0.05), suggesting that certain patients may benefit from prophylactic lysine administration."[1180]
- o Prospective, randomized, double-blind, placebo-controlled, cross-over study of forty-one patients: Treatment of recurrent herpes simplex infections with L-lysine monohydrochloride: The authors report that oral ingestion of 1,248 mg a day of L-Lysine monohydrochloride shows evidence of decreasing the recurrence rate of herpes simplex attacks in their patient population of "nonimmunocompromised hosts", while a dose of 624 mg a day was not effective. Further, they report that "L-Lysine may also be capable of decreasing the severity of symptoms associated with recurrences."[1181]

- **Adenosine monophosphate (AMP):** Based on published trials and clinical experience, Gaby[1182] has been a proponent of AMP in the treatment of herpes simplex virus (HSV) infections, and he reviewed its supporting literature in 2006. Different dosage schemes have been published (see article by Gaby for review and procedure): one scheme involves using AMP administered in a series of intramuscular injections with each intramuscular injection containing AMP 1.5-2.0 mg per kg body weight are administered every other day for a total of 9-12 treatments; Gaby reports using intramuscular AMP injections (usually 100 mg per injection) for a series of 10 injections with good clinical effect. Patients with herpesvirus infections show low levels of AMP in their blood compared with uninfected controls. The antiviral mechanism of AMP is not specifically defined; it may involve modulation of the cyclic adenosine monophosphate-response element, which is a transcription factor complex that participates in the regulation of viral gene expression and virus-induced diseases. Although AMP is a constituent of the human body and is therefore generally safe and nontoxic when administered parenterally/intramuscularly, clinicians might use caution in asthmatic patients given that *inhaled* AMP induces airway obstruction in asthmatic patients (but not in healthy subjects).[1183]
  - o Herpes zoster. The treatment and prevention of neuralgia with adenosine monophosphate: Thirty-two adults were treated with intramuscular injections of gel-sustained adenosine monophosphate (AMP) given three times a week for up to four weeks for acute herpes zoster. Patients reported a reduction in pain soon after the start of treatment; also noted were decreased desquamation time and faster healing of skin lesions. Duration of viral shedding was reduced; indicating both the healing of skin lesions, reduced viral replication, and reduced risk of infectivity. "At the end of the initial four-week treatment period, 88% of AMP-treated patients were pain free, as opposed to only 43% in the placebo group. ... All these patients recovered from pain within three weeks after initiation of treatment. No recurrence of pain or lesions was experienced from three to 18 months after the end of treatment."[1184] Adenosine monophosphate is a natural cellular metabolite, and thus showed no adverse effects or toxicity during or following the treatment. Thus, the anti-herpes effect of AMP is seen against both herpes zoster virus and herpes simplex virus.[1185]

- **Lemon balm (*Melissa officinalis*):** *Melissa officinalis* is available for oral (e.g., tea or tablets) and/or topical use. Like licorice, it has nonspecific antiviral benefits. Possible interference with thyroid function when *Melissa officinalis* is consumed in high doses internally/orally can be monitored via clinical and laboratory assessments. Aqueous extracts from lemon balm (*Melissa officinalis*), peppermint (*Mentha piperita*), prunella (*Prunella vulgaris*), rosemary (*Rosmarinus officinalis*), sage (*Salvia officinalis*) and thyme (*Thymus vulgaris*) exert a direct antiviral effect on free herpes simplex virus.[1186]
  - o Topical application of *Melissa officinalis* L. leaves (70:1) for recurring herpes labialis[1187]: A cream made from *Melissa officinalis* L. leaves (concentrated 70:1) was studied among 66 patients with herpes simplex labialis. Patients had at least four herpes episodes per year. Cream was applied to the affected area four times daily over five days. "The tested formulation is effective for the treatment of herpes simplex

---

[1180] Milman N, Scheibel J, Jessen O. Lysine prophylaxis in recurrent herpes simplex labialis: a double-blind, controlled crossover study. *Acta Derm Venereol*. 1980;60(1):85-7
[1181] McCune MA, Perry HO, Muller SA, O'Fallon WM. Treatment of recurrent herpes simplex infections with L-lysine monohydrochloride. *Cutis*. 1984 Oct;34(4):366-73
[1182] Gaby AR. Natural remedies for Herpes simplex. *Altern Med Rev*. 2006 Jun;11(2):93-101
[1183] "The mechanism of AMP is indirect and occurs via its decay product, adenosine. It stimulates mast cells through its low-affinity receptor A2B to release histamine, which ultimately leads to smooth muscle contraction." Vass et al. Adenosine and adenosine receptors in the pathomechanism and treatment of respiratory diseases. *Curr Med Chem*. 2008;15(9):917-22
[1184] Sklar et al. Herpes zoster. The treatment and prevention of neuralgia with adenosine monophosphate. *JAMA*. 1985 Mar 8;253(10):1427-30
[1185] "The compound displayed an immediate effect upon the healing of the recurrent lesions. Furthermore, twenty-three patients were free of recurrences for varying intervals extending over 2 years." Sklar SH, Buimovici-Klein E. Adenosine in the treatment of recurrent herpes labialis. *Oral Surg Oral Med Oral Pathol*. 1979 Nov;48(5):416-7
[1186] Nolkemper et al. Antiviral effect of aqueous extracts from species of Lamiaceae family against Herpes simplex virus type 1 and 2 in vitro. *Planta Med*. 2006 Dec;72:1378-82
[1187] Koytchev R, Alken RG, Dundarov S. Balm mint extract (Lo-701) for topical treatment of recurring herpes labialis. *Phytomedicine*. 1999 Oct;6(4):225-30

labialis." Benefits included shortening of the healing period, the prevention of a spreading of the infection, prolonged intervals between the periods with herpes outbreaks, and rapid reduction of typical symptoms: itching, tingling, burning, stabbing, swelling, tautness and erythema.

The End

- "It was during the years of my lowest vitality that I ceased to be a pessimist. The instinct of self restoration forbade me a philosophy of poverty and discouragement. As it were, that is how those years appear to me now. I soon discovered life anew…including myself. I turned my will to health, to life, into a philosophy….into the will to power."
- "The time is now past when accidents could befall me; and what *could* now fall to my lot which has not already be my own!? It returns only, it comes home to me at last—mine own Self. And such of it as has been long abroad, and scattered among things and accidents. And one thing more do I know: I stand now before my last summit, and before that which has been longest reserved for me."
- "You have within you the power to merge everything you have lived through – attempts, false starts, errors, delusions, passions, your loves and your hopes – into your highest goal, with nothing left over."
- "At every step one has to wrestle for truth; one has to surrender for it almost everything to which the heart, to which our love, our trust in life, cling otherwise. That requires greatness of soul: the service of truth is the hardest service…"
- "With your love go into your isolation and with your creativity, my brother; and only later will justice limp after you.
- "What makes a person heroic?" Answer: "To simultaneously face one's greatest fear and one's highest hope."
- "My principle article of faith is that one can only flourish among people who share the identical ideas and the identical will."
- "Not around the inventors of new noise but around the inventors of new values does the world revolve."

Friedrich Nietzsche (German classical Scholar, Philosopher and Critic of culture, 1844-1900)

Ceiling of Café de La Pedrera

Education for *la vida*—for life: The educational process begins with the discipline of learning facts and progresses to concept generation, then pattern-recognition, and eventually to pattern-prediction and mastery: "Our culture has truckled to the times, - to the senses. It is not manworthy. If the vast and the spiritual are omitted, so are the practical and the moral. It does not make us brave or free. We teach boys to be such men as we are. We do not teach them to aspire to be all they can. We do not give them a training as if we believed in their noble nature. We scarce educate their bodies. We do not train the eye and the hand. We exercise their understandings to the apprehension and comparison of some facts, to a skill in numbers, in words; we aim to make accountants, attorneys, engineers, but not to make able, earnest, great-hearted men. The great object of Education should be commensurate with the object of life. It should be a moral one; to teach self-trust: to inspire the youthful man with an interest in himself; with a curiosity touching his own nature; to acquaint him with the resources of his mind, and to teach him that there is all his strength, and to inflame him with a piety towards the Grand Mind in which he lives. Thus would education conspire with the Divine Providence." Ralph Waldo Emerson (1803-1882), American philosopher and essayist

How did Colombians overturn laws mandating the destruction of their grains, their mining, (ie, their food and ways of living)?
- Organization, protests and strikes in many cities
- 648 arrests of protesters, 262 detentions (overturned)
- 660 human rights violations
- 485 wounded
- 12 people killed during protests

That is the cost of freedom from GMO monopolization, more accurately described as GMO neocolonization. See reporting at youtube.com/watch?v=9Vz0tiRKvD0

ICHNFM.org • Colombia • Spain • United States

"Early in September, 2013, the Colombian government was forced to partially concede to the demands of a nationwide general strike instigated by farmers of the largely agrarian nation. The three week long protests and blockades that shut down much of the nation were supported by thousands of miners, truckers, students, bus drivers, and Colombian citizens, blocking roads and clashing with police. Close to 650 arrests were made, 485 injuries were reported, 12 people killed, and over 600 cases of human rights violations reported. Coverage of the nationwide protests feature rural peoples and urban demonstrators in the typical contest against body-armor clad, state riot police armed with gas, rubber bullets, flash-bang grenades and batons, beating people and dispersing women and children in clouds of smoke. ... Implementation of seed control was described by Colombian president Juan Manuel Santos as 'having Colombia tuned up to international reality.' This statement is, of course, completely true. The trending international reality is exactly this, trojan horse conquest of national food sovereignty by means of international corporate/government treaties and agreements sponsored by international governing bodies and the bottomless coiffeurs of the companies that benefit directly from such trade agreements. The shift to this international model of farming simply does not make economic or common sense for the people of most nations. Author and self-proclaimed 'economic hitman' John Perkins wrote about this type of imperial foreign occupation by corporate influence in his critical book, '_Confessions of an Economic Hitman_.' It is the newest means of international conquest. The international drive toward the monopolization of seed, the global reduction of seed diversity, and the abolishment of small scale farming is being seen all over the world."
  globalresearch.ca/colombians-successfully-revolt-against-seed-control-and-agricultural-tyranny/5352534

"Tensions have been rising between the Colombian government and the agricultural sector since the regulations imposed by the **U.S.-Colombia Free Trade Agreement**, which went into effect in May 2012. ... But farmers have bristled at the **requirement that they use genetically modified seeds, engineered by international conglomerates like Monsanto and Du Pont, and pay an annual fee to do so**."
  rollingstone.com/politics/news/will-colombias-farmers-get-what-they-want-20131118

Index

12-hydroperoxyeicosatetraenoic acid, 367
12-R-HETE, 367
12-R-lipoxygenase, 372
12-S-HETE, 367
12-S-lipoxygenase, 372
13-S-HODE, 366
15-hydroperoxyeicosatetraenoic acid, 367
15-hydroxy-eicosatrienoic acid, 365
15-lipoxygenase-1, 372
15-lipoxygenase-2, 372
15-S-HETE, 367
2,4-dichlorophenol, 237
2,5-dichlorophenol, 236
2010 ACR guidelines for the diagnosis and assessment of FM, 561
25(OH) vitamin D - testing, 59
2-hydroxyestrone, 523
5-HETE, 367
5-hydroperoxyeicosatetraenoic acid, 366
5-hydroxytryptophan, 583
5-lipoxygenase, 371
5pSPMD, 547
8-lipoxygenase, 372
8-S-HETE, 367
Acacia catechu, 457
Acetaminophen, 565
Acetyl-L-carnitine, 591
Acinetobacter spp, 94
Acupuncture, 592
Acute nontraumatic monoarthritis, 122
Acute red eye, 119
Adipokines, 204
Adipose, 204
ADP, dosing and clinical use, 550
Adrenic acid, 364
Adverse food reactions, 376
ALA, 356
Alginate, 670
Alkalinization, 267
Allergy diagnosis
Alpha-linolenic acid, 356
Alveolar hemorrhage, 639
Alzheimer's disease, 92
Amitriptyline, 563
ANA - interpretation, 78
ANA - overview, 26
Analgesia (natural) - importance and application in basic holistic care, 266, 267
ANCA, 680
Andrographis paniculata, 460
Anesthetics, 298
Anethum graveolens, 457
Anise, 457
Ankylosing spondylitis, 687
Anti-autoantibody interventions, 648
Anticardiolipin antibodies, 641
Anti-CCP antibodies, 81, 601
Anticitrullinated protein antibodies, 81, 601

Anti-double stranded (DS, native) DNA antibodies, 641
Antifibrillarin antibodies, 670
Anti-histone antibodies, 641
Antihistorical, 196
Anti-inflammatory & analgesic treatments, 255
Antimetabolites, 410
Antimicrobial treatment of SIBO, 586
Anti-nuclear antibodies, 641
Antinuclear antibody - interpretation, 78, 79
Antioxidant capacity of fruits/vegetables, 209
Antiphospholipid and Anticardiolipin antibodies, 641
Antiphospholipid/ anticardiolipin/ Hughes syndrome, 85
Anti-Ro antibodies, 641
Anti-Sm (anti-Smith) antibodies, 641
Antiviral (phyto)nutrition, 553
Arachidonic acid, 363
Arachidonic acid metabolites, 365
Armour thyroid, 527
Aromatase, 523
Artemisia annua, 455, 552
Artificial sweeteners, colors and other additives, 212
Aspartame, 212
Atlantoaxial instability, 120, 121
Atlantoaxial instability in AS and RA, 688
Augmentin, 587
Autoimmune hepatitis, 85
Autoimmune thyroid disease, 85
Autointoxication, 412
Autonomization, 224
Avascular necrosis of the femoral head, osteonecrosis, 123
Azithromycin for psoriasis, 625
Babesia, 93
Bacteriophages, 636
Balance shoes, 294
Barrett's esophagus, 655
Bed rest, 254
Beets, 460
Berberine, 455
Berberine, dosing and clinical use, 550
Beta-glucuronidase, 104
Beta-glucuronidase, 435
Betulina, 457
Bile flow, 536
Biochemical individuality, 195
Biochemical Individuality - overview, 216
Bioflavonoids treatment of allergy, 385
Bismuth, 456, 552
Blastocystis hominis, 447
Blastocystis hominis, 550
Body Mass Index, 204
Boerhaavia diffusa, 460
Bone necrosis caused by NSAIDs, 250

Borrelia burgdorferi, 93
Boswellia serrata - importance and application in basic holistic care, 259
Bromocriptine, 521, 522
Brucea javanica, 457
Buchu/betulina, 457
Bystander activation, 401
Cabergoline, 521
Caffeine, 212
Calcium pyrophosphate dihydrate deposition disease, 124, 125
Campylobacter, 93
C-ANCA, 680
Candida albicans, 448
Cannabis sativa and related variants, 261
Caprylic acid, 457
Capsicum annuum, Capsicum frutescens - importance and application in basic holistic care, 260, 626
Carbohydrate loading for supercompensation, 211
Carboxy-methyl-lysine, 559
Carnitine, antiinflammatory effects, 626
Carpal bones myofascial release, 290
Carpal tunnel syndrome - clinical management, 286
Carpal tunnel syndrome - manipulative treatment, 292
Carrageenan, 212
Cartilage destruction caused by NSAIDs, 250
Cat's claw - importance and application in basic holistic care, 259
Cauda equina syndrome, 2, 120
Cayenne pepper - importance and application in basic holistic care, 260, 626
CBC – overview, 25
CCP, 81, 601
Celiac disease, 85
Celiac disease and autoimmunity, 549
Centella asiatica, 666
Cervical Spine: Rotation Emphasis, 280
CH50, 641
Chemistry panel – overview, 25
Chiropractic, 592
Chiropractic model of illness and healing, 152
Chlamydia trachomatis, 93
Chlamydia/Chlamydophila pneumoniae, 93
Chlamydophila pneumoniae, 93, 569
Chlorella, 555, 594
Chlorpyrifos, 236
Chondroitin, 270
Chronic fatigue syndrome, 94
Churg-Strauss syndrome, 676
Citrobacter freundii, 448
Citrobacter rodentium, 448

Clinical criteria for fibromyalgia—description and contrast of the 1990 criteria and the 2010 criteria, 561
Clinical practice involves much more than "diagnosis and treatment", 114
Clove, 457
Coenzyme Q10, 588
Coffee as a gastrointestinal stimulant, 552
Cold and stretch treatment for MFTP, 277
Commiphora molmol, 456
Complement, 84
Complements C3 and C4, 54
Composite seropositivity, 81, 601
Comprehensive parasitology, 26, 102, 451
Compression - use in injury management, 255
Conscious living, 196
Consciousness-raising, 224
Consent to treatment, 110
Contemplation, 194
CoQ-10 in the treatment of allergy, 385
Corrective experience, 224
Cortef, 525
Cortisol, 524
Cosmetics, 594
Counterthrust, 279
CPDD, 125
CPPD, 124, 125
Cranberry, 457
Cranial nerves, 22, 23
C-reactive protein - interpretation, 27
Creatine monohydrate, 591
CREST syndrome, 651
CRP - interpretation, 52
Cryoglobulinemia, 675
Curcumin, 460
Curcumin requires piperine for absorption, 308, 374, 386
Cutaneous dysbiosis/colonization—introduction to assessment, 90
Cyclic citrullinated protein antibodies, 81, 601
Cyclobenzaprine, 565
Cyclooxygenase (COX), 370
Cymbalta, 564
Cytomegalovirus (CMV), 92
Cytomegalovirus (CMV), 631
Cytomegalovirus—Induction of vasculopathy, 661
Cytomel, 527
Daily living, 190
Danazol, 643
DDE, 235
DDT, 235
Deep tendon reflexes, 24
Deglycyrrhizinated licorice, 699
Delta-4-desaturase, 370
Delta-5-desaturase, 370
Delta-6-desaturase, 370
Depuration, 238, 239
Detoxification
Detoxification, 239
Detoxification, 572

Detoxification defects by leaky gut, 434
Detoxification programs are a necessity, 235
Detoxification: Clinical Review, 529
Devil's claw - importance and application in basic holistic care, 259
DGLA, 362
DGLA metabolites by 15-lipoxygenase, 365
DGLA metabolites by cyclooxygenase, 364
DHA, 256, 358
DHEA, 525
DHEA, 685
Diabetes mellitus type 1.5, 85
Dientamoeba fragilis, 448
Diet optimization, 582
Dietary haptenization, 379
Dietary molecular mimicry, 380
Diffuse idiopathic skeletal hyperostosis, 691
Diffuse systemic sclerosis, 651
Diflucan, 587
Dihomo-gamma-linolenic acid, 362
Diindolylmethane, 523
Dill (antimicrobial actions), 457
DIM, 523
Dimercaptosuccinic acid, 539
Dimercaptosuccinic acid, 572
DISH, 691
D-lactic acid, 574
DMSA, 539, 572
DNA methylation, 635
Docere, 131
Docosahexaenoic acid, 358
Docosapentaenoic acid, 358, 364
Docosatrienes, 308, 359
Dostinex, 521
DPA, 358
D-ribose, 591
Drop thrust, 283
Dry needling or injection of local anesthetic or saline
Duloxetine, 564
Dysbiosis
Dysbiosis--introduction to concepts and testing, 86
Educate - importance and application in basic holistic care, 255
Eicosanoid modulation - importance and application in basic holistic care, 267
Eicosapentaenoic acid, 357
Eicosatetraenoic acid, 357
Eicosatetraenoic acid, 363
Eicosatrienoic acid, 362
Elimination and challenge technique, 388
Elongase, 370
Emergencies, 119
Emotional, mental, and social health, 221
Emotional literacy, 224
Endocrinologic activity of adipose, 205

Endolimax nana, 449, 550
Endoplasmic reticulum (ERS), 503
Endotoxin, 405
Endotoxins (lipopolysaccharide) from gram-negative bacteria, 405
Enemas, 459
Enhanced processing of autoantigens, 399
Entamoeba hartmanni, 550
Entamoeba histolytica, 430, 432, 449
Enterococcus, 449
Enteropathic spondylo-arthropathy, enteropathic arthritis, 687
Enthesopathies, 688
Environmental dysbiosis/colonization—introduction to assessment, 90
Enzymes in fatty acid metabolism, 369
EPA - importance and application in basic holistic care, 256
EPA - review, 357
Epstein-Bar virus (EBV), 92, 631
Epstein-Barr virus—Localized infection in skin fibroblasts and endothelial cells, upregulation of cytokine production, 662
Erythromycin, 553
Esophageal dysfunction and GERD in scleroderma, 670
ESR - interpretation, 54
Essential fatty acid, 355, 362
Estrogen, 522
Eucalyptus oil, 446
Exceptional living, 195
Exercise, 201
Facial nerve, 23
Family health history, 13
Fatty Acid / Genetic Expression, 309
Ferritin - interpretation, 54
Ferritin - overview, 26
Fibromyalgia, 557
Fibrosis of the skin and internal organs, 651
Fish oil, EPA with DHA, 256
Five-Part Nutritional Wellness Protocol That Produces Consistently Positive Results, 310
Flax seed oil, 356
Fluconazole, 587
Food allergens, 213
Food allergy, 376
Food allergy diagnosis, 388
Food challenges, 388
Formula SF722, 551
Functional assessment, 19
Gamma strep, 449
Gamma-linolenic acid, 362
Gamma-linolenic acid - importance and application in basic holistic care, 257
Garlic, 456
Gastric ulceration and gastrointestinal bleeding caused by NSAIDs, 250
Gastrointestinal dysbiosis, 430

Gastrointestinal dysbiosis/colonization—introduction to assessment, 88
Gene products NF-kappaB, 373
Genetic Hemochromatosis, 160
Genitourinary dysbiosis/colonization—introduction to assessment, 89
GERD in scleroderma, 670
Giant Cell Arteritis (previously Temporal Arteritis), 119, 674, 677
Giardia lamblia, 449, 450
Ginger, 258, 460
GLA - review, 362
Glossopharyngeal, 23
Glucosamine, 270
Gluten avoidance, SLE treatment, 643
Gotu cola, 666
Gout, 124
Grape seed extract, 308, 374, 386
Green tea, 308, 374, 386
Group A streptococci, 454
Gulf War Illness, 94
Haptenization, 401
Harpagophytum procumbens - importance and application in basic holistic care, 259
Headache and head pain - overview, 171
Helicobacter pylori, 450
Helicobacter pylori, 94
Helicobacter pylori, especially the virulent CagA strain, 663
Hematocolpos, 690
Hemochromatosis, 570
Henoch-Schonlein purpura, 676
Hepatic and renal injury and failure caused by NSAIDs, 250
Hepatitis B virus (HepB, HBV), 92
Hepatitis C virus (HepC, HCV), 92
Hepatobiliary stimulation for IgA-complex removal, 459
Herpes simplex (HSV1, HSV2), 92
HERV, 632
HFE mutation, 167
Hierarchy of Therapeutics, 131
High glycemic foods, 255
HIGH-RISK PAIN PATIENTS, 109
History taking, 8
Holistic conservative care, 244
Hormones in the treatment of allergy, 387
Hospital/physician errors, 253
HTLV (human T-lymphotropic virus), 632
Hughes syndrome, 85
Human herpes virus type-6 (HHV-6), 92
Human immunodeficiency virus (HIV), 92
Human papilloma virus (HPV), 631
HVLA, 279
Hydrogen sulfide, 574
Hypericum perforatum, 456
Hypericum perforatum shows impressive antibacterial action, 552
Hyperinsulinemia, 211
Hyperprolactinemia, 519
Hypoglossal nerve, 23
Hypothyroidism, 568
I3C, 523
Iatrogenic neurosis, 265
Ice/heat, 254
Illustration showing the 9 paired locations of fibromyalgia tender points, 561
Immune complex formation/deposition, 409
Immune complex removal via hepatic and splenic routes, 630
Immunonutrition (against dysbiosis), 458
Immunostimulation by bacterial DNA, 407
Immunotoxicity, 529
Implementing the Five-Part Nutritional Wellness Protocol for the Treatment of Various Health Problems, 312
Inadequacies musculoskeletal education, 246
Increased intestinal permeability/NSAIDs, 250
Individualize treatment - importance, 255
Individuation, 196
Indole-3-carbinol, 523
Inflammation = inflammation, 373
Inflammatory bowel disease--laboratory testing, 85
Informed consent, 110
Inhibition of detoxification by dysbiosis, 419, 421
Insulin resistance, 211
Internal locus of control, 226
Intestinal/mesenteric vasculitis, 639
Intradependence, 224
Introduction to Injection Therapies, 298
Iodine, 527
Iron Overload, 160, 570
Jared Zeff, N.D., 189
Juvenile spondylo-arthropathy, 688
Kawasaki disease, 676
Keratoconjunctivitis sicca, 697
Klebsiella pneumoniae, 430, 450
LA, 362
Labile support surface, 294
Laboratory assessments: general considerations of commonly used tests, 25
Laboratory tests in the evaluation of patients with musculoskeletal complaints, 25
Lactoferrin, 104
Lactoferrin, 436
Lactulose-mannitol assay, 26
Lactulose-mannitol assay evaluates paracellular/pathologic and transcellular/physiologic absorption, 433
LADA, 85
Latent autoimmune diabetes in adults, 85
Laxatives promote eradication of intestinal microbes, 552
Lead, 571
Lead and HTN, 77
Leaky gut, 101
Leaky gut, 418
Leaky gut diagram, 434
Leukotriene B4, 367
Leukotriene B-5, 359
Levothyroxine, 526
Lifestyle habits, 191
Limited cutaneous scleroderma, 651
Linoleic acid, 362
Linoleic acid metabolites formed by lipoxygenases, 366
Linolenic acid, 356
Liothyronine, 527
Liotrix, 527
Lipoic acid, 308, 374, 386
Lipoxygenases (LOX), 371
Liver biopsy in iron overload, 167
Low starch diet, 549
Low-back pain: differential diagnostic considerations, 690
Low-carbohydrate (low fermentation) supplemented Paleo-Mediterranean diet, 548
LOX, 371
LT-C4, 367
LT-D4, 367
LT-E4, 367
L-tryptophan, 577
L-tyrosine and iodine, 527
Lumbar Roll, 284
Lupus, 630
Lyme disease, 93
Lyrica, 564
Madecassol, 666
Magnesium, 584
Manipulation, mobilization, and massage, 266
Manipulation Costovertebral Junction, 282
ManKind Project, 224
Manual Medicine, 278
Mask-like face, 652
Massage - importance and application in basic holistic care, 263
Maximize factors that promote health, 241
Mechanisms of autoimmune induction, 395
Medical history, 13
Melatonin, 200, 590
Mentha piperita, 456, 552
Mercurial myopathy, 571
Mercury, 237, 532, 571
Metabolism of omega-3 fatty acids and related eicosanoids - illustration, 361
Metabolism of omega-6 fatty acids and related eicosanoids - illustration, 368

Methylation of DNA, 635
Metronidazole, 553
MFTP - clinical management, 274
Microbial colonization, 86
Milk thistle, 460
Milnacipran, 564
Minimize factors that promote disease, 241
Mitochondrial dysfunction in autoimmunity, 558
Mitochondrial dysfunction promotes central sensitization, 576
Mitochondrial myopathy, 558
Mitophagy, 560, 575, 577, 580, 587, 588, 589
Mixed connective tissue disease, 651
Mobilization, 266
Molecular mimicry, 395
Monoarthritis, 122
Mononeuritis multiplex, 678
Mononucleosis, 92
Motivation, 193
Motivation, 194
Mucuna pruriens, 520
Multifocal Dysbiosis, 392, 710
Multifocal polydysbiosis, 86
Multiple sclerosis, 93, 94
Muscle strength – grading scale, 24
Musculoskeletal emergencies, 119
Musculoskeletal Manipulation, 278
Mycoplasma, 94
Mycoplasma species, 569
Myelopathy, 2, 120
Myofascial, 274
Myrrh, 456
Nail pitting, 617
Naturopathic model of illness and healing, 129
Naturopathic principles, 130
Neomycin, 586
Neurologic examination, 19
Neuronal autoimmunity, 94
Neuropsychiatric lupus, 119
Neuropsychiatric lupus is a medical emergency, 638
NF-kappaB, 408
NF-kappaB and its phytonutritional modulation, 373
Niacinamide, 270
Nuclear transcription factor kappaB, 373
Nutrigenomics, 217
Nutrition and Physical Degeneration, 206
Nutritional Genomics, 217
Nutritional immunomodulation, 307
Nystatin, 553
Obesity, 204
Objective means for the identification of allergens, 388
Occult infections, 569
Octreotide, 660
Oculomotor, 23
Olfactory, 23
Omega-3 fatty acids - review, 356
Ophthalmic, 23
Opioid epidemic, 245

Oregano oil, 455
Oregano oil, dosing and clinical use, 550
Organic foods rather than industrially-produced foods, 212
Orodental dysbiosis/colonization—introduction to assessment, 88
Orthoendocrinology, 518
Orthomolecular Immunomodulation, 383
Orthomolecular Medicine - overview, 216
Orthopedic/musculoskeletal examination: concepts and goals, 20
Orwellian newspeak, 249
Osteochondritis dissecans, 123
Osteomyelitis, 2, 121
Osteopathic manipulation, 592
Osteopathic Medicine, 149
Overlap syndromes, 651
PABA, 665
Paleo-Mediterranean Diet, 219
Pancreatic enzymes, 273
PAR, 110
Paradigms, 197
Parasites, 102, 447, 451
Parenchymal dysbiosis, 91
Parvovirus B19, 93
Parvovirus B-19 (PvB19), 631
Parvovirus B19—Induction of fibrosis, 662
Patient (mis)education in standard medicine, 565
Penicillin treatment of psoriasis, 624
Pentosidine, 559
Peppermint, 456, 552
Peptidoglycans, 403
Pesticide exposure, 237
Phenolic content, 209
Phospholipase-A2, 370
Physical examination, 19
Physical exertion, 201
Physician errors, 253
Phytochelatins, 541
Phytochemicals, 208
Phytochemicals, 209
Picrorhiza, 460
Plasminogen activator inhibitor, 359
Political and social action, 238
Polyarteritis nodosa, 675
Polymyalgia Rheumatica, 677
Porphyria cutanea tarda, 162
Post-isometric stretching for MFTP, 276
Potaba, 665
Pre-contemplation, 194
Pregabalin, 564
Preparation, 194
Primary biliary cirrhosis, 85
Primary sclerosing cholangitis, 85
Primary/Genetic Hemochromatosis, 160
Primum Non Nocere, 130
Probiotic supplementation, 458, 585
Problems and solutions, 534
Progressive Systemic Sclerosis, 651

Proinflammatory adipose tissue, 205
Pro-inflammatory foods, 255
Prolactin, 519
Prolotherapy, 298
Propolis, 308, 374, 386
Proprioceptive rehabilitation, 266, 293, 300
Prostacyclin, 365
Prostaglandin D2, 365
Prostaglandin E-1, 364
Prostaglandin E2, 307, 365
Prostaglandin E-3, 359
Prostaglandin F2-alpha, 366
Prostaglandin G2, 366
Prostaglandin G-3, 359
Prostaglandin H2, 366
Prostaglandin H-3, 359
Prostaglandin I2, 365
Prostaglandin I-3, 359
Prostaglandin synthase complex, 370
Protect & prevent re-injury, 254
Protein - calculation of daily intake, 206
Protein - importance and application in basic holistic care, 267
Protein per Pound of Body Weight, 207
Protein per Pound of Body Weight, 328
Protein supplements, 207
Proteolytic enzymes, 273, 457
Proteus mirabilis, 430
Pseudomonas aeruginosa, 94, 430
Psoriasis, main chapter, 616
Psoriatic rheumatism, 616
Pyridoxine, 288
Pyridoxine, 519
Qigong, 592
Raynaud's phenomenon in scleroderma, 671, 705
Raynaud's phenomenon, 94, 705
Reactive arthritis, 93, 687
Reasons to avoid the use of nonsteroidal anti-inflammatory drugs (NSAIDs), 246, 249
Referred pain with compression, 274
REFLEXES – grading scale, 24
Relative rest - definition and application in basic holistic care, 254
Renal failure is a leading cause of death in patients with SLE, 638
Renal injury and failure by NSAIDs, 250
Resolvins, 360
Restless leg syndrome, 578
Retinal vasculitis, 639
Review of systems, 12
Rheumatic psoriasis, 616
Rheumatoid Factor - interpretation, 80
Rheumatoid factor - overview, 26
Rib manipulation, 282
Riboflavin, 290
Rifaximin, 578, 587
Rifaximin as treatment for SIBO and IBS, 579
Roger J Williams, 195

ROS: review of systems, 12
Rose Bengal staining, 698
Rosemary, 308, 374, 386
Saccharomyces boulardii, 550
S-adenosylmethionine, 584
Safe patient + safe treatment = safe outcome, 110
Salivary gland biopsy, 698
Salmonella, 93
Savella, 564
Schirmer test, 698
Schober test, 691
Scleroderma, 651
Scleroderma secondary to xenobiotic immunotoxicity, 651
Screening laboratory tests in the evaluation of patients with musculoskeletal complaints, 25
Secondary Hemochromatosis, 160
Secretory IgA, 103
Secretory IgA, 435
Septic arthritis, 121, 125, 126
Septic arthritis, in rheumatoid arthritis, 600
Seropositivity, 81, 601
Serotonin synthesis, 211
Serum 25(OH) vitamin D, 59
Serum IgE and IgG assays, 388
Shigella, 93
Short-chain fatty acids, 104
Short-chain fatty acids, 435
SIBO, in fibromyalgia, 573
Sicca syndrome, 697
Sick role, 265
Silymarin, 168
Sinorespiratory dysbiosis, 88
Sjögren Syndrome/Disease, 697
Skin taping to increase afferent stimuli, 296
Skin-prick testing, 388
SLE, 630
Sleep, 199
Slipped capital femoral epiphysis, 124
Small intestine bacterial overgrowth (SIBO), 573
Small intestine bacterial overgrowth in fibromyalgia, 573
Social history, 13
Sodium benzoate, 212
Somatic dysfunction, 149
Somatostatin analog, 660
Spinal accessory nerve, 23
Spinal cord compression, 2, 120
SPMD, 547
St. John's Wort, 456
Standard Medical Treatment for Fibromyalgia, 563
Staphylococcus aureus, 453
Stearidonic acid, 357
Stool analysis, 103
Streptococcal infections, 94
Streptococcus pyogenes, 454
Stress is a "whole body" phenomenon, 222
Stress management, 221

Superantigens, 398
Supercompensation, 211
Supplemented Paleo-Med. diet, 219, 256
Syndemic obesity, inflammation, cardiometabolic, brain dysfunction, 504
Synthroid, 526
Systemic Lupus Erythematosus, main chapter, 630
Systemic Sclerosis, 651
Syzygium species, 457
Takayasu arteritis, 675
Tartrazine, 212
Television, 191
Temporal arteritis, 119, 677
Testing for Occult Infections and Dysbiosis, 86
Testosterone, 524
Therapeutic dependency - defined, 265
Therapeutic exercise - importance and application in basic holistic care, 266
Therapeutic Interventions, 580
Therapeutic passivity - defined, 265
Thrombocytopenia, 549
Thromboxane A-2, 365
Thromboxane A-3, 359
Thromboxane B2, 365
Thrust vectors, 279
Thyme, 457
Thymus vulgaris, 457
Thyroid, 526, 527
Thyroid glandular, 527
Thyroid hormone, 519
Thyroid stimulating hormone, 64
Thyrolar, 527
Tolle Causam, 130
Toll-like receptors, 408
Toll-like receptors (TLR2 and TLR4), 503
Total microbial load (TML), 631
Toxic oil syndrome, 653
Toxicant Exposure and Detoxification/Depuration, 535
Toxoplasma gondii, 663
Tramadol, 565
Transient synovitis, irritable hip, 123
Treatment for MFTP, 277
Tricycline, dosing and clinical use, 551
Trigeminal, 23
Tripterygium wilfordii Hook F, 520
Triptolide, 520
Trochlear, 23
Truncated self, 226
Tryptophan, 583
TSH: thyroid stimulating hormone - interpretation, 64
Turmeric, 460
Twilight of the Idiopathic Era, 544
Twitch response, 274

Una de gato - importance and application in basic holistic care, 259
Uncaria guianensis and Uncaria tomentosa - importance and application in basic holistic care, 259
Undecenoic acid, 457, 551
Unfolded protein response (UPR), 502
Unhistorical, 196
Uva Ursi, 456
Vancomycin orally administered, 587
Varicocele, 523
Vasculitic Diseases, 672
Vegetarian diet for fibromyalgia, 582
Vestibulocochlear, 23
Vinyl chloride disease, 653
Viruses, part 1—Known/popular "epigenomic" viruses, 631
Viruses, part 2—Human endogenous retroviruses (endoretroviruses, HERVs or ERVs), 632
Viruses, part 3—Bacteriophages of the gastrointestinal bacteria, 636
Viruses, part 4—Bacterial synergism via NFkB activation and immunosuppression, 637
Vis Medicatrix Naturae, 130
Viscous Agents, 298
Visual analog scale, 23
Vitamin B-12 treatment of allergy, 385
Vitamin B-6, 288
Vitamin C, 273
Vitamin C in the treatment of allergy, 385
Vitamin C purge, 551
Vitamin D - antiinflammatory benefits, 375
Vitamin D deficiency, 26, 567
Vitamin D status testing, 59
Vitamin E in the treatment of allergy, 385
Vitex astus-cagnus, 520
Wegener granulomatosis, 674
Wegener's Granulomatosis, 679
Weight optimization, 265
Wellness, 4
Williams, Roger J,, 195
Willow bark, 258
Wobble board, 294
WomanWithin, 224
Work ethic, 198
Xenobiotic Immunotoxicity, 529
Xenobiotics, 571
Xerostomia, 697
Xifaxan, 587
Yellow dye #5, 212
Yersinia, 93
Yoga, 290
Zeff, N.D., 189
Zingiber officinale, 258

DrV's "Functional Inflammology Protocol"
for Disorders of:
❶ Metabolic Inflammation, ❷ Allergic Inflammation, and ❸ Autoimmune Inflammation
Clinical Precision with Nutrition and Functional Medicine

Main Topics in the 4-part Version of this Presentation Series:

1. Introduction and Overview: The Paradigm Shift using the "Functional Inflammology" acronym
2. Metabolic Inflammation: Diabetes Mellitus, Hypertension, Obesity, CardioMetabolic Syndrome; also some mention of Alzheimer's and Parkinson's diseases
3. Allergic Inflammation: Food/General Allergies and Allergic Rhinitis, Asthma, Atopic Dermatitis
4. Autoimmune Inflammation: Exemplified by Psoriasis and Rheumatoid Arthritis

Alex Vasquez, D.C., N.D., D.O., F.A.C.N.

Notices

- Copyright: Except for quotations and images obtained elsewhere, the material and contents of these presentations are copyrighted by Dr Alex Vasquez and have often been excerpted from his books which are also copyrighted. Any unauthorized use of this material—including photocopying or any distribution—is prohibited.
  - No cameras.
  - No recorders.
- Copyright 2012-2014 by Dr Alex Vasquez. All rights reserved and enforced.
- Trademark: The "Functional Immunology/Inflammology Protocol" discussed in this series of videos and notes is Trademarked ® in association with Dr Vasquez's book *Functional Immunology and Nutritional Immunomodulation* and other books and videos.
- Dr Vasquez's views are his own.

Trademark

Inflammation Mastery & Functional Inflammology: Volume 1
Excerpted Presentation Slides • Page 1

Example of effectiveness: 51yoF with "severe aggressive drug-resistant rheumatoid arthritis"

March 2012

CCP Antibodies IgG/IgA	>250	High	units	0 - 19
			Negative	<20
			Weak positive	20 - 39
			Moderate positive	40 - 59
			Strong positive	>59

January 2013

CCP Antibodies IgG/IgA	195	High	units	0 - 19
			Negative	<20
			Weak positive	20 - 39
			Moderate positive	40 - 59
			Strong positive	>59

April 2013

CCP Antibodies IgG/IgA	54	High	units	0 - 19
			Negative	<20
			Weak positive	20 - 39
			Moderate positive	40 - 59
			Strong positive	>59

Dr Vasquez: Introduction

- Education:
  - **Doctor of Chiropractic**, University of Western States (March 1996) Portland, Oregon
  - **Doctor of Naturopathic Medicine**, Bastyr University (September 1999) Seattle, Washington
  - **Doctor of Osteopathic Medicine**, University of North Texas Health Science Center (May 2010) Fort Worth, Texas
  - Read thousands of articles/books; thousands of hours of post-graduate training in seminars, clinics, hospitals; many years of experience with thousands of patients
- Publications and presentations:
  - International lecturer to physicians and clinicians on integrative/functional medicine
  - Several textbooks for doctors and health science students
  - More than 100 articles and letters in professional magazines and peer-reviewed journals
- Current professional activities:
  - Former adjunct faculty for several universities and post-graduate institutions
  - Compiling research, conducting research, authoring books and articles
  - Healthcare product design
  - International seminars and presentations
  - Consulting practice specializing in difficult and complex cases

Dr Vasquez: Articles (~100)

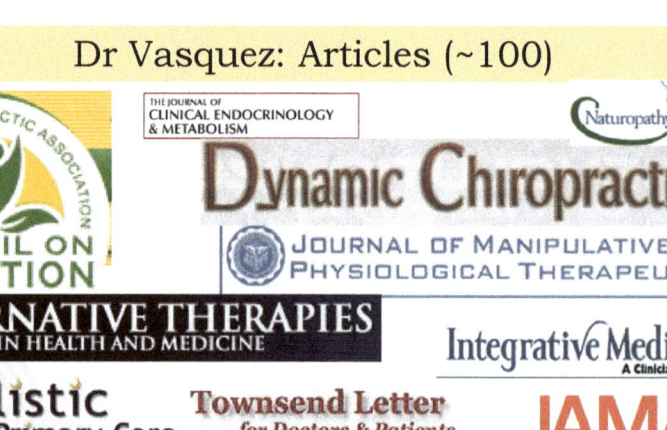

Dr Vasquez: Peer-Reviewed Publications

Peer-reviewed and scientific publications

1. Vasquez A. Reply to "role of Western diet in inflammatory autoimmune diseases" by Manzel et Al. *Current Allergy and Asthma Reports* 2014 Aug;14(8):454
2. Vasquez A. Mitochondrial medicine arrives to prime time in clinical care. *Altern Ther Health Med* 2014 Winter;20 Suppl 1:26-30
3. Gordon CM, Williams AL, Feldman HA, May J, Sinclair L, Vasquez A, Cox JE. Treatment of Hypovitaminosis D in Infants and Toddlers. *Journal of Clinical Endocrinology & Metabolism.* 2008 Apr 15.
4. Vasquez A. Interventions Need to be Consistent With Osteopathic Philosophy. [Letter] *JAOA: Journal of the American Osteopathic Association* 2006; Sep;106(9):528-9
5. Vasquez A. Web-like Interconnections of Physiological Factors. *Integrative Medicine* 2006, April/May, 32-37
6. Vasquez A, Muanza DN. Accolades and Addenda for "Use of Botanicals in Osteoarthritis and Rheumatoid Arthritis": Comment on Article by Ahmed et al. *Evidence-based Complementary and Alternative Medicine.* 2005 published on-line December 15
7. Vasquez A. Subphysiologic Doses of Vitamin D are Subtherapeutic: Comment on the Study by The Record Trial Group. *The Lancet .com* 2005 Published on-line May 6
8. Vasquez A, Cannell J. Calcium and vitamin D in preventing fractures: data are not sufficient to show inefficacy. [letter] *BMJ: British Medical Journal* 2005;331:108-9
9. Vasquez A. Comment: evaluation of presence of aspirin-related warnings with willow bark. *Annals of Pharmacotherapy.* 2005 Oct;39:1763.
10. Vasquez A. Healthcare for our bones: A practical nutritional approach to preventing osteoporosis. [Letter]. *Journal of Manipulative and Physiological Therapeutics* 2005; 28: 213
11. Muanza DN, Vasquez A, Cannell J, Grant WB. Isoflavones and Postmenopausal Women. [letter] *JAMA: Journal of the American Medical Association* 2004; 292: 2337
12. Vasquez A, Manso G, Cannell J. The Clinical Importance of Vitamin D (Cholecalciferol): A Paradigm Shift with Implications for All Healthcare Providers. *Alternative Therapies in Health and Medicine* 2004; 10: 28-37.
13. Vasquez A. Musculoskeletal disorders and iron overload disease: comment on the American College of Rheumatology guidelines for the initial evaluation of the adult patient with acute musculoskeletal symptoms. *Arthritis & Rheumatism: Official Journal of the American College of Rheumatology* 1996; 39:1767-8

Dr Vasquez: Books and Textbooks

Books—partial listing

1. Integrative Orthopedics ('04,'07,'12)
2. Integrative Rheumatology ('06,'07,) revision and expansion: Integrative Rheumatology, Nutritional Immunology, Functional Inflammology (Third Edition, '13pending)
3. Musculoskeletal Pain: Expanded Clinical Strategies ('08, published by IFM)
4. Chiropractic and Naturopathic Mastery of Common Clinical Disorders ('09)
5. Integrative Medicine and Functional Medicine for Chronic Hypertension ('10)
6. Chiropractic Management of High Blood Pressure & Chronic Hypertension ('10), Integrative Chiropractic Management of High Blood Pressure & Chronic Hypertension ('11)
7. Migraine Headaches, Hypothyroidism, and Fibromyalgia ('12)
8. Fibromyalgia in a Nutshell ('12)
9. Foundational Assessments and Wellness Promotion in Integrative Chiropractic and Functional Medicine ('12)
10. Functional Immunology and Nutritional Immunomodulation: Presentation Slides Part 1: Introduction to the Use of Nutrition and Functional Medicine in the Prevention and Treatment of Chronic Inflammation, Allergy, Autoimmunity, and the New FIND SEX Acronym ('12),
11. *International Journal of Human Nutrition and Functional Medicine* ('13) Int J Hum Nutr Funct Med. Org
12. Dr Vasquez's Presentation on Migraine Headaches, Fibromyalgia, and Chronic Fatigue Syndrome ('13)
13. Functional Inflammology, Allergy, Asthma, and Dysbiosis ('13)
14. Selected Topics in NeuroMusculoSkeletal Medicine ('13)

Goals: Personal and practical

▸ My main personal goal is to **outline a "new" way to manage disorders of inflammation-allergy-autoimmunity** beyond both 1) ineffective unscientific treatments, and 2) drug-based treatments that do little other than suppress the end manifestations of immune-metabolic physiologic disturbance.

▸ Achieving this goal:

= better success for you as professionals,

= the delivery of true **authentic healthcare** (rather than perpetuation of **our current system of diseasecare**)

= better care for our shared human society,

= progress for humanity ☺

Goals

1. **Identification**: To review the **seven most important modifiable factors that mediate immune dysfunction**, which are the cause(s) of *or major modifiable contributor(s)* to chronic **inflammation, allergy, and autoimmune disease**.

2. **Recitation**: For clinicians-practitioners to be able to **list these factors from memory** (declarative knowledge) so that they can explain these factors to their clients/patients.

3. **Explanation and implementation**: For clinicians-practitioners to be able to **explain the mechanisms and interventions for each of these 7 factors**.

This means you.

Medical education—nutritionally deficient, drug dependent

1. The tragic irony is that the vast majority of medical doctors—and therefore the largest component of the healthcare delivery system in the world—are untrained in nutrition and therefore incapable/ incompetent to deliver nutrition assessment and treatment to their patients. Raman. *J Clin Gastroenterol*. 2009 Jul; Vetter. *J Am Coll Nutr* 2008 Apr

2. Thus, not surprisingly, medical doctors practice in a way that focuses on 1) the diagnosis, and 2) the drug(s) for the diagnosis. Ely. *BMJ* 1999 Aug

3. The medical profession generally lacks appreciation of how body systems work interactively and interdependently. Vasquez. *Integrative Med*. 2006 Apr

4. **Diagnosis and drugs are the emphasis of medical practice without consideration of the nutritional needs of the patient and without an appreciation of how the body works together as an integrated whole**; this fails to address the *reality* of most diseases and therefore keeps most patients dependent on drugs for the masking of metabolic imbalances better treated with nutritional interventions.

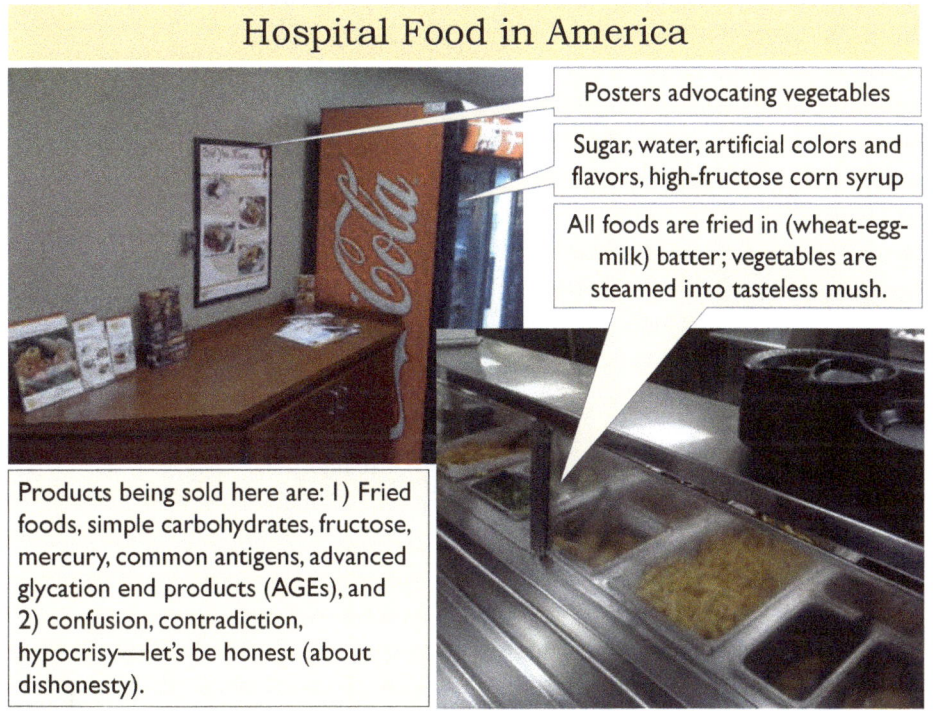

Hospital Food in South America (Bogota, Colombia)

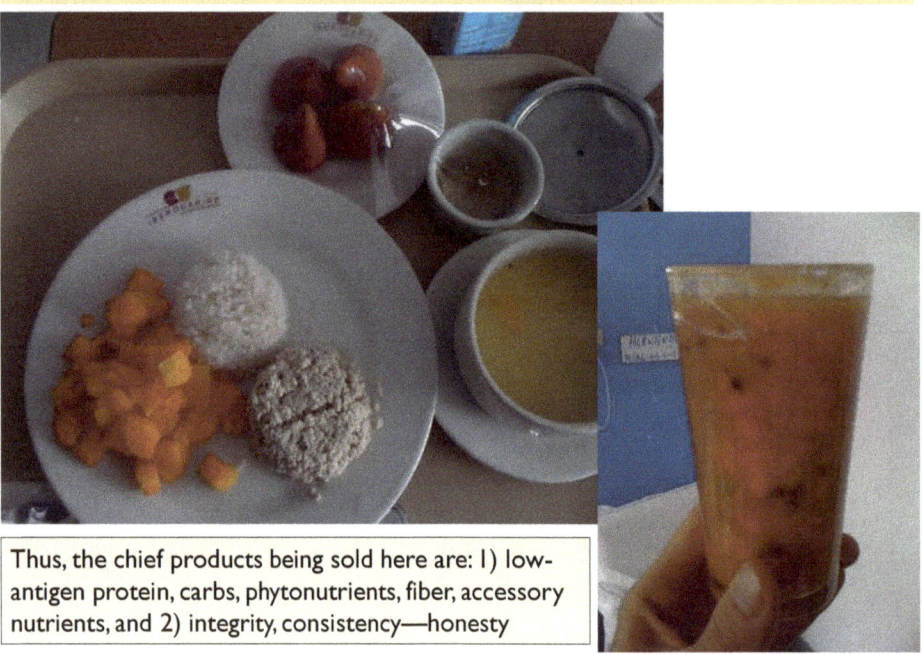

Thus, the chief products being sold here are: 1) low-antigen protein, carbs, phytonutrients, fiber, accessory nutrients, and 2) integrity, consistency—honesty

Evidence-Based Healthcare: Balancing Details & Practicality

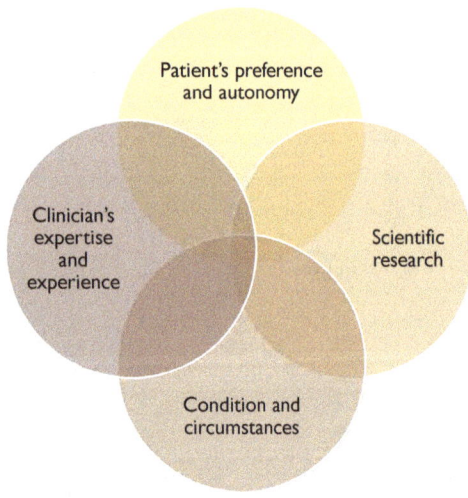

Geyman. *J Am Board Fam Pract.* 1998 Jan
Haynes et al. *Evid Based Med* 2002;7

- This presentation will attempt to blend each of the 4 main components of evidence-based healthcare into a **rational system of clinical intervention.**
  - Too much focus on molecules and research = not enough practical application to help patients.
  - Too much focus on practical applications = failure to understand the scientific basis of treatments and the underlying rationale.
  - Too much reliance on published research = failure to make progress in the present moment.

Medical schools teach students and doctors that 1) most diseases are complex and "idiopathic", and 2) drugs are the answer.

Outcome of Medical Education: Centers on "Diagnosis and Drug"

1. "What is the cause of symptom X?"
2. "What is the dose of drug X?"
3. "How should I manage disease or finding X?"

"Doctors spent an average of less than 2 minutes pursuing an answer, and they used readily available print and human resources. Only two questions led to a formal literature search." Ely et al. *BMJ*. 1999 Aug

What we learn in medical school:

1. Nearly all diseases are **complex and idiopathic**—some mixture of genetics and "unknown environmental factors."
2. We can apply scientific methods to patient assessment and treatment…but this will almost always result in the use of drugs and/or surgery/procedures.
3. Symptom-suppressing with pharmacologic monotherapy ("silver bullet") or polypharmacy is the **goal**, *not simply the means*.

If you took away the prescription pad (or scalpel) from most doctors, how could they practice?

What we must learn *here* today in order to manage chronic inflammatory disorders:

1. **Diseases are complex and understandable**: We will look at the components of each disease.
2. **We can understand the complexity of complex diseases, and we can apply scientific methods to patient assessment**: We will focus on *understanding* and *providing effective treatment* based on that understanding.
3. **"Science" is not synonymous with "drugs" or "scalpel"—many nondrug nonscalpel science-based treatments exist**: We will review and understand each of the 7 major causes of chronic inflammation and immune dysfunction. For many of you, this will be an entirely new approach; so please be willing to accept new information and apply this to your patient care.

Vasquez. *Integrative Med.* 2006 Apr

Inflammation Mastery & Functional Inflammology: Volume 1
Excerpted Presentation Slides • Page 8

"If you came here to get out of trouble, then you are like the man, who —wanting to get out of the rain— jumped into the ocean."

Attributed to William Blake

Protocol applications

This new protocol has a very broad range of clinical applications. This is **because it corrects the underlying physiologic imbalances that are the "common themes" that result in most common clinical dis-orders**, such as:

1. Hypertension, Diabetes mellitus, Metabolic syndrome, Alzheimer's disease and Parkinson's disease, what I call "**Metabolic Inflammation**"
2. Allergies, asthma, eczema,... "**Allergic Inflammation**"
3. Autoimmune disorders including but not limited to rheumatoid arthritis, psoriasis, ankylosing spondylitis, systemic lupus erythematosus,... "**Autoimmune Inflammation**"

Clinical applications—charting with S.O.A.P.

<u>Always start with good clinical care</u>: *Competent care starts with an open-minded, compassionate, information-seeking excellence-aspiring clinician.*

- **Subjective:** History of presenting complaints; patient's concerns,
- **Objective:** Physical exam, lab tests: always assess renal function and other basic biochemical parameters; more complex cases require evaluation of more sensitive markers of metabolic and immune imbalance, imaging, biopsy, procedures—as necessary,
- **Assessment:** Reach an **assessment** of the entire constellation of patient's situation; **diagnosis** and appropriate management of each true disease and concern,
- **Plan:** Informed consent (PARBQ): procedures, alternatives, risks, benefits, questions answered; treatments; follow-up, rescheduling, referral, co-management.

```
Patient name: _____
Date of birth: _____
Date of visit: _____

S.
O.
A.
P.

Doctor: _____
```

Clinical applications—starting with D.I.R.T.

<u>Practice competently and defensively—risk management must be pro-active</u>:

- **Defensive mindset:** Start with the conscious intention to practice defensively and effectively
- **Duration of treatment:** Define and limit the duration of each component of the treatment plan; define the next steps of care (e.g., continued care or laboratory tests) and the date of the return visit.*
- **Interactions—drugs and diseases:** Double-check for interactions of the treatment plan with drugs and the patient's disease(s), especially renal insufficiency
  - High-potassium diet ≠ renal insufficiency
  - Vitamin D ≠ hydrochlorothiazide or other hypercalcemic predisposition/state
  - Calcium and magnesium ≠ tetracycline antibiotics
  - Etc.
- **Referral:** Determine the need for additional consultation,
- **Return visit:** Specify and chart timeframe or date of next visit. *Intentional redundancy
- **Treatment plan, charted, dated, signed:** Treatment plan must be archived in chart and should be given to patient; the clinician must sign and date the chart note and treatment plan.

Let's get started...

Mediterranean Sea, Spain

Main topics for now

- **Disorders of Immune Dysfunction:**
  - **Presentations: Chronic Inflammation, Allergy, Autoimmunity**
  - **Standard Medical Evaluations**
  - **Examples of Common Medical Treatments**
- **Causes of Immune Dysfunction—An Integrated Model:**
  - 7 major modifiable components of immune dysfunction will be presented, validated, and discussed with relevance for their clinical evaluations and interventions.
- Disorders of Immune Dysfunction—Interventions:
  1. Chronic Inflammation: Cardiovascular Disease, Diabetes Mellitus Type-2, and Other Common Inflammatory Syndromes
  2. Allergy: Asthma, Eczema,
  3. Autoimmunity: Rheumatoid arthritis, Psoriasis, Spondylitis, IBD

Immune Dysfunction: Presentations
1) Chronic Inflammation, Allergy, Autoimmunity

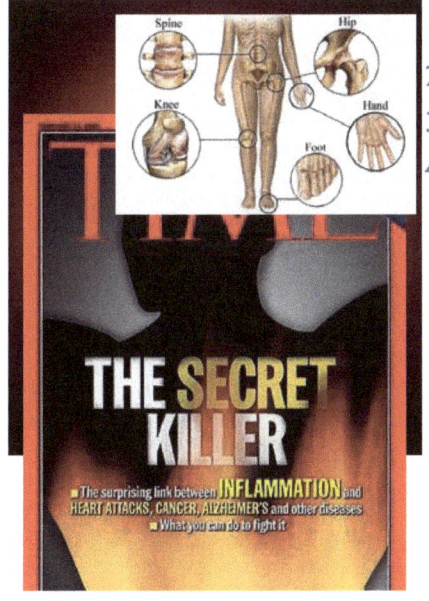

1. Cardiovascular disease,
2. Hypertension,
3. Diabetes Mellitus Type-2,
4. Metabolic Syndrome:
   - Standard medical evaluation: limited physical exam, blood pressure, lipids, glucose, CRP
   - Standard medical treatment: drugs to lower hypertension, lipids, glucose: "*treating the numbers; treat the manifestation of the problem—not the problem*"
   - Comments: fails to address aspects of the disease that can be treated effectively; leaves patients in a downward spiral of poor health.

"ABCD" of hypertension treatment — Cornerstones of "medical" management

- **ACEi**: -pril, renoprotective, teratogenic, hyperkalemia risk, angioedema risk due to preserved bradykinin, cough,
- **ARB**: -sartan, angiotensin-2 receptor blocker, renoprotective, hyperkalemia risk, no cough or vasodilation due to bradykinin, losartan is uricousuric,
- **Alpha-2 agonist**: (clonopin) tricks the CNS into thinking it is in a hypercatecholamine state so that SNS output is reduced; used for acute/severe HTN,
- **Alpha-1 blocker**: -osin, high risk of syncope, also treates BPH, (eg, prazosin)
- **Beta-blocker**: aten**olol** and labet**olol** are the prototypes; also used for some migraines and anxiety; avoid abrupt discontinuation.
- **Calcium-channel blocker**: dihydropyridine class are peripheral vasodilators; many nutritional nondrug means exist for modulating intracellular calcium.
- **Diuretics**: **thiazide** diuretics are first-line outpt tx even though they worsen DM2-MetSyn and promote mineral depletion; Lasix isn't really used for chronic HTN except with fluid overload.
- **Direct vasodilators**: Hydralazine IV is commonly used in acute settings and is safe for PG pts. Other drugs in class: nitroprusside,

While effective at lowering blood pressure numbers, none of these drugs provides hope of actually curing the disease "primary hypertension" by addressing the underlying problems.

DM2-MetSyn: Drug Treatments — Cornerstones of "medical" management

1. **Metformin**: Promoted as initial pharmacologic management due to benefits (reduction of HgbA1c by 2% max; reduction in mortality) and safety (less hypoglycemia); reduces hepatic gluconeogenesis and increases peripheral insulin sensitivity. Causes B-12 deficiency, often misdiagnosed and mistreated as diabetic neuropathy, also depression, fatigue.

2. **Sulfonylurea drugs—glyburide, glipizide, glimepiride**: Stimulate pancreatic insulin production and improve peripheral insulin sensitivity. These drugs increase morbidity and mortality in diabetic patients in a dose-response relationship despite reductions in glucose; they also increase death post angioplasty for MI. CMAJ—Canadian Med Association Journal 2006 Jan; J Am Coll Cardiol. 1999 Jan

3. **Thiazolidinedione drugs—pioglitazone and rosiglitazone**: Improve peripheral insulin sensitivity; reduction of HgbA1c by 1.5% max

4. **Dipeptidyl peptidase 4 (DPP-4) inhibitors**: sitagliptin/Januvia; reduce glucagon and thereby increases insulin secretion, slows gastric emptying.

5. **Insulin**: Basal/bolus insulin lowers glucose; some evidence shows that insulin directly promotes atherogenesis; possible "anti-inflammatory" effects of insulin are difficult to distinguish from glucose-lowering effects, since hyperglycemia is directly pro-inflammatory. Insulin promotes macrophage foam cell formation. Lab Invest. 2012 Apr

6. **Essentially all DM2 patients will also get a "statin" and an ACEi**
   While effective at lowering blood glucose numbers, none of these drugs provides hope of actually curing the disease by addressing the underlying problem(s).

Immune Dysfunction: Presentations
Chronic Inflammation, 2) Allergy, Autoimmunity

1. **Asthma:**
2. **Allergic rhinitis/conjunctivitis:**
3. **Eczema, atopic dermatitis:**
   - Standard medical evaluation: limited physical exam, blood oxygen, spirometry; maybe allergy tests via skin or blood.
   - Standard medical treatment: antihistamines, bronchodilators (beta-agonists), steroids/prednisone, leukotriene blockers (montelukast/zafirlukast), anticholinergics (ipratropium), "**immunoparalytic agents**" **(AV)**: cyclosporin/ciclosporin and tacrolimus block intracellular signaling, (hydroxychloroquine impairs lysosomes and TLR9, cholchicine blocks microtubules and migration as a "mitotic poison")... Drug/suppress the manifestations of immune dysfunction, but never address the problem directly.
   - Comments:, standard medical management of allergy fails to address the underlying causes of immune dysfunction, thereby leaving patients dependent on medications, many of which have high costs and serious adverse effects.

Immune Dysfunction: Presentations
Chronic Inflammation, Allergy, 3) Autoimmunity

1. <u>Rheumatoid arthritis (RA):</u> "idiopathic"
2. <u>Psoriasis:</u> "idiopathic"
3. <u>Other autoimmune syndromes:</u>
   - <u>Standard medical evaluation</u>: clinical evaluation with serum testing for RF, CCP, ESR/CRP, ANA and other routine tests to determine the type—*not the causes*—of the immune dysfunction.
   - <u>Standard medical treatment</u>: NSAIDs, prednisone, methotrexate, sulfasalazine, hydroxychloroquine, "biologics", stem cell transplant; bowel removal for IBD.
   - <u>Comments</u>: None of these drugs addresses the underlying problems—immune activation, inflammation dysregulation.

Drug/medical management of musculoskeletal pain and inflammation: sequence of medicalization

1. ASA, NSAIDs, and APAP,
2. Prednisone
3. Methotrexate
4. Sulfasalazine
5. Hydroxychloroquine
6. "Biologics"—TNFa inhibitors
7. Stem cell transplant

None of the drugs 'traditionally' used against autoimmune diseases provides any hope of actually curing the disease(s).

None of these drugs (perhaps except sulfasalazine) addresses the underlying causative factors that trigger and perpetuate chronic inflammation and autoimmunity.

Medical/drug suppression of inflammation

- "...sustained remission in daily practice as uncommon, being reached by only 17% to 36% of RA patients for up to 6 months. These studies did not evaluate time in remission beyond 6 months."
- "...long-term remission is rare, considering that the probability of a remission lasting 2 years was 6% to 14%."
- ~10% over 2 years is very poor performance!

Medical schools teach students and doctors that 1) most diseases are complex and "idiopathic", and 2) drugs are the answer.

Diabetes type-2	Hypertension	Allergy	Pain & Inflammation
1. Metformin 2. Sulfonylureas 3. TZDs 4. Dipeptidyl peptidase (DPP) 4 inhibitors 5. Insulin 6. Statin 7. ACEi	1. ACEi 2. ARB 3. Alpha-2 agonist 4. Alpha-1 blocker 5. Beta-blocker 6. Calcium-channel blocker 7. **Diuretics** 8. Vasodilators Cornerstones of "medical" management	1. Antihistamines 2. Bronchodilators (beta-agonists) 3. Steroids 4. Leukotriene blockers 5. Anticholinergics (ipratropium) 6. "immunoparalytic agents" (AV): ciclosporin, tacrolimus, hydroxychloroquine, cholchicine "mitotic poison"	1. NSAIDs 2. Prednisone/steroids 3. Methotrexate 4. Sulfasalazine 5. Hydroxychloroquine 6. "Biologics"—notice the misuse of language in labeling these drugs* 7. Opioids 8. "Antidepressants" and antiseizure drugs 9. Anti-neuropathic drugs for GABA receptors

*Marketing antiTNF drugs as "biologics" was brilliant for promoting sales because doing so gives the impression that these drugs are "logical for life" despite the major risks for cancer, infection, and bankruptcy for the patients taking these drugs.

Give them (more) drugs

America, the medicated
We buy more medicine than any other country, a trend that threatens our health and wealth

In medicine, polypharmacy is complimented as "skilled prescribing."

Americans are the most drugged society in human existence: This is accepted and considered OK as long as the drugs come from corporations. "Natural" treatments from nature are generally viewed by the allopathic medical profession as suspect ("alternative" and "unproven"), illegal (cannabis: analgesic, anxiolytic, antinausea) if not evil.

> "Recent estimates suggest that each year more than 1 million patients are injured while in the hospital and approximately 180,000 die because of these injuries. Furthermore, drug-related morbidity and mortality are common and are estimated to cost more than $136 billion a year." Holland, Degruy. *Am Fam Physician*. 1997 Nov

Americans: the most drugged society in human existence

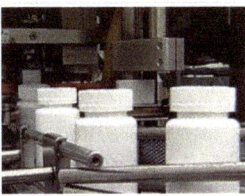

TODAY | April 10, 2013
Pill nation: Are we too reliant on prescription meds?
While modern medicines do help us manage pain and live with chronic illnesses, Americans are taking more prescription medication than ever before, leading medical ethicists to ask whether we are taking too many pills for our own good. NBC's Tom Costello reports.

- **"More than 4 billion prescriptions were written in 2011. That is the most ever.** Everything from sleeping pills to drugs for anxiety and depression—you name it.
- "The question medical ethicists are asking is 'if we are taking entirely too many pills for our own good?
- "Something changed in the 1990s, when it became legal for drug makers to advertise. And that's created a sense on the part of many patients who say 'I saw that ad on television. I think I should be on that medicine.' **Demand for drugs skyrocketed.**"

http://www.today.com/video/today/51490407/#51490407

American healthcare is the highest expense and lowest return-on-investment (ROI) healthcare system in the world

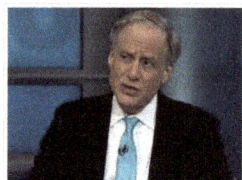

February 22, 2013

Bitter Pill: Inside Time magazine's cover story on medical bills

Time magazine's Jeffrey Kluger breaks down the growing number of medical bills across the country.

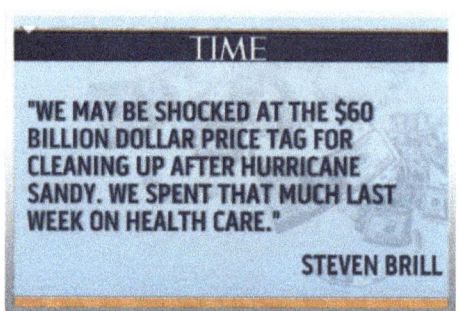

"WE MAY BE SHOCKED AT THE $60 BILLION DOLLAR PRICE TAG FOR CLEANING UP AFTER HURRICANE SANDY. WE SPENT THAT MUCH LAST WEEK ON HEALTH CARE."

STEVEN BRILL

America spends **$60,000,000,000 per week** on healthcare/diseasecare/drugcare.

http://video.msnbc.msn.com/jansing-and-co/50906214#50906214

American healthcare financially incentivizes poor healthcare and poor outcomes

Patients with surgical complications provide greater hospital profit-margins

Posted: 16 Apr 2013 01:18 PM PDT

Privately insured surgical patients with a complication provided hospitals with a 330 percent higher profit margin than those without a complication, report researchers. Medicare patients with a complication produced a 190 percent higher margin. For hospitals, reducing surgical complications may mean reduced financial performance.

- "We found **clear evidence that reducing harm and improving quality is perversely penalized in our current health care system**," Eappen, lead author and chief medical officer of Massachusetts Eye and Ear Infirmary.
- "It's been known that **hospitals are not rewarded for quality**. But it **hadn't been recognized exactly how much more money they make when harm is done**," said senior author Atul Gawande, lab director, professor and a surgeon.
- An estimated **$400 billion is spent on surgical procedures each year in the U.S.** While effective methods to reduce complications have been identified, hospitals have been slow to implement them.

Original study in *JAMA* April 17, 2013 reviewed by Harvard School of Public Health: http://www.hsph.harvard.edu/news/press-releases/patients-with-surgical-complications-provide-greater-hospital-profit-margins/

We can—*must*—address the causes of immune dysfunction and inflammatory imbalance:

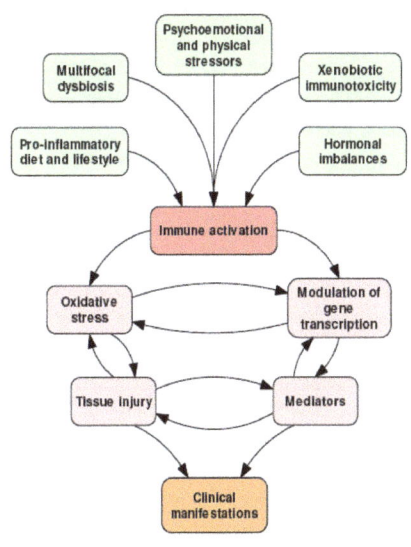

Vasquez A. *Integrative Rheumatology, Second Edition*.

What we will review today:

1. Diseases are complex and understandable:

2. We can apply scientific methods to patient assessment and treatment (even if this means NOT relying on drugs) to correct the underlying imbalances that cause the disease and its manifestations.

3. Symptom-suppressing drugs are NOT the best answer—these patients need a multifaceted approach:

Immune Dysfunction: 7 Main Modifiable Factors

- Non-modifiable mechanisms:
  - "Genes" in the form of DNA

> Note that the standard medical evaluation fails to consider these important modifiable components.

- Modifiable mechanisms:
  1. **Diet**: Pro-inflammatory *versus* anti-inflammatory diets,
  2. **Dysbiosis**: Multifocal polydysbiosis,
  3. **Nutritional immunomodulation**: Therapeutic modulation of immunocyte phenotype via epigenetic mechanisms,
  4. **Mitochondrial dysfunction**: Proinflammatory effects of dysfunctional mitochondria,
  5. **Psychoneuroimmunology**: Stress, paradigms and immune disorders,
  6. **Hormonal imbalance**: Dysendocrinology, orthoendocrinology,
  7. **Xenobiotic immunotoxicity**: Chemical and toxic metal exposures.

Immune Dysfunction: Mechanisms

▸ *How can we remember all of that?*

▸ I have a simple memory aid for you!

Let's memorize these
1. **F**ood and Lifestyle
2. **I**nfection
3. **N**utrition
4. **D**ysfunctional mitochondria
5. **S**tress, p**S**ychology, Lifestyle
6. **E**ndocrine
7. **X**enobiotics/**T**oxins

These are the 7 main modifiable factors in the cause and control of chronic inflammatory disorders.

(Each of these could take 2 hours [2 days] to explore.)

Notice that these 7 factors can be remembered by the acronym:
F.I.N.D. S.E.Xenobiotics or **F.I.N.D. S.E.T**oxins

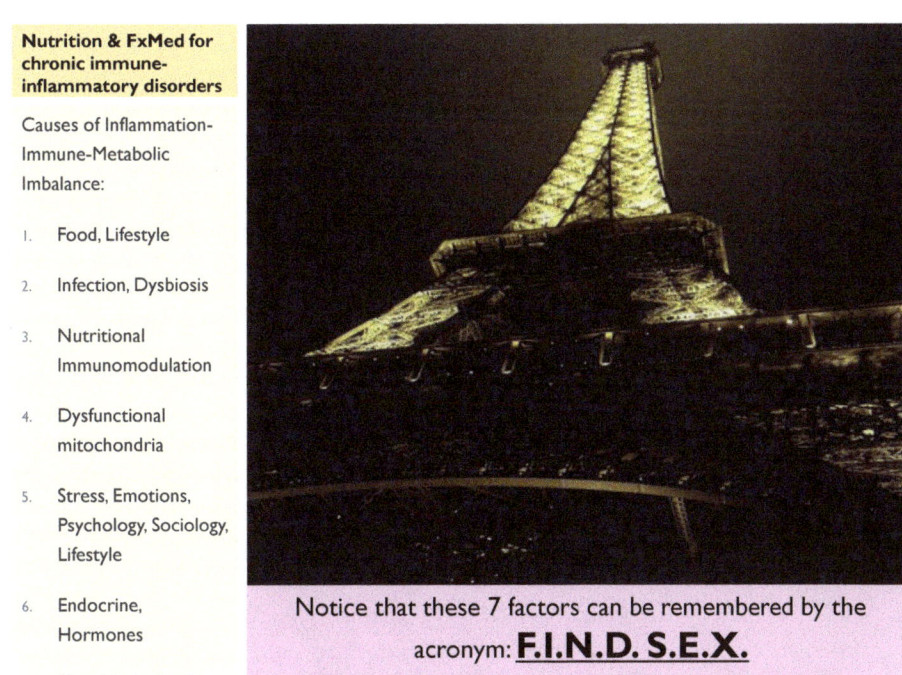

Nutrition & FxMed for chronic immune-inflammatory disorders

Causes of Inflammation-Immune-Metabolic Imbalance:

1. Food, Lifestyle
2. Infection, Dysbiosis
3. Nutritional Immunomodulation
4. Dysfunctional mitochondria
5. Stress, Emotions, Psychology, Sociology, Lifestyle
6. Endocrine, Hormones
7. Xenobiotics, Toxins

Notice that these 7 factors can be remembered by the acronym: **F.I.N.D. S.E.X.**
♥ First presented in Paris in 2012 ♥

Clinical protocol

- **Subjective**—patient's concerns and complaints
- **Objective**—clinical findings
- **Assessment**—diagnoses
- **Plan**—treatments, tests, referral, follow-up
    1. Food and lifestyle
    2. Infection and dysbiosis
    3. Nutritional immunomodulation
    4. Dysfunctional mitochondria
    5. Stress, Sociology-psychology, Lifestyle
    6. Endocrine/hormones
    7. Toxins/Xenobiotics

Patient name: _____
Date of birth: _____
Date of visit: _____

S.

O.

A.

P.

F.I.N.D.S.E.T.

Doctor: _____

Nutrition & FxMed for chronic immune-inflammatory disorders

Causes of Inflammation-Immune-Metabolic Imbalance:

1. Food, Diet
2. Infection, Dysbiosis
3. Nutritional Immunomodulation
4. Dysfunctional mitochondria
5. Stress, Emotions, Psychology, Sociology
6. Endocrine, Hormones
7. Xenobiotics, Toxins

← **Common to each problem**: What we are going to notice is that every clinical disorder characterized by chronic inflammation, allergy, and/or autoimmunity has treatable contributors within each of these 7 categories.

- **Why isn't genetics specifically mentioned?** Because we are focusing on areas where we can take *action*. Although we cannot change the DNA, we *can* change genetic expression, transcription factors, and epigenetic mechanisms such as DNA methylation and histone methylation and acetylation.
- **Oxidative stress and free radicals are important; why aren't these specifically mentioned?** Oxidative balance is an epiphenomenon related to other factors such as dietary intake, nutritional supplementation, mitochondrial function, infections, and toxin exposure.
- We will briefly detail each of these 7 mechanisms now, then apply additional details to each inflammation-immune problem discussed.

Nutrition & FxMed for chronic immune-inflammatory disorders

Causes of Inflammation-Immune-Metabolic Imbalance:

1. **Food, Diet**
2. Infection, Dysbiosis
3. Nutritional Immunomodulation
4. Dysfunctional Mitochondria
5. Style of living, Stress, Sociology, Sleep, Sweat, Spinal Health
6. Endocrine, Hormone Imbalances
7. Xenobiotics, Toxins

What do YOU think of when you think of "food, diet, nutrition"?

- For example, a patient comes to your office and says something like:
  - "Can you tell me how to eat right to stay healthy?"
  - "Doctor, how can I eat better to help treat my disease?"

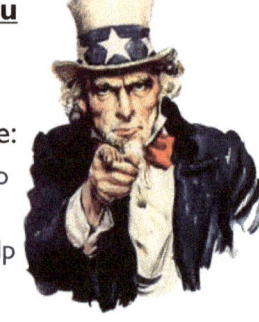

Here are some of the things I think about:
1. Food-induced inflammation
2. Oxidative stress
3. Immune suppression
4. Phytonutrients: antioxidants, antimicrobial, defense stimulatory
5. pH/acid-base balance
6. Sugar/insulin excess, carbohydrate-tailoring
7. GI dysbiosis & SIBO
8. Deficiencies of vitamins, minerals, ALA, GLA, EPA, DHA
9. Allergens and circulating immune complexes
10. NFkB and nutrigenomics
11. GMO-altered foods: increased immunogenicity, chemicals…

Nutrition & FxMed for chronic immune-inflammatory disorders

Causes of Inflammation-Immune-Metabolic Imbalance:

1. Food, Diet
2. Infection, Dysbiosis
3. Nutritional Immunomodulation
4. Dysfunctional Mitochondria
5. Style of living, Stress, Sociology, Sleep, Sweat, Spinal Health
6. Endocrine, Hormone Imbalances
7. Xenobiotics, Toxins

The Solution: 5-Part Nutrition Protocol

1. **Paleo-Mediterranean Diet**: fruits, vegetables, nuts, seeds, berries, high-quality protein; allergy avoidance.
2. **Multivitamin/multimineral**: high potency broad-spectrum
3. **Vitamin D3**: 2,000 – 4,000 – 10,000 IU/d to optimize serum levels
4. **Combination fatty acid therapy (CFAT)**: ALA, GLA, EPA, DHA, Oleic acid
5. **Probiotics**: especially with allergies, IBS, and/or antibiotics

Vasquez A. Five-Part Nutritional Wellness Protocol That Produces Consistently Positive Results. *Nutritional Wellness* 2005 Sept www.InflammationMastery.com/reprints/

Revisiting the Five-Part Nutritional Wellness Protocol: The Supplemented Paleo-Mediterranean Diet

Alex Vasquez, DC, ND, DO

ABSTRACT: This article reviews the five-part nutritional protocol that incorporates a health-promoting nutrient-dense diet and essential supplementation with vitamins/minerals, specific fatty acids, probiotics, and physiologic doses of vitamin D3. This foundational nutritional protocol has proven benefits for disease treatment, disease prevention, and health maintenance and restoration. Additional treatments such as botanical medicines, additional nutritional supplements, and pharmaceutical

---

The Pro-inflammatory Lifestyle (most people)

1. **High-sugar foods**: Immunosuppression + oxidative stress for 4 hours
2. **High-fat foods**: Especially arachidonic acid, linoleic acid, and saturated fats
3. **Fatty acid imbalances**: Insufficiencies of ALA, EPA, DHA, GLA, with excesses of saturated fat, arachidonate, linoleic acid, and trans-fats
4. **Vitamin and mineral deficiencies**, especially magnesium and vitamin D.
5. **Allergens**: molecular mimicry, immune-complexes
6. **Insufficient phytonutrients**: Anti-inflammatory benefits, antioxidants, fiber, nutrigenomic benefits (e.g., salicylate, phytate)
7. **Insufficiency of fiber**: Fiber is "decoy" for bacterial adhesion; lack of fiber = constipation and increased intraluminal pressure; reduced mucosal repair = increased bacterial translocation
8. **Foods that promote bacterial overgrowth of the small bowel**: Sucrose, wheat, potatoes, lactose/dairy
9. **Dysbiosis**: GI is most appreciated, but sinorespiratory and GU are problems
10. **Insufficient exercise**: 1) Adipose is pro-inflammatory and pro-estrogenic, 2) exercising muscle reduces inflammation (myokines) and 3) improves insulin sensitivity for a secondary anti-inflammatory benefit
11. **Xenobiotic/toxin accumulation**: Underdiagnosed pandemic
12. **Emotional stress and toxic relationships**: Promote inflammation, impair wound healing, and promote mucosal immunosuppression which facilitates dysbiosis

Nutrition & FxMed for chronic immune-inflammatory disorders

Causes of Inflammation-Immune-Metabolic Imbalance:

1. **Food, Diet**
2. Infection, Dysbiosis
3. Nutritional Immunomodulation
4. Dysfunctional Mitochondria
5. Style of living, Stress, Sociology, Sleep, Sweat, Spinal Health
6. Endocrine, Hormone Imbalances
7. Xenobiotics, Toxins

"Unhealthy diet" = proinflammatory diet

1. <u>Grains, especially wheat</u>: wheat is highly allergenic and contains subfractions that have direct pro-inflammatory effects; baked wheat contains pro-inflammatory glycosylated amino acids via the "Maillard reaction"; grains in general and wheat in particular are difficult to digest and thereby provide fermentable carbohydrate to intestinal bacteria, promoting bacterial overgrowth of the small intestines which is pro-inflammatory.
2. <u>Simple carbohydrates</u>: Simple sugars cause 2-4 hours of increased inflammation coupled with immune suppression.
3. <u>Lack of fruits, vegetables, nuts, seeds, berries = lack of fiber and phytonutrients</u>: causes constipation/toxicity, deficiency of antioxidants and antiinflammatory agents.
4. <u>Insufficient protein</u>: impairs healing and detoxification.
5. <u>Excess n-6 fatty acids</u>: promotes inflammation and cancer.

Diet-induced proinflammatory state. *JManipulativePhysiolTher* 2002 Mar
Seaman. **Dietary Pursuit of Disease**. *NutritionalWellness.com* 2007 Aug

---

Healthy diet = anti-inflammatory effects

1. **Composition**: primarily of fruits, vegetables, nuts, seeds, berries, and lean protein.
2. **Phytonutrients**: 8,000 compounds that generally have antioxidant and antiinflammatory benefits.
3. **Fiber for bulk/laxation**: Important to cleanse the bowels to avoid GI dysbiosis and to remove toxins.
4. **Low-carbohydrate (CHO) intake**: Avoids immune suppression and oxidative stress from simple CHO intake; lowers insulin levels and Na retention to alleviate HTN.
5. **Low sodium** (water/HTN/inflamm) **chloride** (acidogenic)
6. **Nutrient-dense**: Promotes satiation and supports metabolic needs and physiologic expectations,
7. **Promotes alkalinization**: potassium citrate promotes optimal urine pH of 7.5 to enhance mineral retention, lower cortisol, eliminate toxins, and increase endorphin analgesia.
8. **Sufficient protein and n-3 fatty acids**:
9. **Sun or supplementation for physiologic amounts of vitamin D3**: ~4,000 IU/d for adults

Unhealthy "fast" food = inflammation

- A single meal of <u>egg and sausage muffin sandwiches with 2 hash browns</u> caused an **increase of 150% for NF-kappaB** (from ~190 to ~510 AUC) for approximately **2 hours** and was associated with increases in oxidative stress and the inflammatory marker **CRP**.
  - Hospital food = inflammation = additional treatment with anti-inflammatory drugs, known to have multiple adverse effects, including CKD, ARF, gastric ulceration, DM, infxn, PPI/H2agonsts,

Aljada, *Am J Clin Nutr*, 2004

Increase in intranuclear nuclear factor κB and decrease in inhibitor κB in mononuclear cells after a mixed meal: evidence for a proinflammatory effect[1-3]

Ahmad Aljada, Priya Mohanty, Husam Ghanim, Toufic Abdo, Devjit Tripathy, Ajay Chaudhuri, and Paresh Dandona

Sidebar — Causes of Inflammation-Immune-Metabolic Imbalance:
1. Food, Diet
2. Infection, Dysbiosis
3. Nutritional Immunomodulation
4. Dysfunctional Mitochondria
5. Style of living, Stress, Sociology, Sleep, Sweat, Spinal Health
6. Endocrine, Hormone Imbalances
7. Xenobiotics, Toxins

Unhealthy "fast" food = inflammation

- **How much of the American diet is "fast food"?**
  - VERY IMPORTANTLY: What really matters here is "processed food" not simply "fast food"; so looking strictly at "fast food" is simply the tip of the processed food iceberg.

Figure 2. Percentage of calories from fast food among adults aged 20 and over, by age and race and ethnicity: United States, 2007–2010

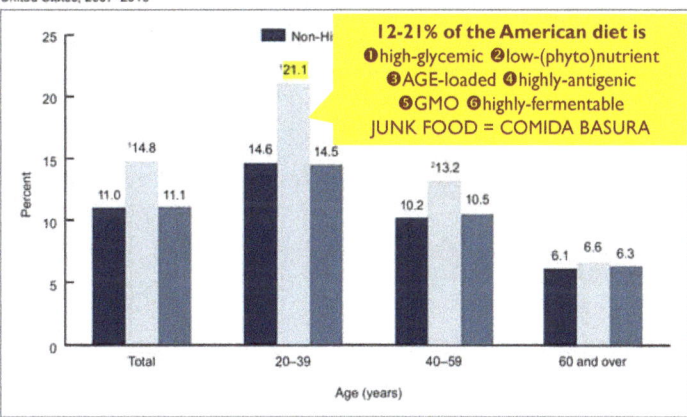

12-21% of the American diet is ❶high-glycemic ❷low-(phyto)nutrient ❸AGE-loaded ❹highly-antigenic ❺GMO ❻highly-fermentable JUNK FOOD = COMIDA BASURA

February 2013   http://www.cdc.gov/nchs/data/databriefs/db114.pdf

Nutrition & FxMed for chronic immune-inflammatory disorders

Causes of Inflammation-Immune-Metabolic Imbalance:

1. Food, Diet
2. Infection, Dysbiosis
3. Nutritional Immunomodulation
4. Dysfunctional Mitochondria
5. Style of living, Stress, Sociology, Sleep, Sweat, Spinal Health
6. Endocrine, Hormone Imbalances
7. Xenobiotics, Toxins

Sugar (simple carbohydrates) = oxidative stress and antioxidant depletion

- "Glucose challenge stimulates reactive oxygen species (ROS) generation by leucocytes." Mohanty. *J Clin Endocrinol Metab.* 2000 Aug
  - 14 normal subjects: Consumed 75g (300kcal) glucose
  - ROS generation increased 240%: Of normal by polymorphonuclear leucocytes (PMNL) and mononuclear cells (MNC),
  - Antioxidant depletion: alpha-Tocopherol levels decreased significantly at 1 h, 2 h, 3 h.

Nutrition & FxMed for chronic immune-inflammatory disorders

Causes of Inflammation-Immune-Metabolic Imbalance:

1. Food, Diet
2. Infection, Dysbiosis
3. Nutritional Immunomodulation
4. Dysfunctional Mitochondria
5. Style of living, Stress, Sociology, Sleep, Sweat, Spinal Health
6. Endocrine, Hormone Imbalances
7. Xenobiotics, Toxins

Sugar (simple carbohydrates) = immune suppression

- "Oral 100-g portions of carbohydrate from glucose, fructose, sucrose, honey, or orange juice all **significantly decreased the capacity of neutrophils to engulf bacteria** …
- Starch ingestion did not have this effect. The decrease in phagocytic index was rapid following the ingestion of simple carbohydrates.
- The greatest effects occurred between 1 and 2 hr postprandial, but the values were still significantly below the fasting control values 5 hr after feeding…
- On the other hand, a fast of 36 or 60 hr significantly increased ($P < 0.001$) the phagocytic index."

Sanchez. *Am J Clin Nutr.* 1973 Nov

Nutrition & FxMed for chronic immune-inflammatory disorders

Causes of Inflammation-Immune-Metabolic Imbalance:

1. Food, Diet
2. Infection, Dysbiosis
3. Nutritional Immunomodulation
4. Dysfunctional Mitochondria
5. Style of living, Stress, Sociology, Sleep, Sweat, Spinal Health
6. Endocrine, Hormone Imbalances
7. Xenobiotics, Toxins

Many/most phytonutrients have antioxidant and antiinflammatory activities that are synergistic and—*in total*—clinically significant

- Diets low in fruits, vegetables, nuts, seeds, berries are low in phytonutrients.
- "We propose that the additive and synergistic effects of phytochemicals in fruit and vegetables are responsible for their potent antioxidant and anticancer activities, and that the benefit of a diet rich in fruit and vegetables is attributed to the complex mixture of phytochemicals present in whole foods."

Liu. Am J Clin Nutr. 2003 Sep

Health benefits of fruit and vegetables are from additive and synergistic combinations of phytochemicals[1-4]

Rui Hai Liu

Nutrition & FxMed for chronic immune-inflammatory disorders

Causes of Inflammation-Immune-Metabolic Imbalance:

1. Food, Diet
2. Infection, Dysbiosis
3. Nutritional Immunomodulation
4. Dysfunctional Mitochondria
5. Style of living, Stress, Sociology, Sleep, Sweat, Spinal Health
6. Endocrine, Hormone Imbalances
7. Xenobiotics, Toxins

Many plants contain "beneficial toxins" that improve human health

- Plants protect themselves from the sun with **antioxidant phytochemicals**.
- Plants protect themselves from consumption/ infection with slightly "toxic" phytochemicals that induce aversion (**bitter taste**) and/or which have **antimicrobial** effects.
- Antimicrobial phytochemicals in plants—such as oregano, garlic, carrots, berberine—have clinically meaningful effects in humans and can be used to treat human diseases.
  - This is also a major means by which a plant-based diet provides microbe-modulating benefits.
  - Thereby, when we change the diet, we change the microbes, and when we change the microbes we change the immune phenotype and inflammatory balance.
- Mild "toxins" in plants also stimulate human defense systems such as **Nrf2-ARE** (antioxidant response element) and **phase-2 detoxification/conjugation enzymes**.

Nutrition & FxMed for chronic immune-inflammatory disorders

Causes of Inflammation-Immune-Metabolic Imbalance:

1. Food, Diet
2. Infection, Dysbiosis
3. Nutritional Immunomodulation
4. Dysfunctional Mitochondria
5. Style of living, Stress, Sociology, Sleep, Sweat, Spinal Health
6. Endocrine, Hormone Imbalances
7. Xenobiotics, Toxins

Excess dietary carbohydrate is the *most common*—3-6 times per day for most people—cause of:

1. Chronic hyperglycemia, type-2 diabetes mellitus: immune suppression, oxidative stress, antioxidant depletion, protein glycosylation (nerve/eye, vascular, and kidney damage),
2. Chronic hyperinsulinemia: promotes dyslipidemia via stimulation of HMG-CoA reductase, promotes atherogenesis,
3. Chronic hypertension, metabolic syndrome: insulin promotes sodium and water retention thus leading to hypertension,
4. Proinflammatory and pro-oxidative state:
5. Mitochondrial dysfunction: synergistic with nutritional deficiencies

---

Nutrition & FxMed for chronic immune-inflammatory disorders

Causes of Inflammation-Immune-Metabolic Imbalance:

1. Food, Diet
2. Infection, Dysbiosis
3. Nutritional

Hyperglycemia→Insulin→Ceramide→InsulinResistance: This is how "*insulin causes insulin resistance*" and how "*hyperglycemia causes hyperglycemia*"—one part of the DM2 story

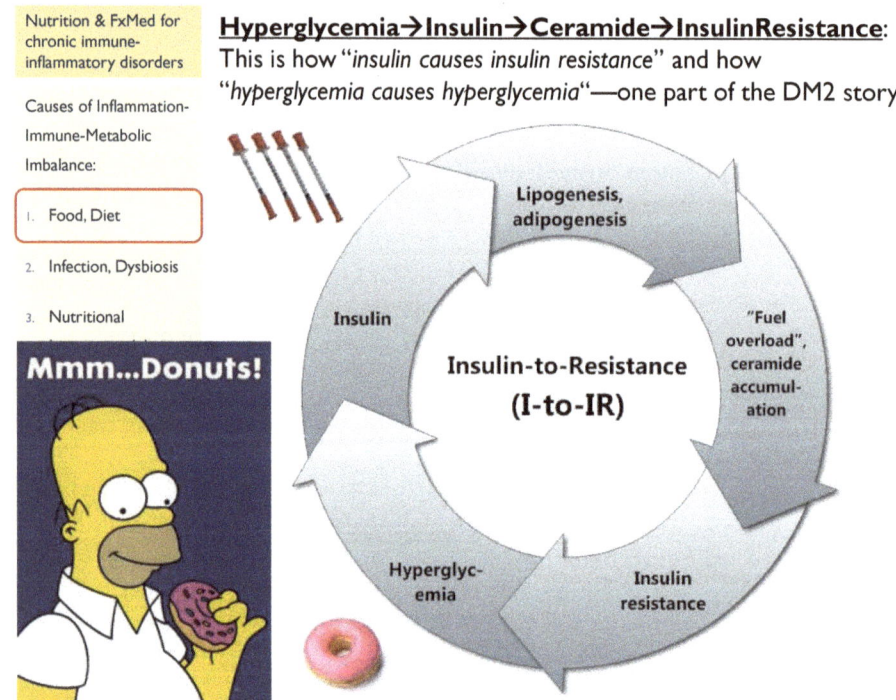

Inflammation Mastery & Functional Inflammology: Volume 1
Excerpted Presentation Slides • Page 27

Nutrition & FxMed for chronic immune-inflammatory disorders

Causes of Inflammation-Immune-Metabolic Imbalance:

1. **Food, Diet**
2. Infection, Dysbiosis
3. Nutritional Immunomodulation
4. Dysfunctional Mitochondria
5. Style of living, Stress, Sociology, Sleep, Sweat, Spinal Health
6. Endocrine, Hormone Imbalances
7. Xenobiotics, Toxins

Microbes + metabolic stress = inflammasome activation → inflambesity/IR/AI

- Microbial debris (PAMP—**P**athogen**A**ssoc**M**ol**P**at) and **obesity-related cellular stress** (DAMP—Damage/DangerAssocMolPat) activate —via cytosolic pattern-recognition NOD*-like receptor (NLR) – the **inflammasome** which activates IL-1 & IL-18 for **chronic inflammation and autoimmunity** via **IL-6, TNF-a, IL-17/Th-17**.

*nucleotide-binding oligomerization domain

Lukens. *Discov Med.* 2011 Jul

Nutrition & FxMed for chronic immune-inflammatory disorders

Causes of Inflammation-Immune-Metabolic Imbalance:

1. **Food, Diet**

Wheat and other antigenic hyperglycemic AGE-loaded highly-fermentable overly consumed (dietary monotony) processed foods are the perfect recipe—the perfect storm—for simultaneous induction of **GI microbial overgrowth**, increased intestinal permeability, and **hyperglycemic metabolic stress**.

Microbes + metabolic stress = inflammasome activation → inflambesity/IR/AI

PAMP + DAMP = inflammasome activation

- "large cytoplasmic complexes called **inflammasomes** that **link** the sensing of **microbial products** and **metabolic stress** to the proteolytic activation of the **proinflammatory cytokines.**" Martinon. The inflammasomes. *Annu Rev Immunol.* 2009 Apr
- Inflammasome:
  - Multiprotein oligomer consisting of caspase 1, PYCARD, NALP and sometimes caspase 5 (also known as caspase 11 or ICH-3).
  - Expressed in myeloid cells; component of the innate immune system.
  - Exact composition of an inflammasome depends on the activator which initiates inflammasome assembly i.e. "customizable" like NFkB.
  - The inflammasome is responsible for activation of inflammatory processes, and has been shown to induce cell pyroptosis, a process of programmed cell death distinct from apoptosis.

Nutrition & FxMed for chronic immune-inflammatory disorders

Causes of Inflammation-Immune-Metabolic Imbalance:

1. Food, Diet
2. Infection, Dysbiosis
3. Nutritional Immunomodulation
4. Dysfunctional Mitochondria
5. Style of living, Stress, Sociology, Sleep, Sweat, Spinal Health
6. Endocrine, Hormone Imbalances
7. Xenobiotics, Toxins

Wheat = inflammation

In this context, it is important to note that a low CHO diet offers further possibilities to target inflammation through omission or inclusion of certain foods. Usually, CHO restriction is not only limited to avoiding sugar and other high-GI foods, but also to a reduced intake of grains. Grains can induce inflammation in susceptible individuals due to their content of omega-6 fatty acids, lectins and gluten [159,160]. In particular gluten might play a key role in the pathogenesis of auto-immune and inflammatory disorders and some malignant diseases. In the small intestine, gluten triggers the release of zonulin, a protein that regulates the tight junctions between epithelial cells and therefore intestinal, but also blood-brain barrier function. Recent evi-

Open access

Klement, Kämmerer. *Nutrition & Metabolism* 2011, 8:75
nutritionandmetabolism.com/content/8/1/75

Nutrition & FxMed for chronic immune-inflammatory disorders

Causes of Inflammation-Immune-Metabolic Imbalance:

1. Food, Diet
2. Infection, Dysbiosis
3. Nutritional Immunomodulation
4. Dysfunctional Mitochondria
5. Style of living, Stress, Sociology, Sleep, Sweat, Spinal Health
6. Endocrine, Hormone Imbalances
7. Xenobiotics, Toxins

Wheat = fermentation, dysbiosis, and small intestinal bacterial overgrowth (SIBO)

- We conclude that the malabsorbed fraction of wheat bread was dependent on the amount ingested, ... Fermentation of wheat bran resulted in a very low breath-hydrogen response compared with lactulose or wheat bread."
Olesen, *Am J Clin Nutr* 1997;66

- "...hydrogen response was increased by all breads."
Hallfrisch, *J Am Coll Nutr.* 1999

Proposal: Given | wheat = proportionate ∝ growth-fermentation
thus ∴ wheat = proportionate ∝ SIBO

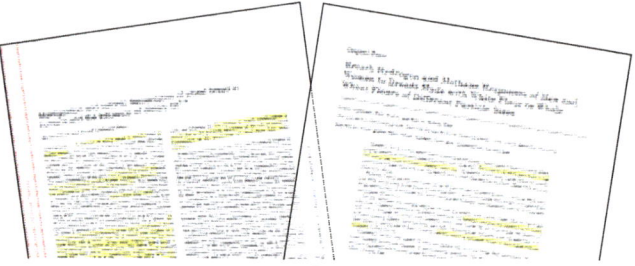

Inflammation Mastery & Functional Inflammology: Volume 1
Excerpted Presentation Slides • Page 29

Is wheat medically justifiable?

- Rather than asking "Why should we/patients avoid wheat?", the question that is more intellectually and scientifically appropriate is, **"What is the medical justification for allowing patients to eat wheat?"**
- Convenience, taste, and habituation (shared completely with alcohol and tobacco) are not sufficient medical and scientific justifications to allow patients to consume proinflammatory antigens, AGEs, and high glycemic load and high glycemic highly fermentable GMO foods.
- The only medical justification for wheat consumption is the prevention/treatment of starvation, and even then treatment duration should be as short as possible.
- "The doctor of the future will give no medication, but will interest his patients in the care of the human frame, diet and in the cause and prevention of disease." Thomas A. Edison (American inventor and businessman, 1847-1931)
- "The doctors of the future will counsel against wheat* consumption just as doctors do at present against alcohol and tobacco." Alex Vasquez

*and fructose and GMO

Nutrition & FxMed for chronic immune-inflammatory disorders

Causes of Inflammation-Immune-Metabolic Imbalance:
1. Food, Diet
2. Infection, Dysbiosis
3. Nutritional Immunomodulation
4. Dysfunctional Mitochondria
5. Style of living, Stress, Sociology, Sleep, Sweat, Spinal Health
6. Endocrine, Hormone Imbalances
7. Xenobiotics, Toxins

Low-carbohydrate diets reduce inflammation,...which was obviously caused/triggered by excess dietary carbohydrate

Effects of a Low–Glycemic Load Diet on Resting Energy Expenditure and Heart Disease Risk Factors During Weight Loss

...lesterol with weight loss. C-reactive protein declined by nearly 50% with weight loss in the low–glycemic load group but remained essentially unchanged in the low-fat group (P = .03 for

CRP -47%

Pereira, JAMA, 2004

Nutrition & FxMed for chronic immune-inflammatory disorders

Causes of Inflammation-Immune-Metabolic Imbalance:

1. Food, Diet
2. Infection, Dysbiosis
3. Nutritional Immunomodulation
4. Dysfunctional Mitochondria
5. Style of living, Stress, Sociology, Sleep, Sweat, Spinal Health
6. Endocrine, Hormone Imbalances
7. Xenobiotics, Toxins

Induction of lipolysis and ketogenesis promotes global histone acetylation via BHB's inhibition of histone deacetylase *Science* 2013 January

Induction of global histone acetylation is associated with induction of a rejuvenative phenotype *Cellular and Molecular Life Sciences* 2001 Dec

> Discuss means (i.e., dosing schedule) and implications corresponding with clinical observations. Kaufman Wlm. Niacinamide therapy for joint mobility; therapeutic reversal of a common clinical manifestation of the normal aging process. *Conn State Med J.* 1953 Jul

Research Article

Rapid reversion of aging phenotypes by nicotinamide through possible modulation of histone acetylation

K. Matuoka[a,*], K.Y. Chen[b] and T. Takenawa[a]

[a] Institute of Medical Science, University of Tokyo, Tokyo 108-8639 (Japan)
[b] Department of Chemistry, Rutgers University, 610 Taylor Road, Piscataway, New Jersey 08854-8087 (USA)

Received 27 August 2001; received after revision 15 October 2001; accepted 15 October 2001

Abstract. Aging appears to be an irreversible process. Here we report that nicotinamide (NAA) can induce rapid and reversible reversion of aging phenotypes in human diploid fibroblasts in terms of cell morphology and senescence-associated β-galactosidase activity. Although NAA seems to enhance the replicative potential of the ... NAD precursor/niacin, NAD analogs, and polyADP-ribosyl polymerase inhibitors) exerted similar effects. Thus, NAD-related metabolism and polyADP-ribosylation are unlikely related to the NAA action. On the other hand, histone acetyltransferase (HAT) activity was elevated in NAA-exposed cells, while in aged cells,

---

Nutrition & FxMed for chronic immune-inflammatory disorders

Causes of Inflammation-Immune-Metabolic Imbalance:

1. Food, Diet
2. Infection, Dysbiosis
3. Nutritional Immunomodulation
4. Dysfunctional Mitochondria
5. Style of living, Stress, Sociology, Sleep, Sweat, Spinal Health
6. Endocrine, Hormone Imbalances
7. Xenobiotics, Toxins

Unhealthy high-carbohydrate diets promote inflammation via several mechanisms, including gastrointestinal dysbiosis (bacterial overgrowth)

- Unhealthy diets with components such as **wheat**/grains, **sugar, and potatoes** promote inflammation via several mechanisms including promotion of **gastrointestinal dysbiosis and small intestine bacterial overgrowth (SIBO).**
  - Proof of this concept is data showing that change to a **plant-based diet evokes clinical improvements in patients** with inflammatory diseases (RA) that correlate with and appear to be dependent on **favorable alterations in gastrointestinal flora—quality, quantity, and activity.**
  - *Hear me now, believe me later*: We don't simply change patients' diets to change their nutrient intake:
    - **We change the diet to change the microbes**.

Healthy diets alleviate inflammation by improving quality & reducing quantity of intestinal bacteria

- "43 RA patients were randomized into two groups: the test group to receive living food, a form of uncooked vegan diet rich in lactobacilli, and the control group to continue their ordinary omnivorous diets."
- "We conclude that a vegan diet changes the fecal microbial flora in RA patients, and changes in the fecal flora are associated with improvement in RA activity."

Peltonen, *Br J Rheumatol*, 1997 Jan

Hear me now, believe me later: "*We change the diet to change the microbes.*"

Healthy diets alleviate inflammation by improving quality & reducing quantity of intestinal bacteria

- "Significant alteration in the intestinal flora was observed when the patients changed from omnivorous to vegan diet.
- This finding of an association between intestinal flora and disease activity may have implications for our understanding of how diet can affect RA."

Toivanen. *Rheumatology*. 2002 Aug

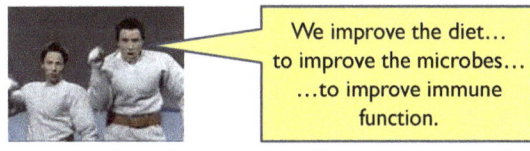

Nutrition & FxMed for chronic immune-inflammatory disorders

Causes of Inflammation-Immune-Metabolic Imbalance:

1. Food, Diet
2. Infection, Dysbiosis
3. Nutritional Immunomodulation
4. Dysfunctional Mitochondria
5. Style of living, Stress, Sociology, Sleep, Sweat, Spinal Health
6. Endocrine, Hormone Imbalances
7. Xenobiotics, Toxins

Excess exposure to (SIBO) and/or absorption (leaky gut) of bacterial debris promotes diabetes:

- "…bacterial components in blood predicts the onset of diabetes mellitus in a large general population." Koch *Nature Reviews Endocrinology* 2012 Jan
- Blood levels of the bacterial marker (16S ribosomal DNA) predict the onset of diabetes and abdominal adiposity in a large general population (n= 3,280) followed for 9 years. The adjusted OR (95% CIs) for incident diabetes and for abdominal adiposity were 1.35 and 1.18, respectively. 16S rDNA was shown to be an independent marker of the risk of diabetes. These findings are evidence for the concept that **tissue bacteria are involved in the onset of diabetes in humans**. Amar. *Diabetologia*. 2011 Dec

16S ribosomal RNA (16S rRNA) is a component of the 30S small subunit of prokaryotic ribosomes; genes coding for it are 16S rDNA.

Nutrition & FxMed for chronic immune-inflammatory disorders

Causes of Inflammation-Immune-Metabolic Imbalance:

1. Food, Diet
2. Infection, Dysbiosis
3. Nutritional Immunomodulation
4. Dysfunctional Mitochondria
5. Style of living, Stress, Sociology, Sleep, Sweat, Spinal Health
6. Endocrine, Hormone Imbalances
7. Xenobiotics, Toxins

Nutritional deficiencies = inflammation, oxidative stress, low-grade immune activation

- **Vitamin and mineral deficiencies are epidemic** in the general population and are pandemic among patients with chronic diseases due to disease effects, malabsorption-maldigestion-hyperexcretion (due to disease or drugs), hypermetabolism and oxidative stress due to inflammation.
  - My research: Vitamin D deficiency was found in 156/157 rheumatology patients in Texas in the southern USA, a region with abundant sunshine,
  - Magnesium deficiency has been noted in ~40% of general and patient populations internationally, with some studies as large as 16,000 subjects.
- **Fatty acid deficiencies of ALA, GLA, EPA, and DHA are commonplace**: the average intake of n3 fatty acids has historically been 7 grams per day and in industrialized nations is currently 1 gram per day; thus patients should be assumed to be deficient in n3 fatty acids.

Nutritional supplementation should be routine

- Most people do not consume an optimal amount of all vitamins by diet alone.
- ...it appears prudent for all adults to take vitamin supplements.
- Physicians should make specific efforts to...ensure that patients are taking the vitamins they should..."

Fletcher, Fairfield. *JAMA*. 2002 Jun

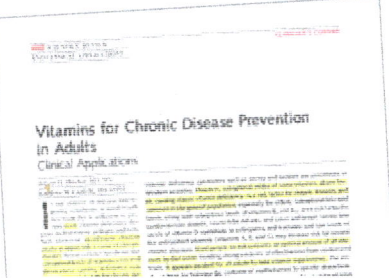

Nutritional supplementation reduces inflammation: *Clinical pearl*: Most micronutrients provide antiinflammatory effects/benefits.

- "RESULTS: At 6 months, C-reactive protein levels were significantly lower in the multivitamin group than in the placebo group (between-group difference = -0.91 mg/L).
- CONCLUSION: In a post hoc analysis of a randomized, double-blind, placebo-controlled study, **multivitamin use was associated with lower C-reactive protein levels**."

Church. *Am J Med*. 2003 Dec

Vitamin D3 supplementation—correction of vitamin D deficiency—causes clinically important reductions in systemic inflammatory activity:

- MMP9 (-68%),
- TIMP-1 (-38%)
- CRP (-23%)

Timms, *QJM*. 2002 Dec

Q J Med 2002; 95:787-796

Original papers — QJM

Circulating MMP9, vitamin D and variation in the TIMP-1 response with VDR genotype: mechanisms for inflammatory damage in chronic disorders?

P.M. TIMMS[1], N. MANNAN[2], G.A. HITMAN[2], K. NOONAN[1], P.G. MILLS[4], ...COURT[3], E. AGANNA[2], C.P. PRICE[3] and B.J. BOUCHER[2]

Mechanisms of vitamin D immunomodulation:

1. VDR is a member of the steroid/thyroid/retinoid receptor gene superfamily of transcription factors and regulates the expression of many genes.
2. **VDR have been detected in over 30 different tissues including circulating monocytes, dendritic cells and activated T cells—"...the highest concentration is in immature immune cells within the thymus and in mature CD8 T lymphocytes..."**
3. Vitamin D "has direct effects on T and B cells and shapes their responses to activation"
4. **Vitamin D inhibits T lymphocyte proliferation, particularly inhibits Th1 cell proliferation and cytokine production.**
5. Vitamin D "decreased secretion of interleukin (IL)-2 and IFNγ by CD4 T cells and promotes IL-5 & IL-10 production.

Mechanisms of vitamin D immunomodulation:

6. **1,25(OH)2D3 downregulates IL-6, an important stimulator of Th17 cells, which are a critical component of autoimmunity.**
7. "In B cells, **vitamin D has been shown to inhibit antibody secretion and autoantibody production.**
8. "1,25(OH)2D3 is one of the most powerful blockers of dendritic cell differentiation and of IL-12 secretion.
9. "interferes with the NFκB-induced transcription of IL-12.
10. "decrease in IL-12 and IFNγ **while IL-10 and transforming growth factor β production is enhanced**, resulting in inhibition of T cell activation.
11. 1,25(OH)2D3 increased the macrophage-specific surface antigens and the lysosomal enzyme acid phosphatase while stimulating the "oxidative burst" function.

Vitamin D receptor activation is necessary for maintaining the integrity of the intestinal mucosal barrier: Kong J. Am J Physiol Gastrointest Liver Physiol. 2008 Jan

- "These observations suggest that VDR plays a critical role in mucosal barrier homeostasis by **preserving the integrity of junction complexes** and the healing capacity of the colonic epithelium.
- Therefore, **vitamin D deficiency may compromise the mucosal barrier,** leading to increased susceptibility to mucosal damage and increased risk of IBD [and probably other autoimmune/autoinflammatory/immune diseases].
- ∴ Vitamin D deficiency probably → leaky gut → microbe/food antigen absorption → immune stimulation → immune activation → inflammation/allergy/autoimmunity

Nutrition & FxMed for chronic immune-inflammatory disorders

Causes of Inflammation-Immune-Metabolic Imbalance:

1. Food, Diet
2. Infection, Dysbiosis
3. Nutritional Immunomodulation
4. Dysfunctional Mitochondria
5. Style of living, Stress, Sociology, Sleep, Sweat, Spinal Health
6. Endocrine, Hormone Imbalances
7. Xenobiotics, Toxins

Deficiencies of vitamins, minerals, fatty acids:
Vitamin C has anti-allergy ☺ and enjoyment-enhancing benefits ☺☺

- Antihistamine effect of supplemental ascorbic acid: "...[blood] histamine levels were depressed 38% following VC supplementation. ...These data indicate that VC may indirectly enhance chemotaxis by detoxifying histamine in vivo." Johnston. *J Am Coll Nutr.* 1992 Apr

- High-dose ascorbic acid increases intercourse frequency and improves mood. *Biol Psychiatry.* 2002 Aug

---

Nutrition & FxMed for chronic immune-inflammatory disorders

Causes of Inflammation-Immune-Metabolic Imbalance:

1. Food, Diet
2. Infection, Dysbiosis
3. Nutritional Immunomodulation
4. Dysfunctional Mitochondria
5. Style of living, Stress, Sociology, Sleep, Sweat, Spinal Health
6. Endocrine, Hormone Imbalances
7. Xenobiotics, Toxins

These fatty acids are anti-inflammatory

- These fatty acids are notably missing from many modern "convenience" diets, and each of these has antiinflammatory effects; thus, "combination fatty acid deficiency" contributes to a pro-inflammatory condition, and CFAT supplementation has a clinically proven antiinflammatory effect:

  1. ALA—n3 alpha linolenic acid from flax oil,
  2. GLA—n6 gamma linolenic acid, borage oil,
  3. EPA—n3 eicosapentaenoic acid from cold water fatty fish,
  4. DHA—n3 docosahexaenoic acid from cold water fatty fish, also algae,
  5. Oleic acid: n9 mostly in olive oil.

  Historical Paleolithic intake of n3 fatty acids was **seven** grams per day; Western/American intake of n3 fatty acids is **one** gram per day. Thus, by definition, nearly everyone is deficient in n3 anti-inflammatory fatty acids.

Nutrition & FxMed for chronic immune-inflammatory disorders

Causes of Inflammation-Immune-Metabolic Imbalance:

1. Food, Diet
2. Infection, Dysbiosis
3. Nutritional Immunomodulation
4. Dysfunctional Mitochondria
5. Style of living, Stress, Sociology, Sleep, Sweat, Spinal Health
6. Endocrine, Hormone Imbalances
7. Xenobiotics, Toxins

Health-promoting fatty acids (ALA, GLA, EPA, DHA, oleic acid) provide clinically meaningful antiinflammatory benefits:

- GLA—dose 500-1,000-4,000 mg/d for proven clinical benefits in RA via activation of PPAR-g and reductions in NFkB and leukotrienes,
- EPA and DHA—therapeutic benefits start at 1,000 mg/d but are more significant at 3,000 mg/d via activation of PPAR-a and reductions in NFkB and prostaglandins, increases in docosatrienes and resolvins.

www.InflammationMastery.com/reprints/

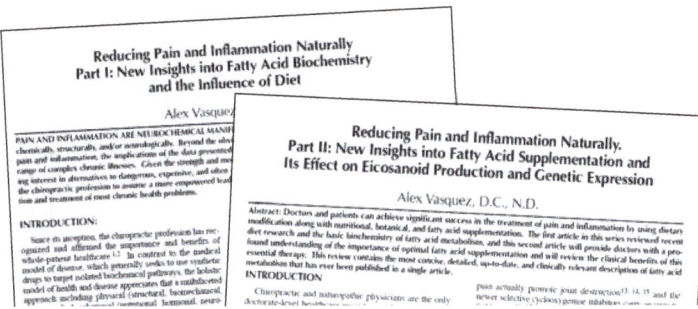

Nutrition & FxMed for chronic immune-inflammatory disorders

Causes of Inflammation-Immune-Metabolic Imbalance:

1. Food, Diet
2. Infection, Dysbiosis
3. Nutritional Immunomodulation
4. Dysfunctional Mitochondria
5. Style of living, Stress, Sociology, Sleep, Sweat, Spinal Health
6. Endocrine, Hormone Imbalances
7. Xenobiotics, Toxins

Health-promoting fatty acids (ALA, GLA, EPA, DHA, oleic acid) provide clinically meaningful anti-inflammatory benefits:

- **Fish oil [EPA & DHA] supplementation** allows patients with inflammatory diseases such as **rheumatoid arthritis** to reduce their need for anti-inflammatory drugs. *Br J Rheumatol.* 1993 Nov
- "CONCLUSION: A diet **low in arachidonic acid** ameliorates clinical signs of inflammation in patients with RA and augments the **beneficial effect of fish oil supplementation**." *Rheumatol Int.* 2003 Jan
- "The children (**mean age, 11.4 months**) with atopic dermatitis (mean duration, 8.56 months) were openly treated with **3 g/day gamma-linolenic acid**, for 28 days… A gradual improvement in erythema, excoriations and lichenification was seen; significant differences were shown for itching, and the use of antihistamines." *J Int Med Res.* 1994 Jan-Feb

CFAT: Combination Fatty Acid Therapy

Molecular Mechanisms of CFAT

1. Precursor competition in cell membranes and enzyme sites (COX and LIPOX),
2. Activation of PPAR-gamma and PPAR-alpha
3. Nutrigenomics exemplified: modulation of gene transcription via downregulation of NF-kappaB
4. Docosatrienes, Resolvins, Protectins, Maresins: Active healing / anti-inflammation
5. Reduction in hypothalamic inflammation via modulation of TLR4
6. Induction of Treg via GLA activation of PPAR-gamma
7. Activation of GPR120—G-protein coupled receptor 120
8. Improved cell membrane dynamics and function
9. Mitochondrial support via DHA-cardiolipin and the inner mitochondrial membrn.
10. Neuro/Psych benefits: improved neurotransmitter synthesis
11. Reduction in intracellular calcium, thus lessening a proinflammatory phenotype
12. Synergistic/cumulative antiinflammatory benefits

Nutrition & FxMed for chronic immune-inflammatory disorders

Causes of Inflammation-Immune-Metabolic Imbalance:

1. **Food, Diet**
2. Infection, Dysbiosis
3. Nutritional Immunomodulation
4. Dysfunctional Mitochondria
5. Style of living, Stress, Sociology, Sleep, Sweat, Spinal Health
6. Endocrine, Hormone Imbalances
7. Xenobiotics, Toxins

Allergenic foods (foods to which the patient is immunologically sensitized) can contribute to systemic inflammation and musculoskeletal pain by many mechanisms:

1. Formation of immune complexes (chains of antigens and antibodies) that can deposit in the joints/vessels/kidneys to cause a localized inflammatory response.
2. Triggering migraine headaches: (neurogenic switching?)
3. Increasing intestinal permeability, which then increases antigen load and systemic inflammation.
4. Adversely altering gastrointestinal flora, which can then promote systemic inflammation, particularly if the intestinal mucosa is compromised by the allergic inflammation.

Inman, *Rheum Dis Clin North Am.* 1991

### Sidebar
Nutrition & FxMed for chronic immune-inflammatory disorders

Causes of Inflammation-Immune-Metabolic Imbalance:
1. **Food, Diet**
2. Infection, Dysbiosis
3. Nutritional Immunomodulation
4. Dysfunctional Mitochondria
5. Style of living, Stress, Sociology, Sleep, Sweat, Spinal Health
6. Endocrine, Hormone Imbalances
7. Xenobiotics, Toxins

Food Allergens: Many patients unknowingly consume foods that promote their allergic reactions—wheat is the best example.

- "60 migraine patients, elimination diets after a 5-day period of withdrawal from their normal diet.
- **The commonest foods causing reactions were:**
    - wheat (78%)—look out for celiac disease,
    - orange (65%),
    - eggs (45%),
    - tea and coffee (40% each),
    - chocolate and milk (37% each),
    - beef (35%),
    - corn, cane sugar, and yeast (33% each).
- When **an average of ten common foods were avoided** there was a dramatic fall in the number of headaches per month, 85% of patients becoming headache-free.

Grant. Lancet. 1979 May

"Food Allergies" and circulating immune complexes (CIC):
Many patients unknowingly consume foods that promote their allergic reactions—wheat is the best example. Mechanisms include increased intestinal permeability (progressive panallergy, exacerbation of dysbiosis-mediated disorders) and formation of immune complexes. Inman, *Rheum Dis Clin North Am.* 1991

- METHODS: N=352 healthy individuals were tested for CICs containing C1q and IgG and gliadin IgG antibodies
- RESULTS: In our study, 15.3% (54/352) of the patients presented with elevated CIC concentrations (above 50 microg/ml) and 6.5% (23/352) of the study population were positive for gliadin IgG antibodies (above 20 U/ml)
- "CONCLUSIONS: The results of this study indicate that certain food antigens (e.g. gluten) could play a role in the formation of CICs." *Scandinavian J Gastroenterol* 2009

NF-kappaB: Pro-inflammatory transcription factor

"Activation of the NF-KB pathway ... plays a central role in inflammation through its ability to induce transcription of proinflammatory genes."
J Clin Invest 2001 Jan

Reducing Pain and Inflammation Naturally - Part IV:
Nutritional and Botanical Inhibition of NF-kappaB,
the Major Intracellular Amplifier of the Inflammatory Cascade.
A Practical Clinical Strategy Exemplifying Anti-Inflammatory Nutrigenomics

Alex Vasquez, DC, ND

www.InflammationMastery.com/reprints/

NF-kappaB: Modulation with (phyto)nutrients

1. Vitamin D3
2. Curcumin (w/ piperine)
3. Lipoic acid
4. Green tea
5. Rosemary
6. Grape seed extract
7. Propolis
8. Zinc
9. Co-enzyme Q-10
10. Selenium
11. Indole-3-carbinol (I3C)
12. N-acetyl-L-cysteine
13. Resveratrol
14. GLA activates PPAR-gamma
15. EPA activates PPAR-alpha
16. Boswellia serrata
17. Harpagophytum procumbens
18. Willow bark

"On the other hand <u>in humans</u> after a dose of 2 g curcumin alone, serum levels were either <u>undetectable</u> or very low. Concomitant administration of **piperine 20 mg produced much higher concentrations** from 0.25 to 1 h post drug ($P < 0.01$ at 0.25 and 0.5 h; $P < 0.001$ at 1 h), the **increase in bioavailability was 2000%.** The study shows that in the dosages used, piperine enhances the serum concentration, extent of absorption and bioavailability of curcumin in both rats and humans with **no adverse effects.**" *Planta Med* 1998 May

Vasquez A. Nutritional and Botanical Inhibition of NF-kappaB, the Major Intracellular Amplifier of the Inflammatory Cascade. Anti-Inflammatory Nutrigenomics. *Nutritional Perspectives* 2005; Jul
http://optimalhealthresearch.com/part4.html

Nutrition & FxMed for chronic immune-inflammatory disorders

Causes of Inflammation-Immune-Metabolic Imbalance:

1. **Food, Diet**

1. GMO-related toxin-proteins and toxic pesticides are measurable in non-pregnant women, pregnant women, and human fetuses.

GMO-altered foods: Increased allergenicity, toxins, changes in gut microbes, gut permeability, cytokine levels, and immunocyte populations…

- **Pesticides associated to genetically modified foods (PAGMF),** are engineered to tolerate herbicides such as glyphosate (GLYP) and gluphosinate (GLUF) or insecticides such as the bacterial toxin bacillus thuringiensis (Bt).
  - GLYP and its metabolite aminomethyl phosphoric acid (AMPA),
  - GLUF and its metabolite 3-methylphosphinicopropionic acid (3-MPPA)
  - Cry1Ab protein: a Bt toxin
- "Serum GLYP and GLUF were detected in NPW and not detected in PW. Serum 3-MPPA and CryAb1 toxin were detected in **PW**, their **fetuses** and **NPW**."
- "This is the first study to reveal the presence of circulating PAGMF in women with and without pregnancy, paving the way for a new field in reproductive toxicology including nutrition and utero-placental toxicities."

Aris A, Leblanc S. *Reprod Toxicol.* 2011 May

Nutrition & FxMed for chronic immune-inflammatory disorders

Causes of Inflammation-Immune-Metabolic Imbalance:

1. **Food, Diet**

1. GMO-related toxin-proteins and toxic pesticides are measurable in non-pregnant women, pregnant women, and human fetuses.
2. Bt pesticide exposure causes IgE and IgG immune responses in humans.

GMO-altered foods: Increased allergenicity, toxins, changes in gut microbes, gut permeability, cytokine levels, and immunocyte populations…

- **Bt pesticide exposure = elevations in IgG and IgE**:
  - Dose-response: Allergic skin sensitization and induction of **IgE and IgG antibodies**, or both."
  - Implication: "…skin sensitization to Bt in pesticides could be a precursor of clinical IgE-mediated diseases…"
  - Concerns: "…**immediate hypersensitivity induced by bacteria and transgenic foods engineered to incorporate pesticidal genes in their genomes.**"

Bernstein et al. Immune responses in farm workers after exposure to Bacillus thuringiensis pesticides. *Environ Health Perspect.* 1999 Jul

Nutrition & FxMed for chronic immune-inflammatory disorders

Causes of Inflammation-Immune-Metabolic Imbalance:

1. **Food, Diet**

   1. GMO-related toxin-proteins and toxic pesticides are measurable in non-pregnant women, pregnant women, and human fetuses.
   2. Bt pesticide exposure causes IgE and IgG immune responses in humans.
   3. Pro-inflammatory immune disturbances including increases in IL-6 and gamma-delta-T-cells.

GMO-altered foods: Increased allergenicity, toxins, changes in gut microbes, gut permeability, cytokine levels, and immunocyte populations…

- **MON810 corn causes increased IL-6 and *gd*-Tcells**:
  - GMO MON810 maize induced increases of serum IL-6, IL-13, IL-12p70, and MIP-1beta and *gamma-delta*-Tcells of mice.
    - We all know that IL-6 = inflammation and generally more CRP/IR/CVD/AzD.
  - "One of the more recurrent alterations in lymphocyte phenotypes observed in this study was an increase in the TCRγδ+ population. … Higher numbers of γδT cells have been observed in **humans** with **asthma**, in IELs of children with untreated **food allergy**, and in the duodenum of children with **juvenile idiopathic arthritis** or **connective tissue disease** with gastrointestinal symptoms." Finamore et al. *J Agric Food Chem.* 2008 Dec
  - Per review in Feb 2013 and previous work dating back decades, we know that **gd-Tcells promote inflammation and autoimmunity**! Su et al. *Clin Dev Immunol.* 2013 Feb

---

Nutrition & FxMed for chronic immune-inflammatory disorders

Causes of Inflammation-Immune-Metabolic Imbalance:

1. **Food, Diet**

   1. GMO-related toxin-proteins and toxic pesticides are measurable in non-pregnant women, pregnant women, and human fetuses.
   2. Bt pesticide exposure causes IgE and IgG immune responses in humans.
   3. Pro-inflammatory immune disturbances including increases in IL-6 and gamma-delta-T-cells.

GMO-altered foods: Increased allergenicity, toxins, changes in gut microbes, gut permeability, cytokine levels, and immunocyte populations…

- **MON810 corn causes increased IL-6 and *gd*-Tcells**:
  - Finamore et al. *J Agric Food Chem.* 2008 Dec
  - "As a subset of T cells that bridge innate and adaptive immunity, **γδ T cells** may display different functions similar to those of CD4+ T-cell subsets such as CTLs, Th1/Th2 cells, Tregs, Th17 cells, and APCs depending on specific microenvironment. They **definitely play important roles in the development of autoimmune diseases** such as RA and SLE through their antigen-presenting capacity, release of proinflammatory cytokines, immunomodulatory properties, interaction with CD4+CD25+Tregs, and promotion of antibody production by providing B-cell help." Su et al. *Clin Dev Immunol.* 2013 Feb

Nutrition & FxMed for chronic immune-inflammatory disorders

Causes of Inflammation-Immune-Metabolic Imbalance:

1. **Food, Diet**

1. GMO-related toxin-proteins and toxic pesticides are measurable in non-pregnant women, pregnant women, and human fetuses.
2. Bt pesticide exposure causes IgE and IgG immune responses in humans.
3. Pro-inflammatory immune disturbances including increases in IL-6 and gamma-delta-T-cells.
4. Longest animal study showed tumors, early death, degenerative and necrotic changes in kidney, liver, pituitary.

GMO-altered foods: Increased allergenicity, toxins, changes in gut microbes, gut permeability, cytokine levels, and immunocyte populations…

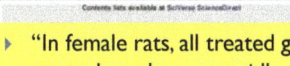

- "In female rats, all treated groups died 2-3 times more than controls, and more rapidly.
- "Females developed large mammary tumors almost always more often than and before controls, the pituitary was the second most disabled organ; the sex hormonal balance was modified by GMO and Roundup treatments.
- "In treated males, liver congestions and necrosis were 2.5-5.5 times higher.
- "Marked and severe kidney nephropathies were also generally 1.3-2.3 greater.
- "Males presented 4 times more large palpable tumors than controls which occurred up to 600 days earlier.
- "These results can be explained by the non linear endocrine-disrupting effects of Roundup, but also by the overexpression of the transgene in the GMO and its metabolic consequences."

Séralini et al. *Food Chem Toxicol.* 2012 Nov

Nutrition & FxMed for chronic immune-inflammatory disorders

Causes of Inflammation-Immune-Metabolic Imbalance:

1. **Food, Diet**

Reasons for retraction:
1. **Unreliable / worthless data**: either as a result of misconduct (e.g. data fabrication) or honest error (e.g. miscalculation or experimental error)
2. **Redundant** publication
3. **Plagiarism**
4. **Unethical** research

Science-based *or* industry-influenced retraction?

- Although the paper by Seralini *et al* showing clear **evidence of harm by GMO corn and pesticides** was published with only minor revisions requested by the journal's chief editor, it was *unscientifically* withdrawn… following the creation of an "associate editor" position at the journal filled by a former employee of **Monsanto**.
- 13 letters published against the Seralini paper: 11 of the authors had undisclosed financial relationships with Monsanto.
- From the BioEthics Forum:
  - "It would have been perfectly appropriate for the journal to have written an editorial expressing its concerns. Instead, it seems the editors may have succumbed to industry pressure to do the wrong thing. The media coverage in the U.S. has been one-sided; criticism of Séralini's study has been widely covered in mainstream press, while information about the conflicts of interest of critics have remained in the alternative press."

http://retractionwatch.com/2014/01/16/journal-editor-defends-retraction-of-gmo-rats-study-while-authors-reveal-some-of-papers-history/
http://www.thehastingscenter.org/Bioethicsforum/Post.aspx?id=6684

Arch Toxicol (2012) 86:805–813
DOI 10.1007/s00204-012-0804-8

GENOTOXICITY AND CARCINOGENICITY

Cytotoxic and DNA-damaging properties of glyphosate and Roundup in human-derived buccal epithelial cells

Verena J. Koller · Maria Fürhacker · Armen Nersesyan · Miroslav Mišík · Maria Eisenbauer · Siegfried Knasmueller

Received: 14 September 2011 / Accepted: 11 January 2012 / Published online: 14 February 2012
© Springer-Verlag 2012

Abstract Glyphosate (G) is the largest selling herbicide worldwide; the most common formulations (Roundup, R) contain polyoxyethyleneamine as main surfactant. Recent ... the herbicide and its formulation. Since we found genotoxic effects after short exposure to concentrations that correspond to a 450-fold dilution of spraying used in agriculture, our findings indicate that inhalation may cause DNA damage in exposed individuals.

Inflammation Mastery & Functional Inflammology: Volume 1
Excerpted Presentation Slides • Page 45

Time to rest and refuel

Barcelona, Cataluña 2013

Nutrition & FxMed for chronic immune-inflammatory disorders

Causes of Inflammation-Immune-Metabolic Imbalance:

1. Food, Diet
2. Infection, Dysbiosis
3. Nutritional Immunomodulation
4. Dysfunctional Mitochondria
5. Style of living, Stress, Sociology, Sleep, Sweat, Spinal Health
6. Endocrine, Hormone Imbalances
7. Xenobiotics, Toxins

Infections & Dysbiosis = inflammation

Important concepts:
- Subclinical infections are common in patients with chronic inflammatory diseases, especially autoimmunity.
- Remember, the microbe(s) alone are not the problem; the patient's total inflammatory load (TIL) must also be addressed, as well as immunorestoration to prevent recurrence of the colonization.

Clinical assessments:
- Culture/sensitivity are helpful; DNA-based assessments are also used.
- **Response to treatment is most compelling and meaningful.**

Therapeutic implementation:
1. Antimicrobials,
2. Immunorestoration,
3. Functional Immunomodulation: Enhance inflammatory tolerance.

Dysbiosis → "*multifocal poly*dysbiosis"

Location Subtypes:
1. **Gastrointestinal**
2. **Orodental**
3. **Sinorespiratory**
4. **Parenchymal**
5. **Genitourinary**
6. **Cutaneous**
7. **Environmental**

Problematic Microbes Include:
Aeromonas hydrophila, Blastocystis hominis, Candida albicans and other yeasts, *Citrobacter rodentium, Citrobacter freundii, Dientamoeba fragilis, Endolimax nana, Entamoeba histolytica,* Gamma strep, *Enterococcus, Giardia lamblia, Hafnia alvei, Helicobacter pylori, Klebsiella pneumoniae, Proteus mirabilis, Pseudomonas aeruginosa, Staphylococcus aureus, Staphylococcus epidermidis, Streptococcus pyogenes,* Group A streptococci

Molecular Mechanisms
1. **Molecular mimicry**
2. Superantigens
3. Enhanced processing of autoantigens
4. **Bystander activation**
5. Peptidoglycans and exotoxins
6. Endotoxins (LPS)
7. Immunostimulation by bacterial DNA
8. Activation of Toll-like receptors and NF-kappaB
9. **Immune complex formation and deposition**
10. **Th17 induction; Treg suppression**
11. Haptenization and Neoantigen formation
12. Damage to the intestinal mucosa
13. Inhibition/alteration of detoxification
14. Antimetabolites
15. Autointoxication, hepatic encephalopathy, intestinal arthritis-dermatitis syndrome
16. Impairment of mucosal and systemic defenses
17. Impairment of mucosal digestion by microbial proteases and inflammation
18. Inflammation-induced endocrine dysfunction

Nutrition & FxMed for chronic immune-inflammatory disorders

Causes of Inflammation-Immune-Metabolic Imbalance:

1. Food, Diet
2. Infection, Dysbiosis
3. Nutritional Immunomodulation
4. Dysfunctional Mitochondria
5. Style of living, Stress, Sociology, Sleep, Sweat, Spinal Health
6. Endocrine, Hormone Imbalances
7. Xenobiotics, Toxins

Dysbiosis subtypes *by location*:

1. **Gastrointestinal**: at least 7 different subtypes of gastrointestinal dysbiosis.
2. **Orodental**: Noted in rheumatoid arthritis.
3. **Sinorespiratory**: Noted in Wegener's vasculitis.
4. **Parenchymal**: Occult infections in liver, joints.
5. **Genitourinary**: Classic in reactive arthritis.
6. **Cutaneous**: Eczema and more.
7. **Environmental**: Exposure to microbial debris/toxins and bioaerosols can induce a pro-inflammatory state that triggers autoimmunity and systemic inflammation.
8. **Microbial**: Yes, es posible que a vezes [it is possible that at times] microbes such as amoeba may be infected with smaller microbes and that one can have environmental dysbiosis induced by a microbe-within-a-microbe. *Eur J Clin Microbiol Infect Dis.* 2005 Mar

Nutrition & FxMed for chronic immune-inflammatory disorders

Causes of Inflammation-Immune-Metabolic Imbalance:

1. Food, Diet
2. **Infection, Dysbiosis**
3. Nutritional Immunomodulation
4. Dysfunctional Mitochondria
5. Style of living, Stress, Sociology, Sleep, Sweat, Spinal Health
6. Endocrine, Hormone Imbalances
7. Xenobiotics, Toxins

Dysbiosis subtypes *by major clinical effect*:

1. **Metabolic**: Chief clinical manifestation is in the realms of impaired function, precocious degeneration or rapid biological aging; molecular mechanisms may include inflammation, but the primary manifestations are those of impaired metabolic function or non-inflammatory pain:
   1. **Diabesity + serum bacterial 16SrDNA**: Amar. *Diabetologia* 2011 Dec
   2. **Raynaud's + H pylori**: Gasbarrini et al *Int J Angiol* 1998 Aug
   3. **Migraine + H pylori**: Faraji et al. *Pain Physician*. 2012 Nov-Dec
   4. **Alzheimer's + HSV1**: Very compelling molecular, infectious, and clinical associations are documented. Itzhaki and Witzhaki. *J Alzheimers Dis* 2008 May, Itzhaki et al. *J Neurovirol* 2008 Jan
   5. **Fibromyalgia + SIBO**: Wallace, Hallegua. *Curr Pain Headache Rep* 2004 Oct, Vasquez *Fibromyalgia in a Nutshell* 2012

2. **Inflammatory**: Vasquez *Integrative Rheumatology* 2007, 2013
   1. **Psoriasis + various microbes**: Noah. *Semin Dermatol* 1990 Dec
   2. **Wegener's vasculitis + *Staph aureus***: Stegeman. *N Engl J Med*. 1996 Jul
   3. **Eczema + *Staph aureus***: Krakowski et al. *Pediatrics*. 2008 Oct
   4. **Hypersensitivity alveolitis + *Candida albicans* (1 case)**: Schreiber et al. *Eur J Med Res*. 2000 Mar
   5. **Chronic arthritis + *Chlamydophila pneumoniae***: Carter et al. *Arthritis Rheum* 2010 May

Dysbiosis Location Subtypes: Gastrointestinal, Orodental, Sinorespiratory, *Tissue*, Genitourinary, Cutaneous, Environmental, Microbial

Date and Time Collected	Date Entered	Date and Time Reported	Physician Name	NPI	Physician ID
08/29/11 09:41	08/29/11	09/03/11 01:35ET	VASQUEZ , A		

Tests Ordered
FSH+TestT+LH+DHEA S+Prog+E2...; CBC With Differential/Platelet; Comp. Metabolic Panel (14); Chlamydia pneumoniae(IgG/M); Thyroxine (T4) Free, Direct, S; TSH; Prolactin; IGF-1; C-Reactive Protein, Cardiac; Homocyst(e)ine, Plasma; Triiodothyronine (T3); Reverse T3; Magnesium, RBC; Cortisol - AM; Venipuncture

```
Chlamydia pneumoniae(IgG/M)
   Chlamydia pneumoniae IgG      >1:256     High           Neg:<1:16
   Chlamydia pneumoniae IgM      <1:10                     Neg:<1:10
   Test Information:
```

- "*Chlamydia trachomatis* and *Chlamydophila* (*Chlamydia*) *pneumoniae* are known triggers of reactive arthritis (ReA) and exist in a persistent metabolically active infection state in the synovium…" *Arthritis Rheum* 2010 May
- "These studies confirm our previous reports concerning the high prevalence of C. pneumoniae in the CSF of MS patients." *Clin Diagn Lab Immunol*. 2002 Nov
- "Because there is as yet no standardisation of serological criteria for persistent infection, we considered antibody titers of > 1/20 in the IgA fraction, together with **IgG titers of 1/64 to 1/256**, to be indicative of persistent infection." *J Clin Pathol*. 2002 May
- Thank you, Bill Beakey DOM, from www.professionalco-op.com for provision of these lab tests.

Nutrition & FxMed for chronic immune-inflammatory disorders

Causes of Inflammation-Immune-Metabolic Imbalance:

1. Food, Diet
2. Infection, Dysbiosis
3. Nutritional Immunomodulation
4. Dysfunctional Mitochondria
5. Style of living, Stress, Sociology, Sleep, Sweat, Spinal Health
6. Endocrine, Hormone Imbalances
7. Xenobiotics, Toxins

Excess exposure to (SIBO) and/or absorption (leaky gut) of bacterial debris promotes diabetes:

- "…bacterial components in blood predicts the onset of diabetes mellitus in a large general population." Koch *Nature Reviews Endocrinology* 2012 Jan
- Blood levels of the bacterial marker (16S ribosomal DNA) predict the onset of diabetes and abdominal adiposity in a large general population (n= 3,280) followed for 9 years. The adjusted OR (95% CIs) for incident diabetes and for abdominal adiposity were 1.35 and 1.18, respectively. 16S rDNA was shown to be an independent marker of the risk of diabetes. These findings are evidence for the concept that **tissue bacteria are involved in the onset of diabetes in humans**. Amar. *Diabetologia*. 2011 Dec

16S ribosomal RNA (16S rRNA) is a component of the 30S small subunit of prokaryotic ribosomes; genes coding for it are16S rDNA.

Dysbiosis: Antimicrobial Botanicals

PHYTOTHERAPY RESEARCH
Phytother. Res. 14, 213–214 (2000)

SHORT COMMUNICATION
Inhibition of Enteric Parasites by Emulsified Oil of Oregano *in vivo*

Gastrointestinal dysbiosis: Additionally or empirically, treatment for gastrointestinal dysbiosis may include the following:

- **Oregano oil**: Emulsified oil of oregano in a time-released tablet is proven effective in the eradication of harmful gastrointestinal microbes, including *Blastocystis hominis*, *Entamoeba hartmanni*, and *Endolimax nana*.[1] An *in vitro* study [2] and clinical experience support the use of emulsified oregano against *Candida albicans* and various bacteria. The common dose is 600 mg per day in divided doses for 6 weeks.

[1] Force et al. Inhibition of enteric parasites by emulsified oil of oregano in vivo. *Phytother Res*. 2000 May
[2] Stiles et al. Inhibition of Candida albicans by oregano. *J Applied Nutr* 1995;47:96–102

© Med Sci Monit, 2011; 17(7): RA164-167
PMID: 21709646

Received: 2010.08.17
Accepted: 2011.02.14
Published: 2011.07.01

Modulating gut microbiota as an anti-diabetic mechanism of berberine

Junling Han[ABCDEF], Huiling Lin[ABCDEF], Weiping Huang[ACDG]

Authors' Contribution:
A Study Design
B Data Collection
C Statistical Analysis
D Data Interpretation
E Manuscript Preparation
F Literature Search
G Funds Collection

Department of Endocrinology and Metabolism, the 187th Hospital of PLA, Haikou, China

Source of support: Self-financing

Summary

Berberine, one of the main constituents of a Chinese traditional herb used to treat bacterial diar-

==Most clinical trials these days are using **berberine 500 mg 2-3 times per day in adults** with DM2 / MetSyn for 3 months with very clear benefits and no adverse effects.==

Nutrition & FxMed for chronic immune-inflammatory disorders

Causes of Inflammation-Immune-Metabolic Imbalance:

1. Food, Diet
2. Infection, Dysbiosis
3. Nutritional Immunomodulation
4. Dysfunctional Mitochondria
5. Style of living, Stress, Sociology, Sleep, Sweat, Spinal Health
6. Endocrine, Hormone Imbalances
7. Xenobiotics, Toxins

Often what we find when working with autoimmune/inflammatory patients is that they are having a _pathogenic inflammatory response_ to a _nonpathogenic_ microbe.

- Remember, we are not looking for classic "infection" here; we are looking to determine which underlying disruptions may be exacerbating inflammation and the patient's symptomatology.
- We have to look beyond the _disease-associated characteristics of the microbe_ to see _the patient's individualized response_ to the microbe.
  - **Dysbiosis = relationship**
  - Dysbiosis in one patient may present with dermatitis, while [what appears to be] the same microbial imbalance in another patient can present as peripheral neuropathy or inflammatory arthritis.

Nutrition & FxMed for chronic immune-inflammatory disorders

Causes of Inflammation-Immune-Metabolic Imbalance:

1. Food, Diet
2. Infection, Dysbiosis
3. **Nutritional Immunomodulation**
4. Dysfunctional Mitochondria
5. Style of living, Stress, Sociology, Sleep, Sweat, Spinal Health
6. Endocrine, Hormone Imbalances
7. Xenobiotics, Toxins

Nutritional Immunomodulation

Important concept: We can favorably influence the number and function of immune cell populations by using nutrients.

- **Our clinical goal:** to reduce inflammation, allergy, autoimmunity.
- **Our mechanistic goal:** to increase number-activity of T-regulatory (Treg) cells and to decrease number-activity of Th1 (cell-mediated inflammation), Th2 (humoral inflammation, autoimmunity), and Th-17 (autoimmunity) cells.

Children & adults eat far too much sodium.

- 75% of adults worldwide eat almost double (4,000 mg/d) daily recommended amount of sodium (<2g/d WHO, <1.5g/d AHA). "In the US, the average intake was about 3,600 mg/d." American Heart Association Meeting Report. March 2013. http://newsroom.heart.org/news/adults-worldwide-eat-almost-double-daily-aha-recommended-amount-of-sodium

- Most pre-packaged meals and snacks for toddlers contain high amounts of sodium. Some toddler meals contain 630 mg of sodium per serving. http://newsroom.heart.org/news/most-pre-packaged-meals-snacks-for-toddlers-contain-too-much-salt

    - Importantly, early exposure to high levels of sodium

        1) condition the nervous system to acclimate/crave additional and unnaturally high levels of sodium,

        2) likely promotes early steps in the development of hypertension, which may not clinically manifest until later childhood or adulthood,

        3) likely affect life-long programing of the immune system.

Sodium induces inflammatory Th-17 cells.

Nutrition & FxMed for chronic immune-inflammatory disorders

Causes of Inflammation-Immune-Metabolic Imbalance:

1. Food, Diet
2. Infection, Dysbiosis
3. Nutritional Immunomodulation
4. Dysfunctional Mitochondria
5. Style of living, Stress, Sociology, Sleep, Sweat, Spinal Health
6. Endocrine, Hormone Imbalances
7. Xenobiotics, Toxins

Sodium drives autoimmune disease by the induction of pathogenic TH17 cells. Kleinewietfeld et al. *Nature* 2013 Mar

> In this investigation, we found that modest increases in NaCl concentration could stimulate an almost logarithmic *in vitro* induction of IL-17A in naive CD4+ cells mediated through p38/MAPK, NFAT5 and SGK1. Importantly, the addition of 40 mM of NaCl to T_H17 differentiation cultures not only increased IL-17A expression but also led to a pathogenic phenotype of T_H17 cells. In line with these findings, common salt added to the diet of mice led to severe worsening of EAE accompanied by increased numbers of T_H17 cells.

Nutrition & FxMed for chronic immune-inflammatory disorders

Causes of Inflammation-Immune-Metabolic Imbalance:

1. Food, Diet
2. Infection, Dysbiosis
3. Nutritional Immunomodulation
4. Dysfunctional Mitochondria
5. Style of living, Stress, Sociology, Sleep, Sweat, Spinal Health
6. Endocrine, Hormone Imbalances
7. Xenobiotics, Toxins

Vitamin A: necessary for Treg induction

Characterization of Protective Human CD4+CD25+ FOXP3+ Regulatory T Cells Generated with IL-2, TGF-β and Retinoic Acid

Ling Lu[1,2], Xiaohui Zhou[1,3], Julie Wang[1], Song Guo Zheng[1*], David A. Horwitz[1*]

1 Division of Rheumatology, Department of Medicine, Keck School of Medicine at University of Southern California, Los Angeles, California, United States of America, 2 Department of Liver Transplantation, First Affiliated Hospital of Nanjing Medical University, Nanjing, China, 3 Immune Tolerance Center Shanghai East Hospital, Tongji University of Medicine, Shanghai, China

Abstract

Background: Protective CD4+CD25+ regulatory T cells bearing the Forkhead Foxp3 transcription factor can now be divided into three subsets: Endogenous thymus-derived cells, those induced in the periphery, and another subset induced ex-vivo with pharmacological amounts of IL-2 and TGF-β. Unfortunately, endogenous CD4+CD25+ regulatory T cells are unstable and can be converted to effector cells by pro-inflammatory cytokines. Although protective Foxp3+CD4+CD25+ cells resistant to proinflammatory cytokines have been generated in mice, in humans this result has been elusive. Our objective, therefore, was to induce human naive CD4+ cells to become stable, functional CD25+ Foxp3+ regulatory cells that were also resistant to the inhibitory effects of proinflammatory cytokines.

Methodology/Principal Findings: The addition of the vitamin A metabolite, all-trans retinoic acid (atRA) to human naive CD4+ cells suboptimally activated with IL-2 and TGF-β enhanced and stabilized FOXP3 expression, and accelerated their maturation to protective regulatory T cells. AtRA, by itself, accelerated conversion of naive to mature cells but did not induce FOXP3 or suppressive activity. The combination of atRA and TGF-β enabled CD4+CD45RA+ cells to express a phenotype and trafficking receptors similar to natural Tregs. AtRA/TGF-β-induced CD4+ regs were anergic and low producers of IL-2. They had potent *in vitro* suppressive activity and protected immunodeficient mice from a human-anti-mouse GVHD as well as expanded endogenous Tregs. However, treatment of endogenous Tregs with IL-1β and IL-6 decreased FOXP3 expression and diminished their protective effects *in vivo* while atRA-induced iTregs were resistant to these inhibitory effects.

Conclusions/Significance: We have developed a methodology that induces human CD4+ cells to rapidly become stable, fully functional suppressor cells that are also resistant to proinflammatory cytokines. This methodology offers a practical novel strategy to treat human autoimmune diseases and prevent allograft rejection without the use of agents that kill cells or interfere with signaling pathways.

Vitamin A: NIH Guidelines

Office of Dietary Supplements
National Institutes of Health

Table 3: Recommended Dietary Allowances (RDAs) for vitamin A

Age (years)	Children (mcg RAE)	Males (mcg RAE)	Females (mcg RAE)	Pregnancy (mcg RAE)	Lactation (mcg RAE)
1-3	300 (1,000 IU)				
4-8	400 (1,320 IU)				
9-13	600 (2,000 IU)				
14-18		900 (3,000 IU)	700 (2,310 IU)	750 (2,500 IU)	1,200 (4,000 IU)
19+		900 (3,000 IU)	700 (2,310 IU)	770 (2,565 IU)	1,300 (4,300 IU)

In Table 3, RDAs for vitamin A are listed as micrograms (mcg) of Retinol Activity Equivalents (RAE) to account for the different biological activities of retinol and provitamin A carotenoids. Table 3 also lists RDAs for vitamin A in International Units (IU), which are used on food and supplement labels (1 RAE = 3.3 IU).

http://ods.od.nih.gov/factsheets/vitamina/ Accessed August 2011

Vitamin D induces regulatory T-cells (1)

Vitamin D is epigenetically active. Burrell. *Discov Med.* 2011

- Most "healthy" subjects were vitamin D deficient at the start of this study.
- Participants received one dose of vitamin D 140,000 IU (nonphysiologic dosing)
- Most patients were not corrected to optimal vitamin D status.
- **Benefit: Significant increase in Treg cells.**

Prietl, *Isr Med Assoc J.* 2010 Mar

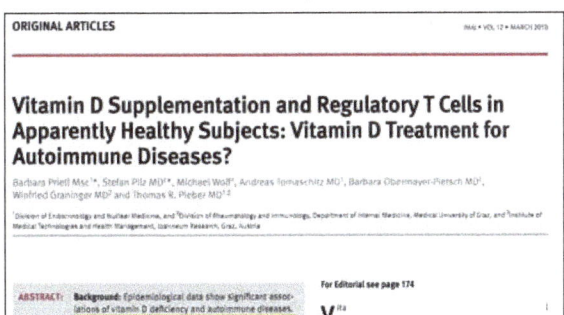

Nutrition & FxMed for chronic immune-inflammatory disorders

Causes of Inflammation-Immune-Metabolic Imbalance:

1. Food, Diet
2. Infection, Dysbiosis
3. Nutritional Immunomodulation
4. Dysfunctional Mitochondria
5. Style of living, Stress, Sociology, Sleep, Sweat, Spinal Health
6. Endocrine, Hormone Imbalances
7. Xenobiotics, Toxins

Vitamin D induces regulatory T-cells (2)

- 15 patients with MS given Vitamin D3 20,000 IU per day for 3 months: Reasonable dose, short duration
- **Treg suppressive function improved** in several subjects, this effect was not significant in the total cohort (P = 0.143).
- **Increased suppressor T-cells**: an increased proportion of IL-10+CD4+T cells was found after supplementation (P = 0.021)
- Note the lack of vitamin A, which must be administered with vitamin D to achieve benefit.

Nutrition & FxMed for chronic immune-inflammatory disorders

Causes of Inflammation-Immune-Metabolic Imbalance:

1. Food, Diet
2. Infection, Dysbiosis
3. Nutritional Immunomodulation
4. Dysfunctional Mitochondria
5. Style of living, Stress, Sociology, Sleep, Sweat, Spinal Health
6. Endocrine, Hormone Imbalances
7. Xenobiotics, Toxins

Vitamin D induces regulatory T-cells (3)

Inflammation Mastery & Functional Inflammology: Volume 1
Excerpted Presentation Slides • Page 55

Vitamin D3: clinical implementation protocol

www.InflammationMastery.com/reprints/

Vitamin D3: clinical implementation

- Rationale: Benefits heart, glucose/insulin/diabetes, anti-inflammatory, immunomodulatory, anti-cancer, mood enhancement.
- Dosing: Infants and children 2,000 IU/d, Adults 4,000-10,000 IU/d to optimize serum 25-OH-vitamin D.
- Safety margin: Very wide.
- Toxicity: Mediated exclusively via hypercalcemia. Periodically monitor serum calcium.
- Cautions/contraindications/considerations: Use lower dose and frequent monitoring in patients with hypercalcemic states, sarcoidosis, and granulomatous diseases (lymphoma).
  - Hepatic/renal insufficiency: Renal insufficiency reduces conversion to 1,25-di-OH-vitamin D; severe ESRD promotes hypercalcemia due to reduced renal excretion.
  - Drugs: HCTZ (hydrochlorothiazide, used for HTN) reduces renal excretion of calcium and promotes hypercalcemia.

www.InflammationMastery.com/reprints/

Probiotics

- Rationale: "Probiotics" in general have been shown/suggested/correlated to have anti-inflammatory and anti-allergy anti-autoimmune activities, and recently two mechanistic explanations have been provided 1) direct via microbe-specific effects, and 2) indirect via the probiotic metabolite butyric acid.
- Dosing: Per product, per diet, billions/trillions organisms.
- Safety/Risks: Very safe; however, legitimate concern exists for exacerbation of SIBO, which can cause D-lactic acidosis and other inflammatory complications; probiotic-induced abscess/sepsis is rare but has been reported.
- Cautions/contraindications/considerations:
    - Pregnancy/lactation: No special precautions.
    - Hepatic/renal insufficiency: No special precautions; benefit shown in these groups.
    - Drugs: Probiotic supplementation should be used nearly anytime antibiotics/antibacterials are administered.

Lipoic acid reduces IL-17 by 35-50% in vitro in patients with multiple sclerosis:

Salinthone, *PLoS One*. 2010 Sep

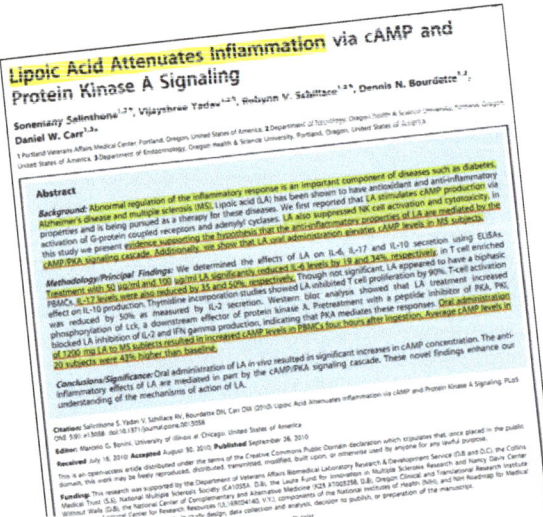

Nutrition & FxMed for chronic immune-inflammatory disorders

Causes of Inflammation-Immune-Metabolic Imbalance:

1. Food, Diet
2. Infection, Dysbiosis
3. Nutritional Immunomodulation
4. Dysfunctional Mitochondria
5. Style of living, Stress, Sociology, Sleep, Sweat, Spinal Health
6. Endocrine, Hormone Imbalances
7. Xenobiotics, Toxins

N3 fatty acids have an anti-inflammatory (metabolic, nutrigenomic) and anti-autoimmune (epigenetic) effect that is mediated in part via induction of Treg cells.

- N3 fatty acids protect against autoimmune diabetes
  - <u>Subjects</u>: 1770 children at increased risk for type 1 diabetes. <u>Results</u>: 1) omega-3 fatty acid intake was inversely associated with risk of IA (hazard ratio [HR], 0.45), 2) omega-3 fatty acid content of erythrocyte membranewas also inversely associated with IA risk (HR, 0.63
- **Conclusion:** Dietary intake of omega-3 fatty acids is associated with reduced risk of [islet autoimmunity] in children at increased genetic risk for type 1 diabetes.

Norris. JAMA. 2007 Sep

Nutri-immuno-epigenomics: GLA activates PPAR-gamma

DCs from other sites. In the present studies, using in vitro and in vivo approaches, we now demonstrate that PPARγ activation enhances iTreg generation through increased RA synthesis from murine splenic DCs and that endogenous PPARγ ligands may play a critical role in regulating iTreg generation.

Es probable que, some of the anti-inflammatory benefit of GLA is derived from GLA's activation of PPAR-gamma with works with/via retinol (vitamin A) for the induction of immunomodulating anti-allergy and anti-inflammatory Treg cells.

1. Housley. PPARgamma regulates retinoic acid-mediated DC induction of Tregs. *J Leukoc Biol.* 2009 Aug
2. Vasquez A. New Insights into Fatty Acid Supplementation and Its Effect on Eicosanoid Production and Genetic Expression. *Nutr Perspect* 2005; Jan

Green tea increases Treg

Nutritional induction of regulatory T-cells

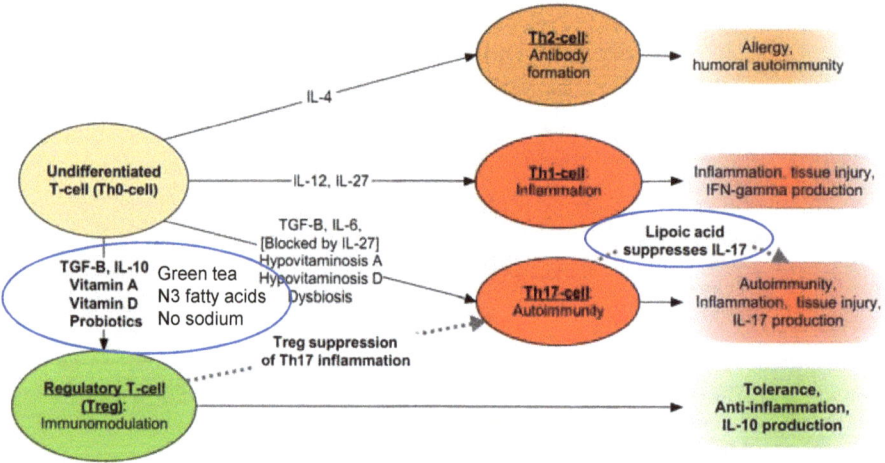

© Vasquez A. *Functional Immunology and Nutritional Immunomodulation: Presentation Slides Part 1* (2012), *Inflammation Mastery and Integrative Rheumatology (Third Edition, 2014)*.

Nutrition & FxMed for chronic immune-inflammatory disorders

Causes of Inflammation-Immune-Metabolic Imbalance:

1. Food, Diet
2. Infection, Dysbiosis
3. Nutritional Immunomodulation
4. Dysfunctional Mitochondria
5. Style of living, Stress, Sociology, Sleep, Sweat, Spinal Health
6. Endocrine, Hormone Imbalances
7. Xenobiotics, Toxins

Tregs—a few additional details:

- What I call "Treg global effectiveness": A factor of number and function; however, "net/overall inflammatory balance" combines many pro- and anti-inflammatory factors, the latter of which includes Tregs as one of many.
- Treg populations by location of development: Thymus-derived natural Tregs (nTreg) and peripheral inducible Tregs (iTreg).
- Treg populations by molecular markers:
  1. **CD4+CD25+FOXp3+Treg = the main "Treg"**
  2. Type-1 T-regulatory cells (Tr1)
  3. T-helper type-3 cells (Th3)
  4. CD8+ regulatory T cells (Tcreg)
  5. $\gamma\delta$Tregs: immunoregulatory functions appear to suppress the activity of CD4+ T cells and dendritic cells; earlier studies have indicated that peripheral $\gamma\delta$-T-cells are more capable than CD4+Tregs in suppressing the proliferation of CD4+effector T cells

Su et al. *Clin Dev Immunol*. 2013 Feb

Nutritional Immunomodulation: Induction of Treg at the expense/suppression of Th-1/2/17

1. Mitochondrial optimization
2. Biotin
3. E-vitamin
4. Sodium avoidance
5. Transgenic food avoidance
6. Probiotics
7. Lipoic acid
8. A-vitamin
9. Infection/dysbiosis clearance
10. D-vitamin
11. Fatty acids: EPA-DHA and GLA
12. IL-6 reduction: create overall antiinflammatory milieu for Treg induction
13. Green tea

What is the new acronym?

Mitochondrial Dysfunction = Inflammation:

© Vasquez A. *Mitochondrial Nutrition and Mitochondrial Medicine (2014)*.

Nutrition & FxMed for chronic immune-inflammatory disorders

Causes of Inflammation-Immune-Metabolic Imbalance:

1. Food, Diet
2. Infection, Dysbiosis
3. Nutritional Immunomodulation
4. **Dysfunctional Mitochondria**
5. Style of living, Stress, Sociology, Sleep, Sweat, Spinal Health
6. Endocrine, Hormone Imbalances
7. Xenobiotics, Toxins

Mitochondria cause Inflammation—Important concepts:

- "Mitochondria participate in the detection of infectious microorganisms and cellular damage to activate innate immune responses."
- "…likely that **accumulation of damaged mitochondria is an important cause of inflammation**."
- "…the removal of mitochondria that have a rather low threshold for permeabilization (mitochondrial "purging")."
- "**Exercise and caloric restriction stimulate autophagy** in most tissues…"

Green, *Science*. 2011 Aug

Nutrition & FxMed for chronic immune-inflammatory disorders

Causes of Inflammation-Immune-Metabolic Imbalance:
1. Food, Diet
2. Infection, Dysbiosis
3. Nutritional Immunomodulation
4. **Dysfunctional Mitochondria**
5. Style of living, Stress, Sociology, Sleep, Sweat, Spinal Health
6. Endocrine, Hormone Imbalances
7. Xenobiotics, Toxins

1. Mitochondrial dysfunction = disease

1. <u>Inflammation</u>: mitochondrial dysfunction contributes to cell senescence, chronic inflammation, and "inflammaging"
2. <u>Allergy</u>: especially asthma,
3. <u>Autoimmunity</u>: especially SLE and RA,
4. <u>Metabolic Syndrome, Diabetes Type-2, Hypertension</u>: mitochondria are required for insulin secretion and reception,
5. <u>Heart failure</u>: failure of energy production,
6. <u>Fibromyalgia</u>: histologic and biochemical evidence of mitochondrial failure, mitophagy,
7. <u>Migraine</u>: biochemical evidence of mitochondrial impairment,
8. <u>Neurodegeneration—Parkinson's and Alzheimer's, et al</u>: I think pretty much everyone should know this by now, especially regarding Parkinson's disease.

Mitochondria cause Inflammation: important concepts:

- Mitochondria have the ability to sense microbial (especially viral) infections and also to contribute to chronic inflammation.
- Dysfunctional mitochondria can be "purged" with **exercise** and **fasting**, and/or their function can be improved with nutritional supplementation, especially **CoQ-10, actyl-carnitine, lipoic acid**.

Therapeutic implementation:
- **Exercise,**
- **Therapeutic fasting, carbohydrate restriction,**
- **Mitochondrial nutritional support: CoQ-10, lipoic acid, acetyl-carnitine, resveratrol, and other nutrients,**
- **Eradicate dysbiosis: LPS, herpes, Chlaym…**

Nutrition & FxMed for chronic immune-inflammatory disorders

Causes of Inflammation-Immune-Metabolic Imbalance:

1. Food, Diet
2. Infection, Dysbiosis
3. Nutritional Immunomodulation
4. Dysfunctional Mitochondria
5. **Style of living, Stress, Sociology, Sleep, Sweat, Spinal Health**
6. Endocrine, Hormone Imbalances
7. Xenobiotics, Toxins

Clinical considerations that start with "S"

- **S**tyle of living—lifestyle
- **S**tress—reduction, management, avoidance
- **S**ocioPsychology—social psychology, socioPolitcs…
- **S**leep—that's when you close your eyes and turn off for a while
- **S**weat—exercise, euadaptation-inducing activity
- **S**pinal health—osteopathic and chiropractic manipulation/adjustment
- **S**pecialized supplementation—above and beyond the basic protocol
  - Selenium for antiviral effects
  - Melatonin for immune and mitochondrial stimulation
  - B6 to lower glutamate and raise GABA, etc.
- **S**urgery—bright lights and cold steel
- **S**tamp your passport and get the heck out of Dodge

Nutrition & FxMed for chronic immune-inflammatory disorders

Causes of Inflammation-Immune-Metabolic Imbalance:

1. Food, Diet
2. Infection, Dysbiosis
3. Nutritional Immunomodulation
4. Dysfunctional Mitochondria
5. **Style of living, Stress, Sociology, Sleep, Sweat, Spinal Health**
6. Endocrine, Hormone Imbalances
7. Xenobiotics, Toxins

Stress, Emotions, Psychology, Sociology:

- We live in a fast-paced stressful world where we paradoxically have more "networks" and activities, yet less meaningful connection with people. "Problems of existence" are generally ignored in preference for entertainment/distraction, shopping, alcohol, drugs. I think many of these issues were best addressed by Fredrich Nietzsche PhD (*Twilight of the Idols*, and *Human, All to Human**) and Nathaniel Branden PhD (*Six Pillars of Self-Esteem*)

  * http://video.google.com/videoplay?docid=-1842405914611103528

Mechanisms:

1. Mucosal immune suppression: reductions in sIgA
2. "Stress eating": people eat more wheat, sugar, alcohol when stressed; these promote inflammation, immune suppression, nutrient loss, oxidative stress, and increased gut permeability.
3. Microbial endocrinology: norepinephrine promotes microbial pathogenicity.
4. Sleep deprivation: promotes inflammation.

Nutrition & FxMed for chronic immune-inflammatory disorders

Causes of Inflammation-Immune-Metabolic Imbalance:

1. Food, Diet
2. Infection, Dysbiosis
3. Nutritional Immunomodulation
4. Dysfunctional Mitochondria
5. Style of living, Stress, Sociology, Sleep, Sweat, Spinal Health
6. **Endocrine, Hormone Imbalances**
7. Xenobiotics, Toxins

Patients with inflammatory and autoimmune disorders have hormonal imbalances:

- Hormones modulate immune and inflammation balance; thus, **hormone imbalances cause immune imbalances.** Anti-inflammatory eumetabolic benefits are derived from optimization of hormone levels and correction of the underlying imbalances:

  1. **Prolactin—high**: promotes inflammation, lymphocyte proliferation,
  2. **Estradiol—high, imbalanced**: drives inflammation, lymphocyte proliferation, autoantibodies, DNA mutation.
  3. **Fasting glucose <85 mg/dL, HgbA1c 4-5%, Insulin <5 microIU/mL,**: Hyperinsulinemia is a marker for chronic hyperglycemia and insulin resistance, which correlate directly with inflammation, oxidative stress, atherosclerosis, visceral adiposity, hypertension, hypercoagulability. Lindeberg *Metabolism* 1999 Oct, Brewer *Diabetes Care* 2008 Jun and discussion with Bill Beakey, Todd LePine, Umahro Cadogan, Maelan Fontes, Kara Fitzgerald, Pedro Bastos.

  1. **Low DHEA**: immunomodulatory
  2. **Low cortisol**: immunomodulatory
  3. **Low testosterone**: immunomodulatory

  Of course, always check thyroid: history, physical, labs x5, treatment response.

  Vasquez A. *Integrative Rheumatology, 3rd Edition*, chapter 4

Nutrition & FxMed for chronic immune-inflammatory disorders

Causes of Inflammation-Immune-Metabolic Imbalance:

1. Food, Diet
2. Infection, Dysbiosis
3. Nutritional Immunomodulation
4. Dysfunctional Mitochondria
5. Style of living, Stress, Sociology, Sleep, Sweat, Spinal Health
6. Endocrine, Hormone Imbalances
7. **Xenobiotics, Toxins**

The "toxins"
- Environmental pollution
- Xenobiotics
- Toxic/heavy metals: mercury, lead,
- Persistent organic pollutants—POPs

The main mechanisms
- Inflammation
  - Molecular haptenization = nonself = autoimmune response
- Mitochondrial dysfunction = inflammation, impaired glucose-insulin signaling, premature cell death, oxidative stress

The disease associations
- Inflammation / allergy / autoimmunity
- Parkinson's disease
- Insulin resistance, diabetes, metabolic syndrome, hypertension

Toxin awareness / detoxification support are necessary!

BPA Among Toxic Chemicals Driving Up Health Care Costs, Experts Say

Lynne Peeples | 01/22/14 07:23 PM ET

Health care spending in the U.S. has surged more than eightfold since the 1960s. Skyrocketing in that same time: Rates of chronic disease, use of synthetic chemicals, and evidence that many of these widely used substances may be wreaking havoc on human health.

"We know that these chemicals are reaching people. We know that chemicals can cause disease," said

huffingtonpost.com/2014/01/22/bpa-health-care-costs_n_4644372.html

 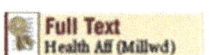

BPA is linked to insulin resistance and other forms of endocrine disruption

- Bisphenol A (BPA), a chemical used in the production of polycarbonate plastics and the linings of aluminum cans,
- BPA exposure was estimated to be associated with 12,404 cases of childhood obesity and 33,863 cases of newly incident coronary heart disease, with estimated social costs of $2.98 billion in 2008. Removing BPA from food uses might prevent 6,236 cases of childhood obesity and 22,350 cases of newly incident coronary heart disease per year, with potential annual economic benefits of $1.74 billion (sensitivity analysis: $889 million-$13.8 billion per year).

Trasande L. *Health Affairs* 2014 Feb

Nutrition & FxMed for chronic immune-inflammatory disorders

Causes of Inflammation-Immune-Metabolic Imbalance:

1. Food, Diet
2. Infection, Dysbiosis
3. Nutritional Immunomodulation
4. Dysfunctional Mitochondria
5. Style of living, Stress, Sociology, Sleep, Sweat, Spinal Health
6. Endocrine, Hormone Imbalances
7. Xenobiotics, Toxins

Xenobiotic/toxin (mercury, lead, chemical persistent organic pollutants [POPs]) cause inflammation:

- **Toxins impair metabolic function**: mercury and lead promote hypertension; mercury promotes drug-resistance by bacteria.
- **Toxins promote insulin resistance**: well-established in diabetes: "…any effort to reduce the external and internal exposure to POPs would be necessary to decrease the social burden of type 2 diabetes. Lee, *Epidemiol Health*. 2012
- **Toxins lower immunity**: Lower IgG
- **Toxins promote autoimmunity**: Higher levels of ANA—antinuclear antibodies. Cooper, *Environ Health Perspect*. 2004 Jul

Toxin awareness / detoxification support are necessary!

Nutrition & FxMed for chronic immune-inflammatory disorders

Causes of Inflammation-Immune-Metabolic Imbalance:

1. Food, Diet
2. Infection, Dysbiosis
3. Nutritional Immunomodulation
4. Dysfunctional Mitochondria
5. Style of living, Stress, Sociology, Sleep, Sweat, Spinal Health
6. Endocrine, Hormone Imbalances
7. Xenobiotics, Toxins

13 pesticides in body of average American:

- "A comprehensive survey of more than 1,300 Americans has found traces of **weed- and bug-killers [herbicides and pesticides] in the bodies of everyone tested**, leading environmentalists in both Canada and the United States to call for far tighter controls on pesticides."
- "The survey, conducted by the U.S. Centers for Disease Control and Prevention, found that **the body of the average American contained 13 of these chemicals.**

The Globe and Mail, Friday May 21, 2004, Page A17
http://www.theglobeandmail.com/life/article927534.ece

Toxin awareness / detoxification support are necessary!

Nutrition & FxMed for chronic immune-inflammatory disorders

Causes of Inflammation-Immune-Metabolic Imbalance:

1. Food, Diet
2. Infection, Dysbiosis
3. Nutritional Immunomodulation
4. Dysfunctional Mitochondria
5. Style of living, Stress, Sociology, Sleep, Sweat, Spinal Health
6. Endocrine, Hormone Imbalances
7. Xenobiotics, Toxins

Everyone in the world has hexachlorobenzene/ perchlorobenzene: fungicide (banned?), industrial pollution continues at 4,000 tons/y in USA.

- **This probably includes you.**
- **"world-wide detectable levels are approaching 100% and average residue levels tend to increase with age.** World-wide HCB levels are higher in females...."

An evaluation of hexachlorobenzene body-burden levels in the general population of the USA. IARC Sci Publ. 1986

Toxin awareness / detoxification support are necessary!

Everyone in the world has hexachlorobenzene/ perchlorobenzene:

Nutrition & FxMed for chronic immune-inflammatory disorders

Causes of Inflammation-Immune-Metabolic Imbalance:
1. Food, Diet
2. Infection, Dysbiosis
3. Nutritional Immunomodulation
4. Dysfunctional Mitochondria
5. Style of living, Stress, Sociology, Sleep, Sweat, Spinal Health
6. Endocrine, Hormone Imbalances
7. **Xenobiotics, Toxins**

- "Persistent environmental pollutant,
- "HCB has **immunotoxic properties** in laboratory animals and probably also in man,
- "**Stimulatory effects** on spleen and lymph node weights and histology,
- "increased serum IgM levels, and an enhancement of several parameters of immune function.
- "Moreover, more recent studies indicate that HCB-induced effects in the rat may be related to **autoimmunity**.
- "In Wistar rats exposed to HCB, IgM **antibodies against several autoantigens were elevated**; in the Lewis rat, HCB differently modulated two experimental models of autoimmune disease.
- "Such a thymus-independent immunopathology is remarkable, as HCB strongly modulates T-cell-mediated immune parameters. This points at a very complex mechanism and possible involvement of multiple factors in the immunopathology of HCB.

Environ Health Perspect. 1999 Oct

Toxin awareness / detoxification support are necessary!

Diabetes mellitus type-2 is linked to accumulation of dioxins/toxins—epidemiology and biologic plausibility:

Nutrition & FxMed for chronic immune-inflammatory disorders

Causes of Inflammation-Immune-Metabolic Imbalance:
1. Food, Diet
2. Infection, Dysbiosis
3. Nutritional Immunomodulation
4. Dysfunctional Mitochondria
5. Style of living, Stress, Sociology, Sleep, Sweat, Spinal Health
6. Endocrine, Hormone Imbalances
7. **Xenobiotics, Toxins**

- "Specifically, we suggest that **aryl hydrocarbon (Ah) receptor functions may antagonize peroxisome proliferator-activated receptor (PPAR) functions**, and hence that the Ah receptor may promote diabetogenesis through a mechanism of PPAR antagonism."

Environ Health Perspect. 2002 Sep;110(9):853-8
http://www.ncbi.nlm.nih.gov/pmc/articles/PMC1240982

Toxin awareness / detoxification support are necessary!

Parkinson's disease strongly linked to persistent organic pollutants (POPs):

> "These findings are not inconsistent [ie, they *are consistent*] with the hypothesis derived from epidemiological work and animal studies that **organochlorine insecticides produce a direct toxic action on the dopaminergic tracts of the substantia nigra** and may contribute to the **development of PD in those rendered susceptible by virtue of cytochrome P-450 polymorphism, excessive exposure**, or other factors."
>
> *J Toxicol Environ Health.* 2000 Feb 25

Toxin awareness / detoxification support are necessary!

*Sidebar:*
Nutrition & FxMed for chronic immune-inflammatory disorders

Causes of Inflammation-Immune-Metabolic Imbalance:
1. Food, Diet
2. Infection, Dysbiosis
3. Nutritional Immunomodulation
4. Dysfunctional Mitochondria
5. Style of living, Stress, Sociology, Sleep, Sweat, Spinal Health
6. Endocrine, Hormone Imbalances
7. Xenobiotics, Toxins

Xenobiotics & toxic metals:

- Toxins lower immunity (lower IgG) and promote autoimmunity via higher levels of ANA—antinuclear antibodies. Cooper, *Environ Health Perspect.* 2004 Jul
- **Mercury**: known to increase ANA production, promote colonization by drug-resistant bacteria, and to increase IgE-mediated allergies.
    - Mercury and acute eczema: "The results of this population-based case-control study in children with **acute eczema** show a strong association between the body burden of mercury and disease state, indicating a possible role for mercury as triggering factor."
    - clear-cut relation between body burdens of mercury and acute but not chronic AE.
    - Children with amalgam fillings = higher urinary mercury,
    - Significantly higher risk for acute eczematous lesions with higher urinary mercury concentrations,
    - **positive and linear association between mercury and serum levels of total IgE.**
    - Perhaps mercury exacerbates allergic disorders by promoting a TH2-cytokine profile and facilitating production of IgE against yet unknown antigens, such as autoantigens.

Weidinger, *J Allergy Clin Immunol,* 2004 Oct

Toxin awareness / detoxification support are necessary!

Nutrition & FxMed for chronic immune-inflammatory disorders

Causes of Inflammation-Immune-Metabolic Imbalance:

1. Food, Diet
2. Infection, Dysbiosis
3. Nutritional Immunomodulation
4. Dysfunctional Mitochondria
5. Style of living, Stress, Sociology, Sleep, Sweat, Spinal Health
6. Endocrine, Hormone Imbalances
7. Xenobiotics, Toxins

Accumulation of "persistent organic pollutants"(POPs) = insulin resistance, MetSyn

- Mechanism: Exposure to and accumulation of toxic chemicals leads to activation of the Aryl hydrocarbon receptor, which causes downregulation (suppressed expression) of GLUT-4 insulin receptors, thus leading to insulin resistance. *J Med Toxicol* 2010; 6:275. *Lancet* 2008 Jan

- Solution: Detoxification programs, or—better yet—*detoxification as a lifestyle.*

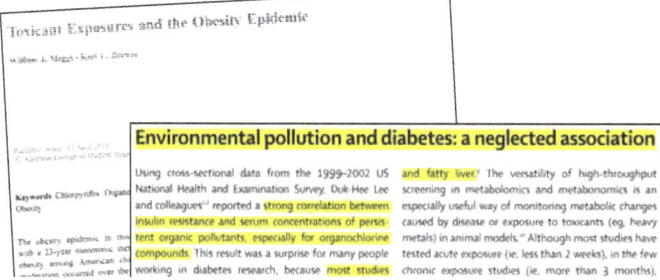

Nutrition & FxMed for chronic immune-inflammatory disorders

Causes of Inflammation-Immune-Metabolic Imbalance:

1. Food, Diet
2. Infection, Dysbiosis
3. Nutritional Immunomodulation
4. Dysfunctional Mitochondria
5. Style of living, Stress, Sociology, Sleep, Sweat, Spinal Health
6. Endocrine, Hormone Imbalances
7. Xenobiotics, Toxins

Common problems in "detoxification"

1. Oxidation: Phase 1
   - Inhibition: too slow
   - Imbalanced: too fast relative to phase 2
2. Conjugation
   - Too slow
   - Unsupported
3. Urinary excretion
   - Hydration
   - Urinary pH
4. Biliary-colonic excretion
   - Insufficient bile flow
   - Enterohepatic recirculation
   - Deconjugation by microflora
   - Constipation
5. Failure to limit/reduce exposure

Vasquez A. *Inflammation Mastery*, chap 4

Deconstructing the phenomena of inflammatory diseases

"IN ORDER FOR A PARTICULAR SPECIES TO MAINTAIN ITSELF AND INCREASE ITS POWER, ITS CONCEPTION OF REALITY MUST COMPREHEND ENOUGH OF THE CALCULABLE AND CONSTANT FOR IT TO BASE A SCHEME OF BEHAVIOR ON IT." FWN. *Will to Power*, 1901, #480

1. D.I.R.T.—Duration of treatment, interactions with drugs/diseases, referral and return visit, treatment plan signed and dated
2. S.O.A.P.—Subjective, objective, assessment, plan
3. F.I.N.D.S.E.X.
    1. Food, Diet
    2. Infection, Dysbiosis
    3. Nutritional Immunomodulation
        1. Mi BEST PLAID FIG
    4. Dysfunctional mitochondria
    5. Style, sleep, sweat, social... surgery
    6. Endocrine
    7. Xenobiotics, Toxins
4. P.A.R.B.Q.—Procedures, alternatives, risks, benefits, questions answered

Clinical protocol—chart note

Patient name: _____

Date of birth: _____

Date of visit: _____

S.

O.

A.

P.

F.I.N.D.S.E.T.D.I.R.T.P.A.R.B.Q.

Doctor: _____

▸ <u>Name the 7 parts of the protocol and implementation of each:</u>

Component	Implementation

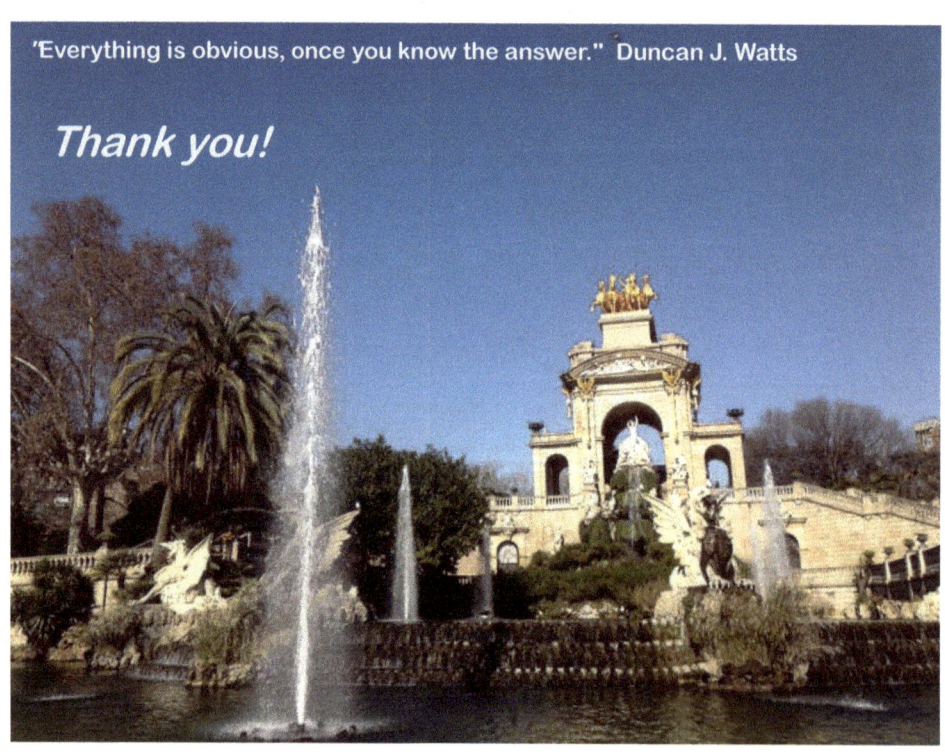

Inflammation Mastery & Functional Inflammology: Volume 1

DrV's "Functional Inflammology Protocol"
❶ Metabolic Inflammation, ❷ Allergic Inflammation, and ❸ Autoimmune Inflammation

Focus on Component #2: Infections and Dysbiosis

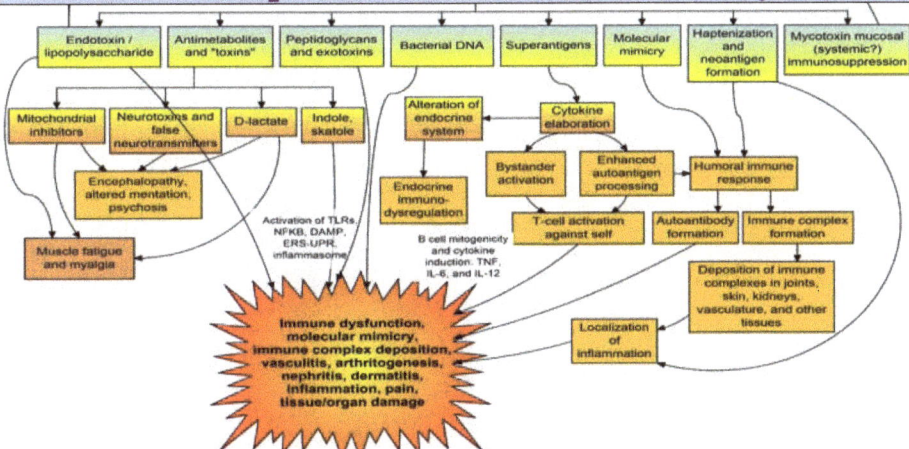

Alex Vasquez, D.C., N.D., D.O., F.A.C.N.

Notices

- <u>Copyright</u>: Except for quotations and images obtained elsewhere, the material and contents of these presentations are copyrighted by Dr Alex Vasquez and have often been excerpted from his books which are also copyrighted. Any unauthorized use of this material—including photocopying or any distribution—is prohibited.
  - No cameras.
  - No recorders.
- Copyright 2012-2014 by Dr Alex Vasquez. All rights reserved and enforced.
- <u>Trademark</u>: The "Functional Immunology/Inflammology Protocol" discussed in this series of videos and notes is Trademarked ® in association with Dr Vasquez's book *Functional Immunology and Nutritional Immunomodulation* and other books and videos.

Trademark

View the recorded version of this presentation

- **Link**: vimeo.com/drvasquez/dysbiosis2014review
- **Password**: DysbiosisMasteryAV
- **Location**: Ponferrada, Espana

Dysregulated Inflammation and Immune Activation *as the Cause of* Inflammation, Allergy, and Autoimmunity:
Nutritional & Functional Medicine Approaches

DrV's Functional Immunology Protocol:
Part 2: Dysbiosis and Chronic Infections as Triggers for Inflammation and Autoimmune Disease: An Introduction to Basic and a Few Advanced Concepts—Molecular Mechanisms of Disease

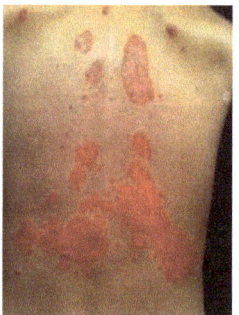

Alex Vasquez, D.C., N.D., D.O.

Inflammation Mastery & Functional Inflammology: Volume 1
Dysbiosis Review Presentation Slides • Page 2

Clinical protocol

- **S**ubjective—patient's concerns and complaints
- **O**bjective—clinical findings
- **A**ssessment—diagnoses
- **P**lan—treatments, tests, referral, follow-up
    1. **F**ood and lifestyle
    2. **I**nfection and dysbiosis
    3. **N**utritional immunomodulation
    4. **D**ysfunctional mitochondria
    5. **S**tress, Sociology-psychology, Lifestyle
    6. **E**ndocrine/hormones
    7. **X**enobiotics/**T**oxins

Copyrights © and Trademarks ®: Except for quotations and images obtained elsewhere, the material and contents of these presentations are copyrighted by Dr Alex Vasquez and have often been excerpted from his books which are also copyrighted. Any unauthorized use of this material—including photocopying or any distribution—is prohibited. The FIND SEX/T acronym is protected by trademark ™ in association with the copyrighted book *Functional Immunology and Nutritional Immunomodulation*.

Prior publications on this topic—Dr Vasquez

- Vasquez A. Reducing pain and inflammation naturally - Part 6: Nutritional and Botanical Treatments Against "Silent Infections" and Gastrointestinal Dysbiosis, Commonly Overlooked Causes of Chronic Health Problems. Nutritional Perspective

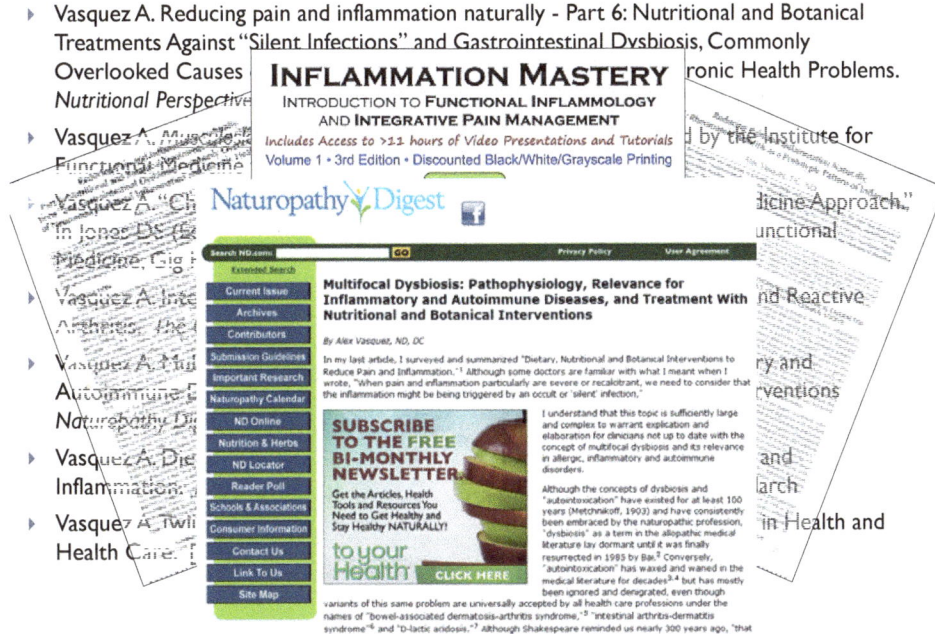

Dysbiosis: Topic Outline

1. **Introduction and definitions**: Terminology, perspectives, locations
2. **Molecular mechanisms**: 18...*and counting toward more...*
3. **Locations**: Introduction to the 7 main loci
4. **Microbes**: Introduction to some of the most common microbes seen in clinical practice and represented in the literature
5. **Additional detail for gastrointestinal dysbiosis**: GI dysbiosis deserves additional attention due to its pathophysiologic quantitative and qualitative preeminence in addition to its greater representation in the research literature
6. **Case reports and clinical examples**: Mostly related to GI dysbiosis
7. **Antidysbiotic Interventions**: Simple as ❶ ❷ ❸

Dysbiosis in Biomedical Literature

THE PROLONGATION OF LIFE

OPTIMISTIC STUDIES

BY

ÉLIE METCHNIKOFF
SUB-DIRECTOR OF THE PASTEUR INSTITUTE, PARIS

THE ENGLISH TRANSLATION
EDITED BY
P. CHALMERS MITCHELL
M.A., D.SC. OXON., HON. LL.D., F.R.S.
Secretary of the Zoological Society of London; Corresponding Member of the Academy of Natural Sciences of Philadelphia

G. P. PUTNAM'S SONS
NEW YORK & LONDON
The Knickerbocker Press
1908

- Concept consolidated by Metchnikoff in 1908
- 180 Medline articles indexed by "dysbiosis" as of August 2010. **471 Medline articles indexed by "dysbiosis" as of April 2013.**
- Other related terms:
  - Dysbacterosis
  - Autointoxication
  - Dermatitis-arthritis syndrome
  - Short bowel syndrome
  - **Bacterial overgrowth of the small bowel, small intestine bacterial overgrowth (SIBO)**
  - Mucosal colonization
  - **Subclinical infection**
- Clinical associations:
  - Autoimmunity of nearly all types
  - "chronic unwellness" → CFIDS FMS, IBS, ...allergy
  - "medically unexplained" and "idiopathic" disorders and syndromes
  - Hypertension, diabetes mellitus

What is Dysbiosis?

- **DrV: "A _relationship_ of non-acute non-infectious host-microorganism interaction that adversely affects the human host"**
- Generally does NOT have signs of infection
  - No fever
  - No redness
  - No swelling, induration, or (acute) lymphadenopathy
- The _location_ of active dysbiosis often has no symptoms/manifestations or such findings are "nonspecific." For example, **many patients with GI dysbiosis have no major clinical GI manifestations**, just as patients with sinorespiratory or genitourinary dysbiosis do not present with manifestations of URI or UTI, respectively.

Patients Have Unique Inflammatory and Metabolic Responses to Dysbiotic Organisms

- **Remember, we are not looking for classic "infection" here; we are looking to determine which <u>underlying disruptions</u> may be exacerbating inflammation and the patient's symptomatology.**

- We have to look beyond the _disease-associated characteristics of the microbe_ to see the **_patient's individualized response_** to the microbe.
  - Dysbiosis in one patient may present with dermatitis, while [what appears to be] the same microbial imbalance in another patient can present as peripheral neuropathy or inflammatory arthritis.

- <u>Often what we find when working with autoimmune/inflammatory patients is that they are having a _pathogenic inflammatory response_ to a _nonpathogenic microbe_.</u>

Clinical example of "*pathogenic inflammatory response* to a *nonpathogenic* microbe"

relate a history of recent infection. In fact, the old aphorism, "psoriasis is a disease of healthy people," seems to be accurate. Our experience has led us to conclude that otherwise apparently healthy psoriasis patients are often found to be harboring pathogenic microorganisms and that their psoriasis improves when they are treated with antibiotics.

Our present view is to consider "colonization" or "carriage" of pathogenic microorganisms the essential feature of active psoriasis. Remove these pathogens, and the psoriasis patient retains an inherited tendency to react, but exhibits no clinical evidence of either skin or joint disease.

Rosengerg, Noah, Skinner. *J Natl Med Assoc* 1994 Apr

Dysbiosis → "*multi*focal *poly*dysbiosis"

Location Subtypes:
1. **Gastrointestinal**
2. **Orodental**
3. **Sinorespiratory**
4. **Parenchymal**
5. **Genitourinary**
6. **Cutaneous**
7. **Environmental**

Problematic GI Microbes Include:
Aeromonas hydrophila, Blastocystis hominis, Candida albicans and other yeasts, *Citrobacter rodentium, Citrobacter freundii, Dientamoeba fragilis, Endolimax nana, Entamoeba histolytica,* Gamma strep, *Enterococcus, Giardia lamblia, Hafnia alvei, Helicobacter pylori, Klebsiella pneumoniae, Proteus mirabilis, Pseudomonas aeruginosa, Staphylococcus aureus, Staphylococcus epidermidis, Streptococcus pyogenes,* Group A streptococci

Molecular Mechanisms
1. **Molecular mimicry**
2. Superantigens
3. Enhanced processing of autoantigens
4. **Bystander activation**
5. Peptidoglycans and exotoxins
6. Endotoxins (LPS)
7. Immunostimulation by bacterial DNA
8. Activation of Toll-like receptors and NF-kB
9. **Immune complex formation and deposition**
10. Haptenization and Neoantigen formation
11. Damage to the intestinal mucosa
12. Inhibition/alteration of detoxification
13. Antimetabolites
14. Autointoxication, hepatic encephalopathy, intestinal arthritis-dermatitis syndrome
15. Impairment of mucosal and systemic defenses
16. Impairment of mucosal digestion by microbial proteases and inflammation
17. Inflammation-induced endocrine dysfunction
18. **Central sensitization**

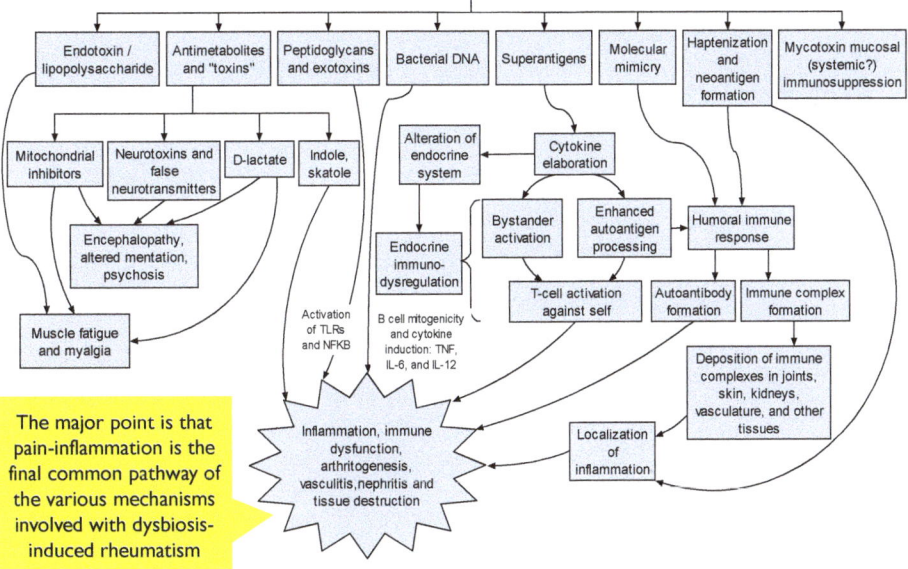

What is Dysbiosis?

- **DrV: "A relationship of non-acute non-infectious host-microorganism interaction that adversely affects the human host"**
- **Generally does NOT have signs of infection:**
  - No fever
  - No redness
  - No swelling, induration, or (acute) lymphadenopathy
- **The *location* of active dysbiosis often has no symptoms/manifestations or such findings are "nonspecific."** For example, many patients with GI dysbiosis have no major clinical GI manifestations, just as patients with sinorespiratory or genitourinary dysbiosis do not present with manifestations of URI or UTI, respectively.

"Dysbiosis" is not so much about the microbe as it is about the effect of that microbe on a susceptible host; i.e., it is about "the *relationship* between host and microbe"

- Understanding **dysbiosis** from this "**relationship model**" rather than from the perspective of earlier models of Microbiology or Pathology (ie, Robbins Pathologic Basis of Disease) should help clinicians **appreciate the requisite role of the patient's "host defense" and "inflammatory balance" and "immune balance"** and therefore why the **effective treatment of dysbiotic pain/inflammation must include treatments that optimize/ normalize/ restore internal homeostatic mechanisms** within the patient in order for treatment to be effective and durable.

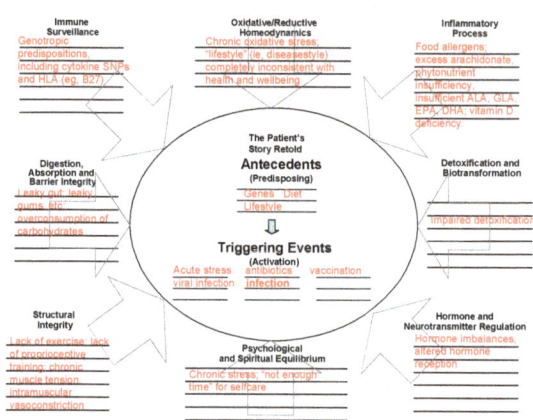

Vasquez A. Musculoskeletal Pain: Expanded Clinical Strategies. Institute for Functional Medicine, 2008

Patients have unique **inflammatory** and **metabolic** responses to dysbiotic organisms

- **Remember, we are not looking for classic "infection" here; we are looking to determine which underlying disruptions may be exacerbating inflammation and the patient's symptomatology.**
- We have to look beyond the *disease-associated characteristics of the microbe* to see the *patient's individualized response* to the microbe.
    - Dysbiosis in one patient may present with dermatitis, while [what appears to be] the same microbial imbalance in another patient can present as peripheral neuropathy or inflammatory arthritis.
- **Often what we find when working with autoimmune/inflammatory patients is that they are having a *pathogenic inflammatory response* to a *nonpathogenic microbe*.**

Often what we find when working with autoimmune/inflammatory patients is that they are having a *pathogenic inflammatory response* to a *nonpathogenic* microbe:
- Wegener's granulomatosis
- Rheumatoid arthritis
- Ankylosing spondylitis
- Dermatomyositis/PM
- Sjogren's syndrome
- Psoriasis
- SLE

You know this is true: Just consider reactive arthritis and short-bowel syndromes as the prototypes.

Dysbiosis: Topic Outline

1. <u>Introduction and definitions</u>: Terminology, perspectives, locations
2. **Molecular mechanisms**: 18...*and counting toward more...*
3. **Locations**: Introduction to the 7 main loci
4. **Microbes**: Introduction to some of the most common microbes seen in clinical practice and represented in the literature
5. **Additional detail for gastrointestinal dysbiosis**: GI dysbiosis deserves additional attention due to its pathophysiologic quantitative and qualitative preeminence in addition to its greater representation in the research literature
6. **Case reports and clinical examples**: Mostly related to GI dysbiosis
7. **Antidysbiotic interventions**: Simple as ❶ ❷ ❸

Dysbiosis: molecular mechanisms and clinical evidence related to pain and inflammation

1. **Molecular mimicry**
2. Superantigens
3. Enhanced processing of autoantigens
4. **Bystander activation**
5. Peptidoglycans and exotoxins from gram-positive bacteria
6. Endotoxins (lipopolysaccharide) from gram-negative bacteria
7. Immunostimulation by bacterial DNA
8. Activation of Toll-like receptors and NF-kappaB
9. **Immune complex formation and deposition**
10. Haptenization and Neoantigen formation
11. Damage to the intestinal mucosa
12. Inhibition/alteration of detoxification
13. **Antimetabolites**
14. Autointoxication, hepatic encephalopathy, intestinal arthritis-dermatitis syndrome
15. Impairment of mucosal and systemic defenses
16. Impairment of mucosal digestion by microbial proteases and inflammation
17. Inflammation-induced endocrine dysfunction
18. **Dysbiosis-induced central sensitization**

> The many variables of dysbiosis-induced disease include the quantity (total microbial load), quality (identity, phenotypic behavior) and variety (various combinations of different microbes) and host factors such as nutritional status, xenobiotic load (quality, quantity, variety), and genetic factors.
>
> These variables combine to create various **patterns of inflammation** that doctors cluster together in named diagnoses which are semispecific (eg, rheumatoid arthritis) or nonspecific (eg, mixed connective tissue disease, seronegative undifferentiated oligoarthritis).

Mechanism #1: Molecular mimicry

Molecular mimicry: Several microbes have peptides and other structures that resemble or "mimic" the peptides and cell structures found in human tissues.

- Thus, when the immune system fights against the microbe, the antibodies and T-cells can "**cross-react**" with the tissues of the human host.
- In this way, the immune system begins attacking the human body, which is otherwise an innocent bystander—the victim of "friendly fire."
- As reviewed by Ringrose, evidence clearly indicates that specific microbial proteins have **amino acid homology** with human proteins and/or that homologous bacterial peptides appear to stimulate (auto)immunity toward similar human peptides.

Wucherpfennig. Mechanisms for the induction of autoimmunity by infectious agents. *J Clin Invest.* 2001 Oct   Ringrose. HLA-B27 associated spondyloarthropathy, an autoimmune disease based on cross-reactivity between bacteria and HLA-B27? *Ann Rheum Dis.* 1999 Oct

Mechanism #4: Bystander activation

Bystander activation: Autoreactive immunocytes that have bypassed thymic deletion are generally kept anergic when the general biochemical milieu of the body is noninflammatory; autoreactive immunocytes can be aroused from quiescence by inflammatory cytokines, molecular signals, microbial debris, and heavy metals.

- Normally, these autoreactive cells are kept anergic, dormant, quiescent, and otherwise inactive through various mechanisms that regulate the immune system; in this way, such autoreactive cells can be considered "bystanders" because they are not really doing anything and are basically "standing by."
- Bystander activation occurs when these cells are awakened by the cascade of inflammatory processes that occur as a result of superantigen exposure, molecular mimicry, immune complex deposition, or xenobiotic immunotoxicity.
- Bystander activation appears to contribute to the development of certain autoimmune conditions, such as drug-induced lupus [1], and it may be a contributing pathogenic mechanism in metal-induced autoimmunity.[2]

[1] Rubin. Drug-induced lupus. *Toxicology*. 2005 Apr. [2] "It is therefore theoretically possible that compounds present in vaccines such as thiomersal or aluminium hydroxyde can trigger autoimmune reactions through bystander effects." Fournie et al. *J Autoimmun*. 2001 May

Mechanism #9: Immune complexes

Immune complex deposition directly contributes to the renal disease, vasculitis, and arthritis common to the pathophysiology of many autoimmune diseases.

- Patients with autoimmune disease commonly have circulating IgM and IgA antibodies against bacteria from the gastrointestinal, genitourinary, oropharyngeal tracts clearly indicating an active immune response against these bacteria and suggesting breaches in mucosal integrity.

Newkirk et al. *Rheumatology* 2005 Nov.   Theofilopoulos, Dixon. *Am J Pathol*. 1980 Aug

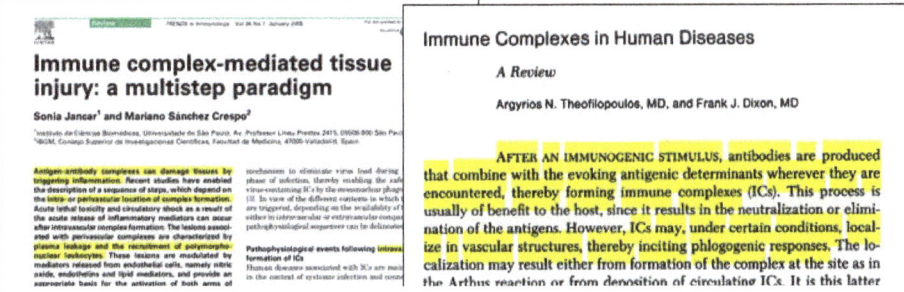

Mechanism #13: Antimetabolites

Antimetabolites: Microbes produce substances that interfere with human cellular physiology with noteworthy inflammatory and mitochondrial consequences.

- Antimetabolites produced from (intestinal) microbes which are associated with human disease and dysfunction include **ammonia, tryptamine, tyramine, octopamine, mercaptates, aldehydes, alcohol, tartaric acid, indolepropionic acid, indoleacetic acid, skatole, indole, putrescine, and cadaverine**. Several of these metabolites—known to impair cellular/mitochondrial function [relevance: fibromyalgia] — are measured in higher amounts in patients with migraine, depression, weakness, confusion, schizophrenia, agitation, hepatic encephalopathy, chronic arthritis and rheumatoid arthritis.

- Degradation of tryptophan by **bacterial tryptophanase** predisposes to "**tryptophan deficiency**" and may result in insufficiency of serotonin which would contribute to **hyperalgesia, depression, impaired adrenal responsiveness** ("hypoadrenalism"), and insomnia; **indole** and **skatole**, which are gut-derived bacterial degradation products of tryptophan, produce an **inflammatory arthritis** that is identical to rheumatoid arthritis in animal models.

Nakoneczna et al. The arthritogenic effect of indole, skatole and other tryptophan metabolites in rabbits. *Am J Pathol.* 1969 Dec. Rogers et al. Arthritogenic properties of lipophilic, aryl molecules. *Proc Soc Exp Biol Med.* 1969 Jun

Mechanism #13: Antimetabolites

Increased D-lactic acid intestinal bacteria in patients with chronic fatigue syndrome. Sheedy et al. *In Vivo.* 2009 Jul-Aug

- "A **significant increase of Gram positive facultative anaerobic faecal microorganisms** in 108 CFS patients as compared to 177 control subjects (p<0.01) is presented in this report.
- ....Further, both E. faecalis and S. sanguinis **secrete more D-lactic acid** than E. coli. ...
- Given the fact that this might explain not only neurocognitive dysfunction in CFS patients but also mitochondrial dysfunction, these findings may have important clinical implications."

Musculoskeletal Pain. Vasquez. 2008 ☺

1. **Bacterial endotoxin/LPS**: causes inflammation, mitochondrial/muscle impairment, increased sensitization to pain.
2. **Bacteria-produced D-lactic acid**: neurotoxin and metabolic poison; causes fatigue, muscle pain, dyscognition.
3. **Bacteria-produced hydrogen sulfide (H2S)**: neurotoxin and metabolic poison; causes fatigue, muscle pain, dyscognition.
4. **Bacteria-produced tryptophanase**: leads to tryptophan deficiency (documented in FM patients) and "serotonin deficiency" (pain, fatigue, carbohydrate cravings, depression) and "melatonin deficiency" (sleep disturbance, mitochondrial impairment, oxidative stress, muscle fatigue).

Mech #18: Central pain sensitization

Commensal microbiota is fundamental for the development of inflammatory pain.

- "...inflammatory hypernociception induced by carrageenan, lipopolysaccharide, TNF-alpha, IL-1beta, and the chemokine CXCL1 was reduced in germ-free mice. Reduction of hypernociception induced by carrageenan was associated with reduced tissue inflammation and could be reversed by reposition of the **microbiota or systemic administration of lipopolysaccharide**.
- Significantly, decreased hypernociception in germ-free mice was accompanied by enhanced IL-10 expression upon stimulation and could be reversed by treatment with an anti-IL-10 antibody.

▶ Therefore, **these results show that contact with commensal microbiota is necessary for mice to develop inflammatory hypernociception.**"

Amaral et al. *Proc Natl Acad Sci.* 2008 Feb

Acute experimental endotoxemia induces visceral hypersensitivity and altered pain evaluation in healthy humans.

- "Growing evidence suggests that systemic immune activation plays a role in the pathophysiology of pain in functional bowel disorders.
- 11 healthy men, mean age 26.6 years received an intravenous injection of either lipopolysaccharide (LPS; 0.4 ng/kg) or saline on 2 otherwise identical study days.
- This report is novel in that it demonstrates that a **transient systemic immune activation results in decreased visceral sensory and pain thresholds and altered subjective pain ratings**. Our results support the relevance of **inflammatory processes in the pathophysiology of visceral hyperalgesia** and underscore the need for studies to further elucidate immune-to-brain communication pathways in gastrointestinal disorders."

Benson et al. *Pain.* 2012 Apr

Dysbiosis: molecular mechanisms and clinical evidence related to pain and inflammation

1. **Molecular mimicry**
2. Superantigens
3. Enhanced processing of autoantigens
4. **Bystander activation**
5. Peptidoglycans and exotoxins from gram-positive bacteria
6. Endotoxins (lipopolysaccharide) from gram-negative bacteria
7. Immunostimulation by bacterial DNA
8. Activation of Toll-like receptors and NF-kappaB
9. **Immune complex formation and deposition**
10. Haptenization and Neoantigen formation
11. Damage to the intestinal mucosa
12. Inhibition/alteration of detoxification
13. **Antimetabolites**
14. Autointoxication, hepatic encephalopathy, intestinal arthritis-dermatitis syndrome
15. Impairment of mucosal and systemic defenses
16. Impairment of mucosal digestion by microbial proteases and inflammation
17. Inflammation-induced endocrine dysfunction
18. **Dysbiosis-induced central sensitization**

The many variables of dysbiosis-induced disease include the quantity (total microbial load), quality (identity, phenotypic behavior) and variety (various combinations of different microbes) and host factors such as nutritional status, xenobiotic load (quality, quantity, variety), and genetic factors.

These variables combine to create various patterns of inflammation that doctors cluster together in named diagnoses which are semispecific (eg, rheumatoid arthritis) or nonspecific (eg, mixed connective tissue disease, seronegative undifferentiated oligoarthritis).

Combinatorial Inflammology

Major variables in the equation

* Genes—cyokine SNP
* Genes—HLA-B27 + molecular mimicry
* Diet ≅ processed food + AGE intake
* Hyperglycemia
* TML—total microbial load
* TXL—total xenobiotic load
* Vitamin D status (AMP, Treg, mucosal permeability)
* Mitochondrial function
* Adiposity/adipokines/estrogen
* Hormonal balance
* Phenotypic immune balance
* Stress, sleep, and psychosocial health
* Structural/spinal integrity

Microbe-Host Interaction determines the "**pattern of inflammation**"

Microbial variables

1. Quantity of total
2. Quantity of individual
3. Diversity of total
4. Phenotypic pathogencity and activity (varies per strain and host stress, nutrition)
5. Molecular mimicry (degree of match to human host)
6. Superantigens
7. Enhanced processing of autoantigens (possibly exacerbated by heavy metals and food antigens)
8. Bystander activation
9. Peptidoglycans and exotoxins
10. Endotoxins (LPS)
11. Immunostimulation by bacterial DNA (ability of human host to clear bacterial DNA)
12. Activation of Toll-like receptors and NF-kappaB (potently influenced by human host's nutritional status)
13. Immune complex formation and deposition (excretion efficiency varies per host)
14. Haptenization and Neoantigen formation
15. Damage to the intestinal mucosa
16. Inhibition/alteration of detoxification (varies per host, influenced strongly by drugs)
17. Antimetabolites such as H2S and D-lactate
18. Impairment of mucosal and systemic defenses
19. Impairment of mucosal digestion by microbial proteases and inflammation
20. Inflammation-induced endocrine dysfunction (also consider microbial endocrinology)

Microbe-Host Interaction determines the **"pattern of inflammation"**

Host variables

1. Host stress: mucosal permeability, hormones/neurotransmitters (inflammation, microbial endocrinology)
2. Host nutrition: immune function, inflammatory balance,
3. Molecular mimicry (degree of match to human host)
4. Enhanced processing of autoantigens (possibly exacerbated by heavy metals and food antigens)
5. Bystander activation: genetic predisposition
6. Immunostimulation by bacterial DNA (ability of human host to clear bacterial DNA)
7. Activation of Toll-like receptors and NF-kappaB (potently influenced by human host's nutritional status)
8. Immune complex formation and deposition (excretion efficiency varies per host)
9. Damage to the intestinal mucosa: other variables include nutritional status, alcohol, other microbes, genetic predisposition, drugs such as NSAIDs
10. Inhibition/alteration of detoxification (varies per host, influenced strongly by drugs)
11. Impairment of mucosal and systemic defenses: genes, nutrients,
12. Impairment of mucosal digestion by microbial proteases and inflammation: dietary selection,

Combinatorial Inflammology

* **Com•bi•na•to•ri•al**: *adjective*. 1. of, pertaining to, or involving the **combination of elements**, as in phonetics or music. 2. of or pertaining to the enumeration of the number of ways of doing some specific task or of arranging items in a specific configuration. 3. *Mathematics*. of or pertaining to **combination, or the modes, properties, etc., of combinations**.

* **In•flam•mol•o•gy**: *noun*. 1. the study of the causes of and various contributors to the (patho)physiologic processes, molecular mechanisms, and clinical and societal consequences of inflammation and inflammatory diseases

Combinatorial Inflammology

Pattern of Inflammation

<u>Clinician's lens</u>: diagnostic paradigm and technology

<u>Clinical presentations</u>: Autointoxication, hepatic encephalopathy, intestinal arthritis-dermatitis syndrome, fibromyalgia, autoimmune diagnosis RA, SLE, GCA

Dysbiosis: Topic Outline

1. **Introduction and definitions**: Terminology, perspectives, locations
2. **Molecular mechanisms**: 18…and counting toward more…
3. **Locations**: Introduction to the 7 main loci
4. **Microbes**: Introduction to some of the most common microbes seen in clinical practice and represented in the literature
5. **Additional detail for gastrointestinal dysbiosis**: GI dysbiosis deserves additional attention due to its pathophysiologic quantitative and qualitative preeminence in addition to its greater representation in the research literature
6. **Case reports and clinical examples**: Mostly related to GI dysbiosis
7. **Antidysbiotic Interventions**: Simple as ❶ ❷ ❸

Dysbiosis: Gastrointestinal...*and elsewhere*

Dysbiosis subtypes (based on location): **"Multifocal dysbiosis"**

1. **Gastrointestinal:** Very common and the most appreciated among clinicians, but not the most clinically relevant for all conditions
2. **Orodental:** A contributor to the inflammatory pathogenesis of rheumatoid arthritis, psoriasis, and cardiovascular disease
3. **Sinorespiratory:** Nasal overgrowth of *Staphylococcus aureus* may be particularly relevant in SLE, psoriasis, and Wegener's granulomatosis
4. **Tissue/ Parenchymal:** Occult bone/mandibular infections, and occult viral hepatitis (more of a true "subclinical infection" than "dysbiosis" *per se*) are relevant for some cases of chronic fatigue and arthritis
5. **Genitourinary:** Particularly relevant for rheumatoid arthritis and "oligoarthritis" and "reactive arthritis" (formerly Reiter's syndrome)
6. **Cutaneous:** Colonization of Behchet's lesions increases the risk for inflammatory arthritis
7. **Environmental:** Exposure to airborne microbial toxins and debris can precipitate systemic inflammation resulting in diagnosis of rheumatic disease such as rheumatoid arthritis or ankylosing spondylitis; the disease remits when the patient is removed from the contaminated environment
8. **(Endo)Microbial:** Microbes (amoebas) can harbor dysbiotic microbes (*Chl.pn*)

Dysbiosis: Gastrointestinal...*and elsewhere*

Clinical assessments:

- ☺ Swab & culture / DNA probe / PCR
- ☺ **Antigen tests** (e.g., stool *H pylori* antigen)
- ☹ **Breath hydrogen/methane** for SIBO
- ☹ Jejunal aspiration
- ☺ **Stool tests must be performed by a specialty lab** familiar with dysbiosis and should be interpreted in context of markers such as sIgA
- ☺ Response to building renovation or water/mold remediation for cases of "environmental dysbiosis"; mold plates
- ☺ **Response to treatment:** subjective (e.g., VAS) and objective markers (e.g., ESR, CRP, disease activity indexes)

Noah. *Semin Dermatol.* 1990 Dec
Vasquez A. *Integrative Rheumatology*.

Dysbiosis: Gastrointestinal...*and elsewhere*

Dysbiosis subtypes (based on location): "Multifocal dysbiosis"

1. **Gastrointestinal**: Very common and the most appreciated among clinicians, but not the most clinically relevant for all conditio...
2. **Orodental**: A contributor to the inflammato... arthritis, psoriasis, and cardiovascular disease
3. **Sinorespiratory**: Nasal overgrowth of *Staph*... relevant in SLE, psoriasis, and Wegener's granu...
4. **Tissue/Parenchymal**: Occult bone/mandibu... hepatitis (more of a true "subclinical infection"... relevant for some cases of chronic fatigu...
5. **Genitourinary**: Particularly relevant... "oligoarthritis" and "reactive arthritis" (for...
6. **Cutaneous**: Colonization of Behchet's lesion... inflammatory arthritis
7. **Environmental**: Exposure to airborne microbial toxins and debris can precipitate systemic inflammation resulting in diagnosis of rheumatic disease such as rheumatoid arthritis or ankylosing spondylitis; the disease remits when the patient is removed from the contaminated environment
8. **(Endo)Microbial**: Microbes (amoebas) can harbor dysbiotic microbes (*Chl.pn*)

1. "Patients are entitled to more than one dysbiotic microbe....
2. ...in more than one location...
3. ...and rapidly the combinations of "patterns of inflammation" increase exponentially—
4. However, they do so within a limited capacity for physiologic expression and
5. clinician's recognition."

Dysbiosis: 1. Orodental

Control of Periodontal Infection Reduces the Severity of Active Rheumatoid Arthritis

Mhd. Khaldoun Al-Katma, DDS, MSD; Nabil F. Bissada, DDS, MSD; Judith M. Bordeaux, DDS, MSD; J. Sue, MD; and Ali D. Askari, MD

"Elimination of bacterial plaque and endotoxins by periodontal therapy may contribute to improvement in the RA by reduced exposure of the joint structures to bacteria and their products."

Culture of mouth, throat, dentures for yeast and bacteria can be performed.

Antibody titers and endotoxin levels correlate with severity of oral microbial overgrowth and gum/gingival permeability.

Li et al. Systemic diseases caused by oral infection. *Clin Microbiol Rev.* 2000 Oct

Amar and Han. The impact of periodontal infection on systemic diseases. *Med Sci Monit.* 2003 Dec

Noah. The role of microorganisms in psoriasis. *Semin Dermatol.* 1990 Dec

Dysbiosis: 1. Orodental

- **Problem**: "CONCLUSIONS: **Gentle mastication is able to induce the release of bacterial endotoxins from oral origin into the bloodstream, especially when patients have severe periodontal disease.** This finding suggests that a diseased periodontium can be a major and underestimated source of chronic, or even permanent, release of bacterial pro-inflammatory components into the bloodstream." Geerts et al. Systemic release of endotoxins induced by gentle mastication: association with periodontitis severity. *J Periodontol*. 2002 Jan

- **Solutions**: Avoid sugar(s), rinse, drink water, drink green tea, ensure abundant intake of vitamins (especially A, D, folate, CoQ-10), …use antiseptic mouthwash, …use plaque-disolving mouthwash, … floss (!), then use antiseptic mouthwash again, preferably with sonic toothbrush… consider antibiotic (amoxicillin prophylaxis 1-2g 1h prior to home dental cleaning for more moderate-severe cases or in patients with immunosuppression, cardiac valve defects, or inflammatory disease. Obviously, refer for dental care and cleaning.

Dysbiosis: 2. Sinorespiratory

Patients with **Wegener's granulomatosis** have a high incidence of sinus colonization with *Staphylococcus aureus*.

- In these patients, *Staphylococcus aureus* produces a superantigen as well as an antigenic acid phosphatase which haptenizes endothelial cells via an electrostatic charge to induce autoimmune vasculitis, nephritis, the production of antineutrophil anticytoplasmic antibody (ANCA), and the formation of immune complexes.

- **Antimicrobial treatment to eradicate *Staphylococcus aureus* frequently results in clinical remission of the "autoimmune" disease, thus proving the microbe-autoimmune link.**

- Increased nasal colonization with *Staphylococcus aureus* has also been documented in other inflammatory/autoimmune diseases, including systemic lupus erythematosus and psoriasis.

Popa et al. *Arthritis Res*. 2002;4(2):77-9

Dysbiosis: 3. Gastrointestinal

Many clinicians find comprehensive stool analysis and comprehensive parasitology to be among the most valuable laboratory assessments they utilize, second only to basic lab tests such as CBC, CRP, UA, and chemistry/metabolic panels.

Problematic microbes include:
- *Aeromonas hydrophila*
- *Blastocystis hominis*
- *Candida albicans* and other yeasts
- *Citrobacter rodentium, Citrobacter freundii*
- *Dientamoeba fragilis*
- *Endolimax nana*
- *Entamoeba histolytica*
- Gamma strep, *Enterococcus*
- *Giardia lamblia*
- *Hafnia alvei*
- *Helicobacter pylori*
- *Klebsiella pneumoniae*
- *Proteus mirabilis*
- *Pseudomonas aeruginosa*
- *Staphylococcus aureus*
- *Staphylococcus epidermidis*
- Group A streptococci, *Streptococcus pyogenes*—especially intracellular

We will review more details about gastrointestinal dysbiosis after introducing the other locations

Vasquez A. *Integrative Rheumatology*.

Vasquez A. *Functional Perspectives* 2006; Jan
OptimalHealthResearch.com/part6.html

Dysbiosis: 4. Parenchymal/Tissue

1. **Viral hepatitis may present with polyarthropathy** while the hepatitis is asymptomatic and serum levels of liver enzymes are within normal limits; in these cases, the underlying dysbiosis/infection is identified with the use of specific serologic testing.

2. **Polyarteritis nodosa is an autoimmune/inflammatory vasculitic syndrome strongly associated with hepatitis B infection**, and 90% of patients with the immune complex vasculitis *cryoglobulinemia* have hepatitis C.

3. A young girl was tentatively diagnosed with **juvenile rheumatoid arthritis before being more accurately diagnosed with "recurrent multifocal osteomyelitis."**

[1] "HCV arthritis should be considered in the differential diagnosis of seronegative arthritis of undetermined etiology even in the setting of normal liver chemistries." Akhtar AJ, Funnye AS. Hepatitis C virus associated arthritis in absence of clinical, biochemical and histological evidence of liver disease--responding to interferon therapy. *Med Sci Monit*. 2005 Jul

[2] Tierney (eds). *Current Medical Diagnosis and Treatment*. 45thEd. Lange : 2006, pp844-850

[3] Robertson, Hickling. *Ann Rheum Dis*. 2001 Sep

Nutrition & FxMed for chronic immune-inflammatory disorders

Causes of Inflammation-Immune-Metabolic Imbalance:

1. Food, Diet
2. Infection, Dysbiosis
3. Nutritional Immunomodulation
4. Dysfunctional Mitochondria
5. Style of living, Stress, Sociology, Sleep, Sweat, Spinal Health
6. Endocrine, Hormone Imbalances
7. Xenobiotics, Toxins

"...Tissue bacteria are involved in the onset of diabetes in humans."

- "...bacterial components in blood predicts the onset of diabetes mellitus in a large general population." Koch *Nature Reviews Endocrinology* 2012 Jan
- Blood levels of the bacterial marker (16S ribosomal DNA) predict the onset of diabetes and abdominal adiposity in a large general population (n= 3,280) followed for 9 years. The adjusted OR (95% CIs) for incident diabetes and for abdominal adiposity were 1.35 and 1.18, respectively. 16S rDNA was shown to be an independent marker of the risk of diabetes. These findings are evidence for the concept that tissue bacteria are involved in the onset of diabetes in humans. Amar. *Diabetologia*. 2011 Dec

16S ribosomal RNA (16S rRNA) is a component of the 30S small subunit of prokaryotic ribosomes; genes coding for it are 16S rDNA.

Dysbiosis: 4. Parenchymal/Tissue

Date and Time Collected	Date Entered	Date and Time Reported	Physician Name	NPI	Physician ID
08/29/11 09:41	08/29/11	09/03/11 01:35ET	VASQUEZ, A		

Tests Ordered: FSH+TestT+LH+DHEA S+Prog+E2...; CBC With Differential/Platelet; Comp. Metabolic Panel (14); Chlamydia pneumoniae(IgG/M); Thyroxine (T4) Free, Direct, S; TSH; Prolactin; IGF-1; C-Reactive Protein, Cardiac; Homocyst(e)ine, Plasma; Triiodothyronine (T3); Reverse T3; Magnesium, RBC; Cortisol - AM; Venipuncture

```
Chlamydia pneumoniae(IgG/M)
   Chlamydia pneumoniae IgG      >1:256    High        Neg:<1:16
   Chlamydia pneumoniae IgM      <1:10                 Neg:<1:10
   Test Information:
```

- "*Chlamydia trachomatis* and *Chlamydophila* (*Chlamydia*) *pneumoniae* are known triggers of reactive arthritis (ReA) and exist in a persistent metabolically active infection state in the synovium..." *Arthritis Rheum* 2010 May
- "These studies confirm our previous reports concerning the high prevalence of C. pneumoniae in the CSF of MS patients." *Clin Diagn Lab Immunol*. 2002 Nov
- "Because there is as yet no standardisation of serological criteria for persistent infection, we considered antibody titers of > 1/20 in the IgA fraction, together with IgG titers of 1/64 to 1/256, to be indicative of persistent infection." *J Clin Pathol*. 2002 May

Dysbiosis: 4. "blood microbiota dysbiosis"

Dysbiosis: 5. Genitourinary/Urogenital

Genitourinary infection with *Chlamydia trachomatis* is well known to cause inflammatory arthropathy—"reactive arthritis"—previously known as Reiter's syndrome.

Kobayashi and Kida. *Intern Med.* 2005 May   Panush, Wallace, et al. Retraction of the suggestion to use the term "Reiter's syndrome" sixty-five years later: the legacy of Reiter, a war criminal, should not be eponymic honor but rather condemnation. *Arthritis Rheum.* 2007 Feb

"Urogenital swab cultures showed a microbial infection in 44% of the patients with oligoarthritis (15% Chlamydia, 14% Mycoplasma, 28% Ureaplasma), whereas in the control group only 26% had a positive result (4% Chlamydia, 7% Mycoplasma, 21% Ureaplasma)."

Erlacher et al. Reactive arthritis: urogenital swab culture is the only useful diagnostic method for the detection of the arthritogenic infection in extra-articularly asymptomatic patients with **undifferentiated oligoarthritis**. *Br J Rheumatol.* 1995 Sep

Dysbiosis: 5. Genitourinary

British Journal of Rheumatology 1995;34:838–842

REACTIVE ARTHRITIS: UROGENITAL SWAB CULTURE IS THE ONLY USEFUL DIAGNOSTIC METHOD FOR THE DETECTION OF THE ARTHRITOGENIC INFECTION IN EXTRA-ARTICULARLY ASYMPTOMATIC PATIENTS WITH UNDIFFERENTIATED OLIGOARTHRITIS

L. ERLACHER, W. WINTERSBERGER, M. MENSCHIK, A. BENKE-STUDNICKA, K. MACHOLD, G. STANEK,* J. SÖLTZ-SZÖTS,† J. SMOLEN and W. GRANINGER

*Department of Internal Medicine III, Division of Rheumatology, *Department of Microbiology and †Department of Dermatology, University of Vienna, Vienna, Austria*

SUMMARY

Reactive arthritis (ReA) is a seronegative oligoarthritis triggered by a preceding extra-articular infection. While evidence of a microbial infection is mandatory for establishing the diagnosis of ReA, the sensitivity of bacteriological and serological tests has not been determined in patients without symptoms of infection. In a retrospective study, we evaluated the usefulness of urogenital swab cultures, serology and stool culture to identify infections in 234 patients with undifferentiated oligoarthritis. One hundred and forty-four patients complaining about joint pain who had no sign or history of inflammatory arthritis served as controls. Urogenital swab cultures showed a microbial infection in 44% of the patients with oligoarthritis (15% *Chlamydia*, 14% *Mycoplasma*, 28% *Ureaplasma*), whereas in the control group only 26% had a positive result (4% *Chlamydia*, 7% *Mycoplasma*, 21% *Ureaplasma*) ($P < 0.001$). A *Chlamydia* IgG-antibody titre $\geq 1:256$ was found in 22% of the patients in the oligoarthritis group and in 9% of the controls ($P < 0.01$). However, for only half of *Chlamydia* IgG-positive patients could a *Chlamydia* infection be confirmed by urogenital swab culture. Twenty-one per cent of patients with oligoarthritis vs 23% of the controls had positive antibody titres for *Salmonella* (not significant), 15% vs 5% for *Yersinia* ($P < 0.05$) and 17% vs 3% for *Borrelia* IgG ($P < 0.01$). In two patients, stool cultures were positive for *Campylobacter*. Urogenital swab culture is a sensitive diagnostic method to identify the triggering infection in ReA. A single determination of antibodies against *Chlamydia trachomatis* is of limited value because of the high prevalence of positive results in the control group.

KEY WORDS: Reactive arthritis, Oligoarthritis, Urogenital swab culture, Serology, Stool culture, *Chlamydia* infection.

This 34yoM presented for consultation on "possible psoriatic arthritis" and was also found to have conjugate seropositivity for RA, as well as thyroiditis.

FECHA	20/08/2011	# 200037
EDAD	33 AÑOS	Sexo M

INMUNOLOGIA

ESTUDIO	RESULTADO
REACCIONES FEBRILES	
PARATIFICO A	NEGATIVO
PARATIFICO B	NEGATIVO
TIFICO O	NEGATIVO
TIFICO H	NEGATIVO
PROTEUS OX - 19	POSITIVO 1:80
BRUCELLA HUDDLESON	NEGATIVO

Método: Aglutinación en placa.

Proteus mirabilis and *Proteus vulgaris* are both strongly correlated with both rheumatoid arthritis and psoriasis.

Vasquez, *Integrative Rheumatology.*

Dysbiosis: 6. Cutaneous

Microorganisms from dermal infections such as acne can incite systemic inflammation either by dermal absorption of bacterial[1] and fungal[2] (super)antigens and by serving as loci for metastatic infections which produce septic arthritis.[3]

- Patients with the autoimmune vasculitic syndrome known as Behcet's disease are more likely to develop arthritis if their skin lesions are infected, thus implicating absorption of an inflammatory immunogen.[4]
- Most (57%) of patients with atopic dermatitis show evidence of IgE-mediated histamine release (i.e., "allergy") to exotoxins secreted from *Staphylococcus aureus*, which commonly colonizes eczematous skin[5].

[1] Delyle et al. Chronic destructive oligoarthritis associated with Propionibacterium acnes in a female patient with acne vulgaris. *Arthritis Rheum*. 2000 Dec [2] Hemalatha et al. *Indian J Med Microbiol* 2004 [3] Schaeverbeke et al. Propionibacterium acnes isolated from synovial tissue and fluid in a patient with oligoarthritis associated with acne and pustulosis. *Arthritis Rheum*. 1998 Oct [4] Diri et al. *Ann Rheum Dis*. 2001 Nov [5] Leung et al. Presence of IgE antibodies to staphylococcal exotoxins on the skin of patients with atopic dermatitis. *J Clin Invest*. 1993 Sep

Dysbiosis: 7. Environmental

Airborne immunogens include fungi, bacteria, actinomycetes, endotoxin, ß(1,3)-glucans, peptidoglycans, microbial volatile organic compounds (MVOC), and mycotoxins.

We may reasonably speculate that a susceptible person might have a systemic inflammatory response from the inhalation of bioaerosols/LPS/etc in the air of their home and/or work environments.

- Bioaerosol health effects and exposure assessment. Douwes et al. *Ann Occup Hyg* 2003 Apr
- Joint symptoms and diseases associated with moisture damage in a health center. Luosujärvi et al. *Clin Rheumatol*. 2003 Dec
- A cluster of inflammatory rheumatic diseases in a moisture-damaged office. Myllykangas-Luosujärvi et al. *Clin Exp Rheumatol*. 2002 Nov-Dec
- Chlamydophila pneumoniae antibodies in office workers with and without inflammatory rheumatic diseases in a moisture-damaged building. Seuri et al. *Eur J Clin Microbiol Infect Dis*. 2005 Mar

Dysbiosis → "*multi*focal *poly*dysbiosis"

Location Subtypes:
1. **Gastrointestinal**
2. **Orodental**
3. **Sinorespiratory**
4. **Parenchymal**
5. **Genitourinary**
6. **Cutaneous**
7. **Environmental**

Problematic GI Microbes Include:
Aeromonas hydrophila, Blastocystis hominis, Candida albicans and other yeasts, Citrobacter rodentium, Citrobacter freundii, Dientamoeba fragilis, Endolimax nana, Entamoeba histolytica, Gamma strep, Enterococcus, Giardia lamblia, Hafnia alvei, Helicobacter pylori, Klebsiella pneumoniae, Proteus mirabilis, Pseudomonas aeruginosa, Staphylococcus aureus, Staphylococcus epidermidis, Streptococcus pyogenes, Group A streptococci

Molecular Mechanisms
1. **Molecular mimicry**
2. Superantigens
3. Enhanced processing of autoantigens
4. **Bystander activation**
5. Peptidoglycans and exotoxins
6. Endotoxins (LPS)
7. Immunostimulation by bacterial DNA
8. Activation of Toll-like receptors and NF-kB
9. **Immune complex formation and deposition**
10. Haptenization and Neoantigen formation
11. Damage to the intestinal mucosa
12. Inhibition/alteration of detoxification
13. Antimetabolites
14. Autointoxication, hepatic encephalopathy, intestinal arthritis-dermatitis syndrome
15. Impairment of mucosal and systemic defenses
16. Impairment of mucosal digestion by microbial proteases and inflammation
17. Inflammation-induced endocrine dysfunction
18. **Central sensitization**

This might be a good time for a rest.

Malaga, Jan 2013

Dysbiosis: Topic Outline

1. <u>Introduction and definitions</u>: Terminology, perspectives, locations
2. <u>Molecular mechanisms</u>: 18…*and counting toward more…*
3. <u>Locations</u>: Introduction to the 7 main loci
4. **<u>Microbes</u>**: Introduction to some of the most common microbes seen in clinical practice and represented in the literature
5. **<u>Additional detail for gastrointestinal dysbiosis</u>**: GI dysbiosis deserves additional attention due to its pathophysiologic quantitative and qualitative preeminence in addition to its greater representation in the research literature
6. **<u>Case reports and clinical examples</u>**: Mostly related to GI dysbiosis
7. **<u>Antidysbiotic Interventions</u>**: Simple as ❶ ❷ ❸

Dysbiosis: Definition, Assessments, Treatment

- **Dysbiosis**: "A *relationship* of non-acute non-infectious host-microorganism interaction that adversely affects the human host"
  - Often what we find when working with autoimmune/inflammatory patients is that they are having a pathogenic inflammatory response to a nonpathogenic microbe.
- **Microbial assessments**: can sample each location:
  - Gastrointestinal, Orodental, Sinorespiratory, Cutaneous, Genitourinary (culture and sensitivity—yes, microscopic—yes, DNA?),
  - Parenchymal (blood tests for antibodies and antigens, rarely biopsy)
  - Environmental (plate and culture, mold count)
- **Treatment for dysbiosis**:
  1. Antimicrobial: no microbe = no dysbiosis
  2. Immunorestoration: effective immune response = better control of microbial colonization = no dysbiosis
  3. Immunomodulation: no pathogenic immune response = no inflammation = no dysbiotic relationship

---

Gastrointestinal Dysbiosis Treatments

Introduction to dysbiosis

Clinical and laboratory assessments

Dysbiotic microbes

❶ Antimicrobial treatments: Diet, Nutrients, Drugs, Botanicals

❷ Immunorestoration: Diet and nutrients

❸ Immunomodulation: Promoting tolerance

Summary, conclusions, and clinical applications

Scientific validation: gut microbes can cause non-GI *systemic* disease:

- The following section of slides provides ❶ scientific evidence and ❷ several example reports from my office of dysbiosis-induced disease.

"Dysbiotic microbes":

- A "dysbiotic microbe" is one that is more likely than others—via molecular structures (eg, antigens, molecular mimicry) or metabolic effects (eg, H_2S, D-lactate) to impair health or cause systemic [inflammatory] disease.

Aeromonas hydrophila

> *Aeromonas hydrophila* can cause colitis and should therefore be eradicated immediately upon detection.

Farraye FA, et al. Segmental colitis associated with Aeromonas hydrophila. *Am J Gastroenterol.* 1989 Apr;84(4):436-8

Blastocystis hominis

> Many infections are asymptomatic
> Can cause abdominal pain, nausea, fatigue, vomiting, diarrhea, weight loss[1],[2] as well as fever, chills, malaise, anorexia, flatus, and eosinophilia[3]
> Fecal leukocytes are occasionally seen[4]
> Can cause colitis [5]

1. O'Gorman et al. *Clin Pediatr* (Phila) 1993 Feb
2. Telalbasic S et al. *Scand J Infect Dis* 1991;23(3)
3. Sheehan et al. *J Clin Microbiol.* 1986;24(4):548-50
4. Diaczok BJ, Rival J. *South Med J* 1987 Jul
5. Russo et al. *Arch Intern Med.* 1988 May

Gastrointestinal Dysbiosis Treatments

Introduction to dysbiosis

Clinical and laboratory assessments

Dysbiotic microbes

❶ Antimicrobial treatments: Diet, Nutrients, Drugs, Botanicals

❷ Immunorestoration: Diet and nutrients

❸ Immunomodulation: Promoting tolerance

Summary, conclusions, and clinical applications

Candida albicans and other yeasts

- Although normal in small amounts ("+1"), excess *Candida* in the intestines is never a sign of optimal health.
- Patients may have mild general symptoms such as **fatigue and dyscognition** ("brain fog"); gas and intestinal bloating following consumption of carbohydrates are common.
- ***Candida* produces an immunosuppressive myotoxin called gliotoxin** as well as an IgA-destroying protease and can cause watery diarrhea, particularly in elderly, ill, and immunosuppressed patients.[1]
- *Candida* is always present in the gastrointestinal tract of women with **recurrent yeast vaginitis**.[2]
- Some people have an inflammatory hypersensitivity to *Candida*, as it can cause **local allergic dermatitis/mucositis**[3], **colitis**[4], and **pulmonary inflammation (hypersensitivity alveolitis** from gastrointestinal colonization).[5]
- Other yeasts such as *Candida parapsilosis* and *Geotrichum capitatum* are occasionally seen and should be eradicated.

Gastrointestinal Dysbiosis Treatments

Introduction to dysbiosis

Clinical and laboratory assessments

Dysbiotic microbes

❶ Antimicrobial treatments: Diet, Nutrients, Drugs, Botanicals

❷ Immunorestoration: Diet and nutrients

❸ Immunomodulation: Promoting tolerance

Summary, conclusions, and clinical applications

Candida albicans and other yeasts—citations

1. Gupta TP, Ehrinpreis MN. *Gastroenterology* 1990 Mar
2. Miles MR, Olsen L, Rogers A. Recurrent vaginal candidiasis. Importance of an intestinal reservoir. *JAMA*. 1977 Oct
3. Ramirez De Knott et al. *Contact Dermatitis*. 2005 Oct
4. Doby T. *J Maine Med Assoc*. 1971 May
5. "We conclude that the disease was induced by C.a.-antigen reaching the lungs from the intestinal tract via the bloodstream." Schreiber J, Struben C, Rosahl W, Amthor M. Hypersensitivity alveolitis induced by endogenous candida species. *Eur J Med Res*. 2000 Mar 27;5(3):126

in the patients flat. After initiation of antimycotic treatment the symptoms resolved completely.
 We conclude that the disease was induced by C.a.-antigen reaching the lungs from the intestinal tract via the bloodstream. It is still a matter of debate whether an additional factor is necessary for the antigen to penetrate the intestinal mucosa.

24yo male with subacute onset of fatigue and dyscognition following severe stress

Bacteriology

Beneficial Bacteria

Lactobacillus species	N	4+
Escherichia coli	I	NG
Bifidobacterium	N	4+

Additional Bacteria

alpha haemolytic Streptococcus	N	3+
gamma haemolytic Streptococcus	N	4+
Citrobacter freundii	P	4+
Klebsiella pneumoniae	P	4+
beta Strep (Not Group A or B)	I	2+

Mycology

Candida krusei	P	4+
Geotrichum capitatum	P	4+

Gastrointestinal Dysbiosis Treatments

Introduction to dysbiosis

Clinical and laboratory assessments

[Dysbiotic microbes]

❶ Antimicrobial treatments: Diet, Nutrients, Drugs, Botanicals

❷ Immunorestoration: Diet and nutrients

❸ Immunomodulation: Promoting tolerance

Summary, conclusions, and clinical applications

Citrobacter rodentium/freundii

- *Citrobacter freundii* is a gram-negative anaerobe; it produces pro-inflammatory endotoxin
- *Citrobacter* species may cause **gastroenteritis** in humans[1]
- **Most strains of *Citrobacter freundii* produce hydrogen sulfide[2] which interferes with mitochondrial function** and energy production and may be a major causative molecule in **ulcerative colitis**.[3]
- Animal studies have shown that this bacterium can induce an intense inflammatory response in the gastrointestinal tract that resembles **inflammatory bowel disease**.[4]
- Gastrointestinal dysbiosis with *Citrobacter freundii* may be causative in so-called "rheumatoid arthritis" in some patients. [author's experience]

Gastrointestinal Dysbiosis Treatments

Introduction to dysbiosis

Clinical and laboratory assessments

Dysbiotic microbes

❶ Antimicrobial treatments: Diet, Nutrients, Drugs, Botanicals

❷ Immunorestoration: Diet and nutrients

❸ Immunomodulation: Promoting tolerance

Summary, conclusions, and clinical applications

Citrobacter rodentium, Citrobacter freundii—citations

1. Lipsky BA et al. *Rev Infect Dis*. 1980 Sep-Oct
2. Lennette EH (editor in chief). Manual of Clinical Microbiology. Fourth Edition. Washington DC; American Society for Microbiology: 1985, page 269. See also http://web.indstate.edu/thcme/micro/GI/general/sld038.htm Accessed 10/27/2005
3. "CONCLUSIONS: Metabolic effects of sodium hydrogen sulfide on butyrate oxidation along the length of the colon closely mirror metabolic abnormalities observed in active ulcerative colitis, and the increased production of sulfide in ulcerative colitis suggests that the action of mercaptides may be involved in the genesis of ulcerative colitis." Roediger et al. *Gastroenterology*. 1993 Mar
4. Higgins et al. *Infect Immun*. 1999 Jun http://iai.asm.org/cgi/reprint/67/6/3031.pdf

---

38-yo woman with periorbital dermatitis

MICROBIOLOGY

Bacteriology Culture

Beneficial flora		Imbalances		Dysbiotic flora	
Bifidobacter	3+	Gamma strep	4+	Klebsiella pneumoniae	3+
E. coli	4+			Citrobacter freundii	1+
Lactobacillus	3+				

INFLAMMATION

	Within	Outside	Ref. Range
Lysozyme	276		<= 600 ng/mL
Lactoferrin	5.3		< 7.3 µg/mL
WBC	None		None - Rare
Mucus	Neg		Neg

Lysozyme: Lysozyme is an enzyme secreted at the site of inflammation in the GI. Elevated levels of fecal lysozyme have been identified in IBD. **Lactoferrin:** Lactoferrin is a quantitative GI specific marker of inflammation used to diagnose and differentiate IBD from IBS and to monitor patient inflammation levels during active and remission phases of inflammatory bowel disease. **WBCs:** Elevated stool levels of white blood cells occur following an infiltration of leukocytes within the intestinal lumen during an inflammatory process. **Mucus:** Mucus in the stool may result from prolonged mucosal irritation or in response to parasympathetic excitability such as spastic constipation or mucous colitis.

IMMUNOLOGY

	Within	Outside	Ref. Range
sIgA		904	40 - 204 mg/dL

sIgA: Secretory IgA is secreted by mucosal-associated lymphoid tissue and represents the first line of defense of the GI mucosa and is central to the normal function of the GI as an immune barrier. Elevated levels of sIgA are associated with an upregulated immune response.

51-year-old man with 4-year history of rheumatoid arthritis and hsCRP of 124 mg/L

TEST	RESULT	LIMITS	LAB
C-Reactive Protein, Cardiac			
C-Reactive Protein, Cardiac	124.00H mg/L	0.00 - 3.00	HD

Comprehensive Parasitology, stool, x2

MICROBIOLOGY

Bacteriology Culture

Beneficial flora		Imbalances		Dysbiotic flora	
Bifidobacter	0+	Gamma strep	1+	Citrobacter freundii	1+
E. coli	2+	Enterobacter sp.	1+		
Lactobacillus	0+				

Mycology (Yeast) Culture

Normal flora	Dysbiotic flora
No yeast isolated	

PARASITOLOGY

Sample 1		Sample 2	
No	Ova or Parasites	No	Ova or Parasites

51-year-old man with 4-year history of RA

TEST	RESULT	LIMITS	LAB
C-Reactive Protein, Cardiac			
C-Reactive Protein, Cardiac	7.58H mg/L	0.00 - 3.00	HD

Relative Risk for Future Cardiovascular Event
- Low <1.00
- Average 1.00 - 3.00
- High >3.00

LAB: HD LabCorp Houston
DIRECTOR: Edward Kott ? MD

Major success!

hsCRP is down from 124 to 7.5.

Major improvement

Continue current plan

Completely N 8.15.05

Dientamoeba fragilis

- *Dientamoeba fragilis* is a flagellate protozoan that can cause **diarrhea, abdominal pain, nausea, vomiting, fatigue, malaise, eosinophilia, urticaria, pruritus and/or weight loss**. It is commonly associated with pinworm infection and may produce a clinical picture that mimics **food allergy, colitis, or eosinophilic enteritis**.

Cuffari et al. Dientamoeba fragilis masquerading as allergic colitis. *J Pediatr Gastroenterol Nutr.* 1998 Jan

Endolimax nana

- *Endolimax nana*, a protozoa, has a world-wide distribution and is commonly considered an harmless commensal of the intestine.[1]
- Intestinal infection with *Endolimax nana* can cause a **peripheral arthropathy** that is clinically similar to **rheumatoid arthritis** and which remits with effective parasite eradication.[2]
- In my own clinical practice, I have seen several cases of intestinal colonization with *Endolimax nana* in patients who presented with **chronic fatigue, myalgia, eczema**, and especially refractory **chronic vaginitis**.

1. http://www2.provlab.ab.ca/bugs/webbug/parasite/artifact/enana.htm as of December 26, 2003
2. "Endolimax nana grew on stool culture. Both the patient's diarrhea and arthritis responded effectively to therapy with metronidazole. The diagnosis of parasitic rheumatism was made in retrospect." Burnstein SL, Liakos S. **Parasitic rheumatism presenting as rheumatoid arthritis.** *J Rheumatol.* 1983 Jun

Gastrointestinal Dysbiosis Treatments

Introduction to dysbiosis

Clinical and laboratory assessments

Dysbiotic microbes

❶ Antimicrobial treatments: Diet, Nutrients, Drugs, Botanicals

❷ Immunorestoration: Diet and nutrients

❸ Immunomodulation: Promoting tolerance

Summary, conclusions, and clinical applications

Entamoeba histolytica

- Induces tissue damage, **amebic colitis**, and **liver abscess**.[1]
- Associated with Henoch Schonlein purpura in a single case report[2]
- **Amebic colitis** may be misdiagnosed as ulcerative colitis.[3]
- May contribute to irritable bowel syndrome, rheumatoid arthritis, fibromyalgia, food allergy, or multiple chemical sensitivity and can exacerbate HIV infection.[4]
- Hepatic infection is associated with induction of antineutrophil cytoplasmic antibodies (ANCA) such as seen with the vasculitic disease Wegener's granulomatosis.[5]

1. Huston. *Trends Parasitol*. 2004 Jan; 20
2. Demircin et al. Henoch Schonlein purpura and amebiasis. *Acta Paediatr Jpn*. 1998 Oct
3. Galland L. Intestinal protozoan infection is a common unsuspected cause of chronic illness. *J Advancement Med*. 1989;2: 539-552
4. Galland L. *J Advancement Med*. 1989;2: 539-552
5. George J, Levy Y, Kallenberg CG, Shoenfeld Y. Infections and Wegener's granulomatosis--a cause and effect relationship? *QJM*. 1997 May
http://qjmed.oxfordjournals.org/cgi/reprint/90/5/367

Gastrointestinal Dysbiosis Treatments

Introduction to dysbiosis

Clinical and laboratory assessments

Dysbiotic microbes

❶ Antimicrobial treatments: Diet, Nutrients, Drugs, Botanicals

❷ Immunorestoration: Diet and nutrients

❸ Immunomodulation: Promoting tolerance

Summary, conclusions, and clinical applications

Gamma strep Enterococcus

- "Gamma strep", *Enterococcus faecalis*, and *Streptococcus faecalis* are somewhat interchangeable terms.[1],[2],[3]
- These terms refer to gram-positive *Enterococcus* species such as *Enterococcus faecalis*, which cause **urinary tract infections, bacteremia, intra-abdominal infections, and endocarditis**.
- Enterococci produce lipoteichoic acid which is proinflammatory in a manner similar to endotoxin from gram-negative bacteria, and these gram-positive bacteria also appear to produce a superantigen.[4]
- "Gamma strep" is commonly identified in stool tests of patients with chronic unwellness and fatigue.

1. "Figure 38: "Gamma *Streptococcus*" : *Enterococcus faecalis*" and "The genus *Enterococcus* was once a part of the *Streptococcus* genus, was considered a "gamma *Streptococcus* species."
http://www.microbelibrary.org/asmonly/details_print.asp?id=1986&lang
2. "Enterococcus faecalis. Synonyms: group D strep, Streptococcus faecalis. Classification: facultative anaerobic, gram+ bacteria, cocci." http://medinfo.ufl.edu/year2/mmid/bms5300/bugs/strfaeca.html
3. "Microscopically, Gram-positive cocci occurring in chains or pairs with individual cells being somewhat elongated can be presumed to be streptococci or enterococci."
http://members.tripod.com/piece_de_resistance/SAARS/bugs/menteroc.htm
4. Lynn et al. Department of Microbiology and Immunology, University of Oklahoma Health Sciences Center. Pathogenicity of Enterococci published in "Gram-Positive Pathogens" edited by Fischetti V et al.
http://w3.ouhsc.edu/enterococcus/lynn_revirew.asp

Inflammation Mastery & Functional Inflammology: Volume 1
Dysbiosis Review Presentation Slides • Page 34

Gastrointestinal Dysbiosis Treatments

Introduction to dysbiosis

Clinical and laboratory assessments

Dysbiotic microbes

❶ Antimicrobial treatments: Diet, Nutrients, Drugs, Botanicals

❷ Immunorestoration: Diet and nutrients

❸ Immunomodulation: Promoting tolerance

Summary, conclusions, and clinical applications

Giardia lamblia

- Causatively associated with **abdominal pain, diarrhea, constipation, bloating, chronic fatigue, and food allergy/intolerance.**[1]
- May contribute to **irritable bowel syndrome, rheumatoid arthritis, food allergy, or multiple chemical sensitivity.**[2]
- Extraintestinal symptoms of gastrointestinal *Giardia* infection can include **fever, maculopapular rashes, geographic tongue, pulmonary infiltrates, lymphadenopathy, polyarthritis, aphthous ulcers, and urticaria.**[3]

1. Galland L, Lee M. #170 High frequency of giardiasis in patients with chronic digestive complaints. *Am J Gastroenterol* 1989;84:1181
2. Galland L. Intestinal protozoan infection is a common unsuspected cause of chronic illness. *J Advancement Med.* 1989;2: 539-552
3. Corsi et al. Ocular changes associated with Giardia lamblia infection in children. *Br J Ophthalmol.* 1998 Jan;82(1):59-62 http://bjo.bmjjournals.com/cgi/content/full/82/1/59

Gastrointestinal Dysbiosis Treatments

Introduction to dysbiosis

Clinical and laboratory assessments

Dysbiotic microbes

❶ Antimicrobial treatments: Diet, Nutrients, Drugs, Botanicals

❷ Immunorestoration: Diet and nutrients

❸ Immunomodulation: Promoting tolerance

Summary, conclusions, and clinical applications

Giardia lamblia—continued

- **Ocular complications** from gastrointestinal infection include iridocyclitis, choroiditis, retinal hemorrhages, anterior and posterior uveitis, retinal vasculitis, and "salt and pepper" retinal degeneration. These complications are most likely due to deposition of **immune complexes** in the retinal epithelium.[1]
- Reported to have caused numerous cases of **reactive arthritis (peripheral arthritis and/or sacroiliitis)** in patients who are either positive or negative for HLA-B27[2]; "beaver fever" is a cause of reactive arthritis.[3]
- Antigen detection appears superior to microscopic examination for detection.[4]

Gastrointestinal Dysbiosis Treatments

Introduction to dysbiosis

Clinical and laboratory assessments

Dysbiotic microbes

❶ Antimicrobial treatments: Diet, Nutrients, Drugs, Botanicals

❷ Immunorestoration: Diet and nutrients

❸ Immunomodulation: Promoting tolerance

Summary, conclusions, and clinical applications

Giardia lamblia—citations

1. "The retinal changes associated with giardiasis are more than likely caused by immune mechanisms. Wania reported that circulating immune complexes were found in all of the patients with ocular complications he examined." Corsi A et al. Ocular changes associated with Giardia lamblia infection in children. *Br J Ophthalmol.* 1998 Jan http://bjo.bmjjournals.com/cgi/content/full/82/1/59

2. Layton et al. Sacroiliitis in an HLA B27-negative patient following giardiasis. *Br J Rheumatol.* 1998 May http://rheumatology.oxfordjournals.org/cgi/reprint/37/5/581

3. "Giardia lamblia infection is rarely associated with adult reactive arthritis. We report the first North American case and review the pediatric and adult literature to date. **Antimicrobial treatment is essential to eradicate the parasite and control the arthritis.**" Tupchong et al. Beaver fever--a rare cause of reactive arthritis. *J Rheumatol.* 1999 Dec

4. "For all patients, microscopy was uniformly negative, but 6 of 13 patients were antigen positive... Giardiasis, an increasing problem in family practice, should be considered early in patients with GI disturbances. New, sensitive immunodiagnostic tests that usually require a single specimen are more useful than microscopy." Chappell CL, Matson CC. Giardia antigen detection in patients with chronic gastrointestinal disturbances. *J Fam Pract.* 1992 Jul

---

Gastrointestinal Dysbiosis Treatments

Introduction to dysbiosis

Clinical and laboratory assessments

Dysbiotic microbes

❶ Antimicrobial treatments: Diet, Nutrients, Drugs, Botanicals

❷ Immunorestoration: Diet and nutrients

❸ Immunomodulation: Promoting tolerance

Summary, conclusions, and clinical applications

Hafnia alvei

▸ *Hafnia alvei* is a gram-negative bacterium capable of causing **reactive arthritis** from gastrointestinal infection; the reactive arthritis associated with *Hafnia alvei* occurs without association with HLA-B27.

Toivanen et al. Two forms of reactive arthritis? *Ann Rheum Dis.* 1999 Dec http://ard.bmjjournals.com/cgi/content/full/58/12/737 See also: Newmark et al. Reactive arthritis associated with Hafnia alvei enteritis. *Arthritis Rheum.* 1994 Jun

Helicobacter pylori

- *H. pylori* is a gram-negative endotoxin-producing rod that causes stomach ulcers and appears to cause reactive arthritis in some patients.[1]
- *H. pylori* colonization is increased in patients with scleroderma.[2]
- *H. pylori* is commonly found in the middle ear of patients with acute otitis media.[3]
- More common in pts with migraine, ITP, Raynaud's.

1. "Our findings suggest that HP may be included in the list of possible arthritis triggering microbes." Melby et al. *Infection*. 1999
2. Yazawa et al. High seroprevalence of Helicobacter pylori infection in patients with systemic sclerosis: association with esophageal involvement. *J Rheumatol*. 1998 Apr
3. "Twelve of 15 smears for MEE were positive for HP by immunohistochemistry and 14 by Giemsa that were Gram-negative." Morinaka et al. Detection of Helicobacter pylori in the middle ear fluid of patients with otitis media with effusion. *Otolaryngol Head Neck Surg*. 2005 Nov

---

Klebsiella pneumoniae

- Many cases of gastrointestinal colonization with this microorganism produce no acute gastrointestinal symptoms such as nausea, vomiting, constipation, or diarrhea. Patients may have mild general symptoms such as fatigue and dyscognition ("brain fog").
- Can cause **diarrhea**[1] and **acute gastroenteritis.**[2]
- Associated with reactive arthritis such as ankylosing spondylitis.[3]
- Gram-negative bacteria, produces endotoxin/lipopolysaccharide that is capable of impairing cytochrome p-450 and **reducing hepatic clearance and urinary/biliary excretion of drugs.**[4] Clinically this is seen as chemical sensitivity.

- Niyogi et al. *Indian J Med Res* 2000 Oct
- Ananthan et al. *Jpn J Infect Dis* 1999 Feb
- Ahmadi K, Wilson C, Tiwana H, Binder A, Ebringer A. Antibodies to Klebsiella pneumoniae lipopolysaccharide in patients with ankylosing spondylitis. *Br J Rheumatol*. 1998 Dec
- Hasegawa et al. Effects of bacterial endotoxin on drug pharmacokinetics. *Nagoya J Med Sci* 1999 May

60yo woman with a history of moderate fatigue, IBS, and recent acute episode of <u>transverse myelitis</u>

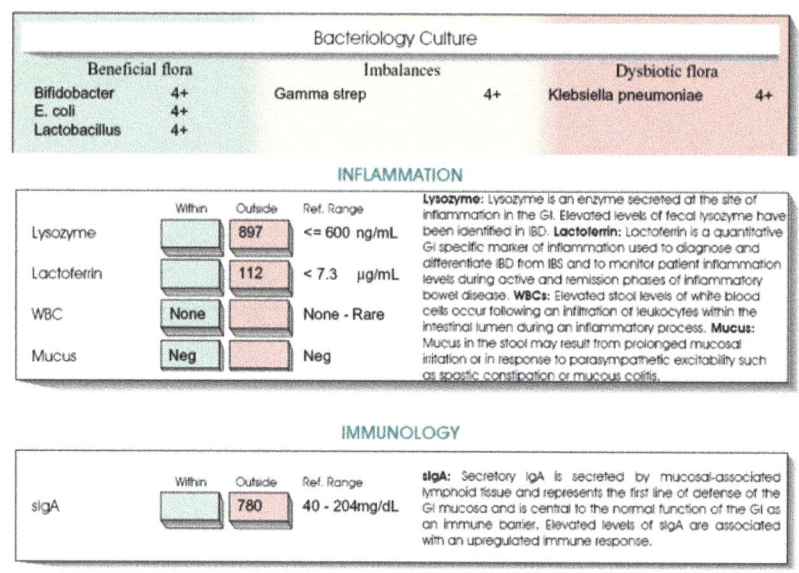

Gastrointestinal Dysbiosis Treatments

Introduction to dysbiosis

Clinical and laboratory assessments

Dysbiotic microbes

❶ Antimicrobial treatments: Diet, Nutrients, Drugs, Botanicals

❷ Immunorestoration: Diet and nutrients

❸ Immunomodulation: Promoting tolerance

Summary, conclusions, and clinical applications

Proteus mirabilis

- Gram-negative bacteria, produces endotoxin/lipopolysaccharide.[1]
- Gastrointestinal and urinary tract colonization is associated with **rheumatoid arthritis**[2, 3] and **ankylosing spondylitis**.[4]

1. Kondakova et al. *Carbohydr Res* 2003 May
2. Ebringer et al. **Rheumatoid arthritis: proposal for the use of anti-microbial therapy in early cases**. *Scand J Rheumatol* 2003
3. Rashid et al. *Clin Rheumatol* 1999
4. Wilson et al. *J Rheumatol* 2003 May;30(5):972-8

Gastrointestinal Dysbiosis Treatments

Introduction to dysbiosis

Clinical and laboratory assessments

Dysbiotic microbes

❶ Antimicrobial treatments: Diet, Nutrients, Drugs, Botanicals

❷ Immunorestoration: Diet and nutrients

❸ Immunomodulation: Promoting tolerance

Summary, conclusions, and clinical applications

Pseudomonas aeruginosa

- Many cases of gastrointestinal colonization with this microorganism produce no acute gastrointestinal symptoms such as nausea, vomiting, constipation, or diarrhea.
- Patients may have mild general symptoms such as fatigue and dyscognition ("brain fog").
- *Pseudomonas aeruginosa* is a gram-negative bacterium, produces endotoxin[1] and can cause antibiotic-associated diarrhea.[2],[3]   Patients with **multiple sclerosis** show evidence of a heightened immune response against *Pseudomonas aeruginosa*, suggesting the possibility of immune cross-reactivity.[4]

1. Bergan T. *Scand J Infect Dis Suppl.* 1981;29
2. Kim et al. *J Korean Med Sci.* 2001 Dec
3. Porco FV, Visconte EB. *Ann Pharmacother.* 1995 Nov
4. Hughes et al. **Antibody responses to Acinetobacter spp. and Pseudomonas aeruginosa in multiple sclerosis**. *Clin Diagn Lab Immunol.* 2001 Nov

---

38yo man with "autoimmune peripheral neuropathy"

Comprehensive Stool Analysis / Parasitology x3

MICROBIOLOGY

Bacteriology Culture

Beneficial flora		Imbalances		Dysbiotic flora	
Bifidobacter	4+	Haemolytic E. coli	4+	Pseudomonas sp.	4+
E. coli	4+	Gamma strep	2+		
Lactobacillus	2+				

Mycology (Yeast) Culture

Normal flora		Dysbiotic flora
Candida glabrata	1+	
Rhodotorula sp.	1+	

Vasquez A. Musculoskeletal Pain: Expanded Clinical Strategies. Institute for Functional Medicine, 2008

Staphylococcus aureus, Staphylococcus epidermidis

- **Any and all GI-overgrowth *Staphylococcus aureus* should be eradicated immediately due to the well-known inflammatory consequences of the toxins and superantigens this bacterium produces.** *Staphylococcus aureus* is a gram-positive bacterium, certain strains of which produce the toxic shock syndrome toxin-1 (TSST-1) that produces scalded skin syndrome, toxic shock syndrome, and food poisoning; other strains of *Staphylococcus aureus* that do not produce TSST-1 are also capable of causing toxic shock syndrome from colonization of bone, vagina, wounds, or rectum.

Staphylococcus aureus, Staphylococcus epidermidis

- Gastrointestinal colonization with *Staphylococcus aureus* is a known cause of **acute colitis**[2],
- Nasal carriage of this bacterium is documented in patients with several autoimmune disorders, including **Wegener's granulomatosis**[3], **systemic lupus erythematosus**[4] and **psoriasis**.[5], [6]
- *Staphylococcus aureus* can trigger **reactive arthritis**.[7]
- *Staphylococcus epidermidis* can trigger **reactive arthritis and sacroiliitis**.[8]
- Patients with **Behcet's syndrome** commonly have skin lesions that are colonized by *Staphylococcus aureus*.[9]
- Most (57%) of patients with **atopic dermatitis** show evidence of IgE-mediated histamine release (i.e., "allergy") to exotoxins secreted from *Staphylococcus aureus*, which commonly colonizes eczematous skin[10]; in other words: most eczema patients are allergic to their own dermal bacteria and can thus be said to have *hypersensitivity dermal dysbiosis*.

Staphylococcus aureus, Staphylococcus epidermidis—citations

[1] Shandera WX, Moran A. "Infectious diseases: viral and rickettsial." In Tierney LM, McPhee SJ Papadakis MA (eds). Current Medical Diagnosis and Treatment. 44th edition. New York: Lange; 2005, page 1356-8

[2] Watanabe H, Masaki H, Asoh N, Watanabe K, Oishi K, Kobayashi S, Sato A, Nagatake T. Enterocolitis caused by methicillin-resistant Staphylococcus aureus: molecular characterization of respiratory and digestive tract isolates. Microbiol Immunol. 2001;45(9):629-34 http://www.jstage.jst.go.jp/article/mandi/45/9/629/_pdf

[3] Popa ER, Stegeman CA, Kallenberg CG, Tervaert JW. Staphylococcus aureus and Wegener's granulomatosis. Arthritis Res. 2002;4(2):77-9 http://arthritis-research.com/content/4/2/077

[4] Medline abstract from Polish research: "In 9 from 14 patients with (64.3%) a.b. very massive growth of Staphylococcus aureus in culture from vestibulae of the nose swab was, in other cultures very massive growth of physiological flora was seen. ...clinical significance of asymptomatic bacteriuria and pathogenic bacteria colonisation of nostrils as a precedence to symptomatic infections needs further investigations." Koseda-Dragan M, Hebanowski M, Galinski J, Krzywinska E, Bakowska A. [Asymptomatic bacteriuria in women diagnosed with systemic lupus erythematosus (SLE)] Pol Arch Med Wewn. 1998 Oct;100(4):321-30.

[5] "The nasal carriage rate of Staphylococcus aureus in psoriatics was higher than the control groups." Singh G, Rao DJ. Bacteriology of psoriatic plaques. *Dermatologica*. 1978;157(1):21-7

[6] "In this study, S aureus was present in more than 50% of patients with AD and PS. We found that the severity of AD and PS significantly correlated to enterotoxin production of the isolated S aureus strains." Tomi NS, Kranke B, Aberer E. Staphylococcal toxins in patients with psoriasis, atopic dermatitis, and erythroderma, and in healthy control subjects. *J Am Acad Dermatol*. 2005 Jul;53(1):67-72

[7] "CONCLUSION--Reactive arthritis may rarely follow Staph aureus infection. HLA-B27 negativity may be associated with a self limited arthritis in these cases." Siam AR, Hammoudeh M. Staphylococcus aureus triggered reactive arthritis. *Ann Rheum Dis*. 1995 Feb;54(2):131-3

[8] "We report an unusual case of a patient with SE bacteriaemia, who developed elbow arthritis, asymmetrical sacroiliitis, keratoderma and restrictive cardiomyopathy." Giordano N, Senesi M, Battisti E, Palumbo F, Mondillo S, Bargagli G, Palazzuoli V, Nardi P, Gennari C. Reactive arthritis by staphylococcus epidermidis: report of an unusual case. *Clin Rheumatol*. 1996;15(1):59-61

[9] "At least one type of microorganism was grown from each pustule. Staphylococcus aureus (41/70, 58.6%, p = 0.008) and Prevotella spp (17/70, 24.3%, p = 0.002) were significantly more common in pustules from BS patients, and coagulase negative staphylococci (17/37, 45.9%, p = 0.007) in pustules from acne patients. CONCLUSIONS: The pustular lesions of BS are not usually sterile." Hatemi G, Bahar H, Uysal S, Mat C, Gogus F, Masatlioglu S, Altas K, Yazici H. The pustular skin lesions in Behcet's syndrome are not sterile. *Ann Rheum Dis*. 2004 Nov;63(11):1450-2

[10] "These data indicate that a subset of patients with AD mount an IgE response to SEs that can be grown from their skin." Leung DY, Harbeck R, Bina P, Reiser RF, Yang E, Norris DA, Hanifin JM, Sampson HA. Presence of IgE antibodies to staphylococcal exotoxins on the skin of patients with atopic dermatitis. Evidence for a new group of allergens. *J Clin Invest*. 1993 Sep;92(3):1374-80 http://www.pubmedcentral.gov/articlerender.fcgi?tool=pubmed&pubmedid=7690780

Streptococcus pyogenes, Group A streptococci

- Intestinal overgrowth of this bacterium, which produces peptidoglycans, can cause dermatosis, inflammatory polyarthritis, tenosynovitis, malaise, fever, and cryoglobulinemia.[1]
- Non-infectious manifestations precipitated by infection with *S. pyogenes* include autoimmune neuropsychiatric disorders (including obsessive-compulsive disorder and Sydenham's chorea), dystonia, glomerulonephritis, and reactive arthritis.[2] Group A streptococci can cause reactive arthritis in humans.[3]
- *Streptococcus pyogenes* is a very likely trigger of psoriasis[4]; chronic penicillin treatment leads to clinical improvement of recalcitrant psoriasis.[5]
- Certain strains of *S. pyogenes* produce an exotoxin that can cause toxic shock syndrome.[6]

Gastrointestinal Dysbiosis Treatments

Introduction to dysbiosis

Clinical and laboratory assessments

Dysbiotic microbes

❶ Antimicrobial treatments: Diet, Nutrients, Drugs, Botanicals

❷ Immunorestoration: Diet and nutrients

❸ Immunomodulation: Promoting tolerance

Summary, conclusions, and clinical applications

Streptococcus pyogenes, Group A streptococci—citations

[1] Ely PH. The bowel bypass syndrome: a response to bacterial peptidoglycans. *J Am Acad Dermatol*. 1980 Jun;2(6):473-87

[2] Hahn RG, Knox LM, Forman TA. Evaluation of poststreptococcal illness. *Am Fam Physician*. 2005 May 15;71(10):1949-54 http://www.aafp.org/afp/20050515/1949.pdf

[3] "We present a patient whose clinical features are more consistent with post-streptococcal reactive arthritis than acute rheumatic fever." Howell EE, Bathon J. A case of post-streptococcal reactive arthritis. *Md Med J*. 1999 Nov-Dec;48(6):292-4

[4] "These findings justify the hypothesis that S pyogenes infections are more important in the pathogenesis of chronic plaque psoriasis than has previously been recognized, and indicate the need for further controlled therapeutic trials of antibacterial measures in this common skin disease." El-Rachkidy RG, Hales JM, Freestone PP, Young HS, Griffiths CE, Camp RD. Increased Blood Levels of IgG Reactive with Secreted Streptococcus pyogenes Proteins in Chronic Plaque Psoriasis. *J Invest Dermatol*. 2007 Mar

---

Gastrointestinal Dysbiosis Treatments

Introduction to dysbiosis

Clinical and laboratory assessments

Dysbiotic microbes

❶ Antimicrobial treatments: Diet, Nutrients, Drugs, Botanicals

❷ Immunorestoration: Diet and nutrients

❸ Immunomodulation: Promoting tolerance

Summary, conclusions, and clinical applications

Streptococcus pyogenes, Group A streptococci—citations

[5] "Total duration of the study was two years. Initially benzathine penicillin 1.2 million units, was given I.M. AST fortnightly. After 24 weeks benzathine penicillin was reduced to 1.2 million units once a month... Significant improvement in the PASI score was noted from 12 weeks onwards. All patients showed excellent improvement at 2 years." Saxena VN, Dogra J. Long-term use of penicillin for the treatment of chronic plaque psoriasis. *Eur J Dermatol*. 2005 Sep-Oct;15(5):359-62 http://www.john-libbey-eurotext.fr/en/revues/medecine/ejd/e-docs/00/04/10/A4/article.md?type=text.html

[6] Chikkamuniyappa S. Streptococcal toxic shock syndrome and sepsis manifesting in a patient with chronic rheumatoid arthritis. *Dermatol Online J*. 2004 Jul 15;10(1):7

Dysbiosis: Topic Outline

1. <u>Introduction and definitions</u>: Terminology, perspectives, locations
2. <u>Molecular mechanisms</u>: 18...*and counting toward more*...
3. <u>Locations</u>: Introduction to the 7 main loci
4. <u>Microbes</u>: Introduction to some of the most common microbes seen in clinical practice and represented in the literature
5. **Additional detail for gastrointestinal dysbiosis**: GI dysbiosis deserves additional attention due to its pathophysiologic quantitative and qualitative preeminence in addition to its greater representation in the research literature
6. **Case reports and clinical examples**: Mostly related to GI dysbiosis
7. **Antidysbiotic Interventions**: Simple as ❶ ❷ ❸

Dysbiosis: 3. Gastrointestinal

Many clinicians find comprehensive stool analysis and comprehensive parasitology to be among the most valuable laboratory assessments they utilize, second only to basic lab tests such as CBC, CRP, UA, and chemistry/metabolic panels.

Vasquez A. *Integrative Rheumatology*.
Vasquez A. *Nutritional Perspectives* 2006; Jan

Problematic microbes include:
- *Aeromonas hydrophila*
- *Blastocystis hominis*
- *Candida albicans* and other yeasts
- *Citrobacter rodentium, Citrobacter freundii*
- *Dientamoeba fragilis*
- *Endolimax nana*
- *Entamoeba histolytica*
- Gamma strep, *Enterococcus*
- *Giardia lamblia*
- *Hafnia alvei*
- *Helicobacter pylori*
- *Klebsiella pneumoniae*
- *Proteus mirabilis*
- *Pseudomonas aeruginosa*
- *Staphylococcus aureus*
- *Staphylococcus epidermidis*
- Group A streptococci, *Streptococcus pyogenes*—especially intracellular

Gastrointestinal Dysbiosis Treatments

Introduction to dysbiosis

Clinical and laboratory assessments

Dysbiotic microbes

❶ Antimicrobial treatments: Diet, Nutrients, Drugs, Botanicals

❷ Immunorestoration: Diet and nutrients

❸ Immunomodulation: Promoting tolerance

Summary, conclusions, and clinical applications

Stool testing via specialty laboratory

- Routine hospital testing and medical lab testsing generally is not detailed enough—they limit the evaulation to true pathogens that cause acute GI infections (eg, salmonella, shigella, enterohemorragic E coli).
  - Even if a microbe is not a true pathogen and is thus not a therapeutic target from a *disease-oriented paradigm*, we as clinicians are still justified in eradicating it from our chronically ill patient from a *wellness-oriented paradigm* because we know that 1) eradicating *potentially* harmful bacteria will do no harm to the patient, and 2) in many cases—indeed *the majority* of cases—patients experience a significant and sustained clinical improvement regardless of their presenting complaint, thus implying a causal relationship between the microbe and the non-infectious illness.

Gastrointestinal Dysbiosis Treatments

Introduction to dysbiosis

Clinical and laboratory assessments

Dysbiotic microbes

❶ Antimicrobial treatments: Diet, Nutrients, Drugs, Botanicals

❷ Immunorestoration: Diet and nutrients

❸ Immunomodulation: Promoting tolerance

Summary, conclusions, and clinical applications

Stool testing via specialty laboratory

- **One of the benefits of specialized stool testing is that it allows the presence of microbes to be determined within a context that evaluates the patient's individualized response.** For example, the finding of a mild degree of *Candida albicans* ("+1" on a 0-4 scale) might be considered insignificant; however if no other pathogens are identified, and the secretory IgA, lactoferrin, and lysozyme levels are elevated, then the clinician is justified in determining that the patient is having a hypersensitivity reaction to an otherwise "benign" yeast. **Remember, we are not looking for classic "infection" here; we are looking to determine which underlying disruptions may be exacerbating inflammation and the patient's symptomatology.** We have to look beyond the *disease-associated characteristics of the microbe* to see *the patient's individualized response to the microbe*. **Often what we find when working with autoimmune/inflammatory patients is that they are having a** *pathogenic inflammatory response* **to a** *nonpathogenic* **microbe.**

GI dysbiosis: Prototype, for IBD and more

- **Prototypic:** When most clinicians—and an increasing number of patients—talk about "dysbiosis" they are talking about "gastrointestinal dysbiosis"—it is the prototype, and it is the form that is most commonly appreciated, and thus has major quantitative importance as well as qualitative importance.
- **Lots of information on this important topic:** This is such a common and important topic that we could talk about it all day and still not cover all the details.
- **Area of greatest focus, especially related to IBD—inflammatory bowel disease:** 180 Medline articles indexed by "dysbiosis" as of August 2010. 471 Medline articles indexed by "dysbiosis" as of April 2013—more than doubled in less than 3 years.

Tamboli, *Gut* 2004

GI dysbiosis: Subtypes

1. **Insufficiency dysbiosis:** This results when there is an insufficient quantity of the "good bacteria." Obviously, this affects Treg/Th17 balance.
2. **Bacterial overgrowth:** Quantitative excess of bacteria/microbes in the gut.[1-3] Effects are due to malabsorption, maldigestion, malnutrition, increased intestinal permeability, impaired detoxification, immunostimulation due to LPS/superantigen/DNA absorption, and mitochondrial impairment due to LPS and antimetabolites such as H2S and D-lactate.
3. **Immunosuppressive dysbiosis:** Some microbes, particularly yeast, produce toxins that suppress immune function. The immunosuppressive mycotoxin produced by *Candia albicans* is called gliotoxin. [4,5]
4. **Allergic/hypersensitivity dysbiosis:** Some people have an exaggerated immune response to otherwise "normal" yeast and bacteria.[6,7]
5. **Inflammatory/hypersensitivity dysbiosis and reactive arthritis:** The best-known example of systemic musculoskeletal inflammation caused by microbial exposure is reactive arthritis.
6. **Amoebas, cysts, protozoas, and other parasites:** In this case when we use the term "parasites" we are not talking about worms/helminths, per se, although these are occasionally found with parasitology examinations. Certain microorganisms are not consistent with optimal health and should be eliminated even though the microbe is not classically identified as a "pathogen" when the clinical picture includes immune dysregulation and "sustained inflammation."

GI dysbiosis: Citations to previous slide

[1] **Lin HC. Small intestinal bacterial overgrowth: a framework for understanding irritable bowel syndrome. *JAMA*. 2004 Aug 18;292(7):852-8**

[2] Zaidel O, Lin HC. Uninvited guests: the impact of small intestinal bacterial overgrowth on nutrition. *Practical Gastroenterology* 2003; 27(7):27-34

[3] "The initial skin changes were frankly vasculitic with "target" lesions, whilst older lesions showed a psoriasiform scale and a tendency to central clearing. The illness was associated with raised levels of IgM and IgG containing circulating immune complexes and deposition of IgM and IgG in the dermis." Fairris et al. A dermatosis associated with bacterial overgrowth in jejunal diverticula. *Br J Dermatol*. 1985 Jun

[4] "Candida albicans is known to produce gliotoxin, which has several prominent biological effects, including immunosuppression." Shah et al. Effect of gliotoxin on human polymorphonuclear neutrophils. *Infect Dis Obstet Gynecol*. 1998

[5] "Based on the recent finding that C. albicans is able to produce an immunosuppressive mycotoxin, gliotoxin, we analyzed vaginal samples of 3 women severely symptomatic for vaginal candidiasis and found that they contained significant levels of gliotoxin." Shah et al. In situ mycotoxin production by Candida albicans in women with vaginitis. *Gynecol Obstet Invest*. 1995

[6] Doby T. Monilial esophagitis and colitis. *J Maine Med Assoc*. 1971 May

[7] "We conclude that the disease was induced by C.a.-antigen reaching the lungs from the intestinal tract via the bloodstream." Schreiber et al. Hypersensitivity alveolitis induced by endogenous candida species. *Eur J Med Res*. 2000 Mar 27;5(3):126

Dysbiosis: 3. Gastrointestinal (simplified, 1998)

Image copyright: Vasquez A. *Integrative Rheumatology*.

Dysbiosis: Topic Outline

1. **Introduction and definitions**: Terminology, perspectives, locations
2. **Molecular mechanisms**: 18…and counting toward more…
3. **Locations**: Introduction to the 7 main loci
4. **Microbes**: Introduction to some of the most common microbes seen in clinical practice and represented in the literature
5. **Additional detail for gastrointestinal dysbiosis**: GI dysbiosis deserves additional attention due to its pathophysiologic quantitative and qualitative preeminence in addition to its greater representation in the research literature
6. **Case reports and clinical examples**: Mostly related to GI dysbiosis
7. **Antidysbiotic Interventions**: Simple as ❶ ❷ ❸

38yo man with "autoimmune peripheral neuropathy"

- 38yo white male with a 5-y history of "idiopathic" peripheral neuropathy…exacerbated by consumption of shellfish, associated with fever
- Some evidence of autoimmunity (slightly elevated ANA) and a family history of autoimmunity.
- Has already spent $10,000 on neurological consultations, MRIs, CT scans, lab tests, and lumbar puncture for CSF analysis.
- Desires cure and preventive healthcare
- **Cardiovascular profile: normal except for elevated fibrinogen and hsCRP at 11 mg/dL**
- Intestinal permeability assessment
    - no gastrointestinal complaints
    - **markedly elevated lactulose: mannitol ratio**
- Stool analysis and parasitology:
    - Elevated sIgA
    - Elevated lysozyme
    - **+4 Proteus miribalis** (later showed Pseudomonas aerugenosa; wife had same)

40yo man with "autoimmune peripheral neuropathy"

Patient:
Age: 40
Sex: M
MRN:

Order Number: 40220637
Completed: April 24, 2003
Received: April 22, 2003
Collected: April 21, 2003

HOUSTON OPTIMAL HEALTH
ALEX VASQUEZ DC ND

Houston, TX 77098

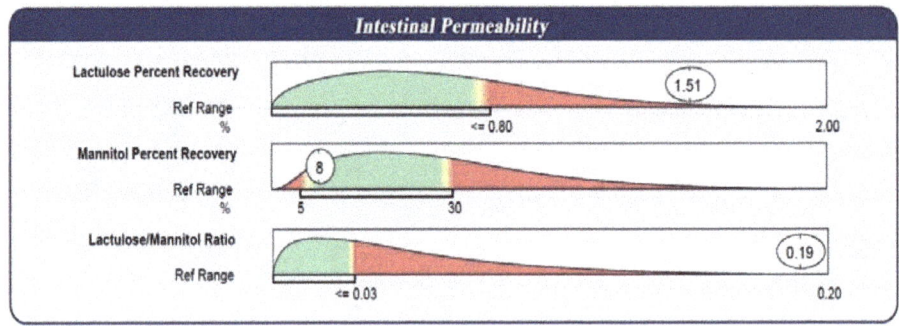

Intestinal Permeability

- Lactulose Percent Recovery: 1.51 (Ref Range % <= 0.80, max 2.00)
- Mannitol Percent Recovery: 8 (Ref Range % 5–30)
- Lactulose/Mannitol Ratio: 0.19 (Ref Range <= 0.03, max 0.20)

40yo man with "autoimmune peripheral neuropathy" (approx. page 91 of Ch1)

Comprehensive Stool Analysis / Parasitology x3

MICROBIOLOGY

Bacteriology Culture

Beneficial flora		Imbalances		Dysbiotic flora	
Bifidobacter	4+	Haemolytic E. coli	4+	Pseudomonas sp.	4+
E. coli	4+	Gamma strep	2+		
Lactobacillus	2+				

Mycology (Yeast) Culture

Normal flora		Dysbiotic flora
Candida glabrata	1+	
Rhodotorula sp.	1+	

38-yo woman with periorbital dermatitis

60yo woman with a history of moderate fatigue, IBS, and recent acute episode of transverse myelitis

51-year-old man with 4-year history of rheumatoid arthritis and hsCRP of 124mg/L

TEST	RESULT	LIMITS	LAB
C-Reactive Protein, Cardiac	124.00H mg/L	0.00 - 3.00	HD

Comprehensive Parasitology, stool, x2

MICROBIOLOGY

Bacteriology Culture

Beneficial flora		Imbalances		Dysbiotic flora	
Bifidobacter	0+	Gamma strep	1+	Citrobacter freundii	1+
E. coli	2+	Enterobacter sp.	1+		
Lactobacillus	0+				

Mycology (Yeast) Culture

Normal flora	Dysbiotic flora
No yeast isolated	

PARASITOLOGY

	Sample 1		Sample 2
No	Ova or Parasites	No	Ova or Parasites

51-year-old man with 4-year history of rheumatoid arthritis and hsCRP of 124mg/L

TEST	RESULT	LIMITS	LAB
C-Reactive Protein, Cardiac	7.50H mg/L	0.00 - 3.00	HD

Relative Risk for Future Cardiovascular Event
- Low: <1.00
- Average: 1.00 - 3.00
- High: >3.00

Major success!

hsCRP is down from 124 to 7.5.

Major improvement

Continue current plan completely N 8.15.05

43yo woman: Obese, cardiometabolic syndrome, tobacco, anxiety, and…now… vasculitis

- Obesity
- Insulin resistance
- Severe anxiety and external locus of control (!!!)
- Cigarette smoking
- ….now complicated by new **leukocytoclastic vasculitis**
  - Are you surprised that her vasculitis is not responding to anti-inflammatory treatment prescribed by her rheumatologist?

43yo woman: Obese, cardiometabolic syndrome, tobacco, anxiety, and…now… vasculitis

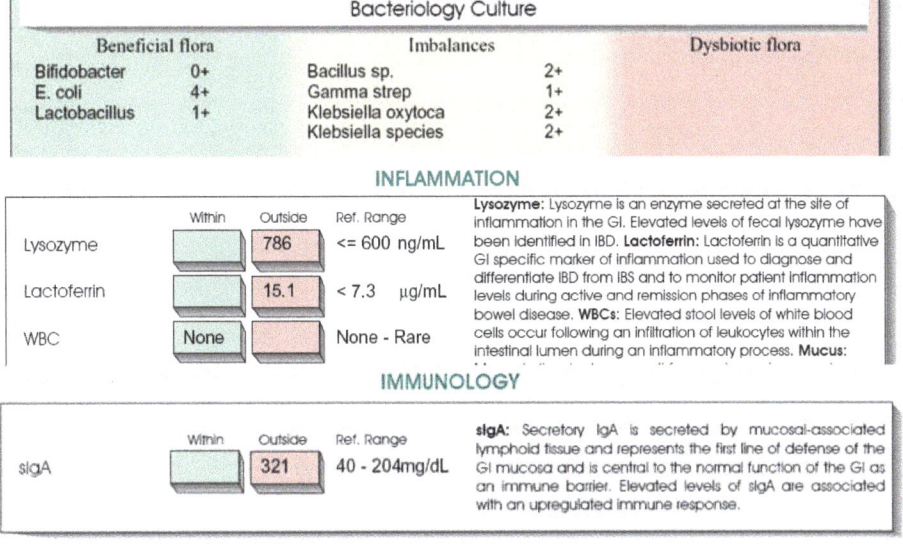

24-31-yo male with subacute onset of severe dyscognition and rapidly progressive "food allergies"

Bacteriology

Beneficial Bacteria

Lactobacillus species	N	(4+)
Escherichia coli	I	*NG
Bifidobacterium	N	(4+)

Additional Bacteria

alpha haemolytic Streptococcus	N	(3+)
gamma haemolytic Streptococcus	N	(4+)
Citrobacter freundii	P	(4+)
Klebsiella pneumoniae	P	(4+)
beta Strep (Not Group A or B)	I	(2+)

Mycology

Candida krusei	P	(4+)
Geotrichum capitatum	P	(4+)

"You can only know what you have lived through.
If you have not lived through something, it is just not true."

Kabir (1440 - 1518)

Got dysbiosis??? *When in doubt, clear 'em out.*

- **Over-reliance on tests (?)**: If you have stool test results, then you can always base treatment on those findings...except when other things are going on that were not picked up by the lab test....

- **(In)complete therapy (?)**: Sometimes the ❶ antimicrobial "one bug, one drug, one cure" model actually works...for a while.
  - I wouldn't know for sure since I've never treated dysbiosis without also implementing ❷ nutritional immunomodulation...
  - ...and ❸ nutritional immunorestoration at the same time.

- **Empiric treatment is well supported by the clinical literature...**
  - ...and does not have to rely on prescription drugs...
  - ...risk benefit ratio...
  - ...informed consent...
  - ...clinical decision-making requires performance in the face of uncertainty: Yes!—this is why doctor's have brains and autonomy.

Dysbiosis: Topic Outline

1. **Introduction and definitions**: Terminology, perspectives, locations
2. **Molecular mechanisms**: 18...*and counting toward more...*
3. **Locations**: Introduction to the 7 main loci
4. **Microbes**: Introduction to some of the most common microbes seen in clinical practice and represented in the literature
5. **Additional detail for gastrointestinal dysbiosis**: GI dysbiosis deserves additional attention due to its pathophysiologic quantitative and qualitative preeminence in addition to its greater representation in the research literature
6. **Case reports and clinical examples**: Mostly related to GI dysbiosis
7. **Antidysbiotic Interventions**: Simple as ❶ ❷ ❸

Gastrointestinal Dysbiosis Treatments

Introduction to dysbiosis

Clinical and laboratory assessments

Dysbiotic microbes

❶ Antimicrobial treatments: Diet, Nutrients, Drugs, Botanicals

❷ Immunorestoration: Diet and nutrients

❸ Immunomodulation: Promoting tolerance

Summary, conclusions, and clinical applications

Antimicrobial treatments

▸ <u>Diet</u>: low-carb plant-based diet

  ▸ Dr Vasquez: "When you change the diet, you change the intestinal microbes."

  ▸ Specific carbohydrate diet: *Breaking the Vicious Cycle* by Gottschall

  ▸ Low-carb plant-based diet is generally the diet of choice for nearly everyone; this is the foundation of the Paleo Diet—just add lean protein.

  ▸ Consumption of sugars promotes bacterial overgrowth and immune suppression—two things we are trying to avoid and overcome in these patients.

  ▸ Carrots are particularly antimicrobial.

▸ <u>Nutrients</u>: ❶ iodine/iodide, ❷ vitamin D3, ❸ vitamin C purge in selected patients

Gastrointestinal Dysbiosis Treatments

Introduction to dysbiosis

Clinical and laboratory assessments

Dysbiotic microbes

❶ Antimicrobial treatments: Diet, Nutrients, Drugs, Botanicals

❷ Immunorestoration: Diet and nutrients

❸ Immunomodulation: Promoting tolerance

Summary, conclusions, and clinical applications

Antimicrobial nutrients: ❶ iodine/iodide,

- Iodine/iodide is one of the most commonly used and widest-spectrum antimicrobial agents ever discovered.
- Broad-spectrum use against all bacteria, viruses, fungi, protozoans, etc.
- Concentration-dependent and time-dependent.
- Orally administered iodine/iodide has been used for the systemic treatment of drug-resistant fungal skin infections. *Pediatric Dermatology 2007v24* and *Journal of European Academy of Dermatology and Venereology 2007v21*
- Oral iodine/iodide is likely to be effective against microbes in the stomach and upper GI,
- Patients should be supplemented with selenium and other antioxidants to protect the thyroid gland when using higher-dose Iodine/iodide

---

Gastrointestinal Dysbiosis Treatments

Introduction to dysbiosis

Clinical and laboratory assessments

Dysbiotic microbes

❶ Antimicrobial treatments: Diet, Nutrients, Drugs, Botanicals

❷ Immunorestoration: Diet and nutrients

❸ Immunomodulation: Promoting tolerance

Summary, conclusions, and clinical applications

Antimicrobial nutrients: ❷ vitamin D3

- Vitamin D is critically important—essential—for endogenous antimicrobial effectiveness.
- **Vitamin D deficiency should be seen as a state of immunosuppression.**
  - Another way of stating that is: **Vitamin D deficiency causes immunosuppression.**

Gastrointestinal Dysbiosis Treatments

Introduction to dysbiosis

Clinical and laboratory assessments

Dysbiotic microbes

❶ Antimicrobial treatments: Diet, Nutrients, Drugs, Botanicals

❷ Immunorestoration: Diet and nutrients

❸ Immunomodulation: Promoting tolerance

Summary, conclusions, and clinical applications

Vitamin D enhances immunity via AMP:

- **Antimicrobial peptides (AMP):**
  - Potent, broad spectrum natural "antibiotics",
  - Able to kill Gram negative and Gram positive bacteria (including strains that are resistant to conventional antibiotics), mycobacteria (including Mycobacterium tuberculosis), enveloped viruses, fungi and transformed or cancerous cells.
  - AMP may also have the ability to enhance immunity by functioning as immunomodulators,
  - These evolutionarily conserved peptides are usually positively charged and have both a hydrophobic and hydrophilic side that enables the molecule to be soluble in aqueous environments yet also enter lipid-rich membranes. *J Am Acad Dermatol.* 2005 Mar

---

Vitamin D enhances immunity via AMP:

Future Microbiol. 2009 November ; 4: 1151. doi:10.2217/fmb.09.87.

The vitamin D–antimicrobial peptide pathway and its role in protection against infection

Adrian F Gombart
Linus Pauling Institute, Department of Biochemisty & Biophysics, Oregon State University, 2011 ALS Bldg, Corvallis, OR 97331-7305, USA, Tel.: +1 541 737 8018, Fax: +1 541 737 0481, adrian.gombart@oregonstate.edu

Abstract

Vitamin D deficiency has been correlated with increased rates of infection. Since the early 19th century, both environmental (i.e., sunlight) and dietary sources (cod liver) of vitamin D have been identified as treatments for TB. The recent discovery that vitamin D induces antimicrobial peptide gene expression explains, in part, the 'antibiotic' effect of vitamin D and has greatly renewed interest in the ability of vitamin D to improve immune function. Subsequent work indicates that this regulation is biologically important for the response of the innate immune system to wounds and infection and that deficiency may lead to suboptimal responses toward bacterial and viral infections. The regulation of the cathelicidin antimicrobial peptide gene is a human/primate-specific adaptation and is not conserved in other mammals. The capacity of the vitamin D receptor to act as a high-

Gastrointestinal Dysbiosis Treatments

Introduction to dysbiosis

Clinical and laboratory assessments

Dysbiotic microbes

❶ Antimicrobial treatments: Diet, Nutrients, Drugs, Botanicals

❷ Immunorestoration: Diet and nutrients

❸ Immunomodulation: Promoting tolerance

Summary, conclusions, and clinical applications

Vitamin D enhances immunity via AMP:

- **Cathelicidin LL-37:** In neutrophils, proteolytic cleavage generates the mature AMP.
  - "LL-37 peptide is a potent killer of different microorganisms with the ability to prevent immunostimulatory effects of bacterial wall molecules such as lipopolysaccharide and can therefore protect against lethal endotoxemia." *Arch Immunol Ther Exp* 2010 Feb
- **Defensins:** Antimicrobial peptides with a characteristic β-sheet-rich fold, expressed by leukocytes and various epithelial cells that come in contact with environmental microbes. Constitutive and inducible depending on the tissue.

"Both cathelicidins and defensins disrupt the integrity of the bacterial cell membrane, resulting in the death of the microbe." *Future Microbiol.* 2009 Nov

---

Gastrointestinal Dysbiosis Treatments

Introduction to dysbiosis

Clinical and laboratory assessments

Dysbiotic microbes

❶ Antimicrobial treatments: Diet, Nutrients, Drugs, Botanicals

❷ Immunorestoration: Diet and nutrients

❸ Immunomodulation: Promoting tolerance

Summary, conclusions, and clinical applications

Vitamin D modulates immune function:

J Clin Virol. 2011 March ; 50(3): 194–200. doi:10.1016/j.jcv.2010.12.006.

Vitamin D and the anti-viral state

Jeremy A. Beard[b], Allison Bearden[a,b], and Rob Striker[a,b,*]

[a]W. S. Middleton Memorial Veterans Administration Hospital, 53705, USA

[b]University of Wisconsin-Madison, Department of Medicine, 53706, USA

Abstract

Vitamin D has long been recognized as essential to the skeletal system. Newer evidence suggests that it also plays a major role regulating the immune system, perhaps including immune responses to viral infection. Interventional and observational epidemiological studies provide evidence that vitamin D deficiency may confer increased risk of influenza and respiratory tract infection. Vitamin D deficiency is also prevalent among patients with HIV infection. Cell culture experiments support the thesis that vitamin D has direct anti-viral effects particularly against enveloped viruses. Though vitamin D's anti-viral mechanism has not been fully established, it may be linked to vitamin D's ability to up-regulate the anti-microbial peptides LL-37 and human beta defensin 2. Additional studies are necessary to fully elucidate the efficacy and mechanism of vitamin D as an anti-viral agent.

Gastrointestinal Dysbiosis Treatments

Introduction to dysbiosis

Clinical and laboratory assessments

Dysbiotic microbes

❶ Antimicrobial treatments: Diet, Nutrients, Drugs, Botanicals

❷ Immunorestoration: Diet and nutrients

❸ Immunomodulation: Promoting tolerance

Summary, conclusions, and clinical applications

Vitamin D: clinical antiviral benefit

- **Vitamin D supplementation improves sustained virologic response in chronic hepatitis C (genotype 1)-naïve patients.**
  - N=72, randomized to Peg-α-2b interferon plus ribavirin "together with vitamin D3 (2000 IU/d, target serum level > 32 ng/mL)" or no vitamin D
  - At week 12, 34 (94%) treated patients and 17 (48%) controls were HCV-RNA negative (P < 0.001).
  - At 24 wk post-treatment (SVR), 31 (86%) treated patients and 15 (42%) controls were HCV-RNA negative (P < 0.001).
- **CONCLUSION: Adding vitamin D to conventional Peg-α-2b/ribavirin therapy for treatment-naïve patients with chronic HCV genotype 1 infection significantly improves the viral response.**

Abu-Mouch et al. *World J Gastroenterol.* 2011 Dec

Gastrointestinal Dysbiosis Treatments

Introduction to dysbiosis

Clinical and laboratory assessments

Dysbiotic microbes

❶ Antimicrobial treatments: Diet, Nutrients, Drugs, Botanicals

❷ Immunorestoration: Diet and nutrients

❸ Immunomodulation: Promoting tolerance

Summary, conclusions, and clinical applications

Vitamin D receptor helps maintain integrity of the intestinal mucosal barrier:

- VDR++ = tight gut   VDR-- = leaky gut

Kong J. *Am J Physiol Gastrointest Liver Physiol.* 2008 Jan

In summary, in this report we presented evidence suggesting that the VDR plays a critical role in preserving the integrity of the intestinal mucosal barrier. VDR is able to enhance the intercellular junctions; it is also required for mucosal wound healing. Mice lacking VDR are much more susceptible to DSS-induced mucosal injury, leading to extensive ulceration and early death. In vitro experiments demonstrate that VDR mediates the activity of $1,25(OH)_2D_3$ that induces junction protein expression and strengthens the tight junction complex. These data are consistent with, and explain at least in part, the observation reported in the literature that vitamin D deficiency is linked to increased incidence of IBD in human population.

Gastrointestinal Dysbiosis Treatments

Introduction to dysbiosis

Clinical and laboratory assessments

Dysbiotic microbes

❶ <u>Antimicrobial treatments</u>: Diet, Nutrients, Drugs, Botanicals

❷ Immunorestoration: Diet and nutrients

❸ Immunomodulation: Promoting tolerance

Summary, conclusions, and clinical applications

Leaky gut promotes dietary and microbial antigen absorption which promotes immune activation (inflammation) and immune sensitization (allergy)

Selenium

 The Journal of Nutrition
Symposium: Micronutrient Regulation of Host-Pathogen Interactions

Selenium and Vitamin E Status: Impact on Viral Pathogenicity[1–3]

Melinda A. Beck*

Department of Nutrition, University of North Carolina, Chapel Hill, NC 27599-7461

Abstract

Selenium (Se), an essential trace element, and vitamin E, a lipid soluble antioxidant, are important mediators for protection against oxidative stress. Recent work has demonstrated that deficiencies in either Se or vitamin E result in increased viral pathogenicity and altered immune responses. Furthermore, deficiencies in either Se or vitamin E results in specific viral mutations, changing relatively benign viruses into virulent ones. Thus, host nutritional status should be considered a driving force for the emergence of new viral strains or newly pathogenic strains of known viruses. J. Nutr. 137: 1338–1340, 2007.

Gastrointestinal Dysbiosis Treatments

Introduction to dysbiosis

Clinical and laboratory assessments

Dysbiotic microbes

❶ Antimicrobial treatments: Diet, Nutrients, Drugs, Botanicals

❷ Immunorestoration: Diet and nutrients

❸ Immunomodulation: Promoting tolerance

Summary, conclusions, and clinical applications

Antimicrobial nutrients: ❸ "vitamin C purge"

Osmotic laxative "purge" for quick removal of excess microbes, alleviation of constipation:

- Safe for the vast majority of patients.
- Dose to effect: laxative effect may start at 5grams for some patients, while others get safe and effective results within about 45 minutes using 30-60grams of vitamin C (buffered ascorbates with mannitol works nicely, gently).
- Treatments that effect changes in water balance and electrolytes are less likely to be well tolerated in patients who are frail, have preexisting electrolyte abnormalities, have renal insufficiency, or cardiac arrhythmias, etc.

Gastrointestinal Dysbiosis Treatments

Introduction to dysbiosis

Clinical and laboratory assessments

Dysbiotic microbes

❶ Antimicrobial treatments: Diet, Nutrients, Drugs, Botanicals

❷ Immunorestoration: Diet and nutrients

❸ Immunomodulation: Promoting tolerance

Summary, conclusions, and clinical applications

Antimicrobial drugs for GI dysbiosis:

- Nystatin: antifungal, natural product, nonabsorbed, very safe,
- Diflucan: antifungal drug, systemic absorption, may cause dizziness, long half-life means patients can take it every other day for 1-2 weeks.
- Rifaxamin: nonabsorbed broad-spectrum antibiotic with successful applications in hepatic encephalopathy, IBS, and fibromyalgia. Very expensive at about $1,500 for 2 weeks of treatment.
- Oral vancomycin: nonabsorbed antibiotic against mostly Gram-positive bacteria *and more* ☺
- Augmentin: Kills up to 90% of gut bacteria.
- Metronidazole/tinidazole: Kills anaerobes and protozoans.

Gastrointestinal Dysbiosis Treatments

Introduction to dysbiosis

Clinical and laboratory assessments

Dysbiotic microbes

❶ Antimicrobial treatments: Diet, Nutrients, Drugs, Botanicals

❷ Immunorestoration: Diet and nutrients

❸ Immunomodulation: Promoting tolerance

Summary, conclusions, and clinical applications

Antimicrobial botanicals:

<u>Oregano</u>: emulsified and time-released

- Effective against
    - Blastocystis hominis,
    - Entamoeba hartmanni,
    - Endolimax nana.
- 6 weeks of supplementation with 600 mg emulsified oil of oregano daily. Force M, Sparks WS, Ronzio RA. *Phytother Res.* 2000 May
- **Combination herbal formulas:**
    - Components reviewed in following slides

Oregano

PHYTOTHERAPY RESEARCH
Phytother. Res. 14, 213–214 (2000)

SHORT COMMUNICATION
Inhibition of Enteric Parasites by Emulsified Oil of Oregano *in vivo*

Mark Force, William S. Sparks and Robert A. Ronzio*
Health Explorations Trust, Scottsdale, AZ, USA (M.F.) and Biotics Research Corporation, P.O. Box 36888, Houston, Texas 77236, USA

Oil of Mediterranean oregano *Oreganum vulgare* was orally administered to 14 adult patients whose stools tested positive for enteric parasites, *Blastocystis hominis*, *Entamoeba hartmanni* and *Endolimax nana*. After 6 weeks of supplementation with 600 mg emulsified oil of oregano daily, there was complete disappearance of *Entamoeba hartmanni* (four cases), *Endolimax nana* (one case), and *Blastocystis hominis* in eight cases. Also, *Blastocystis hominis* scores declined in three additional cases. Gastrointestinal symptoms improved in seven of the 11 patients who had tested positive for *Blastocystis hominis*. Copyright © 2000 John Wiley & Sons, Ltd.

Keywords: oregano; essential oil; *Blastocystis hominis*; enteric parasites; *Endolimax nana*; *Entamoeba hartmanni*.

Gastrointestinal Dysbiosis Treatments

Introduction to dysbiosis

Clinical and laboratory assessments

Dysbiotic microbes

❶ Antimicrobial treatments: Diet, Nutrients, Drugs, Botanicals

❷ Immunorestoration: Diet and nutrients

❸ Immunomodulation: Promoting tolerance

Summary, conclusions, and clinical applications

Bismuth:

▸ Bismuth is commonly used in the empiric treatment of diarrhea (e.g., "Pepto-Bismol") and is commonly combined with other antimicrobial agents to reduce drug resistance and increase antibiotic effectiveness.

Veldhuyzen van Zanten et al. *CMAJ*. 1997;156(11):1565-74
http://www.cmaj.ca/cgi/reprint/156/11/1565.pdf

Gastrointestinal Dysbiosis Treatments

Introduction to dysbiosis

Clinical and laboratory assessments

Dysbiotic microbes

❶ Antimicrobial treatments: Diet, Nutrients, Drugs, Botanicals

❷ Immunorestoration: Diet and nutrients

❸ Immunomodulation: Promoting tolerance

Summary, conclusions, and clinical applications

Thyme (*Thymus vulgaris*):

▸ Thyme extracts have direct antimicrobial actions and also potentiate the effectiveness of tetracycline against drug-resistant *Staphylococcus aureus*.[1] Thyme also appears effective against *Aeromonas hydrophila*.[2]

[1] Fujita M et al. *Microbiol Immunol*. 2005;49(4):391-6

[2] "...thyme essential oil showed the greatest inhibition against A. hydrophila." Fabio et al. *New Microbiol*. 2003 Jan

Gastrointestinal Dysbiosis Treatments

Introduction to dysbiosis

Clinical and laboratory assessments

Dysbiotic microbes

❶ **Antimicrobial treatments**: Diet, Nutrients, Drugs, Botanicals

❷ Immunorestoration: Diet and nutrients

❸ Immunomodulation: Promoting tolerance

Summary, conclusions, and clinical applications

- **Clove (*Syzygium* species)**: Clove's eugenol has been shown in animal studies to have a potent antifungal effect.[1]
- **Anise**: Although it has weak antibacterial action when used alone, anise does show in vitro activity against molds.[2]
- **Buchu/betulina**: Buchu has a long history of use against urinary tract infections and systemic infections.[3]

Gastrointestinal Dysbiosis Treatments

Introduction to dysbiosis

Clinical and laboratory assessments

Dysbiotic microbes

❶ **Antimicrobial treatments**: Diet, Nutrients, Drugs, Botanicals

❷ Immunorestoration: Diet and nutrients

❸ Immunomodulation: Promoting tolerance

Summary, conclusions, and clinical applications

Citations for previous slide:

[1] Chami N, Chami F, Bennis S, Trouillas J, Remmal A. Antifungal treatment with carvacrol and eugenol of oral candidiasis in immunosuppressed rats. *Braz J Infect Dis.* 2004 Jun;8(3):217-26 http://www.scielo.br/pdf/bjid/v8n3/21619.pdf

[2] "Anise oil was not particularly inhibitory to bacteria (inhibition zone, approximately 25 mm); however, anise oil was highly inhibitory to molds." Elgayyar M, Draughon FA, Golden DA, Mount JR. Antimicrobial activity of essential oils from plants against selected pathogenic and saprophytic microorganisms. *J Food Prot.* 2001 Jul;64(7):1019-24

[3] "Buchu preparations are now used as a diuretic and for a wide range of conditions including stomach aches, rheumatism, bladder and kidney infections and coughs and colds." Simpson D. Buchu--South Africa's amazing herbal remedy. *Scott Med J* 1998 Dec;43(6):189-91

Gastrointestinal Dysbiosis Treatments

Introduction to dysbiosis

Clinical and laboratory assessments

Dysbiotic microbes

❶ Antimicrobial treatments: Diet, Nutrients, Drugs, Botanicals

❷ Immunorestoration: Diet and nutrients

❸ Immunomodulation: Promoting tolerance

Summary, conclusions, and clinical applications

- **Dill (*Anethum graveolens*)**: Dill shows activity against several types of mold and yeast.[1]
- **Brucea javanica**: Extract from *Brucea javanica* fruit shows *in vitro* activity against *Babesia gibsoni*, *Plasmodium falciparum*[2], *Entamoeba histolytica*[3] and *Blastocystis hominis*.[4],[5]
- **Acacia catechu**: *Acacia catechu* shows moderate *in vitro* activity against *Salmonella typhi*.[6]

Gastrointestinal Dysbiosis Treatments

Introduction to dysbiosis

Clinical and laboratory assessments

Dysbiotic microbes

❶ Antimicrobial treatments: Diet, Nutrients, Drugs, Botanicals

❷ Immunorestoration: Diet and nutrients

❸ Immunomodulation: Promoting tolerance

Summary, conclusions, and clinical applications

Citations for previous slide

[1] "Antimicrobial testings showed high activity of the essential A. graveolens oil against the mold Aspergillus niger and the yeasts Saccharomyces cerevisiae and Candida albicans." Jirovetz L, Buchbauer G, Stoyanova AS, Georgiev EV, Damianova ST. Composition, quality control, and antimicrobial activity of the essential oil of long-time stored dill (Anethum graveolens L.) seeds from Bulgaria. *J Agric Food Chem*. 2003 Jun 18;51(13):3854-7

[2] Murnigsih T, Subeki, Matsuura H, et al. Evaluation of the inhibitory activities of the extracts of Indonesian traditional medicinal plants against Plasmodium falciparum and Babesia gibsoni. *J Vet Med Sci*. 2005 Aug;67(8):829-31
http://www.jstage.jst.go.jp/article/jvms/67/8/829/_pdf

[3] Wright CW, O'Neill MJ, Phillipson JD, Warhurst DC. Use of microdilution to assess in vitro antiamoebic activities of Brucea javanica fruits, Simarouba amara stem, and a number of quassinoids. *Antimicrob Agents Chemother*. 1988 Nov;32(11):1725-9
http://www.pubmedcentral.gov/articlerender.fcgi?tool=pubmed&pubmedid=2908094

[4] "Dichloromethane and methanol extracts from the Brucea javanica seed and a methanol extract from Quercus infectoria nut gall showed the highest activity." Sawangjaroen N, Sawangjaroen K. The effects of extracts from anti-diarrheic Thai medicinal plants on the in vitro growth of the intestinal protozoa parasite: Blastocystis hominis. *J Ethnopharmacol*. 2005 Apr 8;98(1-2):67-72

[5] "The crude extracts of Coptis chinensis (CC) and Brucea javanica (BJ) were found to be most active against B. hominis." Yang LQ, Singh M, Yap EH, Ng GC, Xu HX, Sim KY. In vitro response of Blastocystis hominis against traditional Chinese medicine. *J Ethnopharmacol*. 1996 Dec;55(1):35-42

[6] "Moderate antimicrobial activity was shown by Picorhiza kurroa, Acacia catechu, ..." Rani P, Khullar N. Antimicrobial evaluation of some medicinal plants for their anti-enteric potential against multi-drug resistant Salmonella typhi. *Phytother Res*. 2004 Aug;18(8):670-3

Gastrointestinal Dysbiosis Treatments

Introduction to dysbiosis

Clinical and laboratory assessments

Dysbiotic microbes

❶ **Antimicrobial treatments**: Diet, Nutrients, Drugs, Botanicals

❷ Immunorestoration: Diet and nutrients

❸ Immunomodulation: Promoting tolerance

Summary, conclusions, and clinical applications

Oral administration of proteolytic enzymes:

- First, orally administered proteolytic enzymes are efficiently absorbed by the gastrointestinal tract into the systemic circulation[1] to then provide a **clinically significant anti-inflammatory benefit** as I reviewed recently.[2]

- Second and more specifically, oral administration of proteolytic enzymes is generally believed to effect a **reduction in immune complexes and their clinical consequences**[3], and immune complexes are probably a major mechanism of dysbiosis-induced disease and are pathogenic in rheumatoid arthritis[4] and many other autoimmune diseases such as systemic lupus erythematosus, dermatomyositis, Sjogren's syndrome, and polyarteritis nodosa.[5]

- Third, proteolytic enzymes have been shown to **stimulate immune function**[6] and may thereby promote clearance of occult infections.

- Fourth, **proteolytic enzymes inhibit formation of microbial biofilms** and increase immune penetration and the effectiveness of antimicrobial therapeutics.[7] Although individual enzymes may be used in isolation, enzyme therapy is generally delivered in the form of polyenzyme preparations containing pancreatin, bromelain, papain, amylase, lipase, trypsin and alpha-chymotrypsin.[8]

Citations

[1] Liebow C, Rothman SS. Enteropancreatic Circulation of Digestive Enzymes. *Science* 1975; 189(4201): 472-474

[2] Vasquez A. Reducing pain and inflammation naturally - Part 3: Improving overall health while safely and effectively treating musculoskeletal pain. *Nutritional Perspectives* 2005; 28: 34-38, 40-42 http://optimalhealthresearch.com/part3

[3] Galebskaya LV, Ryumina EV, Niemerovsky VS, Matyukov AA. Human complement system state after wobenzyme intake. *VESTNIK MOSKOVSKOGO UNIVERSITETA. KHIMIYA.* 2000. Vol. 41, No. 6. Supplement. Pages 148-149

[4] Edwards JC, Cambridge G. Rheumatoid arthritis: the predictable effect of small immune complexes in which antibody is also antigen. *Br J Rheumatol.* 1998 Feb;37(2):126-30 http://rheumatology.oxfordjournals.org/cgi/reprint/37/2/126

[5] Jancar S, Sanchez Crespo M. Immune complex-mediated tissue injury: a multistep paradigm. *Trends Immunol.* 2005 Jan;26(1):48-55 http://www.i3u.org/i3u-papers/MSC-2005-TIMM.pdf

[6] Zavadova E, Desser L, Mohr T. Stimulation of reactive oxygen species production and cytotoxicity in human neutrophils in vitro and after oral administration of a polyenzyme preparation. *Cancer Biother.* 1995 Summer;10(2):147-52

[7] "The enzymes were shown to inhibit the biofilm formation. When appliled to the formed associations, the enzymes potentiated the effect of antibiotics on the bacteria located in them." Tets VV, Knorring Glu, Artemenko NK, Zaslavskaia NV, Artemenko KL. [Impact of exogenic proteolytic enzymes on bacteria][Article in Russian] *Antibiot Khimioter.* 2004;49(12):9-13

[8] Vasquez A. Reducing pain and inflammation naturally - Part 3: Improving overall health while safely and effectively treating musculoskeletal pain. *Nutritional Perspectives* 2005; 28: 34-38, 40-42 http://optimalhealthresearch.com/part3

Nutritional Immunomodulation

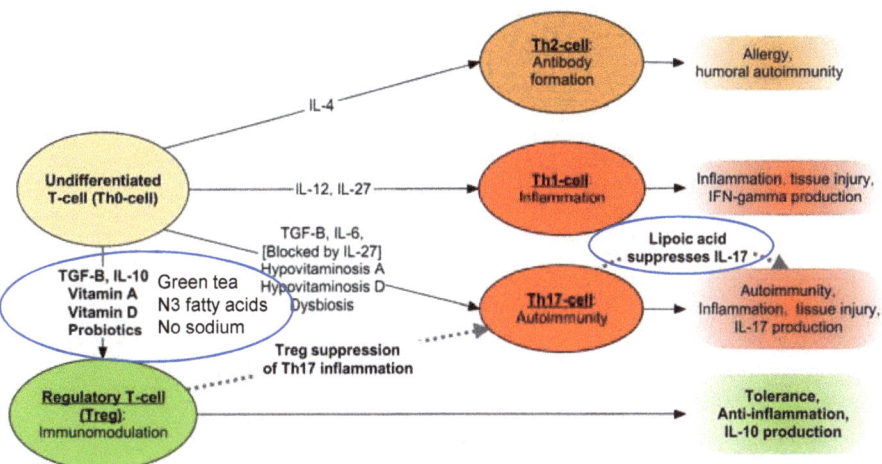

© Vasquez A. *Functional Immunology and Nutritional Immunomodulation: Presentation Slides Part 1* (2012), *Integrative Rheumatology, Nutritional Immunology, Functional Inflammology (Third Edition, 2013 pending)*.

Nutritional Immunomodulation: Induction of Treg at the expense/suppression of Th-1/2/17

Organic/nonGMO

1. Probiotics
2. Lipoic acid
3. A-vitamin
4. Infection/dysbiosis clearance
5. D-vitamin
6. Fatty acids: EPA-DHA and GLA
7. IL-6 reduction: create overall antiinflammatory milieu for Th0 maturation
8. Green tea
9. Sodium avoidance

What is the new acronym?

Dysbiosis: Topic Outline

1. **Introduction and definitions**: Terminology, perspectives, locations
2. **Molecular mechanisms**: 18…*and counting toward more…*
3. **Locations**: Introduction to the 7 main loci
4. **Microbes**: Introduction to some of the most common microbes seen in clinical practice and represented in the literature
5. **Additional detail for gastrointestinal dysbiosis**: GI dysbiosis deserves additional attention due to its pathophysiologic quantitative and qualitative preeminence in addition to its greater representation in the research literature
6. **Case reports and clinical examples**: Mostly related to GI dysbiosis
7. **Antidysbiotic Interventions**: As simple as:
   ❶ **Antimicrobial**: no microbe = no dysbiosis
   ❷ **Immunorestoration**: effective immune response = microbe = no dysbiosis
   ❸ **Immunomodulation**: no pathogenic immune response = no inflammation = no dysbiotic relationship

"Dysbiosis" → "*multi*focal *poly*dysbiosis" — Summary

Location subtypes
- GI
- Oral
- Sinorespiratory
- Parenchymal
- GU
- Cutaneous
- Environmental

Strongest evidence
- Psoriasis
- Fibromyalgia
- "inflammatory arthritis and rheumatic disease"
- Wegener's granulomatosis

Mechanisms of Dysbiosis (4 of 18)
- Molecular mimicry
- Bystander activation
- Immune complex deposition
- Antimetabolites

Assessments
- History of IBS, ppG&B
- Culture, DNA probe, PCR
- Stool tests by specialty lab
- *Response to treatment*

Problematic GI microbes include
- *Aeromonas hydrophila, Blastocystis hominis, Candida albicans* and other yeasts, *Citrobacter rodentium, Citrobacter freundii, Dientamoeba fragilis, Endolimax nana, Entamoeba histolytica,* Gamma strep, *Enterococcus, Giardia lamblia, Hafnia alvei, Helicobacter pylori, Klebsiella pneumoniae, Proteus mirabilis, Pseudomonas aeruginosa, Staphylococcus aureus, Staphylococcus epidermidis, Streptococcus pyogenes,* Group A streptococci

Treatments
- Botanical and/or Pharmaceutical antimicrobials: combination, long-duration may be required
- Overall health optimization
- Diet optimization, esp. low-carb
- Correction of nutritional deficiencies, esp. vitA, vitD, zinc
- Remember: the microbes are only half of the relationship; the other half is the patient!

What Dr V is doing these days for multifocal polydysbiosis

Treatments I am very sure about and implement regularly

See presentation for information

1. _____
2. _____
3. _____
4. _____
5. _____
6. _____

What Dr V is doing these days for multifocal polydysbiosis

Treatments I use after lab testing or per situation

See presentation for information

1. _____
2. _____
3. _____
4. _____
5. _____
6. _____

What Dr V is doing these days for multifocal polydysbiosis

Treatments I use after lab testing or per situation

See presentation for information

1. _____
2. _____
3. _____
4. _____
5. _____
6. _____

Notices

- Copyright: Except for quotations and images obtained elsewhere, the material and contents of these presentations are copyrighted by Dr Alex Vasquez and have often been excerpted from his books which are also copyrighted. Any unauthorized use of this material—including photocopying or any distribution—is prohibited.
  - No cameras.
  - No recorders.
- Copyright 2012-2014 by Dr Alex Vasquez. All rights reserved and enforced.
- Trademark: The "Functional Immunology/Inflammology Protocol" discussed in this series of videos and notes is Trademarked ® in association with Dr Vasquez's book *Functional Immunology and Nutritional Immunomodulation* and other books and videos.

Trademark